Physiology in Childbearing

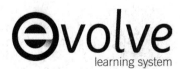
learning system

Evolve Learning Resources for Students and Lecturers.
See the instructions on the inside cover for access to the web site.

Think outside the book...evolve

This book is dedicated to the wonderful people who provide care for mothers and babies throughout the world.

For Elsevier:
Commissioning Editor: Mairi McCubbin
Development Editor: Sheila Black
Project Manager: Kerrie-Anne McKinlay
Designer: Charles Gray
Illustrator: Cactus
Illustration Manager: Gillian Richards

Physiology in Childbearing

with Anatomy and Related Biosciences

THIRD EDITION

Edited by

Dot Stables BA(Hons) MSc MTD DN RM RN

Formerly Lecturer in Applied Biology,
St Bartholomew's College of Nursing and Midwifery,
City University, London, UK

Jean Rankin BSc(Hons) MSc PhD PGCE RM RGN RSCN

Lead Midwife for Education, School of Health, Nursing and Midwifery,
University of the West of Scotland, Paisley and Hamilton;
Supervisor of Midwives – Ayrshire and Arran,
West of Scotland Local Supervising Authority, UK

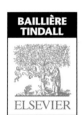

BAILLIÈRE
TINDALL

ELSEVIER

Edinburgh   London   New York   Oxford   Philadelphia   St Louis   Sydney   Toronto   2010

BAILLIÈRE
TINDALL
ELSEVIER

First edition © Harcourt Brace and Company Limited 1999
Second edition © Elsevier Limited 2005
Third edition © Elsevier Limited. 2010. All rights reserved.

ISBN 978-0-7020-3106-9

British Library Cataloguing in Publication Data
A catalogue record for this book is available from the British Library

Library of Congress Cataloging in Publication Data
A catalog record for this book is available from the Library of Congress

Notice

Knowledge and best practice in this field are constantly changing. As new research
and experience broaden our knowledge, changes in practice, treatment and drug
therapy may become necessary or appropriate. Readers are advised to check the
most current information provided (i) on procedures featured or (ii) by the
manufacturer of each product to be administered, to verify the recommended dose or
formula, the method and duration of administration, and contraindications. It is the
responsibility of the practitioner, relying on their own experience and knowledge of
the patient, to make diagnoses, to determine dosages and the best treatment for each
individual patient, and to take all appropriate safety precautions. To the fullest extent
of the law, neither the Publisher nor the Editors assumes any liability for any injury
and/or damage to persons or property arising out of or related to any use of the
material contained in this book.

The Publisher

Contents

Contents

Contributors

Lyz Howie BSc MM RM RGN PGCTLHE
Lecturer (Midwifery), School of Health, Nursing and Midwifery, University of the West of Scotland, Paisley and Hamilton, UK

Barbara V. Novak BA(Hons) MSc RN RSCN RM
Lecturer in Applied Biological Sciences, St Bartholomew's School of Nursing and Midwifery, City University, London, UK

Jean Rankin BSc(Hons) MSc PhD PGCE RM RGN RSCN
Lead Midwife for Education, School of Health, Nursing and Midwifery, University of the West of Scotland, Paisley and Hamilton; Supervisor of Midwives—West of Scotland Local Supervising Authority, UK

Hora Soltani BSc MMedSci PhD
Principal Research Fellow, Centre for Health and Social Care Research, Sheffield Hallam University, Sheffield UK

Dot Stables BA(Hons) MSc MTD DN RM RN
Formerly Lecturer in Applied Biology, St Bartholomew's College of Nursing and Midwifery, City University, London, UK

Margaret Yerby MSc PGCEA RN RM ADM C&G730
Formerly Senior Lecturer, Thames Valley University, London, UK

Most of the authors who contributed to the second edition of this textbook have willingly stayed on board for this third edition. They have updated the amount and depth of knowledge and its application to practice in the different aspects of pregnancy, labour, postnatal and neonatal care as necessary in these fast-growing fields. Dot Stables and Jean Rankin remain author/editors and Hora Soltani, Margaret Yerby and Barbara V. Novak have been joined by Lyz Howie (recently from Princess Royal Maternity Hospital, Glasgow), all writing about their specialist areas. This specialised input will enable students, midwifery practitioners and others caring for women during childbearing to base their decision-making on detailed knowledge and understanding.

As midwives and educators the authors are aware of the increasing need for an in-depth understanding of the physiological processes of childbearing so that early recognition of pathology can prevent morbidity and mortality. They are dedicated to introducing an appreciation of the wider application of biological sciences to the practice of midwifery. Wherever possible the application of theory to practice has been discussed to demonstrate how knowledge of the biological sciences enhances the care given to mothers and babies. The aims of the third edition of this textbook remain:

- to provide a biology textbook for basic and post-basic students and practitioners of normal and abnormal midwifery.
- to enable an understanding of physiology and other biosciences applied to childbearing in order to ensure safe and efficient practice.
- to foster integrated knowledge of applied biosciences and their importance for understanding humanity's place in nature.
- to ensure the safety of mothers and babies, both in the developed world and in those countries where the provision of adequate care is difficult.

The authors are also aware of the importance of the psychological and social aspects of reproduction and how they may affect the physiological well-being of childbearing women. The student should not lose sight of the integration of biology, psychology and sociology when giving health care to women and their families. There are many well-written books on the social and psychological implications of childbearing, to which the student can refer.

Childbearing is a normal biological function that brings about major changes in each system of the woman's body. The changes may occasionally lead to disease, so it is important to understand how the systems function. An understanding of the embryological development of each system also helps students to appreciate problems arising in the neonate. For these reasons a systems approach is used throughout the textbook. Allied biosciences include anatomy, biochemistry, behavioural biology, embryology, evolution, ecology, genetics, microbiology, pharmacology and pathophysiology. Since the first edition there have been rapid advances in the field of genetics, with implications for diagnosis and treatment of diseases with a genetic basis, so the chapter on genetics has therefore been extensively updated.

The book is divided into four sections. Section 1 covers preconception aspects of childbearing and includes cellular structures and functions, genetics, the anatomy and physiology of the male and female reproductive systems, fertility control and infertility. A chapter on preconception care includes wide environmental and lifestyle issues so that the practitioner can select appropriate advice for both the general public and for couples seeking specific information.

Section 2 is divided into three parts. Section 2A is concerned with the development and growth of the fetus, its placenta and membranes. The embryology is quite detailed, but is presented in an easy-to-follow style. Problems of fetal health and growth are covered. Section 2B is about the physiological adaptation of the woman's body to pregnancy. Each system is described in the non-pregnant state, followed by alterations brought about by pregnancy and their significance to health. Section 2C covers pathological states in pregnancy. Each disorder is discussed in depth and management in terms of diagnosis and treatment is outlined.

Section 3 is divided into two parts. Section 3A is about normal labour and includes management that arises from an understanding of physiology. There are chapters about the onset of labour and each of the three stages of labour, and one devoted to the causes and management of pain in labour. Section 3B is concerned with abnormal labour. The effects of the powers, passages and passenger on the progress of labour are considered.

Section 4, which is divided into two parts, considers the mother and baby in the puerperium. Section 4A is about the neonate: two chapters examine the normal neonate and adaptation to extrauterine life and four chapters explore common neonatal disorders and an outline of their management. Section 4B includes chapters on the breast and breastfeeding.

The physiological changes in the puerperium and the pathological conditions that may affect women are presented. The last chapter, which discusses the development of mother–infant relationships in terms of biological theory, has been rewritten to a large extent to include new findings.

We hope that you will find the content of this textbook as fascinating as we do and that your ability to care for mothers and babies will be enhanced by this knowledge.

Hereford and Paisley/Hamilton, 2010

Dot Stables
Jean Rankin

Acknowledgements

The editors would like to thank all the contributors to this third edition as it would not have been possible without their sterling work. We are also grateful for the help of the staff of Elsevier, in particular Sheila Black, whose support made our work so much easier. We would like to mention Gordon Stables, whose unfailing support of our joint effort included providing regular meals and snacks when we editors were working together to streamline this edition.

Dot Stables believes that this book could not have been designed without the many colleagues with whom she has worked during her career in both clinical and education settings, in particular the staff of the Applied Biology Department at St Bartholomew's School of Nursing, City University, whose support allowed her to extend her knowledge of physiology and the allied biosciences, thus providing the foundation from which the chapters could be developed.

Jean Rankin would like to acknowledge Sandra Galloway, Labour Ward Sister in the Ayrshire Maternity Unit, whose passion for midwifery practice and enthusiasm for teaching student midwives has been inspirational.

Section 1

Preconception

SECTION CONTENTS

A major aim of *Physiology in Childbearing* is to enable an understanding of physiology and other biosciences applied to childbearing so that safe and efficient practice is ensured. This first section provides the basic knowledge to underpin the more complex content of the remaining chapters. Chapter 1 introduces basic biochemistry for those who have no previous knowledge of the subject, and the content will act as a reference base. Chapter 2 examines the nature of the cell and its interactions with other cells in some detail. Chapter 3 is about the structure and function of the gene. Huge strides are being made in the subject and its practical applications and the chapter has again been updated to keep the reader informed. Chapters 4 and 5 present the anatomy of the female and male reproductive systems. Chapters 6 and 7 examine the issues of fertility control and infertility. Chapter 8 is about preconception care and examines wide issues such as environment and lifestyle so that the practitioner can select appropriate advice both for the general public and for the couple seeking specific information.

Chapter One

Basic biochemistry

1

Introduction

Chemistry is concerned with the scientific study of elements and how they react when they are combined or are in contact with each other. **Organic chemistry** is based on **carbon compounds** whose molecules are central to the structure and function of all living organisms. This chapter is about the chemical nature of the human body and its metabolic processes.

Energy

The production, storage and release of **energy** are essential to living cells which need a constant supply of energy to function and reproduce. This energy is acquired from breakdown of food molecules, in particular sugars. There are two main types of energy: **kinetic** and **potential**. Kinetic energy is the energy of movement and includes **thermal** (heat) energy. Potential or stored energy is more relevant to biological systems. **Glucose** stores potential energy and is broken down continuously to perform work (Guyton & Hall 2006). **Adenosine triphosphate** (ATP) is important in energy release (Ch. 23).

Catabolic reactions (breakdown of cell products) release large quantities of energy, whereas **anabolic reactions** (such as the manufacture of proteins) are energy-requiring. Cells must have a balance between energy-producing and energy-demanding processes (Rose 1999). All forms of energy are interchangeable and can be expressed in the same unit of measurement. The **SI unit** (International System of Units) for measuring energy is the **joule** (J) or kilojoule (kJ): 1 kJ = 4.2 **calories**.

The chemistry of living organisms

Atoms

Living organisms are made up of **chemical elements**. Over 100 elements are known and each has its own symbol. These elements form a **periodic table** depending on the atomic mass of each element (see below). Elements consist of particles called **atoms**, which are the smallest indivisible part of an element that still retain its chemical and physical properties. Atoms are constructed from three subatomic particles: **neutrons**, **protons** and **electrons** (Sackheim 2008). The **central nucleus** of the atom is made up of neutrons and protons of similar mass, and the very small electrons are arranged in **orbital shells** surrounding the nucleus (Fig. 1.1).

The formation of particles within the atom is maintained by minute **electrical charges**. The neutrons of the nucleus carry no charge, protons carry a positive charge and electrons carry a negative charge. The number of protons is equal to the number of electrons so that most atoms are uncharged. Each element has a different number of electrons and protons which give it its atomic number. Neutrons are heavy and contribute to the **mass** of the element. The number of neutrons and protons together give the element its **mass number**. This determines the atomic mass (**atomic weight**) of an element. Table 1.1 gives values for the six most common elements which make up 99% of living matter.

Radioactive atoms

Variation in the number of neutrons in an atom leads to different forms of the element called **isotopes**, with different mass numbers. In some isotopes the presence of extra neutrons causes them to be unstable. They will break down into a more stable configuration (**decay**) during which they radiate energy and atomic particles. This is **radioactivity** and the isotopes are radioactive.

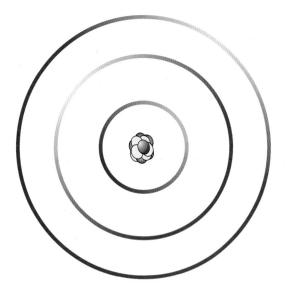

Figure 1.1 • Diagrammatic representation of the structure of an atom showing the nucleus surrounded by electron orbital shells. (From Montague S E, Watson R, Herbert R A 2005, with kind permission of Elsevier.)

Radioactive stable isotopes have been used successfully in medical diagnosis and treatment (Cooper 2006).

Molecules

Atoms are formed into **molecules** by **chemical bonds** of which there are two types: the strong, stable **covalent bond** which is hard to disrupt, and the weaker, less-stable **non-covalent bond**. The making and breaking of these bonds is associated with energy changes; the more stable the bond, the greater the thermal energy needed to disrupt it. These bonds are formed by electrons that can be donated, received or shared by atoms. One bond is formed by one electron, but some atoms have more than one electron that is free to form bonds. The number of available electrons is called the **valency** of the atom. For example, hydrogen has a valency of 1 and carbon a valency of 4.

Covalent bonds

When atoms are joined together by sharing electrons a molecule is formed by covalent bonds. The atoms are held closely together because electrons in their outermost shells move in orbitals that are shared by both atoms. Some atoms require more than one electron to form a bond with another atom. Bonds may be single, such as in a molecule of hydrogen gas, or double, as in a molecule of oxygen gas. Complex molecules are formed by linkage of different atoms depending on their valencies. Molecules can be represented as a molecular formula or structure (Table 1.2).

When more than two atoms form covalent bonds with a central atom, the bonds form a regular structure held in shape by electrical forces. The bonds are always orientated at right-angles to each other. The rigid structures formed are necessary for the structure and function of large biological molecules such as proteins and nucleic acids. The molecular mass of a substance can

Table 1.1 Values for the six most common elements that make up 99% of living matter					
Element	**Atomic number**	**Number of protons**	**Number of neutrons**	**Mass number**	**Atomic mass**
Hydrogen	1	1	0	1	1
Carbon	6	6	6	12	12
Nitrogen	7	7	7	14	14
Oxygen	8	8	8	16	16
Phosphorus	15	15	16	31	31
Calcium	20	20	20	40	40

be calculated by adding together the mass of each of its component atoms. Examples are shown in Table 1.3.

Non-covalent bonds

Many bonds that maintain the complex structures of large molecules are not covalent. The three-dimensional structures are stabilised by much weaker forces called non-covalent bonds. Only small amounts of energy are released in their formation. There are four main types: the **ionic bond**, the **hydrogen bond**, the **van der Waals interaction** and the **hydrophobic bond**.

Ionic bonds (electrovalent bonds)

In ionic bonds, electrons are not shared by atoms but are donated from one atom to another. The number of ionic bonds that can be formed is dictated by valency. Atoms of metallic elements such as sodium, calcium and iron lose electrons readily. The loss or gain of an electron is called **ionisation** and the atom becomes an ion. Electrons carry a negative charge so the atoms that lose an electron become positively charged **cations** such as sodium; this is shown by the addition of a plus sign to

the chemical symbol, Na^+. The atom that receives the electron becomes negatively charged and is known as an **anion**; this is shown by the addition of a minus sign, for example chlorine, Cl^-. An atom or molecule that has lost or gained an electron is said to be **polarised**.

Most ionic compounds are soluble in water because a large amount of energy is set free when ions bind to water molecules. Oppositely charged ions are shielded from each other by the water and do not usually recombine. Molecules with opposite polar bonds (**dipoles**) easily form hydrogen bonds so they attract water molecules. These polar molecules are called **hydrophilic** (water-loving) molecules. Cations are attracted to anions giving rise to compounds called **salts**. For example, when sodium donates an electron to chlorine a well-known salt—**sodium chloride**—is formed:

$$Na^+ + Cl^- \rightarrow NaCl$$

In this form the salt is crystalline and consists of a rigid lattice structure, but if dissolved in water the salt dissociates into free ions which disperse in the solution. The role of **fluids, solutes, acids, bases** and **hydrogen ion concentration** in systemic function is discussed in Chapter 20.

Table 1.2 Examples of molecules					
Atomic element	**Valency**	**Compound**	**Molecular formula**	**Molecular structure**	**Bond type**
H	1	Hydrogen gas	H_2	H — H	Single
O	2	Oxygen gas	O_2	O = O	Double
O	2	Water	H_2O	H H \ / O	Single
N	3	Nitrogen gas	N_2	N ≡ N	Triple
N	3	Ammonia	NH_3	H / H — N \ H	Single
C	4	Carbon dioxide	CO_2	O = C = O	Double
C	4	Methane	CH_4	H H \ / C / \ H H	Single
P	5	Phosphoric acid	H_3PO_4	OH | HO — P = O | OH	Single and double

Hydrogen bonding

Besides covalent and ionic bonds, a weak type of bond can occur between molecules. Normally a hydrogen atom forms a covalent bond with only one other atom. However, molecules containing hydrogen atoms can form an additional bond because they are attracted to each other by a weak **electropositive** charge left on the hydrogen atom when it is drawn to an **electronegative** atom with which it is associating. Hydrogen is the **donor atom** and the electronegative atom is the **acceptor atom**.

The association of oxygen and hydrogen to form water is a good example of this. Although the water molecule is electronically neutral, the positive and negative charges are not distributed uniformly. There is a slight difference between the two ends of the charge in that the hydrogen end of the molecule is slightly positive and the oxygen end of the molecule is slightly negative. Such a molecule is still a dipole. This ability of hydrogen to create weak bonds is essential for the formation of **helical structures**, as in the double helix of **deoxyribonucleic acid** (DNA) (see Ch. 3).

The van der Waals interaction

When two atoms approach closely to each other an attractive force called a **van der Waals interaction** (named after a Dutch physicist) is produced. Transient dipoles are created and that of one atom disturbs the electrons of the other atom, creating a dipole. There is weak attraction between the two dipoles. The bond formed is weaker than a hydrogen bond (Hames & Hooper 2005).

Both polar and non-polar molecules form this type of bond. If the van der Waals attraction between the two atoms balances the repulsion between their electron clouds, the atoms stay in van der Waals contact. Distance is essential in forming this contact and each type of atom has a van der Waals radius at which it is in van der Waals contact with other atoms. These radii are very important in biological systems, especially when the precise shapes of two large molecules complement each other, giving many van der Waals contacts. Examples are **antigen–antibody interactions** (Ch. 29) and bonds between **enzymes** and their **substrates** (Ch. 23).

Hydrophobic interactions

Non-polar molecules contain neither ions nor dipolar bonds. They are insoluble in water and are hydrophobic. The covalent bonds between two carbon atoms or between carbon and hydrogen atoms are the most common non-polar bonds in biological systems. That is why the **hydrocarbons** (Hames & Hooper 2005) found in cell membranes are almost insoluble in water. A hydrophobic interaction is not a separate type of bonding force. It results from the energy needed to insert a non-polar molecule into water. The non-polar molecule cannot form hydrogen bonds and distorts the structure of water to make a cage around it. Non-polar molecules bind together comfortably using the van der Waals interaction.

Chemical equilibrium

Local environmental conditions such as concentration, temperature and pressure will affect the rate at which a chemical reaction occurs and the extent to which it proceeds. When two **reactants** come together, their individual concentrations determine the formation of a product. As the concentrations decrease so does the reaction rate. Some of the products will begin to reverse the process, reforming the reactants.

Eventually the forward and reverse reactions become equal. At this point a chemical mixture is said to be in dynamic **chemical equilibrium**. The **equilibrium constant** (K) defines the ratio of the concentrations of reactants at equilibrium. The presence of a **catalyst** (a substance that aids or speeds up a chemical reaction without being changed itself) may facilitate any reaction.

Composition of the human body

About two-thirds of the human body is made up of water. The other third is composed of six main elements, of which carbon is the most important as it readily combines with other carbon atoms to form larger molecules, and traces of other elements. The chemical elements come together in various combinations to form thousands of components of living tissue. Knowledge of **biochemistry** is essential to the understanding of **physiological**

Table 1.3 The molecular masses of some common chemical compounds

Molecular formula	Calculation	Molecular mass
H_2	1 + 1	2
O_2	16 + 16	32
H_2O	1 + 1+16	18
N_2	14 + 14	28
NH_3	1 + 1+1 + 14	17
CO_2	12 + 16 + 16	44
C_2H_5OH (ethanol)	12 + 12 + 1+1 + 1 +1 + 1+16 + 1	46
$C_6H_{12}O_6$ (glucose)	$(12 \times 6) + (1 \times 12) + (16 \times 6)$	180

processes such as nutrition, respiration and metabolism. The basic substances such as **carbohydrates** (sugars), **lipids** (fats and oils) and **proteins** are discussed in the appropriate chapters.

Proteins are called **polymers** and are formed from long chains of small molecules called **monomers**. Other examples of polymers are plant substances such as starch and cellulose. Other essential substances are the nucleic acids such as DNA. Table 1.4 lists the common elements that make up the basic substances of the human body.

Chemical reactions in the body

As mentioned above, non-covalent bonds are not as stable as covalent bonds, a feature that is essential to the working of the body. They allow complex biological compounds to change during chemical reactions without the need for large amounts of energy. Most chemical reactions in the body require the use of **enzymes** and their associated **cofactors** to act as catalysts. The types of chemical reactions found during metabolic processes are summarised in Table 1.5.

Table 1.4 Elements found in the human body

Element	Atomic symbol	Approximate weight (%)
Oxygen	O	65
Carbon	C	18
Hydrogen	H	10
Nitrogen	N	3
Calcium	Ca	2
Phosphorus	P	1
		TOTAL = 99%
Potassium	K	0.35
Sulphur	S	0.25
Sodium	Na	0.15
Chlorine	Cl	0.15
		TOTAL = 0.9%
Magnesium	Mg	Trace
Iron	Fe	Trace
Zinc	Zn	Trace
Copper	Cu	Trace
Iodine	I	Trace
Manganese	Mn	Trace
Chromium	Cr	Trace
Molybdenum	Mo	Trace
Cobalt	Co	Trace
Selenium	Se	Trace
		TOTAL = 0.1%

Table 1.5 Types of chemical reaction occurring during metabolism

Type	Reaction	Typical processes
Condensation	Combining molecules with the elimination of water	Formation of glycoside, ester and peptide bonds
Hydrolysis	Splitting a molecule with the addition of water	Digestion of carbohydrates, triglycerides and proteins
Dehydration	Removal of water from a molecule	Carbohydrate and fatty acid metabolism
Hydration	Incorporation of water into a molecule	Carbohydrate and fatty acid metabolism
Oxidation	Removal of hydrogen (or electrons)	Conversion of alcohols to aldehydes
Reduction	Addition of hydrogen (or electrons)	Biosynthesis of fatty acids
Carboxylation	Incorporation of carbon dioxide	Carbohydrate synthesis
Decarboxylation	Elimination of carbon dioxide	Fermentation, amine formation
Amination	Incorporation of amino group ($-NH_3$)	Amino acid biosynthesis
Deamination	Elimination of ammonia	Amino acid degradation
Methylation	Incorporation of methyl group ($-CH_3$)	Synthesis of DNA and adrenaline
Demethylation	Removal of methyl group	Amino acid degradation

Main points

- Energy is central to cellular functioning. Kinetic energy is the energy of movement, whereas potential energy is stored in substances such as glucose which can undergo energy-releasing chemical reactions. ATP is the most important substance involved in energy release.

- Living organisms are made up of atoms. The formation within the atom is maintained by minute electrical charges. Neutrons carry no charge, protons carry a positive charge and electrons have a negative charge. The number of protons equals the number of electrons so that most atoms are uncharged.

- Variation in the number of neutrons leads to different isotopes. The presence of extra neutrons makes some isotopes unstable. They transform into a more stable configuration by radiating energy and atomic particles. Radioactive isotopes are used in medical diagnosis and treatment.

- Atoms form compounds by using chemical bonds of which there are two kinds: strong, stable covalent bonds and weaker less-stable non-covalent bonds. The making and breaking of chemical bonds is associated with energy changes. Stable bonds require greater thermal energy to disrupt them.

- Covalent bonds are formed by electrons which may be donated, received or shared by atoms. When two or more atoms share electrons a molecule is formed. When more than two atoms form covalent bonds with a central atom, regular, rigid structures form which are necessary for the functioning of biological molecules.

- Ionic bonds are also involved information of compounds. Electrons are not shared by atoms but are donated from one atom to another. The number of ionic bonds that can be formed is dictated by the valency. The loss or gain of an electron is called ionisation and the atom becomes an ion.

- Atoms that lose an electron become positively charged cations. The atom that receives an electron becomes a negatively charged anion. An atom or molecule that has lost or gained an electron is polarised. Cations are attracted to anions, producing salts.

- Molecules containing hydrogen are attracted to each other by the weak positive charge left on the hydrogen atom when its sole electron is drawn towards the other molecule with which it is associating. Weak hydrogen bonds are essential for the formation of helical structures such as DNA.

- When two atoms approach closely to each other a van der Waals interaction is produced and transient dipoles are created. If the van der Waals attraction between the two atoms balances the repulsion between their electron clouds, the atoms stay in van der Waals contact.

- Non-polar molecules contain neither ions nor dipolar bonds and are hydrophobic. Hydrocarbons found in cell membranes are almost insoluble in water.

- Local environmental conditions affect the rate and extent of chemical reactions. Individual concentrations of reactants determine the formation of a product. As concentrations decrease, so does the reaction rate until some of the products begin to reverse the process, reforming the reactants. When the forward and reverse reactions equalise, the mixture is in chemical equilibrium. Enzymes may speed up reactions.

- The human body is made up of two-thirds water and one-third of six main elements—carbon, oxygen, hydrogen, nitrogen, phosphorus and calcium—and traces of other elements. Basic substances include carbohydrates, lipids, proteins and nucleic acids.

References

Cooper, G.M., 2006. Elements of Human Cancer, second edn. Jones and Bartlett, Boston.

Guyton, A.C., Hall, J.E., 2006. Textbook of Medical Physiology, eleventh edn. Elsevier Saunders.

Hames, D., Hooper, N., 2005. Biochemistry, third edn. Taylor & Francis, Abingdon, Oxford.

Montague, S.E., Watson, R., Herbert, R.A. (eds). Physiology for Nursing Practice, 3rd edn. Baillière Tindall, London.

Rose, S., 1999. The Chemistry of Life, third edn. Penguin, Harmondsworth.

Sackheim, G.I., 2008. An Introduction to Chemistry for Biology Students, ninth edn. Pearson/Benjamin Cummings, San Francisco.

Recommended annotated reading

Rose, S., 1999. The Chemistry of Life, third edn. Penguin, Harmondsworth.
The first edition of this paperback was the author's introduction to the topic of biochemistry. Steven Rose makes the subject fascinating and easy to understand with many good examples.

Sackheim, G.I., 2008. An Introduction to Chemistry for Biology Students, ninth edn. Pearson/Benjamin Cummings, San Francisco.
This is an easy-to-follow, comprehensive textbook that looks at each biochemical structure in depth. There is a chapter on cell structure with a paragraph on each organelle, proteins, DNA, enzymes and antibodies and on all the metabolic processes.

The cell—its structures and function

Physical characteristics of mammalian cells

Living species are made up of a diversity of **cells** which are small membrane-bound units filled with a concentrated aqueous solution of carefully balanced chemicals and **organelles** (Fig. 2.1). Although sharing a common origin, cells show considerable morphological diversity which has evolved to support the functional adaptation and survival of a specific organism. **Eukaryotic cells** are distinguished from **prokaryotic cells** by their membrane-bound nucleus and organelles. Cell survival depends on their specific intracellular biochemistry

which supports their **metabolism** and **homeostasis**. All nucleated mature cells can create copies of themselves by replication and division, which ensures the survival of their **genetic lineage**. The morphological uniqueness and specialised functions are governed by complex **genetic activity**. There are more than 200 different cell types in the human body, assembled into tissue types such as **epithelia**, **connective tissue**, **muscle**, conducting **neural tissue**, non-conducting **neuroglia** and **osteocytes**. The function of different cell types is preserved through communication and co-ordination.

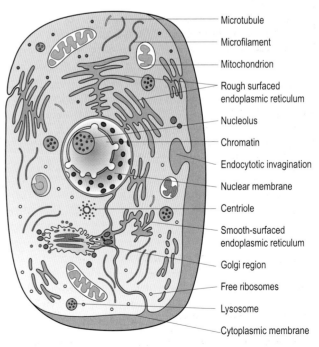

Figure 2.1 • Diagram of the ultrastructure of a cell. (From Hinchliff S M, Montague S E 1990, with kind permission of Elsevier.)

Mammalian cells average 5–20 micrometres (µm) in diameter (Alberts et al 2008). Their microstructure cannot be determined by light microscopy, but electron microscopes and electronic processing can reveal structural details as small as a few nanometres (nm). This has enabled cell biologists to identify complex cellular ultrastructures that are necessary for microstructural and functional integrity. Cells and their microstructural components are sustained, repaired or replaced when necessary by genetic expression and selective assimilation of matter from the **extracellular compartment**.

Cell size and shape

Cells differentiate, modify their structure and activities during their stages of development and aggregate correctly to form specific tissues, organs and systems. Genetic and biochemical controls and communication are fundamental to these processes. Knowledge of the size and appearance of different cells allows conclusions about how their morphological and functional features contribute to the whole body. For instance, resting **lymphocytes** are amongst the smallest of cells, their average diameter being 6 µm, whereas **erythrocytes** are approximately 7.5–9.0 µm in diameter and **columnar epithelial cells** are 20 µm tall and 10 µm wide. Some cells are significantly larger than this; for example, bone marrow **megakaryocytes** average 200 µm in diameter, and mature **ova** may be over 80 µm in diameter (Bannister 2007). Some neurons and multinucleated skeletal muscle cells are relatively large, reflecting their roles as discussed in later chapters.

The external appearance of a cell depends on its functions, interactions with other cells, external environment and the internal structures which mastermind its activities. Cellular dimensions and metabolic activities are also partly determined by the rate of **substrate diffusion** across highly selective **plasma membranes** (Pollard & Earnshaw 2008) which permit rapid diffusion of substrates in both directions over short distances of up to 50 µm. However, as cells increase in size, their mass outstrips their surface area and their shape changes to an irregular or elongated structure as is seen in many neurons. This larger size sustains efficient substrate transport and diffusion, particularly as many physiological processes such as diffusion of gases, ions and nutrient transport depend on cellular surface area.

An increase in cell mass brings problems; for example, the further the cell periphery is from the nucleus, the more difficult is nuclear control of the **cytoplasm** and plasma membrane. This can be overcome to some extent by increasing surface area by either folding the plasma membrane and forming **microvilli**, or other surface protrusions, or flattening the entire body of the cell. Alternatively, nuclear control in larger cells can be enhanced by the presence of multiple nuclei which arise due to fusion of mononuclear cells as seen in skeletal or cardiac muscle or, more rarely, by multiplication of the central nucleus without cytoplasmic division.

Cytoskeleton and cell motility

The **cytoskeleton** is a complex network of specialised proteins organised into filaments and microtubules that extends throughout the cytoplasm. This highly dynamic structure reorganises continuously as the cell changes shape, divides and responds to its environment (Morgan 2007). It is responsible for cellular movement such as cell crawling, the beating of cilia, muscle contraction, migration of **phagocytic leucocytes** from blood to a site of tissue injury, or in response to the presence of pathogens, and changes in cell shape in the developing embryo. The cytoskeleton also provides the machinery for intracellular movement, such as the transport of organelles within the cytoplasm, as well as the segregation of chromosomes at mitosis.

Motility is also observed in the tip(s) of developing dendrites and axons as they grow in response to local conditions and migrate to their synaptic targets. One of the best examples of cell migration is observed in **fibroblasts** during early embryonic development, tissue repair and remodelling when the fibroblasts secrete **collagen** which is essential for the development of the extracellular matrix. As the fibroblasts interact with collagen by means of adhesion plaques they exert traction on the cell matrix. The diverse activities of the cytoskeleton depend on three types of protein filaments: actin filaments, microtubules and the intermediate filaments.

All cells display varying degrees of **motility** which augments their shape and position and facilitates the best conditions for cellular homeostasis by moving the cytoplasm, specific organelles or vesicles from one part of the cell to another. Whilst the exact molecular mechanisms involved in cell motility are unknown, it is unlikely that a single organelle or cytoskeletal component can be responsible for such complex processes (Pollard & Earnshaw 2008). The following interrelated processes are thought to be essential:

1. Cell motility is dependent on adenosine triphosphate (ATP).

2. Cells define their own motility.

3. Cells define their leading edge which adheres to a surface over which the remainder of the cells crawl by dragging themselves towards the leading edge using traction and adhesions as points for anchorage.

4. Microtubules, intermediate and actin filaments unify the cytoskeleton forming a mechanical structure that resists external forces on the migrating cells.

All activities involve actin filaments in different ways, although the plasma membrane of the crawling cell's leading edge appears to organise the actin filaments by providing small aggregates of proteins that promote actin polymerisation (Pollard & Earnshaw 2008; see also below). Biochemical and micro-anatomical environments modulate the speed and direction of cell motility.

Epithelial cells

Epithelial cells are derived from the three embryonic germ layers: the **ectoderm**, the **endoderm** and the **mesoderm** (Alberts et al 2008):

- Ectoderm contributes to the development of epithelia and provides the basis for the epidermis, breast glandular tissue, cornea and the junctional zones of the buccal cavity and anal canal.
- Endoderm forms the epithelial lining of the alimentary canal and its glands, most of the respiratory tract and the distal tract of the urogenital tract.
- Mesoderm gives rise to the epithelium-like cells lining internal cavities such as the pericardium, pleural and peritoneal cavities, the lining of the blood vessels and lymph vessels and the proximal parts of the urogenital tract.

In general, epithelial cells form sheets which line the inner and outer body surfaces and thus provide a covering for the body and its internal organs and serve as selective barriers, facilitating or preventing the transfer of substrates across the surfaces which they cover. Some epithelia, such as the skin, protect underlying tissue from dehydration, chemical or mechanical injury, whilst other epithelia act as sensory surfaces, a function best illustrated by neural tissue, which is a modified form of epithelium.

Classification of the epithelia

The polygonal, diverse shape of epithelial cells is partly determined by their cytoplasmic contents and partly by pressure and the functional demands of the surrounding tissue (Bannister et al 2008). The conventional classification of the epithelia takes into consideration their structural and functional characteristics.

Simple epithelia

Simple epithelia are formed by single layers of cells resting on a basal **lamina** formed of filamentous proteins and proteoglycans. They are subdivided according to the shape of their cells, which may be columnar, cuboidal, pseudostratified or squamous. The cellular shapes are largely related to cell volume. Where cells are small, the volume of the cytoplasm is relatively low, denoting few organelles and low metabolic activity. Conversely, highly metabolic epithelial cells generally form secretory cells containing abundant mitochondria and endoplasmic reticulum and are tall, cuboidal or columnar. Simple epithelia are capable of special functions and help to form cilia, microvilli, secretory vacuoles or sensory features.

Stratified squamous epithelia

Stratified squamous epithelia consist of superficial cells, which are constantly replaced by their regenerating basal layers. These epithelia consist of flattened, interlocking, polygonal cells. Their cytoplasm may sometimes not exceed 0.1 mm in thickness and their nucleus may bulge into the overlying space. As the stratified squamous epithelium is so thin, it is ideally suited to facilitating diffusion of gases and water. However, it is also engaged in active transport, a role indicated by numerous endocytic vesicles. The most critical positions for stratified squamous epithelia are in the lining of the lung alveoli, the glomeruli and the thin segments of the loop of Henle.

Cuboidal and columnar epithelia

Cuboidal and columnar epithelia consist of regular rows of cylindrical cells. Commonly, the free surfaces of columnar cells have microvilli suited to their absorptive role in the small intestine, where they enhance the surface area for absorption of water and nutrients. By contrast, the columnar epithelium of the gall bladder displays a brush border, essential to the concentration and storage of bile. Ciliated columnar epithelium is found in most of the respiratory tract, the lining of fallopian tubes and uterine cervix. Large cuboidal cells are found in the proximal and distal convoluted segments of nephrons, where they form a brush border which selectively reabsorbs substances from the filtrate into the renal medullary interstitium.

Transitional epithelium

The characteristic feature of transitional epithelium is its thickness, formed by an extended arrangement of 4–6 cells held together in a specific arrangement by numerous **desmosomes** (filamentous structures). In stretching, these cells flatten without altering their position relative to each other. Most of these epithelial cells are attached to their basal lamina by slender processes forming a basal structure where they appear cuboidal and uninucleate when relaxed. At the surface of this multilayered epithelium, cells progressively fuse to form larger, and sometimes binucleate, polyploid cells with a plasma membrane covered by glycoprotein particles. This cellular arrangement has two roles:

- It facilitates expansion and contraction, stretching considerably without losing structural integrity.
- It provides an impermeable lining for organs that hold liquid containing toxic metabolic end-products such as urea and uric acid and high concentrations of salts such as potassium and sodium.

Transitional epithelium is invaluable in forming an impermeable lining in the genitourinary tract.

Complex structures derived from epithelium

Complex organ structures derived from epithelia retain familiar cellular complex characteristics; for instance, the capacity of the liver or the placenta to absorb, secrete and transport a diversity of substrates. Similarly, the diverse forms of neural tissue are functional modifications of epithelia. Most neural tissue is differentiated into conducting and non-conducting cells which provide a complex network for processing and managing information by signal transduction.

Cellular organisation

A typical cell includes a single nucleus, cytoplasm and a cellular boundary known as the **plasma membrane**. The different substances making up the cell are collectively known as **cytoplasm** or **protoplasm** and are composed predominantly of water, electrolytes, proteins, lipids and carbohydrates, all of which play crucial roles in shaping the cell and its organelles. These include the cell membrane, the nuclear membrane, the endoplasmic reticulum, Golgi apparatus, mitochondria, lysosomes and centrioles.

The plasma membrane

Plasma membrane is the most common feature of all cells (Alberts et al 2008). An appropriate plasma membrane is crucial to the survival and function of each cell. It encloses the cellular contents, defines cellular boundaries and maintains the essential biochemical differences between the cytosol and the extracellular environment. Plasma membranes are dynamic structures capable of considerable adaptation due to the ability of most of their molecules to move about within the plane of the membranes.

The lipid bilayer

The plasma membrane (Fig. 2.2) consists of a complex lipid bilayer interspersed by a range of protein molecules (Pollard & Earnshaw 2008). This complex arrangement of lipid and specialised proteins is held together predominantly by non-covalent interactions (Ch. 1) which occur in an aqueous environment.

The lipid bilayer is composed almost entirely of fatty acids, made up of **phospholipids** and **cholesterol**. Phospholipids are small molecules constructed mainly from fatty acids and glycerol. The glycerol is joined by two rather than the three fatty acid chains that are characteristic of **triacylglycerols**. The third position (site) on the glycerol molecule is linked to a hydrophilic **phosphate group**, which is in turn attached to a small hydrophilic compound such as **choline**. Each phospholipid molecule has a polar head group and two hydrophobic hydrocarbon tails consisting of fatty acids that differ marginally in length. The differences in the length and saturation of the fatty acid tails allows the phospholipid molecules to stack against one another and construct a functional 'fluid' framework which offers different physical and chemical properties to those of the hydrophobic triacylglycerols (Alberts et al 2008).

The lipid molecules are arranged in a continuous double layer about 5–7 nm thick. The hydrophobic portions

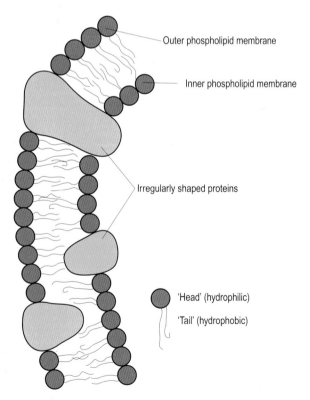

Figure 2.2 • Diagram of the fluid mosaic model of cell membrane structure. (From Hinchliff S M, Montague S E 1990, with kind permission of Elsevier.)

Outer phospholipid membrane

Inner phospholipid membrane

Irregularly shaped proteins

'Head' (hydrophilic)

'Tail' (hydrophobic)

of the phospholipid face each other, whereas the hydrophilic components make up the plasma membrane surface, which is in perpetual contact with the surrounding interstitial and intercellular fluid. This lipid bilayer is highly permeable to lipid-soluble substances, such as hormones, corticosteroids, alcohol, oxygen and carbon dioxide but is relatively impermeable to most water-soluble molecules such as inorganic ions and glucose.

Lipid molecules are insoluble in water which is crucial to their grouping spontaneously to form the bilayers in aqueous solutions whilst dissolving readily in organic solvents. Furthermore, in an aqueous environment these lipid molecules aggregate allowing their hydrophobic tails to be buried in the dry, water-free interior of the plasma membrane. Thus lipid bilayers form sealed compartments ensuring that the hydrophobic tails are not in contact with water. If there is damage to the plasma membranes the lipid molecules rapidly reseal the cavity and avoid exposure of the fatty acid tails to water.

Plasma membrane fluidity is important to the survival of the cellular infrastructure and the capacity of the membrane to sustain selective transport processes and enzyme activities. However, these complex membrane functions are also dependent on the presence within the lipid bilayer of **cholesterol, glycolipids** and **glycoproteins**. Cholesterol molecules stabilise the lipid bilayer rendering it less deformable, reducing its permeability to small water-soluble molecules and preventing the hydrocarbon chains from coming together and crystallising and damaging plasma membrane functional integrity. Glycolipids and glycoproteins act as receptors for extracellular biochemical products.

The membrane proteins

The proteins suspended within, or found on the surface of, the lipid bilayer are mostly glycoproteins, which mediate many of the selective plasma membrane functions. Although these proteins are functionally highly specific they can be classified as **integral** or **transmembrane proteins**, which protrude through the plasma membrane, and **peripheral proteins**, which attach to the inner surface of the membrane.

The transmembrane proteins or integral proteins have a unique orientation in the plasma membrane, reflecting the asymmetrical manner in which the protein is synthesised in the **endoplasmic reticulum** and inserted into the lipid bilayer. Membrane proteins do not flop across the plasma membrane but rotate about an axis perpendicular to the plane of the lipid bilayer. They cross the bilayer more than once folding into distinctive α or β strands (Pollard & Earnshaw 2008).

The asymmetrical construction of lipids and proteins found on the outer and inner surfaces of the membrane facilitates the variety of functions including the control of lipid and protein diffusion. For example, the epithelial cells lining the intestinal tract confine some of the plasma membrane transport proteins to the apical surface of the cells, whereas others are confined to the basal and lateral surfaces. This suggests that cell membranes confine specific proteins to functionally distinctive domains. Whilst many peripheral proteins attach to one of the integral proteins, other proteins form structural links connecting the plasma membrane to the **cytoskeleton** or the extracellular matrix of adjacent cells. A few peripheral proteins serve as specialised ligand-sensitive receptors used for detection and transduction of local chemical signals.

The quantities and types of plasma membrane proteins vary in keeping with cellular functions. For instance, the neural **myelin membrane** serves mainly as an electrical insulation for nerve cell axons; consequently less than 25% of the membrane mass consists of protein. Conversely, **mitochodrial membranes** involved in energy transduction consists of approximately 75% protein. Generally, plasma membrane protein content averages 50% of its total membrane mass (Alberts et al 2008). As protein molecules are much larger than lipid molecules there are fewer of them than lipid molecules in most plasma membranes. There may be 50 lipid molecules for each protein molecule in a membrane that consists of 50% protein by mass.

Concept of selective permeability

Selective permeability of the plasma membrane facilitates free passage of some gases such as oxygen, and water, but restricts the movement of larger ions such as sodium, potassium, calcium, chloride and bicarbonate to their specific protein channels. These open or close in order to regulate transmembrane ion traffic and most integral proteins form **pores** through which the water-soluble substances such as ions **diffuse** passively. The selective passage of many other substances of larger molecular weight, such as glucose and amino acids, is also limited to protein channels, most of which are ion- or substrate-specific. This contrasts with lipid-soluble substances, such as steroid hormones, which diffuse unhindered through the lipid portion of the plasma membranes.

Cells also take up larger molecules and transport them into other cellular regions by **endocytosis**. This involves the invagination of small segments of plasma membrane to create **vacuoles** or **endocytic vesicles**. In addition, many cells ingest extracellular fluid in large endocytic structures defined by Pollard & Earnshaw (2008) as **macropinosomes**. By contrast, the extrusion of organic molecules such as **thyroxine** and **acetylcholine** is achieved by **exocytic vesicles** which fuse with plasma membrane, releasing their content to the cell's exterior.

Plasma membrane excitability and ion transport

The hydrophobic interior of the plasma membranes acts as a barrier to the passage of most polar molecules. This barrier is crucial to cell function allowing the required solutes to be maintained in the cytoplasm and within each of the intracellular membrane-bound organelles at vastly different concentrations to those found in extracellular fluid. Cells selectively transfer water-soluble molecules across their membranes, thereby obtaining essential nutrients, excreting metabolic waste products and regulating intracellular ion concentrations.

The two specialised transmembrane proteins that transport inorganic ions and small water-soluble organic molecules across the lipid bilayer are **ion channels (channels proteins)** and **carrier proteins**. Carrier proteins are coupled to an energy source which facilitates active transport of substrates across the membrane and against a concentration gradient of that substrate. In contrast, channel proteins form a narrow hydrophilic pore, allowing the passive movement of small inorganic ions across the lipid bilayer. This combination of passive permeability and active transport is fundamental to the large differences in the composition of the cytosol compared with the extracellular fluid or the fluid within the membrane-bounded organelles.

By generating ionic concentration differences across the lipid bilayer, cell membranes store **potential energy** in the form of **electrochemical gradients** which drive many of the transport processes, convey electric signals in excitable cells and generate ATP in the mitochondria. In contrast, smaller and more lipid-soluble molecules diffuse more rapidly across the lipid bilayer. Similarly, small non-polar molecules such as oxygen and carbon dioxide readily dissolve in the lipid bilayers and diffuse rapidly across them. Uncharged polar molecules also diffuse rapidly across a bilayer if they are small enough. Water and urea cross rapidly, whereas glycerol, a larger molecule, diffuses less rapidly. Diffusion of the more complex glucose molecules is carrier-dependent.

The lipid bilayers are impermeable to charged molecules (ions) no matter how small they are; their charge and high degree of hydration prevent them from entering the hydrocarbon phase of the bilayer. Therefore ionic transfer is dependent on ion-specific channels that form a continuous pathway across the plasma membrane. The ion-specific channels facilitate passive diffusion of hydrophilic solutes across the cell membrane without coming into direct contact with the hydrophobic lipid bilayer. As most channel proteins are ion-species-specific they play a crucial role in determining ion diffusion efficiency. The advantage of ion channels over carrier proteins is that more than 1 million ions can pass through an open channel each second, a rate 1000 times greater than any carrier protein.

Ion channels

Two important properties distinguish ion channels from single aqueous pores (Alberts et al 2008):

1. They show ion selectivity, permitting some inorganic ions to pass but not others.

2. More importantly, ion channels are not continuously open but use 'gates' that open briefly, usually in response to a specific stimulus closing again once the intracellular electrogradient for a particular ion species has been reached.

The main types of stimuli that cause ion channels to open are **changes in voltage** across the membrane (voltage-gated channels), **mechanical stress** (mechanically gated channels) or the binding of a **ligand** to **specific receptors** (ligand-gated channels). The ligand acts as an extracellular mediator, a neurotransmitter or as an intracellular mediator such as a nucleotide.

Although ion channels are responsible for the electrical excitability of muscle cells and the mediation of electrical signalling in neurons, they are not restricted to electrically excitable cells. They are present in all cell membranes, facilitating diffusion of their specific ion species to maintain the required intracellular electrochemical gradient. The most common forms of ion channels are those permeable mainly to potassium ions, making the plasma membrane much more permeable to potassium than to any other ion; a factor critical in maintaining cell membrane potential and the voltage difference across plasma membranes.

Carrier proteins

In contrast, carrier proteins, which facilitate selective transport of substrates across the plasma membranes, bind their specific solutes and then undergo a series of conformational changes in order to transfer these solutes across the plasma membranes. Each carrier protein has one or more **binding sites** for its substrates permitting full saturation of the carrier sites. When all the binding sites are occupied the rate of transport across the plasma membrane is maximal. However, solute binding can be blocked by competitive inhibitors occupying the same binding sites. These may or may not be transported by the carrier. Non-competitive inhibitors that bind elsewhere can also alter the structure of the carrier protein.

Generally, carrier proteins are classified according to their functional capacity: some are **uniporters**; other more complex proteins are **coupled transporters**, where the transport of one solute depends on the simultaneous transfer of a second solute in the same direction (**symport**) or in the opposite direction (**antiport**). For example, the take-up of glucose from extracellular fluid, where its concentration is high relative to that in the cytosol, is achieved by passive transport by glucose carriers operating as uniporters. Intestinal and kidney epithelial cells take up glucose from the lumen of the intestine and the nephron filtrate, respectively. In both instances the low concentration of glucose in the epithelial cells creates a favourable concentration gradient for the influx of glucose along with sodium.

Within the cell glucose is rapidly phosphorylated to glucose 6-phosphate, which shows no affinity to glucose transporters and is retained in the cytosol for use as a metabolic substrate. As glucose transport is determined by its concentration gradients, higher intracellular versus extracellular glucose concentrations allow its transporters to facilitate glucose efflux into the extracellular compartment.

The sodium–potassium pump

Potassium ion concentration is typically 10–20 times higher in cytoplasm than in extracellular fluid, whereas the reverse is true of sodium ions. Although ion channels play a crucial role in maintaining these differences, fine-tuning of these concentrations is achieved by the highly dynamic **sodium–potassium pumps**. These appear to operate as antiporters, actively pumping sodium out of the cell and potassium into the cell against their steep electrochemical gradients. The sodium gradient produced by these pumps regulates cell volume through its osmotic effects, a mechanism also exploited in the transportation of sugars and amino acids into cells (Fig. 2.3).

Almost one-third of a cell's energy is consumed in fuelling the sodium–potassium pumps. However, in electrically active nerve cells, which are repeatedly gaining small amounts of sodium and losing small amounts of potassium during the propagation of nerve impulses, the energy requirements of the pumps may increase to two-thirds (Alberts et al 2008). ATP is the primary energy required by the sodium–potassium pumps and its supply is facilitated by ATPase, which hydrolyses the ATP molecule thereby releasing its stored energy.

The sodium–potassium pump is a large molecule with binding sites for sodium and ATP on its cytoplasmic surface and a binding site for potassium on its external surface; the molecule is reversibly phosphorylated and dephosphorylated during the pumping cycle. Since the sodium–potassium pump drives three positively charged ions out of the cell for every two it pumps into the cell, it creates an electrical potential with the inside surface of the plasma membrane negative to the outside surface, although this effect contributes only 10% to the

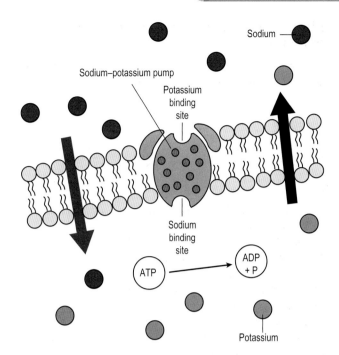

Figure 2.3 • Operation of the sodium–potassium pump. Three sodium ions are moved out of the cell and two potassium ions are moved into the cell. The energy is provided by hydrolysis of one molecule of ATP.

membrane potential. Nevertheless, by controlling the solute concentration inside the cell, the sodium–potassium pump regulates the osmotic forces that influence cell expansion and dehydration. This is important because cells contain high concentrations of solutes, including numerous negatively charged organic molecules (fixed anions) confined within them. Specific cations such as sodium and potassium are required for charge balance, creating a large osmotic gradient that tends to pull water into the cell. This is counteracted by an opposite osmotic gradient caused by a high concentration of inorganic ions, mainly sodium and chloride, in the extracellular fluid. The movement of sodium contributes to intracellular hydration.

Cytoplasm and its organelles

Every living cell uses complex communication pathways to sustain its specific microstructures and functional competence. **Eukaryotic cells** (nucleated) use a diverse range of internal processes supported by elaborate internal membrane machinery and complex arrangements of cell-specific organelles within the cytoplasm.

Cytoplasm

Cytoplasm makes up approximately half of the cell volume. Due to its high protein content (20% by weight), cytoplasm appears more gel-like than an aqueous solution, creating an environment that suspends small molecular structures, large particles and organelles. Organic and inorganic ions dissolve in this gel-like cytoplasm. Also dispersed in the cytoplasm are fat globules, glycogen granules, ribosomes and secretory granules. The most important organelles contained within the cytoplasm are the endoplasmic reticulum, the Golgi apparatus, mitochondria, lysosomes and peroxisomes. Variations in their numbers or densities are found in different cells, although their functions are unchanged across cell types.

Endoplasmic reticulum

The **endoplasmic reticulum** is a network of specialised membranous structures organised into tubular or flat vesicular sacs (Fig. 2.4) which interconnect, ensuring that the entire endoplasmic reticulum forms a continuous framework within the internal cellular space. These specialised reticular membranes also form a barrier between the cytosol and the reticular lumen, mediating the selective transport of molecules between the relevant intracellular compartments.

The endoplasmic reticulum can make up as much as 50% of total cell volume. There are two distinct membrane types: **rough** and **smooth** endoplasmic reticulum. One difference between these two types of organelles is the association of ribosomes on the cytoplasmic surface of the rough endoplasmic reticulum. In addition, the rough endoplasmic reticulum interacts with the nuclear lamina and chromatin (Pollard & Earnshaw 2008). By contrast, the smooth endoplasmic reticulum is composed of more tubular elements, is ribosome-free and commonly located at some distance from the nucleus.

Functionally both the rough and the smooth endoplasmic reticulum are highly dynamic, permitting bidirectional traffic of small substrate-filled vesicles to and from the Golgi apparatus and performing several functions. The rough endoplasmic reticulum plays a central role in the biosynthesis of protein and lipid used in the reconstruction of all organelles, including the Golgi apparatus, nuclear and plasma membranes. The synthesis of membrane lipids such as steroids, phospholipids and triglycerides occurs within both the rough and the smooth endoplasmic reticulum. In addition, the smooth endoplasmic reticulum shows cell-specific functions. For example, in hepatocytes its roles are dedicated to enzyme pathways including the cytochrome P-450 enzymes involved in drug metabolism, whilst in endocrine cells it facilitates steroid synthesis. By contrast, in skeletal and cardiac muscle cells (where it is known as the sarcoplasmic reticulum) it acts as a reservoir for calcium, controlling calcium release into the cytoplasm to support muscle contraction and taking it up again thus facilitating muscle relaxation.

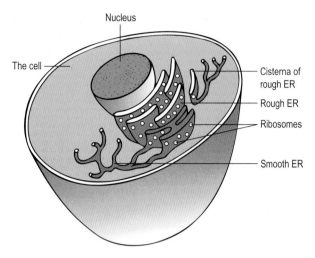

Figure 2.4 ● The endoplasmic reticulum (ER). The rough endoplasmic reticulum and smooth endoplasmic reticulum with their connections are illustrated.

The cytoplasm holds at least two separate groups of **ribosomes** which are best described as particles or granules of no more than 25 nm in diameter, consisting of two-thirds ribonucleic acid (RNA) and one-third protein. All ribosomes are produced in the nucleus under the direction of **deoxyribonucleic acid** (DNA) and each consists of a large (60S) and a small (40S) subunit. All ribosomes play critical roles in protein synthesis for that particular cell.

Membrane-bound ribosomes attached to the external surface of the rough endoplasmic reticulum and the outer nuclear membrane synthesise proteins that are translocated into the **cisternae** of the endoplasmic reticulum and are then transported to the Golgi apparatus. Protein translocation into the cisternae occurs because of specific protein-conducting channels in the membrane whose opening appears to be governed by signal peptides (Alberts et al 2008). By contrast, the unattached free ribosomes are involved in the synthesis of all other proteins encoded by the cell's nuclear DNA and used for intracellular activities such as cytoplasmic filament formation. These proteins are destined for the development or construction of intracellular and extracellular substrates.

Golgi apparatus

The **Golgi apparatus** is a mass of membrane-bound sacs with multiple associated vesicles situated close to the vicinity of the cell nucleus and frequently close to the **centrosomes**. Each Golgi apparatus is adjacent to the endoplasmic reticulum and its membrane is similar in appearance to the smooth endoplasmic reticulum. The apparatus consists of four or more stacked thin, flat vesicles consisting of an entry point (or *cis* face) and an exit (or *trans* face). The entire Golgi apparatus functions in close association with the endoplasmic reticulum. Soluble proteins from the endoplasmic reticulum enter the Golgi apparatus where they are processed and fine-tuned to form lysosomes and secretory vesicles containing enzymes or other cytoplasmic components (Fig. 2.5).

Lysosomes

Lysosomes are cell-specific vesicular organelles dispersed throughout the cytoplasm. They average 250–750 nm in diameter, are surrounded by a membranous lipid bilayer and are filled with large numbers of small granules averaging 5–8 nm in diameter. According to Alberts et al (2008), lysosomes serve as the principal sites for intracellular digestion and processing of materials entering the cells from the extracellular environment prior to their release into the cytoplasm. Lysosomes contain about 40 types of hydrolytic enzymes which are synthesised in the endoplasmic reticulum and transported through the Golgi apparatus to the lysosomes where they are stored as granules until needed.

Lysosomes also degrade unwanted intracellular substances such as proteins, nucleic acid, phospholipids and oligosaccharides, and help to remove damaged structures and foreign particles such as bacteria. These digestive/hydrolytic enzymes **hydrolyse** (Ch. 1) proteins to form amino acids, transform glycogen into glucose, and degrade obsolete parts of the cell such as the mitochondria. This degradation is initiated by the enclosure of organelles in a membrane derived from the endoplasmic reticulum. This creates an **autophagosome**, which then fuses with local lysosomes (Alberts et al 2008). It is unclear what determines the destruction of specific organelles.

Peroxisomes

Peroxisomes are formed by the budding off of membranes from the smooth endoplasmic reticulum. Their size averages 0.15–0.5 μm in diameter. New peroxisomes are formed by growth and fission of existing ones. Since these organelles do not have their own genome or ribosomes, their proteins and lipids are imported from the cytoplasm. All peroxisomes contain oxidases capable of catalysing many reactions, including the **oxidation** of long-chain saturated fatty acids not handled well by mitochondria. Several oxidases combine oxygen with hydrogen ions, thereby forming **hydrogen peroxide**—a highly oxidising substance which, in association with the enzyme catalase, oxidises numerous toxic substances. Given their function, it is not surprising to find peroxisomes involved in cholesterol metabolism, gluconeogenesis within hepatocytes and synthesis of phospholipids within the Schwann cells of the central nervous system. Genetic defects in the peroxisome are, according

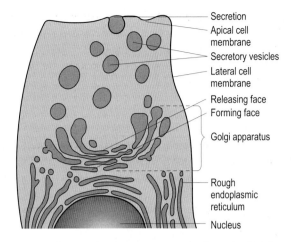

Figure 2.5 • Exocytosis of secretory proteins from the Golgi apparatus. (From Montague S E, Watson R, Herbert R A 2005, with kind permission of Elsevier.)

to Pollard & Earnshaw (2008), responsible for several forms of 'mental retardation'.

Mitochondria

Mitochondria are found in the cytoplasm of most mature cells. Their distinctive structure and variable size reflect the complex nature of their function. These organelles are ellipsoid in shape with an average length of 1–2 μm and width of 0.1–0.5 μm. However, electron microscopic images can be misleading, because, when viewed in a living cell, mitochondria change their shape, fuse, divide and move. Normally a mitochondrion doubles its mass and divides into two during each cell cycle but some mitochondria divide rapidly, whereas others do not divide at all.

Mitochondria have their own double-stranded circular DNA which replicates prior to mitochondrial division. The human mitochondrial genome consists of 16 569 nucleotide pairs (Pollard & Earnshaw 2008; see also Ch. 3) which encode only 13 mitochodrial membrane proteins, two ribosomal RNAs and just enough tRNA (transfer RNA) to translate these genes. The fact that mitochondria usually contain multiple copies of their genome may be a factor that facilitates the rapid growth and division that typically occurs in highly metabolically active cells. Despite the mitochondrial numbers in each cell, their DNA makes up less than 1% of the total cellular DNA. This may be partly attributed to the compactness of mitochondrial DNA with few **intronic sequences** or the presence of untranslated regions between **coding genes** (Ch. 3). Furthermore, the asymmetric distribution of **guanine** and **cytosine** renders one DNA strand heavier due to its guanine content whilst the opposing strand is lighter due to its cytosine content.

The mitochondrion has an outer membrane and an inner membrane, creating two compartments. The outer membrane contains a major integral protein, **porin**, which forms membrane channels thought to facilitate diffusion of substrates of molecular mass less than 50 000 daltons, including metabolites required for ATP synthesis (Pollard & Earnshaw 2008). The highly impermeable inner membrane is arranged into folds known as **cristae**, which increase the surface area considerably, an important feature of mitochondria as the power centres of the cell. The inner membrane consists of 75% protein, which may be significant in supporting the mitochondrial respiratory chain, **adenosine triphosphate** (ATP) synthesis and the transport of oxidative phosphorylation substrates in and out of the mitochondria. As mitochondria provide cells with energy by reducing oxygen and converting **adenosine diphosphate** (ADP) and phosphate to ATP (Ch. 23), in their absence or malfunction cells would be unable to extract energy from nutrients and oxygen, and cellular functions would cease.

According to Pollard & Earnshaw (2008), all 13 of the mitochondrial proteins encoded by nuclear genes are synthesised in the cytoplasm and imported into the mitochondria. These proteins are synthesised by free ribosomes and are thought to be destined for the mitochondria because they possess a mitochondrial signal peptide which binds to a signal receptor on the outer membrane of the mitochondria. The peptide–receptor complexes then move laterally across the outer membrane until they reach a contact site where the outer and inner membranes are joined. There the signal peptide crosses both membranes, using the difference in the membrane potential as the energy source.

The size and shape of mitochondria vary considerably; their appearance varies from globular of no more than a few hundred nanometres in diameter to elongated structures 1 μm in diameter and up to 10 μm in length. The morphology of the mitochondria is constant, however, and arranged to support the functional demands of cells. This is particularly evident in the cristae of the inner membrane, which project into the interior of the organelle and are shelf-like or tubular in structure (Fig. 2.6).

The innermost cavity of the mitochondria is filled with a matrix containing large quantities of dissolved enzymes which are necessary for extraction of energy from nutrients. These enzymes function in association with oxidative enzymes, providing the mechanism for oxidation of nutrients, liberation of energy and formation of carbon dioxide and water. Importantly, the liberated energy is used to synthesise high-energy ATP, which is transported out of the mitochondria into the cytoplasm to support cellular activities. Increased cellular ATP requirements may be responsible for inducing

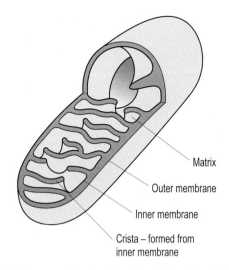

Matrix

Outer membrane

Inner membrane

Crista – formed from inner membrane

Figure 2.6 • Diagram of a mitochondrion. (From Hinchliff S M, Montague S E 1990, with kind permission of Elsevier.)

mitochondrial self-replication. Given that a mitochondrion usually contains multiple copies of its own genome, its efficient replication prior to division is an important mechanism cells use to ensure that their metabolic and energy demands are met. As the mitochondrial genome mutates at a rate 10-fold greater than nuclear DNA does (Nussbaum et al 2004), mitochondrial dysfunction may result in human disorders such as epilepsy, neuropathy and myopathy. However, Pollard & Earnshaw (2008) suggest that many of these disorders can be attributed to mutations in genes for mitochondrial protein encoded by both mitochondrial and nuclear DNA.

The nucleus

The nucleus is the ultimate control centre of the cell and is the largest organelle, measuring approximately 2–10 μm in diameter. Although mainly centrally situated, its position and number(s) can vary with cell type. For example, it is found in the periphery of **adipocytes**, at the base of epithelial and secretory cells and in the centre of the cell body in neurons. Although most cells have only one nucleus, skeletal muscle cells, some myocardial muscle cells and **osteoclasts** can be multinucleated.

Nuclei contain large quantities of DNA which holds the genetic blueprint for the cell type. Thus the nuclear genome determines the characteristics of proteins and enzymes contained in the cytoplasm and controls cytoplasmic activities and cellular reproduction (Pollard & Earnshaw 2008). In addition to the DNA, several other structures are essential to normal nuclear functioning, such as the gel-like **nucleoplasm** and the **nucleoli**; the latter are the site of **ribosomal ribonucleic acid** (rRNA) synthesis. The genetic material, consisting chiefly of DNA, is found in thread-like structures known as chromatin. Prior to cellular reproduction, the chromatin strands shorten and coil into rod-like bodies forming (in humans) 46 recognisable **chromosomes** (see below and Ch. 3).

The outermost part of the nucleus is formed by a complex nuclear membrane composed of two lipid bilayers approximately 20–40 nm apart from each other and enclosing the **perinuclear cisternae**. The outer nuclear membrane is continuous with the cell's rough endoplasmic reticulum, and the intramembranous space of 20–40 nm serves as an extension of the internal compartments of the endoplasmic reticulum. Several thousand **nuclear pores** penetrate the nuclear envelope, making it permeable to substances of low molecular weight. Large complex protein molecules surround these nuclear pores, creating smaller central pores of only 9–10 nm in diameter, although these pores are large enough to permit molecules of up to 44 000 molecular weight to pass through relatively easily. Substrates of molecular weight less than 15 000 pass through the nuclear pores extremely rapidly. The selective transport of large molecules and complexes through the nuclear pores occurs by receptor-mediated processes. Importantly, the membrane porosity permits the movement of messenger RNA into the cytoplasm and entry of enzymes and histones into the nucleus during DNA replication.

The nucleolus (nucleoli)

The nucleolus is the most prominent nuclear subdomain. Most mammalian cell nuclei have 1–5 nucleoli which appear as dense structures visible within the nucleus during the cell's interphase, although their size, shape and number depend on the activity relative to the cell cycle. In cells that are actively synthesising large quantities of different proteins, the nucleoli average 5.0 μm in diameter, whereas the nucleoli are hardly visible in dormant cells. Unlike most organelles, nucleoli do not appear to have a limiting membrane; they have four distinct regions which Pollard & Earnshaw (2008) describe as:

1. A fibrillar centre which contains DNA that is not being transcribed.

2. A dense fibrillar core which contains RNA in a process of transcription.

3. A granular region where the maturing ribosomal particles are assembled.

4. A nuclear matrix which may participate in the organisation of the nucleolus.

Typically the nucleoli usually contain large quantities of RNA and proteins similar to those found in the ribosomes. The proteins appears to be fundamental to the production and assembly of ribosomes as complex macromolecular structures. The functions of many other nucleolar proteins are unknown although, according to Pollard & Earnshaw (2008), nucleoli may be involved in other, undiscovered biological processes. However, nucleoli enlarge considerably when cells actively synthesise protein. At this stage, their increased size enhances the shape of the nucleus, disappearing during mitosis and reassembling again in the daughter cells.

Cell division

Controlled cell division is vital to human reproduction, tissue growth and repair, efficient functioning of the immune defence mechanisms and countless other processes. The cycle of cell division is one of the most fundamental processes by which multicellular species replace cells damaged by wear and tear or lost during programmed cell death (**apoptosis**). To facilitate this, the body must be capable of programmed synthesis and maturation of millions of new cells simply to maintain its status quo. In cases of ill-health, trauma or surgery, loss and corresponding replacement of new cells is fundamental to successful healing and recovery. Conversely, when natural cell division is halted or compromised—as, for example, in exposure to a large dose of ionising radiation—the individual is likely to suffer the consequences of rapid and extensive irreparable cell damage and destruction.

Although details of the cell cycle may vary, certain behavioural requirements of all cells are universal. In the first instance, cells have to co-ordinate various events in the cycle. They must, for example, avoid entering mitosis or meiosis until such time as the chromosomes have been replicated. Failure to comply with this requirement can result in cells that lack a particular chromosome, an aberration which may give rise to cancer at a later stage (Turnpenny & Ellard 2007).

Nucleotide structure of DNA

All cell nuclei, with the exception of mature erythrocytes, contain large amounts of deoxyribonucleic acid (DNA) which holds within its structure the genetic information required for directing all aspects of embryogenesis, growth, development, metabolism, reproduction and apoptosis. Each strand of DNA consists of a chain of nucleotides; these are molecules which contain phosphoric acid, a pentose sugar with five carbon atoms called deoxyribose, and four nitrogenous bases, comprising two purines (adenine and guanine) and two pyrimidines (cytosine and thymine), identified by the single letters A, G, C and T. Different genes have different sequences of these four nucleotides and so code for different biological functions. Given that there are four types of nucleotides, the number of possible sequences in a DNA strand is enormous.

Mitosis and the cell cycle

In order to produce a pair of genetically identical daughter cells, nuclear DNA must be precisely replicated (Fig. 2.7) and the replicated chromosomes must then separate into two genetically identical cells. As the vast majority of cells also double their mass and duplicate all their cytoplasmic organelles in each cell cycle, co-ordination of the many complex cytoplasmic and nuclear processes is fundamental.

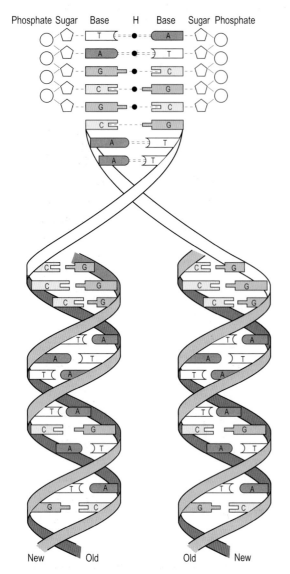

Figure 2.7 • The replication of DNA showing the unwinding of the double helix and the formation of new strands with complementary base pairs. (From Hinchliff S M, Montague S E 1990, with kind permission of Elsevier.)

The duration of the cell cycle (Fig. 2.8) varies greatly from one cell type to another (Alberts et al 2008), although a standard prevails ensuring that cell cycles for all dividing cells follow distinct phases: **interphase**, **mitosis** and **cytokinesis.** Mitosis is the critical process of nuclear division. As cells require time to grow and mature before they can divide, the standard cell cycle is fairly long, extending to 12 h or more in fast-growing mammalian tissue, although in most cells the mitotic phase takes about an hour, which is only a small fraction of the total cell cycle time.

- During **interphase** a cell performs all its normal functions and if necessary prepares itself for division by facilitating DNA replication. The interphase is the longest time of a cell cycle extending from one mitotic phase to the next. It consists of three distinct phases: the G_1 or **gap1** phase, the **S** or **synthesis phase** and the G_2 or **gap2** phase. During the G_1 phase the cells monitor their internal environment and their size, so that when the time is appropriate decisive steps are taken committing the cells to DNA replication, which occurs in the S phase of the cell cycle. The subsequent G_2 phase provides a safety gap, which ensures that DNA replication is complete before mitosis.

- During mitosis the nuclear membrane breaks down and the nuclear contents condense, forming visible chromosomes. The stages of mitosis are **prophase**, **metaphase**, **anaphase** and **telophase** (Fig. 2.9). During prophase, the cell's microtubules reorganise to establish the **mitotic spindle** which eventually separates the chromosomes. Cells appear to pause briefly in metaphase allowing the duplicated chromosomes to align with the mitotic spindle, in preparation for segregation.

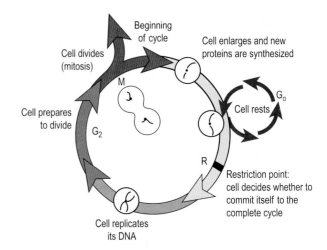

Figure 2.8 • Stages of the cell cycle (reproduced with kind permission of Barbara Novak).

- The segregation of the duplicated chromosomes marks the beginning of the **anaphase**, during which the chromosomes move to the pole of the spindle where they decondense and re-establish new nuclei.

- At this point during telophase the cell membrane contracts and gradually divides by a process commonly known as **cytokinesis**, the critical point of the mitotic phase that terminates the end of the cell cycle.

Although the length of all phases of the cell cycle is variable, the greatest variation appears to occur in the duration of the G_1 phase. A reason for this variability is thought to be the natural need of the cell to replicate. Thus, cells in G_1, if not already committed to DNA replication, can pause in and enter a specialised resting state often referred to as the G_0 phase. Cells

cells are universal; for instance, they must avoid entering mitosis or meiosis until all the chromosomes are replicated. Failure to comply with this requirement can result in cells that evolve with particular chromosomal aberrations which may give rise to cancer at a later stage (Alberts et al 2008, Morgan 2007).

Meiosis

Meiosis (meaning diminution) is a special kind of nuclear division in which the chromosome complement is halved. Meiosis involves two nuclear divisions rather than one (Fig. 2.10). With the exception of the **sex chromosomes** (different in male and female), a **diploid nucleus** contains two similar versions of each of the **autosomes** (alike in male and female). One set of these chromosomes is paternal and one set maternal in origin. These two sets of chromosomes are known as the **homologues**. In most cells the homologues maintain a separate existence as independent chromosomes.

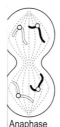
Anaphase

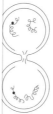
Telophase

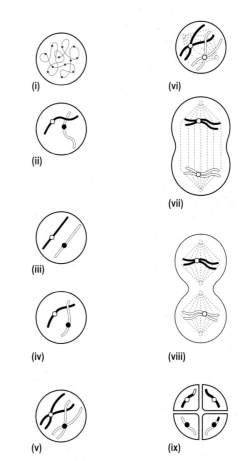

Figure 2.10 The stages of meiosis. (Only one chromosome pair is shown for clarity.) (i) Interphase. (ii) Prophase I: leptotene. (iii) Zygotene. (iv) Pachytene. (v) Diplotene. (vi) Metaphase I. (vii) Anaphase I. (viii) Telophase I. (ix) Second meiotic division. (From Hinchliff S M, Montague S E 1990, with kind permission of Elsevier.)

As a consequence, a mature **haploid gamete** produced by the divisions of a diploid cell during meiosis contains half the original number of chromosomes. This means that only one chromosome from each homologous pair is present, ensuring that either the maternal or the paternal copy of each gene, but not both, is present. Clearly, this specific requirement makes an extra demand on the processes governing cell division. Evidence suggests that mechanisms have evolved permitting the additional sorting of the chromosomes which involves the homologues recognising each other and becoming physically paired prior to lining up on the mitotic spindle. This pairing of the maternal and paternal copy of each chromosome is unique to meiosis.

It is probably only after DNA replication has been completed that the special feature of meiosis becomes evident and this suggests that, rather than separating, the sister chromatids behave as a unit, giving the impression that the earlier chromosome duplication has not occurred. The duplicated homologous pairs form a structure containing four chromatids and this close proximity allows genetic recombination to occur where a fragment of a maternal chromatid is exchanged for a corresponding fragment of an homologous paternal chromatid.

Main points

- Cells are the fundamental units of life. Their morphological and functional features are governed by genetic blueprints contained in their nuclei and in the mitochondria. Numerous physiological processes depend on the size and the surface area of the cell. Cells permit selective but rapid diffusion of substrates over short distances to ensure that metabolic needs are easily sustained.

- In larger cells there is a significant increase in surface area achieved by either folding the plasma membrane and forming microvilli or other surface protrusions or by flattening the entire cell body, generating a larger surface area for selective transport and diffusion.

- The body is composed of a vast variation of cells, most of which display a capacity for motility, generally involving the movement of the cytoplasm and specific organelles from one part of the cell to another. Cell motility is influenced by metabolic demands and environmental factors such as tissue injury.

- Ectoderm, endoderm and mesoderm all contribute to the formation and development of different cells including the epithelia, some of which function as sensory surfaces; others provide an internal and external covering for body surfaces, protecting the underlying tissue from dehydration, chemical or mechanical injury.

- Epithelial cells are classified according to morphological and functional characteristics. Each epithelial cell type is identified by size, shape, cell volume and density. Where cells are small the volume of the cytoplasm is relatively low, containing few organelles, and the metabolic activity is low; large cells have more cytoplasm and organelles and the metabolic activity is high.

- The most obvious feature of any cell is the plasma membrane. It is constructed of a lipid bilayer interspersed with protein molecules; its capability to physically adapt is fundamental to competent cell function.

- Lipid molecules consist of a hydrophilic polar head and a hydrophobic non-polar tail which are arranged into a bilayer enriched by proteins, cholesterol, glycoproteins and glycolipids, each of which contributes to the structure and function of the plasma membrane and the cell. Most plasma membrane functions are carried out by membrane proteins.

- Selective permeability of the plasma membrane facilitates free passage of gases and water but restricts the movement of larger ions to their specific protein channels which can be opened or closed in order to regulate transmembrane traffic.

- The most common form of plasma membrane ion channel is one that is permeable to potassium ions, ensuring that the plasma membrane potential is maintained. The critical concentration of potassium ions may be 10–20 times higher in the cell than in the extracellular fluid, whereas the reverse is true of sodium. These ionic concentration differences are maintained by sodium–potassium pumps.

- Cytoplasm acts as a reservoir for the suspension of small molecular structures, large particles and organelles such as the endoplasmic reticulum, the Golgi apparatus, mitochondria, lysosomes and peroxisomes. The endoplasmic reticulum plays a central role in lipid and protein biosynthesis whereas the Golgi apparatus processes proteins for intra- and extracellular use.

- Lysosomes are filled with a granular protein aggregate which constitutes necessary digestive enzymes. Peroxisomes contain oxidases which are enzymes that can combine intracellular oxygen with hydrogen ions to form hydrogen peroxide which is used to oxidise substances that might otherwise be poisonous to the cell.

- Mitochondria vary in size and shape but their structure is constant, being mainly composed of two limiting membranes. Mitochondria are self-replicating, contain their own DNA and generate ATP, a form of energy essential to normal cellular function.
- The nucleus is the largest structure of the cell, containing large quantities of DNA, which holds the cell's genetic blueprint. The nuclear genome determines the characteristic morphological and functional features of the cell.
- Controlled cell division is vital to human reproduction, tissue growth, repair and other processes. To produce a pair of genetically identical daughter cells the nuclear DNA must be replicated precisely and the replicated chromosomes must be separated into two genetically identical cells.
- Meiosis leads to gamete formation where the chromosome numbers are halved. Ideally, after exchanging genetic material, one of each pair of homologous chromosomes is represented in the mature gamete.

References

Alberts, B., Bray, D., Johnson, A., Lewis, J., Raff, M., Roberts, K., Walters, P., 2008. Essential Cell Biology. Garland Publishing, New York/London.

Bannister, L., et al., 2007. Cells and tissues. In: Bannister, L., Berry, M., Collins, P. et al (Eds.) Gray's Anatomy. Churchill Livingstone, New York.

Morgan, D., 2007. The Cell Cycle. Oxford University Press, Oxford.

Nussbaum, R., McInnes, R., Huntington, W., 2004. Genetics in Medicine. Saunders Elsevier, London.

Pollard, T., Earnshaw, W., 2008. Cell Biology. Saunders Elsevier, London.

Turnpenny, P., Ellard, S., 2007. Emery's Elements of Medical Genetics, thirteen edn. Churchill Livingstone, Edinburgh.

Annotated recommended reading

Cross, R., 2008. Directing directions. Nature 406, 839–840.

This article offers an exploratory account of the role of molecular motors in transporting cargoes to their correct destinations and considers the energy-dependent biochemical processes that enable the molecular motors to support the survival of the cells.

Karp, G., 2002. Cellular and Molecular Biology—Concepts and Experiments. John Wiley, New York.

This textbook offers a refreshing account of the relationship between molecular structures and functions. It details the way chemical energy can be used in running the diverse cellular activities.

Pocock, G., Richards, C., 2006. Human Physiology. Oxford University Press, Oxford.

This book offers a series of concise chapters exploring physiological phenomena involved in controlling body temperature, exercise and acid–base balance and links these to possible sequences of events that contribute to the onset of systemic disorders such as hypertension.

Rothstein, J., 2000. Bundling up excitement. Nature 407, 141–143.

This article considers glutamate, an abundant amino acid in all cells, and reflects on its synthesis, transportation and functions in the brain.

Chapter Three

Structure, organisation and regulation of genes

Introduction

'Life depends on the ability of cells to store, retrieve and translate the genetic instructions to make and maintain a living organism' (Alberts et al 2002). Over the last decade there have been major developments in the science of genetics. The finding that there is a **genetic basis** for many aspects of human disease has led to the search for treatments. The research has involved the **Human Genome Project** which was undertaken to identify the structure and function of all human genes. The study of the human genome is called **genomics**.

With the completion of mapping the human genome in the year 2000 ethical and moral implications became apparent. The rate of development of industries based on **recombinant gene technology**, **cloning** and **gene therapy** has been so fast that the general public and the government have found it difficult to understand the implications. This has led to a sense of fear and distrust of technologies such as genetically modified (GM) foods.

Key discoveries

In 1865 a monk called Gregor Mendel presented a paper on the results of his experiments with garden peas. He had studied varieties of pea that differed in a single characteristic, such as tall and short plants or wrinkled and smooth seeds. He found an **inheritance pattern** where one of two characteristics—for example tall plants—seemed to **dominate** the next generation (i.e. the **first filial (F1) generation**) and these were called **dominant factors**. The opposite characteristic—short plants—disappeared, to reappear in the 'grandchildren' (the **second (F2) generation**); these were called **recessive factors**.

Mendel proposed that each pair of characteristics was controlled by a pair of factors, one of which was inherited from each parent plant. These factors were called **genes** by the Danish botanist Johannsen (Turnpenny & Ellard 2007). Pure-bred pea plants were **homologous** ('homo' means alike) and inherited two identical genes from their parents. The F1 generation resulted from the breeding of a tall plant with a short plant and were all tall plants. However, they inherited two different genes from their parents and were **heterozygous** ('hetero' means different). The alternative versions of genes are called **allelomorphs**, usually shortened to **alleles**.

Mendel's laws

Out of Mendel's work three main principles were developed:

1. The Law of Uniformity. When two homozygotes with different alleles are crossed, all the offspring of the F1 generation are identical and heterozygous. Characteristics do not blend and can reappear in subsequent generations.

2. The Law of Segregation. Each individual possesses two genes for a particular characteristic, only one of which can be passed on in the ovum or sperm to the next generation.

3. The Law of Independent Assortment. Members of different gene pairs segregate to offspring independently of one another.

The third law is not strictly true, because if two genes are situated closely together on the same **chromosome** (see below) they may be **linked** and inherited together.

Mendel's findings were ignored until 1900, but, once the importance of his experiments was recognised, interest in inheritance developed. At that time thread-like structures had been seen in the nuclei of cells. These were the chromosomes and in 1903 two people independently proposed that they carried the hereditary factors known as genes. However, it was only in 1952 that **deoxyribonucleic acid (DNA)** was identified as the universal genetic material. In 1953, the structure of DNA was discovered by James D Watson and Francis HC Crick. However, without Rosalind Franklin, who revealed the power of **X-ray crystallography**, their discovery might not have occurred (Sayre 2000). The correct number of 46 human chromosomes was identified in 1956.

Composition of DNA

Building blocks

Cell nuclei contain large amounts of species-specific DNA. A second form of nucleic acid is **ribonucleic acid (RNA)**. Nucleic acids are long **polymers** of molecules called **nucleotides**, which are composed of several simple chemical compounds bound together in a regular pattern. These building blocks are **phosphoric acid**, a **pentose sugar** with five carbon atoms called **deoxyribose** and four **nitrogenous bases**. These bases comprise two **purines** (adenine and guanine) and two **pyrimidines** (thymine and cytosine) identified by the single letters A, G, T and C. In RNA thymine is replace by **uracil (U)**.

RNA is found in the cytoplasm, particularly concentrated in the **nucleolus**, whereas DNA is found mainly on the 46 chromosomes which are arranged in 23 pairs in somatic cells. One chromosome of each pair originates from the ovum and the other from the sperm. A cell containing two sets of chromosomes is described as **diploid**. Gametes are **haploid**, containing one of each pair of chromosomes. In 22 of the pairs the chromosomes are identical; these pairs are called **autosomes**. The two chromosomes are termed **homologous**. The 23rd pair is the sex chromosomes: two X chromosomes in females and an X and a Y chromosome in males. Maternal and paternal chromosomes become closely apposed during meiosis and exchange segments of DNA between **homologues**, a phenomenon called **crossing over**.

The double helix

DNA molecules consist of a double helix made up of two complementary chains of nucleotides. Two sugar-phosphate strands wind around each other and the base pairs are stacked between these strands, pointing inwards to the centre of the double helix (Turnpenny & Ellard 2007). The two chains are held together by hydrogen bonds between the base pairs. These bonds are easily broken, a feature necessary for DNA replication. The sugar-phosphate molecules form the backbone of the chains.

Pentose sugars

The five carbon atoms in the pentose sugar are numbered with primes, represented as 1′to 5′. The carbon atoms 3′ to 5′ are on the same side of the molecule. The 5′ carbon is always linked to the phosphate molecule and the 1′ carbon to the base. The two strands run in opposite directions as indicated by their 3′ and 5′ carbon atoms and are complementary or **antiparallel** (Fig. 3.1). A purine always pairs with a pyrimidine. A is paired with T by two hydrogen bonds and C is paired with G by three hydrogen bonds. The pairs stack one above the other and the structure is stabilised by two other forms of bond—hydrophobic and van der Waals interactions (Ch. 1)—between adjacent pairs.

DNA holds the instructions for constructing, organising and maintaining the body and must be replicated accurately during **mitosis** (Ch. 2). One of the two strands must be passed on to the next generation by means of ova and sperm.

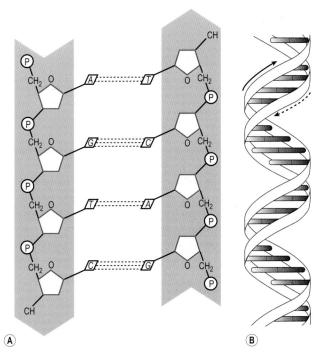

(A) (B)

Figure 3.1 • DNA double helix. (A) Sugar phosphate backbone and nucleotide pairing of the DNA double helix (P, phosphate; A, adenine; T, thymine; G guanine; C, cytosine). (B) Representation of the DNA double helix.

Chromosomes

Chromosomes take up different states depending on the stage of the **cell cycle** (Ch. 2). When the cell is not dividing, chromosomes are extended and their **chromatin** is in the form of long, thin tangled threads known as **interphase** chromosomes. The highly condensed chromosomes in a dividing cell are called **mitotic** chromosomes (Alberts et al 2002), which are much wider than the DNA double helix.

If the DNA of a single human cell were to be stretched out it would be several metres long, yet the total length of the chromosomes placed end to end is less than 0.5 mm. DNA is packaged into chromosomes by coiling and folding (Turnpenny & Ellard 2007). Besides the double helix there is a secondary coiling around spherical molecules called **histones** to form **nucleosomes**. A tertiary coiling of nucleosomes forms the chromatin fibres which are then wound into a tight coil to make the chromosomes.

Circulating lymphocytes from peripheral blood are commonly used to study chromosomes but skin or bone marrow cells can be used. Fetal cells from the chorionic villi or found in amniotic fluid (**amniocytes**) can be sampled. The process of cell division is stopped during mitosis by adding **colchicines**, which prevents the formation of the spindle and arrests the cells in metaphase. Hypotonic saline solution is added, which destroys the cells, releasing the chromosomes. A photograph is taken. The chromosome images are cut out, laid out in a standard fashion, and photographed again to produce a karyotype (Fig. 3.2). Chromosomes are identified by their size, light and dark banding patterns and the position of the centromere.

At that moment DNA replication has taken place and the chromosomes consist of two identical strands called sister chromatids which are held together by a **centromere**. Centromeres consist of lengths of **repetitive DNA** and are responsible for the movement of the chromosomes that takes place in cell division. A chromosome is divided by its centromere into short and long arms. The short arm is referred to as 'p' and the long arm as 'q'. Chromosomes can be classified by the position of their centromeres. If located centrally the chromosome is **metacentric,** if intermediate it is **sub-metacentric** and if found at one end of the chromosome it is **acrocentric**. Acrocentric chromosomes may have stalks with satellites attached to them which contain multiple copies of the genes for **ribosomal RNA**.

The tip of each chromosome arm is called the **telomere**, consisting of many repeats of a TTAGGG sequence which seals the ends of the chromosome to maintain its structural integrity. The length of these sequences is reduced each time the cell divides. This is part of normal cellular ageing; most cells can only undergo 50–60 divisions before becoming senescent.

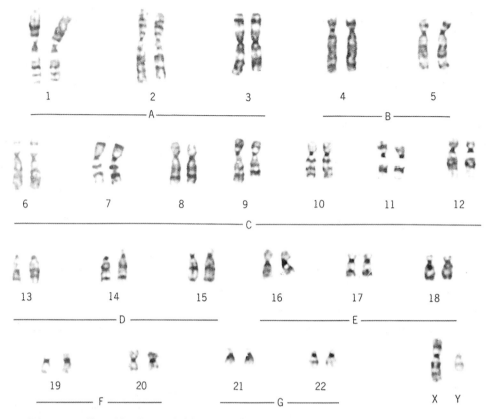

Figure 3.2 • A normal karyotype. (From Henderson C, Macdonald S 2004, with kind permission of Elsevier.)

Genes

The full complement of DNA is called the **genome**. Along the genome about 60–70% of DNA is in the form of single or short repeats of single sequences called low copy sequences, whereas 30–40% consists of highly repetitive sequences that appear inactive. DNA is arranged in discrete segments called **genes** and there may be 25 000–30 000 (far less than was originally conjectured) of these in the human genome. There is a rule of genetics that says 'one gene, one protein'. However, genes often exist in families; for example, those that code for the various types of haemoglobin (Ch. 16) and those that code for antibodies (Ch. 29).

Genes code for **polypeptides**, which include enzymes, hormones, receptors and structural and regulatory proteins (Turnpenny & Ellard 2007). The alternative alleles of any gene are present at a specific place or locus on each of a pair of chromosomes. If both parents contribute an identical allele for a locus, the new individual is **homozygous**. If the two alleles differ, the new individual is **heterozygous**.

Discrete single genes form about 25% of the DNA and are separated from each other by long runs of inactive, repetitive DNA sequences. It is not known why there is so much redundant DNA. The coding sequences of genes are called **exons** and the intervening non-coding sequences **introns**. Exons are usually interrupted by introns. Individual introns can be much larger than the exons and some have been found to contain a gene within a gene.

The role of the environment

Genes act in response to environmental changes (Ch. 15). These may be internal, such as a response to fluctuations in hormone level, or external, such as a response to a meal. The full range of genes inherited by an individual is called the **genotype**. The outward appearance of an individual, i.e. their physical, biochemical and physiological nature, is known as the **phenotype** and results from gene–environment interactions.

From DNA to RNA to protein

Proteins are the working components of the cell. DNA stores the information. RNA (Fig. 3.3) carries out instructions encoded in DNA and synthesises the proteins involved in cellular function (Jorde et al 2006).

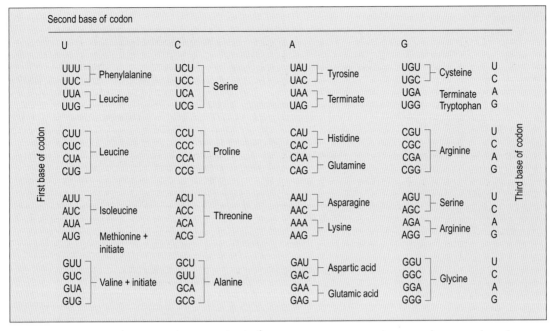

Figure 3.3 • Messenger RNA (mRNA) code words. (From Hinchliff S M, Montague S E 1990, with kind permission of Elsevier.)

The genetic code

Twenty different amino acids are found in proteins, so it became obvious to Watson and Crick that, as there were only four bases, more than one base must be necessary to specify a particular amino acid. Even two bases would not be enough as 4^2 gives only 16 possibilities. However, 4^3 bases allows 64 possibilities of codon to occur with some redundancy. Each group of three nucleotides, called a **triplet codon** (Fig. 3.4), spells out each amino acid. The sequence of amino acids shapes a particular protein. There are also codons at the ends of genes that signify start and stop. The process of reading the DNA code which results in a functional protein product involves two processes: **transcription** and **translation**.

Transcription

There are three types of RNA involved in the production of a protein:

1. **Messenger RNA** (mRNA) copies the genetic code of a stretch of DNA in the form of a sequence of bases that codes for a sequence of amino acids.

2. **Transfer RNA** (tRNA) carries the correct amino acids specified by the DNA to the ribosome and places them in the correct order.

3. **Ribosomal RNA** (rRNA) combines with proteins to make ribosomes, which have binding sites for the molecules needed to make a protein.

In any particular gene only one of the DNA strands acts as a template for a polypeptide and it must be copied before it can be read (Fig. 3.5). This copying is called transcription. It must be accurate as mistakes may lead to an inactive product. The information stored in the gene is transmitted from DNA to mRNA. Every base in the single-stranded mRNA is complementary to the DNA, but uracil replaces thymine. An enzyme called RNA polymerase tacks the bases onto the developing strand in the correct order.

Translation

Following transcription, non-coding introns are excised and the coding exons are spliced together to form mature mRNA. This is transported to the ribosomes in the cytoplasm for translation into a specific protein (Fig. 3.6). In the cytoplasm a particular amino acid is bound to its tRNA for transporting to the ribosome, where it is linked up with others to form a polypeptide chain. The ribosome moves along the mRNA, linking up the amino acids to build the protein.

Mutations

Genes usually produce their product faithfully, but rarely a mutation or alteration in the arrangement or amount of genetic material in a cell arises either naturally or because of the effects of environmental challenges such as radiation, chemical or physical stressors; these are called mutagens. Mutations can be minor changes in DNA such as

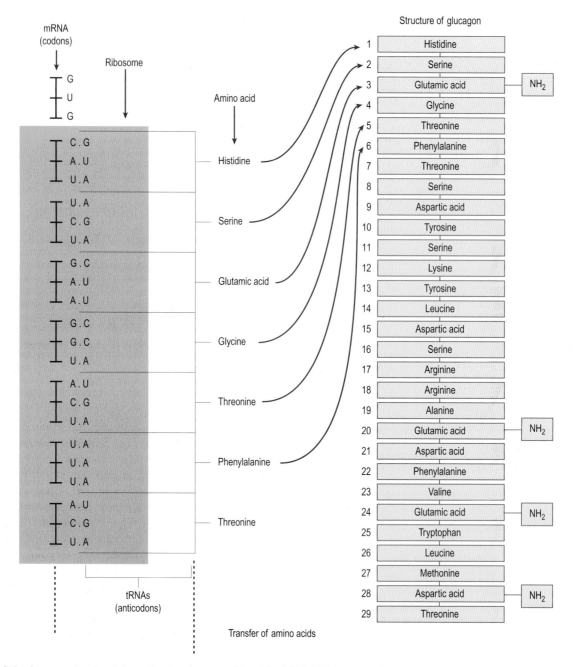

Figure 3.4 • An example of protein synthesis: glucagon. (From Hinchliff S M, Montague S E 1990 with kind permission of Elsevier.)

point mutations (single base substitutions) or **macro-mutations** involving alterations such as **deletions** of large amounts of a chromosome.

Mutations often result in harmful or lethal defects. Point mutations cause amino acid substitutions resulting in faulty protein products. This may cause specific functional defects such as **cystic fibrosis or sickle cell disease**. Macromutations may cause syndromes as multiple changes in a particular chromosome may lead to recognisable changes in the body as seen in Down syndrome (trisomy 21), often including mental retardation. **Nonsense mutations** involve the creation of a stop codon in an abnormal situation. The broken gene does not code for a protein product. In **frameshift mutations** additions or deletions of a nucleotide alter the reading frame of the DNA to the left or the right so that triplet codons do not code for amino acids.

Regulation of gene expression

Every cell in the body (except gametes) has the full complement of genes. The cells making up organs have specialised functions and only a small proportion of the

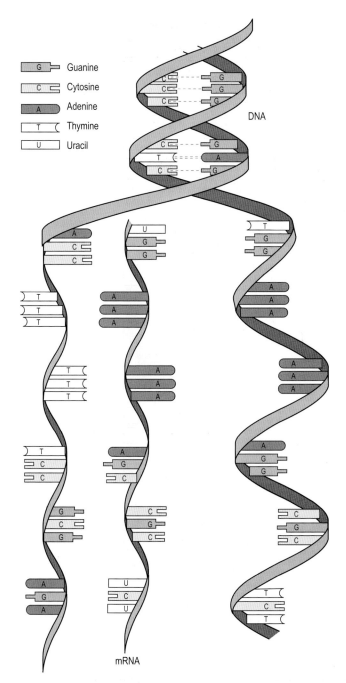

G Guanine
C Cytosine
A Adenine
T Thymine
U Uracil

DNA

mRNA

Figure 3.5 • Transcription of a strand of DNA by messenger RNA (mRNA). (From Hinchliff S M, Montague S E 1990, with kind permission of Elsevier.)

genes will be active in a particular cell. Also, genes make only the amount of their protein product necessary for a particular body function. Imagine a person whose pancreas produced continuous amounts of insulin, regardless of the amount of glucose in the blood! Genes may only function at specific phases of development of an organism and are activated and suppressed as needed (Turnpenny & Ellard 2007).

Patterns of inheritance

Dominant genes

As mentioned above, specific genes may be inherited as dominant, recessive or sex-linked. A dominant allele manifests its effects in heterozygotes as only one copy is needed to affect the phenotype. Except in cases of a new mutation, every child with that particular phenotype receives a copy of one allele from a similar parent. Most genes work normally, but if the gene codes for an abnormality where one parent is affected a child will have a 1 in 2 chance of inheriting the gene and being affected (Fig. 3.7).

Recessive genes

A recessive allele only affects the phenotype in homozygotes. People with one copy of the allele are carriers. If the gene codes for an abnormality, the children of two carriers will have a 1 in 4 chance of being affected or normal and a 1 in 2 chance of being a carrier (Fig. 3.8).

Sex-linked genes

The X chromosome carries a large number of genes involved in development and function. Males only have one X chromosome and are **hemizygous** for X chromosome genes. If there is an abnormal X chromosome gene, boys will be affected by an X-linked disorder. Females are usually heterozygous for such an abnormal X chromosome gene and will not be affected because of the opposing normal allele (Fig. 3.9). However, homozygosity may rarely occur if an affected man and carrier woman have a daughter. These girls will be affected. In females only one X chromosome is functional in each cell and the other is randomly inactivated in the early embryo. This is called lyonisation (Box 3.1).

Genomic imprinting

It has recently been discovered that genes on homologous chromosomes are not expressed equally. Different clinical features can arise depending on whether a gene was inherited from the mother or the father. This is genomic imprinting, which affects only a small proportion of the genome. Prader–Willi syndrome is characterised by short stature, obesity, small gonads and learning difficulty and occurs in about 1 in 20 000 births. In 55% of those affected there is deletion of the proximal portion of the long arm of chromosome 15. A further 15% involves a microscopic deletion. DNA analysis has shown that it is nearly always the paternal homologue

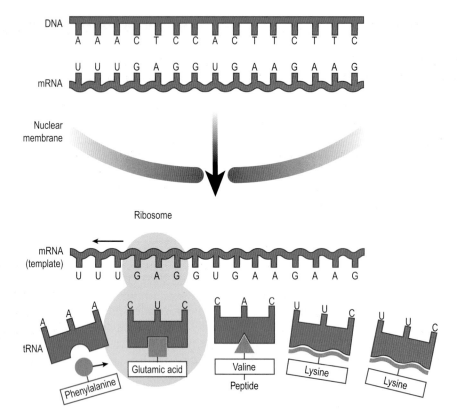

Figure 3.6 • Representation of the way in which genetic information is translated into protein.

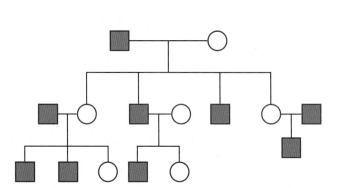

Figure 3.7 • An autosomal-dominant pedigree. (From Henderson C, Macdonald S 2004, with kind permission of Elsevier.)

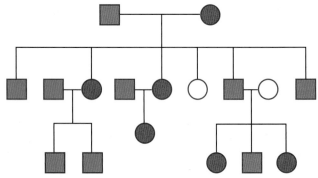

Figure 3.9 • An X-linked pedigree. (From Henderson C, Macdonald S 2004, with kind permission of Elsevier.)

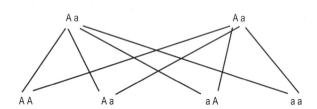

Figure 3.8 • In an autosomal recessive disorder, the disease is only manifest if both parents are carriers of the abnormal gene (a), then there is a one in four chance that a child will have the disease. (From Henderson C, Macdonald S 2004, with kind permission of Elsevier.)

that is deleted. The remaining cases occur because of maternal disomy: two maternal and no paternal chromosome 15 (Turnpenny & Ellard 2007).

Mitochondrial DNA

Each mitochondrion has its own circular double-stranded DNA called **mitochondrial DNA** (mDNA) and is inherited only from the mother. The mitochondria in sperm are situated behind the head of the sperm in the neck, and as only the head enters the ovum mitochondria are

BOX 3.1 LYONISATION

In females one or other of the X chromosomes is inactivated in cells early in embryonic life. Inactivation occurs at around 15 days when the embryo consists of about 5000 cells. Their descendants retain the same activated X chromosome so that half the cells contain one activated X chromosome and half the other. This effect is called lyonisation after its discoverer Dr Mary Lyon. Each female is a **mosaic** of half paternal and half maternal X chromosomes. Abnormal X chromosomes seem

to be preferentially inactivated (Bainbridge 2003, Turnpenny & Ellard 2007).

In females or males with more than one X chromosome, any inactivated X chromosome can be seen during interphase as a dark mass of chromatin called sex chromatin or a **Barr body**. Looking for Barr bodies was used as a method of sex determination by taking a buccal smear, but this method is now obsolete as chromosomal abnormalities can be complex.

left outside with the tail. Mitochondrial DNA codes for only 13 genes, some of which are important in cellular respiration. However, most mitochondrial proteins (about 1500) are coded for in the nuclear genome so that mitochondria rely on both genomes to carry out their functions (Lane 2005). Mitochondrial DNA has a higher rate of spontaneous mutation than nuclear DNA and accumulation of mistakes may be responsible for some of the physical effects of ageing.

Mitochondrial inheritance may cause rare disorders which affect males and females but are transmitted only through their mothers. These disorders, which usually combine muscular and neurological features involving muscular weakness, are known as **mitochondrial myopathies**. Mitochondria are important in tissues with a high energy requirement, so it is not surprising that they are involved in abnormalities of these systems.

Some inherited conditions

Most inherited disorders are a result of nuclear gene mutations, which are either dominant (Table 3.1), recessive (Table 3.2) or sex-linked (Table 3.3). Some may be due to a mutation in mDNA (Table 3.4). Slight differences in a protein brought about by a mutation may cause devastating diseases such as cystic fibrosis or sickle cell disease. Some genes are **pleiotrophic**, underpinning multiple functions, thus an abnormality may affect multiple systems. In the recessive disorder phenylketonuria, low tyrosine levels lead to lack of pigment in hair, skin and eyes due to reduced melanin production.

Chromosomal defects

About 50% of spontaneous abortions result from chromosomal defects occurring during oogenesis. Chromosomal defects may be present in up to 6% of all pregnancies. Numerical or structural changes may affect the autosomes or the sex chromosomes. People with chromosomal defects

Table 3.1 Disorders of systems caused by dominant genes

System	Disorder
Nervous	Huntington's disease
	Neurofibromatosis
Bowel	Polyposis coli
Kidney	Polycystic disease
Eyes	Blindness
Ears	Deafness
Blood	Hypercholesterolaemia
Skeleton	Osteogenesis imperfecta
	Achondroplasia

Table 3.2 Some recessively inherited conditions

System	Disorder
Metabolism	Cystic fibrosis
	Phenylketonuria
Nervous	Friedreich's ataxia
Blood	Sickle cell anaemia
	Beta-thalassaemia
Ears	Congenital deafness
Eyes	Recessive blindness

usually have characteristic phenotypes as, for example, in Down syndrome where the typical features may cause the children to look more similar to each other than to their relatives.

Table 3.3 Some X-linked disorders

System	Disorder
Locomotor	Duchenne muscular dystrophy
Blood	Haemophilia
Brain	Fragile X syndrome
Vision	Childhood blindness

Table 3.4 Some mitochondrial disorders

System	Disorder
Vision	Chronic progressive external ophthalmoplegia
Hearing	Aminoglycoside-induced deafness
Cardiovascular	Hypertrophic cardiomyopathy with myopathy

Numerical chromosomal defects

Many numerical defects arise during **failure of disjunction**, which is an error in cell division where the sister chromatids fail to separate at anaphase. The resulting number of chromosomes may be too many or too few.

- **Polyploidy** means the presence of multiples of the haploid number of 23 chromosomes.
- **Triploidy** is the presence of 69 chromosomes. It may occur because the chromosomes of the second polar body fail to be ejected from the ovum or because of entry of two sperm into the ovum. It occurs in about 2% of fertilisations and the zygote is mostly lost early in development.
- **Monosomy** is when one of a chromosome pair is missing, leaving 45 chromosomes. This is only compatible with survival if the missing chromosome is an X. The resulting female has Turner's syndrome.
- **Trisomy** is the presence of an extra chromosome. The usual cause is non-disjunction so that either the ovum or sperm carries 24 chromosomes instead of 23. At fertilisation this results in 47 chromosomes. The most common condition is Down syndrome where there are three copies of chromosome 21. Non-disjunction occurs with increasing frequency as maternal age increases.
- **Mosaicism** results when the zygote develops into an individual with two genotypes or cell lines. The condition arises due to non-disjunction during early mitosis. The defects seen are less serious than those found in full monosomic or trisomic disorders.

Structural chromosomal defects

Environmental factors may induce breaks in chromosomes, resulting in structural rearrangements called macromutations. Two of these—**inversion** and **translocation**—may be transmitted from parent to child.

- **Translocation** is the transfer of a piece of one chromosome to another non-homologous chromosome. This may be a reciprocal translocation where two non-homologous chromosomes exchange pieces. If the translocation is balanced, the individual receives the normal complement of chromosomal material and there will be no abnormality. However, if the translocation results in extra chromosomal material, abnormality will occur. About 4% of people with Down syndrome receive their third chromosome 21 translocated to another chromosome, often chromosome 14 or 15.
- **Deletion** is the loss of part of a chromosome. Loss of the termination of chromosome 5 causes cri du chat syndrome where affected infants have a weak, cat-like cry, microcephaly, heart defects and mental retardation.
- **Duplication** is where a section of a chromosome is repeated, either within a chromosome, attached to another chromosome or as a separate fragment. This type of defect is less harmful as there is no loss of chromosomal material.
- **Inversion** occurs if a segment of a chromosome breaks free and becomes reattached in reverse position. **Paracentric** inversion involves just one arm of the chromosome whereas **pericentric** inversion involves both arms and the centromere.
- **Isochromosome** is where the centromere divides horizontally instead of longitudinally; this occurs most often in the X chromosomes. Loss of the short arm of chromosome X is associated with features of **Turner's syndrome**.

Application to practice

The Human Genome Project

The **Human Genome Project** involved mapping all human genes to their chromosomes. It began in Utah under the auspices of the US Department of Energy (DOE) who were interested in finding out the mutation rates of DNA in response to exposure to radiation and chemicals. The project began in 1991 and France, UK and Japan soon joined, followed by many other countries. The short-term hope of the project is to enable better diagnosis and counselling for families with genetic disease. In the longer term, the aim is to develop preventive strategies and treatments of genetic disorders. The project was completed in 2000.

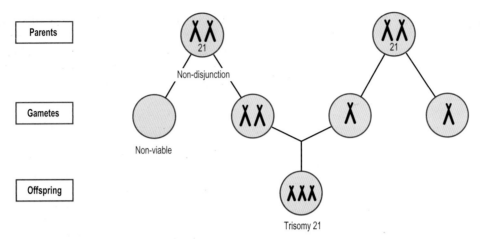

Figure 3.10 • Non-disjunction of chromosome 21 leading to Down syndrome. (From Montague S E, Watson R, Herbert R A 2005, with kind permission of Elsevier.)

Detection of abnormality

Following the production of a karyotype, chromosomes can be identified by their size, banding patterns and the position of the centromere. Gross chromosomal defects can be seen (Fig. 3.10). Single gene defects where the identity of the gene is known can be found by using **gene probes**; these are commercially available synthetic sections of DNA, which are attracted to the appropriate gene and can even identify single base changes.

DNA technologies

Those wishing to learn more about the techniques are referred to either Turnpenny & Ellard (2007) or Jorde et al (2006). Techniques include the use of enzymes called **restriction endonucleases** which cut DNA at a specific point, **polymerase chain reaction** (PCR) and the **Southern blot technique**. DNA technology can be split into two main areas: **DNA cloning** (producing identical copies) and **DNA analysis**. Possible applications include medical cures, increased food production, crime detection and better energy production.

Therapeutic applications of recombinant DNA technology

The medical applications of the new technology include the manufacture of hormones and enzymes; the production of human insulin is already in use. Uses also include pre-implantation genetic screening for disease and the sex of the embryo, fetal screening, screening of adults and gene replacement therapy. Stem cell therapy can be added to this list.

Victor McKusick, the man behind the Human Genome Project, began a catalogue of all known genetic conditions. An on-line version known as the Online Mendelian Inheritance on Man (OMIM) can be accessed by the internet (McKusick 2002). On 16 July 2008 there were 18 831 entries. Non-therapeutic uses, such as selecting attributes for a child or cloning of a person, are causing ethical and moral problems which will increase as the new technology is accepted.

Population screening

The issue of confidentiality and privacy and who accesses medical data about an individual is of supreme importance. If population screening techniques are used, how much information could be requested by employers, providers of insurance, life partners and others? Could a person be penalised for possessing a particular genetic defect which has yet to show its effect (e.g. Huntington's disease)? If carrier detection becomes available, it must be voluntary and there must be adequate counselling services in the event of a positive result.

Gene therapy

Therapeutic uses of recombinant DNA (rDNA) techniques include gene therapy or 'the replacement of a deficient gene product or correction of an abnormal gene' (Turnpenny & Ellard 2007). When the gene enters the new cell, it may change the way the cell works or the chemicals that the cell secretes. Advances in molecular biology leading to the identification of many abnormal human genes and their products have led to possible treatments for some important diseases (Jorde et al 2006).

These recent developments promise a new type of medicine but also bring moral dilemmas. In 2003 concerns about the development of leukaemia in children undergoing gene therapy led to the halting of programmes in some countries. Regulatory bodies have been set up to oversee the technical, therapeutic and safety aspects of gene therapy. Whereas somatic cell therapy which affects only the individual is acceptable, germ cell therapy where changes could be transmitted to future generations is currently considered morally and ethically unacceptable.

There have been successes over the past few years, such as therapy for X-linked SCID (severe combined immune deficiency), factor XI expression in haemophilia and some good effects in cancer and heart disease. But the successes have involved only a few individuals (Jorde et al 2006). Safety and cost may prevent gene therapy treatments becoming widespread.

Important considerations

Before gene therapy trials can take place there are a number of technical aspects to be overcome (Turnpenny & Ellard 2007):

1. The gene involved must have been cloned. This means not only the structural gene but the sequences involved in its expression and regulation.
2. The specific targets—cell, tissue and organ—must be identified and accessible.
3. There must be an efficient vector system to carry the gene into the target cells.
4. There should be no harmful effects, such as malignancy, on the target cells.

Methods of gene therapy

These can be divided into two groups: viral and non-viral (Turnpenny & Ellard 2007).

Viral agents

- **Retroviruses** are RNA viruses that can insert themselves into target cells where their RNA is transformed into DNA and inserted into the cellular genome. They must be rendered inactive prior to use so that they cannot produce infection. The main problem with their use is that only very small stretches of DNA can be introduced.
- **Adenoviruses** are especially suitable for targeting the respiratory tract. They are more stable than retroviruses.

They do not integrate into the genome so there is no risk of mutagenesis. However, their effect is likely to be transient. They contain **oncogenes** which are involved in the production of cancer so there could be a danger of provoking malignancy.

- Other viruses such as the herpes virus, influenza virus and other RNA viruses could produce large quantities of the gene product but are likely to have the same problems already discussed. Viruses elicit an immune response which limits their repeated use.

Non-viral agents

These methods are likely to be safer but differ in their ability to produce sufficient gene product to be useful. They include:

- Direct injection of naked DNA.
- Liposome-mediated transfer—DNA packaged in a lipid bilayer surrounding an aqueous vesicle.
- Receptor-mediated endocytosis where specific receptors on the cell surface are targeted.

Stem cell therapy

After fertilisation the single cell and its early offspring are unspecified cells (**totipotent**) and can form any tissue in the body. When these embryonic stem cells begin to specialise they are usually described in reference to the organ of origin, such as haemopoietic stem cells (Turnpenny & Ellard 2007). The embryo-forming cells can become any tissue type but are not capable of developing into the placenta and membranes.

Stem cells could theoretically be used to treat human diseases. Bone marrow transplantation is a form of stem cell therapy which has been in use for more than 40 years (Turnpenny & Ellard 2007). Stem cell therapy could be used for some genetic disorders, but risks of infection because of immunosuppression and graft versus host disease are high. Stem cells derived from cord blood could overcome these problems (see below).

Some common multifactorial diseases such as diabetes mellitus, Parkinson's disease, Alzheimer's disease, cancer and heart disease may become treatable by specific stem cell transfer in the future, although controlling the environmental risks such as smoking and lung cancer may be more available. There are various sources of stem cell lines: the embryonic inner cell mass, embryonic tissue retrieved after a termination of pregnancy, cord blood and some adult somatic cell lines.

Embryonic cells

Obtaining these cells means in vitro fertilisation and artificial growing of human embryos. There are ethical problems in harvesting cells from developing embryos and President George W Bush banned any funding for research requiring the creation and destruction of human embryos (Ezzell 2002). Taking cells from an aborted fetus may also be considered ethically unsound.

Adult cells

Recent research into adult cells suggests there may be some **multipotent** cells that, even though they appear to be specialised, may have the ability to produce other types of cells (Turnpenny & Ellard 2007). Stem cells become dedicated to producing tissue with a specific function: for instance, blood stem cells are located in the bone marrow and may also circulate in the blood stream in small numbers. They continually replenish red cells, white cells and platelets. Some stem cells found in bone marrow have been able to produce liver cells.

However, when such cells were transplanted into mice, they did not form new cell lines but fused with recipient cells to create giant cells with more than the normal number of chromosomes (Ezzell 2002). Such abnormal cells may not have the ability to change tissue type and could lead to cancer.

Umbilical cord blood

Allogenic (tissues of two unalike individuals) stem cell transplantation has revolutionised the outcome for a wide range of malignant and non-malignant haematological conditions (Lennard & Jackson 2000). Infusion of cord blood, which is very rich in highly proliferative stem cells, has been used with success in children and young adults with some haematological and immunological disorders. The best results were from HLA-matched siblings with a success rate of 63%. The results have been less good with unmatched donor/recipient pairs, only 30% of recipients being alive after 1 year. An advantage of cord blood over other tissue is a reduced incidence of graft versus host reaction. There are cord blood banks in the UK.

In utero transplantation

Stem cell transplantation in utero may treat genetic disorders. The immature fetal immune system will tolerate novel cells, ending the need for a matched donor. Trials are underway for severe combined immunodeficiency disorder (SCID), alpha- and beta-thalassaemia and sickle cell disease (Turnpenny & Ellard 2007). In utero fetal gene therapy has been successful in mice with cystic fibrosis so the possibility for treatment for the human fetus is real; however, because there is a risk of inadvertent germ cell therapy it is considered unacceptable at present. Trials are being carried out in the USA and UK treating cystic fibrosis patients using a liposome–gene complex or an adenovirus vector sprayed into the nasal passages. The presence of the introduced gene appears to cause no harm but also there is no evidence of its effectiveness.

Somatic cell nuclear transfer

Somatic cell nuclear transfer involves placing a somatic cell next to an ovum emptied of its nucleus. The two cells fuse together and the resultant cell may be totipotent. If the newly created ovum were allowed to grow, cells from the inner cell mass would give rise to pluripotent stem cell lines. The donor cell could be from the individual needing treatment, which would solve the problem of tissue rejection. An ethical problem arises because the totipotent cell is a clone of the donor somatic cell.

Conclusion

The moral and ethical issues accompanying gene technology are of major importance to the future of human health and medical treatment. It is essential that countries develop safeguards to ensure that safety, privacy and confidentiality are not at risk. On a national and global scale, how can we ensure that any developments are available to the maximum number of affected people? Biochemistry and its associated disciplines have real power to change the world. It is important to consider how this occurs and in whose interests the changes are made.

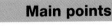

Main points

- The genetic basis for health and disease has led to the search for preventative, palliative and curative treatments. The development of industries based on recombinant gene technology has been so fast that the general public and governments have been barely able to keep up with the implications.

- Gregor Mendel proposed that each pair of characteristics in pea plants was controlled by a pair of factors, one inherited from each parent. He developed three main laws: the Law of Uniformity, the Law of Segregation and the Law of Independent Assortment.

- The correct number of 46 human chromosomes was identified in 1956. A cell containing two sets of chromosomes is referred to as diploid. One chromosome of each pair originates with the ovum and the other with the sperm. Gametes contain 23 chromosomes and are called haploid.

- In 22 pairs called autosomes the chromosomes are identical. The 23rd pair is the sex chromosomes.

- The DNA molecule consists of a double helix made up of two complementary chains of nucleotides packaged into discrete chromosomes by coiling and folding. Chromosomal images can be photographed to produce a karyotype.

- The genome is arranged in genes which carry the code for polypeptides. Discrete single genes called exons are separated from each other by long runs of non-coding repetitive DNA sequences called introns which interrupt the coding sequence of most genes.

- The genotype is the full complement of genes of individuals. The phenotype is their outward appearance and results from an interaction between genes and environment.

- A triplet codon spells out each amino acid in the specific order for a particular protein. The process of reading the code of DNA involves transcription and translation. Genes must make only the amount of their product necessary for functioning and are regulated by being activated and suppressed as needed.

- Genes may be dominant, recessive or sex-linked. A dominant gene affects heterozygotes, whereas a recessive allele only affects homozygotes.

- Males have only one X chromosome and are hemizygous for X. In female cells one X chromosome is deactivated at random, a process called lyonisation. In genomic imprinting, different clinical features arise depending on whether the gene was inherited from the mother or the father.

- Mitochondrial DNA is inherited only from our mothers. Mitochondrial inheritance may cause rare disorders that usually combine muscular and neurological features. These affect males and females and are transmitted by their mothers.

- Slight differences in a protein brought about by a genetic mutation may lead to devastating diseases such as sickle cell disease or cystic fibrosis. Numerical and structural defects may affect the autosomes or sex chromosomes. Environmental factors may induce breaks in chromosomes, resulting in inversions or translocations which may be transmitted from parent to child.

- The Human Genome Project aims to achieve better diagnosis and counselling for families with genetic disease and to develop new preventative strategies and treatments of genetic disorders.

- Developments in gene technology raise questions about the application of genetic engineering to diagnosis and treatment of genetic diseases. Regulatory bodies have been set up to oversee the technical, therapeutic and safety aspects of gene therapy.

- Fetal transplantation of pluripotent stem cells may treat genetic disorders because the fetal immune system will tolerate foreign cells. Infusion of cord blood has been used with some success in some haematological and immunological disorders.

- Cystic fibrosis patients have been treated using a liposome–gene complex or an adenovirus vector sprayed into the nasal passages. Although the introduced gene causes no harm there is little evidence of effectiveness.

- The moral and ethical issues surrounding gene technology are of major importance to medical research but their use must be carefully regulated to avoid controversy.

References

Alberts, B., Johnson, A., Lewis, J., et al., 2002. Molecular Biology of the Cell, fourth ed. Garland Science, London.

Bainbridge, D., 2003. The X in Sex. Harvard University Press, Cambridge, MA.

Ezzell, C., 2002. The child within. Sci. Am. 286 (6), 16.

Henderson, C., Macdonald, S. (Eds.), 2004. Mayes' Midwifery: A Textbook for Midwives, thirteenth ed. Baillière Tindall, London.

Jorde, L., Carey, J., Bamshad, M.J., White, R., 2006. Medical Genetics, third ed. Mosby Elsevier, St Louis.

Lane, N., 2005. Power, Sex and Suicide: Mitochondria and the Meaning of Life. Oxford University Press, Oxford.

Lennard, A.L., Jackson, G.H., 2000. Stem cell transplantation. Br. Med. J. 32, 433–437.

McKusick, V., 2002. Online Mendelian Inheritance in Man (OMIM). <http://www3.ncbi.nih.gov/omom/>.

Montague, S.E., Watson, R., Herbert, R.A. (Eds.), 2005. Physiology for Nursing Pratice, third ed. Baillière Tindall, London.

Sayre, A., 2000 (reprint). Rosalind Franklin and DNA. WW Norton, New York.

Turnpenny, P., Ellard, S., 2007. Emery's Elements of Medical Genetics, thirteenth ed. Churchill Livingstone Elsevier, Edinburgh.

Annotated recommended reading

Bainbridge, D., 2003. The X in Sex. Harvard University Press, Cambridge, MA.

This is a highly readable book on the X chromosome, including lyonisation and its effects on women.

Jones, S., 1996. In the Blood, Gods, Genes and Destiny. Harper Collins, London.

Steve Jones writes clearly and entertainingly about the topic of genetics and its benefits and limitations. This book takes a measured look at the role of genetics in a social world.

Turnpenny, P., Ellard, S., 2007. Emery's Elements of Medical Genetics, thirteenth ed. Churchill Livingstone Elsevier, Edinburgh.

This is an excellent introduction to the complex subject of medical genetics, a subject which will continue to grow in importance as research continues. Students looking for a book on the subject of genetics will find this book excellent, with clearly written text and good diagrams.

Chapter Four

The female reproductive system

Introduction

The male and female reproductive systems ensure the future of the species by producing the gametes, i.e. spermatozoa and oocytes. Although sex is not strictly necessary and some animals reproduce asexually, there is benefit in producing unique combinations by reshuffling genes from two parents. Genetic variability helps to provide adaptation to changing environments. Female mammals also provide optimum conditions for fetal development. Nourishment and protection are ensured until the offspring is able to survive independently. Finally, expulsion from the mother's body at the correct gestation must occur and lactation be initiated.

Sexual differentiation

In the early embryo there is no anatomical difference internally or externally prior to the 7th week of development. Two pairs of genital ducts are present: the **paramesonephric** or **Müllerian** ducts with the potential to develop into female genitalia and the **mesonephric** or **Wolffian** ducts with the potential to develop into male genitalia. A Y chromosome gene called **SRY** (sex-determining region Y gene) is expressed in male embryos (Jones 2002). Under its influence, testes and functioning Sertoli cells are formed in the presence of testosterone (Ch. 5).

If the embryo is XX, ovaries will form and the female ducts develop into female genitalia. The ducts that are not required to develop degenerate. This influence on the indifferent tissues (Moore & Persaud 2008) leads to **homologous structures**, i.e. structures developed from the same origin. Examples include testis and ovary, penis and clitoris. Rarely, instant recognition of the sex of the baby is difficult or impossible without genetic testing.

Anatomy of the female reproductive tract

The soft tissues forming the female internal genitalia are situated in the pelvic cavity. Although the organs are separate structures, they form a continuous tract. The organs are: vulva, vagina, uterus and cervix, uterine tube and ovary. Figure 4.1 is a diagram of the whole female reproductive tract.

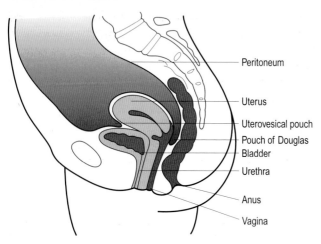

Figure 4.1 • The pelvic organs in sagittal section. (From Henderson C, Macdonald S 2004, with kind permission of Elsevier.)

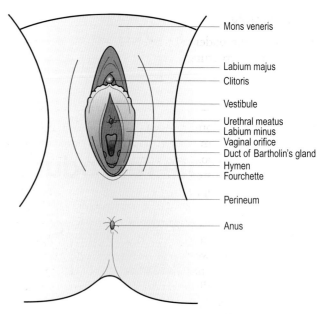

Figure 4.2 • The external genitalia. (From Henderson C, Macdonald S 2004, with kind permission of Elsevier.)

The vulva

Figure 4.2 shows the external organs that constitute the vulva, each of which will be described in turn.

The labia majora

These are two folds containing sebaceous and sweat glands embedded in adipose and connective tissue. They are covered with skin and form the lateral boundaries of the vulval cleft. They are homologues of the scrotum. They unite anteriorly to form the **mons veneris**, an adipose pad over the symphysis pubis. Hair covers the mons veneris and terminates in a horizontal upper border. Posteriorly the labia majora unite to form the **posterior commissure**. Hair grows on the outer surface of the labia majora but not on the inner surface.

The labia minora

These are two delicate folds of skin containing some sebaceous glands but no adipose tissue. On the medial aspect keratinised skin epithelium changes to squamous epithelium with many sebaceous glands. Anteriorly, the labia minora split into two parts. One passes over the clitoris to form its **prepuce** and the other passes beneath the clitoris to form a homologue of the frenulum in the male. Posteriorly, the two labia minora unite to form the **fourchette**. The size of the labia minora varies between women but this is of no significance.

The clitoris

This is the homologue of the male penis. It is composed of erectile tissue and can enlarge and stiffen during sexual excitement. Only the **glans** and **prepuce** are normally visible but the **corpus** can be palpated as a cord-like structure along the lower surface of the symphysis pubis.

The vestibule

This is the cleft between the labia minora onto which open:

• The urethral meatus.
• The vaginal orifice.

Bartholin's glands

Bartholin's glands are two pea-sized glands embedded in connective tissue that are connected to the vestibule by ducts that are 2 cm long. These glands are homologues of **Cowper's glands** in the male. The ducts are lined with columnar epithelium which produces a mucoid secretion onto the vestibule for lubrication during coitus.

Blood supply

The vulva is very vascular, receiving its arterial supply from the internal pudendal arteries, which are branches of the internal iliac arteries, and the external pudendal arteries, which are branches of the femoral arteries. Venous drainage is usually by corresponding veins which accompany the arteries but, from the clitoris, a plexus of veins joins the vaginal and vesical venous plexi.

Lymphatic drainage

Lymphatic vessels form an interconnecting meshwork through the labia minora, prepuce, fourchette and vaginal introitus. These drain into the superficial and deep femoral nodes and the internal iliac nodes.

Nerve supply

Branches of the pudendal nerve and perineal nerve supply the vulval structures.

The vagina

The vagina is a fibromuscular sheath and a potential canal extending from the vulva to the uterus. The walls are normally in apposition. The widest diameter of the vagina is anteroposterior in the lower one-third and transverse in the upper two-thirds. This is important to remember when inserting vaginal speculae. It runs upwards and backwards from the vestibule at 85% to the horizontal, which is parallel to the plane of the pelvic brim when the woman is standing erect. The vagina is surrounded and supported by the pelvic floor muscles.

The posterior wall ends blindly to form the vault of the vagina and is 9 cm long. The cervix projects into the anterior wall of the vagina, shortening it to 7 cm in length. This cervical projection divides the vault of the vagina into four fornices, shallow anterior and lateral fornices and a more capacious posterior fornix.

The entrance to the vagina is partially covered by the membranous **hymen** which has a few perforations to allow menstrual flow. This membrane varies in elasticity and is usually torn at the first coitus and more so at the first birth. Imperforate hymen is a possible cause of failure to menstruate. Once ruptured, remnants are left called **carunculae myrtiformes**. The walls of the vagina fall into transverse folds or **rugae** to allow for distension. These spread out from two longitudinal columns which run sagittally in the anterior and posterior walls.

Layers of the vagina

- Stratified squamous non-keratinised epithelium 10–30 cells deep rests on a basement membrane to form the inner lining of the vagina. This is continuous with the epithelium of the infravaginal cervix. The cells are divided into three layers, derived from the basement membrane and changing as they near the surface. These are the **parabasal cells**, **intermediate cells** and **superficial cells**.
- A layer of vascular connective tissue contains elastic tissue, nerves, lymphatic and blood vessels.
- An involuntary muscle coat whose inner muscle fibres are more oblique than circular while the outer are longitudinal. The vagina varies in size, mainly as a function of muscle tone and contraction in the pelvic floor muscles which are under voluntary control.
- Fascia or loose connective tissue surrounds the vagina.

The epithelium changes with the ovarian and menstrual cycles. There is further development and differentiation during pregnancy in response to circulating oestrogens, **progesterone** and **androgens**. The vaginal epithelium does not secrete mucus but secretions seep between the cells to moisten the vagina. Superficial cells and some intermediate cells contain glycogen. Superficial cells are continuously exfoliated and release their glycogen which is metabolised by **Döderlein's bacillus**, producing lactic acid as a waste product. This results in a normal vaginal acid medium of 4.5, preventing pathogenic organisms from invading. The cells can also absorb drugs, in particular oestrogens.

Relations

The lower half of the anterior wall is in contact with the urethra to which it is tightly bound. The upper half is in close contact with the base of the bladder. The lower third of the posterior wall is separated from the anal canal by the perineal body, the middle third is in apposition with the rectum and the upper third with a pouch of peritoneum called the pouch of Douglas. Laterally the upper third of the vagina is supported by pelvic connective tissue, the middle third by the **levatores ani** and the lower third by the **bulbocavernosus muscle**.

Blood supply

Arterial supply is from the vaginal and uterine arteries, which are both branches of the internal iliac artery. Venous drainage is by rich venous plexi in the muscular layer. These communicate with pudendal, vesical and haemorrhoidal plexi and then to the internal iliac vein.

Nerve supply

Nerve supply to voluntary vaginal muscle is via the pudendal nerve.

Vaginal functions

- Escape of menstrual blood flow.
- Coitus with entry of the male penis.
- Birth of the fetus, placenta and membranes.

The non-pregnant uterus

The uterus develops from the fusion of the two embryonic Müllerian ducts (Johnson 2007). It is a thick-walled, muscular, hollow, pear-shaped organ flattened in its anteroposterior diameter. Its lower third forms the cervix which projects into the vault of the vagina through its anterior wall. The uterus lies in the pelvic cavity in an anteverted and anteflexed position. Its normal measurements are shown in Table 4.1.

Structure

The uterus (Fig. 4.3) consists of the body which is 5 cm long, the narrow **isthmus** 0.5 cm long and the cervix 2.5 cm long. The fundus is the area above and between the **uterine tubes** (Fallopian tubes), and the junction between each uterine tube and the uterus is called the **cornu** (plural cornua). A constriction at the upper end of the isthmus is called the **anatomical internal os** and where the endometrium meets the columnar cervical epithelium is called the **histological internal os**. The cavity has a triangular shape when viewed in coronal section and a capacity of about 10 ml.

Although the cervix is continuous with and part of the uterus, it differs in its structure and function from the body of the uterus and will be described separately. The cervix is barrel-shaped and penetrated by the cervical canal. It is 2.5 cm long and separated from the body of the uterus by the isthmus. It is divided into two equal parts:

Table 4.1 Measurements of the non-pregnant uterus	
Dimension	**Measurement**
Length, including cervix	7.5 cm
Breadth	5.0 cm
Depth	2.5 cm
Average thickness of walls	1.5 cm
Weight	60 g

1. The **supravaginal cervix** lies above the vaginal vault and is surrounded by pelvic fascia, the **parametrium**, except posteriorly where it is in apposition with the **pouch of Douglas**.

2. The cone-shaped **infravaginal cervix** projects into the vagina and is covered by stratified squamous epithelium, continuous with the vaginal epithelium. It joins the columnar epithelium of the cervical canal at the external os, a site called the **squamocolumnar junction**, an important site of cellular change (see Box 4.1).

Lining of the body (corpus)

The mucous lining or **endometrium** builds up from a layer of basal cells. It consists of **stroma** (connective tissue component of an organ) covered by a layer of ciliated cuboid cells. This layer dips down into the stroma to form mucus-secreting tubular cells opening into the uterine cavity (Fig. 4.4). The thickness varies depending on the phase of the menstrual cycle and is thinnest at the isthmus.

Lining of the cervix

The spindle-shaped cervical canal connects the uterine cavity at the internal os with the vagina at the external os. The canal is lined by columnar mucus-secreting epithelium thrown into anterior and posterior folds from which circular folds radiate like branches from a tree trunk (the arbour vitae or tree of life). The epithelium dips into the stroma in a complex system of crypts and tunnels separated by ridges of stroma consisting of 80% collagen, 10% muscle fibres and 10% blood vessels.

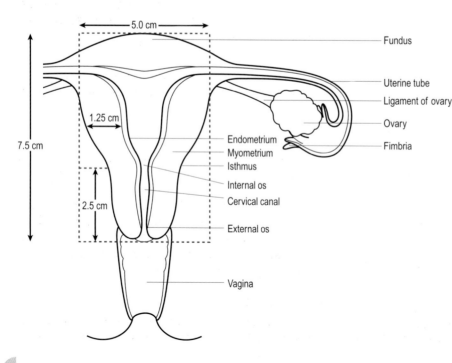

5.0 cm
1.25 cm
7.5 cm
2.5 cm

Fundus
Uterine tube
Ligament of ovary
Ovary
Fimbria
Endometrium
Myometrium
Isthmus
Internal os
Cervical canal
External os
Vagina

Figure 4.3 • The uterus and the left uterine tube and ovary. (From Henderson C, Macdonald S 2004, with kind permission of Elsevier.)

BOX 4.1 THE SQUAMOCOLUMNAR JUNCTION AND CERVICAL SCREENING

The squamocolumnar junction is between the columnar epithelium of the cervical canal and the squamous epithelium continuous with the vaginal epithelium. This may be an abrupt transformation but sometimes the two tissue types merge in a **transformation zone** which is the usual site for cervical carcinoma to arise. The position of this junction is determined by the amount of stroma which is influenced by the levels of the hormones oestrogen and progesterone.

Oestrogen softens the cervical collagen by binding water to the molecules. This increases the volume of stroma which causes the clefts and tunnels to unfold. The squamocolumnar junction is displaced downwards and out of the cervical canal, an event called **eversion**. Exposure of the columnar epithelium causes the tissues to hypertrophy (**squamous metaplasia**) leading to the development of the transformation zone.

In some women the cervical epithelium seems unstable, and cells with nuclear **dyskaryosis** (abnormal appearance of the nucleus) and **cellular dysplasia** (abnormal cell growth) are likely to lead to cervical carcinoma. These abnormalities are due to an infection with the **human papilloma virus** (HPV) types 16, 18 and 6. HPV can be a cause of genital warts. Epidemiological evidence has indicated that up to 30% of sexually active women have been affected by HPV by the age of 30.

Early recognition of these precancerous changes allows surgical treatment to be successful so that screening women on a regular basis can be life-saving. The technique is called **cervical exfoliative cytology** and is offered to antenatal patients who have not been recently screened. A specially shaped spatula such as an Ayres spatula is used to obtain cells from both outside and inside the cervical canal.

The cells are examined under a microscope and reported as:

1. Unsatisfactory: insufficient cells or incorrect processing of the slide.
2. Inflammatory or inconclusive: cells distorted by other infections such as Monilia.
3. Normal.
4. Mild dyskaryosis (CIN1) (CIN means cervical intraepithelial carcinoma).
5. Moderate dyskaryosis (CIN2).
6. Severe dyskaryosis (CIN3).

Over 90% of smears will be reported as normal. Categories 1, 2 and 4 need a repeat smear after 3–4 months following treatment for infection if necessary. Categories 5 and 6 need direct vision examination by colposcopy followed by a tissue biopsy. The extent of surgical treatment will depend on the results of the biopsy and whether the woman wishes to have more children. It will vary from the destruction of the abnormal cells by laser or cryosurgery to cone biopsy to hysterectomy. More serious and likely to lead to death of the woman is invasive carcinoma of the cervix where the cancer has spread beyond the epithelial tissues.

Compound racemose glands secrete cervical mucus that varies in quality and quantity under the influence of the sex hormones.

Muscle layer

The muscle layer or **myometrium** is made up of bundles of smooth muscle fibres. The outer longitudinal layer and the inner circular layer are not well developed in the non-pregnant uterus so that most fibres run obliquely and interlace to surround blood vessels and lymphatic vessels. The proportion of muscle begins to diminish in the isthmus, being replaced by connective tissue until it reaches the 10% muscle content of the cervix.

Peritoneal layer

The peritoneal layer is a double serosal layer known as the **perimetrium**. It covers the anterior and posterior

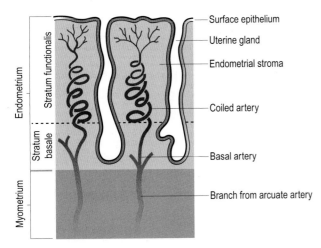

Figure 4.4 • The vascular supply to the endometrium. (From Hinchliff S M, Montague S E 1990, with kind permission of Elsevier.)

surfaces but is absent from the narrow lateral surfaces. It is reflected off the uterus onto the superior surface of the bladder at the level of the anatomical internal os; this is important for understanding the technique of lower segment caesarean section.

Relations

- Anterior: uterovesical pouch and bladder.
- Posterior: pouch of Douglas and rectum.
- Lateral: broad ligaments, uterine tubes and ovaries.
- Superior: intestines.
- Inferior: vagina.

Supports

The structures supporting the uterus are shown in Figure 4.5. Four pairs of ligaments support the uterus, three pairs support its position in relation to the vagina (cardinal, pubocervical and uterosacral ligaments) and one pair maintains uterine anteversion and anteflexion (the round ligaments) (Table 4.2). The broad ligaments are not true ligaments but thickened folds of peritoneum running from the uterus to the side walls of the pelvis.

Blood supply

The blood supply to the uterus is complex and rich and is contributed to by both the **ovarian** and the **uterine** arteries (Fig. 4.6). The uterine artery, which is a branch of the internal iliac artery, enters at the level of the internal os and sends a small branch downwards to join the vaginal arteries in supplying the cervix and the vault of the vagina (Fig. 4.7). The main branch of the uterine artery turns upwards and takes a tortuous path to anastomose with the ovarian artery which enters the broad ligament to supply the ovaries and uterine tubes. Anterior and posterior divisions anastomose with the opposite side of the uterus. Branches leaving these vessels at right angles supply blood to the myometrium; they enter the endometrium as the **basal arteries** (Fig. 4.8).

Venous drainage

This is by the uterine and ovarian veins after the blood has been collected into **pampiniform plexi** (tendril-like), some of which communicate with veins from the bladder.

Lymphatic drainage

Good lymphatic drainage of the uterus protects against uterine infection, especially following birth. There are three communicating networks of vessels and small nodes at the level of the endometrium, myometrium and subperitoneal layer of the uterus. The lymph is collected

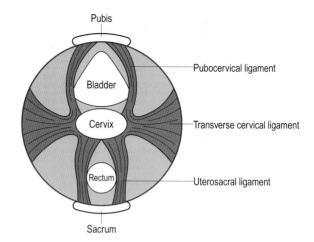

Figure 4.5•The uterine supports seen from above. (From Henderson C, Macdonald S 2004, with kind permission of Elsevier.)

Table 4.2 Ligaments supporting the uterus

Ligament	Origin	Insertion
Cardinal ligaments	Cervix	Side walls of pelvis
Pubocervical ligaments	Cervix	Under bladder to the pubic bones
Uterosacral ligaments	Cervix	Sacrum
Round ligaments	Cornua	Via inguinal canal to labia majora

into major ducts and taken to lumbar and sacral nodes centrally and to inguinal, internal and external iliac nodes laterally.

Nerve supply

The body of the uterus is supplied by autonomic nerves originating in the thoracic 11 and 12 and lumbar 1 vertebrae. Sensation from the body of the uterus is perceived as pain in response to stretch, infection and contraction. The cervix is innervated by the sacral plexus from sacral 2, 3 and 4 vertebral nerves. These pass through the **transcervical** or **Lee-Frankenhäuser nerve plexi**. Pain from the cervix is felt in response to rapid dilatation.

Functions of the uterus

- To receive the fertilised ovum.
- To nurture and protect the developing embryo and fetus.
- To expel the fetus, placenta and membranes.

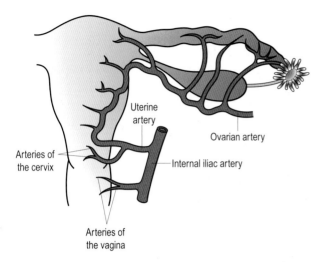

Figure 4.6 • The blood supply to the uterus and its appendages. (From Henderson C, Macdonald S 2004, with kind permission of Elsevier.)

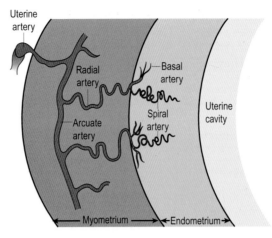

Figure 4.8 • The arterial supply to the uterine endometrium. (From Studd 1989, with permission.)

hollow tubes 10 cm long. Each tube extends from a uterine cornu and travels to the side walls of the pelvis, turning downwards and backwards before reaching them. The tubes lie within the broad ligament and communicate with the uterus at their medial end and with the ovaries at their lateral end. There is a direct pathway between the vagina and the peritoneal cavity, thus a risk of entry of an ascending infection.

Structure

Each uterine tube is divided into four sections:

1. The **interstitial part** is the narrowest part of the tube. Its lumen is only 1 mm in diameter and it runs within the uterine wall.

2. The **isthmus** is a straight, narrow, thick section extending 2.5 cm laterally from the uterine wall.

3. The **ampulla** is the longest and widest section. It extends 5 cm from the isthmus to the side walls of the pelvis. Its lumen is tortuous, relatively thin and distensible.

4. The **infundibulum** or **fimbriated portion** is trumpet-shaped and ends in fimbriae or finger-like processes. It is the lateral 2.5 cm of the tube which turns downwards and backwards. Although the fimbriae have little or no contact with the ovary, they become very active during ovulation and sweep the ovarian surface.

The three layers of the uterine tube are:

1. An inner epithelial layer of cuboid cells arranged in **plicae** (folds), most pronounced in the ampulla. The complexity of the folds and the diameter of the lumen increase from the interstitial portion to the infundibular portion. Many cuboid cells are ciliated whilst others are goblet cells and secrete mucus.

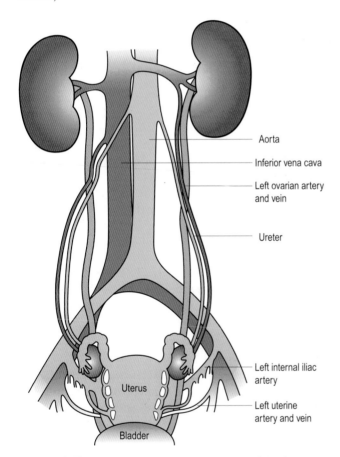

Figure 4.7 • The blood supply to the uterus; note where the ovarian artery terminates. (From Henderson C, Macdonald S 2004, with kind permission of Elsevier.)

The uterine tubes (Fallopian tubes)

The **uterine tubes** develop from the right and left embryonic Müllerian ducts. They are two small, muscular,

2. Involuntary muscle fibres in two layers, inner circular and outer longitudinal, continuous with the fibres in the body of the uterus make up the middle wall. These undergo peristaltic contractions during ovulation.

3. An outer covering of peritoneum on the superior, anterior and posterior surfaces but not on the inferior surface.

Relations

- Anterior, posterior and superior: the peritoneal cavity and intestines.
- Lateral: the side walls of the pelvis.
- Inferior: the broad ligaments and ovaries.
- Medial: the uterus.

Supports

The uterine tubes are held in position by their attachment to the uterus and broad ligaments.

Blood supply, lymphatic drainage and nerve supply

These are shared with the ovaries and are described below.

Functions

- Mucus, cilia and peristaltic movements move the ovum towards the uterus.
- Fertilisation normally takes place within the ampulla.
- The mucus secreted by the uterine tubes may provide nourishment for the ovum.

The ovary

The two ovaries develop from the **embryonic gonadal ridges**. Undifferentiated primitive germ cells that began life on the wall of the yolk sac migrate into the gonadal ridges using amoebic movements at 6 weeks of embryological development (Moore & Persaud 2008). The female ovary is recognisable slightly later than the male testis, at about 10 weeks.

The mature ovaries consist of **interstitial tissue** and **follicles**. They are small almond-shaped glands measuring 3 cm × 2 cm × 1 cm and weighing just 6 g. They have a dull, pinkish-grey, uneven external appearance. They lie in a shallow peritoneal fossa adjacent to the lateral pelvic wall, outside the posterior layer of the broad ligaments and inside the peritoneum. The long axis of each ovary is in the vertical plane but the position is influenced by movements of the uterus and broad ligament.

If the uterus is retroverted they may lie in the pouch of Douglas and cause pain during coitus. The uterine tubes arch over the ovaries.

Macroscopic structure

- The **medulla** is the inner part of the ovary which is directly attached to the broad ligament by the mesovarium. It consists of fibrous tissue containing blood vessels, lymphatics and nerves carried by the infundibulopelvic ligament.
- The **cortex** is the functional part of the ovary and consists of highly vascular stroma in which ovarian follicles are embedded.
- The **tunica albuginea** is a tough fibrous capsule forming the outer part of the cortex.
- The **germinal layer** consists of cuboid cells developed from modified peritoneum and is continuous with the broad ligament. It forms an outer covering for the ovary.

Microscopic structure—the follicles

Tiny sac-like structures called **ovarian follicles** at different stages of maturation are embedded in the ovarian cortex. These stages of maturation (Fig. 4.9) are brought about by neurohormonal changes. The **primordial follicle** contains an immature egg encased in a single layer of squamous-like follicle cells. These cells stay in a state of arrested development at the first **meiotic prophase** and will not complete their development until they are prepared for ovulation (Johnson 2007).

Over 2 million primordial follicles are present in the fetal ovary prior to birth and no mitosis occurs after birth. By the menarche only 200 000 remain, more than 80% having regressed. Only 300–400 will be shed at ovulation. It is not yet understood why these cells behave in this unusual way.

Development of the mature follicle

Each day a few primordial follicles begin to develop but how these are selected is unknown (Johnson 2007). Interactions between the oocytes and the follicular cells lead to oocyte growth. A developing primordial follicle passes through three stages:

1. First it becomes a **primary follicle** or **preantral follicle** and is surrounded by two or more layers of cuboidal **granulosa cells**.

2. Then it becomes a **secondary follicle** or **antral follicle** (Graafian follicle). An outer layer of cells known as the thecal layer develops from the interstitial cells of the stroma.

3. Finally it becomes a **preovulatory follicle**.

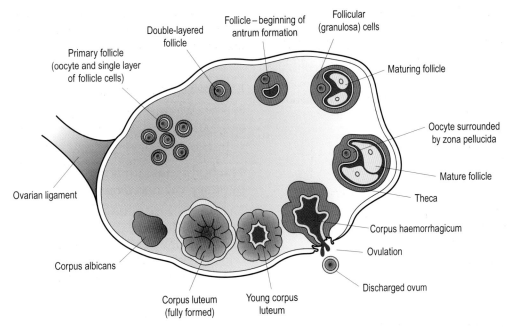

Figure 4.9 Diagrammatic section of an ovary showing stages of follicular maturation. (From Blackburn 2003, with permission.)

Under the influence of the hormones the granulosa and theca cells proliferate and differentiate and the oocyte increases in size by a factor of 300. The granulosa cells divide to become several layers thick, and gap junctions, which allow easy transfer of molecules between cells, develop. Secretion of fluid droplets leads to the formation of a single fluid-filled space called the **antrum** which separates the granulosa cells into distinct layers. A dense layer called the **cumulus** surrounds the oocytes, while a thin outer layer lines the theca.

As the follicle continues to grow, the mature oocyte surrounded by a dense mass of granulosa cells called the **cumulus oophorus** becomes suspended in fluid called the **liquor folliculi**. It is attached to a stalk of granulosa cells which connects the two layers. It then breaks away and floats freely in the fluid. The follicle bulges out from the surface of the ovary. The ovum is next to the outer wall and the stroma overlying it becomes thin. The theca cells differentiate into the **theca interna**, a highly vascularised glandular layer, and the **theca externa**, the dense, fibrous outer capsule of the follicle. Glycoproteins secreted from the cell surface of the oocytes form a translucent layer called the **zona pellucida**.

Each month about 12 growing follicles emerge from the primordial follicles. One or occasionally more of the ripe follicles matures and ruptures and the oocyte escapes. After ovulation the ruptured follicle is transformed into a structure called the **corpus luteum** (yellow body) which, in the absence of a pregnancy, will degenerate in about 6 months into a **corpus albicans** (white body).

Relations

- Anterior: the broad ligaments.
- Posterior: the intestines.
- Lateral: the infundibulopelvic ligaments and the side walls of the pelvis.
- Superior: the uterine tubes.
- Medial: the uterus and ovarian ligament.

Supports

The ovary is held suspended in position:
- To the uterus by the ovarian ligament.
- To the posterior surface of the broad ligament by the mesovarium.
- To the side walls of the pelvis by the suspensory or infundibulopelvic ligament.

Blood supply

The two long, slender ovarian arteries arise high up on the aorta, immediately below the renal arteries, demonstrating the related development of the renal and reproductive systems. Each ovarian artery crosses over the pelvic brim laterally and enters the broad ligament where branches supply the uterine tube and the ovary. Each then anastomoses with its uterine artery to form the uterine blood supply. The right ovarian vein drains directly into the inferior vena cava whereas the left ovarian vein joins the left renal vein which then joins the inferior vena cava.

Lymphatic drainage

Lymphatic drainage is into the lumbar glands.

Nerve supply

The nerve supply of the ovary is well developed via the ovarian plexus. Sympathetic fibres and sensory nerves from the ovary run with the arteries to be relayed to the 10th thoracic segment of the spinal cord. The ovaries, like the testes, are extremely sensitive organs if handled or squeezed.

Functions of the ovary

1. To produce ova.
2. To produce the female steroid hormones oestrogen and progesterone.

Cyclical control of reproduction

The ovarian cycle

In each **menstrual cycle** stromal cells surrounding the developing follicle take on an endocrine function. Developmental changes are much more complex than those that occur during spermatogenesis (Ch. 5). The formation of receptors on follicle cells is in response to cyclical alterations in circulating hormones from the pituitary gland and the ovary itself and occurs in the late preantral and antral phases. There may also be involvement of local intraovarian regulators such as **epidermal growth factor** (EGF). The ovum is prepared for ovulation, fertilisation and implantation. At the same time changes occur within the woman's body, in both reproductive and non-reproductive tissues, to prepare for pregnancy and lactation. These also depend on the cyclical presence of specific hormone receptors on cells.

Ovulation

The ovarian capsule stretches and bursts, the follicle ruptures and the ovum with its surrounding tissues and liquor is flushed into the abdominal cavity where it is picked up by the fimbriae of the uterine tubes. These waft the ovum into the tubal ampulla to await fertilisation. Some women feel a pain at this time called **mittelschmerz**. The follicle now collapses to become the corpus luteum. The lining cells of the follicle, granulosa and theca interna absorb fluid, swell and proliferate until the corpus luteum is about 1–2 cm across.

Neurohormonal control of the ovarian cycle

The cyclical changes that occur are an integrated process but they can be discussed individually to achieve understanding. The following aspects will be considered:

1. The hormonal function of the hypothalamic–pituitary–ovarian axis.
2. Growth and development of the oocytes.
3. The menstrual cycle.
4. Changes in other tissues.

The hormonal function of the hypothalamic–pituitary–ovarian axis

The average ovarian cycle lasts 28 days with ovulation on day 14. However, the cycle shows considerable variation, both from cycle to cycle in an individual woman and between women. The cycle is responsive to stress, disease, allergies, physical activity and nutritional deficiencies. It is usually the duration of the follicular phase leading up to ovulation that is variable.

The hypothalamus
The control of the rhythmicity of the ovarian cycle and menstrual cycle is via the **hypothalamus** and the **anterior pituitary gland** (Fig. 4.10). Hormonal interactions

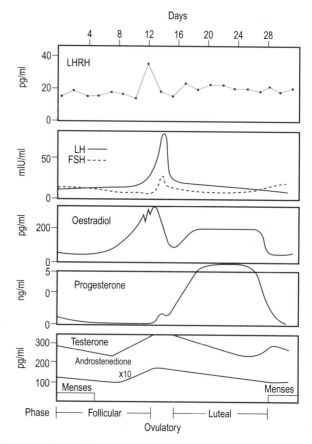

Figure 4.10 ● Profile of plasma hormone levels throughout the menstrual cycle. (From Berne & Levy 1993, with permission.)

between the hypothalamus and the pituitary gland occur by vascular and neuronal pathways (Johnson 2007). The larger anterior pituitary lobe or **adenohypophysis** has no direct neural connections with the hypothalamus, whereas the posterior lobe or **neurohypophysis** consists mainly of axons whose cell bodies are situated in the hypothalamus (Hinson et al 2007). The hormone oxytocin released by the posterior pituitary gland is important in labour.

The anterior pituitary gland

At least five groups of hormone-producing cells are found in the anterior lobe of the pituitary. Their function is regulated by neuronal substances from the hypothalamus (Hinson et al 2007). Those concerned with reproduction include:

- Follicle-stimulating hormone (FSH).
- Luteinising hormone (LH).
- Adrenocorticotrophic hormone.
- Prolactin.

A detailed consideration of the many interactions involved in the cyclical changes can be found in Johnson (2007). Hypothalamic **gonadotrophin-releasing factor** (GnRH) is transferred by a portal blood system to the anterior pituitary gland where it interacts with specific cell receptors to cause the release of the gonadotrophins FSH and LH (Fig. 4.11).

The ovary

Rising plasma levels of the ovarian hormones **oestrogen** and **progesterone** synthesised from cholesterol can reduce the production of GnRH in a negative feedback mechanism, especially oestrogen. There are three main oestrogens: the most important is estradiol, with estrone second and estriol third in potency. If pregnancy does not occur, the corpus luteum degenerates and both FSH and LH begin to rise on day 1 of the cycle and steadily increase towards the late follicular phase.

Ovulation is dependent upon a mid-cycle surge of LH and FSH and occurs 24 h after the surge. Although plasma levels of both hormones rise, the level of LH is higher and appears to be more important in causing ovulation. Generally a single ovum is released in each cycle and the others that have begun developing regress to become **corpora atretica**.

If more than one follicle develops simultaneously **multiple pregnancy** could occur. The frequency of multiple ovulation increases with age and in Black women. Asian women are less likely than Caucasian women to have multiple ovulation. If there is no pregnancy, the corpus luteum begins to regress after 14 days and production of oestrogen and progesterone declines rapidly. When plasma levels of these hormones become low enough, the anterior pituitary begins to produce FSH and LH and the cycle begins again.

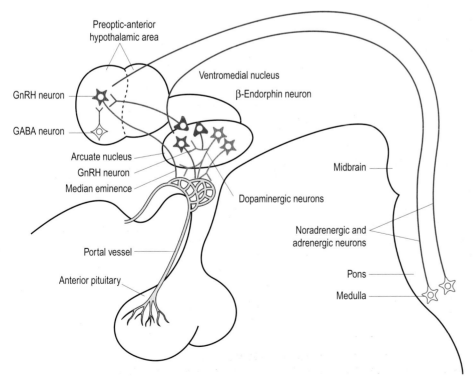

Figure 4.11 • Schematic diagram to show some of the postulated neurochemical reactions that may control GnRH secretion. (From Johnson & Everitt 1995, with permission.)

Preoptic-anterior hypothalamic area

Ventromedial nucleus

β-Endorphin neuron

GnRH neuron

GABA neuron

Arcuate nucleus

GnRH neuron

Median eminence

Dopaminergic neurons

Midbrain

Noradrenergic and adrenergic neurons

Portal vessel

Pons

Anterior pituitary

Medulla

Local control of growth and development of the oocytes

Within the follicle local activities aimed at its growth and development occur. Some are carried out by theca cells, some by granulosa cells and some involve cooperation between both.

Oestrogen and progesterone

During follicle development LH stimulates the theca cells to produce **androstenedione** and **testosterone**. These are transported to the granulosa cells to be converted to oestrogen, which causes proliferation of granulosa and theca cells and further growth of the follicles. The follicle that develops most rapidly may produce larger amounts of oestrogen. This may inhibit the release of FSH by negative feedback to the pituitary gland, preventing further growth of the remaining follicles. Further growth of the dominant follicle results in the estradiol surge that immediately precedes ovulation. Within 12 h progesterone takes over as the dominant hormone produced by the theca and granulosa cells.

Other hormones involved locally

Research into the causes of infertility and the techniques of in vitro fertilisation have led to the realisation that as well as the steroid hormones some peptide hormones have major influences on follicular development. In particular it is worth mentioning two: **inhibin** and **growth hormone**.

Inhibin is known to have an effect on sperm production. It has been found in relatively high quantities in follicular fluid and may be one of the factors that determine the number of follicles released at ovulation. The rise in concentration of inhibin in follicular fluid may be in response to the surge in GnRH from the hypothalamus (Yding Andersen et al 1993).

Growth hormone (GH) may increase the intraovarian production of **insulin-like growth factor 1** (IGF1) which amplifies the response of the granulosa cells to gonadotrophins (Adashi et al 1985). The GH receptor gene and GH-binding sites have been found in human granulosa cells (Carlsson et al 1992). However, GH augmentation does not improve the rate of pregnancies in women who had a poor follicular development response to treatment with gonadotrophin.

Triggering of ovulation

The actions of FSH and oestrogen combine to induce the development of LH receptors on the granulosa cells. This coincides with the FSH and LH surge from the anterior pituitary gland brought about by GnRH from the hypothalamus and ovulation occurs. Ovulation is facilitated by the local release of **prostaglandin E$_2$** (PGE$_2$) and the vasodilatory substances **histamine** and **bradykinin**. PGE$_2$ initiates breakdown of the collagen of the follicular wall, whilst the vasodilatory substances cause local inflammation. Proteolytic enzymes break down the follicular wall, allowing ovulation to occur.

The menstrual (endometrial) cycle

The changing levels and interactions between oestrogen and progesterone lead to alterations in endometrial tissues and selected tissues elsewhere, depending on the presence of hormone receptors in the cells. The endometrium is itself an endocrine organ and secretes oestrogens, progesterone and prolactin; it is not totally dependent on ovarian hormones. The menstrual cycle is divided into three phases: **menstrual**, **proliferative** and **secretory** phases (Fig. 4.12). The menstrual and proliferative phases coincide with the follicular phase of the ovarian cycle and the secretory with the luteal.

Menstrual phase—days 1–5

As the corpus luteum degenerates, plasma progesterone, which has a shorter plasma half-life than oestrogen, falls more rapidly, changing the balance of the two hormones in favour of oestrogen. This causes the endometrium to become unstable. Fluid is lost from the tissues which shrink, compress the spiral arteries and cause endometrial anoxia. Autolysis begins and the upper endometrium sloughs away from the basal layer with bleeding into the tissues.

Oestrogen also increases the excitability of the myometrium which further increases tissue anoxia and expels the sloughed tissue and blood. Menstrual fluid does not normally clot due to high levels of plasmin which breaks down fibrin as it forms. Blood loss is normally between 10 and 80 ml with a mean of 35 ml and an average iron loss of 0.5 mg. At this point the endometrium is thin and poorly vascularised and only the bases of the endometrial glands remain.

The proliferative phase—days 6–14

Rising oestrogen levels cause rapid proliferation of stroma cells with some oedema and the endometrium thickens from 1 to 6 mm by ovulation. The outer epithelium remains one cell thick throughout the cycle. At the same time the glands lengthen and become tortuous. The blood vessels regrow and begin to show a spiral formation. The epithelial cells and the glandular cells begin to synthesise and store glycogen.

The secretory phase—days 15–28

After ovulation the corpus luteum secretes large amounts of progesterone. This acts on the oestrogen-primed

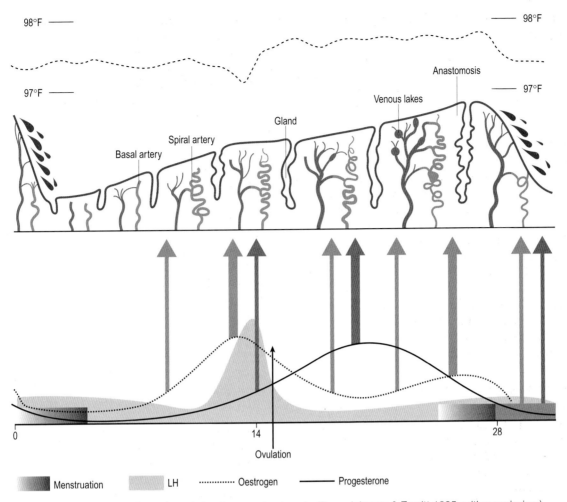

Figure 4.12 Changes in human endometrium during the menstrual cycle. (From Johnson & Everitt 1995, with permission.)

endometrium to convert it into a secretory tissue. The endometrium is now highly vascular and the arteries have developed pronounced spiralling. Venous lakes are formed. The stroma becomes even more oedematous, the cells themselves become larger and there is a further thickening of the endometrium to 6 mm. The endometrial glands secrete glycogen. The endometrial surface becomes folded and prepared for implantation, which occurs 7 days after ovulation. It is completed at 14 days after ovulation when the next menstrual cycle would be due.

Non-endometrial sites of hormone action

The myometrium

Excitability of the myometrium is dependent on the balance between progesterone and oestrogen. Oestrogen increase brings about cyclical changes in the thickness of the myometrium and in muscle excitability. It stimulates spontaneous contractions, while progesterone reduces excitability. High levels of oestrogen also increase myometrial response to oxytocin.

The cervix

The mucus secreted by the cervical glands during the follicular phase is watery and turbid, while that secreted after ovulation is thicker and clearer. Mucus secreted at the time of ovulation will crystallise in a fern-like pattern if left to dry on a glass slide.

The vagina

During the follicular phase the cells of the vaginal epithelium are large and flat with an acidophilic cytoplasm. During the luteal phase they become polygonal and more basophilic. There is an increase in the glycogen content of the vagina, due partly to the secretory activity of the endometrium and partly to activity of the vaginal epithelial cells. Lactobacilli present in the vagina metabolise the glycogen to lactic acid, lowering the pH of the vagina from 6.5 during the follicular phase to 4.5 in the luteal phase.

The uterine tubes

During the follicular phase there is an increase in the number of ciliated cells and in the frequency and co-ordination of the peristaltic contractions of the muscle, reaching a maximum at the time of ovulation. Subsequently, the tubes become more quiescent under the influence of progesterone.

Other actions (Johnson 2007)

Oestrogen causes:
- Development of the typical female shape.

- Growth of the breasts and nipples.
- Development of the adult reproductive organs.
- Control of FSH production by feedback mechanism.
- Maintenance of bone density.
- Reduction of capillary fragility.
- Increase in the ability of the cardiovascular system to withstand high blood pressures.

Progesterone causes:
- Development of the secretory endometrium.
- Development of alveolar breast tissue prior to menstruation.
- Increase of the body temperature by 0.5°C following ovulation.
- Reduction of anxiety.
- Interaction with aldosterone receptors to cause retention of sodium and water.

Main points

- There is no evidence of sexual difference in the embryo prior to the 7th week. If the embryonic genetic make-up contains the SRY gene on the Y chromosome, testes and male genitalia develop. If the genetic make-up is XX, ovaries and female genitalia develop.
- The continuous tract of the female genitalia has a direct opening into the peritoneal cavity from the external environment. This is necessary for fertilisation but increases the risk of pelvic infections.
- The vulva consists of the labia majora, labia minora, clitoris and vestibule onto which opens the urethral meatus and the vaginal introitus.
- The vagina extends from the vulva to the uterus and is lined with stratified, squamous non-keratinised epithelium. Superficial cells release glycogen which Döderlein's bacillus metabolises to produce lactic acid giving a pH of 4.5. This minimises the risk of ascending infection.
- The uterine body endometrium consists of vascular connective tissue containing mucus-secreting glands which open into the uterine cavity. The stroma is covered with a layer of cuboid cells which dip into it to form glands. Endometrial thickness depends on the phase of the menstrual cycle.
- The cervix is divided into the supravaginal cervix and the infravaginal cervix. The cervical canal is lined by columnar mucus-secreting epithelium thrown into anterior and posterior folds from which the arbour vitae radiate.
- In some women the squamocolumnar junction may develop changes that may lead to cervical carcinoma. Early recognition by screening of precancerous changes allows surgical treatment to be life-saving.

- The smooth muscle fibres of the myometrium run mainly obliquely to surround blood vessels and lymphatic vessels. The proportion of muscle diminishes towards the isthmus, being replaced by connective tissue.
- The perimetrium covers the anterior and posterior surfaces but is absent from the narrow lateral surfaces of the uterus. It is reflected off the uterus onto the superior surface of the bladder at the level of the anatomical internal os.
- The uterus receives the fertilised ovum, nurtures and protects the developing fetus and expels the fetus, placenta and membranes.
- The uterine tubes communicate with the uterus at their medial ends and the ovaries at their lateral ends. The inner cuboid epithelium is arranged in plicae. Half the cells secrete mucus and half are ciliated. Fertilisation takes place in the ampulla.
- The ovaries lie in a shallow peritoneal fossa next to the lateral pelvic wall, outside the broad ligaments and inside the peritoneum. They consist of a medulla, cortex, tunica albuginea and germinal layer and produce ova and the female steroid hormones oestrogen and progesterone.
- The mature ovum consists of the haploid cell floating in liquor folliculi, surrounded by the zona pellucida and the corona radiata.
- The ovarian capsule stretches until it bursts and the ovum is expelled into the abdominal cavity to be picked up by the fimbriae of the uterine tube.
- The average ovarian cycle lasts 28 days with ovulation on day 14. The control of the ovarian and menstrual cycles is via the hypothalamus and pituitary gland.

The development of the dominant follicle with its oocyte is a complex process involving local as well as distant hormonal changes.

- The interactions between oestrogen and progesterone lead to alterations in endometrial tissues. The menstrual and proliferative phases of the menstrual cycle coincide with the follicular phase of the ovarian cycle and the secretory phase with the luteal phase.

- Steroid hormones also affect the myometrium, cervix, vagina, uterine tubes and development of secondary sexual characteristics.

References

Adashi, E.Y., Resnick, C.E., D'Ercole, A.J., et al., 1985. Insulin-like growth factors as intra-ovarian regulators of granulosa cell growth and function. Endocr. Rev. 6, 400–420.

Carlsson, G., Bergh, C., Bentham, J., et al., 1992. Expression of functional growth hormone receptors in human granulosa cells. Hum. Reprod. 76, 1205–1209.

Henderson, C., Macdonald, S. (Eds.), 2004. Mayes' Midwifery: A Textbook for Midwives, thirteen ed. Baillière Tindall, London.

Hinson, J., Raven, P., Chew, S. (Eds.), 2007. The Endocrine System. Churchill Livingstone Elsevier, Edinburgh.

Johnson, M.H., 2007. Essential Reproduction, sixth ed. Blackwell Science, Oxford.

Jones, S.Y., 2002. The Descent of Man. Little, Brown, London.

Moore, K.L., Persaud, T.V.N., 2008. The Developing Human—Clinically Oriented Embryology, eight ed. Saunders Elsevier, London.

Yding Andersen, C., Westergaard, L.G., Figenschau, Y., et al., 1993. Endocrine composition of follicular fluid comparing human chorionic gonadotrophin to a gonadotrophin-releasing hormone agonist for ovulation induction. Hum. Reprod. 8, 840–843.

Annotated recommended reading

Bainbridge, D., 2003. The X in Sex. Harvard University Press, Boston, MA.

This is a highly readable, entertaining account of all you need to know about the X chromosome.

Hinson, J., Raven, P., Chew, S. (Eds.), 2007. The Endocrine System. Churchill Livingstone Elsevier.

This is an excellent textbook on the endocrine system. It covers all the endocrine glands in easily readable text.

Johnson, M.H., 2007. Essential Reproduction, sixth ed. Blackwell Science, Oxford.

All the major areas of reproduction are covered in this up-to-date book.

In particular, sexual differentiation and regulation of gonadal function are clearly described.

Chapter Five

5

The male reproductive system

Introduction

An understanding of the anatomy and physiology of the male reproductive system is essential knowledge for the extended role of the midwife. Many aspects of fertility, infertility and preconception care depend on the general and sexual health of both partners.

Anatomy of the male reproductive system

The male genitalia are mainly outside the body cavity, a situation necessary for both production and transfer of

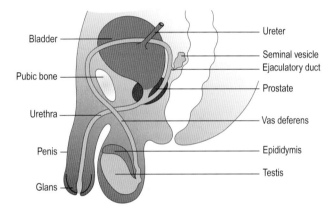

Figure 5.1 • The male reproductive system. (From Henderson C, Macdonald S 2004, with kind permission of Elsevier.)

spermatozoa. The organs are the scrotum, testis, rete and epididymis, ductus deferens, seminal vesicles, prostate gland, bulbourethral glands and penis with the urethra (Fig. 5.1). Unlike the female urinary system where the urethral orifice is separate to the vagina, the male genital and urinary systems share a common outlet through the urethra.

The scrotum and testes

Embryonic development

As discussed in Chapter 4, SRY activity on the Y chromosome converts the indifferent gonad to a testis. In the absence of this factor the gonad develops into an ovary (Jones 2002). It is an efficient process and there are few true **hermaphrodites** who have both testicular and ovarian tissue. Once the gonad is established the SRY gene is switched off. The testicular **Sertoli cells** (see below) also secrete **Müllerian inhibiting hormone** (MIH), which remains active until puberty, when there is a rapid decline in function. The **Leydig cells** (see below) of the testis produce testosterone from 13–15 weeks (Johnson 2007).

In the embryo, the testes develop high up on the lumbar region of the abdominal cavity. In the last few months of fetal life they descend through the abdominal cavity, over the pelvic brim and down the inguinal canal into the scrotal sac outside the body cavity. This descent occurs under the influence of testosterone and is completed in 98% of boys by birth.

The mature testis

At maturity each testis measures 4 cm long and 3 cm in diameter and is surrounded by two coats: the outer **tunica vaginalis**, which is derived from peritoneum, and the inner fibrous capsule, the **tunica albuginea**. One testis sits in each pocket of the **scrotal sac**. The scrotum is a thin-walled sac covered with hairy, rugose skin well supplied with sebaceous glands. The scrotal skin is highly vascularised and has a large surface area.

The temperature of the testes is maintained at 2–3°C below that of the body core to facilitate spermatogenesis. The position of the scrotum relative to the body can be adjusted by a spinal reflex in order to regulate testicular temperature. In a cold environment contraction of the scrotal muscle, the **dartos muscle**, wrinkles the scrotal skin and reduces the size of the sac, whereas the **cremaster muscle**, a skeletal muscle arising from the internal oblique muscle, contracts and lifts the testes nearer to the body. Relaxation of these muscles allows the testes to be held away from the body to facilitate cooling.

Structure

Each testis is divided into 200–300 wedge-shaped lobules by thin fibrous partitions that are extensions of the tunica albuginea (Fig. 5.2). Each lobule contains up to four **seminiferous tubules** which are highly coiled loops. About 80% of the testis by weight consists of seminiferous tubules in which spermatozoa develop. The seminiferous tubules of each lobule converge to form a straight tubule or **tubulus rectus** that conveys the sperm into the **rete testis**, a tubular network on the posterior aspect of the testis. From here the sperm enter the **epididymis** which is in close apposition to the external surface of the testis. Macrophages that phagocytose dead sperm are found in the lumen of the epididymis. Interstitial tissue is packed around the **seminiferous tubules** and contains blood vessels and endocrine cells, the **Leydig cells**, which secrete testosterone.

Blood supply

The testes are supplied by the testicular arteries that arise from the abdominal aorta. The testicular veins form

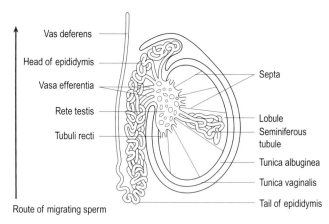

Figure 5.2 • The testis. (From Hinchliff S M, Montague S E 1990, with kind permission of Elsevier.)

a network around the testicular artery called a pampiniform plexus (tendril-like). This absorbs heat from the artery before the blood enters the testis.

Lymphatic drainage

Lymphatic drainage is by the inguinal nodes.

Nerve supply

There is innervation by the autonomic system—both sympathetic and parasympathetic. There is also a rich sensory nerve supply, resulting in much pain and nausea if the testes are struck. The nerve fibres run with the blood vessels and lymphatics in the fibrous connective tissue sheath called the **spermatic cord**.

Function of the testes

- To produce spermatozoa.
- To produce the hormones testosterone and inhibin.

Spermatogenesis (the production of spermatozoa)

Each testis consists of two separate compartments: cells that produce sperm and those that produce hormones. There is a physical barrier consisting of cellular barriers which limit free exchange of water-soluble materials. This barrier develops at puberty and is formed of multiple layers of gap and tight junctions surrounding each Sertoli cell. This is the **blood–testis barrier** (Johnson 2007). Its functions are:

1. To prevent sperm from entering the systemic and lymphatic circulations where they could set up antisperm antibodies, leading to infertility.
2. To maintain distinct chemical environments on either side of the barrier to facilitate sperm development and health.

Seminiferous tubules contain two types of cell: germ cells and Sertoli cells (Fig. 5.3). Primary germ cells are

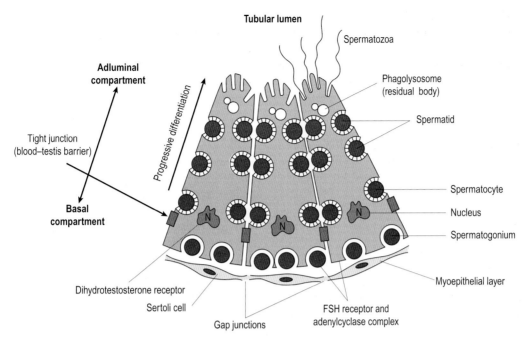

Figure 5.3 • Sertoli cells with developing germ cells at all stages of development from spermatogonia to spermatozoa. (From Tepperman & Tepperman 1987, with permission.)

dormant from the fetal period of life and begin to increase in number at puberty. Sperm production in the seminiferous tubules has three phases:

1. Mitotic proliferation, which produces large numbers of cells.

2. Meiotic division, which generates diversity and halves the chromosome number (haploid).

3. Cytodifferentiation, which packages the chromosomes for effective delivery.

In a functioning testis, germ cells will be present at all stages of development, all originating from **spermatogonia**. Spermatogonia divide by mitosis continuously to ensure a constant supply of cells maturing towards sperm. After undergoing several mitotic divisions they mature, become larger and are known as **primary spermatocytes** but are still diploid cells. Although nuclear division (**karyokinesis**) occurs, cytoplasmic division is incomplete and spermatogonia are linked by cytoplasmic bridges to form a **syncytium**. This persists throughout the meiotic phase and individual cells are only released as mature sperm (Johnson 2007).

Primary spermatocytes undergo the first meiotic division to form two secondary spermatocytes which have only 23 chromosomes—one of each pair. Half will receive the X chromosome and half the Y chromosome. Secondary meiosis results in four haploid cells called **spermatids**.

Spermatids are found in close association with Sertoli cells, which are polymorphic cells attached to a basement membrane but extending into the lumen of the seminiferous tubule. They provide nutrition and support to the sperm and are sometimes called 'nurse cells'. Here the spermatids are transformed from fairly basic cells into highly specialised sperm.

As a sperm matures, excess protoplasm is lost and the chromatin of the nucleus condenses to become the head. One centriole develops into the tail, which is composed of a central filament of two microfibrils surrounded by a circle of nine fibrils. Mitochondria aggregate into the neck region and the Golgi apparatus helps to form the **acrosome cap** which develops over the head of the sperm and contains enzymes called **hyaluronidases** and **proteases**.

The process takes about 70 days and several hundred million sperm per day (about 400 per gram of testis per second) are produced continuously from puberty. As men age, the seminiferous tubules undergo involution and by 70 years extensive atrophy may be present. Germ cells are reduced in number but Sertoli cells remain.

When sperm are fully formed they are pushed along the duct system to the epididymis by the cilia in the lining of the tubuli recti and the smooth muscle in the tubal wall. The columnar epithelium of the epididymis is thought to secrete hormones, enzymes and nutrients to enable sperm maturation. Sperm can be stored in the epididymis for as long as 42 days. This has implications for preconception advice on adverse environmental effects on sperm for at least 2 months before the ejaculation event that fertilises an ovum.

The duct system

The epididymis

The **epididymis** is a comma-shaped, tightly coiled tube about 6 metres long. The head of the comma which caps the superior aspect of the testis receives sperm from the efferent ductules of the testis. Here the sperm become more motile and fertile. However, they do not actively swim until ejaculated into the vagina. During ejaculation, the smooth muscle in the wall of the epididymis contracts strongly, expelling sperm from the tail portion into the ductus deferens.

The vas (ductus) deferens

This muscular tube runs upwards from the epididymis, through the **inguinal canal** into the pelvic cavity. It can be felt where it passes over the pubic bone. Its terminus expands to form the ampulla and joins with the duct from the **seminal vesicle** to form the short **ejaculatory duct**. The two ejaculatory ducts pass into the **prostate gland** and empty into the **urethra**. The wall of the **vas deferens** is composed of an outer layer of loose connective tissue and three layers of smooth muscle which can undergo rapid peristaltic contractions during ejaculation to pass the sperm forward.

This movement is facilitated by the autonomic nerve supply. The cells of the mucosal layer are pseudostratified epithelium arranged in longitudinal ridges. In the extra-abdominal portion, the ductus is accompanied by the **testicular artery**, the **pampiniform plexus** of veins, a nerve plexus, lymphatic vessels and the cremaster muscle. The whole complex is called the **spermatic cord**.

If no ejaculation occurs, the sperm in the epididymis degenerate and phagocytic cells in the epithelial layer remove them. Vasectomy or male sterilisation involves ligating and cutting the vas deferens. Fertility may remain for 6–8 weeks because of viable sperm above the sectioned segment. The operation prevents the presence of sperm in the ejaculate but ejaculation occurs because of the presence of accessory gland fluids.

The urethra

This is the terminal portion of the duct system and serves both urinary and reproductive systems. It is divided anatomically into three regions:

1. The prostatic urethra which exits from the bladder and is surrounded by the prostate gland.

2. The membranous urethra which passes through the urogenital diaphragm.

3. The spongy (penile) urethra which passes through the penis to exit at the external urethral meatus. The spongy urethra is about 15 cm long and is 75% of the total urethral length.

Accessory glands

These include the paired seminal vesicles, the bulbourethral glands and the single prostate gland. They provide a transport medium and nutrients and the bulk of the ejaculate.

The seminal vesicles

The **seminal vesicles** lie behind the prostate gland and are finger-shaped and -sized, i.e. 5–7 cm long. They have a capacity of $3 \, cm^3$. They secrete an alkaline, sticky, yellowish fluid containing fructose, globulin, ascorbic acid and prostaglandins, accounting for 60% of the semen. Sperm and seminal fluid mix in the ejaculatory duct and enter the urethra together during ejaculation.

The prostate gland

The **prostate gland** is situated around the bladder neck and the first part of the urethra. It is about 3 cm in diameter in the normal adult and may involute or hypertrophy after middle age, resulting in urological problems. It produces a thin, acidic, milky fluid which contains enzymes, calcium and citrates. This fluid may act to stimulate motility in the sperm.

Semen

Semen is a milky white sticky fluid mixture of sperm and accessory gland secretions which forms the transport medium and provides nutrients and chemicals that activate the sperm. The **prostaglandins** in semen are thought to decrease the viscosity of the cervical mucus and to cause reverse peristalsis in the uterus, facilitating movement of the sperm up the female reproductive tract. It is relatively alkaline with a pH of 7.2–7.6 which helps to neutralise the acid medium of the vagina to protect the sperm and maintain their motility.

Semen also contains a bacteriostatic chemical called **seminal plasmin** and clotting factors, including **fibrinogen**, which coagulate the semen shortly after it has been ejaculated. Once established in the vaginal vault, the **fibrinolysin** also contained in the semen causes it to liquefy so that the sperm can swim freely into the female duct system. The average ejaculate is about 3–6 ml and contains 60–200 million sperm of which at least 60–80% should be normal and 50% motile after 1 h at 37°C.

The bulbourethral (Cowper's) glands

These are tiny pea-sized glands situated inferiorly to the prostate. They secrete thick, clear mucus that drains into the spongy urethra, acting as a lubricant prior to ejaculation.

The penis

The **penis** is the organ of copulation which normally hangs flaccidly from the perineum in front of the scrotum. It has an attached root and a free shaft that ends in an enlarged tip—the glans penis. Internally it has three long columns of erectile tissue (Fig. 5.4), consisting of two dorsal **corpora cavernosa** side by side and one **corpus spongeosum** containing the urethra. The erectile tissue is a spongy network of connective tissue and smooth muscle full of vascular spaces.

The root of the penis is broad and firmly fixed to the pubic rami by the proximal ends of the corpora cavernosa known as the **crura**. Each crus is surrounded by an **ischiocavernosus muscle**. The terminal glans penis is perforated by the urethral meatus and is very well supplied by sensory nerve endings. It is the main male erogenous zone. In the resting state the glans penis is covered by a folded cylinder of skin known as the **prepuce** or foreskin.

Hormonal control of male reproductive function

Male reproductive function is controlled by hormones from the hypothalamus, anterior pituitary lobe and testes. Gonadotrophin-releasing hormone (GnRH) from the hypothalamus influences the anterior pituitary to produce the same hormones as in the female: follicle stimulating hormone (FSH) and luteinising hormone (LH). In the male, plasma levels of LH are usually three times higher than those of FSH (Hinson et al 2007).

Actions of LH

LH acts on the interstitial tissue to cause synthesis and release of testosterone, and plasma testosterone levels are directly related to plasma LH levels. Testosterone is an **anabolic androgenic steroid** molecule synthesised from cholesterol. It binds loosely to plasma proteins to be taken to its target organs where it acts on intracellular receptors to influence genetic control of production of some proteins that are involved in its functions (Hinson et al 2007) as shown in Table 5.1.

Inhibin is a non-steroidal factor which has been isolated in the testis and may inhibit FSH secretion. It is possibly produced by the Sertoli cells and acts by a negative feedback loop.

Actions of FSH

FSH binds to receptors (FSH-R) on the basolateral surface of Sertoli cells stimulated by the presence of

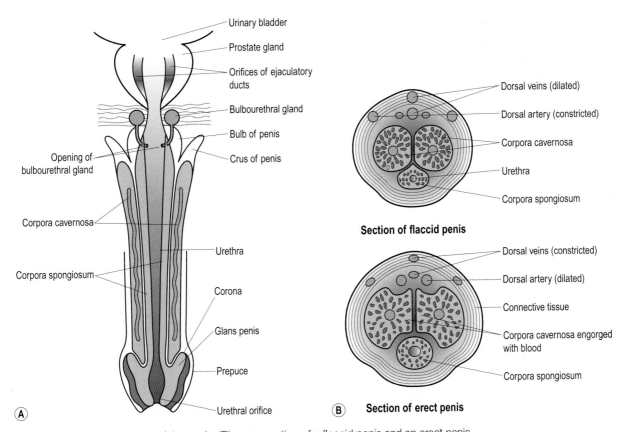

Figure 5.4 • (A) Detailed structure of the penis; (B) cross-section of a flaccid penis and an erect penis.

Table 5.1 Functions of testosterone

Action	Functions
Before birth	Masculinisation of the reproductive tract and external genitalia
	Promotion of testicular descent
Sex-specific tissues	Growth and maturation at puberty
	Maintenance of reproductive tract throughout adult life
	Essential for spermatogenesis
Other reproductive effects	Increased libido and sex drive
	Control of gonadotrophic hormone secretion
Secondary sexual characteristics	Development of male distribution of body and facial hair
	Deepening of the voice due to thickening of the vocal cords and enlargement of the larynx
Other effects	Anabolic effect on protein production
	Growth of the long bones at puberty and fusion of epiphyses
	Increased secretion from sebaceous glands
	Possible role in aggressive behaviour

androgens (Johnson 2007). It seems to act on the later stages of sperm maturation and cannot initiate spermatogenesis in the absence of LH.

The role of prostaglandins in reproduction

The group of chemical messengers known as the prostaglandins are active in multiple sites in the body and are involved in many physiological processes. Some act on smooth muscle, different ones causing bronchodilation or bronchospasm. Prostaglandins also promote pain and inflammation and modulate platelet aggregation. Aspirin is a prostaglandin inhibitor which is why it has so many pharmaceutical uses.

Prostaglandins are fatty acid derivatives of arachidonic acid and are produced and act locally in the body. After they have acted local enzymes rapidly inactivate them so that they do not gain access to the circulatory system.

They are called prostaglandins because they were first isolated in semen and thought to be produced by the prostate gland.

In the reproductive system, prostaglandins:

- Increase uterine activity during menstruation.
- Play a role in ovulation by influencing follicular rupture.
- Promote sperm transport by causing smooth muscle contraction in male and female reproductive tracts.
- Mediate the renal vasodilation in pregnancy.
- Help prepare the cervix for labour by softening it.
- Are probably the final mediator in the regulation of uterine contractions.

The physiology of sexual intercourse

In mammals, fertilisation occurs internally so that sperm must be deposited inside the female body. In humans, there is an enormous psychological and social input to sexual behaviour, and arousal includes both cognitive and emotional aspects. These are equally as important as the physiological context (Haeberle 1983). Masters & Johnson (1966) described the response by both sexes as having four phases: **excitement**, **plateau**, **orgasm** and **resolution**. This is known as the 'EPOR' model (Johnson 2007).

The male response

In the male, two stages can be described: erection and ejaculation.

Erection

Erection is brought about by a spinal reflex triggered by local stimulation of sensitive mechanoreceptors in the tip of the penis (Fig. 5.5). When the man is sexually excited, increased parasympathetic and decreased sympathetic activity cause the arterioles in the erectile tissue of the corpora cavernosa and the corpus spongeosum to dilate and engorge. Normally there is no parasympathetic control over blood vessels and it is the variation in sympathetic stimulation that causes vasodilation and vasoconstriction. Erection is the major instance where both branches of the autonomic nervous system control blood vessels and vasodilation is accomplished much more rapidly then usual.

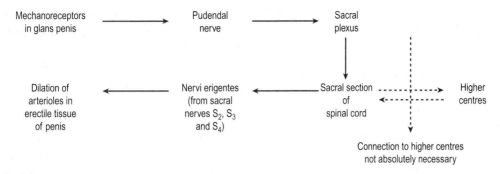

Figure 5.5• The nervous pathways (simplified) involved in the erection reflex. (From Hinchliff S M, Montague S E 1990, with kind permission of Elsevier.)

Ejaculation

Ejaculation is also controlled by a spinal reflex with a patterned sequence of events following the efferent nerve messages. Sympathetic nerve impulses cause sequential contractions of smooth muscle in the prostate, epididymis, ductus deferens, ejaculatory duct and seminal vesicles. This causes **emission** when the genital ducts and accessory glands empty their contents into the posterior urethra. This is followed by the expulsion phase of ejaculation when the semen is expelled from the penis by a series of rapid muscle contractions. The filling of the urethra with semen triggers nerve impulses that activate skeletal muscles at the base of the penis to contract at 0.8 s intervals and expel the semen forcibly.

During ejaculation the sphincter at the base of the bladder is closed so that sperm do not enter the bladder and urine cannot be voided. **Orgasm**, a feeling of intense pleasure accompanied by involuntary rhythmic action of the pelvic muscles and generalised contraction of skeletal muscle throughout the body, occurs followed by resolution with physical and psychological relaxation. Loss of erection follows due to vasoconstriction of the penile arterioles and venous drainage; this varies, depending on circumstances, from a few minutes to several hours. There is an absolute latent or refractory period during which erection cannot occur.

The female response

In the female, there is erection of the **clitoris** and erectile tissue in the **labia minora. Nipples** have erectile tissue and respond to sexual excitement. Lubrication from **Bartholin's glands** facilitates intromission. Orgasm may occur following movement of the penis in and out of the vagina. During the plateau phase vasocongestion of the outer third of the vagina occurs which tightens the introitus around the penis. The uterus is raised upwards, lifting the cervix and enlarging the upper two-thirds of the vagina. This is called ballooning and increases the space for deposition of the ejaculate.

If orgasm occurs, the same pelvic muscle contractions as in the male occur, mostly in the outer third engorged section of the vagina. This region is sometimes called the **orgasmic platform**. The uterus may contract, beginning at the fundus. During resolution, vasocongestion resolves and the cardiac and respiratory changes return to normal. The descriptions of orgasm given by men and women are similar but orgasm appears not to occur with the same regularity in females.

Stimulation of the clitoris can enhance the pleasure and contribute to female orgasm but 10–20% of women appear never to achieve orgasm. Cross-cultural studies suggest that female orgasm may not be reflex but learned. When women are expected to enjoy sex, orgasm is more common (Johnson 2007). Although orgasm is not necessary for fertilisation, contractions of the uterus may aspirate semen and help the sperm on their journey.

Cardiovascular and respiratory changes

In both sexes there are changes in the cardiovascular and respiratory systems. There is a marked increase in heart rate to between 100 and 170 beats/min, systolic blood pressure may increase by 20–40 mmHg. Respiration may double to 40/min and flushing of the chest, neck and face occurs.

Main points

- In the embryo, the testes develop high on the posterior wall of the abdominal cavity, descending into the scrotal sac in late fetal life. Testicular temperature is maintained at 2–3°C below the body core thereby facilitating spermatogenesis.

- The male genital and urinary systems share a common outlet through the urethra.

- The testes produce spermatozoa and the hormones testosterone and inhibin. There is a physical barrier surrounding each Sertoli cell between the tissues that produce sperm and those that produce hormones. This prevents sperm entering the systemic and lymphatic circulations.

- Seminiferous tubules contain two types of cell: germ cells and Sertoli cells. Primary germ cells begin to increase in number from spermatogonia which divide by mitosis continuously from puberty.

- Although nuclear division occurs during mitosis, cytoplasmic division is incomplete and spermatogonia are linked by cytoplasmic bridges to form a syncytium. Individual cells are only released as mature sperm.

- Primary spermatocytes undergo the first meiotic division to form two secondary haploid spermatocytes of which half receive an X chromosome and half a Y chromosome. Secondary meiosis results in four haploid spermatids. Sperm maturation takes about 70 days and several hundred million a day are produced.

- As men age, the seminal tubules undergo involution and there may be extensive atrophy by age 70 years. Germ cells are reduced in number but Sertoli cells remain the same.

- When sperm are fully formed they are pushed along the duct system to the epididymis where they mature and become motile. Sperm can be stored in the epididymis for 42 days.

- Interstitial tissue packed around the seminiferous tubules contains Leydig cells which secrete testosterone.

- The accessory glands of the male reproductive system provide a transport medium and nutrients. The average ejaculate is about 3–6 ml and contains 60–200 million sperm.

- The penis has three long columns of erectile tissue: two dorsal corpora cavernosa and one corpus spongeosum containing the urethra. The glans penis, perforated by the urethral meatus, is well supplied with sensory nerve endings.

- Control of male reproduction is by the hypothalamus, anterior pituitary gland and testes. GnRH influences the anterior pituitary gland to produce FSH and LH. LH acts on the testicular interstitial tissue to produce testosterone. Inhibin may inhibit FSH secretion and prevent sperm manufacture by a negative feedback loop.

- In the reproductive systems prostaglandins increase uterine activity during menstruation, influence follicular rupture and promotion of sperm transport by causing smooth muscle contraction in both male and female reproductive tracts.

- Sexual activity in humans is more than a physiological response. Psychological and social factors are also important. Male and female physiological sexual responses are similar, although psychosexual attitudes differ between the sexes.

References

Haeberle, E.J., 1983. The Sex Atlas. Sheridan Press, London.

Henderson, C., Macdonald, S. (Eds.), 2004. Mayes' Midwifery: A textbook for midwives, thirteenth ed. Baillière Tindall, London.

Hinson, J., Raven, P., Chew, S. (Eds.), 2007. The Endocrine System. Churchill Livingstone, Elsevier.

Johnson, M.H., 2007. Essential Reproduction, sixth ed. Blackwell Science, Oxford.

Jones, S., 2002. Y: The Descent of Men. Little, Brown, London.

Masters, W., Johnson, V., 1966. Human Sexual Response. J&A Churchill, London.

Annotated recommended reading

Hinson, J., Raven, P., Chew, S. (Eds.), 2007. The Endocrine System. Churchill Livingstone, Elsevier.

This is an excellent textbook on the endocrine system. It covers all the endocrine glands in easily readable text and has a specific chapter on the male reproductive tract.

Johnson, M.H., 2007. Essential Reproduction, sixth ed. Blackwell Science, Oxford.

All the major areas of reproduction are covered in this book. In particular, the section on sexual differentiation and regulation of gonadal function is recommended.

Jones, S., 2002. Y: The Descent of Men. Little, Brown, London.

This book is both learned and humorous and contains much information at all levels from molecular to social about being male.

Chapter Six

Fertility control

6

Introduction

Throughout women's lives, from puberty to the menopause, fertility control is of prime concern. Young women who are sexually active may well become pregnant on their first sexual encounter and should take precautions against pregnancy. The human species is not as fertile as some mammals. A **fecundity rate** of 20% has been quoted (Evers 2002); i.e. there is a 1:5 chance of conceiving at the most fertile time.

At birth, the female ovary contains immature ova which remain in limbo until puberty. Under hormonal influence one ovum matures at each ovarian cycle. If more follicles ripen in a cycle, the potential of several ova is lost as partially ripened follicles, including their ova, die. Men produce an almost infinite supply of spermatozoa continuously. Few men take control of their own fertility but should do so as this would help prevent unwanted pregnancies. Reproduction and contraception constitute a significant health issue.

World population

The rate of fertility and the steady rise in world population throughout the 1950s to the 1990s (Fig. 6.1) are directly related to health, environment and poverty. The development of many medical interventions and the greater prosperity of the developed countries have brought about a lower death rate. The trend to have 2.9 children instead of the 6.9 in the 1950s with the lowering death rate has meant that we have an ageing population in Western society with a growth rate declining to 0.1%, whereas population growth in many underdeveloped countries is currently 97% (Nash & De Souza 2002). Despite the graph in Figure 6.1 showing a decline in population in the 21st century, this is misleading and the world population is still expected to increase. It is difficult to predict trends in this area as infertility is increasing and must be compared to the fertility rate at that time (Speidel 2000). Many of the world's population are young and have still to have their families and there is concern that, unless something can be done to slow down this increase in humanity, famine, infections and wars may intervene.

Contraception worldwide

Worldwide, the contraceptive effect of breastfeeding probably has as much impact as all the other forms of contraception put together. However, as education increases

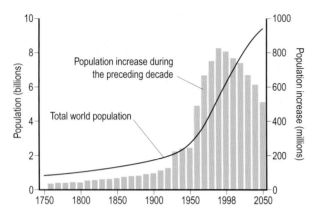

Figure 6.1 ● The rate of fertility and rise in world population related to health, environment and poverty.

Table 6.1	UK use of contraception in year 2002
Sterilisation	Male: 17.0%
	Female: 13.0%
Pill	22%
Injectable implants	3.0%
Intrauterine device	6.0%
Condom	18.0%
Vaginal barrier	1.0%
Other	1.0%
Rhythm	1.0%
Withdrawal	4.0%
Source: United Nations (2003).	

Table 6.2 Methods and their failure rates per hundred woman years (HWY)	
Method	**Failure rate per HWY**
The combined oestrogen with progestogen pill	0.1–7
The progestogen-only pill	0.5–7
Injectable progestogen	0–1
Female barrier methods	2–15
The male condom	2–15
The female condom	Not yet known
The intrauterine device	0.3–4
Spermicidal preparations (used alone)	14–25
Symptothermal method (temperature + cervical mucus)	1–4
Coitus interruptus	25
Male sterilisation	0–0.2
Female sterilisation	0–0.2
The variations in numbers indicate the commitment and skill with which the method is used.	

in under-developed countries, so also will the use of contraception. In the year 2030 it is estimated that 60% of the world's population will live in urban communities. This will mean environmental change, population change and planning for resources. In the UK, 76% of women use some form of contraception (Table 6.1), the most common being the pill and their partner's use of the male condom (Agius & Brincat 2006, Family Planning Association (FPA) 2007).

The effectiveness of contraception

Contraception has been an issue ever since the link was made between sexual behaviour and pregnancy. It certainly occupied the minds of the ancient Egyptians, Greeks and Romans. In modern times contraception has been openly discussed, used and become legal in most countries only during the last 50 years. There are religious, moral and cultural issues to be considered and therefore it is unlikely that one method will ever become universal.

The ideal contraceptive would be 100% effective, painless, easy to use independently of the user's memory, cheap and accessible and without medical control. It would also need to be safe; life-threatening problems from pregnancy should be measured against the safety of any contraception used.

Calculating effectiveness

A mathematical concept used to assess the effectiveness of contraceptive methods is the **failure rate per hundred woman years (HWY)**, i.e. the number of pregnancies if 100 women were to use the method for 1 year (Table 6.2); it is also known as the **Pearl Index** (Guillebaud 2005). In a perfect world this would be truly representative of a method's effectiveness, but it is complicated by factors such as changes in fertility with age, motivation to use the method correctly every time

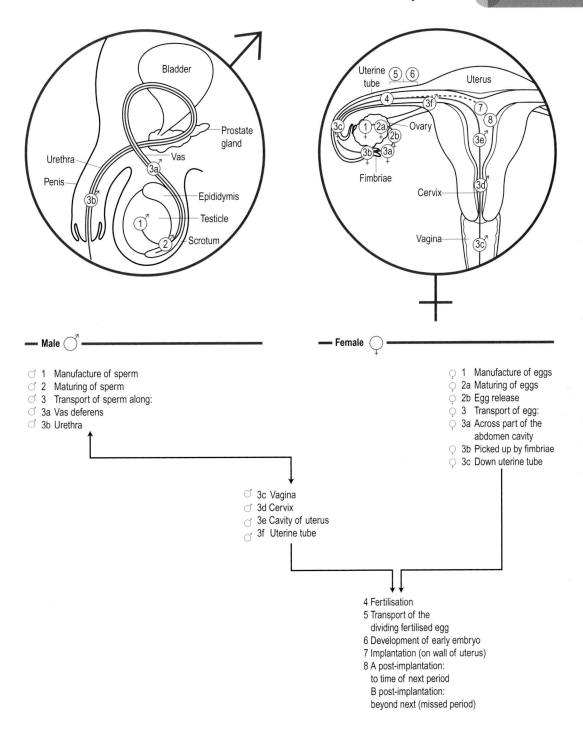

Male ♂

♂ 1 Manufacture of sperm
♂ 2 Maturing of sperm
♂ 3 Transport of sperm along:
♂ 3a Vas deferens
♂ 3b Urethra

♂ 3c Vagina
♂ 3d Cervix
♂ 3e Cavity of uterus
♂ 3f Uterine tube

Female ♀

♀ 1 Manufacture of eggs
♀ 2a Maturing of eggs
♀ 2b Egg release
♀ 3 Transport of egg:
♀ 3a Across part of the
     abdomen cavity
♀ 3b Picked up by fimbriae
♀ 3c Down uterine tube

4 Fertilisation
5 Transport of the
  dividing fertilised egg
6 Development of early embryo
7 Implantation (on wall of uterus)
8 A post-implantation:
    to time of next period
  B post-implantation:
    beyond next (missed period)

Figure 6.2 • The stages of reproduction.

and the infertility of about 10% who will not know it at the time they are using contraception. It is difficult to differentiate between failure of the method and failure of the user to comply with instructions. Failure often occurs in the early months following commencement of any method; developing skills in using the method make it more reliable.

Physiological application of contraception

The stages of reproduction of male and female gametes (Fig. 6.2) offer choices of sites for the development of effective methods of contraception (Fig. 6.3).

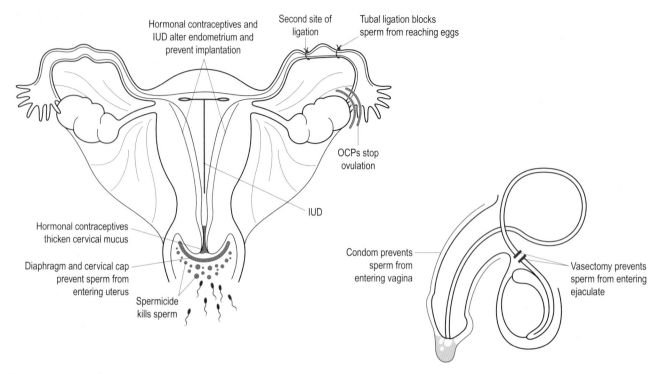

Figure 6.3 • Mechanisms by which contraceptives work.

Prevention of gamete production: ovum

Combined oral contraception (COC)

All the ova available to the woman for reproduction are already present in her ovary at birth. Therefore it is not a matter of preventing ovum production but of preventing their maturation and ovulation by suppressing follicle-stimulating hormone (FSH) and luteinising hormone (LH) at the pituitary level. This, in turn, will prevent the feedback mechanisms between the hypothalamus and the pituitary gland (Coad & Dunstall 2001).

The concept of hormonal control of fertility began in the late 1940s when it was realised that the roots of the wild Mexican yam contained a chemical from which **steroid hormones** could be produced. Unfortunately, natural hormones are expensive to produce and when taken orally are inactivated by the digestive processes. The word **combined** is used because the preparations include oestrogens and progestogens. The synthetic oestrogen is **ethinylestradiol**. The synthetic progestogens used are various and include **norethisterone**, **levonorgestrel** and **gestodene**.

The oestrogen component inhibits FSH release and stops the maturation of the follicle, whereas the progestogen inhibits the release of LH, preventing ovulation. The dose of oestrogen amongst all preparations is a maximum of 20–40 μg. The dose of progestogen is more variable and adds to the contraceptive effect by causing thickening of the cervical mucus (Billings et al 1972) and thinning of the endometrium, making it unsuitable for implantation and reducing the motility of the uterine tubes (Coad & Dunstall 2001).

Since the COC became available in the 1960s it has been beset by media scares, and there is some research evidence to suggest that the higher-dose pills created thrombotic problems in some women. Studies published in 1968 showed a link between the use of COCs and thrombosis. This was thought to be due to the high level of ethinylestradiol in the early pills. However, it has since been realised that a family history of thrombosis or an anticlotting disorder, obesity and cigarette smoking greatly increase the risk of thromboembolism in pill users.

A follow-up of 23 000 women, which included women on the higher-dose pills, found no excessive deaths over a 10-year period. There appeared to be an 80% reduction in ovarian cancer and a 30% reduction in hip fracture at age 75 years when the pill was taken into their forties. Venous thrombosis occurred in 2:100 000 woman years of usage (Kubba et al 2000).

Benefits of the combined pill

• Couples with sexual difficulties because of a fear of pregnancy are relieved of that fear and are able to relax and enjoy a better sex life.

• Reduces premenstrual tension.

- The pill can be used to combat irregular, painful or heavy periods, preventing anaemia.
- Permits men natural coitus without the use of a condom, preventing erectile problems.
- The combined pill may offer protection against ovarian cancer, possibly due to the cessation of ovulation and quiescence of the ovary. A similar protection against cancer of the endometrium has been noticed.
- The pill protects against some forms of pelvic infection by altering cervical mucus and, because it prevents ovulation and tubal infection (salpingitis), it reduces the risk of ectopic pregnancy (British National Formulary (BNF) 2007).

Complications of the combined pill

- **Thromboembolism**—Women who take first- and second-generation pills are at a lower risk of thromboembolism (VTE) than are those taking third-generation pills which contain desogestrel and gestoden. Those containing levonorgestrel or norethisterone, the first- and second-generation pills, are those of first choice (RCOG 2004). There is a three-fold risk of VTE when taking COCs which increases with age. The risk increases further if women suffer from a genetic clotting disorder such as factor V Leiden, a quite common variant of clotting cascade factor V, protein C or protein S deficiency (Kujovich 2007). Acquired risk factors such as pregnancy, surgery, immobilisation and malignancy also increase the risk of VTE (RCOG 2004). Some of the side effects occur because the altered physiology of taking the combined pill mimics that of pregnancy. The risk of arterial or venous thrombosis occurs because of increased clotting factors, platelet aggregation and increased serum lipids. The risk is probably low in slim women under 35 who are normotensive, do not smoke and have no personal or familial history of thrombosis. Women who smoke and are obese are at increased risk of cardiovascular disease and VTE, respectively (WHO 2008). Less serious complications such as weight gain, headaches, water retention and increased blood pressure have been reported.
- **Cancer**—Research indicates that women taking the pill have a reduced incidence of ovarian and endometrial cancer, but women taking oral contraceptives lose the protection that barrier methods give to the cervix. Therefore there is a slightly increased risk of cervical, breast and liver cancer (WHO 2008). While there may have been an increase in breast cancer since the 1960s which may be related to taking oestrogenic compounds, it is possibly due to earlier diagnosis, postponement of the first pregnancy and increased fat consumption, all known risk factors for breast cancer. However, the World Health Organization (WHO 2008) has found a link between women taking the COC and cervical cancer linked to women carrying the human papillomavirus (HPV): 99% of women diagnosed with cancer of the cervix are HPV-positive and one-third are in their twenties (Dyer 2002, Moodley 2004).
- **Hypertension**—The risk increases with age and is more likely in those who smoke.
- **Migraine**—Some women find their migraines improve while they take the pill and some find there is deterioration. However, it is serious if women experience focal migraine with transient weakness, numbness of part of the body or loss of part of the visual field, symptoms which may indicate reduced blood flow to the brain; this is classified as WHO group 4 (see p. 70).
- **Jaundice**—The pill is metabolised by the liver and affects liver function. Most women have a change in bile composition, which may lead to the formation of gallstones. This may be due to an acceleration of the problem rather than being the only cause. A few women may develop jaundice and intense itching of the skin and even fewer women may develop liver tumours.
- **Effect on pregnancy**—Women who have taken the pill may take longer to become pregnant; this would also include the IUCD and injectable contraceptives (Hassan & Killick 2004).
- **Effect on lactation**—Oestrogen suppresses the hormone prolactin secreted by the anterior pituitary gland. Prolactin acts on the alveoli of the breast to stimulate milk production. The result will be diminished milk production and a shorter duration of lactation (see The progestogen-only pill, p. 70).
- **Drug interactions**—Synthetic oestrogens taken orally are well absorbed by the intestinal tract. Unlike natural oestrogens which are rapidly broken down by the liver, synthetic compounds take longer to be metabolised and degraded (Rang et al 2007). The combined pill is probably effective up to 36 h. Other medication may interfere with the contraceptive action of the combined pill. Broad-spectrum antibiotics such as flucloxacillin may impair intestinal absorption, while most anticonvulsant drugs increase liver enzyme production and hasten drug breakdown. Other drugs such as HIV and TB preparations and St John's wort could affect the pill's efficiency. Vomiting and diarrhoea may prevent absorption and the pill should be considered non-effective for that cycle. Oestrogens affect the action of antidiabetic medications (BNF 2007).

WHO classification

In order to define safety in various types of women, the WHO (2008) have devised four categories to guide the practitioner in prescribing the contraceptive pill (Burkman et al 2006):

- Group 1: No restriction of use.
- Group 2: More advantages than risk.
- Group 3: Risk outweighs advantages.
- Group 4: Unacceptable health risk.

Examples:

- Age over 40—group 2.
- Breastfeeding and under 6 weeks postpartum—group 4.
- A non-smoker over 35—group 2.
- A smoker over the age of 35 smoking 15 cigarettes per day—group 4.
- Medical conditions can be categorised: for example, hypertension with no related cardiovascular risk would be group 3 or group 4 (WHO 2008).

The pill should be discontinued if a woman experiences leg pain, abdominal pain, breathlessness and, more serious, with blood-stained sputum, a rise in blood pressure, prolonged headaches, loss or partial sight loss or paraesthesia in a part of the body. Allergic reaction could show as jaundice and result ultimately in liver failure. Discontinuation should also occur before major operative surgery due to the risk of thromboembolism and the consequent inactivity following the operation (Guillebaud 2005).

Prevention of gamete production: spermatozoa

Men typically generate 1000 sperm a minute. The hormones involved are hypothalamic **gonadotrophin-releasing hormone** (GnRH), which controls pituitary production of LH and FSH. LH stimulates the testes to produce testosterone, which together with FSH induces sperm production (see Ch. 5). The process of spermatogenesis is continuous; there is no singular event similar to ovulation. At present, research is focusing on stopping spermatogenesis by reducing feedback mechanisms and the production of GnRH. Altering testosterone levels may well have side effects and there is a fine balance between aggression and sex drive (Guillebaud 2005). Adding a synthetic form of progesterone (progestogen) may allow a lower dose of testosterone to be given without reducing the contraceptive effect. Researchers (Anderson et al 2002) report on the use of implants (Implanon) containing both progestogens and testosterone and, although spermatogenesis was suppressed, this was variable. Guillebaud (2005) suggests that this is the way forward.

Prevention of fertilisation

The progestogen-only pill (POP)

Progestogens thicken cervical mucus and prevent sperm penetration. The endometrium is thinned making embedding inhospitable for the embryo. Uterine tube contractions become less coordinated, so that sperm that have managed to penetrate the cervical mucus find it impossible to journey up the uterine tubes.

The POP is taken continuously without breaks and should be taken at the same time each day to maintain mucus and endometrial changes which inhibit implantation; a pill taken only 3h late would deem to be ineffective contraception (MIMS 2008). This may be why the progestogen-only pill appears less effective than the combined pill. However, Cerazette 75 μg stops ova release in 97% of women (Guillebaud 2005).

The drugs used are similar preparations to those in the COC but progestogen-based in varying doses; the higher the dose the more effective it is (MIMS 2008).

Benefits of the progestogen-only pill

- Cervical mucus thickens after a few hours so that contraceptive protection is achieved after 48h. There is protection against some bacterial pathogens, so that the risk of pelvic inflammatory disease is lessened.
- Milk production is not diminished and little hormone seems to cross into breast milk.
- The very small doses of progestogen used in the pill are unlikely to have an effect on blood vessels and clotting, so this pill is considered a safe option for women who cannot be prescribed the combined pill (BNF 2008).
- Cigarette smokers are likely to develop blood vessel changes. Although stopping smoking is the best option, this pill will not add to the risk.
- Women over the age of 35 have reduced fertility and high motivation to prevent pregnancy. The POP is often prescribed for perimenopausal women.
- Hypertension may indicate the use of the POP. All oestrogen pills are likely to raise blood pressure, which may lead to heart disease.

Side effects of the progestogen-only pill

This form of contraception has been taken by limited numbers of people compared to the combined pill and there have been far fewer studies. Nevertheless the POP has been prescribed for as long as the combined pill and there have been sufficient studies to indicate that no significant problems occur.

- **Bleeding**—Alteration in menstrual bleeding patterns is the most common side effect. The endometrium grows irregularly because progestogens alone are insufficient to balance growth of the lining of the uterus. This usually settles down after the first 3 months but some women find the bleeding troublesome and discontinue the pill.

- **Pregnancy**—There is an extra risk of becoming pregnant whilst taking the POP which is generally attributed to user failure. The motility of the uterine tubes is reduced so that the embryo cannot reach the uterine cavity before it begins to increase in size, causing an ectopic pregnancy, a rare but dangerous complication. This is prevented by the efficacy of Cerazette as this prevents ovulation (Guillebaud 2005, MIMS 2008).

Long-acting progestogen injections

The two preparations available in Britain are Depo-Provera and Noristerat given by deep intramuscular injection. These act similarly to the progestogen-only pill but with a more profound effect on the ovary. The endometrium immediately becomes thinner and theoretically prevents implantation. Depo-Provera is a long-acting injectable progestogen, given every 12 weeks, which contains medroxyprogesterone acetate. Menstrual disturbances occur and there may be a delay in fertility return. There are some reports that bone mineral density is lower than average with long-term use but stabilises after 3 years of use (BNF 2007, Erkkola 2007).

Side effects of long-acting progestogen injections

- Heavy, irregular bleeding may occur and settles after a few months, although some women have no bleeding at all.
- Delayed return of fertility.
- The injections need to be repeated every 12 weeks, 8 weeks for Noristerat.
- Contraindicated if breast cancer diagnosed within 5 years (BNF 2007).

Benefits of long-acting progestogen injections

The concept of informed consent must be a prime consideration. Worldwide, these drugs have been controversial when used in developing countries. It should be noted that:

- Progestogens increase the stability of red cells and women with sickle cell disease may benefit.
- Women who cannot take oral preparations where absorption is poor or the large intestine has been removed may benefit from an injectable preparation.
- The risk of repeated pregnancies may outweigh the side effects of the progestogen injection.
- Beneficial for young girls who may forget the pill.

Emergency contraception (the morning-after pill)

It is not certain how the morning-after pill works as it has not been extensively researched. Its action depends on the stage of the menstrual cycle; for example, if given near ovulation it will prevent ova release (Aschenbrenner 2006). Cervical mucus may change, trapping sperm; changes in the uterine environment may prevent implantation. However, it does not cause an abortion. There have been some reports of nausea, vomiting, dizziness and headache following administration (Ranney et al 2006).

Emergency contraception may be given orally up to 72 h following unprotected intercourse at any time in the menstrual cycle. The pill contains levonorgestrel 750 µg; two tablets are taken together (Aschenbrenner 2006, BNF 2007), although some data suggest the tablets should be taken separately 12 h apart. Controversially, this pill may be given without prescription to those over 16 years of age. Pharmacists are at the front line of counselling these women and giving the morning-after pill without a medical practitioner's intervention. Alternatively, the copper IUD can be inserted up to 5 days, covering the implantation window; antibacterial prophylaxis is recommended (BNF 2007). Emergency contraception should not be used as a contraceptive method (Hale 2007).

Progestogen implants

The contraceptive preparation etonorgestrel 68 mg is contained in small silicone rods which are inserted under the skin of the inner aspect of the upper arm, allowing slow release of the preparation. Implanon is the trade name for these preparations.

Ovulation is stopped a day after insertion and effective contraception will continue for 3 years. Again, this implant may cause irregular bleeding, which may be partly due to its effect on the endometrium; extra hormones could be prescribed orally to settle this (FPA 2006). Once inserted, this contraceptive device can be forgotten; it is not affected by antibiotics and does not have to be metabolised by the liver as it is not a systemic preparation. Some patients experience skin irritation and may have to discontinue its use (BNF 2007). Women with a body mass index of more than 35 kg/m^2 (BNF 2007) may need to change the implant earlier as it may not be as effective in the third year. The Pearl Index over 3 years has been nil (Erkkola 2007).

The contraceptive patch

This is a self-adhesive patch with combined oestrogen and progesterone slowly absorbed through the skin into the blood stream. A new patch is applied weekly for

3 weeks with one patch-free week. This method is effective if used correctly but for some women forgetting to renew the patch might result in pregnancy. Skin reactions have led to discontinuation. Side effects would be as for COC and POP (MIMS 2008).

Vaginal rings

These are rings placed in the vagina which release hormones, effectively blocking feedback mechanisms and preventing pregnancy. They are left in situ for 3 weeks and then removed for 1 week. They are used mainly in the USA and Europe (Erkkola 2007).

Barrier methods of contraception

The female diaphragm

The female diaphragm (Fig. 6.4) is made of polyurethane, and when inserted into the vagina covers the cervix. It must be fitted to the individual and any loss or gain in weight of more than 7 lb (3 kg) necessitates refitting. Cervical and vault caps which adhere to the cervix by suction are less-commonly used (Fig. 6.4). Diaphragms must be used with the addition of a spermicidal preparation and should be left in situ for 6 h for the sperm to be killed (Fig. 6.5).

Benefits of the diaphragm
The diaphragm is an efficient alternative to hormonal contraception and women can take responsibility for avoidance of pregnancy. It may also be protective against some sexually transmitted diseases.

Side effects of the diaphragm
Despite its simplicity, there are a few problems with the diaphragm. Some women may be allergic to the rubber or to the spermicide, and those with a degree of uterine prolapse may find the diaphragm uncomfortable and difficult to maintain in place. The diaphragm predisposes to vaginal candidiasis, especially in diabetic women, and some women may develop recurrent cystitis. Using the diaphragm may be distasteful to women who object to its messiness and the need to handle their bodies or to remember to insert it prior to coitus.

The male condom

These tubular devices have been made from various materials. Historically, sheep's intestines were used, but currently condoms are made from polyurethane and latex. They must be placed on the erect penis prior to sexual contact, as there may be sperm in the fluid released from the tip of the penis following arousal. They are lubricated, therefore there is no need to add lubricant. Oil-based lubricants can damage latex condoms, rendering them ineffective (FPA 2005). After coitus, the penis must be removed from the vagina before the erection is lost and no further genital contact must occur. Condoms are cheap, easily purchased and successful. They are also barriers to various organisms and help in the prevention of the spread of sexual diseases (Fig. 6.6).

The female condom

These were introduced under the trade name of Femidom and are made of polyurethane, which is tougher and finer than rubber. The device lines the vagina with an inner rim that fits into the vaginal fornices and an outer rim around the vulva. They are lubricated to aid penile insertion. They may provide an efficient barrier to sexually transmitted disease and should be as efficient as the diaphragm or condom.

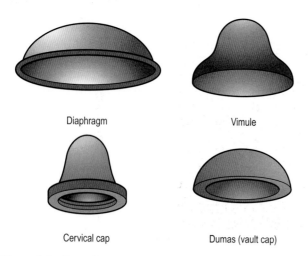

Figure 6.4 ● Examples of female barrier methods. (Reproduced with permission from Cowper & Young 1989.)

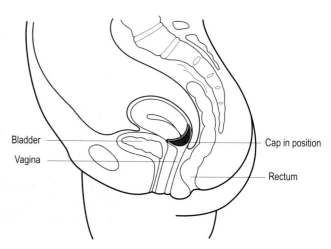

Figure 6.5 ● Diaphragm cap in position. (Reproduced with permission from Cowper & Young 1989.)

Spermicidal preparations

These chemical preparations come in the form of foaming tablets, aerosols, films, creams, pessaries and jellies. While they are efficient at killing spermatozoa, hundreds of millions of sperm may be released per ejaculate so they should not be used alone. Spermicides may reduce the incidence of sexually transmitted organisms such as the gonococcus and spirochaete of syphilis and also viruses. This is because they do not differentiate between the sperm and single-celled micro-organisms, killing them all. Also, some micro-organisms hitch a ride into the female genital tract through the channels in the cervical mucus made by the spermatozoa. The most common spermicidal agent, nonoxynol-9, attaches itself to the spermatozoa and prevents them taking in oxygen. It also destroys the surface tension of the outer membrane of the sperm so that they burst (BNF 2007).

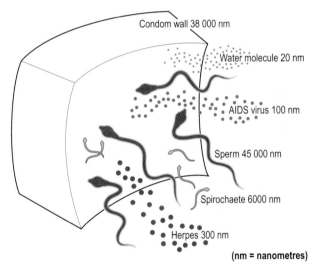

Condom wall 38 000 nm
Water molecule 20 nm
AIDS virus 100 nm
Sperm 45 000 nm
Spirochaete 6000 nm
Herpes 300 nm

(nm = nanometres)

Figure 6.6 • The condom barrier.

Intrauterine contraceptive device (IUCD)

Intrauterine devices for the purpose of contraception began in the 1950s with the development of the plastics industry. Many different shapes have been tried but they must be small enough to insert through the cervix yet large enough to fill the small uterine cavity. This involves a device that can be reduced in diameter during insertion and will recoil to its effective shape once in the uterus (Fig. 6.7). They are widely used and effective, '<2 pregnancies per 100 insertions' and could be an alternative to sterilisation (ESHRE Capri Group 2008).

Third-generation IUCDs are smaller and the plastic holds substances such as copper and progestogens that will prevent pregnancy. A comparison was made between women using the Nova-T (copper) IUCD and the levonorgestrel (progestogen) IUCD (LNG IUCD). There were fewer pregnancies with the LNG IUCD but more spotting in the earlier days of use than with the Nova-T. It is important to counsel women of this and that it improves over time. Fertility returned following removal of both IUCDs. The LNG IUCD was considered an effective contraceptive that could also be used for the treatment of menorrhagia (Andersson 2001). These devices can be left in situ for up to 10 years.

IUCDs work by reducing the likelihood of the sperm being able to swim through the uterine cavity. They also alter the contractility of the uterine tubes, reducing the chances that a fertilised ovum will reach the uterine cavity but increasing the risk of ectopic pregnancy (Andersson 2001). They prevent a fertilised ovum from embedding in the uterus, but also copper has a toxic effect on spermatozoa and ova (Towse 2004).

The Mirena intrauterine system

This device is T-shaped and contains levonorgestrel on its stem. It is suggested that its lifespan could be as long as 7 years although it is recommended to be replaced

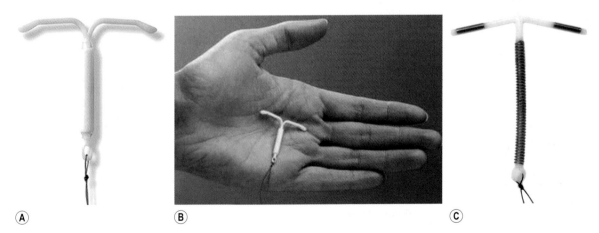

Ⓐ Ⓑ Ⓒ

Figure 6.7 • Examples of intrauterine devices. (A, B) Mirena levonorgestrel-releasing IUD; (C) TTC 380 copper loaded IUD. (Reproduced courtesy of Durbin plc; www.durbin.co.uk.)

after 5 years. It is a highly effective device with levonorgestrel found in the blood stream 15 min after insertion. Its effect is mainly cervical and endometrial but an effect on ovulation has been noted (Erkkola 2007). Some women may suffer severe cramps with any IUCD and severe abdominal pain would need investigation to rule out uterine perforation (MIMS 2008).

Complications from IUCDs

- **Menstrual disorders**—Some women have an increased duration of blood loss. This is not a straightforward lengthening of the menstrual phase of the cycle but an annoying light loss, beginning 2 or 3 days before true bleeding commences and a similar tailing off at the end of the period. The only IUCD without this effect is the progesterone-containing type (Andersson 2001).
- **Infection**—The risk of pelvic inflammatory disease is greatest in those with a sexual transmitted disease when fitted with an IUCD; women with healthy tracts are at no greater risk of ectopic or subsequent infertility (Wilkinson et al 2003).
- **Failure**—Although the IUCD is a very efficient type of contraceptive, it can fail. IUCDs fail because they

have become displaced or expelled from the uterus, so that about 2 people per 100 would become pregnant per year.

- **Fetal abnormalities**—No damage has been seen to a baby conceived with an IUCD in situ, although miscarriage is more common, occurring in about 50% of pregnancies, and ectopic pregnancy may occur. If the IUCD remains in situ and the pregnancy continues, premature onset of labour may occur.

Natural methods

Preventing ejaculation into the vagina

Various techniques of preventing ejaculation into the vagina are practised. Withdrawing the penis from the vagina at climax, termed coitus interruptus, avoiding ejaculation or coitus reservatus and coitus intracrura where the penis is placed between the thighs of the woman are all still used as contraceptive techniques. The more unusual coitus saxonicus, where hard pressure to the male perineum just prior to ejaculation results in retrograde ejaculation into the bladder, is a difficult but effective technique. Anal intercourse is also used

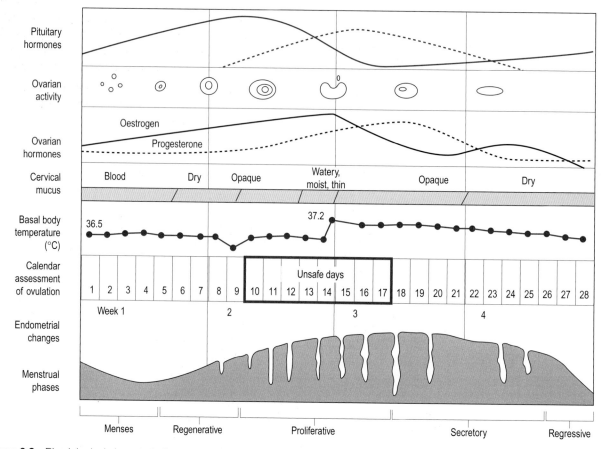

Figure 6.8 • Physiological changes in the menstrual cycle in conjunction with physiological methods of 8 + 78 birth control. (Reproduced with permission from Cowper & Young 1989.)

by some couples. These methods are easy to use and do not need medical supervision, so that, despite their relatively high failure rate, they will continue to be used.

Timing, temperature and cervical mucus

There is a very brief window in each ovulatory cycle when the ovum is available for fertilisation. If intercourse is avoided at that time, it is reasonable to assume that a pregnancy will not occur. In women with a regular menstrual cycle the calendar or timing method has been used successfully (Fehring 2005, Towse 2004).

Ovulation may occur irregularly, so methods of pinpointing it have been developed. These rely on changes brought about by the secretion of progesterone. The first is the change in cervical mucus, the second is the rise in core temperature (Fig. 6.8). A combination of these two, the symptothermal method, is quite successful for highly motivated women. The Persona measures the potential fertile time by measuring levels of LH and breakdown products of oestrogen; used by a dedicated woman it is quite effective, the failure rate being 6 per 100 women years. Its limitation is that cycles need to be between 23 and 25 days (Towse 2004).

Sterilisation

Fertilisation occurs in the ampulla of the uterine tube; the zygote then travels down the tube to the uterus. The aim of female sterilisation is to seal a section of the uterine tube to prevent spermatozoa reaching the ovum (Fig. 6.9). Spermatozoa travel up the vas deferens towards the urethra to be ejaculated into the vagina. The aim of male sterilisation or vasectomy is to remove a section of the vas deferens to prevent the spermatozoa entering the ejaculatory fluid (Fig. 6.10). Other techniques such as flushing the vas with fluid and blocking the cut ends with body tissue have been used (Cook et al 2004). The application of clips has been tried to increase the chances of reversal. These are not difficult operations but must be considered permanent as reversal may not be possible, involving microsurgery. Despite this, recanalisation of the ducts occurs in up to 2 in 1000 men or women, resulting in a pregnancy: 'The effectiveness is lower than the COC in women under 27' (Towse 2004).

Following vasectomy, it may take up to 20 ejaculations to clear spermatozoa from the ducts, and ejaculate should be tested until two clear specimens are obtained. In certain parts of the world where it would be difficult to carry out these tests, 20 condoms are given to the man who is told that when these have been used he can begin unprotected intercourse. There may be a short-term risk of infection or haematoma, but despite multiple studies no statistical link with long-term health problems has been made.

Abortion

For some women abortion may be the only answer to an unwanted or dangerous pregnancy, the most vulnerable women being adolescents and women age 45 plus (Reid 2008). The Abortion Act (1967, C.87) requires that two doctors state that they have formed the opinion that one of four circumstances applies to this pregnancy:

1. Continuing the pregnancy would involve risk to the life of the pregnant woman greater than if the pregnancy were terminated.

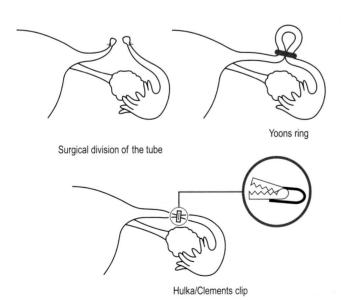

Figure 6.9 • Sterilisation methods. (Reproduced with permission from Cowper & Young 1989.)

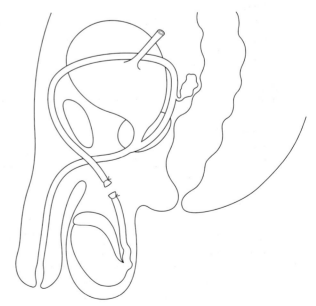

Figure 6.10 • Ligation of the vas deferens. (From Henderson C, Macdonald S 2004, with kind permission of Elsevier.)

2. Continuing the pregnancy would involve risk of injury to the physical or mental health of the pregnant woman greater than if the pregnancy were terminated.

3. Continuing the pregnancy would involve risk of injury to the physical or mental health of the existing child or children of the family of the pregnant woman greater than if the pregnancy were terminated.

4. There is substantial risk that if the child were born it would suffer from such physical or mental abnormalities as to be seriously handicapped.

The British Parliament voted unanimously to maintain legal abortion at 24 weeks (Hansard Debates 2008). The procedure does involve the destruction of the fetus and would be best performed earlier rather than later. Dilatation of cervix and curettage of endometrium (D&C) can be used, followed by vacuum aspiration of the products of conception up to 12 weeks from the last menstrual period. After 12 weeks, prostaglandin induction of uterine contractions is used to expel the fetus. These contractions are painful and the placenta may be retained in the uterus, necessitating evacuation of the uterus.

Future focus

Postnatally it is important to focus the woman's mind on future pregnancy and contraception methods. There are many unplanned pregnancies, in particular to very young woman; therefore education early, even antenatally, could help to focus their minds on future contraceptive methods (Doherty & Smith 2006). Worldwide there is no perfect contraceptive method. Perhaps the saddest result of uncontrolled population growth is the effect on children's health. For this reason it is important to maintain the research into ever simpler and acceptable contraception and to support people in their chosen optimum spacing of their children.

Main points

- The growth of the human population is occurring rapidly and the world population is over 6 billion (2003). The changes are not brought about totally by a surfeit of births. In some countries improving health is reducing the number of children dying and preventing early adult deaths.

- There are religious, moral and cultural issues to be considered, and it is unlikely that one method of contraception could become universal.

- The calculation of the failure rate per hundred woman years (HWY) is used to assess the effectiveness of contraceptive methods.

- All the ova available to the woman are present in her ovary at birth. It is not a matter of preventing ovum production but of preventing their maturation and ovulation. This is the basis for the combined oral contraceptive. Risks of taking the contraceptive pill include its oestrogen content, cigarette smoking, obesity, a sedentary way of life and a family history of thrombosis.

- Progestogen adds to the contraceptive effect by thickening cervical mucus, making the endometrium unsuitable for implantation and by reducing uterine tube motility.

- Other medication that the woman may be taking may interfere with the contraceptive action of the combined pill. Vomiting and diarrhoea may prevent absorption and the pill should be considered non-effective for that cycle. Women with malabsorption disorders should not be prescribed the oral combined pill.

- At present, research is focusing on stopping spermatogenesis by reducing feedback mechanisms and the production of GnRH.

- Milk production is not diminished when women take progestogen only and little hormone seems to cross into breast milk. Alteration in menstrual bleeding patterns, changes in the way that glucose is handled in women who have diabetes and ectopic pregnancy may occur. Methods of progestogen delivery by subcutaneous implant and by release from an intrauterine device are used.

- Barrier contraception methods include the diaphragm, the male condom, the female condom and spermicidal preparations. Some of these methods may prevent the spread of sexually transmitted disease. Natural methods include preventing ejaculation taking place in the vagina, timing, temperature and cervical mucus testing, control of coital frequency.

- Modern methods of postcoital contraception interrupt implantation or even ovulation depending on the time in the menstrual cycle. They include IUCD insertion, taking four tablets of the combined pill and antiprogesterone pills such as RU486.

- Not all requests for terminations of pregnancy are due to lack of prevention as failure occurs in most methods. The 1967 Abortion Act legalises abortion by requiring two doctors to agree that one of four circumstances applies to the pregnancy.

- D&C can be used, followed by vacuum aspiration of the products of conception up to 12 weeks from the last menstrual period. After 12 weeks prostaglandin induction of uterine contractions is used to expel the fetus.

- There is no perfect contraceptive method that could be used globally. Also, there are some countries where for social, cultural or religious reasons contraception is either forbidden or frowned upon. Possibly the saddest result of uncontrolled population growth is the effect on children's health.

References

Abortion Act 1967 (C.87) The UK Statute Law Database. <www.statutelaw.gov.uk/>.

Agius, J.C., Brincat, M., December 2006. 'Conceiving the pill'. The 45th birthday of the oral contraceptive pill in Europe. Malta Med. J. 18 (04).

Anderson, R.A., Kinniburgh, D., Baird, D.T., 2002. Suppression of spermatogenesis by etonogestral implants with depot testosterone potential for long lasting male contraception. J. Clin. Endocrinol. Metab. 87 (8), 3640–3649.

Andersson, K., 2001. The levenorgesterel intrauterine system: more than a contraceptive. Eur. J. Contracept. Reprod. Health Care 6 (Suppl. 1), 15–22.

Aschenbrenner, D.S., 2006. Over the counter access to Emergency Contraception. Am. J. Nurs. 106 (11), 4–36.

Billings, E.L., Billings, J.J., Brown, J.B., Burger, H.G., 1972. Symptoms and hormonal changes accompanying ovulation. Lancet i, 282–284.

British National Formulary (BNF) 2007 7.3. Contraceptives. March. British Medical Association and Royal Pharmaceutical Society of Great Britain.

Burkman, J., Schlesselman, J., Zeiman, M., 2006. Safety concerns and health benefits associated with oral contraception. Am. J. Obstet. Gynecol. 190 (4), S5–S22.

Coad, J., Dunstall, M., 2001. Anatomy and Physiology for Midwives. Edinburgh, Mosby, Ch. 4.

Cook, L.A., VanVliet, H., Lopez, L.M., Pun, M.F.A., Gallo., 2004. Vasectomy occlusion techniques for male sterilization. Cochrane. Database. Syst. Rev. (3) Art no. CD003991. www.cochrane.org/reviews/en/ab003991.html (accessed 24.05.08).

Doherty, E., Smith, A., 2006. Postnatal contraception planning for young women. MIDIRS Midwifery Dig. 16 (2), 237–239.

Dyer, O., 2002. WHO links long term pill use to cervical cancer. Br. Med. J. 324, 808.

Erkkola, R., 2007. Recent advances in hormonal contraception. Curr. Opin. Obstet. Gynaecol. 19 (6), 547–553.

ESHRE Capri Group, 2008. Intrauterine devices and intrauterine systems. Hum. Reprod. Update 14 (3), 197–208.

Evers, L.H., 2002. Female subfertility. Lancet 9327, 151–159.

Fehring, R., 2005. New low- and high tech calendar methods of family planning. J. Midwifery Womens Health 50 (1), 31–38.

FPA, 2005. Your guide to male and female condoms. Leaflet January Sexual Health Direct website: <www.fpa.org.uk>.

FPA, 2006. Your guide to the contraceptive implant. Leaflet March. Sexual Health Direct website: <www.fpa.org.uk>.

FPA, 2007. Contraception: patterns of use. Fact sheet. Sexual Health Direct website <www.fpa.org.uk>.

Guillebaud, J., 2005. What became of the male pill? In: The Pill and other Hormonal Contraception, sixth edn. Oxford University Press, Oxford, Ch. 9.

Hansard Debates. 2008. website: <http://www.publications.parliament.uk/pa/cm200708/cmhansrd/cm080520/debtext/80520-0021.htm>.

Hale, R., 2007. Choices in contraception. Br. J. Midwifery 15 (5), 305–309.

Hassan, M.A.M., Killick, S.R., 2004. Is previous use of the hormonal contraceptive associated with a detrimental effect on subsequent fecundity? Hum. Reprod. 19 (2), 344–351.

Kubba, A., Guillebaud, J., Anderson, R.A., MacGregor, E.A., 2000. Contraception. Lancet 356 (9245), 1913–1919.

Kujovich, J.L., 2007. Factor V Leiden thrombophilia. <www.geneclinics.org/profiles/factor-v-leiden/details.html>.

MIMS, September 2008. The Prescribing Reference for General Practice. Wyndham Heron Limited, Wiltshire.

Moodley, J., 2004. Combined oral contraceptive pill and cervical cancer. Curr. Opin. Obstet. Gynaecol. 16 (1), 27–29.

Nash, J.G., De Souza, R.M., 2002. Making the link: population, health, environment. Population Reference Bureau (PRB) website: <http://www.prb.org>.

Power, J., French, R., Cowan, F., 2007. Subdermal implantable contraceptives versus other forms of reversible contraceptives or other implants as effective methods of preventing pregnancy. Cochrane Database Syst. Rev. 18 (3) CD001326.

Rang, H.P., Dale, M.M., Ritter, J.M., 2007. Pharmacology, sixth ed. Churchill Livingstone, Edinburgh.

Ranney, M.L., Gee, E.M., Merchant, R.C., 2006. Non prescription availability of emergency contraception in the United States: current status controversies and impact on emergency medicine practice. Ann. Emerg. Med. 47 (5), 461–471.

RCOG, 2004. RCOG Guideline No. 40: Venous thromboembolism and hormonal contraception. <www.rcog.uk/resources/public/pdf/vte_hormonal_contraception.pdf> 12.05.08.

Reid, L., March 2008. The midwife and mature contraception. Pract. Midwife 11 (3).

Speidel, J.J., 2000. Environment and health: 1. Population, consumption and human health. Can. Med. Assoc. J. 163 (5), 552–554.

Towse, R., 2004. Fertility and its control. In: Henderson, C., Macdonald, S. (Eds.) Mayes Midwifery: A Textbook for Midwives. Baillière Tindall, Edinburgh Ch. 8, p. 114.

World Health Organization 2008 Medical eligibility criteria for contraceptive use, 3rd edn. website: <http://www.who.int/reproductive-health/publications/mec/coc.html> (accessed 12.05.2008).

Annotated recommended reading

Benangiano, G., Bastianelli, C., Farris, M., December 2006. Contraception today. Ann. N. Y. Acad. Sci. 1092, 1–32.

This publication gives a comprehensive overview of contraception.

British National Formulary (BNF) 2008 7.3: Contraceptives. March, pp 420–430. British Medical Association and Royal Pharmaceutical Society of Great Britain.

This is always a good reference book held in the ward area so it can be used as an immediate check on drug interactions and appropriate dosage. A specific section in the Appendix covers drugs in pregnancy and breastfeeding.

Family Planning Association (FPA) 2008 Website <http://fpa.org.uk>.

This website is useful for anyone: students, midwives and their clients.

It covers all aspects of family planning and abortion.

Towse, R., 2004. Fertility and its control. In: Henderson, C., Macdonald, S. (Eds.) Mayes Midwifery: A textbook for midwives, 13th edn. Baillière Tindall, Edinburgh, Ch. 8, p. 114.

This is a good chapter on family planning which is clearly written with some good diagrams and further references.

Chapter **Seven**

7

Infertility

CHAPTER CONTENTS

Introduction

Considering the size of the world's population, the fertility of humans is quite low compared with other mammals. Fertility in Western couples has steadily decreased since 2001 and was estimated at 1.84 children per woman (Office of National Statistics 2008). After the widely publicised birth of Louise Brown, the first 'test-tube' baby, in 1978, couples could be helped to conceive and sought advice. Midwives will come into contact with families who have had a problem in conceiving and will need to understand infertility, its treatment and its consequent effect on the family and parenting (Allan & Finnerty 2007, Sidebotham 2001).

Defining infertility

NICE Guidelines (NICE 2004) define infertility as 'failure to conceive after regular unprotected intercourse for 2 years in the absence of known reproductive pathology'. For couples who do not conceive, the desire to have a baby may be all-consuming. The couple may blame each other and this could cause marital/partnership disharmony; to seek help, the couple must recognise that a problem exists and a third party has to be brought into their intimate lives. Motherhood brings social status; referral to infertility clinics permits women to verbalise their worries with other women in the same circumstances, whereas contact with fertile women often brings conflict and emotional pressure (Allan 2007). The male suffers too if he is positively diagnosed as subfertile and somehow he feels he has not proved himself as 'manly' (Bainbridge 2007a).

Infertility affects as many as 1 in 6 couples; 80% can be helped by assisted reproductive technology (ART) using their own gametes, and a further 10–15% can be helped by the use of donated gametes (Fishel et al 2000). The Human Fertilisation and Embryology Authority (HFEA) (2008) state that 1.4% of all births in the UK result from infertility treatment. Many couples are delaying their first pregnancy and fertility declines after the age of 30 in both women and men (Balen & Rutherford 2007a, Brosens et al 2004). The age at first birth has risen from 28.6 years in 2001 to 29.2 years in 2006 (Office of National Statistics 2008).

The causes of male and female infertility

The causes of infertility listed in Table 7.1 indicate that investigations should ensure that:

1. Adequate numbers of sperm are deposited around the cervix (postcoital test).
2. The endometrium is in an appropriate state to receive the fertilised ovum (endometrial biopsy).
3. The fallopian tubes are patent (laparoscopy, salpingography).
4. Ovulation occurs (endometrial biopsy, hormonal assays).
5. The woman is psychologically prepared for pregnancy.

Table 7.2 indicates the causes of subfertility, expressed as a percentage (Johnson 2007).

Investigations for infertility

The general health of both partners should be investigated; a body mass index of 19–29 would be ideal; smoking cessation, prescription and recreational drug use and the amount of alcohol consumed each week are other factors (NICE 2004). Hypertensive men treated with calcium channel blockers have poor sperm motility, and insulin-dependent diabetes has been shown to be detrimental to reproduction in the male (Agbaje et al 2007, Balen & Rutherford 2007b).

Frequency and behavioural aspects of coitus and any reproductive history of both partners should be discussed (NICE 2004). Regular spontaneous intercourse is preferable to calculated fertile times and enforced unnatural coupling and its consequent effects on both partners, but this will inevitably change once infertility is diagnosed (Brosens et al 2004).

Male infertility

One in 20 men will be affected by subfertility, mainly caused by dysfunctional spermatozoa thus reducing their fertilising capacity. Environmental factors such as oestrogenic compounds in the drinking water may in part be to blame for lower sperm counts and the increase in cryptorchidism and testicular cancer (Hirsh 2003).

Table 7.1 Causes of infertility

Male	Female
Defective spermatogenesis	**Defective ovulation**
Endocrine disorders: dysfunction of the hypothalamus, pituitary, adrenal glands or thyroid gland	Endocrine disorders: dysfunction of hypothalamus, pituitary, adrenal glands or thyroid gland
Systemic disease such as diabetes mellitus	Systemic disease such as renal disease
Testicular disorders: trauma or environmental	Ovarian disorders: hormonal or polycystic ovarian syndrome or endometriosis
Defective sperm transport	**Defective transport**
Obstruction or absence of seminal ducts	Ovum: because of tubal obstruction or fimbrial adhesions
Impaired secretions from accessory glands	Sperm: because of thick cervical mucus or loss of tubal patency
Ineffective sperm delivery	**Defective implantation**
Impotence due to psychosexual problems	Due to hormone imbalance, congenital anomalies, fibroids or infection
Drug-induced problems by either prescription or recreational drugs	
Physical anomalies	

Table 7.2 Subfertility in UK couples expressed as a percentage

Cause	Approx. percentage frequency
Endometriosis	12
Tubal damage	14
Ovulatory problems	22
Sperm defects	24
Unexplained	28

Semen analysis and sperm deposition

Specimens of semen are obtained into a clean dry glass jar by coitus interruptus or by masturbation following 2 days of abstinence from coitus and examined in the laboratory within 1 h of collection. The alternative to this is a postcoital test, which also assesses the reaction of the sperm on the cervical mucus and could give an indication of the sperm's ability to fertilise the ovum. Semen analysis is more accurate when performed on its own, and ideally an average of three specimens at 2–3-week intervals allows calculation of a semen value.

Normal values for semen (WHO 2002):

- Volume >2 ml.
- Sperm concentration 20 million/ml.
- Motility >50% progressive or >25% rapidly progressing.
- Morphology >15% normal forms.
- Viscosity after liquefaction low.
- White blood cells <1 million/ml.
- Antibodies coating sperm <10%.

Postcoital test

A specimen of cervical mucus taken at the fertile part of the woman's cycle and within 6 h of intercourse is examined. This test can be used to ascertain the following:

- The quality of the cervical mucus.
- The sperm's ability to penetrate the cervical mucus.
- The effectiveness of intercourse.
- The presence of immunological problems.

Defective spermatogenesis

Absence of sperm (azoospermia) is uncommon. It may be due to defective spermatogenesis or damage to the transport ducts. Levels of follicular stimulating hormone and testicular size determine diagnosis. Modern ART can help 75% of these men (Hirsh 2003). Defective spermatogenesis may follow abnormal development of the testes due to poor development of the Sertoli cells. This may be genetic in origin. Late or non-descent of the testes may also have a genetic background and is now treated early in the baby's first year of life by surgery.

Biopsy of the testes and epididymis will show whether sperm are being produced. Two techniques are available: microsurgical epididymal sperm aspiration (MESA) and extraction of individual sperm cells from testicular tissue or testicular sperm extraction (TESA). Chromosomal studies will indicate whether the problem is a chromosomal translocation, which affects the meiotic division of spermatozoa causing aneuploidy in the offspring. While it is possible to assist couples with a genetic disorder, preimplantation chromosomal analysis of the conceptus is necessary to prevent abnormal fetuses being implanted (Ferlin et al 2006, Flinter 2001).

Infection, such as mumps with its complication of orchiditis, may damage the male tubular system. *Chlamydia trachomatis* infection is often asymptomatic and is associated with unexplained male infertility, and certain uropathogenic organisms have been found to affect sperm motility when bacterial counts are high. Treatment with antibiotics and vitamins C and E improves pregnancy rates (Hirsh 2003). Varicoceles, varicose veins of the scrotum, may cause raised testicular temperature and affect the size of the testes, but it is debatable if they are the cause of or are just associated with subfertility (Redmon et al 2002). Sperm production may be improved by eating healthily and by reducing alcohol intake and smoking.

Blood tests for hormone levels sometimes indicate possibilities for treatment. Reduced follicle-stimulating hormone (FSH) may respond to clomifene, while high levels of prolactin may respond to bromocriptine. Treatment with testosterone does not appear to stimulate sperm production. Some authorities recommend that fructose, zinc and acid phosphatase levels in seminal fluid should be measured when the sperm count is reduced. Low levels of fructose and zinc or high levels of acid phosphatase suggest a low-grade vesiculoprostatitis. Antibiotic treatment of prostatic infection may improve sperm count and motility.

Sexual dysfunction

Other causes of infertility include impotence and retrograde ejaculation into the bladder. Some men may benefit from medication such as sildenafil (Viagra) (Hirsh 2003). Artificial insemination by the husband's semen (AIH) may be useful in these cases or intracytoplasmic sperm injection (ICSI) (see below). Intrauterine insemination (IUI) transcervically with prepared partner's sperm with or without ovarian stimulation is also commonly used at the fertile time, 35–38 h prior to luteinising hormone surge (Bensdorp et al 2008).

Female infertility

Specific investigations would include:

- Endocrinology screening on days 1–3 of the menstrual cycle.
- Confirmation of rubella immunity.
- Cervical cytology.
- Screening for infections such as chlamydia.
- Ultrasound to assess the uterus and uterine tubes.
- Hysterosalpingography to assess tubal patency.
- Laparoscopy—observation of pelvic organs (Balen & Rutherford 2007a).

Ovulation

Tests to establish whether ovulation is occurring relate to the physiological changes accompanying ovulation. At ovulation, cervical mucus should become clear, copious and stretchy and show a ferning pattern when dried on a glass slide. Basal body temperature drops slightly and then should rise about 0.3°C. Ovulation predictor kits are available which work by measuring levels of luteinising hormone (LH). Venepuncture will examine the changing relationships of the four hormones oestrogen, progesterone, FSH and LH throughout the cycle. Ultrasound scanning can detect a ripening Graafian follicle and a thickening endometrium.

Depending on the results of investigations and where in the cyclical events the failure of ovulation originates, various drug treatments such as clomifene (BNF 2007) may be successful in stimulating ovulation.

The process of ovulation induction produces many ripe ova for harvesting which may then be used for in vitro fertilisation (IVF) or stored for future use as embryos or ova. Artificial stimulation of the ovary may cause a hyperstimulation syndrome (Buden et al 2005) which is potentially fatal, and produces many ova potentially creating multiple pregnancy which brings its own problems (Balen & Rutherford 2007a).

Polycystic ovarian syndrome (PCOS)

PCOS is the most common cause of anovulatory infertility in the UK (Balen & Rutherford 2007b). The syndrome may be confirmed by the presence of hyperandrogenism, menstrual irregularity and polycystic ovaries. Obesity and insulin resistance are features of the syndrome. These hormone imbalances affect the ovary, thickening the thecal layer, stopping ovulation and creating the menstrual abnormalities. Not all women with PCOS have every symptom, and when presenting with infertility the relevant problem must be treated to enable pregnancy to occur.

Tubal patency

Fertilisation takes place in the outer third of the uterine tube and the zygote takes 4 days to reach the uterine cavity. The normal acidity of the vagina inhibits bacterial growth, and monthly shedding of the endometrium may reduce the risk of chronic infection. Generally, organisms ascend through the cervix and uterus to affect the uterine tubes (salpingitis), the ovaries and the pelvic peritoneum, causing pelvic inflammatory disease (PID). Adhesions may distort the tubes. Alternatively, the endothelial folds lining the tubes may be functionally damaged and blocked with reduced or absent ciliated cells or peristaltic movements. The tubal lumen varies in width at the isthmus and the narrowest part of the uterine tube may be only 100 μm to 1 mm wide (the width of a pencil lead).

The most common organisms implicated in PID are those causing chlamydial infection and gonorrhoea. Women presenting with infertility and diagnosed with PID may have no recollection of an infection. A chlamydial serology screen is useful and a raised titre of more than 1:256 is indicative of tubal damage (Cahill & Wardle 2002). Current and past infections can be treated, if necessary, in both partners. According to a study undertaken in Leeds, the incidence of bacterial vaginosis (BV) is higher in women suffering from tubal infertility (Wilson et al 2002). To investigate and diagnose tubal patency hysterosalpingography can be performed by injecting a radio-opaque contrast medium through the cervix and monitoring its passage through the uterus and uterine tubes using X-rays. A laparoscopy can also examine tubal function and general pelvic structures.

Endometriosis

This is a condition where endometrial tissue that is reactive with the hormonal changes of menstruation is found outside the uterus, causing dysmenorrhoea, pelvic pain, hormonal disturbances and fatigue (Ball et al 2007, Huntington & Gilmour 2005). This condition affects fertility but quite how is not certain (Brosens et al 2004, Tavmergen et al 2007). Recent studies have shown alteration in immunological factors in peritoneal fluid and blood assays. Treatment requires some form of restorative surgery to remove endometrial deposits, as well as pituitary suppressive agents such as analogues of gonadotrophin-releasing hormone to suppress the endometrial deposits (Ball et al 2007). These women do not respond well to ovarian hyperstimulation.

Reproductive technologies

Treatment for infertility

Infertility treatment would be impossible without the ability of the embryologist to manipulate ova and sperm outside the body. Table 7.3 outlines the abbreviations and processes used in assisted conception.

Sperm and ova donation

The donation of ova and sperm is essential in the treatment of infertility for some couples. Donors are carefully selected for health and family history of disease and should be under the age of 35. The National Gamete and Donation Trust was launched in 2000 to

Table 7.3 Terminologies for assisted conception techniques

Term	Explanation
AIH	Artificial insemination by husband treats problems with sperm delivery, antisperm antibodies and where semen has been stored prior to chemotherapy or radiotherapy
AID	Artificial insemination by donor to prevent risk of transmission of an hereditary disease or rhesus incompatibility, where sperm are totally abnormal on semen analysis
ART	Assisted reproductive technology
IVF	In vitro fertilisation: conception takes place outside the body
IVM	Use of immature ova, prior to conception in vitro
GIFT	Gamete intrafallopian transfer: sperm and ova are inserted into the uterine tube for conception to take place in a natural way
ZIFT	Zygote intrafallopian transfer: fertilised ovum replaced into the uterine tube following conception in vitro
ICSI	Intracytoplasmic sperm injection: sperm is manipulated via a pipette into the ova and then implanted into the uterus
MESA	Microsurgical epididymal sperm aspiration: the extraction of sperm from the epididymis
TESA	The aspiration of sperm from the testes
PGD	Preimplantation genetic diagnosis

increase awareness of the need for ova and sperm donation (Klein & Sauer 2002). Sexually transmitted diseases are excluded and the semen is frozen and stored for at least 3 months to ensure that repeated tests for donor HIV are negative. Donors are matched to the physical and mental characteristics of the couple.

HFEA maintains a register of donors so that any child born following sperm or ovum donation has access to details about their biological parentage. All children conceived from donated gametes after April 2005 can trace their biological parents (HFEA 2008).

Assisted conception techniques have resulted in public concern and the report of the Warnock Committee of Enquiry into Human Fertilisation and Embryology (HMSO 1984) led to the Human Fertilisation and Embryology Act 1990. The HFEA was set up by the act to regulate research or treatment involving the creation, keeping and use of human embryos and the storage and donation of human eggs and sperm (HMSO 1990).

This is achieved by a licensing system; all clinics must be licensed and data maintained for analysis.

Principles of in vitro fertilisation

In vitro fertilisation assists in conception by using laboratory techniques to assist sperm and egg to unite and produce an embryo which is then inserted into the uterus. HFEA discusses five phases in the technique of IVF:

- Superovulation.
- Egg recovery; sperm recovery.
- Fertilisation.
- Preparation for pregnancy.
- Embryo transfer.

Superovulation involves using drugs to stimulate development of multiple ova. The investigations necessary to ensure that the phase of egg recovery results in mature ova involve frequent blood tests for estradiol levels and ultrasound scans for follicle tracking. At least six eggs are usually recovered by various methods, including laparoscopy. The ova are placed in a Petri dish in an optimum environment for fertilisation, and donor sperm are added.

The embryos that begin to develop are assessed for quality, and at 24 h embryonic cleavage is noted. About 48 h after the two-cell stage, the embryo is transferred to the uterus. A new technique termed comparative genomic hybridisation (CGH) is being developed in America but has yet to be routinely used in the UK; it would prevent using ova with abnormalities and preventing miscarriage in IVF treatment (Bainbridge 2007b). The HFEA stipulates that no more than two embryos are implanted into the uterus and the remainder are cryopreserved. The woman receives hormones to prepare the endometrial lining for pregnancy. It is possible to observe the ova until the blastocyst stage (about 5 days) which would permit the insertion of one embryo. However, the later the implantation into the uterus, the more risk there is for embryo survival. The delay in implanting the embryo would assist in preimplantation genetic diagnosis, which is not a routine procedure in IVF.

Intracytoplasmic sperm injection (ICSI)

Multiple ova are collected, as in the technique for IVF. Sperm are put into a solution that slows down motility to make them easier to work with. Each egg is sucked into a holding pipette. A microneedle, the diameter of which is seven times smaller than a human hair, is used to inject a sperm directly into the centre of each ovum and then the technique continues exactly as for IVF and embryo transfer (ET). The sperm are collected by electroejaculation technology.

The transfer of genetic disease during ISCI has been a concern, as the natural selection of healthy sperm is bypassed by artificial techniques (Tindall 2003). Why the sperm have been immotile or abnormal should be considered as should the fact that ageing ova may have aneuploidy (Ch. 3), which leads to early pregnancy loss. Infertility may be nature's way of preventing abnormality. Preimplantation genetic diagnosis (PGD) involves polymerase chain reaction (PCR) to define abnormal DNA in the embryo by biopsy of the polar body, blastomere or blastocyst (Bagness et al 2004).

Surrogacy

When infertility treatment with IVF or ICSI fails, the only alternative may be surrogacy. This is accepted more in the USA than in the UK. In Queensland, Australia, it is illegal. The HFEA may need to lay down some guidance to clarify issues. In the USA, surrogate mothers are paid for their services, but in the UK this is banned. Surrogacy has implications on family values and the child's future belief in its adoptive parents such as whether children should be told about their surrogate mother. There are many unanswered questions.

Statistics and conclusions

Assisted reproductive technology (ART) has revolutionised the treatment of infertility and has given many childless couples the healthy baby they desire. This treatment has costs, including monetary, social and psychological aspects, if IVF fails (Bergart 2000). HFEA figures for 2003/2004 showed a success rate of 28.2% for age 35 and slightly lower at 23.6% for age 35–37. There were 29 688 patients treated, with 38 264 IVF cycles, 8251 successful births with 10 242 children, many multiple births being evident from these figures.

Babies born following IVF treatment have problems. Preterm birth and its consequent small-for-dates and high mortality is common in multiple births. There appears to be a higher risk of bleeding, hypertension and diabetes. There is also concern regarding ICSI and genetic abnormality. Tindall (2003) cites an Australian study suggesting that any infant born of any form of ART has double the risk of an abnormality. Despite these facts, couples that are desperate for a baby are determined to surmount all odds and may be slightly 'blinkered' to the pitfalls and what lies ahead for them when embarking on infertility treatment.

Main points

- NICE Guidelines define infertility as failure to achieve a pregnancy after 2 years of unprotected intercourse. The implications are that 1 in 6 couples will be rated as infertile, 80% of these couples can be helped by reproductive technology and a further 10–15% by donated gametes.

- The apparent increase in the incidence of infertility may be because many couples delay first pregnancy and fertility declines after age 30 in both men and women. The average mother's age at first birth is 29.2 years.

- For both men and women, past or present systemic disease must be ruled out as a cause of infertility before proceeding to examination of the reproductive systems.

- Fresh specimens of semen for analysis are obtained following 2 days of abstinence from coitus. The environmental effect on diminishing sperm counts is a worrying problem. Heavy alcohol use causes testicular atrophy, but has not been proven to cause low sperm counts.

- Blood hormone levels may indicate possibilities for treatment of oligospermia. Reduced FSH may respond to clomifene. High levels of prolactin may respond to bromocriptine.

- Tests for establishing the cause of infertility in women include a pelvic examination, tests to establish whether ovulation is occurring, examination of cervical mucus and basal body temperature changes, and detailed blood assays for hormone levels during the menstrual cycle. Ultrasound scanning can detect a ripening Graafian follicle and a thickening endometrium.

- Malformation, infection of the uterus or poor endocrine control of endometrial development may cause infertility. A hysterosalpingotomy can be carried out, preferably just prior to ovulation. Laparoscopy allows examination of the pelvic organs.

- Clinically, women with polycystic ovarian syndrome suffer from irregular menstruation, may be hirsute, overweight, suffer from acne and have endocrine abnormalities. Testosterone and LH may be raised, and there may be insulin resistance.

- A common cause of loss of tubal patency is ascending infection, which, with pelvic adhesions, distorts the uterine tubes. The endothelial folds lining the tubes may be damaged with reduced or absent ciliated cells or peristaltic movements.

- About 40% of patients with endometriosis have involuntary infertility and 10% of women attending infertility clinics have endometriosis.

- IVF treatment consists of a series of steps: superovulation, egg recovery, fertilisation and embryo transfer. The HFEA keeps statistics and registers of all IVF treatments and donors, and regulates all research and storage of ova, sperm or gametes in the UK.

References

Agbaje, I.M., Rogers, D.A., McVicar, C.M., McClure, N., Atkinson, A.B., Mallidis, C., Lewis, S.E., 2007. Insulin dependent diabetes mellitus: implications for male reproductive function. Hum. Reprod. 22 (7), 1871–1877.

Allan, H., 2007. Experiences of infertility: liminality and the role of the fertility clinic. Nurs. Enquiry 14 (2), 132–139.

Allan, H., Finnerty, G., 2007. The practice gap in care of women following successful infertility treatments: unasked research questions in midwifery and nursing. Hum. Fertil. 10 (2), 99–104.

Bagness, C., Yerby, M., Hettle, S., 2004. Genetics, Ch 12, p 172. In: Henderson, C., MacDonald, S. (Eds.) Mayes Midwifery, thirteenth edn. Baillière Tindall, London.

Bainbridge, J., 2007a. Male infertility and emotional wellbeing. Br. J. Mid. 15 (11), 711.

Bainbridge, J., 2007b. Screening eggs for abnormalities: hope for childless couples? Br. J. Mid. 15 (3), 141.

Balen, A., Rutherford, A., 2007a. Management of infertility. Br. Med. J. 335 (7620), 608–611.

Balen, A., Rutherford, A., 2007b. Managing anovulatory infertility and polycystic ovary syndrome. Br. Med. J. 335 (7621), 663–666.

Ball, E., Byrne, H., Davis, C., 2007. The value of two step operative laparoscopy with interval pituitary suppression in the treatment of infertility caused by severe endometriosis. Curr. Opin. Obstet. Gynecol. 19 (4), 303–307.

Bensdorp, A.J., Cohlen, B.J., Heineman, M.J., Vandekerckhove, P., 2008. Intra-uterine insemination for male subfertility. Cochrane Database Syst. Rev. 1.

Bergart, A., 2000. The experience of women in unsuccessful infertility treatment: what do patients need when medical intervention fails? Soc. Work Health Care 39 (4), 45–69.

BNF (British National Formulary). (2007) (53) March. British Medical Association and Royal Pharmaceutical Society of Great Britain.

Brosens, I., Gordts, S., Valkenburg, M., Puttemans, C.R., 2004. Investigation of the infertile couple: when is the appropriate time to explore female infertility? Hum. Reprod. 19 (8), 1689–1692.

Buden, M., Arroliqa, A.C., Falcone, T., 2005. Ovarian hyperstimulation syndrome. Crit. Care Med. Crit. Illn. Pregnancy 33 (10 supplement), S301–S306.

Cahill, D., Wardle, P., 2002. Management of infertility. Br. Med. J. 325, 28–32.

Ferlin, A., Arredi, B., Foresta, C., 2006. Genetic causes of male infertility. Reprod. Toxicol. 22 (Issue 2), 133–141.

Fishel, S., Dowell, K., Thornton, S., 2000. Reproductive possibilities for infertile couples: present and future, Ch. 2, p 17. In: Bentley, G.R., Mascie-Taylor, C.G.N. (Eds.), Infertility in the Modern World. Cambridge: Cambridge University Press.

Flinter, F.A., 2001. Preimplantation genetic diagnosis: needs to be tightly regulated. Br. Med. J. 322 (7293), 1008–1009.

HFEA 2008 Website: www.hfea.gov. uk/docs (accessed April 2008).

Hirsh, A., 2003. Male subfertility. Br. Med. J. 327 (7416), 669–672.

HMSO 1984 Warnock M (Chair) Report of the Committee of Enquiry into Human Fertilisation and Embryology, London.

HMSO, 1990. Human Fertilisation and Embryology Act 1990. Paul Freeman 6.

Huntington, A., Gilmour, J., 2005. A life shaped by pain: women with endometriosis. J. Clin. Nur. 14 (9), 1124–1132.

Johnson, M.H., 2007. Essential Reproduction, sixth edn. Blackwell Science, Oxford.

Klein, J., Sauer, M., 2002. Oocyte donation. Best practice research. Clin. Obstet. Gynaecol. 3, 277–291.

NICE (National Institute for Health and Clinical Excellence) 2004 Assessment and treatment for people with fertility problems. www.nice.org.uk/download. aspx?o=104459 (Accessed April 2008).

Office of National Statistics 2008 UK Population, Fertility. website: www. statistics.gov. (Accessed March).

Redmon, J.B., Carey, P., Pryor, J.L., 2002. Varicocele: the most common cause of male factor infertility? Hum. Reprod. Update 8 (1), 53–58.

Sidebotham, M., 2001. Assisted conception: an issue for midwives. Pract. Midwife 4 (11), 10–12.

Tavmergen, E., Ulukus, M., Goker, E.N.T., 2007. Long term use of gonadotrophin-releasing hormone analogues before IVF in women with endometriosis. Curr. Opin. Obstet. Gynecol. 19 (3), 284–288.

Tindall, G., 2003. Mixed blessings: ethical issues in assisted conception. J. R. Soc. Med. 96, 4–35.

Wilson, J.D., Ralph, S.G., Rutherford, A.J., 2002. Rates of bacterial vaginosis in women undergoing in vitro fertilisation for different types of infertility. Br. J. Obstet. Gynaecol. 109 (6), 714–717.

World Health Organization (WHO) 2002 Laboratory recommendations. World Health Organization, Geneva. http://www.who.org/.

Annotated recommended reading

Barber, D., 2004. Infertility and assisted conception. In: Henderson, C., Macdonald, S. (Eds.), Mayes Midwifery: A Textbook for Midwives, thirteenth edn. Ch. 9, p 129. Baillière Tindall.

This is a good overview of infertility and assisted conception techniques.

HFEA. 2008 Website: www.hfea.gov.uk/docs.

This site provides an excellent coverage of infertility news and new technologies.

NICE (National Institute for Health and Clinical Excellence) 2004 Assessment and treatment for people with fertility problems. www.nice.org.uk/download. aspx?o=104459.

This is an easy to read guideline for the treatment of infertility.

Chapter **Eight**

8

Preconception matters

Introduction

Preconception care is a preventative approach through which biomedical, behavioural and psychosocial risk factors are identified before pregnancy or very early in pregnancy in order to optimise maternal and neonatal health outcomes. The target of preconception interventions is women as well as their partners to ensure a comprehensive approach.

In addition to the purpose of preconception care, this chapter is concerned with the extent to which childbearing can be affected by the lifestyle of individuals and the environment in which they live, as well as with certain interventions and the main challenges in the process of prepregnancy care provision. Concepts from the disciplines of ecology and evolution will be utilised to discuss the implications of radiation, toxic waste and drug ingestion and their interaction with the physiology of conception.

The problems caused by pregnancy-induced disorders are considerable; Moore & Persaud (2008) estimate that between 7% and 10% of birth defects result from the 'disruptive actions of drugs, viruses and other environmental factors'. There are also many cases of multifactorial inheritance where genetic and environmental factors act together in complex ways.

Prepregnancy care provision

A difficulty inherent in the concept of preconceptual care for health professionals is that one-third to half of all babies are conceived accidentally. For most of those who plan their conception, by the time their pregnancy is confirmed, many embryonic organs have been developing and this is the most vulnerable stage of embryogenesis. Embryogenesis is completed by the eighth week of pregnancy and few women attend for their first antenatal visit that early in pregnancy. It is then too late for early preventative strategies such as folic acid intake for elimination of neural tube defects. Ethical considerations limit the conduction of randomised trials to investigate efficacy of preconception counselling. Nevertheless, there is evidence from retrospective, prospective and case control studies to indicate that preconception counselling improves pregnancy outcome.

There has been a progressive reduction in perinatal mortality in the last century, but there should be greater emphasis on prepregnancy care and counselling to reduce these low rates of mortality (Smith 1992) and to minimise perinatal morbidity further. Research suggests that pregnancy outcome is improved markedly when couples are screened and advised prior to conception (Korenbrot et al 2002). The mother's diet and possibly the father's also, immediately prior to and at the time of conception, may influence the developing embryo. There is evidence from animal studies that spermatogenesis is influenced by diet (Smith & Akinbamijo 2000). There are debates concerning appropriate location, timing and format of preconception care provision, and it has been suggested that young girls or women of childbearing age should be opportunistically educated at school or in primary care settings.

Aims of prepregnancy care

Because of the high level of unplanned pregnancies, preconception care should be embraced in the health education of schoolchildren, continued into adult life and special programmes established that are targeted at groups most in need, such as people in lower social class, smokers, obese women or those at high risk of complications (diabetes or epilepsy). The aims of prepregnancy care according to Chamberlain (1992) are:

- To provide the means of ensuring that preventable factors are attended to before pregnancy starts—e.g. rubella inoculation.
- To give advice about the effects of pre-existing disease and its treatment on the pregnancy and unborn child.
- To consider the likelihood and effects of any recurrence of events from previous pregnancies and deliveries.

Chronic diseases

The benefits of preconception care are more evident in pre-existing and chronic diseases. Chapple (2007) identifies certain groups of women who are particularly in need of preconception care and emphasises the importance of a sensitive approach when dealing with them. In addition to their own concerns, they may be fearful of health care professionals' attitude in either condemning their wishes to get pregnant or encouraging termination. Particular conditions for which women should consult specialist care prior to or very early in pregnancy include:

- **Diabetes**—Ray et al (2001) showed that preconception care accompanied with good glycaemic control lowers the risk of fetal abnormalities in diabetic pregnancies. The recent UK Confidential Enquiry

into Maternal and Child Health (CEMACH 2007) suggests dedicated preconception clinics (currently provided in 17% of UK units) in which expert help and advice are available for diabetic women is a most effective way of meeting the needs of these women.

- **Epilepsy**—Antiepileptic medications may be teratogenic, therefore adjusting the required dose under specialist care may help in reducing potential risks.
- **Cardiac diseases**—Collaboration with cardiologists is crucial.
- **Oral anticoagulants**—Changing to injectable medication under clinical specialist care may reduce the risk of teratogenicity.
- **Hypothyroidism**—The thyroid gland is important in human metabolism and the need for thyroid replacement therapy may increase in these women, thus timely intervention could reduce the risk of abnormal neurological development.
- **Phenylketonuria**—A diet reduced in phenylalanine before and during pregnancy can prevent damage to fetal brain development.
- **Mental health**—Minor and major forms of mental health disorders should be screened and supportive care offered.
- **Acne**—The treatment of women with isotretinoin should be stopped because of the risk of teratogenicity.

The healthy gamete

There is no clear demarcation between the health of the gametes immediately prior to conception and the developing embryo. In both instances cells are developing rapidly and are vulnerable to disruption. Even when pregnancies are planned, it is unlikely that a couple will consider the importance of those 100 days of gamete formation (explained by Foresight, an association for the promotion of preconception care—see below). The continuously produced sperm are also at risk of environmental insult. In the female fetus the primary oocytes have already undergone their first reduction division early in the first trimester and no further ova will be generated after the fifth month of gestation. In this arrested stage of development they are relatively resistant to mutagenic damage. Sensitivity increases just prior to ovulation and the mutation rate from radiation may rise sharply.

Following fertilisation, the zygote becomes resistant to genetic injury while undergoing cleavage, but after 16 days intense organogenesis begins. Sensitivity is high but so few cells are present that either the fetus will be affected and aborted spontaneously or not affected and be normal. This may account for a considerable proportion of unexplained pregnancy losses within the first 6 weeks.

General health care

The medical, obstetrical, social and family history of both the man and the woman is taken and known personal or familial health problems are discussed. A gynaecological examination of the woman and screening of blood and urine and, in some cases hair, stool and semen analysis, are carried out. Any infections should be treated, dietary problems discussed and possible work and lifestyle hazards considered.

A general risk assessment through questioning or using technology helps to identify potential problems and develop appropriate individualised care pathways sensitive to the needs of a mother and her baby. The main relevant issues that can be screened by making simple enquiries are summarised by Chapple (2007). Those, in addition to items addressing wider general health issues, are presented below.

Social history

The impact of maternal age on pregnancy outcome at both ends of the reproductive age is important. Teenagers are more likely to be anaemic, or at risk of having growth-restricted infants, preterm labour and higher infant mortality. Most teenage pregnancies are unplanned, therefore they rarely present for preconception care. Early pregnancy counselling could still be helpful. Pregnancies in later life (after 35) are also more likely to be at risk of obstetric complications (e.g. chromosomal abnormalities). However, for physically fit women the risks are lower than previously reported. Some pregnancy outcomes have been shown to be strongly related to the socioeconomic and health status of the mothers, particularly in this age group. These are hypertension, diabetes, placental abruption, preterm delivery, stillbirth and placenta praevia.

Socially disadvantaged women, asylum seekers and women at risk of mental health problems require integrated care from an early stage of pregnancy or ideally before pregnancy (CEMACH 2007). Providing preconception care is, of course, more challenging for such women due to a non-compliance behavioural pattern and reduced access to routine care. However, providing creative outreach services and/or opportunistic care targeting such vulnerable groups can have a huge impact on improving health and reducing maternal health inequalities.

Hair mineral analysis

Hair analysis for mineral content—which involves taking a sample of scalp hair and using equipment that can measure contaminants—is still regarded as fringe research by some practitioners, but studies confirm its usefulness. Both an excess of toxic minerals and a shortage of essential minerals may cause reproductive problems. Some toxins are eliminated from blood and stored in body tissues. Hair grows slowly and will show traces of whatever has passed into the follicle in the previous 6–8 weeks. Hair analysis can therefore be a useful addition to blood and urine tests to screen for minerals. The group Foresight have a fantastic website (Foresight 2008) and the founder of the group has written a small booklet outlining the programme (Barnes 2007). The information includes testing for the following minerals and gives advice depending on the findings:

- Essential minerals: calcium, magnesium, potassium, iron, chromium, cobalt, copper, manganese, nickel, selenium and zinc.
- Toxic minerals: aluminium, cadmium, mercury and lead. The last two are discussed below.

Either supplementation of essential minerals or removal of toxic minerals by methods such as chelation may be offered.

Nutrition and weight

Establishing a balanced diet and a healthy lifestyle prior to pregnancy increases the chance of a successful pregnancy outcome. Prepregnancy weight is positively related to infant birth weight. In developed countries it is rare to find overt malnutrition except in people with eating disorders such as anorexia nervosa.

Poor nutrition

It is not ethically acceptable to experiment on the effects of food restriction on the human fetus. However, retrospective studies during famine provide some information. The Dutch famine of 1944–45 showed that there was more early pregnancy perinatal mortality in undernourished women and that fertility can be reduced by sudden falls in energy intake (Barker 1992). Barker has spent 20 years studying the effects of the fetal environment on adult-onset diseases and has written many journal articles and books, including one aimed at educating parents on the importance of prenatal nutrition (Barker 2003). Perhaps, as a protective measure, nature ensures that women who are too thin or too fat have difficulty in achieving ovulation and fertilisation. There may be a difference in an acute energy deprivation in comparison to a chronic nutritional deprivation. Maternal metabolism adjusts to optimise nutrient availability for the growing fetus.

Obesity

Obesity is a growing problem in industrialised societies, its rate having doubled since the 1980s in the UK. According to UK obesity statistics, 32% of women are overweight and a further 21% are obese. Obesity is associated with increased risk of complications such as gestational diabetes and pre-eclampsia, thrombophlebitis, post-term pregnancy, caesarean delivery, macrosomia and instrumental delivery (Wolfe 1998). Obese women are prone to further development of obesity after pregnancy, particularly the central type of obesity (Soltani & Fraser 2000). This is the pathological type which leads to higher risk of metabolic disorders such as metabolic syndrome, diabetes and cardiovascular disease (Byrne & Wild 2005).

There is no clear guidance with regard to dieting during pregnancy, thus it is very important to adjust maternal diet and weight prior to conception. Prepregnancy weight influences pregnancy outcome. Being undernourished is associated with fetal abnormality and low birth weight, while being obese brings the risk of complications of pregnancy mentioned above.

A guide to ascertaining the optimum weight for a woman is the Quetelet index or body mass index. This is obtained by using the formula of weight (kg) divided by height squared (m^2). The following BMI range is used as a guide:

- Less than 20: underweight.
- 20–24.9: desirable weight.
- 25–29.9: overweight.
- 30 and over: obesity.
- 35 and over: severe obesity.

Specific nutrient abnormalities

Suboptimal dietary deficiencies are common, especially in areas of high unemployment and poverty or women with dietary restriction (vegans or vegetarians).

The importance of nutrition in male fertility has rarely been investigated. Protein, energy and possibly zinc deficiencies may be linked to reduced spermatogenesis (Wharton 1992). There is mounting evidence implicating specific dietary deficiencies affecting the process of organogenesis in the embryo, mainly related to folic acid and zinc.

Although the mechanism is not clear, studies have shown that supplementation with folate/folic acid around conception can prevent neural tube defects (NTD) in the fetus (Schorah & Smithells 1991). It is therefore advised that women planning a pregnancy should take 0.4 mg folic acid as a daily supplement from when they try to conceive until the 12th week in pregnancy (DOH 1993). Women are also encouraged to eat more folate-rich foods (e.g. green beans, peas and dark green leaf vegetables) and avoid overcooking them.

Maternal zinc status is also essential in fetal development. The degree to which maternal zinc deficiency can lead to teratogenic effects in humans is unclear but there is limited evidence that severe maternal zinc deficiency may lead to fetal abnormality (Soltan & Jenkins 1982).

Excessive intake of fat-soluble vitamins is harmful. An epidemiological study in Spain (Martinez-Frias & Salvador 1990) showed an increased risk of birth defects in babies of mothers who had taken high levels of vitamin A (6000–167 000 µg) during the first 2 months of pregnancy. Although its role in causing human abnormalities is not confirmed, in the UK it is advised that women who might become pregnant should avoid vitamin A supplements unless suggested by a doctor or antenatal clinic. Women who are pregnant or might become pregnant are also advised against eating liver or liver products because of its high vitamin A content (National Dairy Council 1994).

Drugs

Drugs may be teratogenic, reduce absorption of nutrients or interfere with normal growth and development. The placenta is not a complete barrier against all chemicals.

Many people are exposed to drugs used to treat medical conditions. These may be essential for treatment and difficult to withdraw or reduce. Sometimes they can be substituted by less toxic drugs or stopped altogether during pregnancy. Women of childbearing age should only take medicines under medical supervision and medical practitioners should be alert to the teratogenic side effects of drugs. People may purchase drugs for minor problems such as pain and indigestion without their doctor's knowledge. The doctor may then prescribe drugs that exacerbate the effects of the over-the-counter drugs. The public should be informed about the danger of taking drugs in pregnancy.

Women are usually advised to discontinue the use of hormonal contraceptives at least 3 months prior to the time they wish to get pregnant. This allows the body to readjust its hormonal system and resume physiological menstrual cycles, as well as regulating the level of minerals and vitamins which may be affected by the contraceptive pill. Mineral and vitamin levels may also be affected by intrauterine devices, especially if they contain copper which can interfere with absorption of zinc and cause zinc deficiency.

Drugs may be taken for recreational reasons because of their mood-altering abilities. It is sometimes difficult to ascertain whether they are being taken and to help people to stop taking them. Such substances include alcohol, tobacco and caffeine as well as addictive drugs such as cocaine and its derivative crack, marijuana and heroin. With appropriate referral systems, preconception counselling would be most effective for women who habitually use drugs, as drug abuse is associated with malnutrition, alcohol abuse, smoking and a higher risk of sexually transmitted diseases.

Smoking and alcohol consumption

The dangers of **smoking** for general health and during pregnancy are well documented. Many harmful chemicals such as polycyclic aromatic hydrocarbons, carbon monoxide, cyanide, lead and cadmium are inhaled in cigarette smoke. The effects of smoking on reproduction are summarised below:

- **Male and female infertility**—Besides experiencing infertility, women who smoke often undergo an early menopause (Jick et al 1977). In men, smoking reduces testosterone levels, reduces the number and motility of sperm and increases the number of abnormal sperm (Evans et al 1981). Alcohol is a direct testicular toxin, causing atrophy of seminiferous tubules and an inhibiting effect on Leydig cells.

- **Low birth weight**—One of the most frequent adverse effects of smoking during pregnancy is reduced fetal growth, which is dose-dependent. Conter et al (1995) carried out a longitudinal study of 12 987 babies: 10 238 from non-smoking mothers, 2276 from mothers smoking 1–9 cigarettes/day and 473 from mothers smoking more than 9 cigarettes/day. The results confirmed the association of smoking during pregnancy with lower birth weight. However, the reduction in birth weight was overcome by 6 months of age and was not permanent.

- **Increased perinatal mortality** (stillbirths or deaths in the first week)—There is an increased risk of sudden infant death syndrome (SIDS) associated with maternal smoking during pregnancy and evidence that household exposure to tobacco smoke has an independent additive effect (Blair et al 1996).

- **Other harmful effects**—Spontaneous abortions, fetal malformations, reduced length of gestation and preterm labour, attention deficit hyperactivity disorder (ADHD) and learning difficulties when school age reached, and reduced immunocompetence.

Alcohol consumption during pregnancy is also hazardous to the growing baby. Drinking alcohol not only affects the mother's health by reducing absorption of vitamins and minerals, it can also damage fetal growth leading to miscarriage, physical defects, low birth weight, preterm birth, hyperactivity, reduced attention span and, in severe cases, fetal alcohol syndrome (known as the most common cause of mental retardation in babies). When alcohol is consumed by mothers, it reaches the fetus quickly and there is no known safe level. It is therefore recommended that women abstain from drinking when deciding to conceive and continue that during pregnancy (American College of Obstetricians and Gynecologists (ACOG) 2008).

Infection

During successful preconception care, any maternal infection should be investigated and treated. Appropriate advice should be given to prevent infection, as it can adversely affect the pregnancy outcome. Commonly, urinary or genital infections may lead to preterm labour or miscarriage. Systemic infections may cause reproductive problems such as infertility and congenital defects (see Ch. 15).

Vaccination to confer immunity to **rubella** may be available, or advice on how to minimise the risk of infection during pregnancy when no vaccine is available. Rubella acquired in the first trimester of pregnancy is associated with a 90% increase in the risk of congenital malformations (Best et al 2002). Although routine screening for rubella is offered to all women in most Western countries, vaccination against rubella is contraindicated during pregnancy. Antenatal screening for rubella can only help to identify the need for postpartum immunisation to protect future pregnancies. Therefore, screening at the preconception period for women who are at risk can play a protective role for their currently planned pregnancy. Following immunisation, pregnancy should be avoided for at least 3 months.

It should also be borne in mind that, due to the recent controversial evidence with regard to the measles, mumps and rubella (MMR) vaccination, there has been a decline in the number of children who have been vaccinated against these diseases. There are also some women who give birth abroad where vaccination against MMR is not widely offered. Therefore, prepregnancy or early pregnancy investigation of rash, particularly in a high-risk group (mentioned above), is important.

Toxoplasmosis caused by the parasite *Toxoplasma gondii*, which is found in soil and vegetation and is able to multiply at refrigerator temperatures (4–6°C or above), and *Listeria monocytogenes* can cause miscarriage, stillbirth or fetal abnormalities. Women planning a pregnancy or already pregnant should be advised on handling cat litter trays to avoid toxoplasmosis and to cook meat thoroughly. To avoid **listeriosis** they should be advised on hygienic food handling and avoid eating soft, ripened cheeses such as Brie and blue-vein types. Cooked chilled meals and ready-to-eat poultry should be reheated until piping hot prior to consumption.

At the preconception clinic, women could be screened for other infections such as sexually transmitted or blood-borne diseases such as Chlamydia, syphilis, HIV and hepatitis B. Most bacteria are too large to cross the placenta but viruses and the spirochaete of syphilis can penetrate the placental membrane to infect the fetus.

Haemoglobinopathies

These include genetic disorders affecting the shape and structure of haemoglobin, leading to a reduction of oxygen-carrying capacity in red blood cells. Sickle cell disease is the most common genetic disorder in the UK (Dick 2006) and is more prevalent in Black Africans and Black Afro-Caribbean ethnic groups. Thalassaemia is less common and the affected people originate mostly from South East Asia, the Middle East, Mediterranean and some European countries (e.g. Italy and Greece). Sickle cell disease or thalassaemia are controlled by recessive genes, thus healthy people who carry only one gene can be haemoglobinopathy carriers. If both parents are carriers, there is a 1 in 4 chance that each pregnancy will be affected with these serious conditions. Ideally, targeted screening should be offered to parents who are at high risk before conception or at an early stage of pregnancy. This provides an opportunity for parents to discuss a range of options, including diagnostic genetic testing, counselling and support in making informed choices.

Environmental issues

With advancing technology and scientific progress, almost everybody is exposed to novel environmental substances, some of which are of concern during pregnancy. It should be emphasised that when harmful prenatal exposure is likely, the woman (or couple) planning a pregnancy should avoid exposure before conception and during pregnancy.

Toxins

Toxins can be natural or manufactured. Natural toxins have evolved alongside humans and a degree of mutual tolerance exists. Manufactured toxins have been developed since the beginning of the industrial revolution and there has been insufficient time for tolerance to develop.

Natural toxins

Many natural toxins were developed by plants as a defence against being eaten. Examples include the tannins and alkaloids found in acorns, or cyanide in apples and apricots—although the flesh is nutritious, the seeds in quantity are poisonous.

Defence systems

Animals, including humans, have developed defence systems against plant toxins. The first line of defence is avoidance mediated by sight, smell and taste. People avoid eating mouldy or rotten food as a defence against bacterial and fungal toxins. Profet (1992) developed

a theory to explain why 80% of pregnant women suffer from nausea and morning sickness during the early weeks of pregnancy. She believes an aversion to bitter-tasting foods protects against possible teratogenic effects of naturally occurring toxins. This has been called the 'prophylaxis hypothesis' by Flaxman & Sherman (2008). They also put forward a 'by-product hypothesis' suggesting that vomiting is a non-functional by-product of conflict over resources between mother and fetus. They conclude that Profet's hypothesis of protection against ingested toxins is most probably correct.

The next line of defence is to expel toxins by vomiting and diarrhoea. People are reluctant to eat foods that have affected them in that way and often develop lifetime avoidance. Stomach acids and enzymes play a part in neutralising some toxins. There are two other cellular defence mechanisms: cells in the epithelial lining of the stomach secrete a thin layer of protective mucus to prevent toxin absorption but, should the toxin breech this mucus layer and damage cells, they are quickly replaced by the high turnover of epithelial tissue cells.

The liver is the main organ responsible for the detoxification of ingested substances. Toxins absorbed by the gastrointestinal tract are taken via the portal vein directly to the liver where a wide range of enzymes can render them harmless. The detoxified substances are then excreted via the kidneys. Although many toxins are potentially damaging, some increase liver enzyme production. Reducing exposure to everyday toxins may reduce the preparedness of liver enzyme systems to a sudden toxic overload (Johns 1990).

Manufactured toxins

The development of the chemical industry has resulted in contamination of the environment by vast quantities of synthetic pollutants such as DDT, polychlorinated biphenyls (PCBs) and polycyclic aromatic hydrocarbons (PAHs) (Colborn et al 1996). The effect of environmental toxins on the formation of the gametes must be researched. American scientists suspected that pesticides such as DDT and other chemical pollutants such as PCBs were disrupting sexual development by mimicking the effect on tissues of oestrogen, causing feminisation of male reproductive organs across species of fish, reptiles, birds and mammals (Colborn et al 1996). The effect was seen in younger rather than older animals. These chemicals were found in high levels in human blood and body fat as well as in human breast milk.

A small study in Canada carried out on herring gulls suggested that air pollution from coal fires and other fossil fuels which release PAHs may trigger inheritable genetic defects. However, the effect is difficult to separate from other forms of pollution such as drinking contaminated water or eating contaminated fish (Cohen 2002).

The role of pollutants as endocrine disruptors and androgen disruptors (which suppress the effects of testosterone) are under investigation but current evidence is worrying scientists (Wakefield 2002). These substances block signals to cells to switch on key developmental genes activated by testosterone. They enter our food chain from the use of fungicides. Scientists found that the fungicide vinclozin stunted sexual development of rat pups in utero. Theoretically, humans could be at risk too. The effect of these substances has been summarised in a readable book by Ashton & Green (2008).

In summary, the harmful effects of toxic waste on animals' reproductive health have been demonstrated in laboratory experiments, but proving this in humans is much more complex and challenging. Nevertheless, the association of high level of toxic substances in human tissue and its association with increasing rates of adverse reproductive health outcomes, alerts us to the importance of regulatory legislation to control chemical wastes and human exposure to them (Alsopp 2006).

Human infertility

Niels Skakkebaek at the University of Copenhagen found male reproductive problems such as reduced sperm counts with an increase in abnormal sperm and a threefold increase in the rate of testicular cancer in Denmark (Carlsen et al 1992). A review of the literature, which included 61 studies of 15 000 men in 20 countries, indicated a fall in sperm count of 50% between 1938 and 1990.

The findings included:

1. The average male sperm count dropped 45% between the 1940s and 1990s.

2. This drop was seen to occur in younger men. The younger the man, the lower the sperm count.

3. The average volume of ejaculate had dropped by 25%.

4. The number of men with an internationally agreed extremely low sperm count of less than 20 million/ml had increased from 6% to 18%.

Skakkebaek is currently trying to find out whether the differences in testicular cancer rates between Denmark and Finland are due to differences in exposure to endocrine disruptors (Wakefield 2002).

A problem with sperm production data is the amount of variation around the world and over time. Earlier results in the 1940s and 1950s may not have been as accurate and artificially high counts obtained. Currently, sperm counts may depend on who donates the sperm and at what time of day (more in the afternoon than morning) (Jones 2003). A survey of potency involving men in four European cities—Edinburgh, Paris,

Copenhagen and Turku in Finland—showed the impact of the combination of physics and chemistry. Both increased testicular temperature due to modern clothing and sedentary occupations such as driving, and chemical pollutants may affect sperm production. However, as in many epidemiological studies, hard evidence is still lacking (Giwercman et al 2007).

Oestrogenic compounds

Sharpe & Skakkebaek (1993) found similar problems and believed that oestrogenic compounds affect fetal testes by preventing development of the full complement of Sertoli cells. This reduces sperm counts, as the number of sperm produced depends on how many can be nurtured by Sertoli cells.

Oestrogenic mimics

There are problems associated with oestrogenic compounds such as PAHs, PCBs, dioxins, phthalates used in plastics, paints and adhesives, breakdown products of alkylphenol polyethoxylates (APEs) used in detergents (nonylphenol) (in domestic cleaners) and organochlorine pesticides such as DDT, aldrin and dieldrin. These problems include:

- In men: increased incidence of prostatic cancer, undescended testicles and penile abnormalities such as hypospadias.
- In women: increased incidence of endometriosis and oestrogen-dependent breast cancer (an increase of 32% between 1980 and 1987 in America).

Leaching from plastics

Soto et al (1991) investigated growth inhibition in cell cultures and examined the role of oestrogen. They had cultures growing in various strengths of oestrogen, including an oestrogen-free culture. In these latter cultures cell division occurred at an unprecedented rate. The scientists suspected that the dishes holding the cultures must be acting as an oestrogenic source.

River pollution

In Britain, anglers found it was difficult to sex the fish they caught. Most appeared to be female or have some female characteristics. Male fish were producing huge quantities of vitellogenin, a substance necessary for egg production that is normally produced by females in response to ovarian release of oestrogen (Sumpter & Jobling 1995). At first, Sumpter postulated that oestrogens in the urine of women taking the contraceptive pill were to blame but no trace of these was found in the water. Having read of the findings of Soto et al (1991), he believed that nonylphenol entering rivers in detergents was responsible.

Milk products

The latest theory attempts to explain the large differences in sperm counts between the Danish men and those in their neighbouring countries. It is possible that drugs used to encourage massive milk production in cattle have contaminated milk and dairy products. Men taking large amounts of dairy produce such as those in Denmark may have much lower sperm counts than men eating less dairy products (Jones 2003).

Unto the third generation

Environmental factors are probably as important in gametogenesis and fetal development. The more rapidly developing cells will be most affected. The effect must be considered over three generations. The ova of today's childbearing woman were developed while she was still in her mother's uterus as were the numbers of Sertoli cells present in the testicles of today's prospective fathers. Around the world 100 000 synthetic chemicals are on sale. Some banned in developed countries such as DDT are still used in Third World countries. Worldwide use of pesticides is increasing annually so the problem is likely to be with us for years ahead.

Heavy metals

Lead

Lead has been known to be toxic to the fetus for at least 100 years. The United Kingdom Lead Regulations (HMSO 1985a) legislate for a woman of reproductive capacity to be withdrawn from a place of work that exposes her to a specific blood level of lead (40 µg/100 ml) and for pregnant women to be suspended from any work involving exposure to lead. Lead is stored in the bones and may enter the fetus along with calcium mobilised from bone to supply fetal skeletal needs. Exposure to lead in early life affects mental development.

Mercury

Organic mercury was shown to be exceedingly toxic when methyl mercury was discharged into the Minamata Bay area of Japan. The mercury entered the food chain in fish, and Nelson (1971) reported that 6% of all births resulted in children with severe neurological abnormalities resembling cerebral palsy.

Pathogen pollution

Another threat is the release of pathogenic organisms into drinking water or the food chain. A current problem is that of the trend to keep cats indoors with the use of a toilet tray. Owners throw cat excrement down their toilet where it, plus its load of *Toxoplasma gondii*, goes into the sewage system. In 1995 the biggest outbreak of toxoplasmosis in humans was traced to the municipal water supply in British Columbia. In California this resulted in a plague affecting sea otters which died (Syufy 2003).

A second example is that of the food poisoning bacterium *Escherichia coli* O157. Reilly of the Scottish Centre for Infection and Environmental Health (Glasgow) believes a percentage of people have contracted the infection from animal manure near camp sites. He believes that animals should be removed from camp sites and venues for pop festivals at least 3 weeks before the use of the field (Randerson 2002).

Radiation

Radiation can be divided into ionising radiation, such as that emitted by X-rays and nuclear medicine, and by atomic weapons testing, and non-ionising radiation, emitted as ultraviolet and infrared rays and by microwaves. Visual display units are now widely used in both the home and the workplace and release low levels of mixed-wavelength radiation.

Ionising radiation

Ionising radiation damages DNA by transferring its energy into living cells (Moore & Persaud 2008). Atoms lose electrons and develop an electric charge. These charged particles penetrate the body and damage molecules, producing free radicals and oxidising agents which break and destroy DNA. An intense dose can kill cells during their actively dividing state.

Diagnostic X-rays

Because of the known dangers of radiation, X-ray examinations of the abdomen, pelvis or hips of women should only be made during the 10 days of a menstrual period to avoid potentially irradiating an early embryo. Modern shorter-wavelength X-rays are safer (Moore & Persaud 2008) and radiology during pregnancy has been reduced because of the development of ultrasound. Shielding the gonads of both men and women whenever possible during diagnostic X-rays helps to prevent possible damage to ovum and sperm.

Natural radiation

Humans are exposed to low-level natural background radiation. This low-level radiation, stemming mainly from natural γ-radiation from uranium in the ground, may be more dangerous than originally thought. High doses are associated with deaths from anaemia, respiratory infections, diseases of the nervous system and problems at birth.

Risks of atomic bomb and chemical weapons

Radiation may damage actively maturing sperm and ova and the rapidly dividing cells of the fetus. In August 1945, following the dropping of atomic bombs at Hiroshima and Nagasaki in Japan by Americans, fetuses were found to be very sensitive to radiation as many babies born to mothers who had survived were born dead or deformed. The critical exposure time seems to be between 8 and 15 weeks post conception (Moore & Persaud 2008). Instances of leukaemia, lung cancer and thyroid cancer have increased amongst atomic bomb survivors.

Chernobyl

Scherbak (1996) called the Chernobyl nuclear reactor accident in the former Soviet Union in 1986 'the worst technogenic environmental disaster in history'. Hot air carried fission products far more reactive than uranium and plutonium into the atmosphere. Amongst the most dangerous were iodine-131, strontium-90 and caesium-137. One-third of the workers who attempted to contain the explosion have developed sexual or reproductive disorders, including impotence and sperm abnormalities with reduced fertilising capacity. There has also been an increase in the number of complicated pregnancies (Scherbak 1996). Radiation has its worst effect on the DNA of rapidly dividing cells such as spermatozoa, the ovum in late menstrual cycle and the early embryo as well as tissues that divide rapidly such as skin cells and epithelial linings.

Urquhart, a statistician, found statistical evidence for a significant increase in babies born with spina bifida, cleft palate and other abnormalities between 1986 and 1989 in five regions of England, mainly in the north and west of the country. Other regions were not affected and there was a similar pattern for infant deaths (Edwards 2002).

Non-ionising radiation (electromagnetic fields)

Non-ionising rays include ultraviolet, infrared, lasers, microwaves, radar and radiofrequency waves. There are three types of electromagnetic field (Falk 2000):

1. High-frequency electromagnetic fields (microwaves) in microwave ovens and mobile phones.

2. Low-frequency electromagnetic fields around high-voltage power lines and domestic electrical equipment. They are linked to electrical currents when the equipment is turned on.

3. Low-frequency electrical fields around domestic electrical equipment. They depend on voltage and are still emitted when the equipment is turned off as long as it is connected to a power source.

There is currently public anxiety about the incidence of leukaemia linked to electromagnetic fields produced by high-voltage power lines and transformer stations. There is little agreement as to whether electromagnetic fields affect human health: some studies believe there are risks and others that the findings are negative. Some studies have revealed clusters of effects, including increased miscarriages, stillbirths and congenital defects. Interpretation of these studies is complicated by the possible effects of work stress as some of the affected women worked uninterrupted for long periods of time (Falk 2000).

Many people are exposed to visual display units (VDUs) at work and at home. VDUs may release low levels of radiation, including X-rays, microwaves, ultraviolet and infrared light. A conference on the health effects of electromagnetic fields held in Stockholm in 1999 found no evidence of danger to reproductive health from electromagnetic fields. The conference concluded that more research with less emotive content is needed (Falk 2000). Meanwhile, caution is advised: for instance, women should avoid standing directly in front of their microwave ovens when they are switched on.

Chemical weapons

Other agents that have devastating consequences on reproduction as well as disabling effects on the developing fetus are chemical weapons. These have been used in many conflicts during the 20th century, most recently by Iraq against its neighbour country Iran and its own Kurdish people (Evison et al 2002).

Main points

- Research suggests that pregnancy outcome is improved markedly when couples are screened and given preconception advice.

- The continuously produced sperm are most at risk of environmental insult. Ova are in a state of arrested development and are relatively resistant to mutagenic damage until just prior to ovulation. During cleavage

the zygote is resistant to genetic injury but after 16 days a period of intense organogenesis begins and sensitivity is high but so few cells are present that an affected fetus will be aborted.

- Any infections should be treated, dietary problems discussed and possible work and lifestyle hazards considered. Long-term health problems should be stabilised prior to conception. In other conditions that are treated with known teratogenic drugs, possible alteration of treatment may be necessary.

- The age of the prospective parents is important as the frequency of all reproductive problems, including the incidence of chromosome abnormalities, increases with maternal age.
- Prepregnancy weight is known to influence pregnancy outcome. Women who are outside the optimal weight range may develop amenorrhoea and infertility.
- Systemic infections may cause reproductive problems such as infertility and congenital defects. Specific organisms can be prevented by vaccination and advice on avoidance of infection.
- Drugs and alcohol may damage sperm or ova or have an adverse effect on nutrient absorption so that essential nutrients are absent at crucial times during embryonic development. The harmful effects of smoking could be explained partly by differences in nutrient intake.
- The development of the chemical industry has resulted in the release into the environment of vast quantities of synthetic chemicals which may disrupt human reproduction. The heavy metals lead and mercury are exceedingly toxic to the developing nervous system of the fetus and young child.
- Environmental factors are important in gametogenesis and fetal development. It is important to look back over three generations. The ova of today's childbearing women were developed while she was still in her own mother's uterus, as were the numbers of Sertoli cells currently present in the testicles of today's prospective fathers.
- Ionising radiation damages DNA. The critical exposure time may be between 8 and 15 weeks of development. Leukaemia, lung cancer and thyroid cancer have increased among atomic bomb survivors.
- A conference on the health effects of electromagnetic fields found no evidence of danger to reproductive health, although it was concluded that more research is needed. Meanwhile, caution is advised.
- Other agents that affect reproduction and have disabling effects on developing fetus are chemical weapons. These have been used in many conflicts during the 20th century, most recently by Iraq during the Iran–Iraq war.

References

ACOG (2008). Tobacco, Alcohol, Drugs and Pregnancy. Patient Education Pamphlet. www.acog.org/publications/patient_education/bp170.cfm. Accessed June 2008.

Alsopp, M., Santillo, D., Kallee, U., Hojsík, M. (2006). Our reproductive health and chemical exposure. Greenpeace Research Laboratories Technical Note 02/2006. Greenpeace International.

Ashton K., Green E. S. 2008 The Toxic Consumer: Living Healthily in a Hazardous World. Sterling, New York.

Barker, D.J.P. (Ed.), 1992. Fetal and Infant Origins of Adult Disease. BMJ Books, London.

Barker, D.J.P., 2003. The Best Start in Life. Century.

Barnes, B., 2007. Preparing for Pregnancy: The Foresight programme. Neal's Yard Press.

Best, J.M., O'Shea, S., Tipples, G., et al., 2002. Interpretation of rubella serology in pregnancy: pitfalls and problems. Br. Med. J. 325, 147–148.

Blair, P.S., Fleming, P.J., Bensley, D., et al., 1996. Smoking and the sudden infant death syndrome: results from 1993–5 case-control study for confidential inquiry into stillbirths and deaths in infancy. Br. Med. J. 313, 195–198.

Byrne, C.D., Wild, S.H., 2005. The Metabolic Syndrome. Wiley, Chichester.

Carlsen, E., Giwercman, A., Keiding, N., Skakkebaek, N., 1992. Evidence for decreasing quality of semen during the past 50 years. Br. Med. J. 305, 609–613.

Chamberlain, G., 1992. ABC of Antenatal Care. BMJ, London.

Chapple, J., 2007. Preconception care (National Knowledge Week). Screen. Spec. Libr.

Cohen, P., 2002. Pollution triggers genetic defects. New Sci. 176 (2373), 8.

Colborn, T., Patterson, J.P., Dumanoski, D., 1996. Our Stolen Future. Little, Brown, Boston.

Confidential Enquiry into Maternal and Child Health (CEMACH), 2007. Diabetes in pregnancy. Are we providing the best care? Find. Nat. Enquiry 6.

Conter, V., Cortinovis, I., Rogari, P., Riva, L., 1995. Weight growth in infants born to mothers who smoked during pregnancy. Br. Med. J. 310, 768–771.

Department of Health (DOH) 1993 Pregnancy, folic acid and you. Heywood: Health Publication Unit. National Dairy Council, Nutrition Service, Maternal and Fetal Nutrition, fact file number 11.

Dick, M. 2006. Sickle cell diseases in childhood: Standards and guideline for clinical care. NHS Antenatal and Newborn Screening Programmes. Published by UK NHS Sickle Cell and Thalassaemia Screening Programme in partnership with the Sickle Cell Society. Accessed on 20.6.08. Available from: http://www.sickleandthal.org.uk/Documents/ClinicalStandardsSummaryOctober2006.pdf.

Edwards, R., 2002. Are hundreds of British baby deaths and defects down to Chernobyl? New Sci. 174 (2349), 6.

Evans, H.J., Fletcher, J., Torrance, M., Hardgreave, T.B., 1981. Sperm abnormalities and cigarette smoking. Lancet i, 627–629.

Evison, D., Hinsley, D., Rice, P., 2002. Chemical weapons. Br. Med. J. 324, 332–335.

Falk R 2000 Health effects of electromagnetic fields. www.niwl.se/wl2000/workshop36article_en.asp.

Flaxman, S.M., Sherman, P.W., 2008. Morning sickness: an adaptive cause or nonadaptive consequence of embryo viability? Am. Nat. 172 (1), 54–62.

Foresight: the Association for Preconceptual Care 2008 www.foresight-preconception.org.uk.

Giwercman, A., Rylander, L., Lundberg, GiwercmanY., 2007. Influence of endocrine disruptors on human male fertility. Reprod. Biomed. 15 (6), 633–642.

HMSO, 1985a. Control of Lead at Work Regulations 1980: Approved Code of Practice—Control of Lead at Work. HMSO, London.

Jick, H., Porter, J., Morrison, A.S., 1977. Relation between smoking and age of natural menopause. Lancet i, 1354–1355.

Johns, T., 1990. With Bitter Herbs They Shall Eat It. University of Arizona Press, Tucson.

Jones, S., 2003. Y: The Descent of Man. Little, Brown, Boston.

Korenbrot, C.C., Steinberg, A., Bender, C., Newberry, S., 2002. Preconception care: a systematic review. Matern. Child Health J. 6 (2), 75–88.

Martinez-Frias, M.L., Salvador, J., 1990. Epidemiological aspects of prenatal exposure to high doses of vitamin A in Spain. Eur. J. Epidemiol. 6, 118–123.

Moore, K.L., Persaud, T.V.N., 2008. The Developing Human, eighth edn. W B Saunders, Philadelphia.

National Dairy Council 1994 Nutrition Service, Maternal and Fetal Nutrition, fact file number 11.

Nelson, N., 1971. Hazards of mercury. Environ. Res. 4, 1–69.

Profet, M., 1992. Pregnancy sickness as adaptation: a deterrent to maternal ingestion of teratogens. In: Barkow, J., Cosmides, L., Tooby, J. (Eds.) The Adapted Mind: Evolutionary Psychology and the Generation of Culture. Oxford University Press, New York, pp. 327–365.

Randerson, J., 2002. Go easy on the manure. New Scientist 175 (2361), 11.

Ray, J.G., O'Brien, T.E., Chan, W.S., 2001. Preconception care and the risk of congenital anomalies in the offspring of women with diabetes mellitus: a meta-analysis. Monthly Journal of the Association of Physicians (QJM) 94 (8), 435–444.

Scherbak, Y.M., 1996. Ten years of the Chernobyl era. Scientific American 1274 (4), 32–37.

Schorah, C.J., Smithells, R.W., 1991. Maternal vitamin nutrition and malformations of the neural tube. Nutr. Res. Rev. 4, 33–49.

Sharpe, R., Skakkebaek, N., 1993. Are oestrogens involved in falling sperm counts and disorders of the male reproductive tract? Lancet 341, 1392–1395.

Smith, N.C., 1992. Detection of the fetus at risk. Eur. J. Clin. Nutr. 46 (Suppl 1), S1–S5.

Smith, O.B., Akinbamijo, O.O., 2000. Micronutrients and reproduction in farm animals. Anim. Reprod. Sci. 60/61, 549–560.

Soltan, M.H., Jenkins, D.M., 1982. Maternal and fetal plasma zinc concentration and fetal abnormality. Br. J. Obstet. Gynaecol. 89, 56–58.

Soltani, H., Fraser, R.B., 2000. A longitudinal study of maternal anthropometric changes in normal weight, overweight and obese women during pregnancy and postpartum. Br. J. Nutr. 84, 95–101.

Soto, A., Justicia, H., Wray, J., Sonnenschein, C., 1991. p-Nonylphenol: an estrogenic xenobiotic released from 'modified polystyrene'. Environ. Health Perspect. 92, 167–173.

Sumpter, J., Jobling, S., 1995. Vitellogenesis as a biomarker for oestrogen contamination of the aquatic environment. Proceedings of the Estrogens in the Environment Conference, Environmental Health Perspectives Supplements.

Syufy F 2003 Sea otters and cat feces. http://cats.about.com/cs/parasiticdisease/a/seaotters.htm.

Wakefield, J., 2002. Boys won't be boys. New Sci. 174 (2349), 42–45.

Wharton, B.A., 1992. Food and biological clocks. Proc. Nutr. Soc. 51, 145–153.

Wolfe, H., 1998. High prepregnancy body mass index: a maternal fetal risk factor. N. Engl. J. Med. 338, 191.

Annotated recommended reading

Colborn, T., Myers, J.P., Dumanoski, D., 1996. Our Stolen Future. Little, Brown, Boston.

If you are anxious about the impact the modern chemical industry has on human reproductive health this seminal book gives an excellent overview that has not been bettered since.

Falk, R. 2000. Health effects of electromagnetic fields. www.niwl.se/wl2000/workshop36article_en.asp.

This summary of a workshop on electromagnetic fields and their effect on health provides an overview of the current research areas on issues affecting reproductive and general health.

Moore, K.L., Persaud, T.V.N., 2008. The Developing Human, eighth edn. W B Saunders, Philadelphia.

This up-to-date embryology textbook has a very good chapter on congenital anatomical anomalies with a section on the importance of environmental factors and another on multifactorial inheritance.

Schettler, T., Solomon, G., Valenti, M., Huddle, A., 2000. Generations at risk: Reproductive Health and the Environment. MIT Press, Boston.

This book is recommended to interested readers. It is a source book on human exposure to toxic chemicals that can have reproduction and development effects.

Wakefield, J., 2002. Boys won't be boys. New Sci. 174 (2349), 42–45.

This article provides a sensible and easy-to-understand update on the research into environmental pollution and problems of human reproduction.

Section 2A

Pregnancy—The Fetus

SECTION CONTENTS

The care of the childbearing woman includes complex screening tests for fetal well-being. The midwife must have knowledge and experience of these procedures in order to inform her clients. This section is concerned with the development and growth of the fetus, placenta and membranes. The topic is presented in some detail because developments in the treatment of infertility and in the detection and management of fetal abnormalities are expanding rapidly. The writing style has been made as easy to follow as possible and the diagrams should clarify three-dimensional concepts. Chapter 9 discusses general points about embryological development, Chapters 10 and 11 look in detail at the development of individual systems, and Chapter 12 examines that important fetal organ, the placenta and membranes, and the nature of amniotic fluid. Chapter 13 explores fetal growth and development while Chapter 14 discusses some common fetal problems. Finally, the very important topic of the causes, diagnosis and management of common congenital defects is discussed in Chapter 15.

Chapter Nine

General embryology

Introduction

This section of the book is about the developmental processes that take the human from one fertilised egg to a fetus ready to be born. In this chapter the general principles of embryology are outlined.

Embryology

Discoveries about the development of the human embryo are gained by research into the development of other species because of the problem of unethical human experimentation (The Human Fertilisation and Embryology Act 1990). There are surprising similarities in the basic machinery of development between species which involves cell division and differentiation, pattern formation, change in form and growth (Wolpert et al 2007).

The study of embryology enables us to understand the causes of congenital abnormalities, which are present in about 6% of live births, of which half are detected at birth and half during the first year of life. At least half of all conceptuses are malformed but are usually aborted spontaneously (Moore & Persaud 2008).

Gametogenesis

Following fertilisation of an ovum by a sperm the resulting zygote regains its full complement of 46 chromosomes. **Gametogenesis** is the formation of the sperm and ova. The primary spermatocytes and primary oocytes are diploid cells, having 46 chromosomes. **Meiosis** results in reduction of chromosomes to the **haploid** 23 found in the mature sperm and ovum (Fig. 9.1). Also independent assortment of maternal and paternal chromosomes amongst the gametes and crossing over between homologues of segments of the maternal and paternal chromosomes occurs (Ch. 3). This recombination of genetic material ensures that each gamete is

Normal gametogenesis

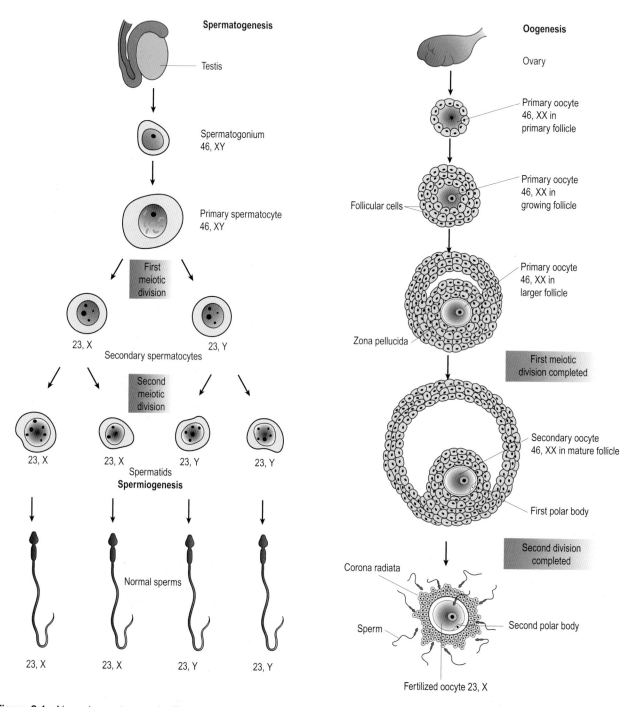

Figure 9.1 • Normal gametogenesis. (Reproduced with permission from Moore 1989.)

a mixture of maternal and paternal genes as is the new zygote.

Oogenesis

Primary **oocytes** are present in a female ovary before birth. **Oogenesis** or the process of transforming oocytes into ova begins before a woman's birth but is not completed until after puberty. By the time a girl is born her **primary oocytes** have undergone the prophase of meiosis. Just before ovulation a surge of follicle-stimulating hormone (FSH) and luteinising hormone (LH) results in maturation of the ovum (Fig. 9.2) and the first meiotic division is completed (Fig. 9.3).

The process results in the formation of a **secondary oocyte** which receives most of the cytoplasm and a non-functional cell called the first **polar body**. The secondary oocyte receives 23 chromosomes, including an X chromosome, and the first polar body receives the other 23 chromosomes. At ovulation the secondary oocyte begins the second meiotic division but becomes arrested in metaphase (Fig. 9.4). If penetrated by a sperm, this division completes and one mature ovum

with a second polar body results. These polar bodies degenerate (Schoenwolf et al 2008).

Spermatogenesis

Spermatozoa are produced in the seminiferous tubules of the testes (Ch. 5). **Primary spermatocytes** begin to increase in number from puberty. In a functioning testis germ cells are present at various stages of development, all originating from **spermatogonia** which divide continuously by mitosis to ensure a constant supply of cells. Spermatogonia divide and grow to become primary spermatocytes, which are diploid cells with 46 chromosomes.

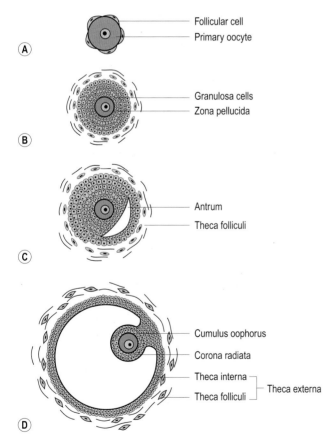

Figure 9.2 • The stages of development in the follicle: (A) primordial follicle, (B) primary follicle, (C) secondary follicle, (D) Graafian follicle. (From Hinchliff S M, Montague S E 1990, with permission.)

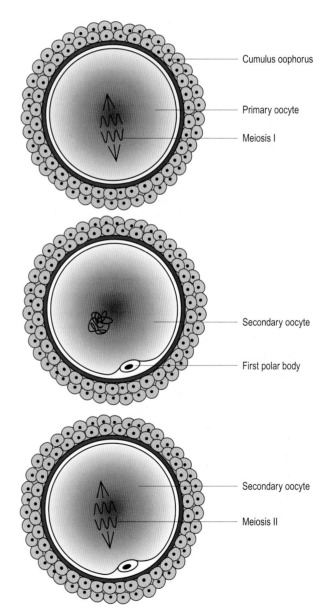

Figure 9.3 • Events within the zona pellucida prior to ovulation. (From Fitzgerald M J T, Fitzgerald M 1994, with permission.)

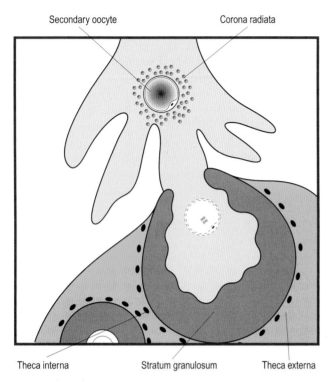

Figure 9.4 • Ovulation. (From Fitzgerald M J T, Fitzgerald M 1994, with permission.)

These undergo the first meiotic division to form two **secondary spermatocytes** which have only 23 chromosomes. Half receive an X chromosome and half a Y chromosome. Secondary meiosis results in four haploid **spermatids** found in close association with the Sertoli cells which provide nutrition and support. The spermatids are transformed into mature **spermatozoa** (Fig. 9.5).

As a sperm matures, excess protoplasm is lost and the nuclear chromatin condenses to become the head of the sperm. One centriole develops into the tail which is composed of a central filament of two microfibrils surrounded by a circle of nine fibrils. Mitochondria aggregate in the neck region and the Golgi apparatus helps to form the **acrosome cap** which develops over the head of the sperm and contains enzymes called hyaluronidases and proteases (Fig. 9.6).

Gamete size

The oocyte is a very large cell, just visible to the unaided eye and usually only one is released at ovulation. It contains all the material necessary for early embryonic growth and development. In sharp contrast, the mature sperm has lost most of its cytoplasm, is very small and millions are released at ejaculation. About 1000 sperm will reach the oocyte and these will all be needed to allow just one to enter to form a diploid zygote, the first cell of a unique human being.

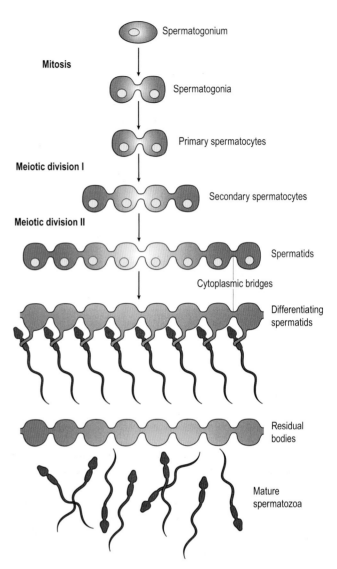

Figure 9.5 • The progeny of a single maturing spermatogonium remain connected to one another by cytoplasmic bridges throughout their differentiation into mature sperm. (Reproduced with permission from Alberts et al 1994.)

Fertilisation

Capacitation

Freshly ejaculated sperm are unable to fertilise an ovum and have to undergo a process of maturation called **capacitation**. The sperm have to penetrate several physical barriers before entering the ovum. While travelling through the female genital tract, usually in the uterus or uterine tubes, glycoproteins are removed from the surface of the acrosome cap. When a capacitated sperm meets the corona radiata of the oocyte the acrosome develops perforations in it and the contents of the acrosomal vesicle are released. This is known as the **acrosome reaction**.

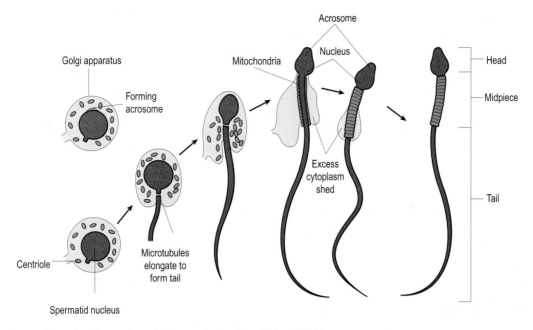

Figure 9.6 • Sperm formation. (Reproduced with permission from Chiras 1991.)

The acrosome reaction

Binding of a sperm of the oocyte's zona pellucida is species-specific. Lytic (digestive) enzymes such as hyaluronidases are released around the oocyte and digest the first physical barrier of cumulus cells embedded in sticky hyaluronic acid. It takes enzymes from many sperm to allow one sperm to enter. These enzymes disperse the corona radiata follicular cells, allowing the head of one sperm to make contact with the zona pellucida. Other enzymes such as acrosin, which produce an opening in the zona pellucida, are released (Wolpert et al 2007). The sperm cell membrane and the sperm nucleus pass into the ovum (Fig. 9.7).

Blocks to polyspermy

Two mechanisms prevent **polyspermy** (the entry of multiple sperm) immediately following the entry of the first sperm, ensuring that the fertilised ovum only contains 46 chromosomes (Fig. 9.8).

- **Fast block**—The electrical resting potential of the oocyte plasma membrane is normally negatively charged at −70 millivolts (mV), at which sperm can readily fuse with the membrane. Immediately after sperm entry sodium channels open in the cell membrane and extra positively charged sodium ions are allowed into the cytoplasm of the ovum. This changes the charge to a positive +20 mV which prevents other sperm from entering. This is a brief reaction and the resting potential soon returns to −70 mV.
- **Slow bock** (cortical reaction)—The brief depolarisation has two other effects. First it allows subcortical granules

lying just under the oocyte's plasma membrane to rupture and release chemicals which bind water into the cytoplasm. The ovum swells and detaches any remaining sperm in contact with it. Secondly, the secondary oocytes are activated to complete the secondary meiotic division and expel the second polar body and the ovum is now mature. Its nucleus is now called the **female pronucleus**. Once the head of the sperm enters the cytoplasm of the ovum its head enlarges to form the **male pronucleus**. The male and female pronuclei fuse and paternal and maternal chromosomes intermingle.

Mitochondrial deoxyribonucleic acid (MtDNA)

The energy-producing mitochondria (Ch. 3) are all inherited from the ovum because sperm mitochondria used in motility are shed with the tail and do not enter the oocyte. In humans MtDNA is circular and very compact, being one of the smallest known in the animal kingdom (Lane 2005).

Results of fertilisation

- The number of chromosomes is restored to the diploid 23 pairs or 46 chromosomes.
- The new individual inherits a unique set of genes from its parents.
- Sex determination occurs.
- Initiation of cleavage stimulates the zygote to begin mitotic cell division.

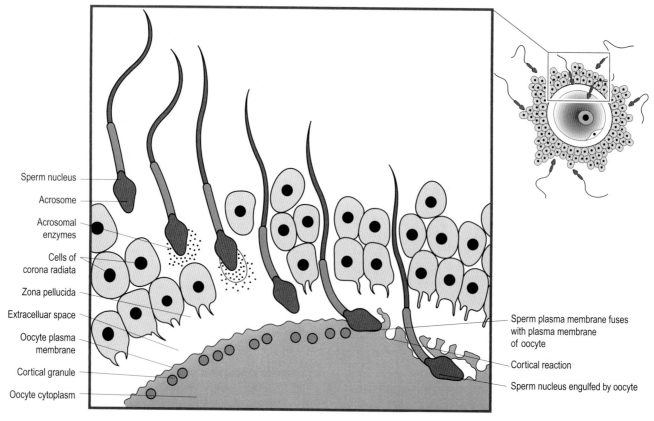

Figure 9.7 • Fertilisation and cortical reaction. (Reproduced with permission from Chiras 1991.)

The embryo

Terminology

The term **conceptus** refers to the products of fertilisation and comprises the embryo with its supporting tissues (adnexi). The developmental process is divided into discrete sections of time. The **preimplantation period** is the time between fertilisation and implantation and lasts about 6 days. The conceptus is called an **embryo** from implantation until the end of the 8th week after fertilisation when it becomes known as a **fetus**. The size of the embryo is expressed as the **crown–rump length**, from the crown of the head to the terminal part of the caudal end. In the fetus, the standing length from crown to heel is used.

General concepts used in embryology

How does one cell develop into millions with hundreds of variations? What instructions does the cell use and what processes carry out the instructions? There are three important concepts towards understanding embryology:

1. A programme of simple instructions can generate complex forms.

2. Most developmental processes depend upon interaction between genetic and environmental factors.

3. Each body system has its own developmental pattern.

Programming the embryo

The information to make an embryo is located in the DNA of the zygote. Although the sperm and ovum contribute 23 chromosomes each, it is the ovum that contributes the organelles and MtDNA. Regulatory genes control development by influencing where and when proteins are made. Developmental processes include (Wolpert et al 2007):

* Pattern formation.
* Differentiation.
* Morphogenesis.
* Development of the germ layers.
* Growth.

Pattern formation

Cells in the embryo seem to 'know' where and when to change shape and position and cell movements are part

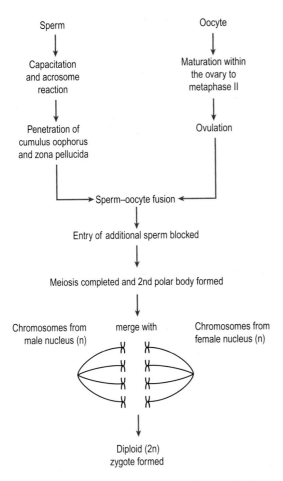

Figure 9.8 • Events in the female reproductive tract leading up to fertilisation. (From Hinchliff S M, Montague S E 1990, with permission.)

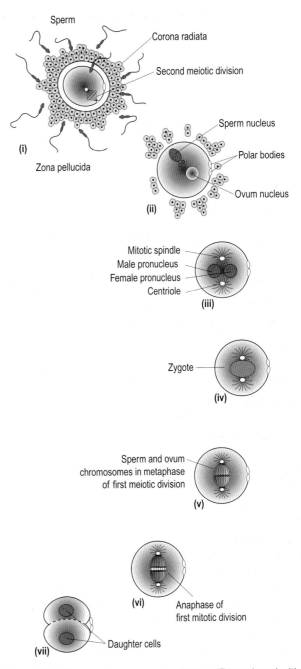

Figure 9.9 • The zygote prepares for division. (Reproduced with permission from Chiras 1991.)

of the embryo's developmental programme. Wolpert (1991) described this as a set of instructions not for describing the final form, but for creating shapes. Consider knitting: the pattern is the code or instruction manual but does not resemble the final article. The knitter must interpret the code and apply energy, order and control and a variety of stitches.

Cellular processes include:

• Somatic cell division where daughter cells receive identical genetic information.
• Cell differentiation to make up the different embryological tissues.
• Induction: cell interaction where one type of cell influences another.
• Migration of cells.
• Programmed cell death to remove redundant cells.

Early cell division—cleavage

Early in pregnancy growth and development are very similar in any human embryo. The exact days when embryonic features develop can be given. Days of development are counted from the moment of fertilisation. Within 24 h the large zygote undergoes mitosis and splits into smaller cells (Fig. 9.9). This is called **cleavage** and the daughter cells are called **blastomeres**. There is synthesis of new DNA but no increase in the amount of cytoplasm so the size of the blastomeres diminishes with each cleavage (Moore & Persaud 2008). The zygote continues its journey down the uterine tube and by the fourth day there are between 16 and 20 cells. Compaction occurs, probably because of cell surface adhesion glycoproteins. The embryo is now called a **morula** (Fig. 9.10). The cells are still totipotent and could contribute to any part of the embryo or even split to form identical fetuses.

Differentiation

In the early embryo there is little cellular difference except in the shape of the cells and they are not specialised. Humans have about 350 different cell types whereas some simpler animals may have only 20 cell types (Wolpert 1991).

Essential proteins

Animals, including humans, appear to have a set of key genes to make proteins from which to construct their bodies. Recognisable versions of human genes were already present in a common ancestor of many species. The embryo builds up different tissue types by combining proteins, of which there are two important classes:

1. **Transmembrane proteins** needed for **cell adhesion** and **cell signalling.**

2. **Gene regulatory proteins.**

Development is led by cell–cell interactions and by differential gene expression. What type of cell develops depends on which path it takes as it migrates. These pathways represent gene activity and are selected depending on extracellular signals (Alberts et al 2008).

Cell–cell interactions

A handful of genetically controlled evolutionary cell–cell signals are used by many organisms to cause cells to differentiate to form a complex multicellular individual. All these signals are genetically controlled:

- Sister cells may differ as a result of asymmetrical cell division.
- Sister cells may compete with each other and inhibit the development of those next to them (lateral inhibition).
- A group of similar cells may be exposed to different signals, called **morphogens**, from outside the group.

Morphogenesis

Regulatory genes

Cells in different parts of the embryo change shape and function to carry out their developing roles. Genes in the cell nuclei interact with environmental factors to bring

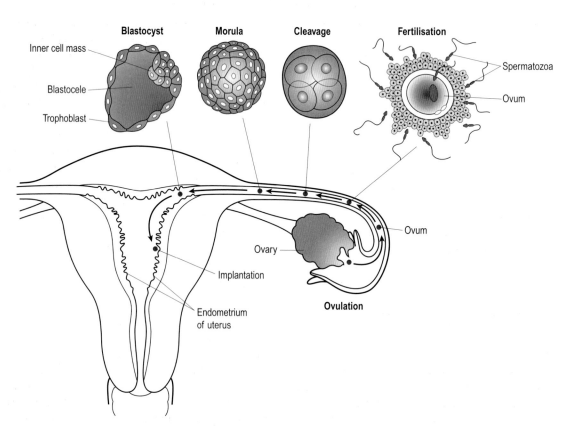

Figure 9.10 • Fertilisation and early embryonic development. (Reproduced with permission from Chiras 1991.)

about this huge variety in cell types making up tissues and organs. Eggs and embryos show **polarity**, which means one end is distinguishable from the other even before organised development has begun. One gene can be mentioned by name for interest and to illustrate the quirkiness of geneticists when naming genes. This is **sonic hedgehog**, so called because it was first found in relation to bristle formation on the thorax of the fruit fly *Drosophila*. Sonic secretes a signal involved in patterning cell migration and differentiation of many cell types of many species (Moore & Persaud 2008).

All vertebrates have a similar basic **body plan** with a segmented vertebral column and the brain at the anterior end. These structures mark the **anteroposterior axis**, i.e. an axis running from head to tail. The vertebrate body also has a distinct **dorsoventral axis** (back to belly) with the mouth on the ventral side. These two axes define the left and right sides with the internal organs such as heart and liver being asymmetrically arranged. There are signalling centres which influence how both nearby cells or cells at a greater distance develop (Wolpert et al 2007).

Finally, although vertebrates are bilaterally symmetrical for many structures such as eyes, ears and limbs, the right to left symmetry is broken to allow differentiation of the internal organs such as the heart, spleen and liver. This left to right specification is different from the other two axes and only develops after they have been set.

Something in the embryonic environment turns on **developmental genes** which control how cells divide, multiply and move around the embryo. Regulatory genes control patterning in the embryo by a cascade of these gene products. The most important discovery was of a discrete portion of DNA with a specific order of genes present in most animals called the **homeobox** (Moore & Persaud 2008).

The homeobox

Genes control **segmentation** in the developing embryo so that the correct positioning of organs occurs. These genes are referred to as **HOM genes** in invertebrates and **Hox genes** in vertebrates, including humans (Carlson 2004). Different homeobox genes are switched on in the order they are positioned in the Hox complex to produce different protein products (Alberts et al 2008, Wolpert et al 2007). These subdivide the embryo into discrete **homeodomains** prior to differentiation into specific tissue types, organs and systems.

Morphogens

Homeobox genes may be switched on sequentially by **chemical gradients**. Cytoplasm with special genetic properties is located at the ends of the zygote. This cytoplasm produces substances that govern the pattern of tissue development. These are called **morphogens** and they spread from a localised source to form a concentration gradient across a developing tissue, activating other genes when they reach specific concentrations. Nusslein-Volhard (1996) writes about *Drosophila* (fruit fly): 'Cells in a developing field respond to a special substance—a morphogen—the concentration of which gradually increases in a certain direction, forming a gradient'.

Induction

Hans Spemann won the only Nobel Prize awarded for embryology for discovering what organises the embryo's development. He demonstrated that a nervous system will only develop if future muscle and adjacent cells move from the outside of the embryo to a situation underneath the outer layer. These migrated cells produce a signal that causes the overlying sheet of cells to develop into a nervous system. This cellular movement is said to induce the development of the nervous system. The influencing tissues are called **inductors** or organisers. The inductor needs to be near but not necessarily in contact with the tissue to be induced. It is generally accepted that some signal passes from inductor to induced tissue. There needs to be a sufficiently large community of cells for induction to occur. This is referred to as the **community effect**.

Cell communication

Cells communicate with each other in different ways. In some tissues the inductor may be a **diffusible molecule** passing directly from one tissue to another. In other tissues the message is mediated by an **extracellular matrix** (ECM) secreted by the inductor and which comes into contact with the reacting tissue. The ECM is a network of mesodermal cells which provides pathways for cells to crawl along and their chemical products appear and disappear in the ECM. Some tissues react to **direct physical contact** between the inducing and reacting tissues (Moore & Persaud 2008) and cells receive cues from their neighbours about where they should be and how they should behave. **Tissue-specific proteins** create cell recognition and accumulation. The originators of a group of cells may specify where it travels to and the tissue it forms.

Programmed cell death

Programmed cell death or **apoptosis** (Greek for shedding leaves) plays a major part in the final pattern of cells, especially in the formation of body cavities (Wolpert et al 2007). It is controlled by mitochondrial gene products (Lane 2005). Cells in some tissues are overproduced and those that are not needed commit suicide (Alberts et al 2008). Cell death is a normal feature of the development of the nervous system, limbs, skeleton and heart as the following examples explain:

- In limb formation, cell death helps to achieve the final shape, such as the disappearance of webbing between the fingers.
- In the developing brain and nervous system over 50% too many axons arrive at target cells. The first to arrive make the best connections and send signals back in the form of nerve growth factor (NGF) which sustains neurons. There is no room for new arrivals which cannot obtain nourishment and die.
- Too many cells are made in the development of tubes such as blood vessels and the tube is hollowed out by cell death.

Development of the embryo

The blastocyst

The group of cells continues cleaving for the first 4 days. The first three cleavages are synchronous but later cleavages are asymmetrical. There is also polarisation, with internal cells differing from external cells. The inner cells divide less frequently and remain large and round, whereas the outer cells in contact with the zona pellucida become flattened. At this point the cells lose their **totipotency** and begin to differentiate. They are destined to become specific parts of the embryo.

On the 5th day the zona pellucida is digested by uterine secretions and the embryo 'hatches'. Fluid accumulates in the space between the peripheral and central cells of the morula and it becomes the hollow **blastocyst**. The inner cell mass of the blastocyst is the **embryoblast** and will become the embryo. The flattened outer cells are called the **trophoblast** and will form the placenta.

Implantation

On the 6th day the embryoblast begins to implant into the endometrium, most commonly on the posterior wall of the uterus. Where the trophoblastic cells make contact with the endometrium they undergo rapid DNA synthesis and become cuboid in shape to form the cytotrophoblast. The daughter cells shed their plasma membranes to form a mass of protoplasm with nuclei and organelles called a **syncytium**. The mass of tissue is called the **syncytiotrophoblast** (Fig. 9.11), which produces enzymes that attack the endometrium and hormones that allow the pregnancy to continue.

The effects of enzymatic erosion

As the enzymes erode the endometrium, the uterine glands release their content to nourish the embryo and the blastocyst begins to enlarge. Nutrition is also provided by the stroma cells which undergo changes known as the **decidual reaction** and become swollen with glycogen and lipid. The change commences at the implantation site and spreads within a few days throughout the whole endometrium except for the lining of the cervix. The endometrium is now known as the **decidua**.

At the implantation site new blood capillaries fed by branches of the spiral arteries and drained by the endometrial veins develop and dilate (Fig. 9.12). The conceptus is completely embedded in the compact layer of the endometrium by the 12th day and is covered by the overlying uterine epithelium. Erosion of these sinuses results in maternal blood entering the syncytiotrophoblast to collect in a labyrinth of little pockets called **lacunae**. **Human chorionic gonadotrophin** (hCG) is secreted into the lacunae by the trophoblast, enters the maternal circulation and maintains the corpus luteum. This ensures the continued production of oestrogen and progesterone for maintenance of the pregnancy until the placenta produces sufficient at 12 weeks.

Development of the germ layers

The bilaminar embryonic disc

The following descriptions should be studied with the accompanying diagrams, remembering that they are two-dimensional sections through a three-dimensional embryo. By the 2nd week of development the cells are well organised and the inner cell mass forms a flattened disc consisting of two layers known as the **bilaminar embryonic disc** (Fig. 9.13). The inner layer or **epiblast** is composed of tall columnar epithelium and the outer layer or **hypoblast** is composed of low cuboidal epithelium.

The margins of the epiblast create a thin epithelial layer, the **amnion**, and the epiblast and amnion form the amniotic sac. The sac grows more rapidly than the embryo and comes to surround the embryo. The cell margins of the hypoblast also divide rapidly to form branched cells that line the cavity of the blastocyst. This lining is called the **extraembryonic mesoderm**. Spaces develop within the mesoderm and coalesce to become the **extraembryonic coelom** (coelom means cavity).

This cavity splits the mesoderm into a **visceral layer** which is included in the **umbilical vesicle** formerly known as the **yolk sac** (Fig. 9.14) but renamed as it contains no yolk (Moore & Persaud 2008), and a **parietal layer**, which contributes to the **chorion** together with the trophoblast. The visceral and parietal extraembryonic mesoderms are linked by a **connecting stalk** that develops into the

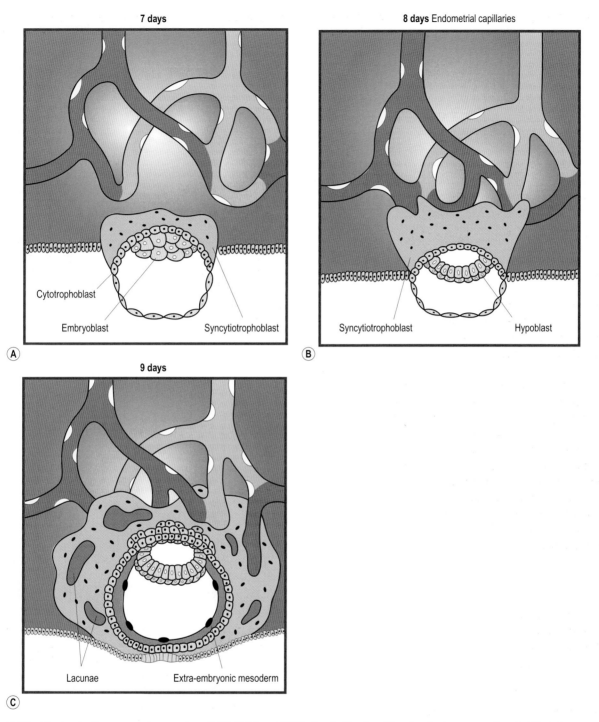

7 days

Cytotrophoblast

Embryoblast   Syncytiotrophoblast

(A)

8 days Endometrial capillaries

Syncytiotrophoblast   Hypoblast

(B)

9 days

Lacunae   Extra-embryonic mesoderm

(C)

Figure 9.11 • The implanting conceptus on days 7 (A), 8 (B) and 9 (C) after fertilisation. The developing conceptus rapidly makes contact with endometrial capillary loops (uterine glands are not represented). (From Fitzgerald M J T, Fitzgerald M 1994, with permission.)

umbilical cord. Towards the end of the 2nd week the flattened disc becomes ovoid. The cranial (head end) part of the hypoblast thickens to form the **prechordal plate**, the future site of the mouth and an important organiser of the head region (Moore & Persaud 2008).

The trilaminar embryo

During **embryogenesis** cells migrate through the embryo, differentiating into specific cell types to form organs and systems. The formation of the **primitive**

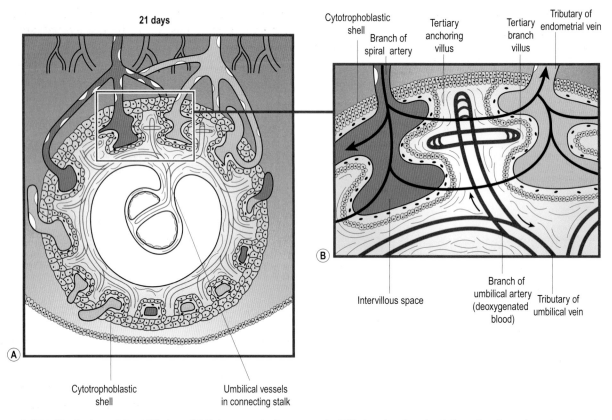

Figure 9.12 • Chorionic vesicle at 21 days. (B) Enlargement of upper part of (A) showing the circulation of embryonic and maternal blood. (From Fitzgerald M J T, Fitzgerald M 1994, with permission.)

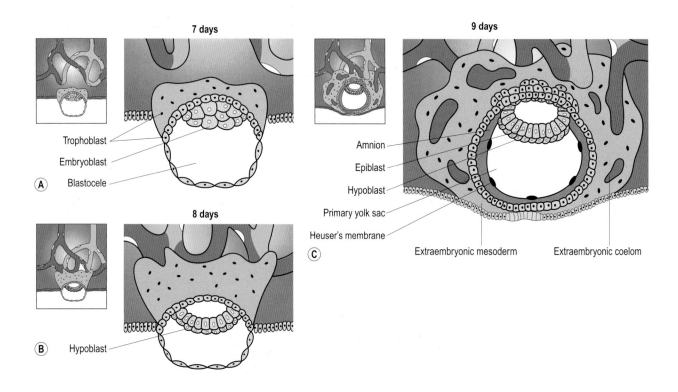

Figure 9.13 • (A–C) Early steps in differentiation of the blastocyst. (From Fitzgerald M J T, Fitzgerald M 1994, with permission.)

streak, **gastrulation** and formation of the **notochord** are important in creating the body plan (Figs. 9.15, 9.16). They will be described separately although they occur simultaneously and are interlinked in the embryo.

The primitive streak

At the beginning of the 3rd week a thick linear band of embryonic epiblast appears caudally (towards the rear) in the dorsal aspect of the embryonic disc. This primitive streak results from epiblastic cells heaping up

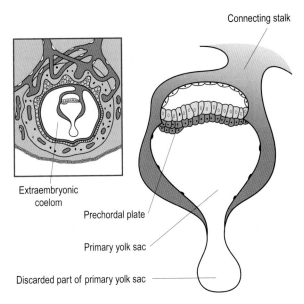

Figure 9.14 • Prechordial plate, connecting stalk and reduction of primary yolk sac. (From Fitzgerald M J T, Fitzgerald M 1994, with permission.)

and migrating to the centre of the embryonic disc. It is the site of enormous cell activity when the first wave of migration forms the middle layer of the embryo and the basic body plan is laid down with cranial and caudal ends. The primitive streak elongates by adding cells to its caudal end and the cranial end enlarges to form a **primitive node** (Fig. 9.17).

The primitive streak continues to form mesodermal cells until the end of the 4th week, by which time it has retreated to the caudal end of the embryo. If it persists it can give rise to a multitissued tumour called a **sacral teratoma**. Embryonic mesodermal cells migrate in three directions: laterally to the margins of the embryonic disc, cranially alongside the notochord and caudally around the cloacal membrane (see below).

Gastrulation

Wolpert (1991) wrote 'It is not birth, marriage or death, but gastrulation which is the truly important event in your life'. **Gastrulation** is a process of invagination by which the inner cell mass becomes the trilaminar embryo. It begins in the 1st week with the formation of the hypoblast, continues during the 2nd week with the formation of the epiblast and is completed during the 3rd week. It ends when the three primary germ layers of **ectoderm, mesoderm** and **endoderm** are in situ and the embryo is a trilaminar disc. A human is just a complex elaboration of these three layers.

Epiblastic cells dip through the primitive streak and spread laterally beneath it. At this time movement is occurring simultaneously over many parts of the embryo. Sheets of cells stream past each other contracting and expanding. Some of the cells displace the

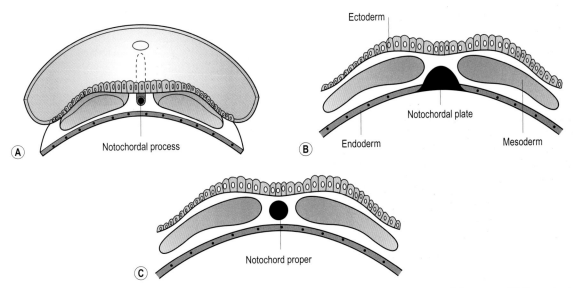

Figure 9.15 • Transverse sections taken rostral to the primitive node, showing (A) the hollow notochordal process, (B) the notochordal plate fused with the endoderm, (C) the notochord proper. (From Fitzgerald M J T, Fitzgerald M 1994, with permission.)

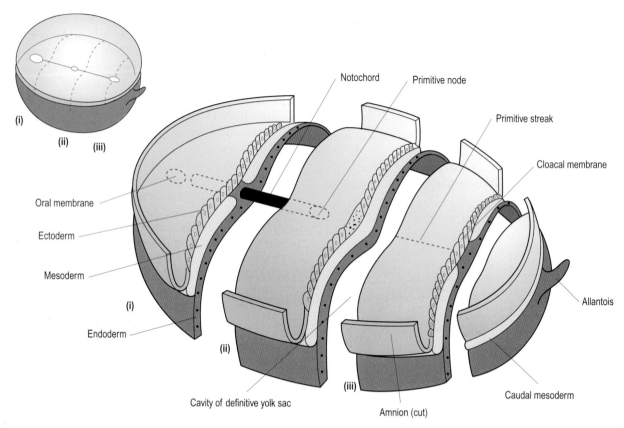

Figure 9.16 • Stereosections of the trilaminar embryonic disc, viewed obliquely from above. (From Fitzgerald M J T, Fitzgerald M 1994, with permission.)

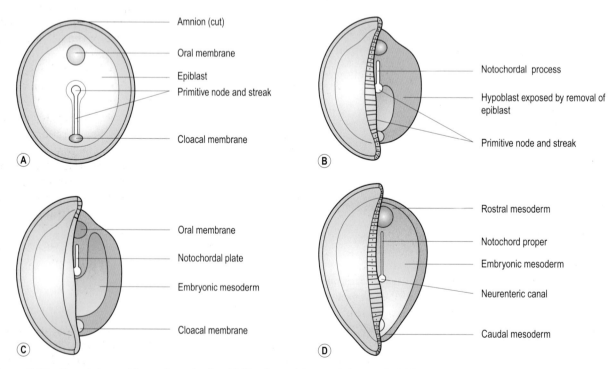

Figure 9.17 • Dorsal views of the embryonic disc. (A) The floor of the amniotic sac. (B–D) The epiblast has been removed from the right side to show migration of the embryonic mesoderm over the surface of the hypoblast. (From Fitzgerald M J T, Fitzgerald M 1994, with permission.)

underlying hypoblast to form the embryonic endoderm, whilst the rest form the embryonic mesoderm or **mesenchyme**. Epiblastic cells that remain on the surface form embryonic ectoderm. The endoderm migrates inside the wall of the umbilical vesicle and a finger of the umbilical vesicle becomes pinched off and extends into the connecting stalk to form the allantois.

Development of body cavities

Late in the 2nd week fluid-filled spaces appear in the cranial half of the embryonic mesoderm. These coalesce during the 3rd week to form the 'U'-shaped **embryonic coelom**. The bend of the U at the cranial end forms the **pericardial coelom**. This is divided by the **septum transversum** from the caudal two arms of the U which form the **pericardioperitoneal canals** (pleural canals) leading to two branches of the **peritoneal coelom**. The end result is the development of three body cavities: a pericardial cavity around the heart, two smaller **pleural canals** and a large **peritoneal cavity**. The first two are divided from the peritoneal cavity by the **diaphragm**.

Formation of the notochord

The notochordal process grows out cranially from the primitive knot beneath the ectoderm until it reaches the prechordial plate. Where the prechordial plate is firmly attached to the ectoderm and remains bilaminar it forms the **oropharyngeal membrane** or future site of the mouth. Caudal to the primitive streak is a circular area which also remains bilaminar called the **cloacal membrane** or future site of the anus and urogenital orifices. The notochord, a rigid cellular rod stretched out along the embryo, develops from the notochordal process. Mesodermal cells gather around it to form the **vertebral column** and it is almost completely formed by the end of the third week. It disappears once it is surrounded by the vertebral bodies.

Organogenesis

From 3 weeks the embryo enters the vulnerable stage of organogenesis which is complete by 8 weeks (Fig. 9.18) Organs are made up of cell types that originate from different sources and obey different instructions. From about day 20 to day 30 the dorsal surface of the embryo looks segmented with the appearance of **paired somites** which are distinct blocks of embryonic tissue on either side of the notochord (Wolpert et al 2007). Somite formation begins at the anterior end of the embryo and proceeds posteriorly with each pair of somites being formed simultaneously. From the somites develop the vertebral column and the segmentally innervate muscles of the trunk. Somites are still visible at 6 weeks but have differentiated by 8 weeks.

Differentiation of the germ layers

Figure 9.19 summarises the tissues and organs developing from the three layers.

Ectoderm

- Tissues derived from neuroectoderm include the central and peripheral nervous systems, the retina of the eye and the posterior lobe of the pituitary gland.
- Tissues derived from surface ectoderm include the outer layer of the skin (the epidermis) with its hair follicles and cutaneous glands, including the breasts, the lens of the eye, the special sense cells of the inner ear, the anterior lobe of the pituitary gland and the enamel of the teeth.

Neurulation

Neurulation is development of the brain and nervous system (Figs. 9.20–9.23). The notochord induces its overlying ectoderm to thicken and form a neural plate. These cells are called the **neuroectoderm** and differ from the remaining surface ectoderm. A flat sheet of cells on the upper surface of the embryo folds up into a tube which will develop into the brain and spinal cord. On about day 18 the neural plate develops a midline neural groove with lateral neural folds. At the beginning of the 4th week the folds come together to form the neural tube.

Fusion of the folds begins at the level of the 4th pair of somites and proceeds simultaneously in cranial and caudal directions. Cells near to the crests of the neural folds escape from the neural tube during closure and come to lie on either side to form the neural crest. The two open ends of the neural tube are termed **neuropores**. The cranial neuropore closes at about day 25 and the caudal neuropore at about day 27. The neural tube becomes the brain and spinal cord. The neural canal within the tube becomes the **ventricular system** of the brain and the central canal of the spinal cord. This early closure of the neural tube has implications for the causation and prevention of open neural tube defects.

Mesoderm

Nearest the midline axis of the embryo is the **paraxial mesoderm** which segments to form the somites. Next to the somites but not undergoing segmentation is the **intermediate mesoderm** and outside that is the **lateral plate**. The lateral plate is divided into **somatic mesoderm** lying

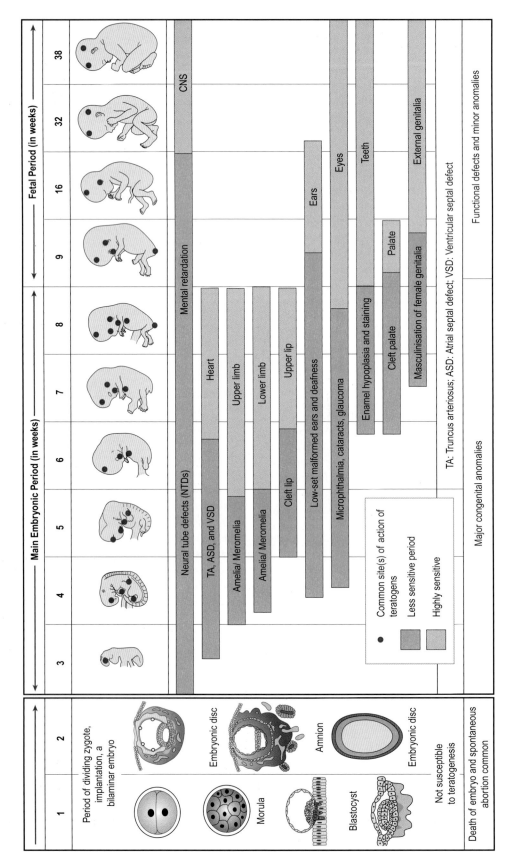

Figure 9.18 • Schematic illustration of critical periods in human prenatal development, showing periods of sensitivity to teratogens. (Reproduced with permission from Moore 1989.)

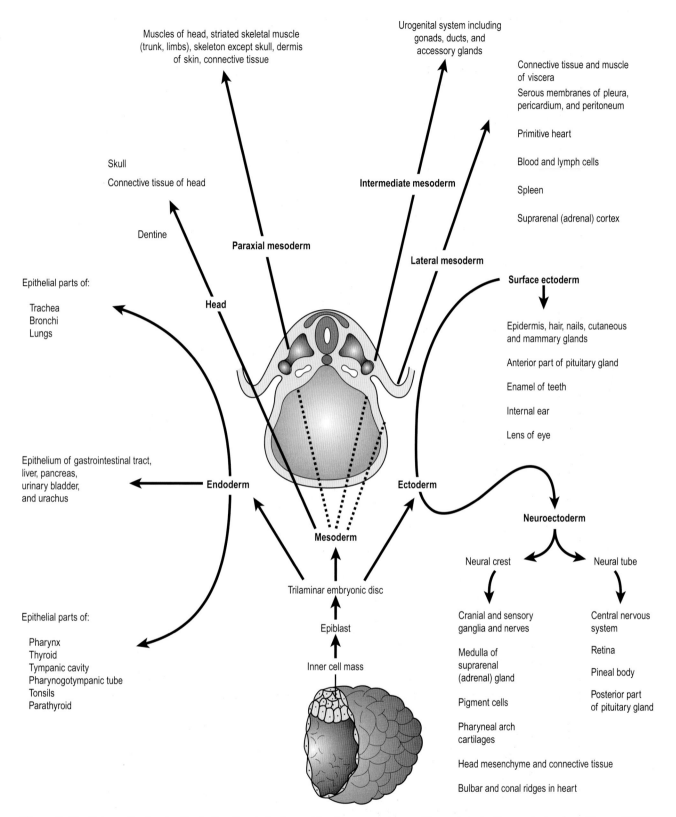

Muscles of head, striated skeletal muscle (trunk, limbs), skeleton except skull, dermis of skin, connective tissue

Urogenital system including gonads, ducts, and accessory glands

Connective tissue and muscle of viscera

Serous membranes of pleura, pericardium, and peritoneum

Primitive heart

Blood and lymph cells

Spleen

Suprarenal (adrenal) cortex

Skull

Connective tissue of head

Dentine

Intermediate mesoderm

Paraxial mesoderm

Lateral mesoderm

Surface ectoderm

Epithelial parts of:

Trachea
Bronchi
Lungs

Head

Epidermis, hair, nails, cutaneous and mammary glands

Anterior part of pituitary gland

Enamel of teeth

Internal ear

Lens of eye

Epithelium of gastrointestinal tract, liver, pancreas, urinary bladder, and urachus

Endoderm

Ectoderm

Neuroectoderm

Mesoderm

Neural crest

Neural tube

Trilaminar embryonic disc

Epiblast

Inner cell mass

Epithelial parts of:

Pharynx
Thyroid
Tympanic cavity
Pharyngotympanic tube
Tonsils
Parathyroid

Cranial and sensory ganglia and nerves

Medulla of suprarenal (adrenal) gland

Pigment cells

Pharyneal arch cartilages

Head mesenchyme and connective tissue

Bulbar and conal ridges in heart

Central nervous system

Retina

Pineal body

Posterior part of pituitary gland

Figure 9.19 • Schematic drawing illustrating the derivatives of the three germ layers. (Reproduced with permission from Moore 1989.)

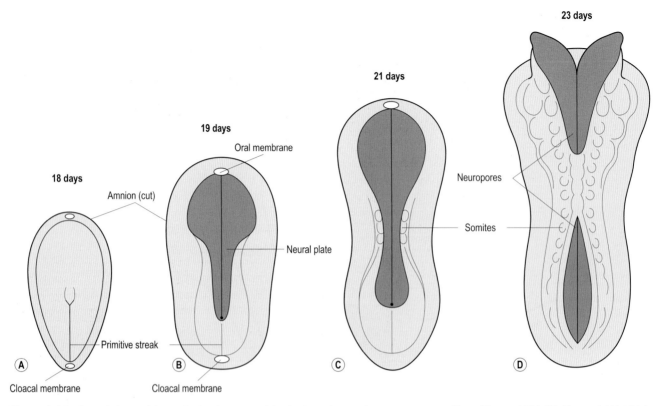

Figure 9.20 • Dorsal views of the early development of the brain and central nervous system. (From Fitzgerald M J T, Fitzgerald M 1994, with permission.)

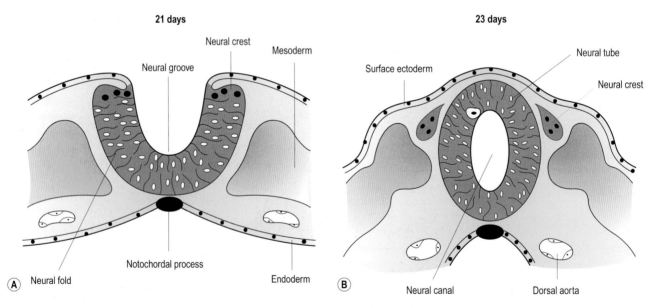

Figure 9.21 • (A, B) Transverse sections of the mid-region of embryos (C) and (D) in Figure 9.20. (From Fitzgerald M J T, Fitzgerald M 1994, with permission.)

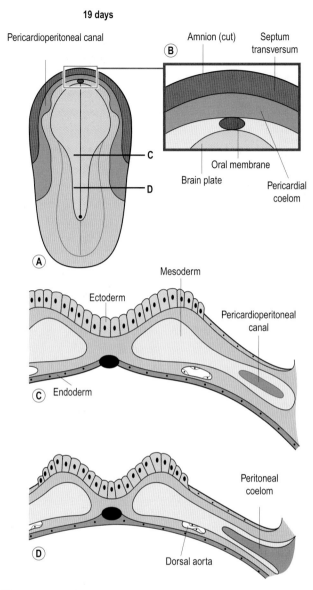

19 days

Pericardioperitoneal canal

B Amnion (cut) Septum transversum

Oral membrane

Brain plate

Pericardial coelom

A

B

Mesoderm

Ectoderm

Pericardioperitoneal canal

C Endoderm

D

Peritoneal coelom

Dorsal aorta

Figure 9.22 • (A) Dorsal view of a 19-day embryonic disc. (B) Enlargement of the rostral part of (A). (C, D) Transverse sections at the levels indicated in (A). (From Fitzgerald M J T, Fitzgerald M 1994, with permission.)

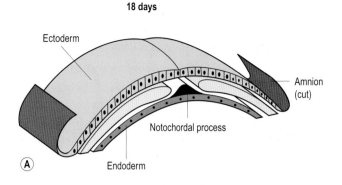

18 days

Ectoderm

Amnion (cut)

Notochordal process

A Endoderm

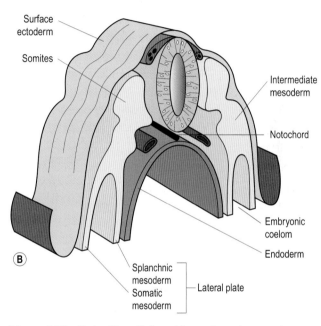

Surface ectoderm

Somites

Intermediate mesoderm

Notochord

Embryonic coelom

Endoderm

B

Splanchnic mesoderm

Somatic mesoderm

Lateral plate

Figure 9.23 • Early differentiation of the embryonic mesoderm. (From Fitzgerald M J T, Fitzgerald M 1994, with permission.)

just beneath the body wall and **splanchnic mesoderm** lying next to the endoderm of the umbilical vesicle.

Tissues derived from mesoderm are:

- From the paraxial mesoderm cranial to the somites: part of the skull and the muscles of the face and jaws.
- From the somites: the vertebral column and the skeletal musculature of the trunk and connective tissue or dermis of the skin.
- From the intermediate mesoderm: the kidneys and ureters, the gonads, the ductus deferens and the uterus and uterine tubes.

- From the somatic mesoderm: the limb skeleton and muscles, the sternum and anterior part of the ribs.
- From the splanchnic mesoderm: the cardiovascular system and blood, the spleen and smooth muscle of the gastrointestinal tract.

Endoderm

- Tissues derived from endoderm include the epithelial linings of the alimentary tract and its glands, the liver, the pancreas, the epithelial lining of the lower respiratory tract and of the bladder and urethra.

Folding of the embryo

Folding of cell sheets forms the basis of early development of organs as described under neurulation. Folding

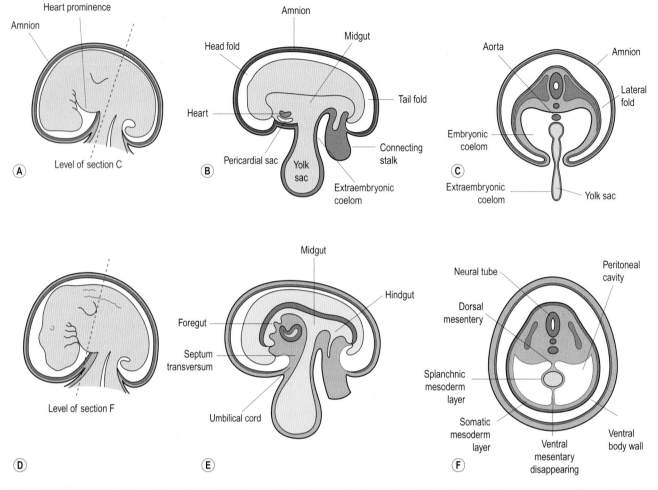

Figure 9.24 • Drawings illustrating embryonic folding and its effects on the intraembryonic coelom and other structures. (Reproduced with permission from Moore 1989.)

of the embryo changes its shape and the relationships of the organs (Figs. 9.24, 9.25). Neurulation is a good example. A flat sheet of cells on the upper surface of the embryo folds up into a tube which develops into the brain and spinal cord. Events in the longitudinal and transverse planes are described separately.

Longitudinal folding

Longitudinal folding brings about flexion and development of the head and tail folds (Figs. 9.26, 9.27) and an hour-glass constriction and partial extrusion of the umbilical vesicle. The portion of the umbilical vesicle retained in the embryo becomes the gut whilst that extruded becomes the **vitelline duct** which remains attached to the gut at the **vitellointestinal communication** and

eventually disappears. When flexion is completed the brain overhangs the developing heart and the heart is ventral to the foregut. The midgut faces into the vitelline duct and the hindgut extends from the vitellointestinal communication to the cloacal membrane.

Transverse folding

The lateral margins of the embryonic disc form the lateral body folds which turn the embryo from a disc into a cylinder. The peritoneal coelom on each side initially opened into the extraembryonic coelom. Transverse folding directs these two openings ventrally and, with the constriction of the umbilical vesicle, the two openings communicate across the midline to form the peritoneal cavity.

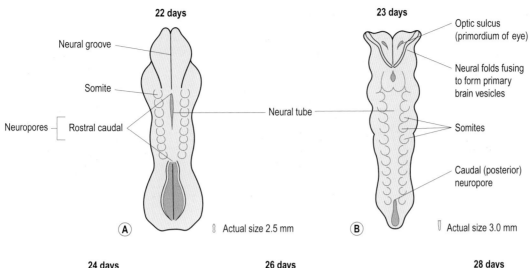

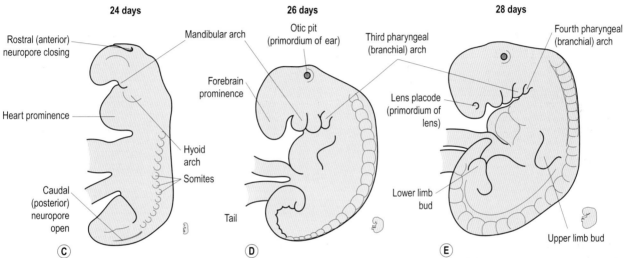

Figure 9.25 • (A, B) Dorsal views of embryos early in the 4th week showing 8 and 12 somites, respectively. (C–E) Lateral views of older embryos showing 16, 27 and 33 somites, respectively. The rostral neuropore is normally closed by 25–26 days and the caudal neuropore by the end of the 4th week. (Reproduced with permission from Moore 1989.)

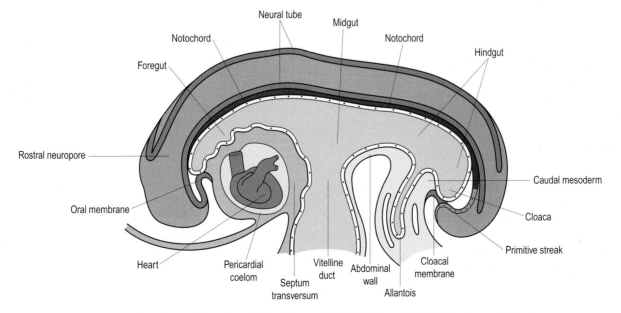

Figure 9.26 • Longitudinal section of a 25-day embryo. (From Fitzgerald M J T, Fitzgerald M 1994, with permission.)

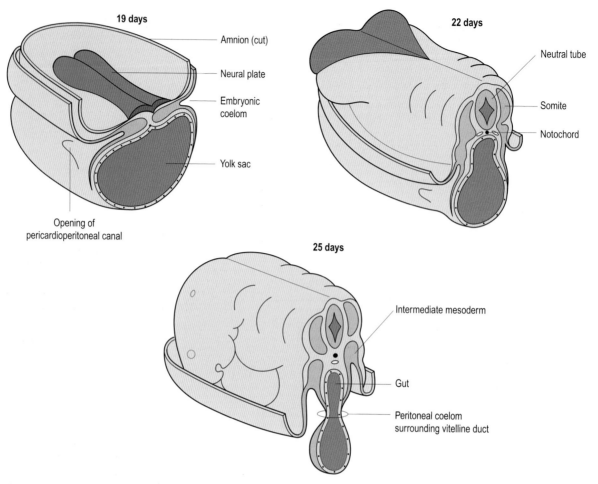

19 days

Amnion (cut)

Neural plate

Embryonic coelom

Yolk sac

Opening of pericardioperitoneal canal

22 days

Neutral tube

Somite

Notochord

25 days

Intermediate mesoderm

Gut

Peritoneal coelom surrounding vitelline duct

Figure 9.27 • Schematic transverse sections depicting formation of the lateral body folds. (From Fitzgerald M J T, Fitzgerald M 1994, with permission.)

Main points

- Gametogenesis allows the independent assortment of maternal and paternal chromosomes amongst the gametes.

- The oocyte contains all the material necessary for embryonic growth and development. When one of the millions of sperm enters a secondary oocyte, the first diploid cell of a new human is formed.

- When a capacitated sperm meets the corona radiata of the oocyte the acrosome reaction occurs. Lytic enzymes disperse the follicular cells of the corona radiata, allowing the head of the sperm to contact the zona pellucida.

- Other enzymes produce an opening in the zona pellucida. The sperm cell's nucleus passes into the oocyte. Mitochondria and other organelles are inherited from the ovum.

- During embryogenesis a programme of simple instructions generates complex forms. Most developmental processes depend on interaction

between genetic and environmental factors. Embryonic cells change shape and position to form body systems. Cellular processes include cell division, cell differentiation, cell migration and programmed cell death.

- Mitotic cleavage splits the large zygote into smaller cells called blastomeres. By the 4th day after fertilisation there are between 16 and 20 cells and the conceptus is called a morula. The cells at this stage are totipotent and if separated there is potential for identical individuals.

- Regulation of embryonic development is by a cascade of gene products. Homeobox genes switched on sequentially by chemical gradients produce proteins which control segmentation so that correct positioning of the organs occurs.

- During early development some embryonic tissues influence the development of adjacent tissues. These influencing tissues are called inductors or organisers.

- Cleavage carries on during the next 4 days. There is also polarisation with internal cells differing from external cells. The inner cells divide less frequently and remain large and round whereas the outer cells in contact with the zona pellucida become flattened.

- On the 5th day the zygote hatches as the zona pellucida is digested by uterine secretions. Fluid accumulates in the space between the peripheral and central cells and the morula becomes a blastocyst. The inner embryoblast becomes the embryo and the flattened outer trophoblast becomes the placenta.

- On the 6th day the embryo begins to implant into the endometrium. Where trophoblast cells touch the endometrium they become cuboid forming the cytotrophoblast. Daughter cells form the syncytiotrophoblast which produces enzymes that erode the endometrium and hormones such as hCG to maintain the corpus luteum and continued production of oestrogen and progesterone until the placenta produces them at 12 weeks. At the implantation site new blood capillaries develop.

- During embryogenesis cells migrate throughout the embryo to differentiate into specific tissues forming organs. Formation of the primitive streak, gastrulation and formation of the notochord are important in creating the body plan.

- From day 20 to day 30 the dorsal embryonic surface develops paired somites from which the vertebral column and segmentally innervated muscles of the trunk develop.

- Embryonic ectoderm gives rise to the epidermis, central and peripheral nervous systems, the eye and the inner ear.

- Embryonic endoderm gives rise to the epithelial lining of the gastrointestinal and respiratory tracts, parenchyma of the tonsils, thyroid and parathyroid glands, thymus, liver and pancreas.

- Embryonic mesoderm gives rise to all skeletal muscles, blood cells and the lining of blood vessels, all visceral smooth muscle coats, all linings of body cavities, the reproductive and excretory systems and most of the cardiovascular system.

- During neurulation a flat sheet of cells on the upper surface of the embryo folds into a tube which develops into the brain and spinal cord.

- Folding of cell sheets forms the basis of the early development of organs. Both longitudinal and transverse folding occur.

References

Alberts, B., Johnson, A., Lewis, J., et al., 2008. Molecular Biology of the Cell, fifth edn. Garland Science Inc, USA.

Carlson, B.M., 2004. Human Embryology and Developmental Biology, third edn. Elsevier, Mosby.

Human Fertilisation and Embryology Act, 1990. HMSO, London.

Lane, N., 2005. Power, Sex and Suicide: Mitochondria and the Meaning of Life. Oxford University Press, Oxford.

Moore, K.L., Persaud, T.V.N., 2008. The Developing Human Clinically Oriented Embryology, eighth edn. Saunders Elsevier.

Nusslein-Volhard, C., 1996. Gradients that organise embryo development. Sci. Am. August, 38–43.

Schoenwolf, G.C., Bleyl, S.B., Brauer, R., Francis-West, P.H., 2008. Larsen's Human Embryology, fourth edn. Elsevier Churchill Livingstone.

Wolpert, L., 1991. The Triumph of the Embryo. Oxford University Press, Oxford.

Wolpert, L., Jessell, T., Lawrence, P. et al., (Eds.), 2007. Principles of Development, third edn. Oxford University Press, Oxford.

Annotated recommended reading

Moore, K.L., Persaud, T.V.N., 2008. The Developing Human Clinically Oriented Embryology, eighth edn. Saunders Elsevier.

This updated textbook clearly describes embryo development week by week and provides an excellent source for understanding the origin of congenital defects. The illustrations are excellent and it is probably the best book for degree students to peruse.

Nusslein-Volhard, C., August 1996. Gradients that organise embryo development. Sci. Am. August 38–43.

This clearly written and well-illustrated seminal article is of interest to anyone wishing to understand how the early embryo develops the axes that lead to the final body plan.

Schoenwolf, G.C., Bleyl, S.B., Brauer, R., Francis-West, P.H., 2008. Larsen's Human Embryology, fourth edn. Elsevier Churchill Livingstone.

This book examines both molecular biological and clinical aspects of embryology with applications linked to an advancing knowledge base.

Chapter Ten

10

Embryological systems 1—trunk, head and limbs

Introduction

This chapter and the next explain when and how normal systems develop and are a knowledge base for the understanding of congenital abnormalities. Explanations will be kept simple as the student is not expected to be an expert.

The trunk

Skeletal features

The vertebral column

There are three phases in the development of the vertebral column (Fig. 10.1): **precartilaginous**, **cartilaginous** and **bony** (Moore & Persaud 2008).

Precartilaginous phase

Precursors of the vertebrae called **sclerotomes** are derived from the **somites**. Mesenchymal cells surround the **notochord** to form the segmented **mesenchymal vertebral column**. The cranial end of each mesenchymal vertebra is thinner than the caudal end because of a relative sparseness of cells. The cells at the interface between the two tissues form an **intervertebral disc** and the remainder of the condensed structure merges with the vertebra caudal to it to form the **centrum**. This is formed from parts of two sclerotomes and is an intersegmental structure. From the upper part of the centrum a pair of **neural arches** grows and surrounds the neural tube, giving rise to pairs of costal and transverse processes.

Cartilaginous phase

Chondrification centres appear in the centrum and neural arch late in the 5th week. In the 12 thoracic

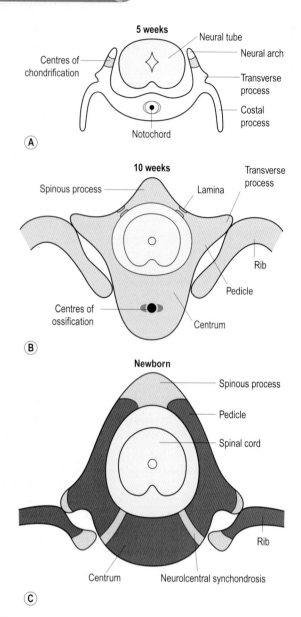

Figure 10.1 • (A) Blastemal vertebra with centre of chondrification (shaded dark), (B) cartilaginous vertebra with centres of ossification (shaded dark), (C) bony vertebra. (From Fitzgerald M J T, Fitzgerald M 1994, with permission.)

vertebrae the cartilaginous coastal processes which will develop into the ribs become detached from their parent neural arches by the formation of synovial joints. Synovial joints also appear between the costal and transverse processes. The remaining costal processes are incorporated into the vertebrae.

Bony phase

During the 8th week **ossification centres** appear in the centrum and neural arches and in the ribs. Ossification of the skeleton is not completed until the 25th year.

Ribs and sternum

As the lateral body folds in the 4th week, the somatic mesoderm is penetrated by the thoracic costal processes. These induce the mesoderm to add to their tips, completing the formation of the prechondrial ribs. Two sternal bars develop in the ventral part of the somatic mesoderm which meet in the midline and unite to form a prechondrial sternum. The **xiphisternum** often remains bifid. The ventral ends of the seven cranial costal processes fuse with the sternum and cartilage persists at the junction as the costal cartilages (Moore & Persaud 2008).

Soft tissues

During the 4th week the somites subdivide into three kinds of mesodermal primordia: **myotomes, dermatomes** and **sclerotomes** (Schoenwolf et al 2008).

Myotomes

Myotomes give rise to all the muscles that link the vertebrae and skull together and to the muscles of the abdominal and thoracic walls. Spinal nerves divide into **dorsal** and **ventral** rami. Dorsal rami supply the muscles with motor fibres and ventral rami supply the muscles and their overlying dermatome with sensory fibres. Limb muscles are not formed from myotomes.

Dermatomes

The dermatomes merge with each other to form the **dermis** layer of the skin. Each dermatome is accompanied by sensory nerve fibres derived from the level of the spinal cord at which the dermatome originated. That is why neurologists divide the body surface into regions called **dermatomes**.

The skin and mammary glands

The dermis develops from the dermatomes but the **epidermis** and its appendages are derived from surface ectoderm which begins as a single cuboidal layer but becomes two-layered in the 2nd month. The superficial layer is shed leaving the underlying germinal layer to form the structures of the skin. In the 3rd month the epidermis becomes stratified and its basal layer sends pegs down into the dermis to form the root sheath of the hair follicles. **Lanugo**, which is very soft fine hair, grows all over the body. True or **vellus hair** is derived from a second set of hair follicles and replaces lanugo which is shed shortly before birth.

During the 5th month the sebaceous glands bud into the dermis from the root sheath and the sweat glands grow down from the epidermis. The sebaceous glands produce a secretion which, when mixed with peridermal cells and lanugo, becomes the vernix caseosa. The mammary glands appear in the 6th week as paired strips of longitudinal ectodermal thickening on the ventral surface of the embryo called the mammary ridge. In humans only one pair of breasts forms from the thoracic part of the ridge and the rest of the ridge disappears.

The skull

The skull forms from mesenchyme around the developing brain. It consists of the neurocranium which encloses the brain and the viscerocranium making up the bones of the face. The base of the skull or **chondrocranium** develops out of cartilage whereas the **vault bones** (Ch. 24) develop from membrane (Moore & Persaud 2008). Intramembranous ossification begins from the 4th month, separate ossification centres giving rise to the parietal bones, frontal bones, occipital bone and the squamous part of the temporal bones.

The viscerocranium

All the facial bones ossify in membrane, starting with the mandible early in the 6th week. Detailed development of the face is given later.

The teeth

Tooth buds form from thickened ectoderm called the **dental lamina**: 10 in the upper jaw and 10 in the lower jaw. These are responsible for the deciduous (milk) teeth. Later the dental lamina forms the buds of the permanent dentition. The permanent molars do not have precursors in the deciduous dentition but develop from a backwards extension of the dental lamina. The crowns of the teeth begin when cells called **odontoblasts** form predentine which later calcifies to become dentine. Calcification signals cells called **ameloblasts** to lay down enamel on the surface of the dentine. The central cells constitute the pulp of the tooth which is richly supplied with blood and sensory nerve endings as many of us can testify!

Deep to the level of enamel production the outer and inner enamel epithelia fuse to form the **epithelial root sheath**. Predentine and dentine are induced to form the root of the tooth. The mesoderm of the dental sac produces a specialised form of bone called cement and the **periodontal ligament** which anchors the cement to the wall of the tooth socket. Eruption of the deciduous teeth occurs between 6 months and 2 years after birth.

The brain

Chapter 26 describes the complex adult brain and central nervous system. The neural tube cranial to the 4th pair of somites develops into the brain (Moore & Persaud 2008). The human nervous system begins to form 19 days after fertilisation and is the earliest system to differentiate. By 19 days three expansions are present (Fig. 10.2). These primary brain vesicles are:
- Forebrain—**prosencephalon**.
- Midbrain—**mesencephalon**.
- Hindbrain—**rhombencephalon**.

From 4 weeks the major regions of the brain are distinct and neurons begin to differentiate from the epithelium of the neural tube. The thalamus and **hypothalamus** are differentiated by the 5th week (Fig. 10.3). By the end of the 8th week the head is equal to half the length of the embryo and controls first movement of the limbs.

The changing shape of the brain

The brainstem buckles and a cervical flexure appears at the junction of the brainstem and spinal cord. A midline flexure moves the mesencephalon to the summit of the brain. The rhombencephalon folds on itself, causing the walls of the neural tube to expand into the 4th ventricle. The dorsal region of the prosencephalon expands on either side to form the cerebral hemispheres or **telencephalon**. Within the cerebral hemispheres the neural tube dilates to form the **lateral ventricles**.

The remainder of the prosencephalon which straddles the midline is known as the **diencephalon**. The 3rd ventricle, a cavity within the diencephalon, communicates with the 4th ventricle through the **aqueduct of Sylvius**. An outgrowth from the diencephalon becomes the two retinas and optic nerves. The cranial end of the rhombencephalon gives rise to the **pons** and the **cerebellum**, while the caudal end becomes the **medulla oblongata**.

The forebrain

Neurons migrate from the ventricular zone of the telencephalon to the surface to form the cerebral cortex. The frontal, parietal, occipital and temporal lobes are present by 12–14 weeks. Two **commissures** of nerve fibres link the two cerebral hemispheres. The anterior commissure links the olfactory regions and the larger corpus callosum links areas of the cerebral cortex.

Other brain structures

The diencephalon gives rise to the **pineal gland**, the paired thalami and the hypothalamus. The **basal ganglia**

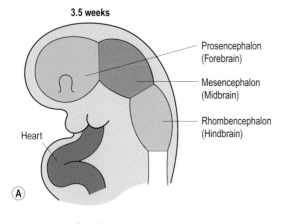

3.5 weeks

- Prosencephalon (Forebrain)
- Mesencephalon (Midbrain)
- Rhombencephalon (Hindbrain)
- Heart

(A)

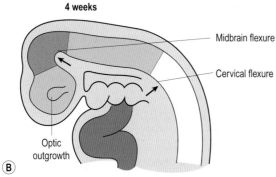

4 weeks

- Midbrain flexure
- Cervical flexure
- Optic outgrowth

(B)

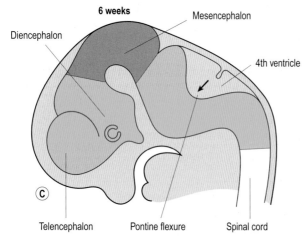

6 weeks

- Diencephalon
- Mesencephalon
- 4th ventricle
- Telencephalon
- Pontine flexure
- Spinal cord

(C)

Figure 10.2 • Early development of the brain. (From Fitzgerald M J T, Fitzgerald M 1994, with permission.)

develop immediately below the thalamus and help control body movement.

Blood supply to the brain

The arterial blood supply develops from cranial segments of the **dorsal aortae**, comprising two internal carotid arteries and two **vertebral arteries**. The internal carotid arteries branch to form the **anterior, middle** and **posterior cerebral arteries**. Each vertebral artery

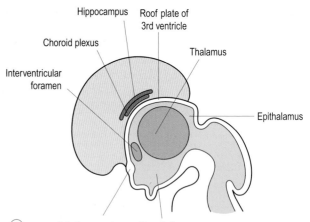

- Hippocampus
- Roof plate of 3rd ventricle
- Choroid plexus
- Thalamus
- Interventricular foramen
- Epithalamus
- Anterior commissure
- Hypothalamus

(A)

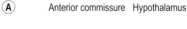

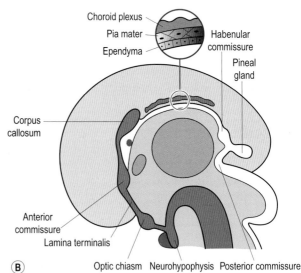

- Choroid plexus
- Pia mater
- Ependyma
- Habenular commissure
- Pineal gland
- Corpus callosum
- Anterior commissure
- Lamina terminalis
- Optic chiasm
- Neurohypophysis
- Posterior commissure

(B)

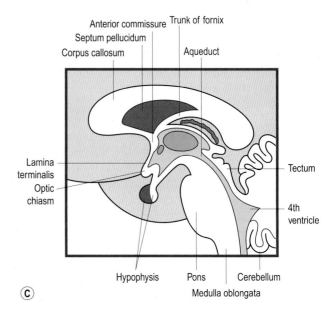

- Anterior commissure
- Trunk of fornix
- Septum pellucidum
- Corpus callosum
- Aqueduct
- Lamina terminalis
- Tectum
- Optic chiasm
- 4th ventricle
- Hypophysis
- Pons
- Cerebellum
- Medulla oblongata

(C)

Figure 10.3 • Median sections of the brain (A) at 8 weeks, (B) at 12 weeks, (C) postnatal. (From Fitzgerald M J T, Fitzgerald M 1994, with permission.)

gives off a branch to supply the cerebellum and medulla oblongata before uniting with its partner to form the **basilar artery**. This gives off two pairs of arteries to the cerebellum and upper brainstem before dividing into two terminal branches that link up with the ends of the internal carotid arteries to form the intercommunicating **circle of Willis**. The venous drainage is discussed in Chapter 24.

The spinal cord

Following the closure of the neural tube and the formation of the somites, neural crest cells form clusters corresponding to the somites. Corresponding levels of the neural tube develop from the primitive streak during a process of secondary neurulation. At first the neural tube is solid but becomes canalised by caudal extension of the neural canal.

Zones of the spinal cord

During the 5th week three zones can be distinguished in the side walls of the neural tube. From within outwards these are the **ventricular**, **intermediate** and **marginal zones**.

- The ventricular zone is where neuroepithelial cells divide. After several cell divisions daughter cells move out of the ventricular zone; the first ones become neurons and the last become the connective tissue cells called **neuroglia**.
- The intermediate zone is the forerunner of the grey matter of the spinal cord. Cells called **neuroblasts** from the ventricular zone differentiate into neurons. **Glioblasts** enter the intermediate zone and become **astrocytes**, the structural support of the central nervous system (CNS) and oligodendrocytes form the **myelin sheaths**. Phagocytic microglial cells develop from blood monocytes and migrate from the capillary bed to the CNS during the 3rd month.
- The marginal zone is the forerunner of the white matter of the spinal cord. Small neurons invade the marginal zone and emit axons alongside the grey matter to form pathways that link different levels of the spinal cord.

During the 6th week an accumulation of neuroblasts in the dorsolateral plate gives rise to the sensory **dorsal horn** of grey matter. The dorsal horn communicates with neural crest cells outside the neural tube to form **dorsal root ganglia**. Large accumulations of cells in the ventrolateral plate form the motor **ventral horn** of grey matter. Axons emerging from the ventral horn form the **ventral nerve roots**, joining with peripheral processes to form mixed spinal nerves.

During weeks 7–10 the spinal cord is formed. The neural canal shrinks to become the central canal of the spinal cord. Cells left behind in the ventricular zone develop cilia and become the lining cells of the central canal called **ependymal cells**. The discrete ascending and descending columns of the spinal cord white matter are finalised.

Cells from the neural crest

Neural crest calls are **pluripotent** and give rise to the following cell types, many of which are involved in the regulation of body systems:

- The dorsal root ganglia cells.
- Autonomic ganglion cells.
- The chromaffin cells of the adrenal medulla.
- The Schwann cells that produce myelin sheaths.
- The pia mater and arachnoid mater (cerebral membranes).
- The skin melanocytes.
- The connective tissue in the wall of the heart and great vessels.
- The parafollicular cells of the thyroid gland.
- The glomus cells of the carotid and aortic bodies.
- Much of the craniofacial skeleton.
- The odontoblasts of the developing teeth.

Structures of the head and neck

Pharyngeal apparatus

The pharyngeal apparatus is described in great detail in Moore & Persaud (2008). It consists of:
- **Pharyngeal arches.**
- **Pharyngeal pouches.**
- **Pharyngeal grooves.**
- **Pharyngeal membranes.**

Pharyngeal arches

Head and neck mesoderm originates from two sources: the paraxial mesoderm and the neural crest. The pharyngeal arches (formerly branchial) begin to develop early in the 4th week. During the 5th week a side view of the embryo shows five pairs of arches numbered I, II, III, IV and VI in craniocaudal sequence. In mammals a pair numbered V may be transient or never develop (Schoenwolf et al 2008).

These arches are the remnants of the gill (branchial) arches found in fishes. In mammals there are no gill arches and the pharyngeal arches are linked by mesoderm (Fig. 10.4). On the surface ectoderm there are

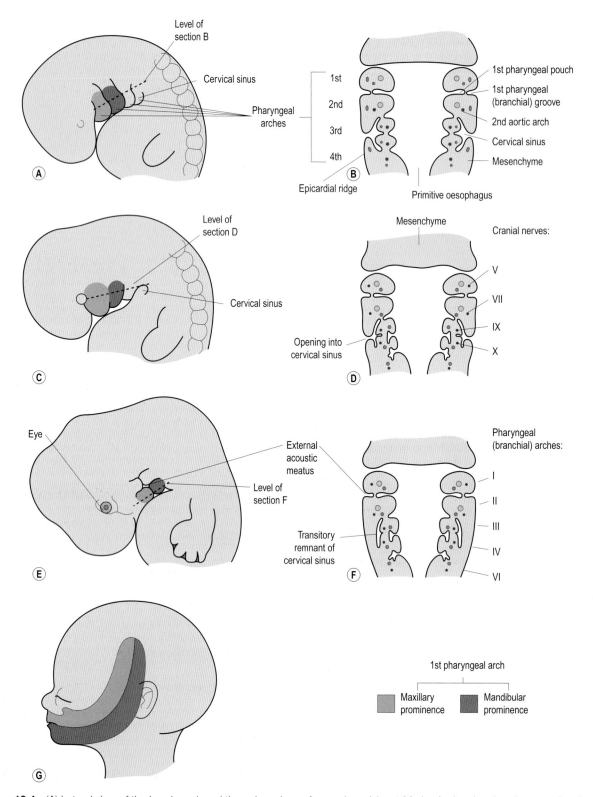

Figure 10.4 • (A) Lateral view of the head, neck and thoracic regions of an embryo (about 32 days), showing the pharyngeal arches and cervical sinus. (B) Diagrammatic section through the embryo at the level shown in (A) illustrating growth of the second arch over the third and fourth arches. (C) An embryo of about 33 days. (D) Section of the embryo shown in (C), illustrating early closure of the cervical sinus. (E) An embryo of about 41 days. (F) Section of an embryo at the level shown in (E), showing the transitory cystic remnant of the cervical sinus. (G) Drawing of a 20-week fetus illustrating the area of the face derived from the first pair of pharyngeal arches. (Reproduced with permission from Moore 1989.)

thickenings called placodes; three of these are the nasal placode, lens placode and otic placode whilst another four contribute sensory ganglion cells to the cranial nerves. Most malformations of the head and neck happen during transformation of pharyngeal arch structures to their final form.

The structure of the pharyngeal arches

Every arch contains the following structures:

1. Migrated neural cells surrounding a central core of mesenchyme cells.
2. Unsegmented mesoderm which forms muscle and bone.
3. A branch of the dorsal aorta on the same side as the pharyngeal arch.
4. A nerve carrying motor fibres called branchial efferents to support the striated muscles.
5. An external covering of ectoderm.
6. An internal covering of endoderm.

Pharyngeal pouches and grooves

Pockets called pharyngeal pouches develop from endoderm between the pharyngeal arches. There are four well-defined pairs and a rudimentary 5th pair. The primitive pharynx develops from the foregut and widens cranially. It is lined by endoderm covering the internal surfaces of the pharyngeal arches. Externally the pharyngeal arches are separated by pockets of ectoderm called pharyngeal grooves.

Derivatives of the pharyngeal arches

First pharyngeal arch

The 1st pair or **mandibular arches** are involved in the development of the face. The cartilage of this arch forms **Meckel's cartilage** which serves as a template for the **mandible**. During the 6th week the mandible develops around the ventral portion of the cartilage by ossification of surrounding membrane and the cartilage mostly disappears. The dorsal end of Meckel's cartilage is incorporated into the middle ear to form the **malleus** and **incus**. From the dorsal part of each mandibular arch the **mandibular prominence** and the **maxillary prominence** develop.

Second pharyngeal arch

The 2nd pair or **hyoid arches** have a much smaller skeletal component than the 1st pair. Their dorsal ends form the **stapes** of the middle ear and the **styloid process** of the temporal bone. The ventral ends form part of the hyoid bone. Most of the mesoderm migrates to form the muscles of facial expression. The sensory facial nerve supplies the muscles formed from the hyoid arches.

Third pharyngeal arch

The third pair forms the posterior part of the tongue and the lower half of the hyoid bone. The **stylopharyngeus muscle** running from the styloid process to the pharynx is the only muscle formed from this arch. It is innervated by the **glossopharyngeal nerve** which also carries the sensory fibres for taste in the posterior part of the tongue. The artery of this arch persists as part of the carotid artery.

Fourth and sixth pharyngeal arches

These form the cartilages, ligaments and muscles of the larynx. The nerve supply to the muscles is via the vagus nerve through laryngeal and pharyngeal branches. The left artery of the 4th arch contributes to the aorta, while the right one forms most of the right subclavian artery.

Derivatives of the pharyngeal pouches

Derivatives of the pharyngeal pouches are:

- First pouch: the **Eustachian tube** and the **middle ear cavity**.
- Second pouch: the **tonsils**.
- Third pouch: the **thymus gland** and **inferior parathyroid gland**.
- Fourth/fifth pouches: **superior parathyroid gland, parafollicular** and **C cells** of the **thyroid gland**.

The thyroid gland is the first endocrine gland to develop, arising during the 4th week from a thickening of endoderm on the floor of the **pharynx**. Two lobes are formed, joined by an isthmus. By 7 weeks the thyroid gland reaches its final destination in the neck.

The tongue develops from five tongue buds on the floor of the pharynx at the end of the 4th week. Two distal tongue buds develop on each side of the median tongue bud and overgrow it to form the anterior or oral two-thirds of the tongue. The posterior part of the tongue develops from mesoderm in the third and fourth pharyngeal arches.

Derivatives of the pharyngeal grooves

The first pharyngeal groove is the only one that contributes to final structures. It forms the **external canal of the ear**. The others form a deep ectodermal depression called the **cervical sinus** during the 5th week. The cervical sinus is obliterated by the 7th week giving the neck a smooth contour.

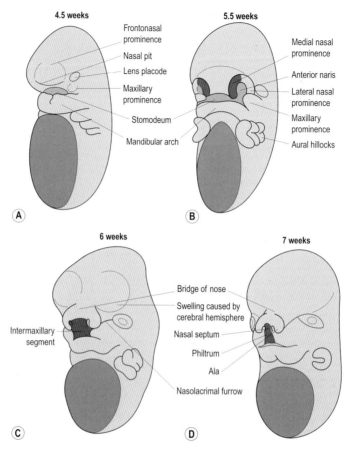

Figure 10.5 • Development of the face. Medial nasal processes and intermaxillary segment are shaded dark. (From Fitzgerald M J T, Fitzgerald M 1994, with permission.)

The face

The development of the face is complex and it is not possible to cover every detail (Fig. 10.5). The primitive mouth begins as a slight depression of the surface ectoderm called the **stomodeum**. It is separated from the foregut by the **oropharyngeal membrane** which ruptures about day 24 to bring the digestive tract into contact with the amniotic cavity. Early in the 4th week, five prominences emerge around the stomodeum: the **frontonasal** prominence, two pairs of mandibular and two pairs of **maxillary prominences**. These merge with each other and are covered by surface ectoderm.

The mandibular prominence forms the lower jaw or mandible and the maxillary prominence gives rise to the upper jaw or **maxilla**, the **zygomatic bone** and the squamous portion of the temporal bone, as well as the outer parts of the upper lip. Mandibular arch mesoderm forms the muscles of mastication which are inserted into the mandible. These muscles are innervated by the mandibular branch of the trigeminal nerve. The skin of the face and mucous membranes are formed from mandibular arch ectoderm. They receive a somatic sensory

nerve supply from three branches of the **trigeminal nerve**: ophthalmic, maxillary and mandibular.

By the end of the 4th week bilateral thickenings of the ectoderm called **nasal placodes** appear. The formation of the nose, palate and upper lip begins early in the 5th week when the two nasal placodes recede into **nasal pits** whose openings become the nostrils. A week later the frontonasal prominence extends onto both sides of the nasal pits to form the medial and lateral nasal prominences. The two medial nasal prominences merge across the midline to form the **intermaxillary segment**. During the 7th week this produces three midline structures: the lower border of the nasal septum, the **philtrum** of the upper lip and the **primary palate**. If these structures fail to develop cleft lip and palate result.

The ears

The outer and middle ear

The **pinna** (auricle) of the ear develops from six **aural hillocks**, three on the first pharyngeal arch and three on the second. It begins in the upper part of the neck and is displaced cranially during development of the mandible. The first pharyngeal cleft gives rise to the **external acoustic meatus** (outer ear canal). The middle ear cavity extends outwards from the first pharyngeal pouch during the 5th week. Where it makes contact with the outer ear canal a thin layer of mesoderm forms the **tympanic membrane** (ear drum). The ear ossicles develop from the dorsal ends of the 1st and 2nd pharyngeal arches.

The inner ear

At the end of the 3rd week an **otic placode** develops on either side of the head. These sink below the surface to form **otic vesicles** which develop into the **vestibular** and **cochlear sacs**. Three plate-like extensions of the vestibular sac become the **semicircular canals** and the remainder of the sac becomes the **utricle**. From the cochlear sac the **cochlea** with the **organ of Corti** arises and the rest becomes the **saccule**. A shell of chondrified mesoderm surrounds the membranous labyrinth and ossifies into the bony labyrinth. The **vestibulocochlear nerve** originates from neural crest cells. The inner ear, tympanic cavity and ossicles are almost fully sized at birth but the outer ear is short and easily damaged by insertion of objects into the canal.

The eyes

In the 4th week two important events occur in the development of the eye (Fig. 10.6):

1. The **optic vesicles** develop as an outgrowth of the diencephalon, remaining attached to it by the **optic stalk**.

2. Under the inducing influence of the optic vesicles the lenses develop as an in-growth of surface ectoderm—the **lens placode**.

As the lens vesicle sinks inwards, the optic vesicle becomes a double-walled optic cup by invagination. This creates the **optic fissure** on the under-surface of the optic cup and stalk. Before the lips of the optic fissure come together during the 6th week, it is infiltrated by mesenchyme (Fig. 10.7). Within the cup the mesenchyme produces a gelatinous secretion that fills the **vitreous component** of the eye. During the 5th and 6th weeks a shell of mesenchyme covers the outer surface of the optic cup and differentiates into the vascular **choroid coat** of the eyeball and the outer fibrous coat consisting of the **sclera** and **cornea**. The six extraocular muscles develop from mesoderm. The cells in the

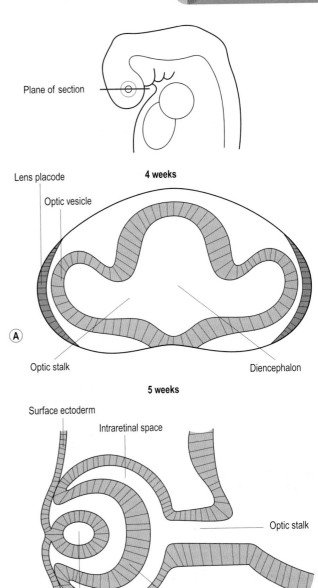

Figure 10.6 • Early development of the eye. (From Fitzgerald M J T, Fitzgerald M 1994, with permission.)

posterior wall of the **lens vesicle** elongate and lay down **primary lens fibres**. **Secondary lens fibres** are laid down later by cells migrating into the interior from the margins of the lens.

The optic cup

The outer epithelium of the optic cup accumulates **melanin pigment** and becomes the pigmented layer of the **retina**. Around the rim of the cup the outer and inner layers form the **ciliary body** and the **iris**.

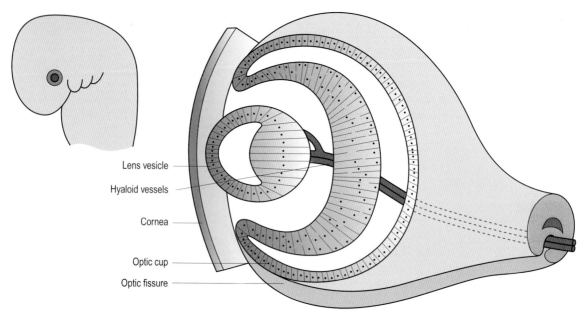

Lens vesicle

Hyaloid vessels

Cornea

Optic cup

Optic fissure

Figure 10.7 • The eye at 6 weeks, showing the optic fissure. (From Fitzgerald M J T, Fitzgerald M 1994, with permission.)

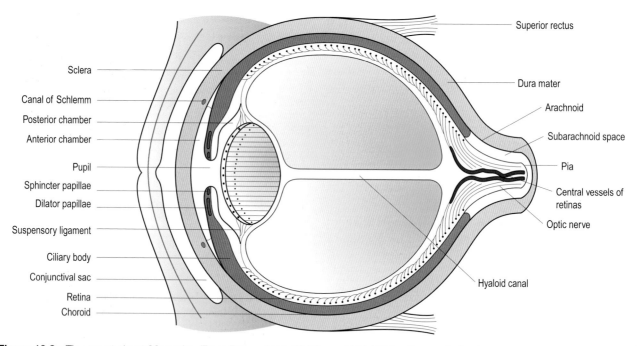

Sclera

Canal of Schlemm

Posterior chamber

Anterior chamber

Pupil

Sphincter papillae

Dilator papillae

Suspensory ligament

Ciliary body

Conjunctival sac

Retina

Choroid

Superior rectus

Dura mater

Arachnoid

Subarachnoid space

Pia

Central vessels of retinas

Optic nerve

Hyaloid canal

Figure 10.8 • The eye at about 20 weeks. (From Fitzgerald M J T, Fitzgerald M 1994, with permission.)

The ciliary muscles develop from ectomesenchymal cells in the ciliary body and the sphincter and dilator pupil muscles develop from the posterior epithelium of the iris. The inner epithelium of the optic cup becomes the nervous layer of the retina. The axons of these neurons converge on the optic stalk to form the **optic nerve** which is an extension of the CNS white matter.

The ciliary processes secrete **aqueous humour** between the cornea and the lens. Between the iris and cornea is the anterior chamber and between the iris and lens the posterior chamber. Aqueous humour moves from posterior to anterior chamber through the pupil and then into a small vein encircling the eye at the anterior margin of the choroid coat called the **canal of Schlemm**. The eye is complete by 20 weeks (Fig. 10.8).

The eyelids and lacrimal apparatus

The eyelids develop from mesodermal folds lined by surface ectoderm that grow to meet each other during the second week. From the 3rd to the 6th months the eyelids are fused, allowing clinicians to estimate the gestational age of a very premature baby. The **lacrimal glands** develop from the outer part of the conjunctival sac and are exocrine glands. It is said that newborns do not produce tears but there is a continuous lacrimal secretion to protect the cornea.

The limbs

When the author was studying for her BA, a visiting lecturer (Lewis Wolpert) asked, 'How do limbs know when to stop making one bone and change to two and then to form the multiple bones of the wrist band hand and how do the two arms end up the same length?' In other words what controls development? This encounter fired the author's interest in embryology!

Development of the limbs

The limbs form from the somatic mesoderm of the lateral body wall in the typical **craniocaudal developmental pattern** (Moore & Persaud 2008) (Figs. 10.9–10.13).

Minute upper limb buds appear in the middle of week 4 at the level of the cervical somites. The lower limb buds appear 2 days later at the level of the lower lumbar somites.

Development of the limbs is regulated by **Hox genes** (Wolpert et al 2007). Proliferation of somatic mesodermal cells is induced in each limb by the **apical ectodermal ridge** (AER), a thickening of surface ectoderm over the limb bud (Schoenwolf et al 2008). This covers the whole surface at first but is later confined to the growing tip of the limb. The limb bud is covered with loose mesenchyme. Cell division in the mesenchyme is restricted to a progress zone immediately below the AER. Daughter cells separate out from this zone to add to the limb's length.

The skeleton is the first part of the limb to demonstrate differentiation and is seen as a condensation of mesenchymal cells in the proximal part of the limb bud. Joint formation occurs by the transverse splitting of precartilaginous rods rather than the coming together of separate limb elements. A gene product similar to sonic hedgehog (see Ch. 9) is known to act on the developing cartilage. It is called Indian hedgehog! (Carlson 2004).

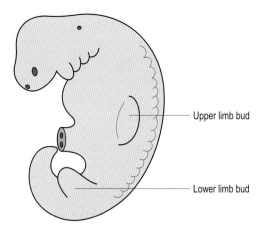

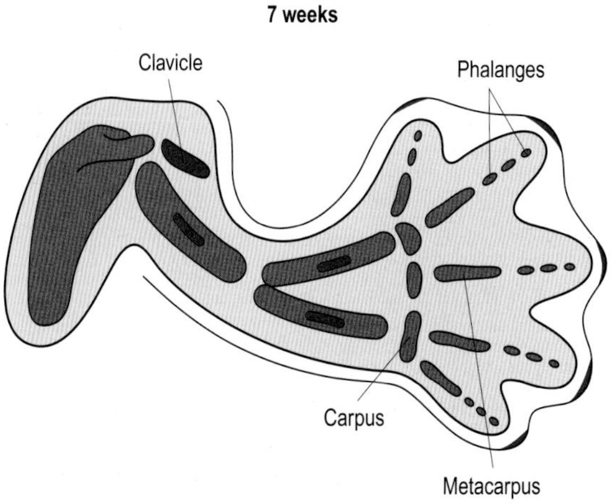

Figure 10.9 • Limb buds at 4 weeks. (From Fitzgerald M J T, Fitzgerald M 1994, with permission.)

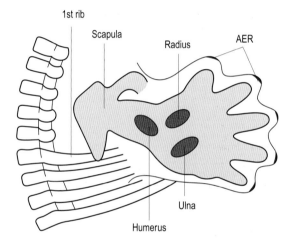

Figure 10.10 • Transilluminated 6-week embryo.

Figure 10.11 • Upper limb skeleton at 7 weeks. Centres of ossification (red) have appeared in the clavicle and in three major long bones. (From Fitzgerald M J T, Fitzgerald M 1994, with permission.)

135

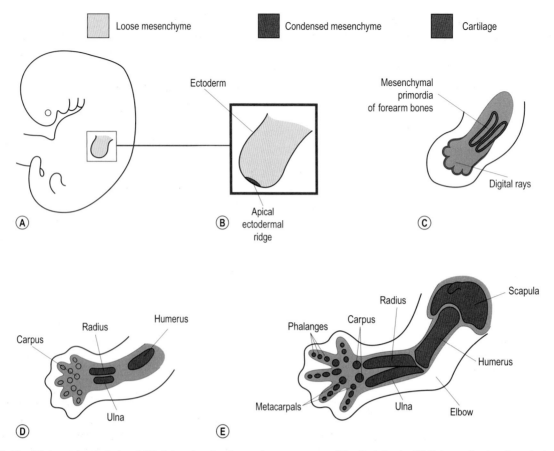

Loose mesenchyme   Condensed mesenchyme   Cartilage

Ectoderm

Mesenchymal primordia of forearm bones

Apical ectodermal ridge

Digital rays

(A)   (B)   (C)

Carpus   Radius   Humerus

Ulna

(D)

Phalanges   Carpus   Radius   Scapula

Metacarpals   Ulna   Humerus   Elbow

(E)

Figure 10.12 • (A) An embryo at about 28 days, showing the early appearance of the limb buds. (B) Schematic drawing of a longitudinal section through an upper limb bud. The apical ectodermal ridge has an inductive influence on the mesenchyme and appears to give it the ability to form specific cartilaginous elements. (C) Similar sketch of an upper limb bud at about 33 days, showing the mesenchymal primordia of the limb bones. The digital rays are mesenchymal condensations that undergo chondrification and ossification to form the bones of the hand. (D) Upper limb at 6 weeks showing the cartilage models of the bones of the upper limb arches. (Reproduced with permission from Moore 1989.)

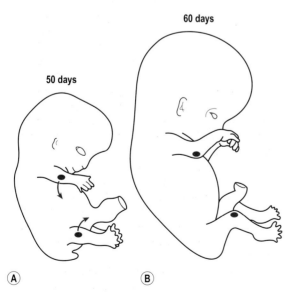

60 days

50 days

(A)   (B)

Figure 10.13 • Positions of the extensor aspects (red marks) of elbow and knee (A) before and (B) after rotation of the limbs. (From Fitzgerald M J T, Fitzgerald M 1994, with permission.)

Formation of the hands and feet

During the 5th week the hands and feet develop as flat limb plates. The AER breaks up into five ridges that mark the positions of the future digits. Each of these lays down a rod of mesoderm called **digital rays**. Webs of loose mesenchyme connect the rays but apoptosis (programmed cell death) (Wolpert 2007) creates **interdigital clefts**.

Development and rotation of the limbs

The limb skeleton passes through the precartilaginous, cartilaginous and ossification stages except the clavicle which develops from membrane. During the 5th week condensations of the limb mesenchyme form a rough skeletal plan. By the end of the 6th week the skeleton is fully cartilaginous. Ossification centres are present in the limb long bones by the 12th week. Ossification of the ankle bones begins late in fetal life but the wrist bones remain cartilaginous until after birth. At first the limbs grow out laterally from the trunk but during the 8th week the limbs rotate to their normal position. Elbow and knee creases appear.

Muscles and nerves of the limbs

The skeletal muscle of the limbs develops from cells that migrate from the nearest somites, whereas tendons develop from somatic mesoderm already present in the limb buds. Spinal nerves called **ventral rami** invade the limbs prior to rotation. They are mixed nerves carrying both motor and sensory fibres. The 31 pairs of spinal nerves are named by the first letter of the name and the number of the vertebra from above downwards:

- Cervical: C1–8.
- Thoracic: T1–12.
- Lumbar: L1–5.
- Sacral: S1–5.

There is also one coccygeal nerve. The upper limbs receive nerves from vertebrae C5 to T1 whilst the lower limbs are invaded by nerves from vertebrae L2 to S2.

Blood supply to the limbs

The limb buds are invaded early by branches of the **intersegmental** blood vessels. A single axial artery is later replaced by new blood vessels. In the upper limb these are **axillary**, **brachial** and **interosseous** arteries with the brachial artery branching into the **radial** and **ulnar** arteries supplying the forearm and hand. In the lower limb the **popliteal** and **peroneal** arteries replace the axial artery with the **femoral** artery developing to join the popliteal artery. The femoral artery branches into the anterior and posterior tibial arteries to supply the lower leg and foot.

Main points

- Three phases—the precartilaginous, cartilaginous and bony phases—lead to the development of the vertebrae.
- Myotomes give rise to the muscles of the head and trunk. Dermatomes merge with each other to form the dermis of the skin. Each dermatome is accompanied by sensory nerve fibres derived from the level of the spinal cord at which the dermatome originated.
- Fetal sebaceous glands produce a secretion that, when mixed with peridermal cells and lanugo, becomes the vernix caseosa. Mammary glands appear in the 6th week as paired longitudinal strips of ectodermal thickening on the ventral surface of the embryo.
- The skull is divided into the neurocranium which encloses the brain and the viscerocranium making up the bones of the face. Ossification gives rise to the parietal bones, frontal bones, occipital bone and squamous portion of the temporal bone of the vault.
- Twenty tooth buds form from thickened ectoderm called dental lamina. These form the basis of the deciduous teeth. Later the dental lamina forms the buds of the permanent dentition.
- The human nervous system is the first system to differentiate. By 19 days three primary brain vesicles are present: the prosencephalon, mesencephalon and rhombencephalon. Frontal, parietal, occipital and temporal lobes are present by 14 weeks.
- Two commissures of nerve fibres link the right and left cerebral hemispheres: the anterior commissure connects the olfactory regions and the corpus callosum links matched areas of the cerebral cortex.

- At first the neural tube is solid but it becomes canalised by caudal extension of the neural canal. During weeks 7–10 the spinal cord is finalised.
- Five mesodermal pairs of pharyngeal arches develop on the future head and neck region. The 1st pair is involved in development of the face, the 2nd forms the stapes of the middle ear and the styloid process of the temporal bone, part of the hyoid bone and the facial expression muscles. The 3rd pair forms the posterior part of the tongue and the lower half of the hyoid bone. The 4th and 6th form the cartilages, ligaments and muscles of the larynx.
- Derivatives of the 1st pharyngeal pouches are the Eustachian tube and the middle ear cavity. The 2nd pouch forms the tonsils. The 3rd pouch forms the thymus gland and inferior parathyroid gland and the 4th/5th pouches form the cells of the thyroid gland.
- The primitive mouth begins as a slight depression of the surface ectoderm called the stomodeum. It is separated from the foregut by the oropharyngeal membrane which ruptures at about day 24 allowing the fetus to swallow liquor amnii.
- The pinna of the ear develops from six aural hillocks, three on the 1st pharyngeal arch and three on the 2nd. The first pharyngeal cleft gives rise to the outer canal. The middle ear cavity extends outwards during the 5th week to make contact with the outer ear canal. Between them a thin layer of mesoderm forms the eardrum.
- Between the 3rd and 6th weeks development of the eye takes place. The eyelids develop during the 2nd month but are fused between the 3rd and the 6th months.

- The limbs form from the somatic mesoderm of the lateral body wall in a craniocaudal pattern. Upper limb buds appear in the middle of the 4th week at the level of the lower cervical somites and lower limb buds appear 2 days later at the level of the lower lumbar somites.
- Development of the limbs is regulated by Hox genes. Proliferation of somatic mesodermal cells is induced in each limb by the apical ectodermal ridge (AER). Cell division in the limb bud mesenchyme is restricted to a progress zone immediately below the AER.
- During the 5th week the hands and feet develop as flat limb plates. Five epidermal apical ridges mark the positions of the future digits. At first the limbs grow out laterally from the trunk but they rotate into their normal position during week 8.

References

Carlson, B.M., 2004. Human Embryology and Developmental Biology, third (updated) edn. Elsevier Mosby, Philadelphia PA.

Moore, K.L., Persaud, T.V.N., 2008. The Developing Human: Clinically Oriented Embryology, eighth edn. Elsevier Saunders, Philadelphia PA.

Schoenwolf, G.C., Bleyl, S.B., Brauer, R., Francis-West, P.H., 2008. Larsen's Human Embryology, fourth edn. Elsevier Churchill Livingstone, Edinburgh.

Wolpert, L., 2007. Principles of Development, third edn. Oxford University Press, Oxford.

Wolpert, L., Jessell, T., Lawrence, P. (Eds.), et al., 2007. Principles of Development, third edn. Oxford University Press, Oxford.

Annotated recommended reading

Carlson, B.M., 2004. Human Embryology and Developmental Biology, third (updated) edn. Elsevier Mosby, Philadelphia PA.

This is a slightly more difficult book to read but Chapter 10 on limb development is especially good.

Moore, K.L., Persaud, T.V.N., 2008. The Developing Human: Clinically Oriented Embryology, eighth edn. Elsevier Saunders, Philadelphia PA.

This updated textbook clearly describes embryo development week by week and provides an excellent source for understanding the origin of congenital defects. The illustrations, as before, are excellent.

Schoenwolf, G.C., Bleyl, S.B., Brauer, R., Francis-West, P.H., 2008. Larsen's Human Embryology, fourth edn. Elsevier Churchill Livingstone, Edinburgh.

This book examines both biological and clinical aspects of embryology. Each chapter is about a specific embryological stage and the clinical applications of the advancing knowledge base.

Chapter Eleven

Embryological systems 2—internal organs

Introduction

The previous chapter examined the skeletal system and formation of the nervous system, including the special senses. This chapter is concerned with the development of the internal organs whose purpose is to keep an individual alive and to perpetuate the species.

The cardiovascular system

The cardiovascular system develops early in the embryo from the end of the 2nd week before it becomes too big to receive nourishment by diffusion. From the end of the 3rd week the embryo must obtain nutrients from the maternal circulation. The cardiovascular system is able to pump blood around embryonic vessels early in the 4th week.

Vasculogenesis and angiogenesis

The formation of the embryonic vascular system during the 3rd week involves **vasculogenesis** which is the formation of vascular channels from cells called angioblasts (Fig. 11.1). **Angiogenesis** is the formation of new vessels by budding and branching from pre-existing vessels.

To summarise blood vessel formation from about 17 days:

- Mesenchymal cells in the extraembryonic mesoderm lining the **umbilical vesicle** differentiate into central **angioblasts** which join together to form **blood islands** which are associated with the umbilical vesicle (yolk sac).
- Small cavities appear within the blood islands.
- Peripheral angioblasts flatten to form endothelial cells that arrange themselves around the cavities in the blood island to form endothelium.
- These endothelial-lined cavities fuse to form networks of endothelial channels (vasculogenesis).
- Vessels sprout into adjacent areas by endothelial budding and fuse with other vessels.

Blood cells develop from **multipotent stem cells** in the mesoderm of the **umbilical vesicle** and **allantois** at

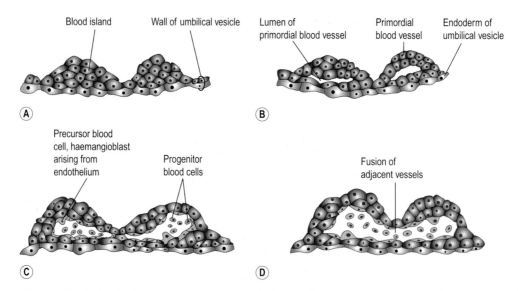

Blood island   Wall of umbilical vesicle   Lumen of primordial blood vessel   Primordial blood vessel   Endoderm of umbilical vesicle

Ⓐ   Ⓑ

Precursor blood cell, haemangioblast arising from endothelium   Progenitor blood cells   Fusion of adjacent vessels

Ⓒ   Ⓓ

Figure 11.1●Sections of blood islands showing progressive stages in the development of blood and blood vessels. (From Moore K L, Persaud T V N 2008, with permission.)

the end of the 3rd week and later in specialised sites along the aorta (Wolpert et al 2007). Later blood cells develop in the liver, spleen, bone marrow and lymph nodes (Moore & Persaud 2008).

All red cells contain the pigment **haemoglobin**, but in cells made in the umbilical vesicle and liver the haemoglobin is fetal haemoglobin which takes up and releases oxygen and carbon dioxide more readily than does adult haemoglobin. Red cells produced by the bone marrow are mature and contain adult haemoglobin.

The primordial cardiovascular system

The heart and great vessels develop from mesenchymal cells in the **cardiogenic area** and by 22 days the heart begins to beat (Fig. 11.2).

Three parts of the embryonic arterial system develop:

1. A pair of **umbilical arteries** carry blood to the placenta.

2. **Vitelline arteries** arise from the **dorsal aortas** linking up with the newly developed capillary bed. These eventually become the **mesenteric arteries** supplying the gut.

3. **Intersegmental arteries** supply blood to the somites and neural tube.

As the pharyngeal arches form during the 4th and 5th weeks they are supplied by paired **aortic arches** arising from the aortic sac and terminating in the dorsal aortas running the length of the embryo. The paired dorsal aortas soon fuse to from a single dorsal aorta (Fig. 11.3).

About 30 branches of the dorsal aorta, called the **dorsal intersegmental arteries**, carry blood to the

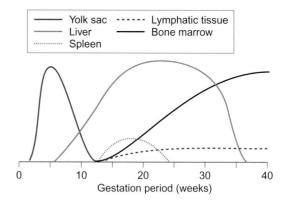

Legend:
—— Yolk sac   - - - - Lymphatic tissue
—— Liver   —— Bone marrow
········· Spleen

0   10   20   30   40
Gestation period (weeks)

Figure 11.2●Sites and times of haemopoiesis. (From Fitzgerald M J T, Fitzgerald M 1994, with permission.)

somites and their derivatives. Those in the neck join to form a **vertebral artery** on either side of the neck. In the thorax they become the **intercostal arteries**. Most of the abdominal branches become **lumbar arteries** but the 5th pair of lumbar intersegmental arteries remains as the **common iliac arteries**. The sacral intersegmental arteries become the **lateral sacral arteries**.

Three pairs of veins drain into the tubular heart of the 4-week embryo:

1. **Umbilical veins** form in the body stalk but only the left one persists to carry oxygenated blood to the embryo.

2. The **vitelline veins** carry blood from the umbilical vesicle to the heart tube.

3. **Common cardinal veins** return poorly oxygenated blood from the embryo.

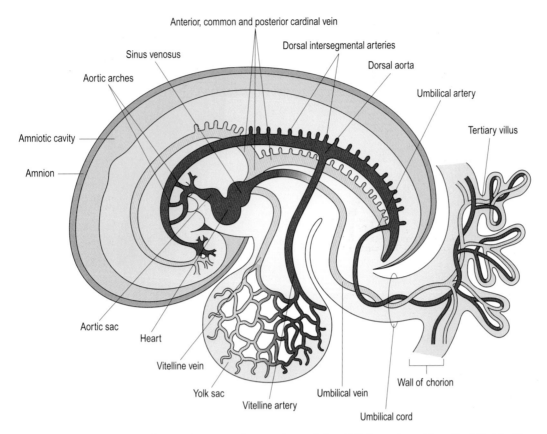

Anterior, common and posterior cardinal vein

Dorsal intersegmental arteries

Sinus venosus

Dorsal aorta

Aortic arches

Umbilical artery

Amniotic cavity

Tertiary villus

Amnion

Aortic sac

Heart

Vitelline vein

Wall of chorion

Yolk sac

Umbilical vein

Vitelline artery

Umbilical cord

Figure 11.3 Diagram of the primitive cardiovascular system in an embryo of about 20 days, viewed from the left side. Observe the transitory stage of paired symmetric vessels. Each heart tube continues dorsally into a dorsal aorta that passes caudally. Branches of the aortae are: umbilical arteries, establishing connections in the chorion; vitelline arteries to the yolk sac; and dorsal intersegmental arteries to the body of the embryo. Vessels on the yolk sac form a vascular plexus that is connected to the heart tubes by vitelline veins. The anterior cardinal veins return blood from the head region. The umbilical vein carries oxygenated blood and nutrients from the chorion to the embryo. The arteries carry poorly oxygenated blood and waste products to the chorionic villi for transfer to the maternal blood. (Reproduced with permission from Moore 1989.)

Development of the heart

The **primordium** (primitive form) of the heart is visible at 18 days and begins to beat at 22 days. Before the head fold develops, cardiogenic mesoderm occupies the floor of the pericardial coelom and gives rise to a pair of **endothelial heart tubes**. These unite to form a single heart tube and a **primordial myocardium** develops (Fig. 11.4). A **pericardial sac** forms around the heart tube. The tubular heart elongates and forms a series of alternating dilatations and constrictions (Fig. 11.5):

- **Truncus arteriosus**.
- **Bulbus cordis**.
- **Ventricle**.
- **Atrium**.
- **Sinus venosus**.

Because the bulbus cordis and the ventricle grow faster than the other regions, the heart tube buckles to form a twisted 'U' shape called the **bulboventricular loop**. The **atrioventricular canal** divides the primordial atrium and

ventricle. The truncus arteriosus is continuous with the aortic sac from which the aortic arches arise. The sinus venosus receives the umbilical, vitelline and common cardinal veins mentioned above.

Blood flow through the early heart

Blood flows via veins from the umbilical vesicle, embryo and chorionic villi to the venus sinosus and into the primitive atrium. The blood then passes through the atrioventricular canal into the primordial ventricle. The ventricle contracts and blood is pumped through the bulbus cordis and truncus arteriosus into the aortic arches. It then passes into the dorsal aortas to return to the umbilical vesicle and early placenta.

Partitioning of the heart

Partitioning of the heart begins in the middle of the 4th week. The primitive atrium is partitioned into two by the growth and fusion of two septa: the **septum primum** from the dorsocranial wall and the **septum secundum** from

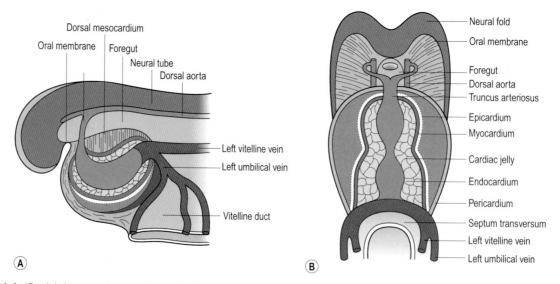

Figure 11.4 • 'Straight' heart tube. (A) Viewed from the left, (B) ventral view. (From Fitzgerald M J T, Fitzgerald M 1994, with permission.)

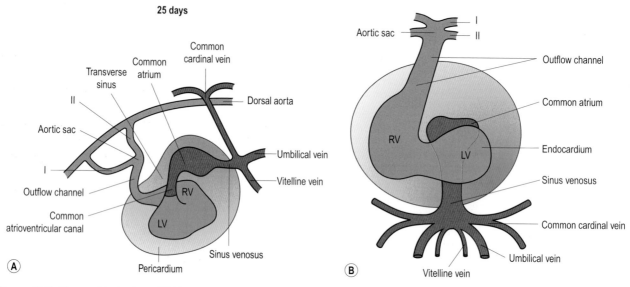

Figure 11.5 • The ventricular loop. (A) Viewed from the left, (B) ventral view. I, II, 1st and 2nd aortic arches; LV, RV, presumptive left and right ventricles. (From Fitzgerald M J T, Fitzgerald M 1994, with permission.)

the ventrocranial wall. An opening with a flap-like valve formed by the septum secundum is left between the atria to accommodate a left-to-right shunt of blood across the atria. This is the **foramen ovale** which closes at birth.

Division of the primitive ventricle begins at the end of the 4th week with the development of a ridge of tissue called the **interventricular septum**. An **interventricular foramen** closes at the end of the 7th week and the pulmonary arterial trunk taking blood to the lungs then communicates with the right ventricle and the aorta carrying blood to the body with the left ventricle. Formation of two atria and two ventricles completes the fetal circulation.

Valves and their supporting **papillary muscles** and **chordae tendinae** and the tissue forming the **conducting system** of the heart begin developing at about 5 weeks and are in place by the end of organogenesis. Development of the heart and great vessels is complex, leading to the possibility of many different types of malformation.

The lower respiratory tract

Development of the laryngotracheal tube

A median **laryngotracheal groove** appears on the floor of the primitive pharynx in the middle of the 4th week. This is converted by the development of a septum to the **laryngotracheal tube** with an opening into the pharynx.

142

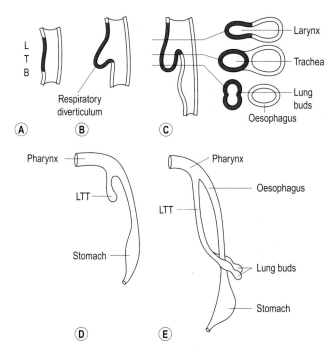

Figure 11.6 • Early development of lower respiratory tract. (A) At 24 days; L, T, B, presumptive epithelial linings of larynx, trachea, bronchial tree. (B) At 25 days. (C) At 26 days. (D) At 4 weeks. (E) At 5 weeks. LTT, laryngotracheal tube. (From Fitzgerald M J T, Fitzgerald M 1994, with permission.)

The epithelial lining of the cranial end of this tube, the laryngeal cartilages and the vocal cords develop from the 4th and 6th pharyngeal arches (Carlson 2004). The cranial epithelium becomes the epithelial lining of the **larynx** and **trachea** and the caudal part lines the **bronchial tree**. **Tracheo-oesophageal folds** grow towards each other to form a septum that divides the cranial part of the foregut into the laryngotracheal tube and the oesophagus (Fig. 11.6).

Development of the lungs

The lung buds develop as a bulge in the caudal part of the laryngotracheal tube during the 4th week. It splits to form two bronchial buds which give rise to the **primary bronchi**. The bronchial buds invaginate the **pericardio-peritoneal canals** which become the pleural cavities. Epithelium covering the outside of the bronchial buds becomes the **visceral pleura** and the epithelium lining the pericardioperitoneal canals becomes the **parietal pleura**. The connections between the two pleural cavities and the pericardial cavity containing the heart become closed off. The two primary bronchi divide into secondary and lobar bronchi and then into segmental bronchi lined with cuboid epithelium to serve three lobes in the right lung and two in the left lung (Fig. 11.7). During the 7th month respiratory **bronchioles** become more abundant and terminate in **alveolar ducts** and **sacs**.

From 5 to 17 weeks the developing lungs are in the **pseudoglandular period**, resembling an exocrine gland and respiration is not possible. In the **canalicular period**, from 16 to 25 weeks, air passages become patent and blood capillaries surround the future alveoli. From 24 weeks until birth alveoli develop in the **terminal sac period** and respiration and survival become possible. Budding of the alveolar ducts and sacs continues for the first 8 years of life. This is the **alveolar period** (Carlson 2004, Moore & Persaud 2008).

At first terminal sacs are lined by **type 1 alveolar cells** which take part in gas exchange. By 24 weeks **type 2 alveolar cells** are found which secrete **surfactant**. This lowers surface tension between the alveolar epithelium and inspired air. Babies born before 34 weeks may develop **respiratory distress syndrome** because of insufficient surfactant production.

The diaphragm

The diaphragm is complex with five elements contributing to its formation:

- The third to fifth somites contribute cells that form the muscles of the diaphragm.
- Ventral extension of the pleural sacs forms diaphragmatic connective tissue.
- Oesophageal mesentery supplies connective tissue around the oesophagus and inferior vena cava.
- The septum transversum gives rise to the fibrous tissue of the central tendon.
- The pleuroperitoneal membranes contribute connective tissue surrounding the central tendon.

The alimentary tract

The primitive gut begins to form during the 4th week when the dorsal part of the umbilical vesicle becomes incorporated into the embryo. The endoderm of this primitive gut gives rise to most of the epithelial lining and glands of the digestive system. By the middle of the 4th week the alimentary tract consists of **foregut**, **midgut** and **hindgut**, each with different arterial blood supply (Carlson 2004, Schoenwolf et al 2008). The epithelial linings of the cranial and caudal ends of the gut, the **stomodeum** and the **anal pit** are derived from ectoderm. The muscular and fibrous parts of the digestive tract form from splanchnic mesoderm.

The foregut

By the 5th week the foregut is visibly divided into the oesophagus, stomach and proximal duodenum (Fig. 11.8).

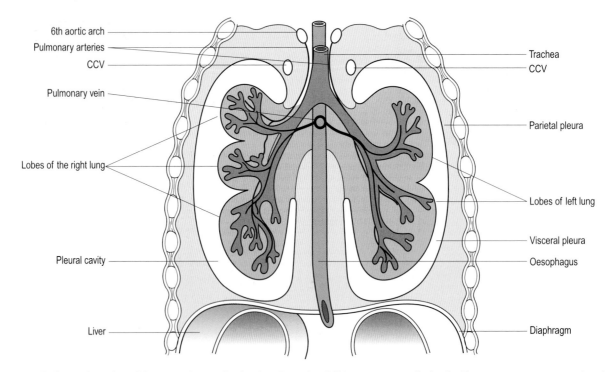

Figure 11.7 ● Coronal section of the posterior mediastinum at 7 weeks. CCV, common cardinal vein. The septum transversum has been incorporated into the diaphragm. (From Fitzgerald M J T, Fitzgerald M 1994, with permission.)

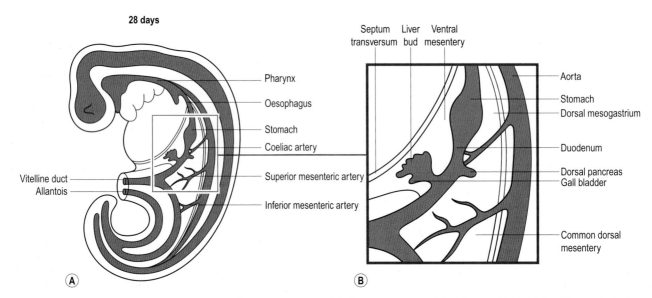

Figure 11.8 ● (A) Digestive system at 4 weeks. (B) Enlargement from (A). (From Fitzgerald M J T, Fitzgerald M 1994, with permission.)

The oesophagus

Although the **oesophagus** is part of the alimentary tract, it is in close proximity to the respiratory tract and is a thoracic structure. As the thoracic cavity lengthens and the heart and lungs descend into it, the oesophagus also lengthens. The upper and lower parts of the oesophagus differ in origin. Pharyngeal arch mesoderm contributes striated muscle to its upper part and this is supplied by the recurrent laryngeal branches of the vagus nerve. Splanchnic

mesoderm contributes smooth muscle to its lower part and the nerve supply is autonomic from the neural crest.

The stomach

The stomach begins as a spindle-shaped dilatation of the caudal end of the foregut. It is attached to the dorsal wall of the abdominal cavity by the dorsal mesentery. During the 5th and 6th weeks the dorsal border elongates to form the convex **greater curvature** of the stomach whilst

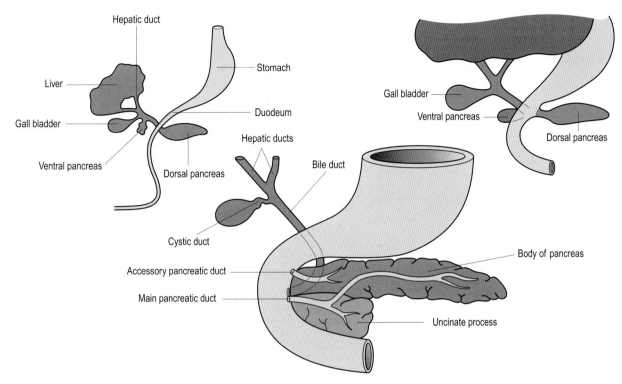

Figure 11.9 • Development of duct systems of liver, gall bladder and pancreas. (From Fitzgerald M J T, Fitzgerald M 1994, with permission.)

the ventral border forms the concave **lesser curvature**. The stomach now rotates clockwise on its axis through 90° taking the **dorsal mesentery** to the left. This rotation ensures that the liver becomes a right-sided organ and the spleen a left-sided organ (Schoenwolf et al 2008).

The duodenum

The **duodenum** develops from the caudal part of the foregut and the cranial end of the midgut. The junction of the two parts is just distal to the common bile duct.

The liver, gall bladder, pancreas and spleen

About day 24 the endoderm thickens directly caudal to the **septum transversum** to form the **hepatic diverticulum** or liver bud, which grows out of the duodenum (Fig. 11.9). The liver bud gives off the **gall bladder** and **biliary duct system**. The hepatic diverticulum divides into left and right hepatic buds which develop into the **lobes** of the liver. The stalk of the gall bladder becomes the **cystic duct** and the stalks of the hepatic buds become the **hepatic ducts**. The **bile duct** is formed by the union of the conjoined hepatic ducts with the cystic ducts. The hepatic buds produce a network of **hepatocytes** arranged in branching and anastomosing plates.

The **pancreas** develops as two separate structures. The smaller ventral pancreas arises from the hepatic diverticulum which will become the bile duct, to form

the uncinate process of the pancreas. The larger dorsal pancreas arises from the duodenum to form the head, body and tail. The main **pancreatic duct** enters the duodenum with the bile duct.

The **spleen** develops from mesenchymal cells between the layers of the dorsal mesentery. It appears about the 5th week on the left side of the abdomen. The spleen is seeded by **haematopoietic cells** from the wall of the umbilical vesicle and manufactures both fetal red and white blood cells in the middle trimester of pregnancy.

Development of the veins of the liver

The vitelline veins infiltrate between the hepatocytes to form the **liver sinusoids**. The **portal vein**, which drains the entire gut below the diaphragm, also develops from segments of the two vitelline veins. During the 5th week the right umbilical vein disappears while the left one enlarges to receive returning placental blood. During weeks 6–8 a large vascular shunt called the **ductus venosus** diverts oxygenated blood from the left umbilical vein to the right hepatic vein, ensuring that the highly metabolic liver receives sufficient oxygen and nutrients.

The midgut

The derivatives of the midgut are the **small intestine**, the **caecum** and **vermiform appendix**, **ascending colon** and the right half of the **transverse colon**. During the

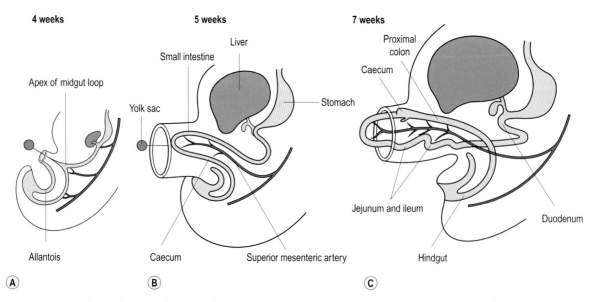

Figure 11.10 (A) Intestine at 4 weeks. (B) Entry of midgut loop into umbilical cord. (C) Counterclockwise rotation through 180° carries caecum and proximal colon to a cranial position. (From Fitzgerald M J T, Fitzgerald M 1994, with permission.)

6th week the midgut lengthens and, because of the rapid growth of the liver and kidneys, there is insufficient room in the abdominal cavity. The gut is found in the umbilical cord (Fig. 11.10) which is called physiological umbilical herniation of the midgut (Moore & Persaud 2008).

As it enters the umbilical cord, the midgut twists on itself in a counter-clockwise direction when viewed from the front. By 10 weeks the peritoneal coelom has increased sufficiently in size to allow the intestines to slide back into the abdomen. The small intestine returns first and the colon follows to frame it. The caecum and appendix enter last to lie on the right side below the liver.

The hindgut: the rectum and anal canal

The hindgut extends from the midgut to the **cloacal membrane**. The **cloaca** will form the bladder and urethra by the 7th week with development of the **urorectal septum**, formed by migration of cells from the **urogenital tubercle**. It forms the **urogenital sinus** ventrally and the **rectum** and upper **anal canal** dorsally (Fig. 11.11; see also below). The upper half of the anal canal is lined by columnar epithelium continuous with the rectum, whereas the lower half develops from the anal pit and is lined with stratified epithelium continuous with the epidermis of the surrounding skin.

The urorectal septum fuses with the cloacal membrane by the end of the 6th week to form the **dorsal anal membrane** and the larger **urogenital membrane**. The anal membrane ruptures at the end of week 7 to form the anal orifice. Imperforate anus occurs in 1 in 5000 births. The mesoderm of the urogenital septum persists as the **perineal body**.

The urinary and genital tracts

The urinary and genital systems are closely related and develop from intermediate mesoderm, with the urinary system developing before the genital system. During embryonic folding the intermediate mesoderm is carried ventrally and loses contact with the somites. A longitudinal ridge of mesoderm on either side of the primitive aorta is called the **urogenital ridge**. Part of this ridge, the **nephrogenic cord**, gives rise to the urinary system and the **gonadal** or **genital ridge** gives rise to the genital system.

The kidneys and ureters

Three pairs of kidneys appear in succession during development:

- The **pronephros** appears in the 4th week. It persists in some fishes but is non-functional in mammals and disappears.
- The **mesonephros** exists between weeks 4 and 8 and is found in amphibians but again disappears in mammals.
- Finally, the **metanephros** or mammalian kidney appears (Fig. 11.12).

Development of the collecting system

The metanephros develops from the **metanephric diverticulum**, a dorsal bud from the mesonephric (Wolffian) ducts and a mass of **metanephric mesoderm**. The stalk of each metanephric diverticulum becomes the **ureter**. As this advances towards the kidney it acquires a lumen

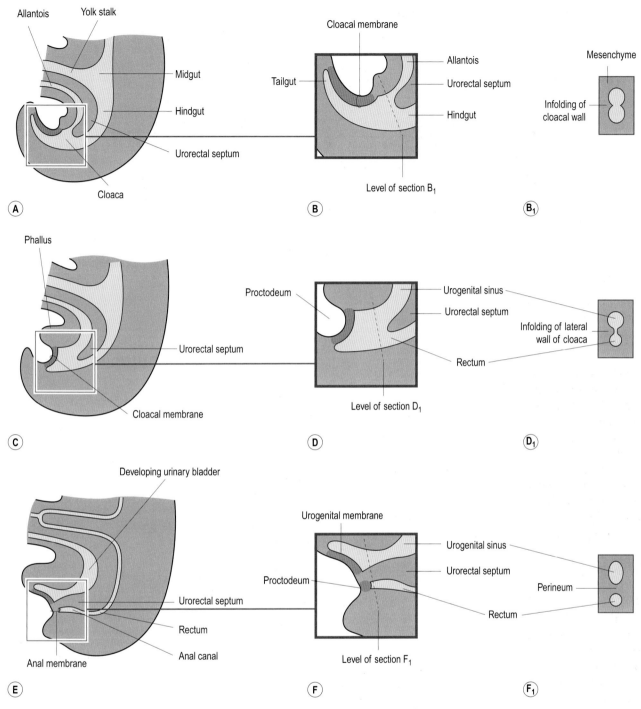

Figure 11.11 • Drawings illustrating successive stages in the partitioning of the cloaca into the rectum and urogenital sinus by the urorectal septum. (A, C, E) Views from the left side at 4, 6 and 7 weeks respectively. (B, D, F) Enlargements of cloacal region. (B₁, D₁, F₁) Transverse sections of the cloaca at the levels shown in (B), (D) and (F) respectively. Note that the tailgut (shown in B) degenerates and disappears as the rectum forms from the dorsal part of the cloaca (shown in C). (Reproduced with permission from Moore 1989.)

by apoptosis and its tip hollows out to become the **renal pelvis**. The ureteric bud keeps dividing to form generations of **collecting tubules** (Fig. 11.13). The first four generations enlarge to become the **major calyces** and the next four become the **minor calyces** of the kidney. The remaining generations form the collecting tubules.

The cells of the intermediate mesoderm surrounding the kidney form a **metanephric cap** over the renal pelvis. A cluster of metanephric cells gathers at the tip of each collecting tubule to form a **nephron**. The kidneys ascend into the abdomen to come into contact with the **adrenal glands** by the 8th week. The fetal kidney

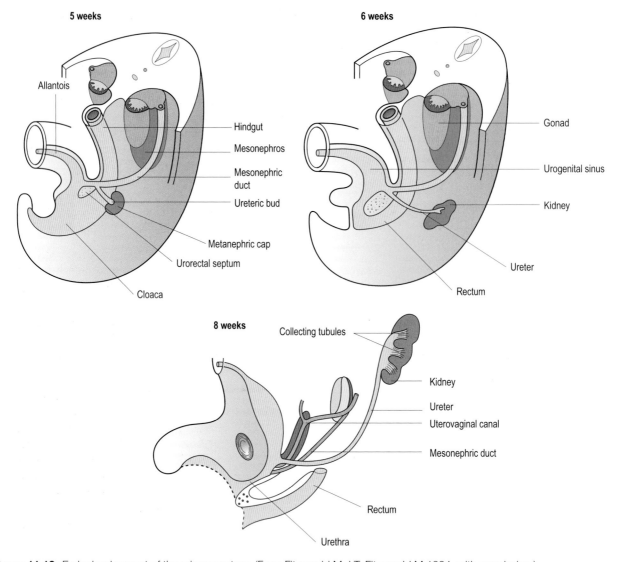

Figure 11.12 • Early development of the urinary system. (From Fitzgerald M J T, Fitzgerald M 1994, with permission.)

produces small amounts of urine from 9 weeks and is more functional from 15 weeks with excretion of urine into the amniotic cavity. Renal arteries develop to supply blood.

The bladder and urethra

Between the umbilicus and the cloacal membrane, caudal mesoderm forms a midline swelling called the **genital tubercle**. Migration of cells from this forms the **urogenital sinus** which gives rise to the bladder and urethra. The urogenital sinus has three parts:

1. A **vesical part** expands to form the bladder and receive the two ureters.

2. A narrow **pelvic part** forms the lining epithelium of the prostatic and membranous parts of the **urethra**.

In females the pelvic part lines the whole of the short urethra.

3. A **phallic part** extends ventrally beneath the **penis**. At first the urethra opens on the underside of the penis behind the developing **glans** but during the 4th month a glandular urethra opens at the tip of the glans. The **prepuce** is an outgrowth of skin from the glans.

As the bladder enlarges, the caudal parts of the mesonephric ducts are incorporated into its dorsal wall so that the ureters open into the urinary bladder.

The suprarenal glands

The cortex and medulla of the **suprarenal glands** are formed from separate tissues. The cortex develops

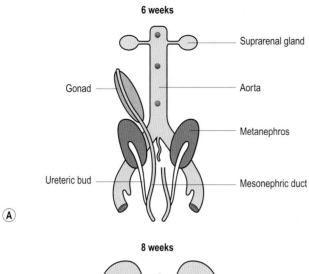

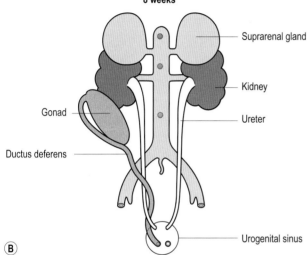

Figure 11.13•Renal ascent. (A) At 6 weeks, (B) at 8 weeks. (From Fitzgerald M J T, Fitzgerald M 1994, with permission.)

and female (Fig. 11.14) but soon differentiate into recognisable male and female from the 7th week (Fig. 11.15).

Testes and the male genital tract

In the presence of the SRY (sex-determining region Y) gene at about day 50 intermediate mesoderm forms the **tunica albuginea**. The sex cords become **testicular cords** and the primordial germ cells become **prospermatogonia**. The testicular cords are gathered into lobules separated by testicular septa derived from the tunica albuginea. The inner ends of the cords are linked together in a network called the **rete testis**. Two sets of endocrine cells form in the lobules:

1. Sertoli cells are the most numerous and produce a **Müllerian duct inhibitory factor** which causes regression of the paramesonephric ducts during week 9.

2. Leydig cells secrete **testosterone** which ensures the survival and growth of the **Wolffian ducts** and the formation of the epididymis, ductus deferens and ejaculatory duct.

The testes descend gradually from their original site in the lumbar region into the scrotal sac, usually by term. They are accompanied by a pocket of peritoneum called the **processus vaginalis** which becomes the **tunica vaginalis** on completion of descent. The testes are accompanied by the ductus deferens, testicular blood vessels, nerves and lymphatics which constitute the spermatic cords. In females the Wolffian ducts disappear by programmed cell death without any ovarian influence. Remnants found in the broad ligament may form **parovarian cysts**.

from mesoderm and the medulla develops from neural crest cells. The medullary **chromaffin cells** are modified sympathetic ganglion cells whose chief secretion is adrenaline (epinephrine).

The reproductive system

The gonads can be identified about the 5th week and develop from three sources. The gonadal ridges on the medial side of the mesonephros include cells from two sources, the **coelomic epithelium** and underlying **intermediate mesoderm**. The epithelium releases a chemical that attracts a third source of cells, **primordial germ cells**, which become ova or sperm. About 100 are present on the caudal surface of the umbilical vesicle during the 4th week. These migrate into the interior of the gonadal ridge and are enclosed in columns of epithelial cells called **sex cords**. At first the indifferent gonads are the same in male

Ovaries and the female genital tract

In the absence of SRY no tunica albuginea forms. The sex cords accumulate in the outer cortex of the gonadal ridge and this becomes filled with **primordial follicles** consisting of an oocyte derived from primordial germ cells, an inner shell of follicular cells and an outer shell—the theca. The number of primordial follicles reaches a maximum of 6–7 million in the 15th week. Programmed cell death reduces this number drastically so that 2 years after birth only 1 million remain and at puberty only 300 000. The ovary descends from the abdominal lumbar region into the pelvis after the 12th week.

The upper and middle sections of the Müllerian tubes form the epithelial lining of the uterine tubes and the lower segments fuse into one during the 9th week to become the **uterovaginal canal** which eventually forms the epithelial lining of the uterus. The muscle

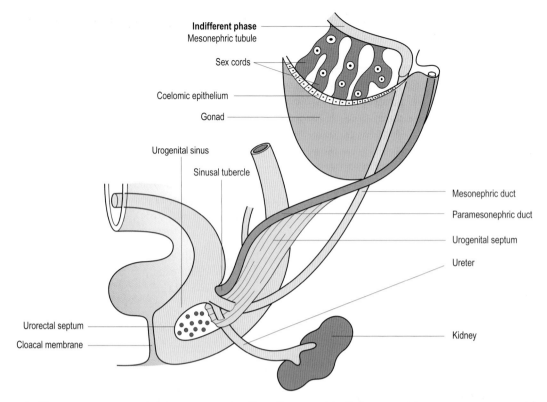

Figure 11.14•Indifferent gonad and genital ducts at 4 weeks. (From Fitzgerald M J T, Fitzgerald M 1994, with permission.)

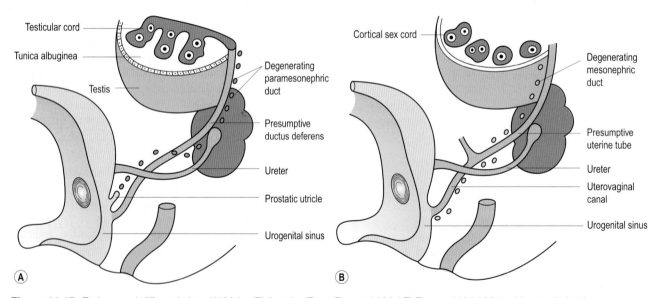

Figure 11.15•Early sexual differentiation. (A) Male, (B) female. (From Fitzgerald M J T, Fitzgerald M 1994, with permission.)

walls of the uterine tubes and uterus are formed from splanchnic mesoderm.

The vagina

If the Müllerian system develops, a small tubercle called the Müllerian eminence gives rise to the **vaginal plate**. This lengthens along the dorsal wall of the urogenital sinus. The lumen of the vagina is formed by canalisation from below upwards and extends around the cervix to form the fornices. The hymen is left as a partition between the vagina and the vestibule.

The external genitalia

Early in the 3rd month it is not possible to see a sexual difference. Externally the phallic urethra is an open groove flanked by paired inner urogenital folds and outer genital swellings derived from mesenchyme.

- In males the matching pairs come together under the influence of testosterone. The urogenital folds unite below the urethral groove to complete the spongy urethra and the genital swellings form the two halves of the scrotum. A line of union at the junction of the two halves of the scrotum is called the scrotal raphe and the line of union of the urogenital folds is marked by the urethral raphe.
- In females the matching pairs stay apart and there is growth in situ of the urogenital folds and genital swellings. The phallus forms the clitoris with a small glans at its tip. The urethral groove and the phallic part of the urogenital sinus remain open as the vestibule and the urogenital folds become the labia minora while the genital swellings become the labia majora.

Estimation of embryonic age

By 8 weeks the embryo is recognisably human although the head is rounder and very large in proportion to the body. The rest of pregnancy is concerned mainly with growth and maturation. The usual calculation of embryonic age is made by ascertaining the date of the first day of the last menstrual period (LMP). However, it is unusual to know the exact day of fertilisation and there are other ways of estimating the age of an embryo if spontaneously or therapeutically aborted. External features and measurements are useful and careful ultrasound scanning can confirm the age of a viable embryo in utero. At 4 weeks after fertilisation (6 weeks from the first day of the LMP) the embryo and its sac measure 5 mm long. A week later discrete embryonic features can be visualised and crown–rump measurements can be made.

Main points

- The cardiovascular system is in place from the end of the 3rd week and nutrients are obtained from the maternal circulation. Blood is pumped round blood vessels by a heart early in the 4th week. Early in the 3rd week blood islands appear in the mesoderm lining the umbilical vesicle.
- Three sets of arteries develop: two umbilical arteries carry blood to the placenta, vitelline arteries arising from the dorsal aortas become the three mesenteric arteries of the gut and intersegmental arteries supply blood to the somites and neural tube.
- Two umbilical veins form in the body stalk to link with the arteries in the placental capillary bed. Two umbilical vesicle veins become the vitelline veins and two main common cardinal veins develop from the fetus.
- A median laryngotracheal groove appears on the floor of the primitive larynx in the middle of week 4. A septum converts this into the laryngotracheal tube with a laryngeal opening into the larynx. Tracheo-oesophageal folds form a septum dividing the cranial part of the foregut into the laryngotracheal tube and the oesophagus.
- Lung buds split to form two bronchial buds which divide into secondary bronchi serving the three lobes of the right lung and two lobes of the left lung. During the 7th month respiratory bronchioles terminate in alveolar ducts and sacs lined by type 1 alveolar cells. At the end of the 6th month type 2 alveolar cells which secrete surfactant appear.
- The primitive gut begins to form during the 4th week when the dorsal part of the umbilical vesicle becomes

incorporated into the embryo during folding. By the middle of the 4th week the alimentary tract consists of foregut, midgut and hindgut.
- The stomach begins as a spindle-shaped dilatation of the caudal end of the foregut. During the 5th and 6th weeks the dorsal border elongates to form the greater curvature of the stomach while the ventral border forms the lesser curvature.
- On day 24 the hepatic diverticulum or liver bud grows out from the duodenum and gives off the gall bladder and biliary duct system. Left and right hepatic buds develop into the lobes of the liver. The gall bladder stalk becomes the cystic duct and the stalks of the hepatic ducts become the hepatic ducts. The bile duct is formed from the union of hepatic and cystic ducts.
- The pancreas develops as two separate structures. The smaller ventral pancreas arises from the hepatic diverticulum to form the uncinate process of the pancreas. The larger dorsal pancreas arises from the duodenum to form the head, body and tail.
- The spleen appears about the 5th week and develops from mesenchymal cells. It is seeded by haematopoietic cells from the umbilical vesicle and produces both red and white blood cells in the middle trimester of pregnancy.
- Derived from the midgut are the small intestine, the caecum and appendix, ascending colon and right half of the transverse colon. During the 6th week there is physiological herniation of the midgut but there is return of the intestines to the abdominal cavity by the 10th week.

- The cloaca forms the bladder and urethra with development of the urorectal septum. The anal membrane ruptures at the end of the 7th week to form the anal orifice.
- The urogenital ridge gives rise to the nephrogenic cord, primordium of the urinary system. The part giving rise to the genital system is called the genital ridge. Three pairs of kidneys appear in succession during development. The last is the metanephros or permanent mammalian kidney.
- The gonadal ridge includes cells from two sources: the coelomic epithelium and underlying intermediate mesoderm. The epithelium releases a chemical that attracts the primordial germ cells which will form ova or sperm. The gonads are identical in males and females up to the 7th week.
- Two pairs of genital ducts are present: the Wolffian ducts are forerunners of the male genital tract and the Müllerian ducts are forerunners of the female genital tract. In the absence of the trigger SRY gene all fetuses become female. SRY triggers formation of the testes.
- Early in the 3rd month the phallic urethra is an open urethral groove flanked by paired urogenital folds and outer genital swellings. In males testosterone influences the matching pairs to come together to complete the spongy urethra and the genital swellings form two halves of the scrotum. In females the urethral groove and the phallic part of the genital sinus remain open. The urogenital folds become the labia minora whilst the genital swellings become the labia majora. The phallus forms the clitoris with a small glans at its tip.
- By 8 weeks the embryo is recognisably human. The remaining intrauterine life is concerned mainly with growth and maturation.

References

Carlson, B.M., 2004. Human Embryology and Developmental Biology, third (updated) edn. Elsevier Mosby, Philadelphia PA.

Moore, K.L., Persaud, T.V.N., 2008. The Developing Human: Clinically Oriented Embryology, eighth edn. Elsevier Saunders, Philadelphia PA.

Schoenwolf, G.C., Bleyl, S.B., Brauer, R., Francis-West, P.H., 2008. Larsen's Human Embryology, fourth edn. Elsevier Churchill Livingstone, Edinburgh.

Wolpert, L., 2007. Principles of Development, third edn. Oxford University Press, Oxford.

Annotated recommended reading

Moore, K.L., Persaud, T.V.N., 2008. The Developing Human: Clinically Oriented Embryology, eighth edn. Elsevier Saunders, Philadelphia PA.

This updated textbook clearly describes embryo development week by week and provides an excellent source for understanding the origin of congenital defects. The illustrations, as before, are excellent.

Schoenwolf, G.C., Bleyl, S.B., Brauer, R., Francis-West, P.H., 2008. Larsen's Human Embryology, fourth edn. Elsevier Churchill Livingstone, Edinburgh.

This book examines both molecular biological and clinical aspects of embryology with applications linked to an advancing knowledge base.

Chapter Twelve

12

The placenta, membranes and amniotic fluid

CHAPTER CONTENTS

Introduction

To survive and grow during intrauterine life the embryo is essentially in a parasitic relationship with the mother (Carlson 2004). It obtains nutrients and oxygen and disposes of waste products through the complex organ called the placenta. This organ is the defining characteristic of all mammals and is a key feature to the transfer of information from mother to fetus and vice versa. It has developed to ensure that the fetus is well protected during its development but problems and malfunctions can arise. By understanding the development and function of the placenta treatments to save babies lives may be possible (Gluckman & Hanson 2005).

Implantation

The embryo obtains nutrients and oxygen and disposes of waste products via its mother's circulation through the **placenta**. The placenta is derived from embryonic trophoblast cells and a few inner cell mass mesodermal cells. The initial trophoblastic cells called collectively the **cytotrophoblast** give rise to the **syncytiotrophoblast** (trophoblast without cells) that has undergone nuclear division without forming daughter cells. This structure invades the uterine lining allowing the embryo to embed by the 10th day when a plug of blood clot and cellular debris closes over its point of entry. The syncytiotrophoblast at the embryonic pole of the **zygote** forms a thick multinucleated layer.

Maternal endometrial capillaries surrounding the embryo swell to form **sinusoids** which are eroded by the invasive syncytiotrophoblast. Small spaces called **lacunae** appear in the syncytiotrophoblast and become filled with a mixture of blood from the sinusoids and secretions from the eroded endometrial glands. This fluid is the **embryotroph** and passes to the embryonic disc by diffusion (Carlson 2004, Moore & Persaud 2008). The lacunae fuse to form the **intervillous spaces** of the placenta through which maternal blood begins to flow.

In normal pregnancy decidual and myometrial arteries undergo changes to convert them to **uteroplacental arteries**. Two types of **migratory cytotrophoblast** (MC) cause this:

1. Endovascular MC invades spiral arterioles on the decidua and myometrium and replaces arterial endothelium, destroying muscle and elastic tissues in the tunica media. The tissues are replaced by maternal fibrinoid. The migration takes place in two waves: at 6–10 weeks and at 14–16 weeks.

2. Interstitial (stromal) MC destroys the ends of decidual blood vessels, promoting blood flow into the lacunae. The maternal arteries are functionally denervated so that they are completely dilated and unresponsive to pressor substance or autonomic neural control. Local prostacyclin maintains vasodilation of the uterine radial arteries.

Soon mesodermal tissue from the developing embryo migrates through the primitive streak and joins trophoblast extensions to form the connecting stalk. This mesoderm gives rise to the umbilical blood vessels and the structure becomes the umbilical cord. By the end of the second week trophoblastic cells have formed finger-like projections called **primary chorionic villi** all round the embryo. The embryo, its umbilical vesicle and the early amniotic sac are suspended in the **chorionic sac** which consists of a layer of mesoderm nearest the embryo, the cytotrophoblast and the syncytiotrophoblast nearest the endometrium. The amniotic sac is nearest to the uterine wall and is divided from the chorion by a fluid-filled cavity, the **extraembryonic coelom**.

Development of the chorionic villi

Early in the 3rd week a core of loose connective tissue developed from embryonic mesenchyme invades each primary chorionic villus to form the **secondary chorionic villi**. Some of the mesenchymal cells in the core differentiate into fetal blood capillaries, forming mature **tertiary chorionic villi**. By 15–20 days there is a functioning **arteriocapillary venous network** connected to the embryonic heart vessels. By the end of the 3rd week fetal blood circulates through the chorionic villi and an exchange of substances between maternal and fetal circulations begins (Figs 12.1, 12.2).

Formation of the cytotrophoblastic shell

At the same time the cytotrophoblastic cells proliferate and extend through the syncytiotrophoblast to form a **cytotrophoblastic shell**. This attaches the chorionic sac to the maternal endometrium by specialised chorionic villi called **stem** or **anchoring villi**. From the sides of the

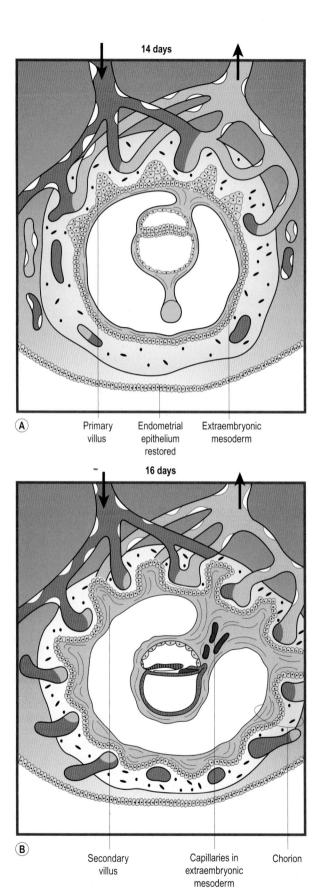

(A)   Primary villus | Endometrial epithelium restored | Extraembryonic mesoderm

(B)   Secondary villus | Capillaries in extraembryonic mesoderm | Chorion

Figure 12.1 • Formation of chorionic vesicle. (From Fitzgerald M J T, Fitzgerald M 1994, with permission.)

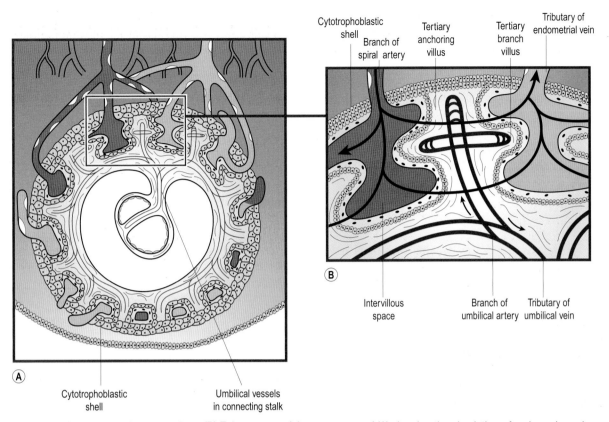

Figure 12.2 • (A) Chorionic vesicle at 21 days. (B) Enlargement of the upper part of (A) showing the circulation of embryonic and maternal blood. (From Fitzgerald M J T, Fitzgerald M 1994, with permission.)

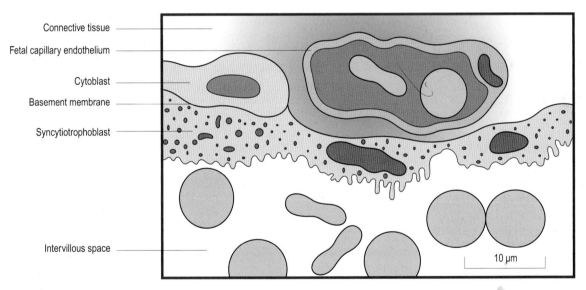

Figure 12.3 • Structure of the placental membrane. All erythrocytes are coloured grey. (From Fitzgerald M J T, Fitzgerald M 1994, with permission.)

stem villi branch villi grow through and it is here that the main exchange of materials between maternal and fetal circulations occurs.

Until about 20 weeks the placental membrane (Fig. 12.3) consists of four layers separating the two circulations: syncytiotrophoblast, cytotrophoblast, connective tissue of the mesenchyme core and the endothelium of the fetal capillary (Moore & Persaud 2008). Maternal and fetal circulations do not mingle unless there is damage to the villi. As pregnancy advances, this placental membrane becomes thinner and many fetal capillaries lie very close to the syncytiotrophoblast.

Later placental development

Once the conceptus has implanted, the decidual reaction spreads outwards from the embedding site and the endometrium becomes the decidua because it is shed at the end of pregnancy. Three regions of the decidua based on their relation to the implantation site are described:

1. The **decidua basalis** lies beneath the conceptus, forming the maternal component of the placenta.

2. The **decidua capsularis** overlies the conceptus.

3. The **decidua vera** or parietalis is the name of the remaining uterine lining.

As the conceptus grows the decidua capsularis bulges into the uterine cavity and eventually fuses with the decidua vera. By 22 weeks the decidua capsularis has degenerated and disappeared (Fig. 12.4).

The entire surface of the chorionic sac is covered by villi until the 8th week. As the sac grows the chorionic villi associated with the decidua capsularis become compressed, reducing their blood supply and degenerate to become the **chorion laeve** (smooth) which becomes the **chorionic membrane**. The chorionic villi of the decidua basalis branch to form the **chorion frondosum** or fetal part of the placenta. By 16 weeks the placenta reaches its full thickness and no new lobes or stem villi develop. Circumferential growth continues with branching of villi. The size and number of maternal capillaries increases, as does the surface area for gas exchange. Cellular proliferation stops at 35 weeks but cellular hypertrophy continues until term and there is scope for the fetus to signal to the placenta if its needs are not being met (Gluckman & Hanson 2005).

The mature placenta

Appearance

The placenta is a flattened discoid organ about 20 cm in diameter. It is 2.5 cm thick at the centre and thins out towards its circumference where it is continuous with the chorion. It is about one-sixth of the baby's weight at term. There are two distinct surfaces (Fig. 12.5): the **maternal surface** attached to the decidua and the **fetal surface** covered with amnion into which the umbilical cord inserts.

At delivery the maternal surface is dark red because it contains maternal blood. Part of the decidua basalis will have been separated with it during delivery. The surface is formed of about 20 **cotyledons** (lobes) separated by **sulci** (grooves). The decidua dips down into these sulci to form septa. The lobes are made up of **lobules**, each containing a tertiary villus and its branches.

Because of the presence of the amnion the fetal surface is a shiny greyish white. From the insertion of the umbilical cord, branches of the single umbilical vein and two arteries spread out and dip down into the tissue. The amnion can be peeled off the surface, leaving the chorionic plate which is the portion continuous with the chorion.

The membranes

The **amnion** and **chorion** grow until about 28 weeks and then increase their size by stretching. They resist rupture as the fetus grows mainly due to the strength of the amnion. Rupture of the membranes during labour is probably brought about by increased intrauterine pressure as contractions reduce the intrauterine space and the amniotic fluid cannot be compressed. The amnion and chorion are not fused and contain up to 200 ml of amniotic fluid between them.

The outer chorion adheres closely to the decidua but the amnion moves over it aided by mucus. This may lead to rupture of the amnion with the formation of amniotic bands which may constrict or amputate fetal limbs (Blackburn 2007). The chorion is a thick, opaque, friable membrane which varies at term from 0.02 to 0.2 mm thick. It consists of four layers of tissue (Fig. 12.6) which atrophy as pregnancy advances. The cells of the chorion laeve are metabolically active, producing enzymes that can reduce the level of locally produced progesterone and a protein that can bind progesterone. The chorion also produces prostaglandins, oxytocin and platelet-activating factor, stimulators of myometrial activity.

The inner amnion is tough, smooth and translucent and lines the chorion and the surface of the placenta, continuing over the outer surface of the umbilical cord. At term it is about 0.02–0.5 mm thick and consists of five layers (Fig. 12.6). It is lined with non-ciliated epithelial cells which may help in the formation and regulation of amniotic fluid. The amnion also produces prostaglandins, in particular PGE_2, which may help to initiate the onset of labour. A rising ratio between estradiol and progesterone may regulate the activity of prostaglandin which may play an important part in the onset of labour by increasing the number of myometrial oxytocin receptors (Johnson 2007).

The umbilical cord

The umbilical cord or **funis** is usually attached to the centre of the placental fetal surface. It is 1–2 cm in diameter and varies in length from 30 cm to 90 cm with an average of 50 cm. There are normally two **umbilical arteries** and one **umbilical vein** surrounded by a mucoid connective tissue called **Wharton's jelly**. The umbilical

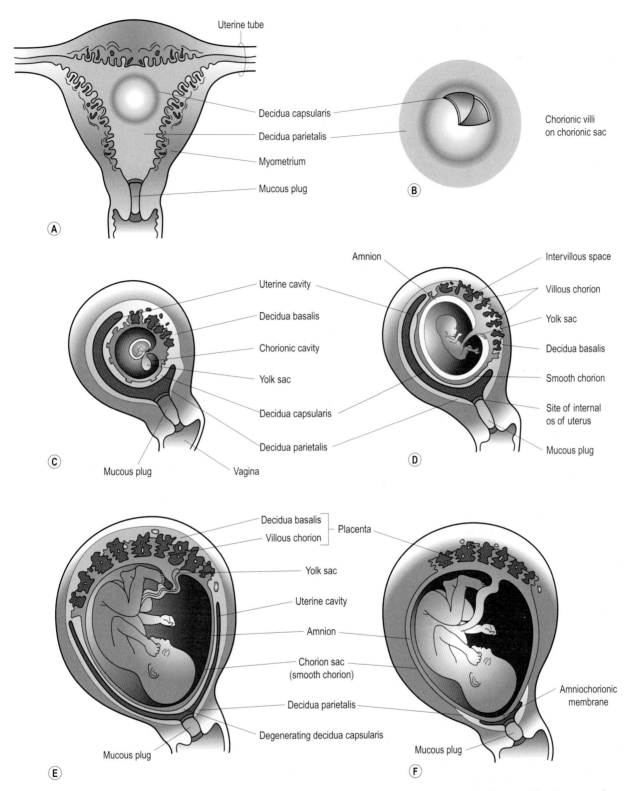

Figure 12.4 • (A) Drawing of a frontal section of the uterus showing the elevation of the decidua capsularis caused by the expanding chorionic sac of an implanted 4-week embryo. (B) Enlarged drawing of the implantation site shown in (A); the chorionic villi have been exposed by cutting an opening in the decidua capsularis. (C–F) Drawings of sagittal sections of the decidua. In (F) the amnion and chorion are fused with each other and the decidua parietalis, thus obliterating the uterine cavity. Note that the chorionic villi persist only where the chorion is associated with the decidua basalis; here they have formed the villous chorion. (From Moore K, Persaud T V N 2008, with permission.)

vein is longer than the arteries which spiral round it. The vessels are longer than the cord and non-significant loops of vessel called **false knots** may be seen. Rarely a **true knot** may be present and the blood vessels may become occluded, causing fetal distress, especially during labour.

The umbilical vesicle (yolk sac) and allantois

By 9 weeks the umbilical vesicle has shrunk to a pear-shaped remnant about 5 mm in diameter. Once its functions in producing blood cells during weeks 3–5 are completed, it becomes detached from the gut and remains present in the umbilical cord (Coad & Dunstall 2005). The **allantois**, which is an important structure

for exchange of gases and removal of urinary waste but is never a prominent structure in the human embryo as in birds and some mammals (Carlson 2004), degenerates forming the **urachus** (median umbilical ligament) that connects the umbilicus to the urinary bladder. In 2% of adults the urachus persists as a **Meckel's diverticulum** of the ileus.

The placental circulation

The placental villi form a huge surface for substance exchange between maternal and fetal circulations. Maternal blood enters the intervillous space in spurts via 80–100 endometrial spiral arteries. It flows slowly over the surface of the villi and substances are exchanged in both directions. The maternal blood reaches the floor of the **intervillous space** where it drains into the endometrial veins (Figs 12.7–12.9). Anything interfering with the uteroplacental circulation will result in fetal hypoxia and may interfere with growth or cause death. An analogy for the placental circulation is taking a shower. If you stand under the shower, your body is the tertiary villus, the shower head is the spiral arteriole delivering blood and the shower drainage is the endometrial vein.

Deoxygenated blood leaves the fetus and passes into the two umbilical arteries which take it to the placenta. Here within the chorionic villi the fetal blood is brought very close to maternal blood from which it picks up oxygen. The oxygenated blood enters the umbilical vein which returns it to the fetus. The fetal circulation is described in detail in Chapter 48.

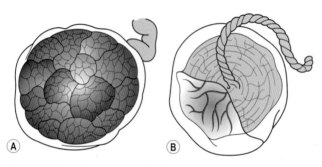

Figure 12.5 • The placenta. (A) The maternal surface, showing cotyledons, (B) the fetal surface. (From Henderson C, Macdonald S 2004, with kind permission of Elsevier.)

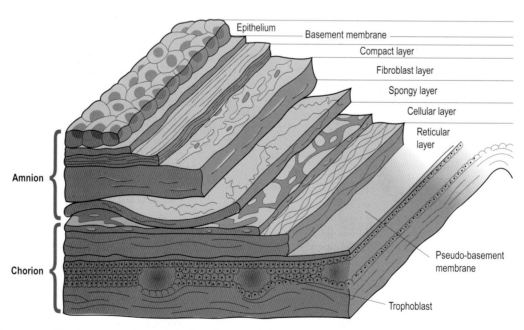

Figure 12.6 • Layers of the human amnion and chorion. (Reproduced with permission from Blackburn & Loper 1992.)

Anatomical variations of the placenta

Placentas may be abnormally shaped and it is important to examine the placenta and seek medical aid if it appears incomplete.

Succenturiate lobe

Sometimes a separate placental lobe is linked by blood vessels to the main placenta. Failure to deliver this succenturiate lobe may lead to infection and haemorrhage. Each placenta must be checked for a hole in the membranes with blood vessels leading away from it (Fig. 12.10).

Battledore placenta

The umbilical cord is inserted into the edge of the placenta, giving it the appearance of a battledore (a bat used to play a medieval game similar to badminton).

Velamentous insertion of the cord

The umbilical cord insertion is into the membranes outside the placental boundary. Rarely the umbilical vessels cross the internal os, a condition known as vasa praevia. If these vessels rupture during labour, the fetus may have a massive haemorrhage.

Circumvallate placenta

An opaque thickened ridge is seen on the fetal surface of the placenta which forms because of doubling back of

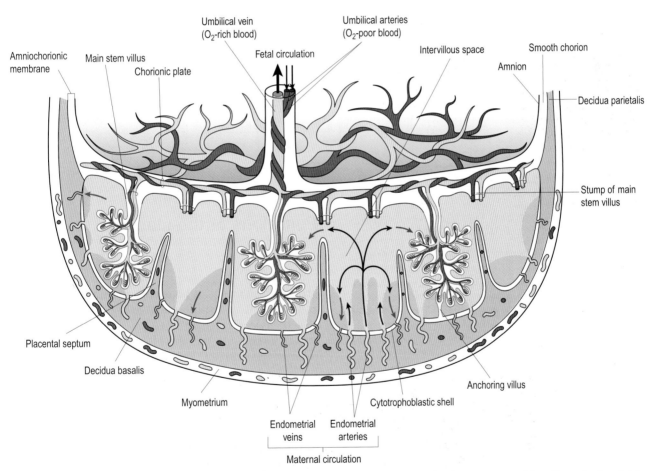

Figure 12.7 • Schematic drawing of a transverse section through a full-term placenta, showing: the relation of the villous chorion (fetal part of the placenta) to the decidua basalis (maternal part of the placenta; the fetal circulation; and the maternal placental circulation). Maternal blood flows into the intervillous spaces in funnel-shaped spurts from the spiral arteries, and exchanges of material between the mother and the embryo/fetus occur. The inflowing arterial blood pushes venous blood out of the intervillous space into the endometrial veins, which are scattered over the entire surface of the decidua basalis. Note that the umbilical arteries carry poorly oxygenated fetal blood (shown in dark grey) to the placenta and that the umbilical vein carries oxygenated blood (shown in light grey) to the fetus. Note also that the cotyledons are separated from each other by placental septa, projections of the decidua basalis. Each cotyledon consists of two or more main stem villi and their many branches. In this drawing only one stem villus is shown in each cotyledon but the stumps of those that have been removed are indicated. (Reproduced from Moore N 1989, with permission.)

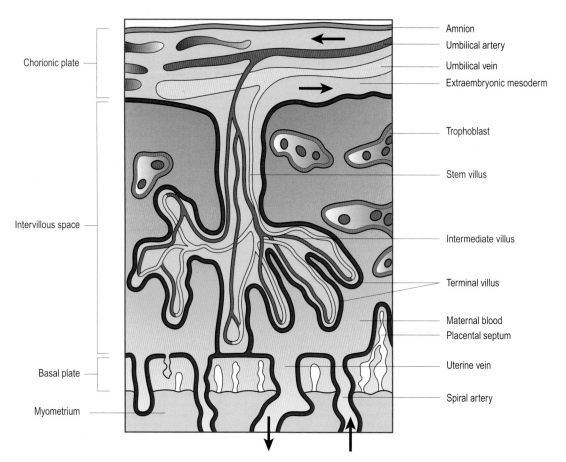

Figure 12.8 • Diagrammatic section through the placenta. The arteries carry deoxygenated blood; the veins carry oxygenated blood. Arrows indicate direction of blood flow. (From Fitzgerald M J T, Fitzgerald M 1994, with permission.)

the membranes (Fig. 12.11). The membranes may leave the placenta nearer to the centre than normal. It is associated with an increased risk of growth retardation.

Bipartite and tripartite placenta

A placenta may be divided into two or three fairly equal lobes.

Infarcts and calcification

Infarcts are patches on the maternal surface of the placenta caused by localised death of placental tissue resulting from an interruption of blood supply. They are red when newly formed and degenerate into white fibrous patches. Any placenta may contain them but they are more commonly associated with pregnancy hypertension.

Calcifications appear as small, gritty, greyish white patches on the surface of the placenta, especially if the pregnancy is post term. These are deposits of lime salts and are of no significance. The major placental pathologies of abruptio placentae and placenta praevia are discussed in Chapter 31.

Functions of the placenta

The key placental function is **transport of nutrients** to the fetus and **waste products** away from the fetus. The placenta also produces **hormones** and **protects** the fetus against environmental hazards. It has an **immunological role** in preventing fetal rejection. These functions are energy consuming and the placenta utilises about one-third of the nutrients devoted to the fetoplacental unit (Chard 2000).

Endocrine function

Although the maternal part of the placenta and the decidua secrete the hormones **prolactin**, **relaxin** and **prostaglandins**, decidual production of these hormones probably influences pregnancy most. **Pregnancy-associated placental protein A (PAPP-A)** is produced by the decidua as well as by placental trophoblast. These decidual hormones target the fetoplacental unit and bind to the fetal membranes and trophoblast.

The fetoplacental hormones alter maternal metabolic processes to benefit the fetus. They can be divided into

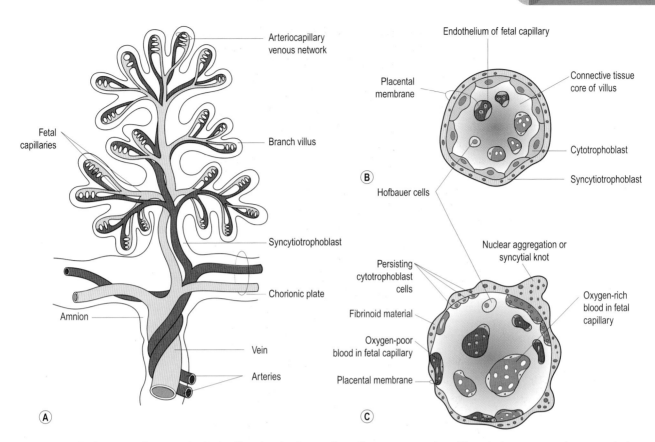

Figure 12.9 • (A) Drawing of a stem chorionic villus showing its arteriocapillary venous system. The arteries carry poorly oxygenated fetal blood and waste products from the fetus, whereas the vein carries oxygenated blood and nutrients to the fetus. (B, C) Drawings of sections through a branch villus at 10 weeks and full term, respectively. The placental membrane, composed of extrafetal tissues, separates the maternal blood in the intervillous space from the fetal blood in the capillaries in the villi. Note that the placental membrane becomes very thin at full term. Hofbauer cells are thought to be phagocytic. (Reproduced from Moore N 1989, with permission.)

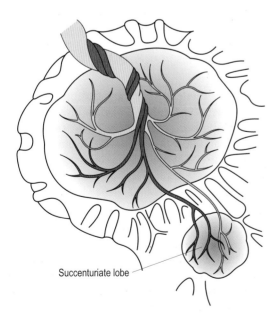

Figure 12.10 • Succenturiate placenta. (From Henderson C, Macdonald S 2004, with kind permission of Elsevier.)

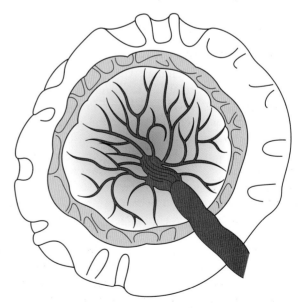

Figure 12.11 • Circumvallate placenta. (From Henderson C, Macdonald S 2004, with kind permission of Elsevier.)

two groups: **steroid hormones** and **protein hormones**. Steroid hormones such as estriol are made by sending a series of molecules backwards and forwards between fetus and placenta until the final hormone structure is reached. Steroid hormones are found in higher concentrations in fetal blood than in maternal blood.

The placenta produces specific protein hormones in substantial amounts as well as small quantities of every protein in the adult body (Chard 2000). The manufacture of protein hormones does not appear to need fetal input but may be linked to the amount of active trophoblastic tissue. They are found only in maternal blood and are implicated in changing maternal physiology. There does not appear to be a feedback mechanism for controlling their production. The syncytiotrophoblast produces its own **luteinising hormone releasing hormone (LHRH)** which controls **human chorionic gonadotrophin** (hCG) production in the same cell.

The protein hormones

The main placental protein hormones are:
- Human chorionic gonadotrophin (hCG).
- Human placental lactogen (hPL).
- Schwangerschaftsprotein 1 (SP$_1$).
- Pregnancy-associated protein A (PAPP-A).
- Pregnancy-associated protein B (PAPP-B).
- Placental protein 5 (PP5).

The above hormones are analogous to some anterior pituitary hormones (see Box 12.1). For example, hCG has a similar structure to LH and hPL is similar to prolactin and growth hormone.

The steroid hormones: oestrogens

Three oestrogens are important: **estrone**, **estradiol** and **estriol**. In the non-pregnant woman estriol is derived from estradiol and estrone, whereas in pregnancy it is synthesised by the fetoplacental unit. The fetal liver and suprarenal glands are important in estriol production and estriol is a direct measure of fetal well-being. **Pregnenolone sulphate**, the precursor of all fetoplacental steroids, is converted to oestrogens by placental enzymes. The steps are:

1. Acetate to cholesterol.
2. Cholesterol to pregnenolone.
3. Pregnenolone to dehydroepiandosterone.
4. 16-Hydroxylation of dehydroepiandosterone to 16-hydroxydehydroepiandosterone.
5. 16-Hydroxydehydroepiandosterone to estriol.

Oestrogen levels in normal pregnancy

Most tissues and organs are affected by oestrogens in pregnancy. Oestrogens are growth stimulators and cause hypertrophy and hyperplasia of uterine muscle as well as growth and development of breasts. In a normal pregnancy maternal serum levels of all three hormones rise but the curve for estriol is the most useful, showing a steep rise from 34 to 36 weeks. This late surge may not occur if pregnancy pathology affects the fetus. Then the curve may flatten out or even fall away. Serial assays of estriol have been used previously in monitoring fetal well-being but are not thought to be useful.

The steroid hormones: progesterone

Progesterone is produced by the syncytiotrophoblast. Some is sent to the maternal circulation and some to the fetus. Production is via cholesterol through pregnenolone to progesterone. Progesterone is broken down into the inactive substance pregnanediol and excreted in maternal urine.

The function of progesterone in pregnancy

Ovarian progesterone plays a part in ovum transport and implantation. It is involved in endometrial development in the second part of the menstrual cycle and the decidual reaction is caused by progesterone secretion for 48 h followed by superimposed oestrogen. Progesterone has a sedative effect on uterine muscle contractibility. With relaxin it may alter membrane potential in myometrial cells to reduce contractile impulses. Progesterone relaxes all smooth muscle during pregnancy, leading to many of the minor disorders of pregnancy. It competes with aldosterone for binding sites in the kidney, leading to urinary sodium loss. Aldosterone secretion is increased to counteract this. There is little evidence that in women a fall in progesterone initiates the onset of labour and the oestrogen:progesterone ratio does not appear to alter significantly in humans (Johnson 2007).

Progesterone levels in normal and abnormal pregnancy

It used to be thought that progesterone levels were indicative of fetal well-being and that low levels caused spontaneous abortion, but progesterone treatment was unsuccessful and low levels follow rather than cause fetal compromise. There is no agreement on normal levels as they fluctuate throughout pregnancy but the average is from 275 nmol/ml at 32 weeks to 450 nmol/ml at term (Klopper 1991). Progesterone is stored in body fat and may act as a buffer against transient low production.

Transfer of substances

The fetus is completely dependent on the mother for respiration, nutrition, excretion and protection and the placenta acts as the fetal lungs, alimentary tract, kidneys and endocrine system. The placenta grows throughout

BOX 12.1 PLACENTAL PROTEIN HORMONES

Human chorionic gonadotrophin

Human chorionic gonadotrophin (hCG) is a glycoprotein consisting of two subunits, a small α (alpha) subunit and a larger β (beta) subunit, joined by a disulphide bond. The β subunit is probably the biologically active one. In early pregnancy there is a rapid increase in hCG production, the urinary rate doubling every 36–48 h (Klopper 1991). The curve flattens out at 9 weeks then declines. The lower level is maintained until just before term when there is another rise. Plasma concentration rises from 7 to 100 IU/ml (international units/ml). Pregnancy test kits contain antibodies which bind to the β subunit which can be detected in maternal blood 9 days after fertilisation.

The hCG influences the ovary to produce extra oestrogen and progesterone which maintains pregnancy. The amount of hCG also appears to influence the level of placental progesterone production. However, no association has been found between insufficient hCG production and spontaneous abortion. A placental abnormality called **hydatidiform mole,** in which many of the chorionic villi develop into nodular swellings, produces large amounts of hCG (Ch. 31).

Human placental lactogen

Human placental lactogen (hPL) is produced by the syncytiotrophoblast and consists of 190 amino acids, of which 163 are found in human growth hormone. It is the only placental protein that does not contain carbohydrate. Maternal blood levels of hPL rise from 0.3 μg at 10 weeks to 5.4 μg at 36 weeks. There is then a fall until delivery which may correspond to a fall in functioning placental tissue. Maternal plasma hPL has been used to check placental function.

In pregnancy hPL probably acts as a growth promoter affecting carbohydrate metabolism. It causes the mobilisation of free fatty acids and antagonises the action of insulin. Pregnant women must manufacture more insulin and, where the insulin reserve is poor, carbohydrate metabolism may be compromised, especially in diabetic women, i.e. hPL is diabetogenic.

Schwangerschaftsprotein 1 (SP₁)

SP₁ is a glycoprotein present in large amounts. It can be detected in early pregnancy and is easily measured in late pregnancy. Like hPL, there is a steady rise until 36 weeks followed by a steady decline until delivery but the large subject-to-subject variation makes it useless as a test of placental function. This hormone may affect immunosuppression, preventing fetoplacental rejection.

Pregnancy-associated proteins A and B

A series of **pregnancy-associated proteins** were discovered in the early 1970s. Of these, **PAPP-A** and **PAPP-B** are produced by the trophoblast. PAPP-A is a large zinc-binding glycoprotein detectable in maternal plasma early in pregnancy with a rising concentration as pregnancy progresses right up to the onset of labour. Low levels may be associated with poor fetal growth and may be involved in preventing rejection of the fetoplacental unit by the cellular lymphocyte component of the maternal immune system. PAPP-B is the largest placental glycoprotein and rises throughout pregnancy with the steepest part of its concentration curve after 30 weeks. It has been used as a check of placental well-being in diseases such as pre-eclampsia and diabetes mellitus.

Placental protein 5

This is a small glycoprotein with different properties from the others. It is found in the stroma of the chorionic villi as well as in the syncytiotrophoblast. It may inhibit the proteolytic activity of trypsin and may inhibit protease activity in the placenta.

pregnancy, weighing about 300 g at 28 weeks and about 900 g at term. As the fetus grows rapidly in the second half of pregnancy, the placenta keeps pace with fetal needs by increased maternal and fetal blood flow (Chard 2000).

New villi are formed until term when their surface area exposed to maternal circulation is about 11 m². By late pregnancy there is thinning of the syncytium in small areas known as **vasculosyncytial membranes**. There are fewer microvilli and the syncytium is closely applied to the capillary basement membrane. A large number of **intracellular vesicles** enable transfer of macromolecules such as immunoglobulins.

Mechanisms of transfer

Substances such as gases, nutrients, waste materials and drugs are transported across the placental membrane by usual cellular membrane systems (Fig. 12.12).

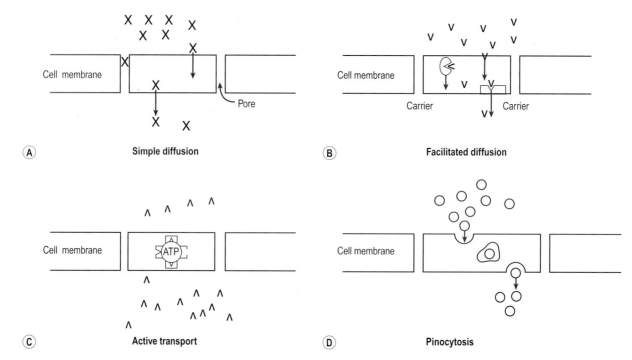

Figure 12.12 • Mechanisms of placental transfer. (Reproduced with permission from Blackburn & Loper 1992.)

- Simple diffusion of lipid-soluble substances.
- Water pores transfer water-soluble substances.
- Facilitated diffusion of substances such as glucose by carrier proteins.
- Active transport mechanisms against a concentration gradient of ions such as calcium and phosphate, of amino acids and of some vitamins.
- Endocytosis (pinocytosis) of macromolecules.

Transport across the placenta increases as pregnancy progresses and the placenta increases in size and becomes modified in structure. The rate of transfer is influenced by increased maternal and fetal blood flow and increased fetal demands. It is also influenced by maternal nutritional status, exercise and disease. Hypertension decreases nutrient transfer and alcoholism impairs placental uptake of glucose and amino acids.

Respiration

The major respiratory gases, oxygen and carbon dioxide, are moved between mother and fetus by simple transfer down a partial pressure concentration gradient. This is made more complex by maternal and fetal differences in haemoglobin concentration and type. If there is interruption to blood flow by maternal or fetal disease, respiratory exchange may be compromised.

Fetal oxygen supply

Most oxygen (O_2) in maternal and fetal blood is bound to haemoglobin in the form of **oxyhaemoglobin** (HbO$_2$).

Maternal blood arrives in the intervillous spaces of the placenta saturated with oxygen at a partial pressure of about 50 mmHg. Fetal blood arrives in the placenta with low O_2 content and a low partial pressure of 20 mmHg rising to only 30 mmHg after oxygenation. Therefore O_2 diffuses readily down the partial pressure gradient from mother to fetus. The diffusion gradient is enhanced in three ways (Guyton & Hall 2006):

1. By an increased affinity for O_2 of fetal haemoglobin (HbF) which combines more readily with O_2 than does adult haemoglobin (HbA).

2. The haemoglobin concentration in fetal blood is about 50% more than in the mother's blood.

3. The Bohr effect means that haemoglobin can carry more oxygen at a low P_{CO_2} than at a high P_{CO_2} (see excretion of CO_2 below).

Fetal systemic P_{O_2} is much lower than that of an adult and parts of the fetal vascular tree are extremely sensitive to O_2. Because of this, after the onset of respiration at birth, a rise in P_{O_2} leads to closure of the ductus arteriosus and constriction of the umbilical vessels.

Carbon dioxide

Most fetal metabolic processes are aerobic and depend on a constant oxygen supply. The fetus produces carbon dioxide (CO_2) for excretion. The much higher lipid solubility of CO_2 over O_2 results in a much more rapid transfer of the gas over cell membranes.

Nutrition

The fetus needs **amino acids** for cell building, **glucose** for energy, **calcium** and **phosphorus** for bones and teeth and iron and other minerals for the formation of blood. Simple forms of nutrients such as amino acids, glucose and fatty acids pass from maternal to fetal blood through the walls of the villi. The placenta selects substances and will deplete maternal supplies if necessary. Water, electrolytes and water-soluble vitamins diffuse across the cell membranes from mother to fetus.

Carbohydrate transfer

Glucose is a principal substrate for energy production which the fetoplacental unit utilises for the synthesis of macromolecules not obtained from the mother. The main form of glucose transport is facilitated diffusion via a carrier protein molecule. Some glycogen is stored in the placenta and may help supply its own needs. The healthy placenta has a capacity for glucose transfer that far exceeds fetal needs. The transfer is affected by maternal blood glucose levels and by insulin.

Amino acid transfer

Fetal proteins are synthesised from amino acids obtained via carrier systems from the maternal circulation. The fetus accumulates amino acids against a concentration gradient and the placenta contains more amino acids than either maternal or fetal circulations (Stacey 1991).

Lipid transfer

The fetus synthesises fatty acids from carbohydrate and short-chain organic acids, compensating for their absence in the diet of strict vegetarians. The fetus also probably obtains and stores fatty acids from the mother by passive transfer. Cholesterol also crosses the placenta.

Vitamin transfer

As **vitamins** cannot be synthesised in the body, the fetus is dependent on its mother for their supply. The lipid-soluble vitamins A, D and E pass from maternal to fetal blood down a concentration gradient. Water-soluble vitamins such as vitamin C appear to be transferred to the fetus against a gradient and cannot be passed back to the maternal circulation.

Trace element transfer

Small amounts of crucial trace elements, including iron, zinc and copper, are transferred to the fetus.

Water and electrolyte transfer

Water balance is achieved by diffusional gradient brought about by hydrostatic pressure and colloid osmotic pressure (see Ch. 1). Solutes such as sodium, potassium, calcium and phosphate are also freely transferred between maternal and fetal fluid circulations. The fine balance maintained between maternal and fetal fluid compartments can be disturbed by administration of hypotonic intravenous solutions such as 5% Dextrose to the mother, especially if it contains the **antidiuretic oxytocin**. Transfer of water to the fetus results in fetal **hyponatraemia**.

Excretion

Besides carbon dioxide, the placenta also passes other metabolic by-products such as urea, uric acid and bilirubin to the maternal circulation for excretion.

Protection

The placental membrane is a barrier against most bacteria, which are too large to penetrate it, but the organisms causing syphilis and tuberculosis can cross the barrier resulting in **transplacental infection**. Most infections that cause fetal abnormality, however, are viral such as rubella, first recognised in 1941. Drugs with a small molecular structure may cross to the fetus and some cause fetal abnormalities. Other drugs such as antibiotics may be beneficial in treating intrauterine infections such as fetal syphilis. Towards the end of pregnancy there is a transfer by pinocytosis of immunoglobulin G (IgG), conferring passive immunity for the first 3 months of extrauterine life.

Immunological role

The trophoblast appears to have immunological properties that make it inert so that maternal antibodies do not reject the fetus as foreign tissue (see Ch. 29).

Amniotic fluid

Production of amniotic fluid

Amniotic fluid (liquor amnii) is an alkaline, clear, pale straw-coloured fluid consisting of about 98% water with organic and inorganic substances in solution.

Sources of amniotic fluid

* Before keratinisation of the fetal skin there is free exchange of fluid and solutes between the fetus and the amniotic cavity.
* Amniotic fluid may be secreted by the amniotic membrane cells which are separated by intracellular channels leading to the amniotic cavity. Between 4 and 8 weeks of gestation amniotic fluid increases to about 20 ml.
* From the 11th week the fetus excretes urine into the amniotic fluid and the volume increases to 350 ml at

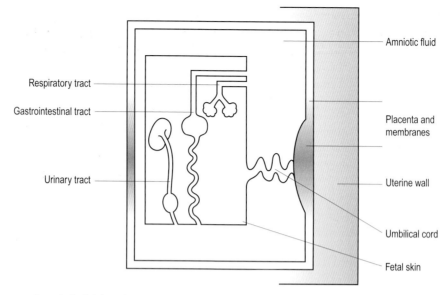

Figure 12.13 • Pathways of amniotic fluid production and exchange. (Reproduced with permission from Wallenburg 1977.)

20 weeks, 700–1000 ml by 37 weeks and declines slightly until term.

- Fluid is also secreted by the fetal respiratory and gastrointestinal tracts.
- Diffusion from maternal interstitial fluid across the amniochorionic membrane from the decidua is probably the main source (Moore & Persaud 2008).

Circulation of amniotic fluid

Amniotic fluid is in a constant state of circulation and the water content changes every 43 h (Moore & Persaud 2008). The fetal gastrointestinal tract is a major pathway for its removal. It is swallowed by the fetus and absorbed into its bloodstream; large amounts diffuse across the placenta into the maternal circulation and some is excreted by the fetus into the amniotic sac. In the second half of pregnancy the chief sources of amniotic fluid are the fetal kidneys, which contribute 700 ml/day and fetal lungs which contribute 350 ml/day (Fig. 12.13).

Content of amniotic fluid

During the first half of pregnancy the fetal skin is not a barrier to fluid and is a site for water and solute transfer. The composition of amniotic fluid in early pregnancy is similar to fetal tissue fluid. After keratinisation of the fetal skin at 17 weeks, the continuity between amniotic fluid and fetal extracellular fluid is lost and the pattern of content and flow changes.

In the latter half of pregnancy osmolality decreases to about 90% of maternal plasma and the composition of amniotic fluid resembles that of dilute urine (Blackburn 2007).

Mature amniotic fluid contains electrolytes, proteins and protein derivatives such as urea and creatinine, carbohydrates, lipids, hormones, enzymes, desquamated fetal cells, vernix and lanugo. Sodium and chloride content decreases and urea, uric acid and creatinine increase as the fetal kidney matures. Increasing amounts of phospholipids from the lungs appear as the fetal lungs mature.

Regulation of amniotic fluid quantity

Decidual prolactin and **prostaglandins** (PGE$_2$) from the amnion may regulate amniotic fluid volume. Concentration of prolactin in amniotic fluid is up to 10 times that of maternal circulation, increasing sharply in the second trimester and declining to a lower plateau after 34 weeks. Prolactin may regulate amniotic fluid volume by controlling electrolyte exchange across the chorioamniotic membrane. PGE$_2$ may regulate amniotic fluid by removing it into the maternal circulation to counterbalance the large volume of fetal urine produced in the second half of pregnancy.

Functions of amniotic fluid

Amniotic fluid is critical to the normal development of the fetus. Amniotic fluid (Moore & Persaud 2008):

- Permits symmetric external growth of the embryo and fetus.
- Acts as a barrier to infection.
- Permits normal fetal lung development.
- Prevents adherence of the amnion to the embryo and fetus.

- Cushions the embryo and fetus against injuries.
- Helps control the embryo's body temperature by maintaining a constant environmental temperature.
- Enables the fetus to move freely, aiding muscular development.
- Assists in maintaining homeostasis of fluid and electrolytes.

Clinical implications: abnormalities of quantity

Moore & Persaud (2008) relate abnormalities of the fetus to abnormalities of amniotic fluid quantity. In fetal conditions such as renal agenesis or urethral obstruction with obstruction to urine flow amniotic fluid volume is very low (oligohydramnios). If the fetus cannot swallow, as in oesophageal atresia or anencephaly, there is in excess of 2000 ml of amniotic fluid (polyhydramnios).

Polyhydramnios

One of the most common anomalies found on ultrasound examination is polyhydramnios. It affects up to 1.5% of all pregnancies. Polyhydramnios may be chronic or acute:

- Chronic polyhydramnios is more common and is gradual in onset from about the 30th week of pregnancy.
- Acute polyhydramnios is rare, occurs at about 20 weeks of pregnancy and is associated with monovular twins and occasionally with severe fetal abnormality.

Diagnosis

Polyhydramnios can be suspected if:

- The uterus is large for gestational age.
- There is easy ballottement of the fetus.
- Fetal parts are difficult to find.
- The fetal heart is muffled.
- Maternal symptoms include breathlessness, vulval varicosities, oedema and gastric problems.

Diagnosis is confirmed by ultrasound examination. In 60% of cases there is no known cause. Fetal causes are associated in 20% of cases and 20% with maternal causes (Box 12.2).

Complications

Polyhydramnios is associated with an increase in maternal and fetal mortality. Maternal complications include pregnancy-induced hypertension and respiratory discomfort. Fetal mortality is associated with conditions incompatible with life and morbidity with minor abnormalities and preterm birth. Obstetric complications include unstable lie, malpresentation, cord presentation and prolapse, preterm labour, premature rupture of membranes (PROM), placental abruption and postpartum haemorrhage.

BOX 12.2 THE CAUSES OF POLYHYDRAMNIOS

Fetal causes

- Multiple pregnancy
- Central nervous system anomalies: anencephaly, hydrocephaly, spina bifida
- Gastrointestinal anomalies: oesophageal atresia, small bowel atresias, diaphragmatic hernia
- Cardiac anomalies
- Haematological anomalies: α-thalassaemia, fetomaternal haemorrhage
- Skeletal malformations: achondroplasia, osteogenesis imperfecta
- Chromosome/genetic abnormalities
- Intrauterine infections: rubella, syphilis, toxoplasmosis

Maternal causes

- Diabetes mellitus
- Rhesus isoimmunisation

Placental causes

- Placental chorioangioma
- Circumvallate placenta syndrome

Management

Diagnostic tests include:

- Ultrasound examination to detect fetal and placental abnormalities and to confirm gestational age.
- Studies of **fetal karyotype** to rule out chromosomal or genetic abnormalities.
- Fetal swallowing studies.
- Screening for intrauterine infection.
- Maternal antibody screening and diabetic screening.

Maternal comfort will be improved by resting in bed in an upright position to aid breathing. She may require antacids to relieve heartburn and nausea. Amniotic fluid may be removed to conserve pregnancy.

Oligohydramnios

Oligohydramnios occurs when the amount of amniotic fluid is less than 500 ml at term. It may be much less than this and affects 4% of pregnancies.

Diagnosis

The condition may be suspected on abdominal examination if the following findings are present:

- The uterus appears smaller than expected for gestational age.

- The mother has noticed a reduction in fetal movements.
- The uterus feels compact and fetal parts are easily felt.

Ultrasound examination confirms the absence of normal amniotic fluid pockets.

Causes

Oligohydramnios may be associated with severe fetal growth retardation, usually associated with maternal disease such as hypertension or chronic renal disease (see Box 12.3 for list).

Complications

Prognosis is poor, especially because of PROM and fetal abnormalities. Pulmonary hypoplasia affects 60% of fetuses deprived of amniotic fluid for several weeks. It is generally lethal with small, immature lungs, poor surfactant levels and pulmonary hypertension. Oligohydramnios is often associated with amnion nodosum. Yellow–grey nodules consisting of desquamated fetal epidermal cells, lanugo and vernix are found in and on the amnion and on the fetal surface of the placenta, probably because of its close application to the fetus.

Management

Management depends on the length of gestation, the maturity of the fetus, fetal and maternal health and the relative risks of conservative management or delivery. The means of delivery is aimed at achieving maximum safety for mother and fetus. There is some evidence that maternal hydration can increase the volume of amniotic fluid (NICE 2006).

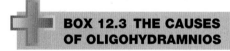

BOX 12.3 THE CAUSES OF OLIGOHYDRAMNIOS

Post-term pregnancy (more than 42 weeks)

Intrauterine growth retardation

Premature rupture of membranes (PROM)

Fetal renal anomalies: renal agenesis (Potter's syndrome), urethral obstruction, prune belly syndrome, multicystic, dysplastic kidneys

Fetal non-renal anomalies: triploidy, thyroid gland agenesis, skeletal dysplasia, congenital heart block, twin–twin transfusion syndrome

Chronic abruptio placentae

Amnioinfusion, where saline or Ringer's lactate solution is infused into the amniotic cavity via a needle inserted through the abdominal wall, has been used and can be repeated if necessary (serial amnioinfusion). This procedure can be performed either antenatally or in labour to:

- Replace fluid in conservative treatment of PROM.
- Prevent the development of fetal lung hypoplasia.
- Decrease cord compression and reduce fetal distress during labour.
- Dilute meconium.

In the United Kingdom NICE (2006) state that this invasive procedure has not been adequately researched and should only be carried out in centres specialising in invasive neonatal medicine, that parents should be informed of the risks and benefits and that any incidence should be part of a clinical trial to acquire more evidence.

Diagnostic uses of amniotic fluid

Biophysical profile

Biophysical profile (BPP) is a non-invasive test of fetal well-being using ultrasound imaging. It is not clear whether there is any benefit to this testing. Further research is suggested. Four variables are measured (Lalor et al 2007):

- Fetal tone.
- Somatic movements.
- Breathing movements.
- Amniotic fluid volume.

Fetal heart rate monitoring can be added as a modification.

Amniocentesis

Cellular and biochemical components of amniotic fluid change with gestational age and provide useful indicators of fetal well-being and maturity (Blackburn 2007). Although the procedure is considered safe there are possible complications of abortion, infection, haematoma, leakage of amniotic fluid or preterm labour. Amniotic fluid analysis can be used as follows:

- Cells can be used for genetic and chromosomal studies.
- α-Fetoprotein can assess the likelihood of neural tube defects or as part of a triple test for Down syndrome.
- Creatinine levels increase as the fetus matures.
- Bilirubin estimates can monitor red blood cell haemolysis in rhesus incompatibility.
- The ratio of the phospholipids lecithin and sphingomyelin can be used to assess lung maturity.
- Enzyme studies of cultured cells can help diagnose many inborn errors of metabolism.

Main points

- The placenta is derived from extraembryonic trophoblast with a few inner cell mass mesodermal cells. The cytotrophoblast gives rise to the syncytiotrophoblast which invades the endometrium to allow embedding. Lacunae fuse to form intervillous spaces. These become filled with a mixture of maternal blood and endometrial gland secretions.

- In pregnancy decidual and myometrial arteries become dilated and unresponsive to circulatory pressor substances or autonomic neural control. By the end of the 3rd week fetal blood circulates through the capillaries of the chorionic villi.

- About the 8th week of pregnancy the chorionic villi of the decidua capsularis degenerate and form the chorion laeve which becomes the chorionic membrane. The villi of the decidua basalis branch to form the fetal part of the placenta. The outer chorion and the inner amnion form the fetal sac.

- The placenta produces protein hormones and steroid hormones. These hormones alter maternal metabolism to benefit the fetus.

- The levels of the protein hormones SP_1, PAPP-A and PAPP-B rise as pregnancy progresses. SP_1 and PAPP-A may be important in preventing immunological rejection of the fetus by the mother.

- hCG stimulates ovarian production of oestrogen and progesterone to maintain pregnancy whilst hPL probably promotes growth by mobilising free fatty acids and antagonising insulin which is why it is diabetogenic.

- The fetal liver and suprarenal glands are important in the production of estriol. Plasma estriol levels rise steeply from 34 to 36 weeks.

- Syncytioblastic progesterone is sent to both maternal and fetal circulations. It relaxes maternal smooth muscle and may be responsible for some minor disorders of pregnancy. Prostaglandin activity is regulated by an increasing estradiol:progesterone ratio. Prostaglandins may increase the number of myometrial oxytocin receptors.

- Fetal growth depends on placental transfer of nutrients and oxygen. This increases as the placenta grows in size. Oxygen and carbon dioxide cross the syncytiotrophoblast and fetal capillary epithelium down a partial pressure concentration gradient. Nutrients, trace elements and vitamins pass from maternal to fetal blood through the walls of the villi.

- The placenta excretes urea, uric acid and bilirubin into the maternal circulation.

- Water and solute balance is achieved by diffusional gradients and are freely transferred between maternal and fetal circulations.

- Many bacteria are too big to penetrate the placental membrane but those causing syphilis and tuberculosis do so, as does the rubella virus. Drugs of small molecular structure may cross the placenta and cause fetal abnormalities. Other drugs such as some antibiotics may be beneficial.

- Mature amniotic fluid contains electrolytes, proteins, urea and creatinine, carbohydrates, lipids, hormones, enzymes, desquamated fetal skin cells, vernix and lanugo.

- Sodium and chloride content decrease and urea, uric acid and creatinine increase as the fetal kidneys mature. Increasing amounts of phospholipids are present as the fetal lungs mature.

- Amniotic fluid is constantly being replaced and the fetal gastrointestinal tract is a major pathway for its removal. Prolactin and prostaglandins may regulate amniotic fluid volume.

- Amniotic fluid provides space for fetal growth and movement and protects the fetus from injury and infection. A constant temperature is maintained.

- Polyhydramnios may be acute or chronic and affects 1.5% of pregnancies. Chronic polyhydramnios is much more common. Causes include multiple pregnancy, fetal anomalies, diabetes mellitus and placental abnormalities. Acute polyhydramnios is associated with monovular twins.

- Obstetric complications of polyhydramnios include unstable lie, malpresentation, cord presentation and prolapse, premature rupture of the membranes, placental abruption and postpartum haemorrhage. Diagnostic tests include ultrasonography, fetal karyotyping, TORCH studies, infection screening, antibody screening and testing for diabetes mellitus.

- Maternal comfort can be improved by bed rest in an upright position to aid breathing. Antacids will help heartburn and nausea. Amniotic fluid may be removed to conserve pregnancy.

- Causes of oligohydramnios include post-term pregnancy, intrauterine growth retardation, fetal renal anomalies and chronic abruptio placentae. Fetal complications include pulmonary hypoplasia which may be lethal. Amnioinfusion is used as an experimental treatment antenatally and in labour.

- Biophysical profile could be an accurate predictor of fetal danger but so far does not show effects on pregnancy outcome.

- Cellular or biochemical components of amniotic fluid provide useful indicators of fetal well-being and maturity. There are risks to amniocentesis of abortion, infection, haematoma, haemorrhage, leakage of amniotic fluid and preterm labour.

References

Blackburn, S.T., 2007. Maternal, Fetal and Neonatal Physiology: A Clinical Perspective. Elsevier Saunders, St Louis MO.

Carlson, B.M., 2004. Human Embryology and Developmental Biology, third edn. Elsevier Mosby, Philadelphia PA.

Chard, T., 2000. The placenta as patient. Yearb. Obstet. Gynaecol. 8, 61–73.

Coad, J., Dunstall, M., 2005. Anatomy and Physiology for Midwives. Mosby, St Louis MO.

Gluckman, P., Hanson, M., 2005. The Fetal Matrix: Evolution, Development and Disease. Cambridge University Press, Cambridge, UK.

Guyton, A.C., Hall, J.E., 2006. Textbook of Medical Physiology, eleventh edn. Elsevier Saunders, Philadelphia PA.

Henderson, C., Macdonald, S. (Eds.), 2004. Mayes' Midwifery: A Textbook for Midwives, thirteenth edn. Baillière Tindall, London.

Johnson, M.H., 2007. Essential Reproduction, sixth edn. Blackwell, Oxford.

Klopper, A., 1991. Placental metabolism. In: Hytten, F., Chamberlain, G. (Eds.) Clinical Physiology in Obstetrics. Blackwell Scientific, Oxford.

Lalor, J.G., Fawole, B., Alfirevic, Z., Devane, D., 2007. Biophysical profile for fetal assessment in high risk pregnancies.

Cochrane Collab. Database Syst. Rev. (2) Wiley.

Moore, K.L., Persaud, T.V.N., 2008. The Developing Human: Clinically Oriented Embryology, eighth edn. Elsevier Saunders, Philadelphia PA.

National Institute for Health and Clinical Excellence (NICE), 2006. Therapeutic amnioinfusion for oligohydramnios during pregnancy (excluding labour). Interventional Procedure Guidance 192.

Stacey, T.E., 1991. Placental transfer. In: Hytten, F., Chamberlain, G. (Eds.) Clinical Physiology in Obstetrics. Blackwell Scientific, Oxford.

Annotated recommended reading

Johnson, M.H., 2007. Essential Reproduction, sixth edn. Blackwell Publishing, Oxford.

This is an excellent book on the physiology of reproduction and describes events in easily understood and well-researched style.

Lalor, J.G., Fawole, B., Alfirevic, Z., Devane, D., 2007. Biophysical profile for fetal assessment in high risk pregnancies. Cochrane Collab. Database Syst. Rev. 2008 4 (2) Wiley.

Reviews in the Cochrane Database provide an excellent start to studying the subject in depth and this one on biophysical profile is typical.

Moore, K.L., Persaud, T.V.N., 2008. The Developing Human: Clinically Oriented Embryology, eighth edn. Elsevier Saunders, Philadelphia PA.

The layout, diagrams and content of this book are excellent. It clearly describes the formation of the placenta, membranes and amniotic fluid.

Chapter Thirteen

Fetal growth and development

Introduction

The general organising principles of embryology, the development of systems and the structure and function of the placenta have been discussed in previous chapters. From the beginning of the 9th week of intra-uterine life most of the organs are in place even though they may be non-functional. The fetal period is mainly concerned with an increase in size and maturation of the systems.

The fetal period

Care must be taken to avoid confusion when calculating fetal age. Traditionally this has been calculated from the first day of the **last menstrual period** (LMP). Following the use of ultrasound scanning, it is more common to calculate fetal age by using the estimated day of fertilisation. The date of birth is about 266 days or 38 weeks after fertilisation and 280 days or about 40 weeks from the first day of the LMP. It is usual to use **post-fertilisation age** when describing organ development and this method will be used throughout this chapter.

Fetal growth

Moore & Persaud (2008) state that 'during the fetal period (9th week until birth) differentiation of tissues and organs formed during the embryonic period occurs'. Wolpert et al (2007) define growth as 'an increase in size, which occurs by cell multiplication, increase in cell size and deposition of extracellular material'. Apoptosis (cell death) is also important in determining overall growth rate.

Tissues may grow by:

- Cell proliferation or **hypertrophy**: increased cell numbers.
- Cell enlargement or **hyperplasia**: increased cell size.
- Accretion of extracellular material such as bone matrix.

From fertilisation, during cleavage and blastula formation, there is little growth and cells become smaller with each cleavage division. From weeks 9 to 24 there is remarkable growth and then growth slows but remains constant from 30 to 36 weeks when it slows again (Johnson 2007). In early pregnancy growth is mainly by

✚ BOX 13.1 CONTROL OF FETAL SIZE

Growth of the fetus is multifactorial, involving both genetic and environmental factors. Fetal growth involves the accumulation of protein early in development which reaches a maximum of 300 g by week 35. Fat deposition exceeds the amount of protein by week 38, most of which is subcutaneous. The human baby has the most subcutaneous fat of any animal and this may be related to ensuring brain growth does not suffer. The relative amount of water in fetal tissues decreases. If the fetus grows too large there may be difficulty in delivery but if it remains too small health patterns in both childhood and later life may be compromised. Intrauterine growth retardation is discussed in Chapter 14.

The mother adapts to fetal needs by increasing calorie intake and modifying metabolic activity. These changes seem to occur in response to signals from the fetoplacental unit. However, the mother also seems to be able to limit fetal growth. Her height is linked to her uterine capacity and small women appear to have small babies but the mechanism is not clear. It may be that the placenta limits the amount of nutrients transferred to the fetus in late pregnancy.

Additional maternal influences include parity with primiparous women having smaller babies by about 200 g than multiparous women and adolescent mothers have smaller babies than fully mature mothers. Gluckman & Hanson (2005) believe this is due to the effect of a first pregnancy on the uterine vascular bed. They give the analogy of elastic bands being easier to stretch after some use. The uterine blood vessels which are small and tortuous before pregnancy respond to placental oestrogens and progesterone by becoming relaxed and more dilated. This improves fetal nutrition and the baby grows larger. They suggest this is also seen in multiple pregnancies when each baby obtains less nutrition than a singleton baby and is therefore smaller.

Haig (1993) first suggested that how big a baby grows is determined by conflict between maternal and paternal genes (see also Abu-Amero et al 2006, Wolpert 2007). The insulin-like growth factors IGF1 and IGF2 closely resemble the simple insulin molecule and appear to have a key role in embryonic and fetal growth. In humans IGF2 is inherited on chromosome 11. The IGF2 gene inherited from the father makes a growth factor which helps the fetus to grow whilst the maternal gene is programmed to be non-functional. This phenomenon is called **genomic imprinting**, i.e. expressed in a parent-specific manner regardless of Mendelian inheritance (Wolpert 2007).

However, evidence for maternal constraint of fetal growth is found in the size of foals from horse crosses between a large shire horse and a smaller Shetland pony. If the mother is a shire horse, the newborn foal is similar in size to a normal shire foal, but if the mother is a Shetland pony the newborn is much smaller than a normal shire foal would be. After birth both foals achieved a similar size, midway between shires and Shetlands (Gluckman & Hanson 2005, Wolpert et al 2007). The size of the fetus may be constrained by the size of the intrauterine environment (Gluckman & Hanson 2005).

The fetus also contributes to growth control by its genetic inheritance and by its sex; male fetuses grow larger than females on average. Synthesis of the IGFs increases throughout pregnancy. IGF1 is a major direct endocrine stimulus whilst IGF2 may have a more indirect effect by stimulating placental growth and transport mechanisms (see Ch. 12).

---

hyperplasia. This is followed by a period of simultaneous hyperplasia and hypertrophy (Bogin 2001). After 34 weeks growth is mainly by hypertrophy (Blackburn 2007). **Growth** and **maturation** of the systems are directly linked to the ability of the fetus to survive after birth, a concept known as **viability**.

Control of cell growth and proliferation

Growth factors (insulin-like growth factors 1 and 2—IGFs or somatomedins) and other **signalling proteins** play a key role in controlling cell growth and proliferation.

Without these signals cells commit apoptosis (cell suicide), brought about by activation of an internal cell death programme (Wolpert et al 2007). However, the mechanisms of embryonic cell division are poorly understood. Placental, fetal and maternal factors determine fetal growth (Box 13.1).

Key events in the fetal stage of development

The details of developmental stages are adapted from Moore & Persaud (2008) and are given in Table 13.1.

Table 13.1 Fetal development based on weeks from fertilisation

Weeks	Developmental feature
9	The fetal head measures half the crown–rump length
10	Intestinal cells have all re-entered the body cavity
12	Fetal length has more than doubled The upper limbs have attained their relative length in comparison to the trunk but the lower limbs remain short The mature forms of the external genitalia appear There is a decrease in red cell formation in the liver and onset in the spleen The formation and excretion of urine begins The beginning of fetal muscle movement occurs The eyelids fuse
13–16	This is a period of very rapid growth
16	The head is now smaller in comparison to the trunk and the lower limbs have reached their correct proportions The skeleton can be seen clearly on X-ray films The face is more human, the eyes pointing anteriorly rather than laterally The external ears have moved to their positions on the sides of the head
17–20	Growth slows down Fetal movements are felt by the mother The skin is covered by vernix caseosa, to protect it from amniotic fluid Lanugo has developed all over the body Head and eyebrow hair become visible Highly metabolic brown fat is formed
21–25	Surfactant production in the lungs begins Towards the end of this period survival becomes possible The skin lacks subcutaneous fat and is wrinkled The skin appears red because of blood capillaries just under the surface The fetus now has periods of sleep and activity and responds to sound
26–29	The lungs are capable of breathing and allowing gas exchange The nervous system controls rhythmic breathing movements and body temperature Intrauterine respiratory movements occur The eyes re-open Head and lanugo hair are well developed White, subcutaneous fat is laid down under the skin At 28 weeks erythropoiesis ends in the spleen and begins in the bone marrow
30–34	The papillary light reflex is present Body fat expands to 8% of total body weight The skin is opaque and smooth From 32 weeks most fetuses will survive Lanugo disappears from the face The fetus begins to store iron
35–38	The grasp is firm Most fetuses are plump At 36 weeks head and abdominal circumferences are equal. Later the abdominal circumference becomes greater. Growth slows towards term By 38 weeks body fat is 16% of body weight Breast tissue is present in both sexes The testes are in the scrotum in males The nails reach the tips of the fingers Lanugo disappears from the body

Note that there is no line of week or measure when a fetus can be said to be viable. Dimensional variations increase with age, making the judgement of gestational age less accurate (Figs 13.1, 13.2). It is still unlikely that a fetus of less than 22 weeks or weighing less than 500 g could survive.

Fetal size

Before birth it is usual to measure the fetus as sitting height or crown–rump length. Table 13.2 is based on post-fertilisation age and is derived from Moore & Persaud (2008).

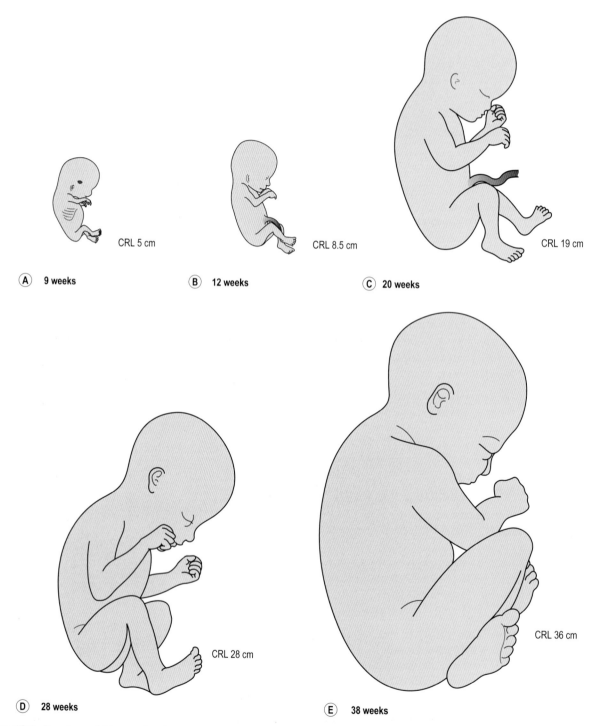

CRL 5 cm

CRL 8.5 cm

CRL 19 cm

(A) **9 weeks**

(B) **12 weeks**

(C) **20 weeks**

CRL 28 cm

CRL 36 cm

(D) **28 weeks**

(E) **38 weeks**

Figure 13.1•Drawings of fetuses at various stages of development. CRL, crown–rump length. (Reproduced with permission from Moore 1989.)

Estimation of fetal age and assessment of fetal growth

Growth curves

If a series of measurements is taken, these can be plotted on a graph and used to calculate growth. Growth can be viewed as a motion through time (Bogin 2001) and, if measurements are taken and plotted at regular intervals, a curve called a distance curve (Fig. 13.3) results. It is more usual to plot a distance curve when monitoring fetal growth. To show how the rate of growth alters over time, the speed or velocity of growth is plotted, generating a velocity curve showing how the rate of growth alters (Fig. 13.4).

Maternal weight and fetal growth

Maternal weight gain has traditionally been used to assess fetal well-being in pregnancy, and continued weight gain is thought to be a favourable sign. However, weight gain varies widely from weight loss to a gain of 23 kg or more. Many factors affect maternal weight gain, including the presence of oedema, maternal metabolic rate, dietary intake, gastrointestinal problems, smoking and the size of the fetus.

Table 13.2 The average size of the fetus related to weeks of gestation

Age in weeks	Crown–rump length in mm	Weight in grams
10	61	14
12	87	45
14	120	110
16	140	250
18	160	320
20	190	460
22	210	630
24	230	820
26	250	1000
28	270	1300
30	280	1700
32	300	2100
36	340	2900
38	360	3400

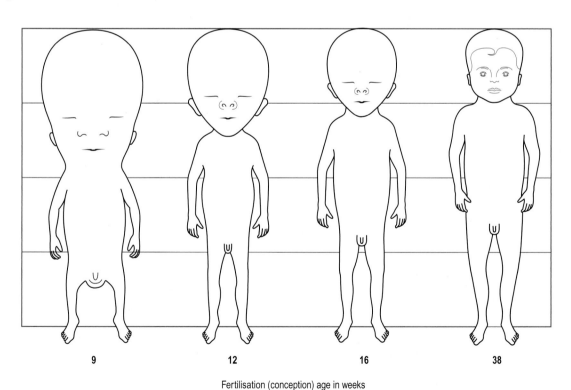

| 9 | 12 | 16 | 38 |

Fertilisation (conception) age in weeks

Figure 13.2 • The changing proportions of the body during the fetal period. At 9 weeks the head is about half the crown–rump length of the fetus. By 38 weeks the circumferences of the head and the abdomen are approximately equal. After this the circumference of the abdomen may be greater. All stages are drawn to the same total height. (Reproduced with permission from Moore 1989.)

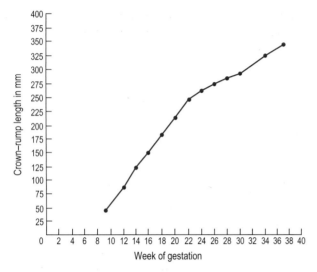

Figure 13.3 • An example of a distance curve using data from fetal crown–rump measurements.

Table 13.3 Distribution of maternal weight gain in pregnancy	
Component of fetal weight	**Gain in grams**
The fetus	3400
The placenta	600
The amniotic fluid	600
The uterus	900
The breasts	500
Fat stores	3500
Blood volume	1500
Extracellular fluid	1000
Total	12000

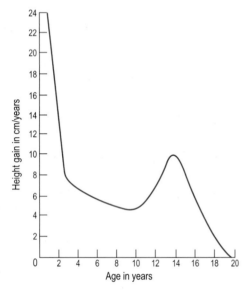

Figure 13.4 • An example of a velocity curve demonstrating the growth of the body from birth to age 18 years.

Attempts to control maternal weight gain in order to reduce the size of the fetus and make delivery easier have been unsuccessful and had little effect on fetal size. The only components of maternal weight gain available for manipulation are maternal fat and extracellular fluid and it may be that neither obesity nor oedema can be influenced by regular weighing. An average weight gain appears to be about 12 kg and should be 2 kg in the first 20 weeks and 0.5 kg/week until term. Components of normal weight gain are shown in Table 13.3.

Poor weight gain has been associated with **intrauterine growth retardation** (IUGR) but is not a sensitive indicator and babies with IUGR are delivered when weight gain has been normal. Daily fluctuations in a woman's weight can be up to 1% of total body weight and there are better ways of assessing the fetus.

Uterine **fundal height** is the most common way to assess fetal growth. The measurements are made in centimetres from the upper border of the symphysis pubis to the top of the fundus of the uterus. Errors may occur if the woman is too thin or obese or has too much or too little abdominal muscle tone. Breech presentation or transverse lie can also result in error. Fundal height can be plotted against a standard curve.

Ultrasound

The gestational age is calculated from the mother's LMP or taken from an early first or second trimester scan. Plotting of later measurements must be accurate to avoid wrong diagnosis. The success rate of ultrasound in detecting IUGR can be as high as 95%. Ultrasound measurements can also be plotted against a normal curve. Linear and non-linear measurements can be used.

Linear measurements

Crown–rump length is used to estimate gestational age in the first trimester. The measurement between the two biparietal eminences is called the biparietal diameter (BPD) (Fig. 13.5). The correct position of the fetal head must be located (Fig. 13.6). This is a useful estimate of gestational age in the second trimester but is less accurate later in pregnancy. Femur length can also be used to assess gestational age.

Non-linear measurements

Measurement of the head circumference (HC) is preferred in the third trimester when moulding of the head

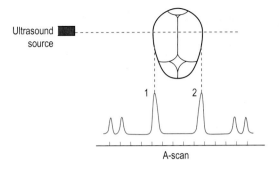

Figure 13.5 • Measuring the biparietal diameter by ultrasound; 1 and 2 indicate the parietal eminences. (From Henderson C, Macdonald S 2004, with kind permission of Elsevier.)

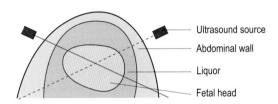

Ultrasound source
Abdominal wall
Liquor
Fetal head

Figure 13.6 • A diagram showing the abdominal wall and the fetal head. (From Henderson C, Macdonald S 2004, with kind permission of Elsevier.)

may alter the BPD. Abdominal circumference (AC) is measured at the level of the bifurcation of the hepatic vein in the centre of the fetal liver. A reduction of AC suggests a reduction in liver size due to depleted stores.

Ratios

- HC:AC compares the status of the brain to the liver. A raised ratio suggests IUGR.
- Femur:AC ratio compares the length of the femur which is minimally affected by IUGR to the AC. A raised ratio suggests IUGR.

Doppler wave form analysis

Measuring the velocity of blood in the umbilical cord using Doppler ultrasound has been suggested as an additional means of assessing fetal well-being (Ch. 14).

Multiple pregnancies

Multiple pregnancy is the term used to describe the development of more than one fetus in utero at the same time. In spontaneous pregnancy the presence of twins is about 1 in 100 but this increased to epidemic proportions in the 1990s with **assisted reproductive techniques** (ART). Because of the economic, social and ethical dilemmas affecting parents, policies in **ovum**

induction and **in vitro fertilisation** aim to reduce the number of fetuses returned to the uterus and so reduce the incidence of multiple pregnancy (Aurell et al 2006).

Types of twin pregnancy

Dizygotic (DZ)

About two-thirds of twin pregnancies are **dizygotic** (binovular, non-identical or fraternal twins) which results from the shedding and fertilisation of two separate ova by two separate sperm. Two babies develop who are genetically no more related than normal siblings but share the uterus at the same time. There is an inherited aspect so that the incidence of recurrence in families is three times that of the rest of the population. Also, this type of twinning varies between ethnic groups so that the incidence is 1 in 500 in Asians, 1 in 125 in White populations and as high as 1 in 20 in some African populations (Moore & Persaud 2008). DZ twins have separate placentas, two chorions and two amnions (dichorionic–diamniotic). They may be the same sex or different sexes. The incidence of congenital malformation is only slightly greater than normal.

Monozygotic (MZ)

About one-third of twinning occurs when a single fertilised ovum divides into two separate fetuses. These are **monozygotic** (uniovular or identical) twins. About one-third of monozygotic twins are **dichorionic** (each has its own chorion) and two-thirds share one placenta and one chorion. In 95% of these each baby has its own amnion (**monochorionic–diamniotic**). In the remaining 5% the babies share one amnion (**monochorionic–monoamniotic**) (Fig. 13.7). About 1% of monoamniotic twins are conjoined (Siamese twins) (Sebire et al 2000).

MZ twinning usually begins in the blastocyst at the end of the 1st week when the embryoblast divides into two embryonic primordia. If the embryonic disc does not divide completely or the adjacent embryonic discs fuse, conjoined twins may develop (Carlson 2004, Moore & Persaud 2008).

MZ twins are identical in their genetic make-up, having developed from one fertilised ovum and are always of the same sex, except in very rare abnormalities of the sex chromosomes. Any physical differences between them are environmentally induced. There is a connection between the two fetal circulations via the placenta. The high incidence of errors of development and of congenital malformations may be linked to the cause of the twinning. MZ twinning begins in the blastocyst, about the end of week 1. It results from the division of the **embryoblast** into two embryonic **primordia**.

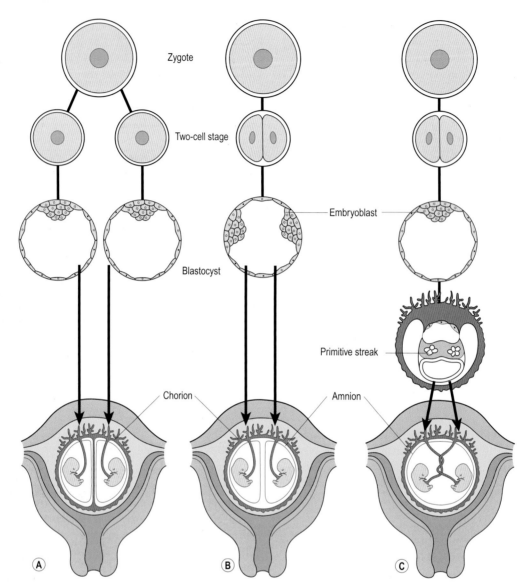

Figure 13.7 • Three kinds of monozygotic twins. (A) Dichorionic–diamniotic. (B) Monochorionic–diamniotic. (C) Monochorionic–monoamniotic. (From Fitzgerald M J T, Fitzgerald M 1994, with permission.)

The incidence of multiple pregnancies

Since the advent of infertility treatment by stimulation of ovulation multiple births have become more common. In naturally occurring pregnancies twins occur in 1 in 90 pregnancies, triplets in about 1 in 90^2, quadruplets in 1 in 90^3 and quintuplets in 1 in 90^4 pregnancies (Moore & Persaud 2008). The differences in twinning rates results from variations in dizygotic twinning and the incidence of monozygotic twinning is constant at 3.5 per 1000 across all nationalities. Other factors influencing the frequency of dizygotic twinning include:

- Maternal age: the incidence increases with maternal age.
- Parity.

- Conception soon after discontinuing oral contraceptives; if these have been taken for more than 6 months and conception occurs within a month of discontinuation, the chances of a twin pregnancy double.

Ultrasound scanning has shown that the incidence of twin pregnancy at conception may be double the number of eventual twin births. One embryo may be reabsorbed (**vanishing twin syndrome**) or rarely remains between the membranes as a fetus papyraceous (paper fetus). The earlier the ultrasound scan, the higher the probability of only one baby surviving to the end of pregnancy.

Triplets and higher-order pregnancies

Drugs to induce ovulation such as **clomifene citrate** have led to a 10% risk in pregnancies with multiple fetuses being conceived. In the United Kingdom triplet births have doubled since 1989. The implications for maternity and neonatal care of these high-risk pregnancies are a cause for concern. The outcome of such pregnancies can be poor and some centres have advocated fetal reduction to ensure survival of fewer fetuses but there is a danger that all fetuses could be lost.

When the figures on fetal survival in triplets and higher-order births are contrasted with selective feticide, it is difficult to support a decision to reduce fetal numbers if there are three or more fetuses (Dodd & Crowther 2003). Dickey et al (2002), using 50 women in their research population, found a high incidence of spontaneous fetal reduction before 12 weeks of gestation in 36% of twins, 53% of triplets and 65% of quadruplets.

Diagnosis of twin pregnancy

It is apparent that the earlier the diagnosis of twins is made, the more successful the outcome. Perinatal losses may be much larger when the diagnosis is made after 28 weeks. Since the development of routine ultrasound scanning the incidence of undiagnosed twins at delivery is rare. However, not all midwives work in countries where access to scanning is easy or possible. It is important to be able to diagnose a multiple pregnancy by clinical examination. A family history of twinning should alert the professional carer to the possibility but vigilance is needed in all pregnancies.

Abdominal examination

Inspection
This method is unlikely to diagnose twins before 20 weeks of pregnancy but the uterus may appear larger than expected for gestational age. The uterus may look large and broad and fetal movements may be obvious all over the abdomen.

Palpation
The fundal height may be greater than expected for the period of gestation. The presence of two fetal poles in the fundus may be an identifying feature. Location of three poles suggests the presence of at least twins. Multiple limbs may also be felt. A later clue is the apparent smallness of the fetal head in relation to the size of the uterus. Lateral palpation may find two fetal backs or the presence of fetal limbs on both sides of the uterus.

Auscultation
It has been stated that hearing two fetal hearts simultaneously with a difference of 10 beats/min is diagnostic of twins. Practically, this is difficult to achieve as the fetal heart of a singleton can be heard over a wide area.

Ultrasound
Ultrasound diagnosis of multiple pregnancy can be made as early as 5 weeks following the LMP. However, it may not be possible to confirm a twin pregnancy until after 12 weeks because of the likelihood of vanishing twin syndrome (Moore & Persaud 2008). Ultrasound diagnosis should be made to ascertain the number of placentas and types of membranes present. Diagnosis of monoamniotic twins is essential because of the higher risk of abnormalities so that management can be planned (Sebire et al 2000).

Complications of pregnancy

Sebire et al (2001) analysed more than 400 000 pregnancies in the United Kingdom and found that obstetric complications were more frequent in multiple births than in singleton births. These included pre-eclampsia, antepartum haemorrhage, anaemia, delivery by caesarean section, preterm delivery, admission of babies to neonatal intensive care units, postpartum haemorrhage and maternal infections. The incidence of complications increased with the number of fetuses present.

Fetal problems

Abortion
Loss of pregnancy by abortion is more common, possibly due to fetal abnormality in early pregnancy and overdistension of the uterus in later pregnancy.

Single fetus demise
Before 14 weeks single fetal demise will probably cause no problems for the survivor. Later there may be transfer of **thromboplastin** released from the tissues of the dead twin. This may cause arterial occlusion, brain damage and renal cortical necrosis. A serious maternal problem is the onset of **disseminated intravascular coagulation** (DIC) about 3 weeks after fetal death.

Congenital malformations
Congenital malformations are more likely to occur in twin pregnancies. Although the incidence is about the same in monozygotic and dizygotic twins, abnormalities in dizygotic twins tend to be minor while those in monozygotic twins tend to be multiple and lethal. The most common in all sets of twins are cleft lip and palate, central nervous system defects and cardiac defects. In monozygotic twins conjoined twins and **fetal acardia** occur.

Monoamniotic twins
When monoamniotic twins are present the perinatal mortality is as high as 50%, mainly because of umbilical cord entanglement. Other causes of loss are **twin-to-twin**

transfusion syndrome, congenital abnormalities and pre-term birth. Ultrasound scanning should be carried out regularly to diagnose any problems and plan management. The babies are best delivered by caesarean section to avoid cord entanglement.

Conjoined twins

Conjoined twins occur in about 1% of monozygotic twin pregnancies (Fig. 13.8); this means in about 1 in 900 twin pregnancies and 1 in 40000 live births. In conjoined twins 70% will be female and the reason is unknown. Partial or complete duplication of just the upper or lower part of the body may occur with associated malformations (Craven & Ward 1996). Table 13.4 shows the different types of conjoined twins.

A diagnosis can be made by ultrasound and suspicion should be raised in the following cases:

- Monoamniotic twins.
- Twins that face each other.

- The heads are at the same level and in the same plane.
- The thoracic cages are in close proximity.
- Both fetal heads are hyperextended.
- There is no change in fetal positions on a later scan.

Table 13.4 Classification of conjoined twins by the site of union

Name	Percentage occurrence	Description
Thoracopagus	40	Joined at the chest
Omphalopagus	35	Joined at the anterior abdominal wall
Pygopagus	18	Joined at the buttocks
Ischiopagus	6	Joined at the ischium
Craniopagus	2	Joined at the head

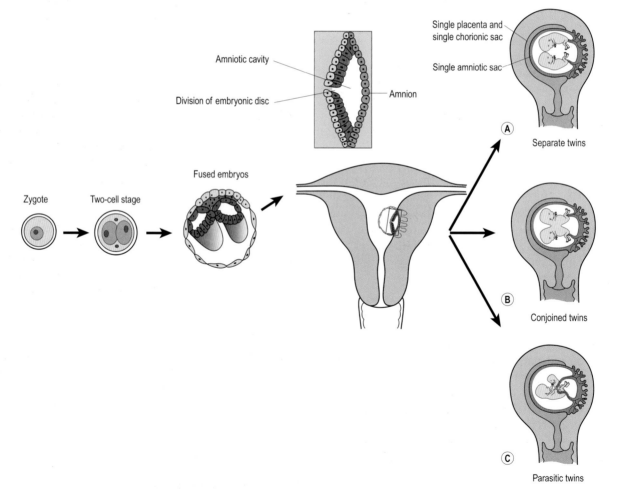

Figure 13.8 • Diagrams showing how some monozygotic (MZ) twins develop. This method of development is very uncommon. Division of the embryonic disc results in two embryos with one amniotic sac. (A) Complete division of the embryonic disc gives rise to twins. Such twins rarely survive because their umbilical cords are often so entangled that interruption of the blood supply to the fetuses occurs. (B, C) Incomplete division of the disc results in various types of conjoined twins. (Reproduced with permission from Moore 1989.)

Once the diagnosis is confirmed delivery by caesarean section is planned but the outcome is poor. About one-third of conjoined twins are stillborn and another third die within 24h. Surgical separation of conjoined twins is the only means by which independent lives can be achieved. The presence of shared organs may make it impossible to save both babies.

Acardiac twinning

This is a malformation occurring in about 1% of monozygotic twins where one twin has no heart and the circulation for both is maintained by the heart of the second twin. The acardiac twin is non-viable and circulatory overload may cause heart failure in the normal twin, giving a mortality rate of 35%.

Twin–twin transfusion syndrome (TTTS)

TTTS affects between 15% and 35% of monozygotic twins. Vascular communications across the placenta occur between the fetuses causing a circulatory imbalance. This results in **hypovolaemia**, **oliguria** and **oligohydramnios** in the donor twin who is small, pale and anaemic. If anaemia is severe the donor may develop **hydrops fetalis** and heart failure. **Hypervolaemia**, **polyuria** and **polyhydramnios** occur in the recipient who is large and **polycythaemic** and may develop **circulatory overload** and **congestive cardiac failure** (Moore & Persaud 2008). Fetal loss up to 80% occurs without treatment (Roberts et al 2007).

Prenatal diagnosis is made when the following conditions are present:

- Same sex twins.
- Diamniotic-monochorionic membranes.
- A 20% difference in estimated fetal weights.
- A discrepancy in the amniotic fluid surrounding the fetuses.
- Fetal hydrops in one or both twins.

Attempts to treat the problem antenatally may reduce the mortality to 40%. These include bed rest and preterm delivery, **amnioreduction** (selective removal of amniotic fluid), occlusion of the vascular anastomoses by **laser coagulation**, and selective ending of the life of one fetus and septostomy (creating a hole between the two chorionic membranes). Evidence shows that laser treatment is associated with fewer babies dying when compared to amnioreduction but if there is no expert available to perform laser surgery amnioreduction has to be the method of choice (Roberts et al 2007).

Polyhydramnios

Polyhydramnios is associated with monozygotic twins and with fetal abnormality. Acute polyhydramnios occurs in mid-pregnancy and usually leads to abortion.

The author remembers an evening when two women, both with monozygotic twins, were being cared for in the same room. Both women delivered identical twin boys within half an hour of each other. All four babies were under 300g and all died.

Intrauterine growth retardation

Most twins show discordant growth with one twin obtaining more nourishment than the other. This is a feature of placental mass and occurs more frequently in dizygotic twins. Genetic syndromes and TTS may also result in discordant growth.

Maternal problems

Detailed accounts of the following maternal problems are given in other chapters.

Exacerbation of minor disorders

The presence of more than one fetus means a higher level of pregnancy hormones and more pressure from the growing uterus. This tends to exacerbate all minor disorders of pregnancy, in particular morning sickness, nausea and heartburn.

Anaemia

The rate of anaemia in multiple pregnancy is about double that in singleton pregnancies. Both **iron deficiency** and **folic acid deficiency** occur. Early in pregnancy iron is utilised in the growth of tissues, in particular the expansion of maternal plasma volume with formation of extra maternal red blood cells. After 28 weeks fetal demands further deplete the iron stores.

Pregnancy-induced hypertension

Hypertension is more common in women with a multiple pregnancy. Both hypertension and oedema may develop because of the increased blood volume but often respond to rest. A more worrying occurrence is the onset of pre-eclampsia with proteinuria, vasoconstriction and reduced blood volume.

Antepartum haemorrhage

There is a significant increase in antepartum haemorrhage. **Placenta praevia** may occur because of the large placental site and **abruptio placentae** because of polyhydramnios. If the membranes rupture early sudden decrease in uterine size may detach the placenta.

Complications of labour

Fetal malpresentations

At the commencement of labour Farooqui et al (1973) found that in 39.6% of twins the presentation was vertex–vertex, in 27.7% vertex–breech, with vertex–transverse, breech–breech, breech–vertex, breech–transverse and other combinations being equally distributed amongst the remaining 33.2% (Table 13.5). In effect these figures are not always significant as after delivery of the first twin the lie, presentation and position of the second twin may change and must be checked and altered if necessary before proceeding with the delivery.

Locked twins

Locked twins occur in 1 in 1000 twin labours. Typically the babies will have presented in a breech–vertex pattern with the head of the first breech twin obstructed by the head of the second vertex win. If diagnosed before the onset of labour, a situation that should be checked in every breech–vertex combination, an elective caesarean section should be performed.

If the body of the first baby has already been born, an attempt to free the head should be made. This may be successful as the babies are usually small; otherwise an emergency caesarean section is performed. The author has seen two deliveries with locked twins; in one case vaginal manipulation was successful and both babies survived. Unfortunately in the second instance vaginal manipulation was unsuccessful and both babies died during caesarean section. It is pleasant to report that the 40-year-old woman that lost her babies had a healthy baby girl, born by caesarean section, within a year.

Umbilical cord problems

Problems affecting the umbilical cord are more common in multiple pregnancies. These include:
- The presence of a single umbilical artery.
- Cord prolapse.
- Velamentous insertion of the cord.
- Vasa praevia.
- Umbilical cord entanglement.

Table 13.5 Fetal presentation in twins by percentage occurrence

Fetal presentation	Percentage
Vertex–vertex	39.6
Vertex–breech	27.7
Vertex–transverse	7.2
Breech–breech	9
Breech–vertex	6.9
Breech–transverse	3.6
Other combinations	6.9

Preterm onset of labour

Labour may begin spontaneously before term or may be induced for maternal or fetal complications. It is unusual for a twin pregnancy to go beyond term. Crowther (2000) reviewed six trials of hospital admission for bed rest in uncomplicated multiple pregnancies and found no evidence that bed rest could prevent preterm birth or fetal mortality. If labour threatens early, a tocolytic drug may be given in an attempt to stop uterine activity.

Mode of delivery

Many obstetricians believe that indications for a caesarean section should include **breech presentation** or **transverse lie** of the first twin. However, in 75% of twin pregnancies, the first twin presents by the vertex and there is no contraindication to vaginal delivery. The second twin should deliver easily as long as the lie is longitudinal. If the lie of the second twin is oblique or transverse, most can be easily converted to longitudinal lie by external cephalic version. Labour may be prolonged by poor uterine action because of uterine overdistension which can be remedied by oxytocin infusion. Epidural analgesia is the first choice as it does not affect the fetuses and allows any unforeseen manipulative manoeuvres to be made.

In cases where there are three or more babies in utero, delivery by caesarean section is probably advisable. It never ceases to amaze the author that the Dionne quintuplet identical girls were born vaginally in their parents' home and all survived. Sextuplets have survived and grown into healthy children in Britain (cared for once home by one of the author's students).

Postpartum haemorrhage

Poor uterine tone and the presence of a large placental site predispose women giving birth to multiple fetuses to **postpartum haemorrhage**, a life-threatening condition, especially if the woman's haemoglobin level is low. Prevention of haemorrhage is a priority. An intravenous infusion of oxytocin should be in situ and intramuscular Syntometrine 1 ampoule or intravenous ergometrine 500 µg administered.

Undiagnosed twins

If the head of the baby appears small in contrast to the known size of the uterus before delivery or the baby itself appears small, a second twin should be suspected and the uterus palpated. If an oxytocic drug has already been given, delivery of the second twin needs to be quick as its life may be in danger. The second baby may be asphyxiated and need active resuscitation.

Postnatal care of mother and babies

Care of the babies

Following birth, once the babies are breathing well, care will depend on their size and maturity. **Premature** or **small-for-gestational-age** babies will need appropriate care. Some twins may not need any special care other than helping the mother to care for them. The babies may be breastfed if the mother wishes.

Care of the mother

Involution of the uterus may be painful because of the increased muscle bulk and analgesia should be offered. If the mother decides to breastfeed both babies a high-protein, high-calorie diet will be needed. Anaemia should be treated and postnatal exercises geared at improving muscle tone of the abdominal wall and pelvic floor encouraged.

Main points

- Following the use of ultrasound scanning it is more common to calculate the age of the fetus using the estimated day of fertilisation. From weeks 9 to 24 there is remarkable growth and then growth slows but remains constant from 30 to 36 weeks when growth slows again.
- Continued maternal weight gain is thought to be associated with fetal growth but is affected by many factors. Poor weight gain is weakly associated with intrauterine growth retardation. Serial fundal height measurements can be used to assess growth.
- The mother adapts to fetal needs by increasing calorie intake and modifying metabolic activity. These changes seem to occur in response to signals from the fetoplacental unit. The mother also seems to be able to limit fetal growth. Her height is linked to her uterine capacity and small women appear to have small babies.
- Additional maternal influences include parity with primiparous women having smaller babies by about 200 g than multiparous women and adolescent mothers have smaller babies than fully mature mothers. This may be due to the effect of a first pregnancy on the uterine vascular bed.
- How big a baby grows may be determined by conflict between maternal and paternal genes. The insulin-like growth factors appear to have a key role in intrauterine growth. In humans the IGF2 gene inherited from the father makes a growth factor which helps the fetus to grow whilst the maternal gene is non-functional. This is called genomic imprinting.
- However, the size of the fetus may be constrained by the size of the intrauterine environment. The fetus also contributes to growth control by its genetic inheritance and by its sex; male fetuses grow larger than females.
- Two-thirds of twin pregnancies are dizygotic and the babies are only as alike as any other two siblings. Ethnic origin, maternal age, parity and conception soon after discontinuing oral contraception influence the frequency of dizygotic twinning.
- About one-third of monozygotic twins are dichorionic and two-thirds share one placenta and chorion. In 95% of these each baby has its own amnion and in 5% the babies are monoamniotic. About 1% of the latter are conjoined. Monozygotic twins are identical genetically. There is a higher incidence of serious congenital abnormalities in monozygotic twins.
- The outcome of higher-order multiple pregnancies can be poor and some centres have advocated multifetal reduction to ensure survival of two or three fetuses. The procedure may lead to loss of all fetuses.
- The earlier the diagnosis of twins is made, the more successful the outcome. Perinatal losses may be much larger when the diagnosis is made after 28 weeks. In countries with no access to ultrasound scanning, midwives must diagnose multiple pregnancies by clinical examination.
- Obstetric complications include abortion, pre-eclampsia, antepartum haemorrhage, anaemia, caesarean section delivery, preterm delivery, low birth weight, stillbirth, babies needing special care, postpartum haemorrhage and maternal infection. Most complications are more common as the number of fetuses in utero increases.
- When monoamniotic twins are present perinatal mortality can be as high as 50%, mainly because of umbilical cord entanglement, twin–twin transfusion syndrome, congenital abnormalities, conjoined twins and preterm birth. Delivery by caesarean section will help reduce the danger of cord entanglement.
- The outcome for conjoined twins is poor. The presence of shared organs may make it impossible to save both babies. In acardiac twinning, circulatory overload may cause the death of the normal twin.
- Twin-to-twin transfusion syndrome (TTS) may be dealt with by amnioreduction, laser obliteration of the vascular anastomoses or septostomy. Laser occlusion gives the best results if done in a specialist unit.
- Most twins show discordant growth because one twin gets less nourishment. Genetic syndromes and TTS may also result in discordant growth. The smaller twin is more at risk of perinatal complications.
- Maternal complications of multiple pregnancies include exacerbated minor disorders of pregnancy, iron and folic acid deficiency, pregnancy-induced

hypertension, pre-eclampsia and antepartum haemorrhage. Fetal malpresentations in labour may occur.

- If locked twins are diagnosed before the onset of labour an elective caesarean section should be performed. If the body of the first twin has been born an attempt at vaginal manipulation to free the head should be made. If unsuccessful urgent caesarean section is necessary.
- In multiple pregnancies labour may begin before term or may be induced for maternal or fetal complications. A recent review found no evidence that bed rest prevented preterm onset of labour or perinatal mortality.

- In 75% of twin pregnancies the first twin presents by the vertex and there is no contraindication to vaginal delivery. Labour may be prolonged by poor uterine action but a Syntocinon infusion can be started. The presence of a large placental site predisposes to postpartum haemorrhage. Care of the babies will depend on their size and maturity.
- The mother may breastfeed both babies but will need a high-protein, high-calorie diet. Anaemia should be treated and postnatal exercises geared at improving muscle tone of abdominal wall and pelvic floor. If there are three or more fetuses present an elective caesarean section is the commonest mode of delivery.

References

Abu-Amero, S., Monk, D., Apostolidou, S., et al., 2006. Imprinted genes and their role in human fetal growth. Cytogenetic Genome Res. 113 (4), 262–270.

Aurell, R., Tur, R., Torelio, M.J., et al., 2006. Clinical strategies to avoid multiple pregnancies in assisted reproduction. Gynecol. Endocrinol. 22 (9), 473–478.

Blackburn, S.T., 2007. Maternal, Fetal and Neonatal Physiology: A Clinical Perspective. W B Saunders, Philadelphia.

Bogin, B., 2001. Patterns of Human Growth. Cambridge University Press, Cambridge.

Carlson, B.M., 2004. Human Embryology and Developmental Biology, third edn. Elsevier Mosby, Philadelphia PA.

Craven, C., Ward, K., 1996. Placental causes of fetal malformation. Clin. Obstet. Gynaecol. 39 (3), 588–606.

Crowther, C.A., 2000. Hospitalisation and bed rest for multiple pregnancies. Cochrane Review. Cochrane Library, Issue 3. Update Software 2003, Oxford.

Dickey, R.P., Taylor, S.N., Lu, P.Y., et al., 2002. Spontaneous reduction of multiple pregnancy: incidence and effect on

outcome. Am. J. Obstet. Gynecol. 186, 77–83.

Dodd, J.M., Crowther, C.A., 2003. Reduction of the number of fetuses for women with triplet or higher order multiple pregnancies. Cochrane Database Syst. Rev. 2003, Issue (2) Art. No. CD003932. DO1: 10. 1002/14651858.CD003932.

Farooqui, M.O., Grossman, J.H., Shannon, R.A., 1973. A review of twin pregnancy and perinatal mortality. Obstet. Gynaecol. Surv. 28, 144–153.

Gluckman, P., Hanson, M., 2005. The Fetal Matrix, Evolution, Development and Disease. Cambridge University Press, Cambridge, UK.

Haig, D., 1993. Genetic conflicts in human pregnancy. Q. Rev. Biol. 68 (4), 495–519.

Henderson, C., Macdonald, S. (Eds.), 2004. Mayes' Midwifery: A Textbook for Midwives, thirteenth edn. Baillière Tindall, London.

Johnson, M.H., 2007. Essential Reproduction, sixth edn. Blackwell Publishing, Oxford.

Moore, K.L., Persaud, T.V.N., 2008. The Developing Human: Clinically Oriented Embryology, eighth edn. Elsevier Saunders, Philadelphia PA.

Roberts, D., Neilson, J. P., Kilby, M., Gates, S., 2007. Interventions for the treatment of twin–twin transfusion syndrome. The Cochrane Collaboration, The Cochrane Database of Systematic reviews 2007 Issue 2. Wiley.

Sebire, N.J., Souka, H., Skentou, L., et al., 2000. First trimester diagnosis of monoamniotic twin pregnancies. Ultrasound Obstet. Gynaecol. 16 (3), 223–225.

Sebire, N.J., Jolly, M., Harris, J., et al., 2001. Risk of obstetric complications in multiple pregnancies: an analysis of more than 400,000 pregnancies in the UK. Prenat. Perinat. Med. 6 (2), 89–94.

Wolpert, L., Jessel, T., Lawrence, P., Meyerowitz, E., et al., 2007. Principles of Development, third edn. Oxford University Press, Oxford.

Annotated recommended reading

Abu-Amero, S., Monk, D., Apostolidou, S., et al., 2006. Imprinted genes and their role in human fetal growth. Cytogenet. Genome Res. 113 (4), 262–270.

For those interested in genetic control of growth this is the most up-to-date paper I could find and is well worth a read.

Craven, C., Ward, K., 1996. Placental causes of fetal malformation. Clin. Obstet. Gynaecol. 39 (3), 588–606.

This excellent paper is still relevant and informative about the relationship between the placenta and developmental abnormalities of fetal structure, including problems in twins such as

acardia, conjoined twins and twin–twin transfusion syndrome.

Moore, K.L., Persaud, T.V.N., 2008. The Developing Human: Clinically Oriented Embryology, eighth edn. Saunders Elsevier, Philadelphia PA.

Chapter 7 discusses the fetal period from the 9th week until birth. The diagrams and photographs make this an excellent visual guide to developmental stages.

Sebire, N.J., Souka, H., Skentou, L., et al., 2000. First trimester diagnosis of monoamniotic twin pregnancies. Ultrasound Obstet. Gynaecol. 16 (3), 223–225.

This article, although a few years' old, still gives a clear and relevant discussion on aspects of abnormal conditions of twin and multiple pregnancies and is well worth tracking down.

Sebire, N.J., Jolly, M., Harris, J., et al., 2001. Risk of obstetric complications in multiple pregnancies: an analysis of more than 400,000 pregnancies in the UK. Prenat. Perinat. Med. 6 (2), 89–94.

This article, although a few years' old, still gives a clear and relevant discussion on aspects of abnormal conditions of twin and multiple pregnancies and is well worth tracking down.

Chapter Fourteen

Common fetal problems

CHAPTER CONTENTS

Introduction

This chapter covers a variety of topics concerning fetal danger. Although there is a blurred line between concepts applied to the fetus and the neonate, this chapter is concerned with the fetus. The following problems are discussed in relation to the neonate in Chapters 48–53.

Intrauterine growth retardation

Before discussing **intrauterine growth retardation** (IUGR), it is useful to understand some definitions:

- A **low-birth-weight baby** (LBW) is a baby who weighs 2500g or less at birth.

- A **very-low-birth-weight baby** (VLBW) is a baby who weighs less than 1500g at birth.
- A **light-for-dates** or **small-for-gestational-age** (SGA) baby is one whose birth weight is below the 10th centile for its gestational age but is not necessarily growth restricted.
- A **large-for-gestational-age** (LGA) baby is one whose birth weight is above the 90th centile for gestational age.
- A **preterm infant** is a baby born before 37 completed weeks of pregnancy (from LMP) irrespective of the birth weight. A preterm infant may also be SGA or LGA.

There are two categories of fetuses which appear SGA:

1. The fetus shows early departure from normal limits of growth that continues until delivery and is small because of conditions such as chromosomal abnormality or intrauterine infection.

2. The fetus shows arrest of previously normal growth caused by a factor outside the fetus such as maternal disease or placental pathology.

The term IUGR should be used only for the second category where growth is known to be arrested. Wrong classification of IUGR does not allow for fetuses that are small and healthy. This may lead to inappropriate interference in the course of pregnancy.

Complications of IUGR

In the antepartum and intrapartum periods there is an increase in the number of stillbirths, oligohydramnios and fetal distress. Neonatal complications including meconium aspiration syndrome, persistent fetal circulation, hypoglycaemia, hypocalcaemia, hyperviscosity syndrome and poor temperature control will be discussed in Section 4A of the book.

Factors adversely affecting fetal growth

Fetal growth depends on interacting factors such as genetic determinants, maternal health and nutrition, availability of growth substrates and an effective maternal blood supply to the placenta (Blackburn 2007). The essential substrates are oxygen, glucose and amino acids. Any decrease in substrate availability due to pathological conditions affecting mother, placenta and fetus will result in poor growth.

Fetal growth retardation may be **asymmetric** or **symmetric**. Asymmetric growth is when fetal weight is reduced out of proportion to length and head circumference and the fetus has little subcutaneous fat. The factors involved are usually maternal in origin. Symmetric growth retardation is due either to a congenital or genetic defect or to decreased growth potential in the fetus. The babies have the normal amount of subcutaneous fat for their size and the head circumference and length are in proportion to the weight.

Maternal conditions are:

- Hypertension.
- Chronic renal disease.
- Diabetes mellitus with vascular lesions.
- Sickle cell anaemia.
- Severe cardiac disease.
- Severe malnutrition.
- Smoking.
- Alcohol ingestion.

Fetoplacental problems include:

- Chromosomal abnormalities.
- Intrauterine infections.
- A history of a previous growth-retarded fetus.
- Multiple pregnancy.
- Small placental site and inadequate changes in uterine spiral arteries.
- Placental infarcts.
- Placenta praevia.

Maternal malnutrition

Although maternal malnutrition and low weight gain in pregnancy have been weakly associated with IUGR (Ott 2001) this is more likely to occur in developing countries. Severe protein calorie malnutrition, especially in the second half of pregnancy, will reduce birth weight; babies born in the Dutch famine of 1944–45 had a reduced birth weight in proportion to their length (Gluckman & Hanson 2005).

Smoking

Smoking is a prime cause of IUGR (Ott 2001). Tobacco smoking affects the fetoplacental unit in all three trimesters. Cigarette smoke contains many toxins which can affect cell proliferation and differentiation, in particular nicotine. Increased risk of miscarriage, fetal growth retardation, stillbirth, preterm birth and placental abruption has been reported (Jauniaux & Burton 2007). Also, carboxyhaemoglobin causes a sustained reduction in oxygen to the fetus with a prolonged effect on growth (Longo 1977). Birth weight reduction is between 120 and 430 g.

Alcohol consumption

Fetal alcohol syndrome (FAS) was first recognised in America. Alcohol has a low molecular weight and crosses the placental barrier. It is a known teratogen and fetal damage has been associated with any drinking. It is not possible to state how much alcohol causes the abnormalities associated with FAS so it is wise to abstain from drinking any alcohol during pregnancy. In a few women alcohol-induced malnutrition will add to the fetal problems.

The characteristic features of FAS are not all present in a particular infant:

- Deficient overall growth.
- Facial abnormalities: small eyes with inner epicanthic folds; poorly formed nasal bridge giving the nose a retroussé appearance; poor or absent vertical groove in a narrow top lip; ears that are large and simple in formation; and cleft palate.
- Musculoskeletal abnormalities: congenital hip lesions and thoracic cage abnormalities.
- Genitourinary abnormalities: undescended testes, male urethral abnormalities, hypoplastic labia in females; and kidney abnormalities.
- Cardiac abnormalities are common, mainly atrial or ventricular septal defects.
- Poor coordination of movement and learning difficulties.
- Alcohol withdrawal symptoms.

Placental insufficiency

In **placental insufficiency** the placenta is usually small with a reduction in the number of stem and villous capillaries and reduced uteroplacental blood flow with incomplete penetration by trophoblastic cells (Robinson et al 2000). There appears to be a failure in vascular invasion of the myometrial spiral arteries with increased risk of morbidity and mortality. These findings are also present in maternal conditions such as pre-eclampsia (Lyall & Robson 2000).

Multiple pregnancy

Poor fetal growth occurs in about 21% of twins, mainly due to abnormal placentation (see Ch. 13).

Genetic factors and chromosomal aberrations

The prevalence of genetic and chromosome disorders amongst babies with IUGR is higher than normal with an incidence of congenital abnormalities of between 5% and 27% compared to 0.1–4% in babies with normal growth (Ott 2001). It is particularly common in babies with trisomies such as Down syndrome. The majority of these babies have symmetric growth retardation.

Diagnosis and management of IUGR

The first step in managing IUGR is to identify those women at risk, then to differentiate the small, healthy babies from those with genuine IUGR (Robinson et al 2000). Monitoring at-risk fetuses allows management decisions to be made. Using a combination of clinical and ultrasound methods should enable a diagnosis to be made in 95% of cases.

Ultrasound

Ott (2006) stated that a combination of **Doppler velocity wave form analysis** of fetal vessels and ultrasonic estimation of fetal weight by measuring abdominal circumference appears to be the best method of identifying and evaluating IUGR. Soregaroli et al (2002) found a correlation between umbilical Doppler velocimetry abnormalities and an increased incidence of perinatal complications. The more abnormal the umbilical arterial blood flow, the more the fetal risk.

Measuring fetal subcutaneous fat

The research of Gardeil et al (2000) included 137 pregnant women. They found a correlation between babies with less than 5 mm of subcutaneous fat at 38 weeks and a low height:weight ratio (**ponderal index**). There were more instances of neonatal morbidity in those babies than in the control group with a subcutaneous fat measurement greater than 5 mm.

Other tests of placental function

Many tests have been shown to be of no value in assessment of placental function and are of historical value only. These include serial estriol estimation, human placental lactogen assays, contraction cardiotocography (CTG) stress testing and monitoring daily fetal movements. Measuring serial fundal height is of value in selecting women for referral to ultrasound screening. Doppler assessment combined with non-stress CTG may be important in diagnosing and managing IUGR (Ott 2006).

Fetal biophysical profile

Four fetal variables are combined to try to reduce the incidence of false-positive diagnoses. These are **fetal movement, tone, breathing movements** and **amniotic fluid volume**. In addition a 20-min CTG is carried out. Lalor et al (2007) reviewed five trials involving 2974 women with high-risk pregnancies and found no reduction either in the number of babies who died or in those with low Apgar scores. However, fetal biophysical profile was associated with a significant increase in induction and caesarean section. They suggest more evaluation of the method is needed.

Delivery of the baby

Once fetal lung maturity is achieved and, preferably after 34 weeks, the baby should be delivered. Excluding congenital malformations, intrapartum asphyxia is a major cause of morbidity and mortality. There is an increased risk of low 5-min Apgar scores and later neurological deficits. Asphyxia must be prevented:

- Direct fetal monitoring by scalp electrode.
- Care with analgesia and epidural anaesthesia may be best.
- The second stage of labour should be short and low forceps used if necessary.
- A paediatrician should be present at delivery.

Most of these babies now survive the neonatal period but they remain smaller than their age cohorts for several years. A major concern is that chronic intrauterine malnutrition may lead to a permanent decrease in brain cells. Small size at birth and low ponderal index are linked to coronary heart disease, high blood pressure and diabetes in later life (Barker 1998, Gluckman & Hanson 2005).

Rhesus isoimmunisation and ABO incompatibility

Rhesus isoimmunisation (RhD incompatibility)

Readers should ensure they understand blood group inheritance before reading on. The fetus inherits a gene for the **rhesus factor** from each parent and as rhesus D is a dominant gene if one or two genes are inherited the baby will be rhesus positive (Rh+). Only if the baby inherits two recessive d genes will the blood group be rhesus negative (Rh−) (Fig. 14.1).

If the mother is Rh− and the fetus Rh+, **haemolysis** of fetal red cells may occur (Fig. 14.2). This rarely affects the first baby as there are no spontaneous anti-D antibodies present in a woman's blood prior to her first pregnancy. This may happen if fetal red blood cells cross the placental barrier during that pregnancy or if she has been transfused accidentally with Rh+ blood.

During pregnancy and labour there is normally no mixing of maternal and fetal circulations. When the placenta separates, the chorionic villi tear and there is a risk of **fetomaternal haemorrhage** (FMH); usually between 0.5 ml and 5 ml of fetal blood enters the maternal circulation. If the fetus is Rh+ the production of antibodies will be stimulated and memory cells will mount a secondary response should the mother become pregnant with a second Rh+ baby. This process is called **isoimmunisation**.

Spontaneous or therapeutic abortion, amniocentesis, antepartum haemorrhage or external cephalic version may lead to an FMH and antibody formation. The problem arises in subsequent pregnancies because anti-D antibodies cross the placenta and haemolyse fetal red cells. Some protection occurs if the mother and fetus are ABO incompatible, as the naturally occurring anti-A or anti-B will destroy fetal red cells before the maternal immune system can respond to the rhesus factor.

Prevention of maternal isoimmunisation

In the past **haemolytic disease of the newborn** led to fetal or neonatal death from rhesus haemolytic disease but this is now largely preventable if three conditions are met:

1. Rhesus-positive blood should never be transfused if a woman's blood group is unknown.

2. Unnecessary risk of FMH should be avoided, for example by placental localisation prior to amniocentesis. Abdominal palpation of women with an antepartum haemorrhage should be kept to a minimum.

3. If there has been a risk of FMH, **anti-D immunoglobulin** (rhesus D antibodies) must be administered to the mother within 72 h; this confers passive immunity for about 3 months. The antibodies will coat and destroy any fetal red cells in the maternal circulation.

The dose of anti-D immunoglobulin (Ig) is normally 250 IU (international units) before 20 weeks of pregnancy and 500 IU after 20 weeks. Occasionally the FMH is so large that one dose of anti-D is insufficient to prevent isoimmunisation. The number of fetal red cells in maternal blood is estimated by means of a Kleihauer test and, if a second dose is needed, the laboratory will inform the doctor.

Antenatal management: anti-D prophylaxis

Every pregnant woman has her blood tested for ABO and rhesus types early in pregnancy. Any rhesus-negative women will be screened for RhD antibodies. If the test is negative further screening will be carried out.

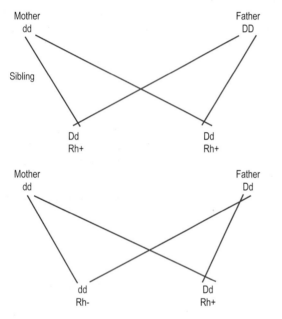

Figure 14.1 • Inheritance of the rhesus factor. (From Henderson C, Macdonald S 2004, with kind permission of Elsevier.)

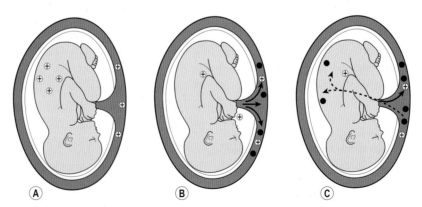

Figure 14.2 • Antibody formation. (A) Transfer of rhesus antigen (+) to the maternal circulation. (B) Antibody formation (•) in the rhesus negative mother. (C) Transfer of the rhesus antibody to the fetus. (From Henderson C, Macdonald S 2004, with kind permission of Elsevier.)

It is now recommended that all non-sensitised women should receive anti-D prophylaxis of at least 500 IU, usually at 28 and 34 weeks of pregnancy. Because some fetomaternal bleeds are undetected in pregnancy, some authorities recommend the use of antepartum RhD Ig prophylaxis (NICE 2007).

Failure to adhere to protocols of anti-D Ig administration means there are still incidences of women becoming sensitised and their babies developing haemolytic disease of the newborn (Percival 2004).

- Not testing the size of an FMH to ensure an appropriate dose of anti-D Ig was given.
- Some women do not receive anti-D Ig, including those who attend accident and emergency departments with bleeding in early pregnancy.
- Not administering anti-D Ig for abdominal trauma in 80% of cases.
- Using an inadequate dose of anti-D Ig following antepartum haemorrhage.
- Not managing sensitising events occurring after 20 weeks gestation.
- Not understanding Kleihauer test results, with a negative result interpreted as a reason not to give anti-D Ig.
- Postnatal omissions resulting because of confusion with women who had recently received antenatal treatment with anti-D Ig.

Wickham (2001) suggested that more research is needed into the midwife's role if a policy of routine administration were to be adopted. Since the 1990s it has become possible to test the fetal RhD status antenatally. This was done by chorionic villus sampling and amniocentesis but these procedures were invasive and not always accurate, especially in multi-ethnic populations. More comprehensive testing is possible by obtaining fetal cells from maternal plasma—a non-invasive prenatal diagnosis. This may avoid unnecessary administration of prophylactic anti-D Ig and prevent the rare possibility of a human blood-derived product with the risk of hepatitis C and rare viruses not yet identified (Avent 2008).

Care at delivery

When a mother is rhesus negative, the umbilical cord is clamped immediately to minimise the amount of placental blood with possible maternal antibodies entering the baby's circulation. Cord blood is taken for testing by using a syringe and needle directly into a placental vein to avoid the risk of contamination by maternal blood and Wharton's jelly which would make interpretation of the results difficult. The needle is removed prior to transferring the blood into a bottle to avoid haemolysis. Cord blood is tested for ABO and rhesus type, **direct Coombs test** looking for maternal antibodies on fetal red cells, and a haemoglobin estimate to check for haemolysis. If the mother has rhesus antibodies, the cord blood is also tested for serum bilirubin level.

Management if rhesus antibodies are present during pregnancy

If antibodies are detected, the titre is checked. Although titre does not relate directly to the fetal condition, it indicates a necessity to carry out an amniotic fluid test. The amount of bilirubin excreted from red cell haemolysis can be measured by optical density to allow judgements about further management. It is best to avoid amniocentesis until after 26 weeks when the fetus is considered viable.

The fetus is monitored for oedema and hepatosplenomegaly (enlarged liver and spleen) by ultrasound. Intravenous immunoglobulin may maintain the fetus until fetal transfusion of O-negative packed cells can be given (Percival 2004). If the fetus is considered mature enough to survive and it is considered dangerous to continue the pregnancy, the baby is delivered when all facilities, including pathology laboratory, are available.

Rhesus haemolytic disease

All babies whose mothers have rhesus antibodies should be transferred to a neonatal intensive care unit until the results of the cord blood tests are known. Depending on the percentage of red blood cells destroyed this disease varies in severity:

1. **Congenital haemolytic anaemia** occurs if haemolysis is minimal. Hepatosplenomegaly will be present but jaundice will not be severe. If the baby's haemoglobin (Hb) level is low a transfusion of packed cells can be given.

2. In **ictarus gravis neonatorum** (severe jaundice of the newborn) there has been fetal haemolysis and the baby's haemoglobin is low. Because the placenta transfers bilirubin to the mother for excretion, the baby is not usually jaundiced at birth. After delivery when the baby's liver has to cope with excessive bilirubin, jaundice rapidly develops. Treatment includes restoring the Hb level, reducing the bilirubin level and removing maternal antibodies.

3. In **hydrops fetalis** severe intrauterine anaemia results in congestive cardiac failure. The baby and placenta are pale and oedematous and the baby may be stillborn. If the baby is alive an immediate transfusion of packed cells will allow tissue oxygenation. Bilirubin and maternal antibodies are removed by an exchange transfusion via an umbilical catheter.

Principles of exchange transfusion

Umbilical vein catheterisation should only be carried out in a specialist unit by an experienced doctor who

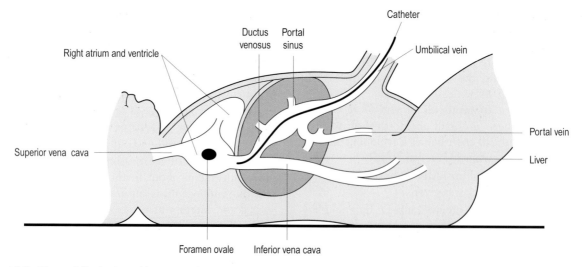

Figure 14.3 • The umbilical vein and its connections in the neonate. The position of the umbilical venous catheter is shown. Note how easy it would be to push it accidentally into the right atrium. (Reproduced with permission from Wallis & Harvey 1979.)

should be aware of the correct direction and position for the catheter.

- Blood is drawn out into a syringe via an umbilical vein catheter (Fig. 14.3).
- This blood is discarded into a waste container.
- Blood, warmed to body temperature, is drawn into this syringe. The blood is cross-matched for compatibility with blood from the baby's mother.
- This blood is injected slowly. The process is repeated until twice the baby's blood volume has been exchanged.

ABO incompatibility

In this condition the mother is blood group O and the baby either group AO or BO. Maternal blood contains unprovoked anti-A and anti-B antibodies even in the first pregnancy and these cross over the placenta to haemolyse fetal red cells. The first child can be affected but jaundice which appears in the first 24 h is usually mild. Treatment will depend on the rate of bilirubin rise in the neonate's blood.

Maternal infection in pregnancy

Microbes are small organisms that live in and on the human body. They can be divided into five major classes: **bacteria**, **viruses**, **algae**, **fungi** and **protozoa**. Some are helpful **commensal organisms** like the lactobacillus that increases vaginal acidity. However, many are **pathogens** causing serious infections against which the immune system develops defence mechanisms. Systemic infections may cause reproductive problems such as infertility and congenital defects and some infections are specific to the genital tract. Some organisms that cause genital tract disease will be outlined, followed by systemic disorders that may damage the fetus.

Suppression of cell-mediated immunity

Although the maternal immune system alters in pregnancy, most women are not immunocompromised. However, the suppression of cell-mediated immunity means that some infections are more severe, especially viruses such as poliomyelitis and influenza and **opportunistic pathogens** associated with HIV such as *Pneumocystis carinii* and *Toxoplasma gondii*. Pregnancy may also reactivate latent cytomegalovirus (CMV) and herpes.

Sexually transmitted diseases

The control of **sexually transmitted diseases** (STDs) is a difficult public health problem. In men they may cause few problems but in women pelvic inflammatory disease (PID) and decreased fertility are frequently seen. Also, pregnant women may pass the STD to the fetus, resulting in birth defects or stillbirth (Moodley & Sturm 2000). About one-third of cases in developed countries affect teenagers because young people often have more than one sexual partner. Many STDs have no symptoms or vague non-specific symptoms and social stigma means that people are less likely to seek treatment. The presence of a second disease often complicates treatment; for example, asymptomatic chlamydial infection may remain after gonorrhoea has been treated.

Bacterial infections

Gonorrhoea

This human disease is still one of the most widespread and symptoms differ between men and women. In women the initial symptoms are mild vaginitis which may go unnoticed while in men the organism causes a painful infection of the urethral canal. The organism can also cause a severe eye infection in neonates.

The causative organism, *Neisseria gonorrhoeae* (Fig. 14.4), is easily killed outside the body and is transmitted by intimate bodily contact. Severe complications include PID and damage to heart valves and joint tissues. Most cases respond to the antibiotic penicillin but **penicillin-resistant strains** of the organism are evolving. Other antibiotics that may be of use are spectinomycin or ceftiaxone. Newman et al (2007) suggest the use of quinolones or cephalosporins and other classes of antimicrobials to combat the ability of the organism to develop resistance.

Syphilis

Syphilis is more serious than gonorrhoea but better controlled as penicillin is very effective against the causative spirochaete *Treponema pallidum* (Fig. 14.5). In those who are allergic to penicillin erythromycin is advocated. The organism enters the body through a break in the skin or mucous membrane. In men infection is usually on the penis while in women it may be hidden in the vagina or on the cervix. In about 10% of cases the infection is extragenital, usually in the oral region. The disease can be transmitted across the placenta to cause congenital syphilis.

The organism multiplies within 2–6 weeks at the entry site to form a primary lesion or **chancre** which soon heals. It then spreads throughout the body and a **generalised skin rash** appears—the secondary stage. About 25% of people undergo a spontaneous cure, 25% remain symptomless although the organism is still present and 50% will develop the tertiary stage with possible fatal involvement of the cardiovascular and/or the central nervous systems. Because the symptoms are noticeable in both sexes, sufferers usually seek treatment. In Great Britain, pregnant women are screened for syphilis and offered treatment to prevent or treat fetal infection.

Chlamydia

Infection with the intracellular organism *Chlamydia trachomatis* is the most common STD. There are various serotypes of this organism. One strain causes severe eye infections but others can cause venereal diseases. Chlamydia is asymptomatic in about 80% of cases but can cause **non-gonococcal urethritis** in men and is the major cause of PID in women. In men testicular swelling and prostate inflammation can occur and in women fallopian tubes may be damaged or blocked by destruction of epithelial lining cells, leading to adhesions (Sönmez et al 2008). Infertility may result in both sexes.

Normally **tetracycline** would be the antibiotic of choice but this cannot be used in pregnancy as it has adverse effects on fetal teeth and bones. **Erythromycin** is a good alternative (Moodley & Sturm 2000). Chlamydia is often present in people with gonorrhoea and treatment to eradicate both organisms should be given.

Group B streptococcus

One in three women in Great Britain may have vaginal carriage of **group B streptococcus** at some time during their pregnancy. Maternal infection is asymptomatic but the organism is the most common cause of overwhelming

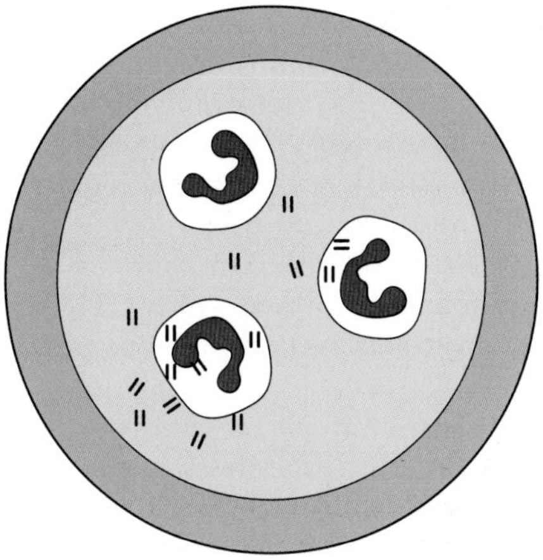

Figure 14.4 • Diagrammatic representation of the organism of *Neisseria gonorrhoeae*. (From Henderson C, Macdonald S 2004, with kind permission of Elsevier.)

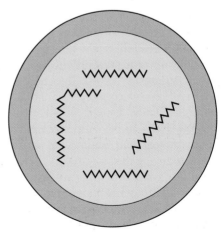

Figure 14.5 • Diagrammatic representation of the organism of *Treponema pallidum*. (From Henderson C, Macdonald S 2004, with kind permission of Elsevier.)

sepsis in neonates. The prevalence is between 0.6 and 3.7 per 1000 live births and infant mortality may be as high as 50%. Screening and treating these women is difficult because of recurrence of infection, but intrapartum antibiotic administration appears to reduce the risk of neonatal infection (Smaill 2003).

Viral infections

Acquired immune deficiency syndrome

Currently more than 22 million people have died from **acquired immune deficiency syndrome** (AIDS) and 42 million people are thought to be infected with the **human immunodeficiency virus** (HIV), most of them living in developing countries (Wilson 2003), especially in sub-Saharan Africa where it is still gaining momentum (Barnett & Whiteside 2006). More than 1.5 million of the infected people are children under the age of 15 years (Brocklehurst & Volmink 2002).

HIV is a **retrovirus** which carries its genetic information as **ribonucleic acid** (RNA) unlike most organisms which contain **deoxyribonucleic acid** (DNA). Cells of the immune system (Ch. 29) containing **CD4 molecules** are its targets. These include T lymphocytes, monocytes and macrophages. On entering a cell the viral RNA is converted to DNA and takes over the cell to produce more viruses.

This disease is not strictly sexually transmitted. The retrovirus is transferred by blood from one person to another so skin or mucous membrane lesions must be present for transmission to occur. This disease is almost always eventually fatal and there is no cure as yet although treatment can be effective for a number of years. Promiscuity is a key factor in the spread of HIV as is blood contamination of needles shared by drug addicts. These types of transmission are called **horizontal transmission**.

After sexual transmission the next most important cause is mother-to-child transmission (MTCT) or **vertical transmission**. The child can be infected prenatally, at the time of delivery or postnatally through breast feeding (Barnett & Whiteside 2006). Infection at the time of delivery is the most common. Factors that increase the risk of transmission include a high maternal viral load and a low CD4 count. Antiretroviral drugs may decrease the viral load and inhibit viral reproduction in the fetus thus reducing the risk of MTCT. A single dose of **nevirapine** given to the mother in labour and to the neonate within 72 h costs little and has been effective but this is not available to the most vulnerable.

As HIV infection may not be obvious at birth but present with recurrent infections and failure to thrive months or years later, it is difficult to assess the risk for MTCT. Studies show that there is a risk of transmission during breast feeding and it may be best in developed countries to advise women not to breast feed. However, most cases occur in developing countries so the risk of transmission has to be weighed against the risks of not breast feeding where there is no access to artificial milk and homes are unhygienic. It may be possible to use nevirapine for longer periods in breast feeding populations (Brocklehurst & Volmink 2002). Medically, HIV has been spread by blood transfusion and by **factor VIII** used to treat **haemophilia** or (in some countries) used in mass vaccination.

Those caring for a multicultural society need to be aware of the risk factors of viral transmission through contamination with blood and body fluids. The following recommendations are valid:

1. Avoid mouth contact with penis, vagina and rectum.

2. Avoid sexual activities that may result in tears in the linings of rectum, vagina and penis.

3. Avoid sexual activity with individuals from high-risk groups. These include male and female prostitutes, homosexual or bisexual individuals and intravenous drug users.

4. If unprotected sexual intercourse takes place with a member of a high-risk group, a blood test should be taken to ascertain whether infection has occurred. If the test is positive, future sexual partners should be protected by using a condom.

The search for a cure

As the T-cell population falls over a few years, production of antibodies falls, the immune system becomes crippled and the person becomes ill with opportunistic infections. Unfortunately the **mutation rate** of HIV is high, resulting in so many **variants** that no vaccine against them all can be developed. Trials of vaccines against viral subunits have proved futile.

Scientists working on vaccines realised they had concentrated on **antibody stimulation** and ignored **cellular immunity** (Ch. 29). **Cytotoxic lymphocytes** (CTLs) kill cells that have foreign protein attached to their surfaces (Clayton 2003). CTLs may account for a group of Nairobi prostitutes who have no virus or HIV antibodies in their blood although they are at high risk. These women appear to have a high CTL response and researchers are trying to find a way to provoke such a response.

Until a successful vaccine is developed, a way to minimise the risk of sexual transmission is needed. In parts of the developing world men refuse to wear condoms and Stone (2003) believes that a method is needed over which women have control. He discusses **microbicides** aimed at destroying causative organisms in situ. These could be gels, foams, creams or impregnated sponges placed in situ prior to sexual activity but no safe medication has been developed (Barnett & Whiteside 2006) although governments and the World Health Organization have noted the value. Two problems need addressing: first such products may also kill sperm; second it is more difficult to protect anal epithelium which is more fragile than vaginal epithelium. Also the drug may dissipate through the bowel rather than remaining in situ.

TORCH organisms and pregnancy risk

TORCH is a word derived from the first letters of a series of infections that can cross the placenta to affect the fetus. These are **Toxoplasmosis, Others, Rubella, Cytomegalovirus** and **Herpes**. Most will cause congenital abnormality if acquired in the first trimester and neonatal infection, often affecting the lungs, liver, spleen and brain if acquired later in pregnancy.

Rubella

In 1941 Gregg in Australia described an association between maternal rubella (German measles) and **congenital cataracts**. Rubella infection during the first few weeks of pregnancy inhibits cell division in the embryonic eyes, ears, heart and brain. After the 3rd month the most common defect is deafness. An infant born with congenital rubella is highly infectious and must be isolated from other women and infants but not from their own mothers (Percival 2004). Rubella vaccination of girls has been carried out in the UK and levels of infection are reduced to a low level. Pregnant women are screened and can be offered vaccination in the postnatal period. Those working with mothers and babies should also be screened and offered vaccination if needed.

Varicella

Varicella (chicken pox) is a childhood illness transmitted by respiratory droplets. If it occurs in pregnancy a woman may develop **adult respiratory distress syndrome** (ARDS) with a mortality rate of up to 35%. Preterm labour is common, as is **herpes zoster** (shingles).

Fetal varicella syndrome with developmental abnormalities may occur if maternal infection is in the first trimester. This includes **low birth weight, eye lesions, undeveloped limbs, skin scars** and **psychomotor retardation**. Infection in the third trimester may cause neonatal infection with **pneumonitis, hepatitis** and **disseminated intravascular coagulation** (DIC). Hyperimmune varicella zoster immune globulin (VZIG) can be offered to women who have been in contact with chicken pox or shingles as can acyclovir. Ultrasound to diagnose fetal abnormalities can be used.

Cytomeglovirus (CMV)

This double-stranded DNA virus is a member of the herpes virus family and is transmitted by contact with infected blood, saliva and urine or by sexual contact. Studies have shown that in developed countries up to 60% of women of childbearing age tested have had a primary infection with CMV. It is often asymptomatic but there may be non-specific symptoms such as malaise and fever, usually in immunocompromised people. If the primary infection occurs in pregnancy, abortion, preterm labour, intrauterine growth retardation or fetal death may occur. The greatest risk to the fetus is in the first 20 weeks although organs develop normally. However, damage to the fetal liver and nervous system may occur. If the baby is born with symptoms the prognosis is poor.

Toxoplasmosis

The causative organism is a protozoon, *Toxoplasma gondii*, found in dog and cat faeces and in uncooked meat. Infection is usually asymptomatic and occurs in 1 in 500 pregnant women. About 36% of their babies will be affected. **Microcephaly, hydrocephaly** and **hepatosplenomegaly** may occur. Screening in pregnancy could be offered and treatment is with **spiramycin**. Umbilical cord blood may be tested to see if the fetus is infected. Some women may consider termination of pregnancy.

Herpes simplex

Genital infection with type 1 or type 2 *Herpes simplex virus* (HVS-1 and HVS-2) may lead to serious neonatal infection, especially HVS-2 (Moodley & Sturm 2000). An infected baby may develop localised lesions, encephalitis or generalised herpes infection including septicaemia, pneumonitis, **liver dysfunction** and **coagulopathy** (Garland & Jones 2001). This is a difficult problem as many women show no signs of clinical infection. The first diagnosis may be made on appearance of neonatal infection by clinical signs and viral isolation.

If the woman gives a history of infection the mode of delivery should be discussed. In the past, caesarean section has been used to prevent exposure of the fetus to the virus. Trials of the antiviral drug **acyclovir** to reduce viral shedding have been inconclusive. A large number of surveys have shown that caesarean section does not protect completely against neonatal infection, and intrauterine infection may have occurred (Moodley & Sturm 2000). There has been no increase in neonatal infection when abdominal deliveries are not performed.

The delivery method may be based on the clinical appearance of the genital tract at the onset of labour. If no active lesions are present a vaginal delivery may be completed. However, if the woman has acquired a new infection there is a high risk of viral transmission and delivery by caesarean section should be considered. Use of techniques that break the baby's skin such as scalp electrodes should be avoided. Two strategies for the future include the search for a vaccine but this is yet another adapting virus against which it is difficult to develop a vaccine, and mass screening which is not cost effective if the incidence of neonatal infection is low.

Listeriosis

The food-borne pathogen *Listeria monocytogenes* is a bacterium found throughout the environment which may cause abortion, fetal disease or death. Cook–chill products have been implicated in the transmission of infection. Diagnosis in women or neonates is by culturing the organism from blood and/or cerebrospinal fluid and it is susceptible to penicillin and erythromycin. Health education on safe preparation of food would help to reduce the incidence of infection.

Hepatitis B (serum hepatitis)

The hepatitis B virus (HBV) is an important cause of morbidity and mortality worldwide. It can be transmitted sexually or parenterally through blood or blood products and by vertical transmission to the fetus. Other body fluids have been implicated in transmission but blood is the main source of spread. This includes contamination of medical equipment and sharing of needles and syringes by drug addicts and needle-stick injuries in health workers. Tattooing and acupuncture can also be risk activities.

As in many viruses the structure includes a **central core** carrying the genetic material, an **outer envelope** and an **outer surface**. There are three sites that can stimulate antibody production: the **surface antigen HBs Ag** (formerly Australia antigen), the **envelope antigen HBe Ag** and the **core antigen HBc Ag**. Virus particles can be found in blood and body fluids of infected people. Long-term infection can lead to chronic hepatitis, cirrhosis of the liver and liver cancer. It is more commonly carried by people from Asia, Sub-Saharan Africa, the Caribbean, Central and South America and immigrants from these regions have a 1 in 10 risk as against a background rate in the UK of 0.1%. The risk factors for HIV are shared by HBV.

Antenatal screening of all pregnant women is recommended with treatment of the affected neonate and precautions taken by birth attendants. The presence of HBe Ag indicates that the disease is highly infectious and there is a 25% risk of transmission to the baby. If women are HBe Ag positive or have had a late pregnancy infection the babies are given hepatitis B vaccine, the first dose within 24 h of birth, repeated at 1 month and 6 months of age to protect them against long-term dangers. If women have become infected during pregnancy or do not have HBe Ag present the baby should receive **hepatitis B specific immunoglobulin** (HBIg) at birth in a different site from the vaccination.

Hepatitis C (HVC)

HVC infection also causes viral hepatitis and occurs worldwide. The main route of admission is by skin inoculation, blood and blood products. Vertical transmission is low but higher rates may be seen in women who are HIV and HCV positive. There is no evidence to support transmission in breast milk.

Main points

- Optimal birth weight depends on an interaction between fetal growth potential and intrauterine environment. Genetic determinants, maternal health and nutrition and availability of substrates interact to create fetal growth.
- Growth potential differs between individuals and races. Some fetuses may be small but healthy, making diagnosis of intrauterine growth retardation problematic.
- Associated maternal conditions are hypertension, cardiac disease, chronic renal disease, diabetes mellitus, sickle cell anaemia, smoking and alcohol abuse. Placental conditions include small placental size, inadequate changes in the spiral arteries and placental infarcts.

- IUGR increases the risk of stillbirth, oligohydramnios and fetal distress. Neonatal complications include meconium aspiration syndrome, hypoglycaemia, hypocalcaemia and poor temperature control. Genetic and chromosomal disorders are common in babies with symmetric IUGR.
- A combination of clinical and ultrasound observations makes a diagnosis possible in 95% of cases. Fundal height measurements may select women for ultrasound screening such as Doppler velocimetry.
- Oligohydramnios is a late sign of fetal malnutrition and indicates a need to expedite delivery. Fetal biophysical profile may be a better indicator than the non-stress cardiotocography at predicting a low 5-min Apgar score.

- Once fetal lung maturity is achieved the baby can be delivered. It may take several years for the baby to reach comparative size with its age cohorts. Some studies have suggested an increased incidence of minimal brain dysfunction; others have found no difference with age cohorts.
- Rhesus haemolysis of fetal red cells rarely affects the first baby as there are no spontaneous anti-D antibodies. If the first fetus is Rh+ these may develop if a fetomaternal haemorrhage (FMH) occurs. If an FMH is likely anti-D immunoglobulin should be administered to the mother within 72 h.
- In Rh− women with a high titre of antibodies a direct test for bilirubin in amniotic fluid should be made so that decisions can be made on further management of the pregnancy. Some authorities recommend the prophylactic antenatal use of anti-D immunoglobulin.
- At delivery, cord blood is tested from all babies of Rh− women for ABO and rhesus type, direct Coombs test and haemoglobin estimation. If the mother has rhesus antibodies, cord blood bilirubin levels are checked.
- Although naturally occurring anti-A antibodies and anti-B antibodies occur and first babies can be jaundiced within the first 24 h, the jaundice is usually mild.
- Systemic infections may cause infertility or congenital defects during pregnancy. Because of the suppression of cell-mediated immunity some infections such as poliomyelitis and influenza may be more severe. Pregnancy may reactivate cytomegalovirus and herpes infections.
- If untreated, sexually transmitted diseases such as gonorrhoea and syphilis can have long-term serious health consequences and pregnant women may transmit the infection to the fetus, causing birth defects or stillbirth. Both diseases are usually easy to treat, responding to penicillin or other antibiotics.

- Contamination of the baby with *Chlamydia trachomatis* may cause severe neonatal illness. The organism responds to erythromycin.
- Infection with group B streptococcus is common and is most often responsible for overwhelming neonatal sepsis with a high mortality rate. Screening and treating women in pregnancy is difficult because of a high recurrence rate but antibiotic treatment of labouring women may be useful.
- Women who are HIV positive may pass the virus across the placenta to the fetus or contaminate their baby during the birth process. A third way of transmission is via breast feeding.
- Anti-retroviral drugs may decrease the viral load and inhibit viral reproduction in the fetus thus reducing the risk of vertical transfer. A single dose of nevirapine given to the mother in labour and to the neonate within 72 h costs little and has been effective but is not available to the most vulnerable.
- TORCH organisms can cause fetal abnormality if acquired during the third trimester. If acquired later in pregnancy neonatal infection, often affecting the lung, liver, spleen and brain may occur.
- The hepatitis B virus is transmitted by blood and sexual intercourse and by vertical transmission to the fetus. Long-term infection can cause chronic hepatitis, liver cirrhosis and liver cancer. Antenatal screening ensures that vulnerable babies are treated.
- Hepatitis C is another blood-borne virus but is more difficult to transmit than hepatitis B virus. There is no evidence to support transmission in breast milk.
- Maternal genital infection with type 1 or type 2 herpes simplex virus may lead to serious neonatal infection. Trials of antiviral agents are inconclusive. Delivery by caesarean section may not protect completely against neonatal infection because of transplacental infection.

References

Avent, N.D., 2008. RHD genotyping from maternal plasma: guidelines and technical challenges. Methods Mol. Biol. 444, 185–201.

Barker, D.P.J., 1998. Mothers, Babies and Health in Later Life. Harcourt Brace, Edinburgh.

Barnett, T., Whiteside, A., 2006. AIDS in the Twenty-First Century: Disease and Globalisation, second edn. Palgrave Macmillan, Great Britain.

Blackburn, S.T., 2007. Maternal, Fetal and Neonatal Physiology: A Clinical Perspective. W B Saunders, Philadelphia.

Brocklehurst, P., Volmink, J., 2002. Antiretrovirals for reducing the risk of mother-to-child transmission of HIV

infection. Cochrane Database Syst. Rev. (1) Update Software 2003, Oxford.

Clayton, J., 2003. Beating the odds. New Sci. 177 (2381), 34–37.

Gardeil, F., Greene, R., Stuart, B., Turner, M.J., 2000. Sonographic measurement of subcutaneous fat in the fetal abdomen: a new predictor of growth restriction? Contemp. Rev. Obstet. Gynecol. March, 7–11.

Garland, S., Jones, C., 2001. Herpes simplex virus in pregnancy. Obstet. Gynecol. 3 (2), 108–111.

Gluckman, P., Hanson, M., 2005. The Fetal Matrix: Evolution, Development and Disease. Cambridge University Press, Cambridge, UK.

Henderson, C., Macdonald, S., 2004. Mayes' Midwifery: A Textbook for Midwives, thirteenth edn. Baillière Tindall, London.

Jauniaux, E., Burton, G.J., 2007. Morphological and biological effects of maternal exposure to tobacco smoke on the feto-placental unit. Early Hum. Dev. 83 (11), 699–706.

Lalor, J.G., Fawole, B., Alfirevic, Z., Devane, D., 2007. Biophysical profile for fetal assessment in high risk pregnancies. Cochrane Database Syst. Rev. 2008 Review 2. Wiley.

Longo, L.D., 1977. The biological effects of carbon monoxide on the pregnant woman, fetus and newborn infant. Am. J. Obstet. Gynecol. 129, 69–103.

Lyall, F., Robson, S.C., 2000. Defective extravillous trophoblast function and pre-eclampsia, Ch. 7. In: Kingdom, J., Jauniaux, E., O'Brien, S. (Eds.) The Placenta: Basic Science and Clinical Practice. RCOG Press, Dorchester.

Moodley, P., Sturm, W., 2000. Sexually transmitted infections, adverse pregnancy outcome and neonatal infection. Semin. Neonatol. 5 (3), 255–269.

National Institute for Health and Clinical Excellence (NICE), 2007. Pregnancy (Rhesus Negative Women): Routine Anti-D. Appraisal Document. NICE, London.

Newman, L.M., Moran, J.S., Workowski, K.A., 2007. Update on the management of gonorrhoea in adults in the United States. Clin. Infect. Dis. 44 (Suppl. 3), S84–S101.

Ott, W.J., 2001. The ultrasonic diagnosis and evaluation of intrauterine growth restriction. Ultrasound Rev. Obstet. Gynecol. 1, 205–215.

Ott, W.J., 2006. Sonographic diagnosis of fetal growth restriction. Clin. Obstet. Gynecol. 49 (2), 295–307.

Percival, P., 2004. Jaundice and infection. In: Fraser, D.M., Cooper, M.A. (Eds.) Myles Textbook for Midwives, fourteenth edn. Elsevier Churchill Livingstone, Edinburgh, pp. 863–889.

Robinson, J.S., Moore, V.M., Owens, J.A., McMillen, I.C., 2000. Origins of fetal growth restriction. Eur. J. Obstet. Gynecol. Reprod. Biol. 92, 13–19.

Smaill, F., 2003. Intrapartum antibiotics for Group B streptococcal colonisation.

Cochrane Database Syst. Rev. (1) Update Software, Oxford.

Sönmez, S., Sönmez, E., Yasar, L., et al., 2008. Can screening Chlamydia trachomatis by serological tests predict tubal damage in infertile patients? New Microbiol. 31 (1), 75–79.

Soregaroli, M., Bonera, R., Danti, L., et al., 2002. Prognostic role of umbilical Doppler velocimetry in growth-restricted fetuses. J. Matern. Fetal Med. 11, 199–203.

Stone, A., 2003. Protect and survive. New Sci. 177 (2381), 42–44.

Wickham, S., 2001. Routine antenatal anti-D: an overview of the evidence. MIDIRS Midwifery Digest 11 (2), 201–203.

Wilson, C., 2003. World without AIDS. New Sci. 177 (2381), 38–41.

Annotated recommended reading

Gluckman, P., Hanson, M., 2005. The Fetal Matrix: Evolution, Development and Disease. Cambridge University Press, Cambridge, UK.

This book is an eye-opener for anyone wishing to find out about the long-term effects of fetal disadvantage. It is well written and opened up a new field of preventive medicine.

Moodley, P., Sturm, W., 2000. Sexually transmitted infections, adverse pregnancy outcome and neonatal infection. Semin. Neonatol. 5 (3), 255–269.

This paper provides an excellent overview of the effects of sexually transmitted diseases on mothers and babies.

Ott, W.J., 2006. Sonographic diagnosis of fetal growth restriction. Clin. Obstet. Gynecol. 49 (2), 295–307.

This is an excellent article on ultrasonography methods of monitoring fetal growth.

Percival, P., 2004. Jaundice and infection, Ch. 46. In: Fraser, D.M., Cooper, M.A. (Eds.) Myles Textbook for Midwives, fourteenth edn. Elsevier Churchill Livingstone, pp. 863–889.

This is an extremely well-written and -researched chapter on both causes and management of jaundice and a comprehensive look at infections in pregnancy and neonates.

Wickham, S., 2001. Routine antenatal anti-D: an overview of the evidence. MIDIRS Midwifery Digest 11 (2), 201–203.

This is an informative review of research into the use of antenatal anti-D prophylaxis. It discusses the changing role of the midwife when new technology or treatments are introduced.

Chapter Fifteen

Congenital defects

15

Introduction

Congenital defects which are present at birth may be visible, involve obvious changes in organs or be hidden such as changes in protein molecules, for example haemoglobin or cell receptors. Moore & Persaud (2008) outline four clinically significant types of **congenital anomalies**:

- **Malformation**: A morphologic defect of an organ, part of an organ or larger region of the body that results from an intrinsically abnormal developmental process. Intrinsic implies that the developmental potential is abnormal from the beginning such as a chromosomal abnormality of a gamete at fertilisation.

- **Disruption**: A morphological defect of an organ, part of an organ or larger region of the body that results from extrinsic breakdown or interference with an originally normal developmental process. Environmental causes such as teratogens, for example drugs and viruses, should be considered.

- **Deformation**: An abnormal form, shape or position of a body part resulting from mechanical causes such as in oligohydramnios.

- **Dysplasia**: An abnormal organisation of cells into tissues because of dyshistogenesis or cellular disturbance.

Congenital defects occur in 2–3% of all live births and account for most severe illness during infancy and childhood and 25% of childhood deaths. However, most are minor and of no functional significance. The percentage of diagnosis increases as children develop and reaches 6% in 2-year-olds and 8% in 5-year-olds (Moore & Persaud 2008).

General causes of congenital abnormalities

The major causes of congenital abnormalities are (Carlson 2004):

- Unknown cause: 50%
- Multifactorial (genetic + environment): 25%
- Chromosomal anomaly: 10%
- Single gene defect: 8%
- Major environmental cause: 7%.

Genes

An introduction to genetics, including causation of fetal abnormalities, is presented in Chapter 3 and the role of genes in embryogenesis is found in Chapter 8. About 18% of fetal anomalies are caused by chromosomal and genetic factors. Mutations may occur in the DNA of protein coding genes or in the homeobox regulatory genes.

Teratogens

Teratology is the study of the causes, mechanisms and patterns of abnormal fetal development. Gregg's finding in 1941 that rubella virus caused a syndrome of abnormalities (Ch. 14) was the first clear evidence of **teratogenesis**, and the terrible effects of the drug thalidomide between 1957 and 1962 convinced scientists of the environmental effect on a fetus that up until the 1940s had been thought to be totally protected from the outside world. Teratogens reach the fetus by crossing the placenta and causing **DNA mutations**.

Malformation of a particular structure is usually caused only during the sensitive period of its development (Moore & Persaud 2008), and the earlier a teratogen is present the more generalised the effect. If malformations occur in the first 17 days when the germ layers are being formed they are usually so complex as to be fatal. Between 3 and 8 weeks survival with major defect is likely. Following completion of **organogenesis** their effects are greatly reduced except in the brain and sensory organs where cell differentiation continues. Later in pregnancy some teratogens, especially microorganisms may destroy already formed tissues.

Environmental and genetic interaction

The rate of new mutations can be increased by environmental factors such as microbial, biochemical and dietary factors, smoking, alcohol ingestion, radiation and many chemicals. These may interfere with embryonic development at very precise times during organogenesis. Some factors such as the rubella virus are easily associated, but others, such as environmental pollution, are more difficult to ascertain. These interactions are discussed in Chapter 8.

Drugs

Medicinal drugs may be dispensed by practitioners or bought over the counter from a chemist. Recreational drugs such as cocaine and heroine may be bought illegally on the streets. These drugs may damage gametes or may prevent nutrient absorption such that essential

Table 15.1 Drugs known to cause fetal defects

Drug	Effect
Thalidomide	Limb deformities, heart defects
Warfarin	Limb defects, central nervous system defects, retarded growth
Corticosteroids	Cleft palate and congenital cataract
Anticonvulsants such as phenytoin	Lip and palate deformities, mental retardation
Androgens	Masculinisation in female fetus
Oestrogens	Testicular atrophy in male
Diethylstilbestrol	Vaginal and cervical cancer at puberty
Cytotoxic drugs (especially folic acid antagonists)	Neural tube defects, cleft palate
Tetracycline	Staining of bones and teeth, thin tooth enamel, impaired bone growth

Source: British National Formulary 2003.

nutrients are absent at crucial times (Table 15.1). Taking medicinal drugs is common in pregnancy and several studies have shown that pregnant women may take up to four types of drug during their pregnancy, 50% of these in the first trimester (Moore & Persaud 2008).

Thalidomide, a drug taken for morning sickness around 1960, caused **major limb reduction deformities** and other problems (Fig. 15.1). The effects of taking thalidomide in early pregnancy are still being seen in South America where the drug is prescribed for leprosy. While care is taken to avoid prescribing it to pregnant women, people offer their drugs to friends and relatives, some of whom will be pregnant.

Prenatal screening for congenital defects

In an ideal world congenital defects could be prevented. However, most women are seen for the first time when their pregnancies are already underway. **Preconception advice** (Ch. 8) will help to reduce the number of abnormal embryos conceived. Early diagnosis is essential so that a couple can be offered the choice of termination of pregnancy. Many defects can now be identified in specific populations. Techniques include ultrasonography, chorionic villus sampling, amniocentesis and maternal serum screening.

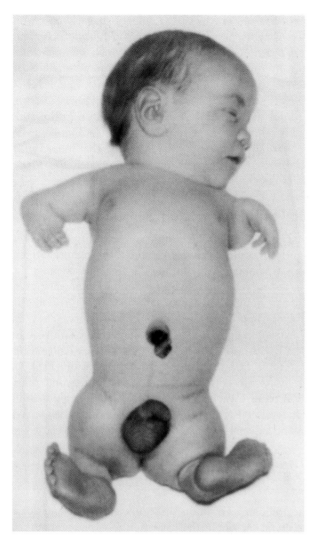

Figure 15.1 • Newborn male infant showing typical malformed limbs (meromelia—limb reduction) caused by thalidomide ingested by his mother during the critical period of limb development. (Reproduced with permission from Moore 1963.)

Turnpenny & Ellard (2007) discuss the above techniques and how they may revolutionise the diagnosis of embryonic and fetal malformations and genetic disease. However, Abramsky & Chapple (2003) consider the human side of prenatal screening and late pregnancy diagnosis of fetal abnormality, including parents' own perspective. Medical technology may have raced ahead with little consideration of the ethical, legal and emotional dilemmas raised by an increased ability to detect fetal defects. Couples may not want to terminate the pregnancy and early diagnosis offers a chance to plan for the baby's treatment after birth.

Ultrasonography

Most women are offered an **ultrasound scan** (USS) in pregnancy. The embryonic sac can be seen as early as 6 weeks following conception. USS screening is probably best carried out at 18–20 weeks' gestation so that an accurate fetal age can be confirmed. Most obstetricians feel the advantages of routine screening far outweigh the disadvantages. Sullivan & Kirk (2003) give a very detailed account of USS by trimester and also discuss women's experiences and attitudes to scanning.

How ultrasound works

Ultrasound imaging depends on the differences in tissue structure between organs. Sounds at a very high pitch (frequency of 3–10 MHz) are produced by a transducer. Because of its frequency, high-pitched sound travels in a narrow beam. These sound waves pass into the body until they reach a tissue and are reflected back. The sound echoes are detected electronically and transmitted onto the screen as a dot. The more dense the tissue, the stronger the echo and the whiter the visual display. Weaker echoes produce various shades of grey. Fluid-filled areas reflect no echoes, producing a black area.

Various types of display modes are used, each with its advantages. **M-mode ultrasonography** shows changes in a structure with time. **B-mode ultrasonography** shows the anatomy of a two-dimensional plane of scanning and can be used in real time. **Doppler ultrasonography** produces flow pattern information of the heart and blood vessels. With **endosonography** an endoscope can be inserted into the vagina to bring it closer to the fetus and receive a higher-resolution image. Real-time B-mode ultrasonography is most often used. Common defects diagnosed by mid-trimester fetal anomaly ultrasound include:

* Anencepahaly, microcephaly and hydrocephaly.
* Neural tube defects.
* Gastrointestinal defects such as atresia or omphalocele.
* Renal agenesis and polycystic kidneys.
* Body defects associated with chromosomal defects.

Obtaining fetal tissue for genetic testing

All invasive techniques carry a risk of infection, haemorrhage and fetal loss. The risks must be weighed against the likelihood of fetal abnormality being present.

Cells obtained by **amniocentesis** or **chorionic villus sampling** can be used for **karyotyping** for chromosomal abnormalities such as Down syndrome, **genetic analysis** using gene probes as in cystic fibrosis and **sexing the embryo** if there is a family history of X-linked disorders such as Duchenne muscular dystrophy. **Enzyme assay** for detection of inborn errors of metabolism is available in many disorders. These invasive tests should be carried out at a specialist centre.

Amniocentesis

A sample of amniotic fluid is withdrawn from the amniotic cavity through a transabdominal needle using ultrasound to avoid the placenta. This is usually carried out at 14–16 weeks when sufficient amniotic fluid is present. If carried out earlier the small amount of fluid present makes it difficult and there may be insufficient cells obtained to study. A further problem is that the **desquamated cells** (those shed by the fetus into the amniotic fluid) obtained are difficult to culture and it may take up to 3 weeks before the chromosomes can be counted. There is a 1% chance of miscarriage and the long waiting period for the results is distressing to the parents.

Chorionic villus sampling

Chorionic villus sampling (CVS) involves obtaining a small amount of tissue (10–40 mg) from the chorionic villi using a cannula or biopsy forceps. Because placental tissue originates from the zygote its genetic make-up is the same as that of the fetus. CVS can be performed transvaginally until about 13 weeks' gestation and can be carried out as early as 6 weeks, although no earlier than 10 weeks is recommended. It can also be carried out transabdominally. The cells are healthy and rapidly dividing so that results of karyotyping can be obtained quickly.

Most women prefer to have the earlier test but maternal tissue may be mistaken for fetal tissue, leading to incorrect diagnoses and sex determination. At worst a decision to abort a normal child could occur. Also, the spontaneous abortion rate following chorionic villus sampling is higher than that following amniocentesis, depending on the skill of the practitioner.

Fetal blood sampling

A needle is guided to the base of the umbilical cord using ultrasound visualisation and a sample of fetal blood is removed (**cordocentesis**). The blood can be used for screening for blood disorders such as haemophilia and haemoglobinopathies, karyotyping for chromosome analysis, DNA analysis and assessment of anaemia in rhesus isoimmunisation. However, the use of this technique has declined because there are improved molecular and cytogenetic tests that allow more diagnoses to be made from chorionic villi or amniotic fluid. Again there is a risk with a fetal loss rate of around 1% (Sullivan & Kirk 2003).

Maternal serum screening

This is carried out to search for the small amounts of **maternal serum α-fetoprotein** (MSAFP) present.

Normal values of MSAFP are highest in early pregnancy, decreasing as pregnancy advances. Multiple pregnancy, fetal death and open fetal defects such as **spina bifida** or **exomphalos** and **Turner's syndrome** associated with a **cystic hygroma** are associated with raised levels of MSAFP. Low levels are associated with Down syndrome if found with a low level of unconjugated estriol and a high level of human chorionic gonadotrophin. Following the finding of an abnormal MSAFP, the fetus can be examined by ultrasound and/or amniocentesis carried out to check the AFP level.

Fetal cells in the maternal circulation

Fetal blood cells, including nucleated red cells not found in adults, can be detected in maternal blood from 6 weeks with numbers increasing as pregnancy progresses. This has led to research into using those cells as a non-invasive diagnostic tool for detecting fetal chromosomal or genetic abnormality. They can be extracted and studied by **polymerase chain reaction** (PCR) with multiple copies of their DNA being stimulated or by **fluorescence in situ hybridisation** (FISH) to test for some conditions such as trisomies and rhesus blood types (Wachtel et al 2001). There is a possibility that fetal cells from a previous pregnancy may survive making a diagnosis unsafe.

Examples of some disorders

The following common disorders are representative of the major factors in the causation of congenital defects. The disorders to be discussed are:

- Chromosomal disorder: Down syndrome (Fig. 15.2).
- Dominant genetic disorder: Huntington's disease.
- Recessive genetic disorder: cystic fibrosis.
- X-linked genetic disorder: Duchenne muscular dystrophy.
- Genetic predisposition with environmental trigger: neural tube defects (NTDs).

Environmental factors such as pollution and infections such as rubella are discussed in other chapters.

Down syndrome

The natural incidence of Down syndrome or trisomy 21 is about 1 in 800 births but increases with maternal age (Fig. 15.3) where the incidence may be as high as 1 in 40. Many more are conceived and, even without action, three-quarters may be aborted spontaneously. About 95% are caused by **non-disjunction**, but **translocation** 14/21 (Ch. 3) may occur in women of any age and may be inherited.

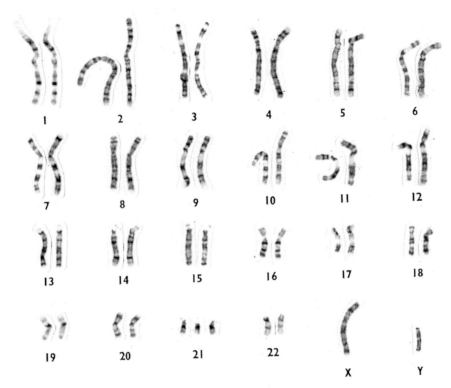

Figure 15.2 • A banded karyotype of Down syndrome (trisomy 21). (From Kelnar C, Harvey D, Simpson C 1995, with permission.)

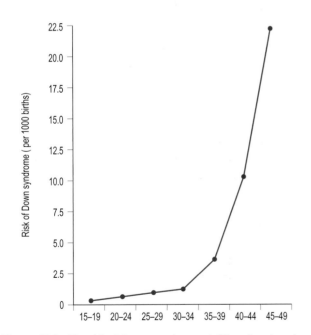

Figure 15.3 • The risk of Down syndrome at different maternal ages. (From Kelnar C, Harvey D, Simpson C 1995, with permission.)

The features of Down syndrome are easily recognised (Fig. 15.4) and include:

- A small head with flattened occiput and a broad flat nose.
- A small mouth cavity with thick gum margins and protruding tongue.
- Epicanthic folds.
- Bruhfield's spots, which are white flecks seen in the iris.
- Short hands with incurving little fingers.
- A single palmar crease.
- A wide deviation of the great toe with a plantar crease between the first and second toes.
- Dry skin.
- Hypotonic muscles.

Other features include heart defects, duodenal atresia, reduced intelligence, inadequate immune system and a tendency to develop leukaemia.

By age 40 many Down syndrome people have developed Alzheimer's disease.

Detection of trisomy 21

There has been controversy about the lack of inter-hospital agreement and availability of the safest and most cost-effective screening tests for Down syndrome. There is also debate on whether testing in the first or second trimester is more effective because many fetuses identified in the first trimester would be spontaneously aborted. It has been general to test for fetal anomalies in the second trimester although first trimester

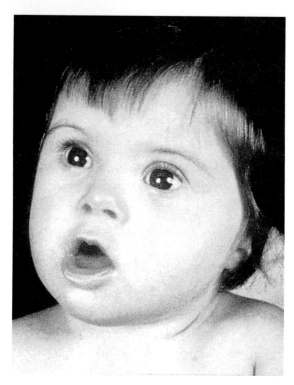

Figure 15.4 • Down syndrome. (From Henderson C, Macdonald S 2004, with kind permission of Elsevier.)

diagnosis is now common because of improvements in ultrasound (Ndumbe et al 2008). A combination of biochemical tests on maternal serum and ultrasound findings linked to maternal age could indicate the presence of an affected fetus (Falcon et al 2006).

The biochemical indicators are:

- Low maternal serum α-fetoprotein (AFP).
- High serum free beta-subunit human chorionic gonadotrophin (β-hCG).
- Low unconjugated estriol (uE3).
- Low serum PAPP-A.

Ultrasonography

The main ultrasound marker is **nuchal translucency** where an increased skin-fold thickness at the back of the neck is a recognised clinical feature. Although increased nuchal translucency is associated with chromosomal defects, it is not a clear indicator of Down syndrome. Other ultrasound markers such as **duodenal atresia** and **cardiac septal defects** may avoid false-positive tests.

Ndumbe et al (2008) suggest that biochemical markers such as serum PAPP-A, β-hCG, AFP and uE3 combined with sonographic measurement of nuchal translucency and the presence or absence of the nasal bone can achieve a detection rate of 97.5% with a false-positive rate of 5% for Down syndrome.

Huntington's disease

Huntington's disease, caused by a dominant gene, occurs in about 1 in 2000 births. The gene was found in 1983 on the terminal band of the short arm of chromosome 4. The gene codes for a protein called **huntingtin** whose role is unknown but may be involved in apoptosis (cell death). Huntington's disease affects the **basal ganglia** and **cerebral cortex**, causing progressive cell death which results in involuntary movement called **chorea**, which begins in the arms and face and eventually affects the whole body. Dementia follows with impaired memory and judgement. It affects all races, the average age of onset is 40 years and the mean duration of the disease is 10–15 years.

Onset of the disease is earlier if the gene is inherited on the paternal chromosome rather than the maternal chromosome; the juvenile cases (before the age of 20) that are seen inevitably inherit the disease from their fathers and have more severe symptoms, but the mode is not understood. The disease tends to commence earlier in succeeding generations (Turnpenny & Ellard 2007). There is no treatment for halting or delaying symptoms and death occurs from cerebral degeneration.

Because the onset is delayed until an affected person has children or even grandchildren genetic presymptomatic testing is offered. This should be as part of a well-planned and carefully monitored counselling package. More women than men appear to take up the offer of testing and the degree of psychological disturbance in those with positive results has been less than expected. Prenatal diagnosis is possible but only 25 or so such tests have been carried out per year in the UK (Turnpenny & Ellard 2007).

Cystic fibrosis

Cystic fibrosis (CF) is a recessive inherited disease of the **exocrine glands** with production of thick mucus that obstructs the gastrointestinal tract and the lungs. Although the disease mainly affects White populations of whom 1 in 2500 newborns are affected in the UK and 1 in 25 people carry the gene, slightly different mutations of the gene occur in Black (1 in 15 000) and Asian populations (1 in 31 000) (Turnpenny & Ellard 2007).

The gene is located in the middle of the long arm of chromosome 7 and codes for a transmembrane regulator protein, the **cystic fibrosis transmembrane regulator** (CFTR). CFTR controls the entry of sodium and chloride ions into cells so that they and their secretions lack water. The resulting thick mucus obstructs and dilates the ducts of the pancreas and the lungs, destroying their structure and function. In the lung secondary bacterial

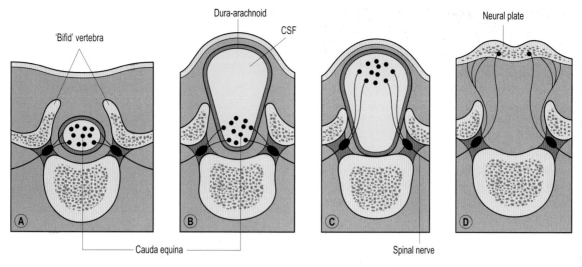

Figure 15.5 • Variants of spina bifida. (A) Spina bifida occulta. (B) Meningocele. (C) Meningomyelocele. (D) Myelocele. (From Hinchliff S M, Montague S E 1990, with permission.)

infection is common with progressive involvement of the bronchial tree, beginning in the alveolar ducts and resulting in large cystic dilations of all bronchi.

Genetic markers allow the prenatal diagnosis of CF and carriers can be detected in over 70% of families with a history of CF. More than 1000 mutations of this gene have been found, not all of which cause severe disease. One that is present in about 95% of cases in the UK is called **DF508**. There is now a national newborn screening test for cystic fibrosis in the UK (NHS 2008).

Modern treatments have increased life expectancy up to 30 years and can be very expensive with the likely need for a heart–lung transplant. As this disease is caused by the absence of a single protein molecule there has been a search for gene replacement therapy. Lee & Southern (2007) compared trials of CFTR delivery by nebuliser with those given a placebo and found no evidence to support the use of these agents as a treatment for cystic fibrosis. They recommended that more studies be carried out.

Duchenne muscular dystrophy

Duchenne muscular dystrophy (DMD) is the most common and most severe type of muscular dystrophy. It occurs only in boys, affecting 1 in 3500 and occurs equally in all nationalities. Sufferers usually die before they have children. It is an X-linked disorder where the abnormal gene is carried on the short arm of the X chromosome. The normal allele codes for a muscle protein called **dystrophin** which is absent in boys with DMD.

DMD can begin as early as age 3 years with slow motor movement and progressive weakness. Muscle bulk diminishes and muscle fibres are replaced by fat

and connective tissue. Muscle weakness begins in the pelvic girdle and the boys develop a waddling gait. There is hypertrophy of the calf muscles in about 80% of cases. Most boys are confined to a wheelchair by age 11. The heart and respiratory muscles finally become affected and death is by respiratory or cardiac failure with survival beyond 25 years being rare (Jorde et al 2006). About 8–10% of female carriers have some degree of muscle weakness.

Fetal diagnosis is possible but not on routine screening. Women with an affected son are offered screening in subsequent pregnancies. This is another disorder that may respond to gene therapy in the future. A similar but much milder condition is called **Becker muscular dystrophy** and is carried by mutations in the same gene and can be diagnosed in the same way. It also may respond to gene therapy (Turnpenny & Ellard 2007).

Neural tube defects (NTDs)

Most major brain defects are the result of defective closure of the anterior neuropore of the neural canal about week 4 from conception. This may result in **anencephaly** with absence of the forebrain and covering skull. Life following birth is not possible although some babies live a few hours or days. Failure of the caudal neuropore at the end of the 4th week results in spinal cord defects such as spina bifida (Fig. 15.5).

Severe NTDs involve the tissues lying over the spinal cord: the meninges, vertebral arch, muscles and skin (Moore & Persaud 2008). **Spina bifida occulta** may have no external signs or clinical symptoms. The defect usually involves vertebra L5 or S1. Severe spina bifida involves protrusion of the spinal cord and meninges through defects in several vertebral arches. These abnormalities occur only 4 weeks after conception and long before most women present for antenatal care. If an NTD is detected counselling concerning the termination of pregnancy is offered.

Terminology

- If the protruding sac contains only meninges and cerebrospinal fluid, it is called **spina bifida cystica**.
- If the spinal cord and nerve roots are included in the sac (75% of fetuses), it is called **spina bifida with meningomyelocele** (Fig. 15.6) Meningomyeloceles may be covered with skin or with a thin, easily ruptured membrane and may be associated with talipes (Fig. 15.7).
- When the spinal cord is only a flattened mass of nervous tissue, the condition is called **myeloschisis**.
- A **meningocele** may be found at the cervical part of the spine. (Fig. 15.8).

It is better to prevent the occurrence of NTDs. There was a suspicion that folic acid deficiency (Hibbard & Smithells 1965) was implicated in the cause of NTDs. Two intervention studies (Laurence et al 1981, Smithells et al 1980), where folate had been given to women who had had a previous pregnancy resulting in a fetus with an NTD, suggested that supplementation might prevent recurrence. This led to a randomised double-blind trial being conducted at 33 centres in seven countries. The results were so clear that the research group recommended that folic acid supplementation be given to all women who were likely to bear children.

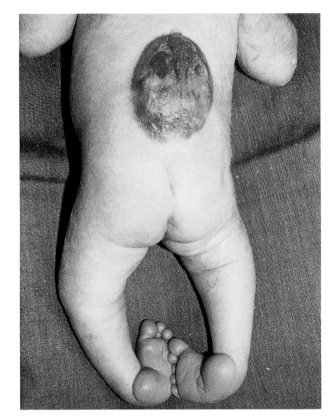

Figure 15.7 • Myelomeningocele with bilateral severe talipes. (From Kelnar C, Harvey D, Simpson C 1995, with permission.)

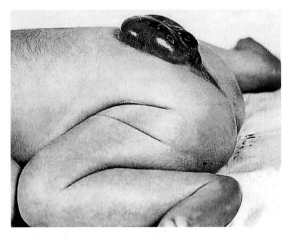

Figure 15.6 • Meningomyelocele. The 'frog leg' posture is characteristic of combined femoral and sciatic nerve paralysis with preservation of hip flexion by the iliopsoas muscle. (From Hinchliff S M, Montague S E 1990, with permission.)

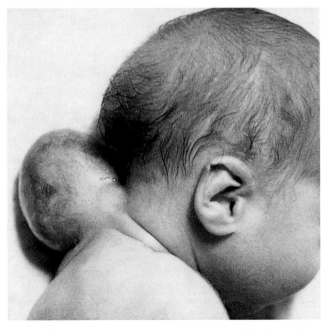

Figure 15.8 • Cervical meningocele. (From Kelnar C, Harvey D, Simpson C 1995, with permission.)

Main points

- Congenital defects account for most severe illness during infancy and childhood and 25% of childhood deaths. During organogenesis the embryo is vulnerable to disruption of development by environmental processes.

- Teratogens lead to genetic mutations. Drugs may damage sperm or ova or may affect embryonic nutrient absorption. Drugs may be teratogenic and interfere with normal development.

- Screening for congenital defects may involve ultrasonography, amniocentesis and chorionic villus sampling. Fetal tissue can be used for karyotyping for chromosomal errors, embryonic sexing if there is a history of X-linked disorders and enzyme assay for detecting inborn errors of metabolism.

- The incidence of Down syndrome (trisomy 21) increases with maternal age and can reach 1 in 40. The risk of a mother carrying a Down syndrome baby is estimated by using a combination of maternal serum biochemical tests and ultrasound findings. Fetal karyotyping is carried out if the fetus is at high risk.

- The onset of Huntington's disease (HD) is earlier if the gene is inherited on the paternal rather than the maternal chromosome and the juvenile cases (before the age of 20) that are seen inevitably inherit the disease from their fathers.

- As the onset of HD is delayed until people have had their own children genetic presymptomatic testing raises ethical and moral issues.

- Cystic fibrosis is much more common in White populations but does occur in other ethnic groups. The gene codes for the cystic fibrosis transmembrane regulator (CFTR) which controls the entry of sodium and chloride into the cell. Neonatal screening is offered.

- Modern treatments have increased life expectancy up to 30 years and can be very expensive with the likely need for a heart–lung transplant. There have been trials of gene replacement therapy by nebuliser but there are no significant findings yet to support the treatment.

- The X-linked disorder Duchenne muscular dystrophy is so severe that sufferers die before they have children. Fetal diagnosis is possible and women who have borne an affected son can be offered screening for subsequent pregnancies.

- A similar but much milder disorder affecting the same gene is Becker muscular dystrophy which can be diagnosed in the same way.

- Most major abnormalities of the brain are the result of defective closure of either the anterior neuropore (anencephaly) or the posterior neuropore (spina bifida) during the 4th week from conception. Research has shown that diet, in particular folic acid deficiency, has been clearly implicated in their cause.

References

Abramsky, L., Chapple, J., 2003. Prenatal Diagnosis: The Human Side, second edn. Nelson Thomas, Cheltenham UK.

Carlson, B.M., 2004. Human Embryology and Developmental Biology, third edn. Elsevier Mosby, Philadelphia.

Falcon, O., Auer, M., Gerovassili, A., Spencer, K., Nicolaides, K.H., 2006. Screening for trisomy 21 by fetal tricuspid regurgitation, nuchal translucency and maternal serum free beta-hCG and PAPP-A at 11 + 0 to 13 + 6 weeks. Ultrasound Obstet. Gynecol. (2), 151–155.

Henderson, C., Macdonald, S. (Eds.), 2004. Mayes' Midwifery: A Textbook for Midwives, thirteenth edn. Baillière Tindall, London.

Hibbard, E.D., Smithells, R.W., 1965. Folic acid metabolism and human embryopathy. Lancet i, 1254.

Jorde, L.B., Carey, J.C., Bamshad, M.J., White, R.L., 2006. Medical Genetics, third edn. Elsevier Mosby, St Louis, Missouri.

Laurence, K.M., James, N., Miller, M.H., et al., 1981. Double-blind randomised controlled trial of folate treatment before conception to prevent recurrence of neural-tube defects. Br. Med. J. 282, 1509–1511.

Lee, T., Southern, K.W., 2007. Topical cystic transmembrane conductance regulator gene replacement for cystic fibrosis-related lung disease. Cochrane Database of Syst. Rev. (2) Art. No. CD005599. OI:10.1002/14651858. CD005599.pub2.

Moore, K.L., Persaud, T.V.N., 2008. The Developing Human: Clinically Oriented Embryology, eighth edn. Elsevier Saunders, Philadelphia.

Ndumbe, F.M., Navti, O., Chilaka, V.N., Konje, J.C., 2008. Prenatal diagnosis in the first trimester of pregnancy. Obstet. Gynecol. Surv. (5), 317–328.

NHS, 2008. Antenatal and Newborn Screening Programme. www.nsc.nhs.uk/.

Smithells, R.W., Shephard, S., Schorah, C.J., et al., 1980. Possible prevention of neural-tube defects by periconceptional vitamin supplementation. Lancet i, 339–340.

Sullivan, A., Kirk, B., 2003. Specialised fetal investigations, Ch. 23. In: Fraser, D.M., Cooper, M.A. (Eds.) Myles Textbook for Midwives, fourteenth edn. Churchill Livingstone, Edinburgh.

Turnpenny, P., Ellard, S., 2007. Emery's Elements of Genetics, thirteenth edn. Elsevier Churchill Livingstone, Edinburgh.

Wachtel, S.S., Shulman, L.P., Sammons, D., 2001. Fetal cells in maternal blood. Clin. Genet. (2), 74–79.

Annotated recommended reading

Lee, T., Southern, K.W., 2007. Topical cystic transmembrane conductance regulator gene replacement for cystic fibrosis-related lung disease. Cochrane Database of Syst. Rev. (2) Art. No. CD005599. OI:10.1002/14651858. CD005599.pub2.

The Cochrane Database offers a wide number of reviews on childbearing subjects. This one is an excellent overview of the new technology of gene replacement for cystic fibrosis.

Moore, K.L., Persaud, T.V.N., 2008. The Developing Human: Clinically Oriented Embryology, eighth ed. Elsevier Saunders, Philadelphia.

This textbook clearly describes embryo development week by week and provides an excellent source for understanding the origin of congenital defects. The illustrations are excellent.

Sullivan, A., Kirk, B., 2003. Specialised Fetal Investigations Ch. 23. In: Fraser, D.M., Cooper, M.A. (Eds.) Myles Textbook for Midwives, fourteenth edition. Churchill Livingstone, Edinburgh.

This is an excellent chapter which explains fetal testing clearly and is especially good on the topic of ultrasonography.

Turnpenny, P., Ellard, S., 2007. Emery's Elements of Genetics, thirteenth edn. Elsevier Churchill Livingstone, Edinburgh.

This book is excellent in its coverage of congenital abnormalities, especially chromosome abnormalities and single gene defects. The suggested implications and treatments are up to date. The diagrams and photographs are excellent.

Section **2B**

Pregnancy—The Mother

SECTION CONTENTS

Pregnant women develop an altered physiology to compensate for the needs of the developing fetus; this section is about those physiological adaptations. In anticipation of students who enter midwifery by the direct route, each system is first described in the nonpregnant state, then the adaptations brought about by pregnancy are discussed; finally their significance to health is discussed. Related systems have been grouped as far as possible. The chapters also provide revision for qualified nurses who enter the midwifery profession. The haematological system (Ch. 16) and the cardiovascular system (Ch. 17) are integral to the support of the growing fetus. Three other systems involved in gas exchange, acid–base control (pH) and fluid balance are the respiratory system (Ch. 18), the renal system (Ch. 19) and fluid balance (Ch. 20). Chapters 21–23 examine the organs of the digestive tract and nutrition, while Chapters 24 and 25 explore the musculoskeletal system. The relationship between the nervous, endocrine and immune systems provides much knowledge about human health. The relatively new science of psychoneuroimmunology is gaining ground. However, to foster understanding, each system is given its own space in Chapters 26–29.

Chapter Sixteen

16

The haematological system— physiology of the blood

CHAPTER CONTENTS

Blood as a tissue

In small-cell organisms, diffusion of substances is sufficient to maintain the metabolic needs of the cell. However, multicellular organisms need more advanced mechanisms other than diffusion to enable the transport of substances. During evolution of multicellular organisms this has been achieved through the cardiovascular system and the circulation of blood.

Blood is a fluid connective tissue, which communicates between internal cells and the body surface, and between the various specialised tissues and organs. In an adult human, blood will normally comprise 6–8% of body weight; this is 5–6 litres in a man and 4–5 litres in a woman.

If a sample of blood is placed in a test-tube and prevented from clotting, the heavier cellular elements settle and the plasma rises to the top. The **haematocrit**, or packed cell volume fraction, essentially represents the percentage of total blood volume occupied by erythrocytes. White cells and platelets form only 1%, settle on top of the red cells and can be seen between the two main layers as a thin cream-coloured layer called the **buffy coat**. The haematocrit averages 45% and the plasma averages 55% of the total volume. Table 16.1 details the specific properties of blood.

Table 16.1 Specific properties of blood

Property	Value
Specific gravity (relative to water)	1.026
Viscosity (relative to water)	1.5–1.75 (cells contribute equally to viscosity)
pH	7.35–7.45
H^+ concentration	35–45 nmol/L

Functions of blood

Blood has three general functions.

1. **Transportation:** Blood transports oxygen from the lungs to the cells and transports carbon dioxide from the cells to the lungs, nutrients from the gastrointestinal tract, hormones from endocrine glands and heat and waste products away from the cells.
2. **Regulation:** Blood is involved in the regulation of acid–base balance, body temperature and water content of cells.
3. **Protection:** Clotting factors in blood protect against excessive loss from the cardiovascular system. White blood cells protect against disease by producing antibodies and performing phagocytosis. In addition, blood also contains interferons and complement proteins that help protect against disease.

Constituents of blood

Blood has a characteristic constituency of living cells suspended in a plasma matrix. It is a sticky, viscous, dark red, opaque fluid consisting of 55% plasma and 45% cells. More than 99% of the cellular component consists of erythrocytes (red blood cells or RBCs). White cells and platelets are present in small quantities. Blood also contains many chemicals in suspension. If blood is exposed to the air it solidifies into a clot and exudes a clear fluid called serum.

Plasma

Plasma is the liquid portion of the blood which acts as the transport medium of substances being carried in the blood. Water comprises approximately 90% of the plasma volume, with the remainder containing protein 8%, inorganic ions 0.9% and organic substances 1.1%. The characteristic straw colour of plasma is produced

Table 16.2 Outline of blood constituents and function

Constituent	Function
Water	Transport medium of nutrients, wastes, gases Heat distributor
Plasma protein—albumin	Transports many substances Large contribution to colloid oncotic pressure
Plasma protein globulins—α and β	Transport substances, involved in clotting
Plasma protein globulins—γ	Antibodies
Plasma protein—fibrinogen	Inactive precursor for fibrin
Electrolytes	Osmotic distribution of fluid between compartments

by bilirubin, the waste product of haemoglobin breakdown. Table 16.2 outlines the constituents and function of plasma.

Serum is blood plasma without fibrinogen and other clotting factors. Protein molecules are too large to pass into the interstitial fluid at the capillary beds; therefore, there is a higher protein content in plasma than in interstitial fluid (i.e. 8% compared with 2%). Most of the protein that does pass into interstitial fluid is taken up by the lymphatic system and returned to the blood. The main plasma proteins are presented in Table 16.3.

The functions of plasma proteins are to:

• Prevent fluid loss from blood to tissues by exerting colloid osmotic (**oncotic**) pressure. This is mainly due to the presence of the protein albumin. If plasma protein levels fall due to either reduced production or loss from the blood vessels then osmotic pressure is also reduced. Fluids will then move into the tissues (oedema) and body cavities. This may occur in diseases of the liver and kidneys, burns, inflammation and allergic disorders.

• Transport bound substances to prevent them from being metabolised until they reach their target tissue: for instance, albumin binds bilirubin. Some substances can displace others and compete for binding sites. An example of this is the displacement of bilirubin from albumin by aspirin or sulphonamides.

• Aid in clotting and fibrinolytic activities.

• Assist in prevention of infection: γ-globulins (also known as immunoglobulins—see Ch. 29) function as specific antibodies for specific protein antigens such as microbial agents and pollen.

Table 16.3 Plasma proteins

Name	Origin	% of total
Albumin	Synthesised in the liver	60
Fibrinogen	Synthesised in the liver	4
Globulins α and β	Synthesised in the liver	36
Globulin γ	Synthesised in the immune system	Trace

Table 16.4 Outline of the cellular constituents of blood

Constituent	Function
Erythrocytes (red cells)	Oxygen and carbon dioxide transport
Leucocytes (white cells)	Defence against micro-organisms
Platelets	Haemostasis

- Help regulate acid–base balance by acting in buffering systems.
- Act as a protein reserve that forms part of the amino acid pool.
- Contribute about 50% to the total viscosity of blood.

Other proteins found in the blood in small quantities are hormones, enzymes and most of the clotting factors. There is also a series of plasma proteins called **complement** that assist in the inflammatory and immune mechanisms. Albumin is the smallest of the plasma proteins with a molecular mass of 69000 and is just too large to pass through the capillary walls in normal circumstances. If the glomerular capillaries in the kidney are damaged, albumin can be lost from the blood in large quantities.

The cellular components of blood

Three major cell types are present in blood, each having a very different function: red cells (**erythrocytes**), white cells (**leucocytes**) and platelets (**thrombocytes**) (Table 16.4).

Under normal circumstances, the proportions of these cells remain constant within narrow limits. However, the body may adjust these levels to maintain health. A simple routine test can measure the cellular content of blood. This is normally carried out on most people at some point in their life, either as part of health screening or to diagnose illness.

Haemopoiesis is the term used for blood cell formation. Embryonic blood cells appear in the bloodstream as early as the 3rd week of development. All blood cell types are descended from a single type of bone marrow cell called a pluripotent stem cell or **haemocytoblast**, which is an undifferentiated cell capable of giving rise to the precursor of any of the blood cell types. These include the red cells and megakaryocytes (leading to platelets). The pluripotent stem cells branch to form myeloid stem cells, which leads to the production of granulocytes and monocytes in the bone marrow. Lymphoid stem cells leave the bone marrow to reside in the lymphoid tissues and produce lymphocytes. Each person has about 1500g of red bone marrow in the body. Two-thirds of the production is white cells and one-third is red cells (Fig. 16.1).

Red blood cells

The major function of erythrocytes or red blood cells (RBCs) is the carriage of oxygen, picked up in the lungs, to all the cells of the body. Erythrocytes contain large amounts of the protein haemoglobin with which oxygen and, to a lesser extent, carbon dioxide reversibly combine. The shape and size of the red cells are significant for this function. Erythrocyctes are biconcave discs (circular and flattened, thinner in the middle than round the edge) and are 7.5 micrometres (μm) in diameter. This provides a high surface-to-volume ratio well suited to the exchange of gases, and allows the volume of the cell to readily alter with the osmotic shifts of water between cell and plasma. The plasma membrane is strong and conveniently pliant, which allows the cells to become deformed as they squeeze through torturous and narrow capillary vessels whose diameter may be smaller than the RBC.

Erythrocytes are normally measured per cubic mm (mm^3, which is the same as $1\,\mu$l of blood) and average 5 million. This value may also be reported as 5.0×10^{12}/L. Women have a range of 4.3–$5.2/mm^3$ and men have a higher range of 5.1–$5.8/mm^3$ (Table 16.5). RBCs are the main cellular contributor to blood viscosity. Therefore any increase in this range will also raise the viscosity of blood, which may occur in circumstances such as a slower flow of blood or a move to an area of high altitude. Any subsequent decrease, such as is seen in normal pregnancy, will lower viscosity and blood will flow more rapidly.

Erythrocytes are completely dedicated to the transport of oxygen and carbon dioxide. Haemoglobin (Hb) is the oxygen-carrying capacity of the erythrocytes and is measured in grams per 100ml of blood (g/100ml or g/dl). The normal range of values is 14–20 g/dl in infants, 12–16 g/dl in females and 13–18 g/dl in males. Haemoglobin also picks up about 20% of carbon dioxide (CO_2) returning from the tissues to form carbaminohaemoglobin, but most of the CO_2 is in solution in the blood.

211

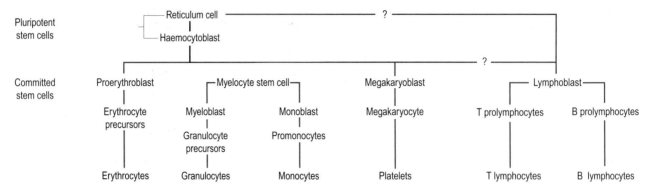

Figure 16.1 • Summary of the major stages of haemopoiesis. (From Hinchliff S M, Montague S E 1990, with permission.)

Table 16.5 Red cell laboratory values	
Parameter	**Value**
Red cell count	$5.1–5.8 \times 10^{12}$/L (males) $4.3–5.2 \times 10^{12}$/L (females)
Haemoglobin	13–18 g/dl (males) 12–16 g/dl (females) 14–20 g/dl (infants)
Mean cell haemoglobin concentration (MCHC)	32 g/dl
Mean cell volume (MCV)	85 femtolitres (1 fl = 1000 million millionths of a litre)

Figure 16.2 • The structure of haemoglobin. Haemoglobin is a protein with four subunits (two α polypeptides and two β polypeptides). Each subunit contains a haem group with an iron atom. (From Jones et al, with permission.)

Haemoglobin

Haemoglobin is a red-coloured pigment found in red cells. Each red cell contains 30 pg (picograms) of haemoglobin. This is reported as the mean cell haemoglobin or MCH. Another measure reported is the mean cell concentration of haemoglobin (MCHC), which is 32 g/dl. Haemoglobin is made up of the protein **globin** bound to the red **haem** pigment. Globin is rather complex. It consists of four polypeptide chains—two alpha (α) and two beta (β)—each bound to a ring-like haem group (Fig. 16.2). Each haem contains one iron ion (Fe^{2+}) that can combine reversibly with one oxygen molecule to form the bright red **oxyhaemoglobin** (HbO_2). The iron–oxygen interaction is very weak and the two can be easily separated without any damage. Once the oxygen has been released in the tissues, it becomes darker red and is known as **deoxyhaemoglobin**.

Each haemoglobin molecule can carry four molecules of oxygen. These are picked up one at a time and each binding changes the configuration of globin and increases the affinity of the haemoglobin molecule for oxygen. The affinity for the fourth molecule of oxygen is 20 times that of the first affinity. This aspect of oxygen uptake will be examined in greater detail when respiration is considered.

The pigment haem is made up of ring-shaped organic molecules called **pyrrole rings**. Four of these join together to form a larger ring and the nitrogen atom of each pyrrole ring holds a ferrous iron atom centrally. The globin proteins consist of long chains of amino acids. There are four types of globin chain, each with slight differences in amino acids: α (alpha), β (beta), δ (delta) and γ (gamma). They can be varied in pairs to form different types of haemoglobin, three of which are found normally:

- HbA, the major adult haemoglobin: 2α2β
- HbA_2, the minor adult haemoglobin: 2α2β
- HbF, fetal haemoglobin: 2α2γ.

At birth HbF makes up two-thirds of haemoglobin content and HbA one-third. From the age of 5 years the adult ratio is established, i.e. HbA is greater than 95%, HbA$_2$ is less than 3.5% and HbF is less than 1.5%. Other fetal haemoglobins have substitutions for the β chains which can persist and may be life-saving in thalassaemia. Abnormal β chains are made in sickle-cell disorders.

Formation of erythrocytes

Mature red blood cells develop from haemocytoblasts within the erythroid tissue in the bone marrow. After 3–5 days the cells pass into the circulation as cells called **reticulocytes** because they still contain rough endoplasmic reticulum and clumped ribosomes. These structures disappear when the cell is mature, which normally takes 4 days. Three or four mitotic cell divisions are involved so that each haemocytoblast gives rise to 8 or 16 red cells. There is a gradual build-up of haemoglobin made at the ribosomes which appears in the cell. Other organelles and the nucleus are extruded from the cell. There is a reduction in cell size and a change in cell shape. Reticulocytes normally comprise less than 2% of the red cells in the blood of an adult. The formation of erythrocytes is called **erythropoiesis** and the dietary substances required are summarised in Table 16.6.

The life span of red cells

About 1% of erythrocytes are replaced each day. Production is stimulated by the hormone **erythropoietin**, which originates in the kidney. This is a glycoprotein produced when the kidney cells are hypoxic: for example, during haemorrhage, haemolytic crises, at altitude and following exercise. Erythropoietin can only stimulate committed cells and there will be an increase in reticulocytes in the blood if the need is drastic. Red blood cells live for about 120 days and are finally ingested and destroyed by macrophages, mainly in the spleen. As the cells circulate, their plasma membrane becomes progressively more damaged until it ruptures. Having no nucleus, they have no mechanism of self-repair. They are fragmented to produce protein and haem, which is mostly reclaimed in the body stores for reuse. The remainder of the haem portion is degraded and bilirubin is excreted as bile (Fig. 16.3).

Very defective cells such as those found in sickle-cell disease may be haemolysed in the circulation. The haemoglobin, which has a molecular mass of 68 000 and is small enough to be excreted in the urine, is released into the plasma. Special plasma proteins called **haptoglobins** bind to free haemoglobin to form larger molecules and prevent it from being excreted. If this mechanism becomes saturated, haemoglobin will appear in the urine (**haemoglobinuria**).

Table 16.6 Dietary substances needed for erythropoiesis

Substance	Utilisation
Protein	Synthesis of the globin part of haemoglobin and for cellular proteins
Iron	Contained in the haem portion of haemoglobin
Vitamin B$_{12}$ (hydroxycobalamin)	Needed for DNA synthesis
Folic acid	Needed for DNA synthesis
Vitamin C (ascorbic acid)	Facilitates absorption of iron

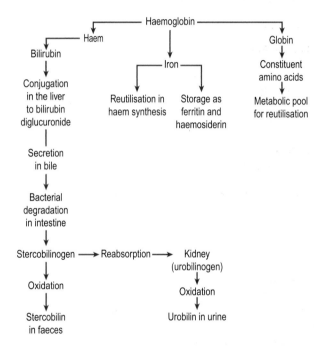

Figure 16.3 • A summary of haemoglobin breakdown. (From Hinchcliff S M, Montague S E 1990, with permission.)

Iron metabolism

Absorption

A typical British mixed diet usually contains about 14 mg of iron daily but normally only 1–2 mg (5–10%) is absorbed. The composition of the diet determines how much iron is available for absorption (Robinson 2002). There are two distinct forms for absorption: iron attached to haem and inorganic iron. Iron attached to haem is found in the haemoglobin and myoglobin protein found in animal products. It is absorbed much more efficiently than non-haem iron and is not affected by factors affecting the absorption of non-haem iron. In most foods, iron is present in its ferric form and has to be converted to ferrous iron in order to be absorbed.

Absorption is enhanced if reducing agents that can aid this conversion are available. Hydrochloric acid found in the gastric juice performs this function, as can ascorbic acid (vitamin C). In grain foods iron forms a complex with phytates and only small amounts of soluble iron are available. The iron in eggs is bound to phosphates in the yolk and is poorly absorbed. The amount of iron absorbed depends on the rate of red cell production, the extent of iron stores, the content of the diet and whether or not iron supplements are given. Intestinal absorption of iron is facilitated when there is erythroid hyperplasia, rapid turnover of iron and a high concentration of unsaturated transferrin, as occurs in pregnancy.

Serum iron, transferrin and total iron-binding capacity

Non-pregnant women have a serum iron content of 13–27 μmol/L but this shows immense individual variability and fluctuates hour to hour. The process for the changes is not fully understood. A low concentration of serum iron usually indicates iron-deficiency anaemia. The **total iron-binding capacity** (TIBC) is 45–72 μmol/L. A low concentration of TIBC is associated with iron-deficiency anaemia. **Transferrin** is the protein that specifically binds iron and is usually between 1.2 and 2 g/L. TIBC is usually one-third saturated with iron. Transferrin rises to 4.7 g/L by the second trimester and TIBC increases to 90 μmol/L. This is also seen in women taking oestrogen-containing oral contraceptives. Oestrogen probably causes the change. TIBC returns to normal within 3 weeks of delivery.

Serum ferritin

Ferritin is a glycoprotein with a high molecular mass and is found in cells where it holds two-thirds of the iron store. It is also present in small amounts in the plasma in a wide range of 15–300 μg/L. It is stable, not affected by iron ingestion and is a good indicator of iron stores, especially in the lower range as in iron-deficiency anaemia in pregnancy.

Marrow iron

Occasionally it is useful to examine bone marrow to assess iron stores. Marrow is taken by aspiration from the iliac crest. A stainable iron–protein complex called **haemosiderin**, which is similar to ferritin, may be seen. No stainable iron will be seen if the serum ferritin has fallen below 40 μg/L. In the absence of iron supplementation, no stainable iron is seen in 80% of women at term. The developing erythrocytes can also be examined for signs of iron deficiency. The presence of infection, especially urinary tract infection, can block the incorporation of iron into haemoglobin as the microbes may utilise iron in their own metabolic processes.

Folate metabolism

Folate is a vitamin found widely distributed in nature. It is found in leafy green vegetables such as spinach and in mushrooms and oranges. Liver is a good source. Folic acid is destroyed by prolonged boiling or by the addition of bicarbonate of soda to the cooking water. Some drugs act as folic acid antagonists and prevent its absorption. A typical Western diet contains 500–800 μg daily and normal daily needs are 100–200 μg. This excess intake partly compensates for the loss in cooking.

Folates are absorbed in the duodenum and jejunum and then stored in the liver. Deficiency is more likely to be seen in the winter months when the foods containing folic acid may be difficult to obtain. It is more common in certain socially and economically deprived groups. It was identified and synthesised in the 1940s. The metabolism of folic acid is the basis for cellular use of folate and it is essential for cell growth and division. Tissue that is active in reproduction and growth is more dependent on the efficient turnover and supply of folate coenzymes and during pregnancy folate metabolism is increased.

Blood groups

Red blood cells, like all cells, have **glycoproteins** in their plasma membranes which are genetically coded for and therefore inherited. These can act as **antigens** (see Ch. 29), provoking an immune reaction if incompatible blood enters the circulation. The red cells are agglutinated and destroyed. There are over 400 different antigens found on the surface of red cells. Some of these antigens cause a more vigorous reaction than others and the two most commonly problematic are those of the ABO system and the rhesus (Rh) system.

The ABO system

The ABO blood groups are based on the presence of two red cell antigens (known as **agglutinogens**) called type A and type B. These types are co-dominant (i.e. neither gene masks the presence of the other so that both proteins are expressed). A person inheriting both antigens will have blood group AB. If neither antigen is inherited, then blood group O arises. Therefore four blood groups are possible depending on the surface antigens present on the red cells: i.e. A, B, AB and O.

A unique factor associated with the ABO system is the presence of preformed antibodies (known as **agglutinins**) in the plasma within 2 months of birth with no previous sensitisation event. A baby cannot have antibodies against any antigen carried on its own red cells or the cells would be destroyed. Therefore a baby who has neither the A nor the B antigen on its red cells will have both anti-A and anti-B antibodies in the serum, while a baby with the blood group AB will have neither antibody present in the serum. Those with blood group A will have anti-B antibodies and those with blood group B will have anti-A antibodies.

The rhesus (Rh) system

There are eight types of Rh antigens but only three are common. These are called the C, D and E agglutinogens. A gene codes for each type and there are two alleles to each gene, giving CDE/cde as the full range of alleles. Rhesus D is by far the most clinically important antigen. The word rhesus is used because agglutinogen D was originally identified in rhesus monkeys.

About 85% of people in the Western world are rhesus positive (Rh+), which means they have the Rh agglutinogen on their red cells, and 15% are rhesus negative (Rh−) and do not have the agglutinogen on their red cells. In Japan 99.7% of people are Rh+ and only 0.3% are Rh −. Unlike the ABO system, there are no spontaneously occurring anti-Rh antibodies and these are only formed if there is a sensitisation event with the presence of Rh+ red blood cells in the circulation of a Rh− person. There is a problem associated with the rhesus factor in pregnancy; this is discussed in Chapter 14.

White cells

These cells are the **leucocytes** and can be referred to as WBCs. Taking all the types together, the average number of WBCs in the circulation is 4000–11 000 per cubic mm which can also be reported as 4–11×10^9/L. They account for only 1% of the cellular content of the blood. An increase in WBCs is called **leucocytosis** and a decrease is **leucopenia**. The white cells present in the blood represent only a small part of the body's total white cell content as the majority of the cells are in the tissues.

The reason for the wide variation in the normal count is that cells enter and leave the circulation constantly in response to physiological factors such as exercise. The newborn baby has approximately double the white cell count of an adult, which decreases to reach adult levels by about 5–10 years of age. These cells are part of the immune defence system (see Ch. 29) and are protective against bacteria, viruses, parasites, toxins and tumour cells. Some white cells undergo **diapedesis**, which means that the cells can slip out of capillaries with an amoebic action in response to positive **chemotaxis** (chemical call).

Types of white cell

Granulocytes (polymorphonuclear leucocytes) contain granules that have a lobed nucleus and substances that can fight infection in their cytoplasm. They are 10–14 micrometres (μm) in diameter. Granulocytes can be further divided into three groups, categorised by the size of their granules and the way they take up Wright's stain. All these granulocytes are phagocytic.

1. **Neutrophils** contain granules of varying sizes that stain violet because they take up both acidic red dyes and basic blue dyes. Neutrophils have the most lobular nuclei and are the most common types of granulocytes, accounting for more than 50% of all white cells. Neutrophils are chemically attracted to sites of inflammation and will ingest and destroy bacteria and some fungi.

2. **Eosinophils** have large granules which are stained red by acidic dyes. The nucleus usually has two lobes. Eosinophils make up about 1–4% of the white cell population. The most important role of this type of cell is to attack parasitic worms such as tapeworms and round worms. When such a worm enters the body the eosinophils surround it and release enzymes from their granules onto the parasite's surface to digest it from the outside. Eosinophils are also involved in dealing with allergy attacks by destroying antigen–antibody complexes.

3. **Basophils** have large granules that take up a basic dye and stain blue-black. The nucleus usually has two or three lobes. These are the rarest of the white cells, accounting for only 0.5% of the population. Their large granules contain histamine, which is an inflammatory substance that acts as a vasodilator and draws other white blood cells to the site of inflammation. Cells similar to basophils that are present in connective tissue are called **mast cells**. Both types of cells release histamine when they bind to immunoglobulin E (IgE). The immune system is discussed in full in Chapter 29.

The production of granulocytes

Granulocytes arise from myeloid precursor cells in the red bone marrow, a process that takes about 14 days. This time can be reduced considerably if cells are urgently required, such as when infection is present. There is also a pool of granulocyte cells in the bone marrow where there can be 50 cells for every granulocyte in the circulation. During **granulopoiesis**, there is progressive condensation and lobulation of the nucleus. Granules develop in the cell cytoplasm and there is loss of organelles such as mitochondria.

Within 7 h of reaching the circulation, half of the granulocytes will have left to meet tissue needs and will not return to the blood. The normal survival of these cells in the tissues is about 4–5 days. Dead cells are eliminated from the body in faeces and respiratory secretions. Dead neutrophils form the pus at infection sites.

Agranulocytes

These include lymphocytes and monocytes and do not contain visible cytoplasmic granules.

Lymphocytes

Lymphocytes are produced in the bone marrow and immature cells migrate to the thymus and other lymphoid tissue to divide again and mature. These are round cells with large round nuclei and are the second most common type of leucocyte. Even though a large numbers of lymphocytes exist in the body, only a small number are found in the circulation. The majority of lymphocytes are often present in lymphoid tissue and are involved in immune reactions.

Monocytes

Monocytes are large cells that are produced in the bone marrow. Mature cells spend about 30 h in the blood and then migrate to the tissues where they develop into macrophages. Macrophages are also phagocytic although they respond more slowly than the neutrophils. They are also greatly involved in regulating the immune response by activating B and T lymphocytes (see Ch. 29).

Platelets

Platelets are small non-nuclear cellular elements produced in the bone marrow. They are colourless discoid bodies and have a diameter of only 2–4 μm. There are about $150–400 \times 10^9$/L.

Production of platelets (**thrombopoiesis**) occurs in the bone marrow. They are formed inside the cytoplasm of large cells called megakaryocytes and bud off from the cell surface (Fig. 16.4). Each megakaryocyte takes about 10 days to mature and produces about 4000 platelets. At any time two-thirds of the body's platelets are in the circulation and one-third in the spleen. The life span of a

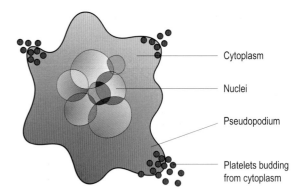

Figure 16.4 • Diagram of megakaryocyte showing platelet budding. (From Hinchcliff S M, Montague S E 1990, with permission.)

platelet is 7–10 days and they are destroyed by macrophages, mainly in the spleen but also in the liver.

Platelets are complex and have many functions other than being involved in the clotting process of blood. They are able to phagocytose small particles such as viruses and immune complexes. They store and transport **histamine** and **serotonin** which are released when platelets are damaged. This affects the tone of smooth muscle in blood vessel walls. Platelets probably supply the endothelial cells of the blood vessels with nutrition and these cells atrophy in platelet deficiency. They secrete **platelet-derived growth factor** (PDGF) which stimulates proliferation of smooth muscle walls to help healing after injury.

Haemostasis

If the endothelium of blood vessels is smooth and uninterrupted, blood flow is maintained. However, if a blood vessel is damaged a series of reactions occurs in order to maintain haemostasis and minimise blood loss. The mechanism is fast, localised and carefully controlled. Many blood coagulation factors normally present in plasma are involved. Some substances involved in the blood clotting process are released from platelets and injured tissues. Haemostasis involves three phases: vascular spasm, platelet plug formation and coagulation of blood (Fig. 16.5). This is followed (30–60 min) by dot retraction and the removed of unnecessary dots by fibrinolysis.

Vascular spasm

Vasoconstriction after injury is brought about by direct injury to vascular smooth muscle, compression of the vessel by extravasated blood, chemicals released by endothelial cells and platelets and reflexes triggered by pain receptors. A strongly constricted artery can significantly reduce blood loss for up to 30 min. This allows

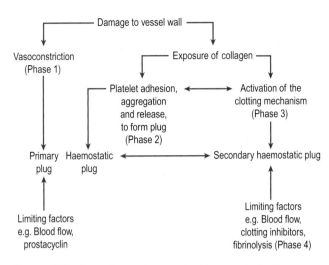

Figure 16.5 • An outline of the events of haemostasis. (From Hinchcliff S M, Montague S E 1990, with permission.)

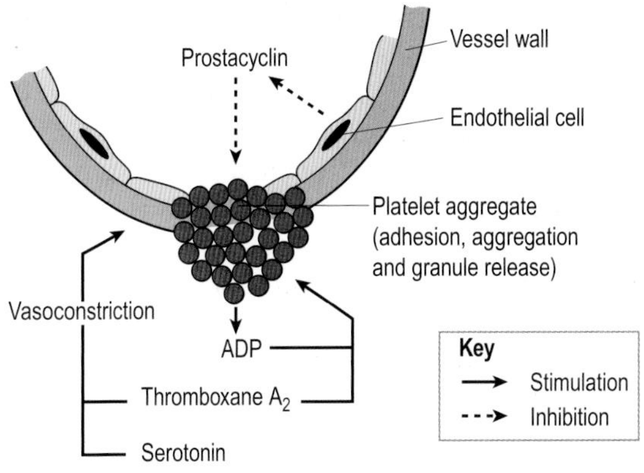

Figure 16.6 • Summary of events in the formation of a platelet plug. (From Hinchcliff S M, Montague S E 1990, with permission.)

time for platelet plug formation and blood clotting to occur. A blunt injury crushes tissue and is more efficient at causing vascular spasm than a sharp cut.

Formation of a platelet plug

Normally platelets do not stick to each other or to the endothelial lining of blood vessels. Damage or disruption of the endothelium exposes underlying collagen fibres. This causes platelets to swell, form spiky processes and stick to the exposed area. Once the platelets have adhered to the endothelium, lipids in the platelet plasma membrane release a short-lived prostaglandin derivative called thromboxane A_2. Degranulation of platelets occurs and other chemicals are released. These are serotonin, which enhances vascular spasm, and adenosine diphosphate, which attracts more platelets. Within 1 min a platelet plug forms (Fig. 16.6). Prostacyclin (PGI_2) limits the process by confining platelet aggregation to the immediate area of damage.

Coagulation

There are three critical events in coagulation of blood:

1. Prothrombin activator is formed.
2. This converts the plasma protein prothrombin to thrombin.
3. Thrombin causes fibrinogen molecules to form a fibrin mesh. This traps blood cells and seals the hole in the blood vessel.

Over 30 different substances affect the process. There are factors that enhance clot formation, called **procoagulants** (see Table 16.7); those that inhibit

Table 16.7 Procoagulant factors

Factor	Name	Function
I	Fibrinogen	Converted to fibrin mesh
II	Prothrombin	Converted to thrombin which converts fibrinogen to fibrin
III	Thromboplastin	Catalyses thrombin formation
IV	Calcium ions	Needed at all stages
V	Platelet accelerator	Affects both intrinsic and extrinsic methods
VI	No substance	
VII	Serum prothrombin conversion accelerator (SPCA)	Extrinsic pathway conversion
VIII	Antihaemophilic factor	Intrinsic mechanism (absence = haemophilia A)
IX	Plasma thromboplastin component (PTC, Christmas factor)	Intrinsic mechanism (absence = haemophilia B)
X	Stuart-Power factor	Both extrinsic and intrinsic pathways
XI	Plasma thromboplastin antecedent (PTA)	Intrinsic mechanism (absence = haemophilia C)
XII	Hageman factor	Intrinsic mechanism
XIII	Fibrin stabilising factor (FSF)	Cross links fibrin to make it insoluble

clot formation are called **anticoagulants**. Most of the clotting factors or procoagulants are plasma proteins synthesised in the liver, except factors III and IV. Many need the presence of vitamin K: factors II, VII, IX and X. The factors are released into the blood where they remain inert until the clotting cascade is triggered.

Clotting may be initiated by either of two pathways. These are the intrinsic and extrinsic pathways; in the body both pathways are usually triggered by the same tissue-damaging events. The intrinsic pathway only initiates clotting of blood outside the body, whereas the extrinsic pathway initiates clotting of blood that has escaped into the tissues. Clot formation is normally complete within 3–6 min. The extrinsic pathway involves fewer steps and is more rapid than the intrinsic pathway. In severe trauma the extrinsic mechanism can clot blood within 15 s.

Clot retraction and fibrinolysis

After 30–60 min a platelet-induced process called **clot retraction** occurs. A contractile protein, **actomyosin**, works in the same way as it does in muscle cells. Serum is squeezed out, the clot is compacted and the torn edges of the blood vessel are drawn together. This is the beginning of healing. PGDF released by degranulation of the platelets stimulates smooth muscle and fibroblasts to divide and rebuild the muscle wall.

Unnecessary clots are removed by **fibrinolysis**. If this did not occur the blood vessels would become occluded. Yet another of the plasma proteins, **plasminogen**, is activated to produce plasmin which is a protein-digesting enzyme. Large amounts of plasminogen may be incorporated into a big clot but remain inactive, producing plasmin only as necessary. Plasminogen activators are released from endothelial cells when clot is present. Factor VII and thrombin are also potent plasminogen activators.

Factors limiting clot growth or formation

* Rapid removal of coagulation factors.
* Inhibitors of activated clotting factors.

Any tendency to clot in rapidly moving blood is usually unsuccessful because any activated clotting factors are diluted and washed away. **Heparin** is a natural anticoagulant normally contained in the granules of the leucocytes—mast cells and basophils. Endothelial cells also produce heparin. Small amounts released into the plasma normally prevent inappropriate blood coagulation.

Maternal haematological adaptations to pregnancy

Blood volume and composition

Total blood volume is a combination of plasma volume and red cell volume. The average increase in total blood volume during pregnancy is between 30% and 50% with an increase above 50% in multiple pregnancies. Plasma volume and total red cell mass are under separate control and bear no fixed relation to one another (Gordon 2007). The increase in blood volume relates to an increase in cardiac output and is noted as early as the 6th week of pregnancy. Most increase takes place before 32–34 weeks and thereafter there is relatively little change. The increase in blood volume may be due to a hormonal mechanism. Plasma volume increases by about 50% while red cell mass increases by 18%. This difference results in hypervolaemia, haemodilution and a fall in Hb level often referred to as **physiological anaemia** (Figs 16.7–16.9).

Plasma volume

The aetiology of plasma expansion is poorly understood but is thought to be related to the effects of nitric

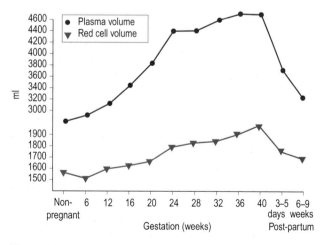

Figure 16.7 • Mean total plasma and red cell volume during normal pregnancy. (Reproduced with permission from Lund & Donovan 1967.)

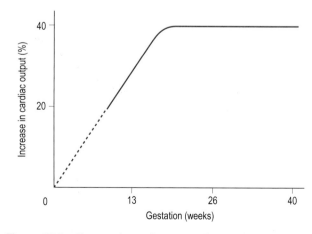

Figure 16.8 • Changes in cardiac output throughout pregnancy. (Reproduced with permission from Hytten & Chamberlain 1991.)

oxide-mediated vasodilation on the renin–angiotensin–aldosterone system and subsequent sodium and water retention (Blackburn 2007). The increase in plasma volume is positively correlated with the birth weight of the baby. Women with multiple pregnancy have an increase greater than women with a singleton pregnancy and the amount increases with the number of fetuses in the uterus. Multigravid women have a further increase of plasma volume, which is mirrored by the greater weight of their babies.

The benefits of the hypervolaemia are to fulfil the extra demands on the circulation in pregnancy. For instance, the basal metabolic rate increases by 20% in pregnancy with the production of more heat. Blood flow to the skin is increased and this allows heat to be lost. The increased blood volume also helps to maintain blood pressure when blood may be sequestered in the lower part of the body in the third trimester. This helps to safeguard the woman against haemorrhage at delivery. The decrease in viscosity with increase in cardiac force leads to a decreased resistance to blood flow, which is essential for placental perfusion.

Red cells

In previous research the increase in red cell content of the blood in a normal pregnancy has been difficult to ascertain because many of the women had been given iron supplements. The range of change in RBC volume

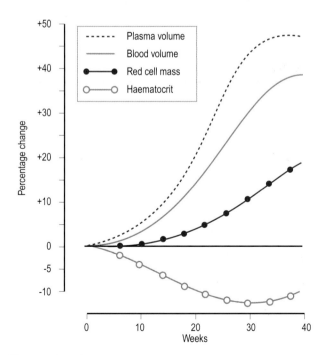

Figure 16.9 • Changes in plasma volume, blood volume, red cell mass and haematocrit during normal pregnancy. (Reproduced with permission from Rosso 1990.)

varies from a moderate rise (30–35%) above non-pregnant values and is influenced by the woman's iron stores (Blackburn 2007). The red cell mass should increase as oxygen needs of the body increase. Therefore an increase in red cell mass of 18% should be adequate to meet the 15% increase in oxygen requirements in pregnancy. The nature of the increase in red cell production is not fully understood but there is a three-fold increase in erythropoietin in plasma in the second trimester. This increase is thought to be related to progesterone, prolactin and human placental lactogen (hPL), rather than by hypoxaemia (Blackburn 2007). There is also a slight rise in the production of HbF, which reaches a peak at 20 weeks and returns to normal 8 weeks after delivery.

Changes in red cell values in pregnancy

- The red cell count increase is less than the plasma increase, resulting in a reduction in red cell count from the normal $4.2–4.5 \times 10^{12}$/L in early pregnancy to $3.6–3.8 \times 10^{12}$/L by term.
- The haemoglobin level falls about 2 g/dl from a normal level of 13 g/dl to about 11 g/dl. The haematocrit falls in parallel with the fall in red cell count.
- Mean cell haemoglobin concentration (MCHC)—the average concentration of haemoglobin in each red cell—changes little in a normal pregnancy. There is a slight progressive fall in some women who are not given iron therapy.
- Mean cell volume (MCV) is a more sensitive haematological measure of iron status in pregnancy. In normal pregnancy with sufficient iron present there is an increase in red cell size. In pregnancy complicated by iron deficiency an early sign is a reduction of cell size.

Iron requirements during pregnancy

In order to meet the expansion in red cell mass and the needs of the fetus and placenta, extra iron is needed in pregnancy. The total requirements are calculated as between 700 and 1400 mg throughout pregnancy. Table 16.8 presents an overview of the distribution of iron requirements in pregnancy. Overall, the requirement is for 4 mg/day but this rises from 2.8 mg/day in the non-pregnant woman to 6.6 mg/day in the last few weeks of pregnancy. The needs can be met only by mobilising iron stores in addition to achieving maximum absorption from dietary iron.

Set against this need is the iron saved during pregnancy and breastfeeding because of amenorrhoea, which is 250–480 mg in total. Box 16.1 provides an overview of the issues surrounding iron supplementation in pregnancy.

Table 16.8 The distribution of the extra iron in pregnancy

Tissue usage	Requirements (mg)
Expansion of the red cell mass	570
Fetus	270–370
Placenta	35–100
Blood loss at delivery	100–250
Breastfeeding (6 months)	100–180
Loss from skin, faeces, urine	270

Folate metabolism in pregnancy

Folates together with iron have a central role in the nutrition of pregnancy. Requirements for folates are increased in pregnancy to meet the needs of the growing fetus and placenta, and for the increased maternal tissues of the growing uterus and red cell mass. The placenta transports folates actively to the fetus even if maternal folate status is deficient. Maternal folate metabolism is altered early in pregnancy before fetal demands act directly.

White cells

The total white cell count rises in pregnancy and is due to an increase in neutrophils with an elevation in mature leucocyte forms (Blackburn 2007). The neutrophil count rises in the menstrual cycle at the time of the oestrogen peak and continues to rise if fertilisation of the ovum occurs. A peak is reached at 30 weeks and then a plateau is maintained until delivery. There is a further rise in labour and the count returns to normal by the 6th postnatal day. Circulating oestrogen is probably the cause of the extra neutrophil production.

There is a slight rise in eosinophils in ratio to the increased white cell count. A sharp fall in circulating eosinophils occurs during labour. These are absent at delivery

BOX 16.1 IRON SUPPLEMENTATION IN PREGNANCY

Iron deficiency, the most common cause of anaemia in pregnancy worldwide, can be mild, moderate or severe. Severe anaemia can have very serious consequences for mothers and babies, but there is controversy about whether treating mild or moderate anaemia provides more benefit than harm (Reveiz et al 2007). It has been suggested that routine intake of iron supplements with and without folic acid during pregnancy improves maternal health and pregnancy outcomes (Péna-Rosas & Viteri 2006). Those who favour supplementation recommend prophylactic iron supplements to all women from as early as 16 weeks of pregnancy onwards while others prefer supplementation only if there is an established iron deficit.

In evolutionary terms, women are adapted to the needs for iron in pregnancy but humans have changed their diet since the beginning of the agricultural revolution about 10 000 years ago. Previously people ate a high-protein diet based on fishing and hunting but changed to a mixed diet with grains and a much lower intake of fish and meat. Women at high risk of iron deficiency due to dietary factors are adolescents consuming a low-calorie diet, vegetarians and vegans. In modern times, Western women now have fewer pregnancies that are often spaced out over time. This should prevent the continuous depletion of iron from the stores made by repeated pregnancies.

Iron requirements in pregnancy are significantly higher than in the non-pregnant state (Bothwell 2000). Although iron requirements are reduced in the first trimester due to the absence of menstruation, they rise steadily thereafter. The amount of iron that can be absorbed from an optimal diet is less than the demands of pregnancy. Unicef/WHO (1999) report that approximately 50% of women already enter pregnancy with insufficient iron stores to supply the increased maternal and fetal needs. In developing countries this may be due to dietary deficiency but also to chronic infection such as malaria. Iron supplementation during pregnancy will improve health status in these populations and may even be life-saving.

Prevention and treatment of iron-deficiency anaemia is essential. Women are more at risk in the third trimester when the fetus obtains iron from maternal stores by active transport across the placenta. Resulting iron deficiency may have an adverse effect on exercise tolerance, cerebral function and fetal and neonatal development. Many advocates of iron supplementation recommend that it would be safer, more practical and less expensive to give all women iron supplements from early pregnancy because of the potential health risks and treatment.

Numerous reviews of the literature have been carried out on this important issue. Enkin et al (2000)

BOX 16.1 (CONTINUED)

conclude that most pregnant women in developing countries show haematological changes indicating iron and folate deficiency. It remains common practice for pregnant women to routinely receive iron and folate supplementation and iron supplementation is essential when there is evidence of genuine iron deficiency (Allen 2002). Data provide evidence that iron supplementation restores normal values for non-pregnant women (Sloan et al 2002) and it may also prevent low haemoglobin at birth or at 6 weeks postpartum. The number of available trials is limited and inconclusive and further controlled trials are needed to investigate treatment of iron deficiency. Controlled trials of iron supplementation have consistently demonstrated positive effects on maternal iron status at delivery but have not demonstrated reductions in factors associated with maternal anaemia such as increased risk of preterm delivery and infant low birth weight (Scholl & Reilly 2000).

The therapeutic approach to iron supplementation suffers from real or perceived problems of compliance (Péna-Rosas & Viteri 2006). Oral iron preparations themselves may cause gastrointestinal upsets such as nausea, constipation and diarrhoea and women may not comply with therapy. The interaction between iron intake and zinc absorption remains unclear. Oral preparations may reduce the bioavailability of zinc, important in pregnancy, and fetal growth may be adversely affected.

Ideally, women should have good iron stores before conception with prevention and control of iron-deficiency anaemia involving good dietary advice, preferably before or early in pregnancy (Hercberg et al 2001). Dietary advice should also include the role of vitamin C in enhancing iron absorption and of the tannins in coffee and tea in inhibiting its absorption.

There is still a considerable amount of information to be explored about the benefits of maternal iron supplementation on the health and iron status of the mother and her child during pregnancy and postpartum. The current situation remains controversial. Women diagnosed with iron deficiency will require iron therapy during pregnancy and prophylactic iron supplements may be considered on a general or selective basis.

and return to normal by the 3rd postnatal day. The basophil and monocyte counts appear to remain unchanged.

Although the lymphocyte count remains unchanged in pregnancy with no change in circulating T cells and B cells, there is profound depression of cell-mediated immunity. This picture is also seen in women taking oral contraceptives containing oestrogen. Oestrogen may increase the number of glycoproteins on the cell surface, leading to impaired response to stimuli. Human chorionic gonadotrophin from the placenta and prolactin from the anterior pituitary are known to suppress lymphocyte function. There is no apparent impairment to the production of immunoglobulins or to humoral-mediated immunity. The depression of cell-mediated immunity is essential to the survival of the fetus but may increase susceptibility to viral infections such as rubella, poliomyelitis and influenza. Worldwide, the increased susceptibility in immune women to malaria leads to an infected placenta with increased fetal mortality.

Haemostasis in pregnancy

The major changes occur in the haemostatic components of blood and some of these are unique to pregnancy. Adaptations lead to a hypercoagulable state during pregnancy. Adequate haemostasis depends on a complex interaction between blood vessel wall, platelets, coagulation factors and fibrinolysis. Haemostasis in health has three main functions: to keep the circulating blood inside the vascular tree, to maintain the fluidity of blood and to arrest bleeding following injury to vessels (Sherwood 2006).

The following changes are seen in pregnancy as detailed in Blackburn (2007):

- Platelet count decreases slightly in relation to the haemodilution. No change in function has been reported.
- There are increased levels of coagulation factors VII, VIII and X and a marked increase in plasma fibrinogen from as early as the 3rd month of gestation. Plasma fibrinogen levels may double in late pregnancy and labour due to increased synthesis. Factor VII may increase 10-fold (also seen in women taking oestrogen/progesterone contraceptives) and the activity of factor VIII doubles.
- These changes are consistent with a continuous low-grade coagulation activity with fibrin deposition in the intervillous space of the placenta and in the walls of the spiral arteries supplying the placenta. As pregnancy progresses, a fibrin matrix replaces the smooth muscle and elastic lamina of the spiral arteries. This allows expansion of the lumen to accommodate an increase in blood volume and decrease the pressure of arterial blood flowing to the placenta. This hypercoagulability is advantageous following placental separation to help in control of blood loss and to prevent haemorrhage. Following delivery, a fibrin mesh very rapidly covers the placental site. The fibrinogen

used represents up to 10% of the total circulating fibrinogen.

- Fibrinolytic activity decreases during pregnancy, remains low in labour and delivery and returns to normal as early as 1 h after placental delivery. These changes help to combat the hazards of haemorrhage at delivery. However, the fact that they occur early in pregnancy and are accompanied by venous stasis predisposes women to thromboembolic episodes.

Intrapartum and immediate postpartum periods

The decrease in blood and plasma volume during the immediate postpartum period corresponds to the amount of blood loss with delivery (Blackburn 2007). Blood volume lost at delivery is possibly 500 ml for a singleton pregnancy and up to a 1000 ml for a multiple pregnancy or following a caesarean section. The normal response to blood loss in non-pregnant women is a drop in blood volume compensated for by vasoconstriction. Over the next few days, the blood volume expands back to near normal values because of increased plasma volume. As a result, there is a fall in the haematocrit proportional to the blood loss. In the normal healthy pregnant woman the response to blood loss is modified because of the hypervolaemia of pregnancy. After the acute blood loss at delivery there is no compensatory increase in blood volume, which remains relatively stable. There is a gradual fall in plasma volume primarily due to diuresis. The red cell mass increase during pregnancy gradually reduces to normal values as red cells come to the end of their life span. The haematocrit gradually increases and blood volume returns to non-pregnant levels.

Main points

- Blood is a fluid connective tissue carrying oxygen and nutrients to the body cells and carbon dioxide and metabolic waste from the cells. Blood volume is about 5–6 litres in a man and 4–5 litres in a woman.
- The functions of blood are: internal transport of substances for respiration, nutrition and excretion; maintenance of water, electrolyte and acid–base balance; metabolic regulation; protection against infection; protection from haemorrhage; and maintenance of body temperature.
- Blood consists of two components: 55% plasma and 45% cells.
- Plasma proteins prevent fluid loss, transport substances around the body, are involved in clotting and fibrinolytic activities, assist in prevention of infection, help regulate acid–base balance, act as a protein reserve and contribute half of total blood viscosity.
- Haemopoiesis is the term for blood cell formation. A pluripotent stem cell in the red bone marrow gives rise to progenitor cells for the three main types of cell, i.e. red cells, white cells and platelets. Each cell type performs a different function. Erythrocytes are involved in transport of gases to and from cells, leucocytes are involved in the defence of micro-organisms and platelets are involved in haemostasis.
- Red blood cells live about 120 days. They are finally fragmented and destroyed by macrophages in the spleen. Protein and haem are produced and enter the body stores while bilirubin is excreted in bile.
- White cells account for 1% of the blood's cellular content.
- Platelets are produced in the bone marrow. In the clotting process they form a platelet plug. Platelets phagocytose small particles such as viruses and immune complexes, store and transport histamine and serotonin, supply the endothelial cells of the blood vessels with nutrition and secrete PDGF, which stimulates proliferation of smooth muscle cells to help healing.
- Blood flow depends on a smooth endothelial surface lining blood vessels. If a vessel is damaged a series of reactions occurs in order to maintain haemostasis and minimise blood loss. Haemostasis involves vascular spasm, platelet plug formation and blood coagulation.
- The ABO blood groups are based on the presence of two red cell antigens, type A and type B. The O blood group arises if neither antigen is inherited; if both are inherited, group AB results.
- Only three rhesus antigens are common, i.e. C, D and E agglutinogens. Rhesus D is by far the most clinically important antigen. About 85% of people in the Western world are Rh+ and 15% are Rh −. There are no spontaneously occurring anti-Rh antibodies. These are formed if there is a sensitisation event.
- Total blood volume is a combination of plasma volume and red cell volume. The increase in blood volume in pregnancy relates to an increase in cardiac output. In pregnancy red cell mass or total volume of red cells increases by 18% while plasma volume increases by about 50%. This difference results in hypervolaemia, haemodilution and a fall in Hb level, often referred to as physiological anaemia.
- The increase in plasma volume is related to the birth weight of the baby. The decrease in viscosity with increase in cardiac force leads to a decreased resistance to blood flow, essential for placental perfusion.

- Extra iron is needed in pregnancy to meet the expansion in red cell mass and the needs of the fetus and placenta. There is no agreement on whether women need iron supplements if well nourished.
- Requirements for folic acid are increased during pregnancy to meet the needs of the growing fetus and placenta, and the increased maternal tissues of the growing uterus and red cell mass.
- The total white cell count rises in pregnancy, mainly due to an increase in neutrophils. The lymphocyte count remains unchanged with no change in circulating T cells and B cells. There is depression of cell-mediated immunity, which may be essential to the survival of the fetus but may increase susceptibility to viral infections.

- Major changes occur in the haemostatic components of blood during pregnancy, leading to a hypercoagulable state. Fibrinolytic activity is decreased during pregnancy, remains low in labour and delivery and returns to normal within 1 h of delivery. These changes help to combat haemorrhage at delivery but are accompanied by venous stasis and predispose women to thromboembolic episodes.
- After the acute blood loss at delivery, the blood volume does not increase as usual in haemorrhage. There is a gradual fall in plasma volume primarily due to diuresis. The red cell mass gradually reduces to non-pregnant levels as red cells come to the end of their life span.

References

Allen, L.H., 2002. Anemia and iron deficiency: effects on pregnancy outcome. Am. J. Clin. Nutr. 71 (5), 1280S–1284S.

Blackburn, S.T., 2007. Maternal, Fetal and Neonatal Physiology: A Clinical Perspective, fourth edn. Elsevier Saunders, St Louis MO.

Bothwell, T.H., 2000. Iron requirements in pregnancy and strategies to meet them. Am. J. Clin. Nutr. 72 (1), 257S–264S.

Enkin, M., Keirse, M.J.N.C., Neilson, J., 2000. A Guide to Effective Care in Pregnancy, third edn. Oxford University Press, Oxford, pp 39–46.

Gordon, M.C., et al., 2007. Maternal physiology in pregnancy. In: Gabbe, S.G., Simpson, J.L., Niebyl, J.R. (Eds.) Obstetrics: Normal and Problem Pregnancies, fifth edn. Churchill Livingstone, London.

Hercberg, S., Preziosi, P., Galan, P., 2001. Iron deficiency in Europe public health. Nutrition 4 (2B), 537–545.

Péna-Rosas, J.P., Viteri, F.E., 2006. Effects of routine oral iron supplementation with or without folic acid for women during pregnancy. Cochrane Database Syst. Rev. (3) 2006, Art. No. CD004736. DOI:10.1002/4651858. CD004736.pub2.

Reveiz, L., Gyte, G.M., Cuervo, L.G., 2007. Treatments for iron-deficiency anaemia in pregnancy. Cochrane Database Syst. Rev. (2) 2007, CD003094.

Robinson, F., 2002. The nutritional contribution of meat to the British diet: recent trends and analyses. Nutr. Bull. 26 (4), 283–293.

Scholl, T.O., Reilly, T., 2000. Anemia, iron and pregnancy outcome. J. Nutr. 130 (2S), 443S–447S.

Sherwood, L., 2006. Human Physiology: From Cells to Systems, sixth edn. Blackwell Science, Oxford.

Sloan, N.L., Jordan, E., Winikoff, B., 2002. Effects of iron supplementation on maternal haematological status in pregnancy. Am. J. Public Health 92 (2), 288–293.

UNICEF/WHO, 1999. Prevention and control of iron deficiency anaemia in women and children. Report of the UNICEF/WHO Regional Consultation. WHO, Geneva.

Annotated recommended reading

Blackburn, S.T., 2007. Maternal, Fetal and Neonatal Physiology: A Clinical Perspective, fourth edn. Elsevier Saunders, St Louis MO.

This text provides a detailed description of the major changes that occur in the body systems during pregnancy. There is an extensive review of the literature of the haematological and cardiovascular system, extending from classical research studies to the more recent research findings.

Sherwood, L., 2006. Human Physiology: From Cells to Systems, sixth edn. Blackwell Science, Oxford.

This textbook presents a detailed overview of human anatomy and physiology as related to the haematological system. The text is well illustrated with diagrams and pictures and is relevant for undergraduates in a health-related profession.

Chapter Seventeen

17

The cardiovascular system

Introduction

The cardiovascular system, consisting of the heart and blood vessels, is designed to meet the crucial homeostatic needs of the cells and tissues by maintaining an adequate blood supply during varying physiological circumstances. For instance, blood can be preferentially directed to individual systems as required. Flow increases to the muscles during exercise and to the gastrointestinal system following food intake. Centres in the brain control the system as a whole, although local events and reflexes may modify the end result.

There are three main roles for the cardiovascular system:

1. Delivery of nutrients and oxygen.

2. Removal of metabolic waste and carbon dioxide.

3. Dissipation of heat from active tissues and redistribution of heat around the body.

Circulatory pathways

Blood flows through a network of blood vessels that extend between the heart and peripheral tissues. The circulation of blood can be subdivided into two distinct circuits, which both begin and end in the heart. The **pulmonary circulation** takes deoxygenated blood from the right side of the heart to the lungs and returns oxygenated blood from the lungs to the left side of the heart. The **systemic circulation** takes oxygenated blood from the left side of the heart to all the tissues and returns deoxygenated blood to the right side of the heart. Exchange of nutrients and metabolic waste products takes place in the systemic circulation. In a normal adult at rest the amount of blood circulated through the heart is 5 litres per minute (L/min), which is the same as the amount of blood in the circulation.

The force required to move blood around the body comes from the heart, which is essentially two separate pumps: the left side supplies the systemic circulation and the right side supplies the pulmonary circulation. As a general principle, veins carry blood **to** the heart: oxygenated in the pulmonary circulatory system and deoxygenated in the systemic veins (Fig. 17.1). Arteries carry blood **away** from the heart: deoxygenated in the pulmonary circulatory system and oxygenated in the systemic circulation.

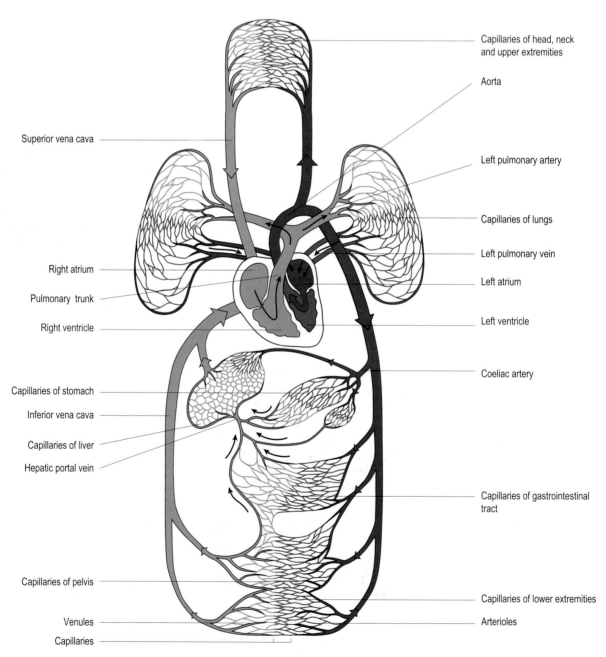

Figure 17.1 • A general plan of the circulatory system. (From Montague S E, Watson R, Herbert R A 2005, with kind permission of Elsevier.)

Anatomy of the heart

Description

The heart lies in the mediastinum of the thoracic cavity between the two lungs enclosed in their pleural sacs. It is positioned with two-thirds of its mass to the left of the body's midline. It is shaped like a blunt cone with its apex pointing downwards and to the left. The heart covers about 12–14 cm from the second to the fifth intercostal space; its base, which points upwards towards the right shoulder, is about 9 cm wide. The heart of an adult normally weighs about 300 g.

Layers

The myocardium, endocardium and pericardium make up the three layers of the heart.

The **myocardium** or contractile wall of the heart consists mainly of cardiac muscle. Connective tissue forms a dense fibrous network which reinforces the myocardium and anchors the muscle fibres. This fibrous network limits the spread of electrical action potentials to specific pathways.

The inner lining or **endocardium** consists of squamous epithelium resting on connective tissue. This also covers the valves and the tendons that hold them in place. It is continuous with the endothelial lining of the blood vessels entering the heart.

The heart is enclosed in a fibroserous sac called the **pericardium**, which protects it and anchors it to the large blood vessels, diaphragm and sternal wall. It has two layers: an outer fibrous layer and an inner serous pericardium. The serous pericardium is also composed of two layers: the outer parietal layer and the inner visceral layer next to the myocardium called the **epicardium**. Between the visceral and parietal layers of the serous pericardium is the **pericardial cavity**, which is filled with **pericardial fluid**. This provides a friction-free area within which the heart can pump.

Chambers and valves

There are four **chambers** in the heart: two superior atria and two inferior ventricles. The right ventricle forms most of the anterior surface of the heart while the left and largest ventricle forms the apex and the inferior posterior aspect of the heart. These chambers are separated by valves and septa: the interatrial septum and the interventricular septum. The valves are attached to papillary muscles by the **chordae tendinae**, which anchor them in the closed position. The valves direct and control the flow of blood through the heart by opening as the associated chamber contracts and closing as the chamber relaxes. The valves ensure a one-way flow of blood through the heart (Fig. 17.2).

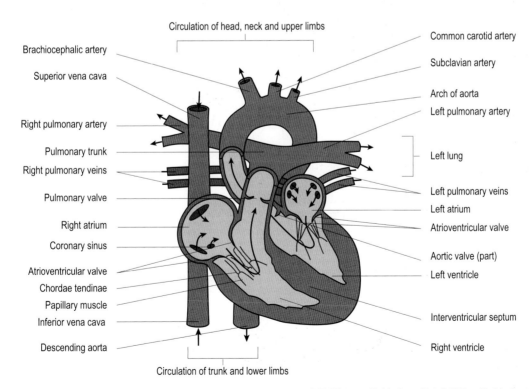

Figure 17.2 • The direction of blood flow within the heart. (From Montague S E, Watson R, Herbert R A 2005, with kind permission of Elsevier.)

The atrioventricular valves

The **tricuspid** valve separates the right atrium from the right ventricle. The **mitral** or **bicuspid** valve separates the left atrium from the left ventricle.

The semilunar valves

The **pulmonary** valve separates the right ventricle from the pulmonary artery. The **aortic** valve separates the left ventricle and the aorta.

The coronary circulation

Oxygen is carried to the cardiac muscle by the right and left coronary arteries, which originate from the aorta just beyond the aortic valve. The right coronary artery supplies the right atrium, right ventricle and portions of the left ventricle. The left coronary artery divides near its origin into:

- The left anterior descending branch, supplying the anterior part of the left ventricle and a small part of the right ventricle.
- The circumflex branch, which supplies blood to the left atrium and upper left ventricle.

Blood returns from the left side of the heart to the right atrium via the coronary sinus and blood returns from the right side of the heart via small anterior cardiac veins.

Pulmonary and systemic circulations

The **pulmonary circulation** takes deoxygenated blood from the right atrium to the lungs via the pulmonary trunk, which divides into two pulmonary arteries, one directed to each lung. The arteries further subdivide until the capillary level where they unite into venules and then veins. Oxygenated blood is then returned to the left atrium from the lungs via four pulmonary veins.

In the **systemic circulation**, oxygenated blood leaves the left ventricle via the aorta and is diverted to all the tissues and cells around the body through smaller arteries and arterioles. At tissue level the blood reaches capillaries, merging with venules to form veins. These veins unite to return deoxygenated blood to the right atrium through two large veins called the venae cavae: the inferior vena cava collects blood from the lower body and the superior vena cava collects blood from the upper body.

Physiology of the heart

Cardiac muscle combines properties of both skeletal and smooth muscle (see Ch. 25). It is striated like skeletal muscle but individual muscle cell membranes have very low electrical resistance. Structures called **intercalated discs** (Fig. 17.3) allow action potentials to pass easily from one cardiac muscle cell to another so that the muscle mass can function as a whole. Intercalated discs contain anchoring units called **desmosomes** to hold the fibres together. Gap junctions between the muscle cells allow easy movement of ions to facilitate the spread of action potentials. The action potential is prolonged, allowing the electrical impulse to travel over the whole atrial and ventricular mass so that the cardiac muscle contracts as a unit. There is then a prolonged refractory period where relaxation phase occurs and no further contraction can begin. This is when the heart chambers refill with blood.

Both atria contract together, propelling blood into each ventricle. Both ventricles then contract together, propelling blood into the pulmonary and systemic circulations. As the atria contract, the ventricles are relaxed so they can fill up with blood. As the ventricles contract, the atria are relaxed and fill up with blood ready for the next cycle.

The electrical conducting system (nodal system)

The electrical conducting system of the heart has the following components:

- Sinoatrial (SA) node.
- Atrioventricular (AV) node.
- Atrioventricular bundle of His.
- Left and right branch bundles.
- Purkinje fibres.

The **SA node**, located in the right atrium, initiates the action potential that causes contraction. It then spreads through both atria and enters the **AV node** at the base of the right atrium. This, plus the **bundle of His**, provide

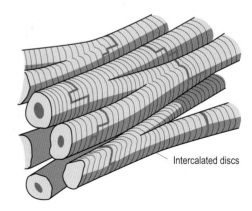

Figure 17.3 • The structure of cardiac muscle showing the intercalated discs. (From Montague S E, Watson R, Herbert R A 2005, with kind permission of Elsevier.)

the only conduction link to the ventricles. There is a 0.1 s delay in conduction, allowing the atria to complete contracting and emptying their blood into the ventricles. The wave now spreads via the left and right branch bundles, which lie on either side of the interventricular septum, to the **Purkinje fibres** and the ventricular muscle. The spread is simultaneous and there is coordinated contraction.

The cardiac cycle

The cardiac cycle is taken from the end of one contraction to the end of the next (Fig. 17.4). It produces two distinct sounds in a single beat, 'lub-dup'. The first heart sound is produced by the closure of the atrioventricular valves at the beginning of ventricular contraction or **systole**. The second sound is produced by the closure of the semilunar valves at the beginning of ventricular relaxation or **diastole**. The **heart rate** is the number of cycles or beats per minute (bpm). At an average heart rate of 72 bpm, each cardiac cycle lasts approximately 0.8 s with approximately 0.4 s being in systole and 0.4 s in diastole.

Control of the heart rate

Intrinsic control

The intrinsic conduction system of the heart allows the heart muscle to beat on its own with no external control. The heart's electrical conduction system has **autorhythmicity**. The SA node acts as a pacemaker and in the absence of any nervous or hormonal influences initiates a rate of 100 bpm. Other parts of the conducting system also have autorhythmicity. The unopposed AV node can initiate a rate of 40–60 bpm and the rest of the system will initiate a rate of 15–40 bpm.

Extrinsic control

The heart rate can also be externally influenced by the autonomic nervous system, hormones such as adrenaline (epinephrine), stretching the atria, temperature and drugs.

Nervous control

In the medulla oblongata the **cardiovascular centre (CVC)** receives input from baroreceptors, chemoreceptors and higher centres in the brain such as the cortex and hypothalamus (Fig. 17.5). The CVC can be subdivided into the **cardiac centre**, affecting heart function, and the **vasomotor centre**, affecting blood vessels, but these probably function interactively. Both sympathetic fibres (from the CVC) and parasympathetic fibres (from the vagus nerve) innervate the SA node. Sympathetic activity causes the heart rate to increase and parasympathetic activity causes the heart rate to decrease (Fig. 17.6). This parasympathetic influence, dominant at rest, is sometimes known as the **vagal brake**. This explains why a normal resting heart rate averages 70 bpm compared with the unopposed SA node rate of 100 bpm.

Hormonal control

Adrenaline (epinephrine) stimulates β_1 receptors in cardiac muscle and causes the heart rate to increase in response to stress. The hormones noradrenaline (norepinephrine) and thyroid hormone also enhance the effect of the sympathetic nervous system to increase heart rate.

Stretch

Stretching of the atrial walls can be caused by increased venous return or increased blood volume. Atrial stretching can increase the heart rate by 10–15%. This is the **Bainbridge reflex** and occurs because the stretch receptors in the atrial walls send impulses to stimulate sympathetic output.

Stroke volume

Excess blood also stretches the ventricles (**ventricular end-diastolic volume (VEDV)**). The more the ventricles are stretched before contraction, the greater the force of contraction and the greater the amount of blood leaving the heart. This is **Starling's law of the heart**. The amount of blood leaving each ventricle during one contraction is called the **stroke volume (SV)** and is normally 70 ml. A ventricle does not empty completely

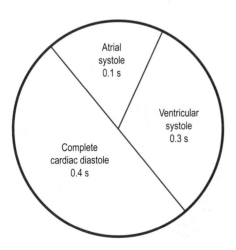

Figure 17.4 • The cardiac cycle.

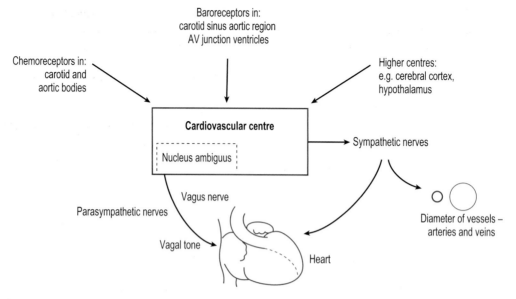

Figure 17.5 • Diagrammatic representation of afferent and efferent pathways associated with the cardiovascular control centre. (From Hinchliff S M, Montague S E 1990, with permission.)

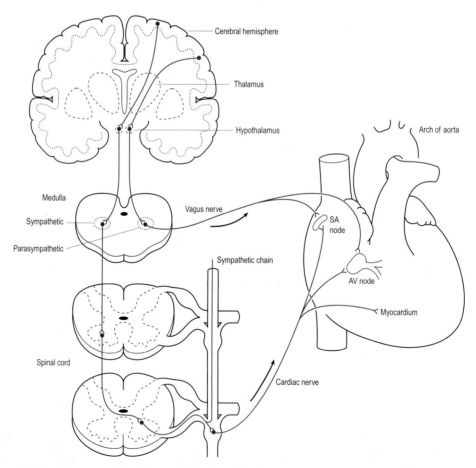

Figure 17.6 • Sympathetic and parasympathetic innervation of the heart (based on Tortora & Anagnostakos 1981).

when it contracts. The blood left in the ventricle at the end of systole is the **ventricular end-systolic volume** (VESV). Typical values for an adult at rest are SV = 70 ml, VEDV = 135 ml and VESV = 65 ml and can be represented by the following equation:

$$SV = VEDV - VESV \qquad (17.1)$$

In health, adding the atrial contents to the remaining blood in the ventricle brings about the extra VEDV of the next cycle. This increases the contraction force, causing the ventricle to empty more completely and thus maintaining SV at a constant level.

Cardiac output

The volume of blood pumped by each ventricle per minute is called cardiac output (CO), usually expressed in L/min. It is also the volume of blood flowing through either the systemic or pulmonary circuit per minute. The CO is determined by multiplying the heart rate, the number of beats per minute (bpm), by the stroke volume, the blood ejected by each ventricle with each beat:

$$CO = HR \times SV \qquad (17.2)$$

Thus if each ventricle has a rate of 72 bpm and ejects 70 ml of blood with each beat, from Eqn (17.2) the cardiac output is:

$$CO = 72 \,bpm \times 0.07 \,L/beat = 5.0 \,L/min$$

These are approximate values for a healthy adult at rest. Since the total blood volume is also approximately 5 litres, this means that essentially all the blood is pumped around the circuit once each minute. Cardiac output may reach 35 L/min in well-trained athletes during periods of strenuous exercise (i.e. total blood volume pumped around the circuit seven times a minute). Sedentary individuals can reach cardiac outputs of 20–25 L/min. The difference between the cardiac output at rest and the *potential* cardiac output is called the **cardiac reserve**.

In response to being stretched the atria secrete a hormone called **atrial natriuretic factor** (ANF) or **atrial natriuretic peptide** (ANP). This is a potent diuretic that causes the kidney to excrete excess sodium and water, resulting in a decrease of blood volume and blood pressure.

Other influences (Fig. 17.7)

- Alterations in core body temperature influence heart rate: there will be an increase in heart rate with an increase in temperature, whereas lowering of core body temperature will decrease the heart rate. This latter is seen in people with hypothermia. The changes in body temperature alter the rate of electrical discharge (Fig. 17.7).

- Drugs such as isoprenaline or adrenaline (epinephrine) can increase the heart rate. Drugs acting as β-adrenergic blockers such as propranolol will decrease the heart rate.

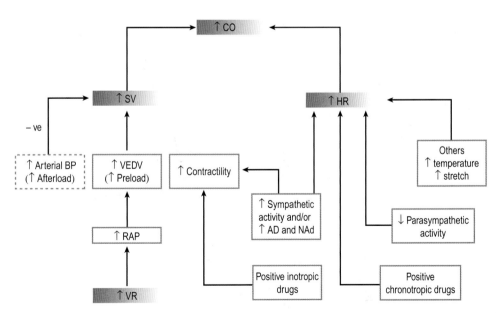

Figure 17.7 • Main factors that can alter cardiac output. An increased arterial blood pressure (i.e. an increased afterload) causes a decrease in stroke volume and consequently a decrease in cardiac output. CO, cardiac output; SV, stroke volume; HR, heart rate; VEDV, ventricular end-diastolic volume; RAP, right atrial pressure; VR, venous return; Ad, adrenaline; NAd, noradrenaline. (From Hinchliff S M, Montague S E 1990, with permission.)

- A raised arterial blood pressure may decrease SV because the ventricles must exert force against a greater load. A normal heart will self-adjust to counter this by increasing the force of ventricular contraction. If the blood pressure is chronically raised, the left ventricle will hypertrophy and fail.

The vascular system

The vascular system delivers blood to all tissues as needed and returns blood to the heart (Figs 17.8, 17.9). To achieve this the system must be able to adapt to local needs. A change from pulsatile arterial blood flow to a steady

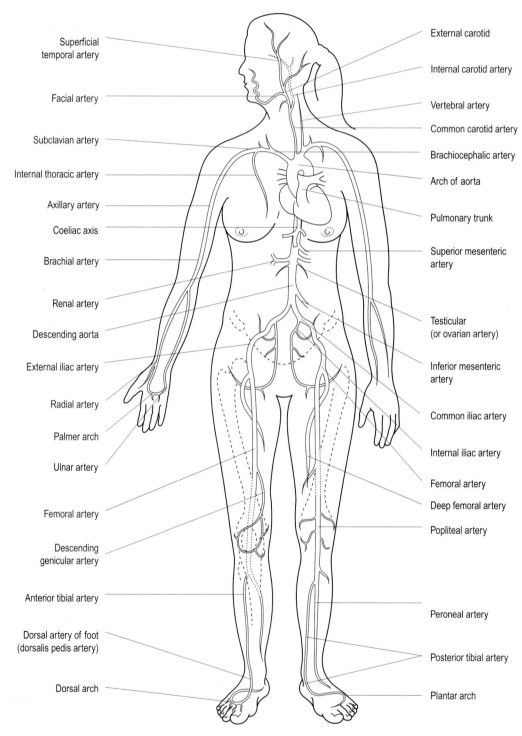

Superficial temporal artery

Facial artery

Subclavian artery

Internal thoracic artery

Axillary artery

Coeliac axis

Brachial artery

Renal artery

Descending aorta

External iliac artery

Radial artery

Palmer arch

Ulnar artery

Femoral artery

Descending genicular artery

Anterior tibial artery

Dorsal artery of foot (dorsalis pedis artery)

Dorsal arch

External carotid

Internal carotid artery

Vertebral artery

Common carotid artery

Brachiocephalic artery

Arch of aorta

Pulmonary trunk

Superior mesenteric artery

Testicular (or ovarian artery)

Inferior mesenteric artery

Common iliac artery

Internal iliac artery

Femoral artery

Deep femoral artery

Popliteal artery

Peroneal artery

Posterior tibial artery

Plantar arch

Figure 17.8 • Major arteries of the human body (anterior view). (From Hinchliff S M, Montague S E 1990, with permission.)

capillary flow is necessary to allow the effective exchange of nutrients and waste to occur at the capillary beds.

In the systemic circulation, blood leaves the left side of the heart via the **aorta**, which subdivides into smaller arteries. The smallest are **arterioles**, branching into **capillaries** where the exchange of gases, nutrients and metabolic wastes occurs. Capillaries unite to form

venules and these unite to form larger veins. Finally, the two largest veins, the **inferior vena cava** returning blood from the lower part of the body and the **superior vena cava** returning blood from the upper part of the body, enter the right atrium of the heart.

In the pulmonary circulation a single pulmonary artery leaves the right ventricle and divides into two

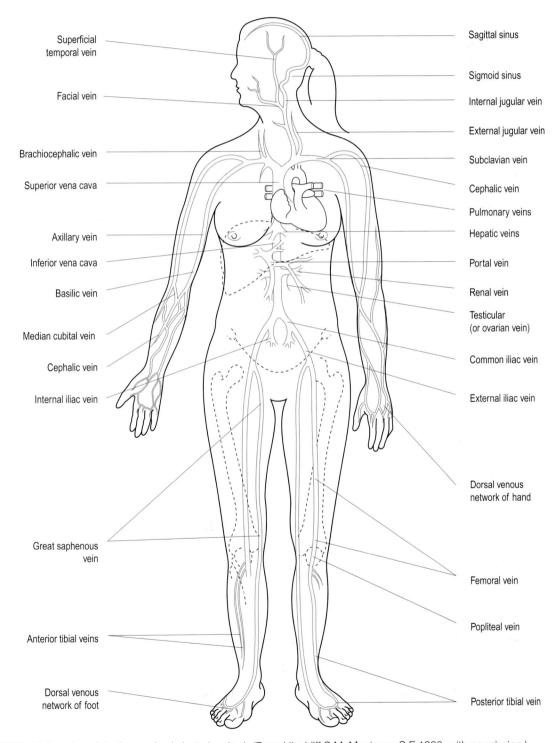

Figure 17.9 • Major veins of the human body (anterior view). (From Hinchliff S M, Montague S E 1990, with permission.)

branches, which deliver deoxygenated blood returning from the tissues to each lung for oxygenation. The division into smaller arteries, arterioles, capillaries, venules and veins is the same as in the systemic circulation. Four pulmonary veins deliver oxygenated blood back to the left atrium.

Structure of blood vessels

The structure of the blood vessels varies depending on their specific functions but the walls of the blood vessels, with the exception of the capillaries, contain the same three layers of tissue (Fig. 17.10):

1. **Tunica intima** is the innermost layer, called the endothelium, which is a single layer of extremely flattened epithelial cells. A basement membrane and some connective and elastic tissue support this layer, which is only found in capillaries.
2. **Tunica media** is the middle layer and consists mainly of smooth muscle and elastic tissue. This is the layer that gives rise to the variation throughout the vascular system.
3. **Tunica adventitia** is the outer layer and is composed of fibrous connective tissue, collagen and fibroblasts.

The arterial system

Elastic arteries (conducting arteries)

Large arteries contain more elastic tissue and can passively expand and recoil to accommodate changes in blood volume. This allows blood to be kept under a continuous pressure rather than starting and stopping with the pulsatile heart beat. When the heart contracts, blood is forced into the aorta and distends these vessels. When the heart rests, the large arteries return to their normal diameters. They have large diameters: that of the aorta is about 2.5 cm.

Muscular arteries (distributing arteries)

These medium-sized arteries distribute blood to all tissues. They have an average diameter of about 0.4 cm and still remain distensible so that resistance to flow is low. As they branch further and become smaller, the amount of elastic tissue decreases and the smooth muscle component increases.

Arterioles

Arterioles are the smallest arteries, less than 0.3 cm in diameter, with a thicker wall mainly composed of

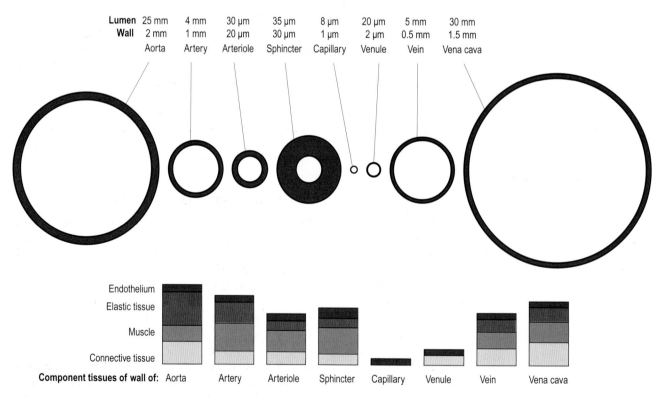

Figure 17.10 • The variations in size and components of the walls of the various blood vessels in the circulatory system. (From Hinchliff S M, Montague S E 1990, with permission.)

muscle tissue in concentric layers. The total resistance to blood flow is mainly determined by the diameter of the arterioles, which also determines the distribution of blood flow to different tissues. The **precapillary sphincters** are specialised regions near the junction between the terminal arterioles and the capillaries. They consist of smooth muscle fibres arranged in a circular manner around the vessels, which control the amount of blood flowing into a capillary bed. This action may also play a part in the formation of tissue fluid (see below).

Capillaries

Capillaries form a dense network of very narrow short vessels. Red blood cells pass through them in single file and may have to fold to negotiate their lumen. They are the exchange vessels where gases, nutrients and metabolic waste products pass between individual cells and the vascular system. Approximately 50 million capillaries are present in the body but at rest only 25% may be patent. Some modified, wider capillaries are known as **sinusoids**. They are found mainly in the liver, bone marrow, lymphoid tissues and endocrine organs and are lined by phagocytic white cells. Blood flows slowly through sinusoids to allow modification of its content: for instance, in the liver when nutrients are extracted.

The microcirculation

Each cell must have access to a capillary supply if it is to remain healthy. Substances need to travel a very short distance to enable adequate **diffusion**. Different tissues have varying amounts of capillaries, depending on their metabolic needs. There may also be **arteriovenous shunts**, connections between the arteries and veins that bypass the capillaries. Blood can flow rapidly through the shunts but this mechanism does not allow exchange of nutrients and gases. They facilitate dissipation of heat from the body via the skin if needed.

The venous system

Veins return blood from the capillary beds to the heart passively along a pressure gradient. As the veins become fewer and larger, resistance to flow decreases. Vein walls have the same three layers as arteries but they are thinner and more distensible than arteries. Some veins, such as those in the legs, have folds in the endothelium which act as valves to ensure that blood flows in one direction towards the heart. These valves may be damaged if overstretched by high pressures, for instance in pregnancy, and this may lead to oedema and varicose veins. The larger part of the circulating blood, about 60%, is contained in the venous system. Veins are sometimes known as capacity vessels and can change their capacity by altering the diameters of the vessels.

The physiology of circulation

Blood vessel diameter

Changes in blood vessel diameter regulate blood pressure and blood flow to the tissues. Altering the degree of smooth muscle contraction in the tunica media changes the blood vessel diameter. Increasing contraction of the circular muscle fibres reduces blood vessel diameter (**vasoconstriction**). When the muscle relaxes, the diameter increases (**vasodilation**). The smooth muscle of the blood vessel walls is normally in a state of contraction known as **vasomotor tone**. Control of the smooth muscle involves nervous and chemical factors.

Nervous control

Sympathetic nerve fibres from the vasomotor centre innervate the smooth muscle in the tunica media. These nerve endings are more densely distributed in the arterioles, precapillary sphincters and venules. Sympathetic nerve discharge increases muscle contraction, causing vasoconstriction. A decrease in the frequency of nerve impulses brings about vasodilation. Vasoconstriction from increased sympathetic activity increases total vascular resistance, increases venomotor tone and reduces venous capacity and venous return.

Chemical control

Vascular smooth muscle is influenced by hormones and locally produced metabolites. Adrenaline (epinephrine) and noradrenaline (norepinephrine) cause vasoconstriction. Angiotensin II, formed by the action of renin (produced by the kidney) on angiotensinogen, is also a potent vasoconstrictor. Histamine and plasma kinins are released from inflamed local tissues and cause vasodilation of small vessels. Local prostaglandins may also be involved in vasodilation.

Endothelial mediated regulation

The endothelium produces a factor, **endothelial-derived relaxing factor** (EDRF), that causes relaxation of vascular smooth muscle and vasodilation. One form of EDRF is **nitric oxide** (NO), which is a free radical. It acts as a chemical messenger, carrying signals from cell to cell. Nitric oxide is released from the endothelial cells and diffuses into the muscle wall of the blood vessel. This local chemical control is extremely important when there is a localised increase in metabolism. Local chemicals largely mediate control of circulation to the brain and the heart. A major factor is the level of oxygen in the blood. The blood flow to the skin is mainly under sympathetic nervous control.

Blood pressure

There are a few facts about the nature of a fluid that may help the reader to understand the concepts involved in blood pressure.

Fluid pressure

Hydrostatic pressure is the force a liquid exerts against the walls of its container. In the vascular system this is the pressure the blood exerts on the blood vessel walls, which is called **blood pressure** (BP). Pressure will also vary with the height of the liquid column. This is related to gravity. When a person is standing up the venous pressure in the feet is greater than that in the head. A third factor that influences hydrostatic pressure is the distensibility of the container. Pressure is less in a distensible container compared to a rigid container. The heart generates a head of pressure that is highest in the aorta and falls throughout the vascular system along the path to the tissues.

Fluid flow

The flow of a fluid through a vessel is determined by the pressure difference between the two ends of the vessel and the resistance to flow. **Resistance to flow** is a measure of the ease with which a fluid flows through a tube. In the vascular system this is described as vascular resistance but for practical purposes most resistance is generated in the small peripheral vessels. This is referred to as **peripheral resistance** (PR). It is affected by:

- **Viscosity**, which is the thickness of a fluid. In blood, viscosity is affected by the ratio of red cells and plasma proteins to plasma fluid. Viscosity increases when there is an increase in cell content or a reduction in plasma fluid, such as in dehydration. An increase in plasma fluid will decrease viscosity. The greater the viscosity, the more force is required to move the fluid along the vessel.
- **Blood vessel length**—the longer the blood vessel, the greater the resistance to flow.
- **Arteriolar diameter**—small changes in diameter can lead to large changes in PR. The smaller the diameter, the greater the resistance. This is because particles in the fluid are more likely to collide with the vessel walls.
- **The lining** also affects flow. A smooth lining in a blood vessel will create a smooth **laminar** flow whilst a rough lining will cause a **turbulent** flow.

Blood pressure is the force exerted on the wall of a blood vessel by the blood it contains. It is measured in millimetres of mercury (mmHg). There is a typical value for different parts of the vascular tree, i.e. for arterial blood pressure, capillary blood pressure, venous blood pressure and so on. These gradients facilitate blood flow around the systems. The pressure in the systemic circulation falls during the blood's journey from the aorta to the right atrium. Pressures in the pulmonary circulation are lower than in the systemic circulation but there is still a falling gradient from right ventricle to left atrium.

Venous return

Blood pressure in the capillary beds is very low so a mechanism is needed to ensure blood return to the right atrium. Blood pressure in the venules is greater than the pressure in the right atrium but gravity opposes venous return when a person is upright and blood may pool in the feet and legs. In contrast, blood returning from the head is aided by gravity when in the upright position and dizziness may occur due to a temporary reduction in brain blood supply if a person stands up too quickly. If venous return to the heart is impeded, cardiac output will fall.

There are several mechanisms to ensure adequate blood flow:

- Increasing **venomotor tone** will reduce the capacity of the venous system.
- The **skeletal muscle pump**: contractions of the skeletal muscles, especially in the limbs, squeezes the veins and pushes the blood towards the heart. Venous valves prevent backflow most effectively when a person is walking. Standing still means the muscle pump cannot act and venous return is not as good. People may faint if they stand still for long periods.
- The **respiratory pump**: as a person breathes in, pressure in the thorax and the right atrium is lowered, which increases the pressure gradient and assists venous return.

The arterial blood pressure is of most value clinically because it ensures an adequate blood supply to the tissues. The main parameter affecting blood pressure is the relationship between cardiac output and peripheral resistance. This can be represented by the following simple equation:

$$BP = CO \times PR \qquad (17.3)$$

Arterial blood pressure

Arterial blood pressure changes throughout the cardiac cycle. Contraction of the ventricles during systole ejects blood into the aorta and raises the arterial pressure. This is the **systolic pressure** and is determined by the stroke volume and the force of the contraction. Systolic pressure will be raised if the arterial walls are stiffer because the vessels cannot distend to accommodate the extra blood. As the heart relaxes during diastole, blood leaves the main arteries and the blood pressure falls. This is the **diastolic pressure**, which is affected by peripheral resistance. Diastolic pressure therefore depends on the level of systolic pressure, the elasticity of the arteries and the viscosity of blood. If the heart rate is slow, diastolic pressure will fall as there is more time for extra blood to flow out of the artery. An increase in heart rate will raise the diastolic pressure.

Pulse pressure and mean arterial pressure

Each ventricular contraction initiates a pulse of pressure through the arteries. The difference between the systolic and diastolic pressure is called the **pulse pressure**. A typical blood pressure would be 120/70 mmHg, giving a pulse pressure of 50 mmHg, i.e. $120 - 70 = 50$ mmHg. The main factors influencing pulse pressure are stroke volume and the rigidity of the arteries.

An average or mean value for arterial pressure is useful as it represents the pressure driving the blood through the arteries. **Mean arterial pressure (MAP)** is more useful as a guide to tissue perfusion than the usual systolic/diastolic BP reading. It is estimated by:

Mean arterial pressure (MAP) = Diastolic pressure +One-third of the pulse pressure

(17.4)

For example, using Eqn (17.4), a blood pressure of 120/70 mmHg gives:

$$MAP = 70 + (\tfrac{1}{3} \text{ of } 50) = 87 \text{ mmHg}$$

The regulation of blood pressure

Neural, chemical and renal controls act to modify blood pressure by influencing cardiac output, peripheral resistance and/or blood volume.

Neural system

The neural system can either alter blood distribution or maintain adequate systemic blood pressure. The system operates by spinal reflex. The vasomotor centre sends sympathetic nerve impulses via vasomotor efferent fibres to the muscular walls of the arterial system and acts mainly on the arterioles. The more impulses from these neurons, the more constricted are the arterioles. The vasomotor centre activity is modified by baroreceptors and chemoreceptors.

Baroreceptors are situated in the tunica adventitia of the internal carotid artery (especially in the carotid sinus), the transverse section of the aortic arch and the largest vessels in the neck and thorax. These provide a short-term feedback mechanism responding to changes in posture and in activity levels. Nerve fibres run from the baroreceptors via the glossopharyngeal cranial nerve (IX) and the vagal nerve (X). The nerve endings respond to stretching of the arterial wall. The normal action of these nerves on the CVC is inhibitory. They slow the heart rate and decrease the force of ventricular contraction as well as causing arterial vasodilation.

Chemoreceptors are situated in the aortic arch and carotid bodies. They respond to a fall in blood oxygen or an increase in blood acidity. The main effect is on the respiratory system but in severe hypoxia they stimulate sympathetic activity, which increases heart rate and blood pressure. Brain centres such as the cortex and the hypothalamus also affect blood pressure.

Chemical control

Hormones from the adrenal medulla, namely adrenaline (epinephrine) and noradrenaline (norepinephrine), act to increase sympathetic activity (the flight or fight response). Antidiuretic hormone (from the posterior pituitary) is released into the circulation to retain fluid during pain and low blood pressure. Some drugs such as morphine, alcohol and nicotine will also increase the blood volume by preventing renal excretion of fluid.

The renal system

The kidneys respond to altered blood volume by altering the amount of urine excreted via the **renin–angiotensin mechanism** (see Chs 19 and 20). A reduction in blood pressure and kidney blood flow results in the excretion of renin by the kidney juxtaglomerular apparatus. Renin acts on angiotensinogen to release angiotensin I, which is then converted to angiotensin II by enzymes. Angiotensin II is a powerful vasoconstrictor and also triggers the release of aldosterone from the adrenal cortex to cause retention of sodium and increased excretion of potassium. Water is retained passively by the increased amount of sodium. Blood volume has a direct effect on blood pressure: the higher the volume, the higher the blood pressure.

Blood pressure values

Blood pressure is highly variable both between individuals and within an individual. It is difficult to quote a normal blood pressure for a population but it is possible to find a typical value for an individual. Both physiological and genetic factors and a range of external influences can affect blood pressure. It is therefore of more value to consider a normal range. Normal adult blood pressure is considered to be between 100/60 mmHg and

150/90 mmHg. Maturation and growth, as well as age, sex and race, can influence blood pressure. Blood pressure readings from 250 000 healthy people presented in Table 17.1 illustrate the range.

The formation of tissue fluid

In the tissues, blood contained in the capillaries is separated from both the interstitial fluid and intracellular fluid of the cells. Capillary walls consist of a single layer of endothelial cells resting on a basement membrane. Slit-like spaces are present between the cells. These are known as pores and represent only a small proportion of the total surface area of the capillary wall. Water and solutes diffuse to and from the blood and interstitial fluid. Although there is a high rate of substance diffusion between the two compartments, the fluid content of the plasma and the interstitial fluid changes very little. The volume of fluid moving out of the capillaries is equal to the amount returned. The hydrostatic pressure

Table 17.1 Blood pressure values		
Age in years	**BP systolic**	**BP diastolic**
Newborn	80	46
10	103	70
20	120	80
40	126	84
60	135	89

on each side of the capillary wall and the osmotic pressure of protein in the plasma and tissue fluid help to ensure this equilibrium (Fig. 17.11).

Hydrostatic pressure

Hydrostatic pressure is the force of water pushing against the cell membrane. In the vascular system it is generated by the blood pressure. In the capillaries a hydrostatic pressure of 25 mmHg is sufficient to push water across the capillary membrane into the extracellular space. It is partly balanced by **osmotic pressure**. The excess water moves into the lymph system.

Blood pressure falls from the arteriolar end of the capillary to the venous end. Fluid, with its dissolved solutes, will also cross the capillary wall. It is forced out at the arteriolar end and returns in the blood at the venous end. Capillary hydrostatic pressure (HP_c) is higher at the arteriolar end (about 25–35 mmHg) than at the venous end (10–15 mmHg). Hydrostatic pressure in the interstitial space (HP_{if}) has usually been rated as 0 mmHg because there is very little fluid present. This is because most of it is drawn into the lymphatic system. This pressure may have a negative value of about −8 mmHg (Marieb & Hoehn 2008). The net hydrostatic pressure is $HP_c − HP_{if}$.

Osmotic pressure

Osmosis is the movement of water down a concentration gradient across a semipermeable membrane. The water moves from high water content to lower water content. Osmosis is directly related to hydrostatic pressure and solute concentration but not to particle size. Osmotic pressure is created by the presence of large

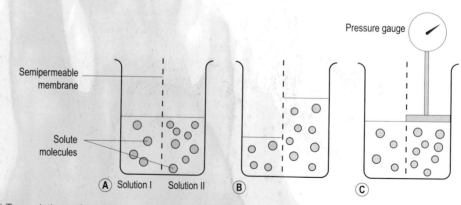

Figure 17.11 • (A) Two solutions of equal volume but differing concentrations are separated by a semipermeable membrane. Solution I is less concentrated than solution II. Soluble molecules are too large to pass through the pores in the semipermeable membrane, but solvent molecules can pass through freely. (B) Solvent has moved across the semipermeable membrane from solution I to solution II, until the concentration of the two solutions is equal. This movement of solvent is called osmosis. Osmotic pressure is the pressure required to stop the movement of solvent by osmosis (C). The greater the difference in concentration between the solutions on either side of the semipermeable membrane, the greater is the pressure required to halt the osmotic movement of solvent across the membrane. (From Hinchliff S M, Montague S E 1990, with permission.)

non-diffusible substances in a fluid. In blood this is provided by plasma proteins (mainly albumin molecules), which apply osmotic pressure if the water concentration surrounding them is lower than the water concentration on the opposite side of the capillary membrane (Fig. 17.12). Capillary osmotic pressure (OP_c) is about 25 mmHg while interstitial fluid, which contains few proteins, has a much lower pressure at $OP_{if} = 0.1–5$ mmHg. The net osmotic pressure is $OP_c − OP_{if}$.

Fluid will leave the capillary where the net hydrostatic pressure is greater than the net osmotic pressure. Hydrostatic forces dominate at the arteriolar end at about 35 mmHg while net osmotic pressure is about 25 mmHg (+10 mmHg). Osmotic pressure dominates at the venous end of the capillary with a net hydrostatic pressure of 13 mmHg and a net osmotic pressure of 23 mmHg (−10 mmHg). Therefore, fluid is forced out of the circulation at the arteriolar end of the capillary beds and forced back in at the venous end (Fig. 17.13).

About 1.5 ml/min is lost from the circulation, picked up from interstitial fluid by the lymphatic system. This fluid, with any lost protein, is returned to the vascular system. The opening of precapillary sphincters will increase capillary pressure and force fluid into the tissues. Their closure will decrease capillary pressure, ensuring that osmotic force draws fluid back into the capillary. In the pulmonary circulation the same mechanism applies but the pressures are much lower.

Diffusion

Movement of substances always occurs along a concentration gradient, from high to low concentration. Oxygen and nutrients will pass from blood to the interstitial fluid and then to cells. Carbon dioxide and waste products of metabolism will flow from the cells into the capillary blood to be eliminated from the body.

Maternal adaptations to pregnancy

During pregnancy, physiologically significant but reversible changes occur in the maternal cardiovascular system (Blackburn 2007). A series of adaptive mechanisms are activated early in pregnancy possibly as early as 5 weeks. These changes are necessary to meet the extra maternal and fetal demands imposed by pregnancy (Gordon 2007). The uteroplacental circulation allows the exchange of gases, nutrients and waste products between mother and fetus. The fetal requirements place an increased load on the cardiovascular system, added to by the increased circulating blood mass, placental circulatory system and gradual increase in body weight. Under normal circumstances these changes are tolerated well but if cardiovascular disease exists the changes could be dangerous for the mother and fetus. On the other hand, no change occurring could compromise

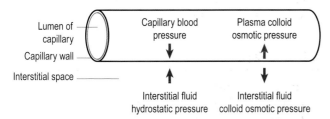

Figure 17.12 Forces affecting fluid movement across the capillary wall. (From Hinchliff S M, Montague S E 1990, with permission.)

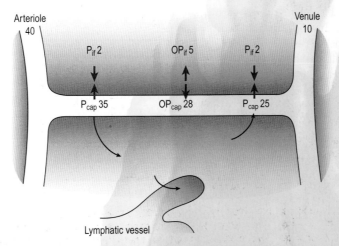

Figure 17.13 • Diagram summarising the forces contributing to the formation and reabsorption of tissue fluid in the systemic circulation (all figures refer to pressures in mmHg). NB: P_{cap} is the only pressure for which magnitude alters. P_{cap}, capillary blood pressure; P_{if}, interstitial fluid pressure; OP_{cap}, plasma colloid osmotic pressure; OP_{if}, interstitial fluid colloid osmotic pressure. (From Hinchliff S M, Montague S E 1990, with permission.)

fetal health, as there may be a possible link between low blood volume and poor fetal growth (see Ch. 13).

Haemodynamic changes

The timing of the adaptive mechanisms and other changes in maternal physiology remains an enigma as to why they are initiated early in pregnancy before there is any physiological need for them. Current evidence suggests that the hormonal and immunological alterations act together very early to begin the process of haemodynamic adaptation. The most important haemodynamic changes in the maternal circulation during pregnancy are the increase in blood volume and cardiac output, and the decrease in peripheral vascular resistance (Blackburn 2007). Other changes occur in the position and size of the heart, heart rate, stroke volume and distribution of blood flow.

Size and position of the heart

As pregnancy progresses, the heart is pushed upwards by the elevation of the diaphragm and rotated forward so that the apex is moved upwards and laterally, appearing in the fourth rather than the fifth intercostal space. The heart volume increases from 70 to 80 ml (about 12%) between early and late pregnancy. There is little increase in wall thickness and the increased venous filling increases the heart size rather than muscle hypertrophy (Gordon 2007).

The increase in atrial size related to the increase in venous return has been associated with more production of ANP in pregnancy. ANP has a diuretic effect and this helps to cope with the increased blood volume of pregnancy. Normal and anatomical and physiological changes may characteristically alter some heart sounds. Systolic or diastolic murmurs can be detected from as early as 12–20 weeks and may mimic pathology. Systolic murmurs are common because of the increased cardiovascular load (Blackburn 2007). In non-pregnant women, a diastolic murmur would indicate disease but in pregnant women it may not be significant because of increased blood flow through the tricuspid or bicuspid (mitral) valves. During pregnancy there is an enhanced myocardial performance with a slight increase in myometrial contractility, probably due to lengthening of the myocardial muscle fibres (Gilson et al 1997).

Cardiac output

Cardiac output (CO) is one of the most significant haemodynamic changes occurring during pregnancy (Blackburn 2007). One of the most dramatic changes in CO is the rapid increase early in the first trimester of pregnancy with an estimated 50% increase by 8 weeks. The increase is not solely to supply uterine blood flow, as the early increase occurs before the uterus has enlarged significantly. The increased CO is achieved by an increase in both heart rate and stroke volume. Changes in heart rate and stroke volume are reported early between 4 and 8 weeks gestation with an initial average increase in heart rate of 15 bpm. The rise in CO early in pregnancy is primarily due to an increase in stroke volume (Abbas et al 2005). There is a small increase in stroke volume that occurs progressively during the first and second trimesters (peaking between 16 and 24 weeks) to about 30% above the non-pregnant rate. Stroke volume declines during the latter stages in pregnancy and returns to prepregnant levels by term (Bridges et al 2003). As pregnancy progresses to term the heart rate which increases more slowly becomes the more dominant factor in determining CO (Monga 2004).

Heart rate is the determinant of CO that has the widest range of values from rest to maximal exercise providing the circulatory system with stability. The maternal heart rate increases progressively during pregnancy, averaging 10–20% (average 10–20 bpm) by 32 weeks and returning to near baseline levels by term. Twin pregnancies have an earlier acceleration in heart rate with a maximum increase at term of 40% above non-pregnant levels (Cunningham et al 2005). There is an even greater increase in CO associated with multiple pregnancy.

The growing uterus provides the primary influence on changes in CO with selected maternal positions. A change from the left lateral recumbent position to supine position can lead to a 25–30% decrease in CO (Bamber 2003). In the supine position the uterine mass compresses the inferior vena cava, leading to this decrease in CO. This syndrome, referred to as **supine hypotension**, is associated with increased heart rate in response to the decreased output. There is somewhat less compression of the vena cava in the sitting position and the most favourable position for venous return is the lateral recumbent position (Tsen et al 2005).

Total blood volume

The increase (between 30–50%) in total blood volume, due to a rise in plasma volume and red cell volume occurring simultaneously, probably explains the increase in CO. Uterine blood rises from 100 ml/min at the end of the first trimester to 500 ml/min at term. Again, this does not parallel the early changes in CO. Red cell mass or total volume of red cells increases by 18%, while plasma volume increases about 50%. The difference results in haemodilution of pregnancy and a fall in Hb level, often referred to as physiological anaemia.

Arterial blood pressure

The slight decrease in systolic blood pressure (BP) accompanied by the greater decrease in diastolic blood pressure leads to an increase in pulse pressure. This is probably due to hormonal vasodilation (Blackburn 2007). It is important to accurately measure BP using the correct size of cuff and standardised technique, e.g. the cuff must be level with the left atrium. Recording a woman's BP when she is lying in a supine position may have a considerable effect by resulting in a profound fall in BP (supine hypotension).

In normal healthy women, a general pattern in BP recordings is noted during pregnancy. There is relatively little change in systolic pressure but there is a marked fall in diastolic pressure, which is lowest at mid-pregnancy and rises thereafter to approximately non-pregnant levels at term. Therefore, there is a raise in pulse pressure for most of pregnancy. At the beginning of labour BP rises slightly and uterine contractions are associated with a rise in mean BP of 10 mmHg, which mirrors the rise in CO in labour.

Age and parity can affect blood pressure. As parity increases, regardless of age, both the systolic and diastolic BP decrease with the greatest difference being between the first and second pregnancy. As age increases (after 35 years of age), systolic blood pressure remains unchanged but diastolic BP increases.

Systemic vascular resistance

Changes in CO during pregnancy are accomplished without an increase in arterial pressure. This is because of the marked decrease in systemic vascular resistance (SVR), especially due to general relaxation of peripheral vascular tone in early pregnancy (Blackburn 2007). SVR (mean arterial pressure divided by cardiac output) decreases by 5 weeks, usually reaches its lowest level by 16–34 weeks and then progressively increases to term. The later change is presumed to be due both to the establishment of new vascular beds such as the low-resistance uteroplacental circulation and to a decreased peripheral vascular resistance.

Pulmonary arterial pressure

During pregnancy the pulmonary artery pressure remains unaltered, implying a large decrease in pulmonary vascular resistance, which mirrors the gestational pattern in CO. The pulmonary circulation has a great capacity for high rates of blood flow without pressure changes and cardiac output may increase four to six times in pregnancy before pulmonary arterial pressure becomes elevated. Reductions in pulmonary resistance are achieved by pulmonary arteriolar vasodilation, capillary recruitment and possibly by arteriovenous shunting.

Venous pressure

Venous pressures during pregnancy do not change significantly. Venous pressure does increase markedly in the femoral veins in pregnancy with no similar rise in right atrial pressure. This finding indicates venous obstruction between the two points (Blackburn 2007). In pregnancy this is brought about by:

- Simple mechanical pressure by the weight of the uterus on the iliac veins and on the inferior vena cava.
- Pressure of the fetal head on the iliac veins.
- Hydrodynamic obstruction due to the outflow of blood at relatively high pressure from the uterus.

The rate of blood flow in the leg veins is much reduced. This contributes to a risk of varicosities developing in the leg veins and vulva as well as haemorrhoids in susceptible women. Another side effect is the development of gravitational oedema.

Regional distribution of increased blood flow

The uterus

The increased circulation of pregnancy mainly targets the uterus. Estimating blood flow to the placental site has been attempted but this has been difficult to measure due to inaccessibility of the uterus and the complex blood supply. It is generally believed that the uterine vascular bed is widely dilated so that oxygen consumption is dealt with by increases in extraction rather than by increases in blood flow. This is a feature of the changes in the uterine blood vessels. Both steroid hormones and the renin–angiotensin system may contribute to the uterine blood flow of pregnancy.

The kidneys

Renal blood flow rises in early pregnancy to about 400 ml/min above non-pregnant levels; this may fall towards the end of pregnancy (see Ch. 19).

The skin

Blood flow to the skin, particularly that of the hands and feet, is greatly increased in pregnancy. Women feel warm and often complain about the heat. Temperature is increased in both the fingers and toes.

Peripheral vasodilation

Increased blood supply to the hands may cause increased fingernail growth. The hair does change character although the rate of hair growth does not appear to be increased. In non-pregnant women, 85% of hairs are actively growing with the remainder in the resting stage prior to falling out. During pregnancy there are 95% of hairs in the growing stage. Therefore by the end of pregnancy the woman has more over-aged hairs that fall out after delivery, leading to the common anxiety of hair coming out 'in handfuls' in the puerperium (de Swiet 1998). Increased blood supply to the nasal mucous membrane increases nasal congestion. Nose bleeds may occur as does increased snoring.

The liver

The research into increased blood flow through the liver is not clear, but it is likely because of the increased metabolic rate during pregnancy (see Ch. 23).

The breasts

Mammary blood flow is probably increased (see Ch. 54).

Control of cardiovascular changes

Control of cardiovascular changes is partly hormonal, with increased circulating levels of oestrogen, progesterone and prostaglandins, and partly mechanical, with changes of growth and development of organs necessitating increased blood supply. Vasodilation of peripheral blood vessels is the primary haemodynamic alteration followed by increases in circulating blood volume and CO. The primary stimulus for generalised vasodilation during pregnancy is more likely to be caused by an EDRF such as nitric oxide of pregnancy rather than being induced by prostaglandins or the hormones of pregnancy (de Swiet 1998, Monga 2004). An increase in physical activity levels has an impact on the cardiovascular system. Box 17.1 provides an overview of the issues related to exercise during pregnancy.

BOX 17.1 EXERCISE AND THE CARDIOVASCULAR SYSTEM

Pregnancy involves anatomical and profound physiological changes unique to pregnancy. This raises important fundamental questions, including the ways in which pregnancy alters a woman's ability to exercise and to what extent exercise influences the course of pregnancy and development of the fetus. Many research studies have investigated the additional impact that exercise has on the changes normally occurring in the body during pregnancy. However, available data are insufficient to infer important risks or benefits for the mother or infant (Kramer & McDonald 2006). The remaining gaps in the existing knowledge mainly focus on concerns related to safety aspects for the woman and her fetus. It is also important to ascertain how the impact of exercise undertaken by serious training on a regular basis differs from the more gentle exercises performed by most pregnant women.

All types of exercise place increased demands on the cardiorespiratory function, which continues to be an area of interest for researchers. Other areas of interest related to exercise in pregnancy include:

- The redistribution of weight.
- The hormone changes of pregnancy.
- Pregnancy and birth outcomes.
- Hyperthermia and fetal normality.
- Hypoxia and the fetus.

Physiological responses to exercise include a redistribution of blood, changes in cardiac output and stroke volume, increased oxygen consumption and alterations in venous pooling. During submaximal exercise, minute ventilation, cardiac output and heart rate are greater in pregnant women than in non-pregnant women (O'Toole 2003). The theoretical redistribution of weight may also affect venous return and blood may be redirected to the exercising skeletal muscles and to the skin for heat dissipation (Hartmann & Bung 1999). Many women spontaneously reduce their level of physical activity. This may be due to the increased amount and distribution of weight gained, which alters the normal balance of the body and shifts the centre of gravity upwards and forwards. As a result, the pelvis tilts forward and down to keep the trunk upright. Spinal changes may be characterised by further developing lumbar lordosis to help bear the weight of the growing fetus.

Uterine blood flow is reduced by exercise (Warnes 2004) and this may be counteracted by an increased oxygen extraction in fit women. Evidence based on animal and human studies suggests that the fetus may experience transient hypoxia resulting in a reduction in the fetal heart rate (FHR) during maternal exercise. The range of FHR in the healthy fetus is normally between 120 and 160 beats/min (bpm) and any reduction below 110 bpm is usually associated with fetal distress. Findings from numerous studies suggest that FHR changes during maternal exercise are transient and do not interfere with normal fetal development and growth. However, there is need for further research in this area, since a reduction in heart rate is assumed to reflect fetal distress.

BOX 17.1 (CONTINUED)

Exercise can improve circulation, posture and attitude to nutrition as well as reduce complaints of constipation and varicose veins. Women who exercise regularly are reported to gain psychological benefits both during and following pregnancy (Rankin 2002). Review of controlled trials indicates that regular aerobic exercise during pregnancy appears to improve (or maintain) physical fitness and body image (Kramer & McDonald 2006). On the basis of the current state of research, physical exercise and sport can be recommended during pregnancy so long as women are aware of the contraindications and follow guidelines for safe exercise.

Main points

- The cardiovascular system has three main roles: delivery of nutrients and oxygen; removal of metabolic waste and carbon dioxide; and distribution of heat around the body. Blood flows in two distinct circuits: the pulmonary circulation and the systemic circulation.

- The myocardium (middle and contractile layer), endocardium (inner layer) and pericardium (outer layer) make up the three layers of the heart. There are four chambers in the heart, two superior atria and two inferior ventricles, separated by septa and valves. Valves direct and control the flow of blood through the heart.

- Oxygen is carried to the cardiac muscle by the right and left coronary arteries.

- Cardiac muscle is specialised tissue. The cardiac cycle is taken from the end of one contraction to the end of the next and lasts approx. 0.8 s. Cardiac output is about 5 L/min increasing to 35 L/min under extreme conditions.

- The structure of blood vessels depends on their specific functions. Muscle contraction will bring about vasoconstriction and muscle relaxation causes vasodilation. The smooth muscle of the blood vessel walls is normally in a state of contraction, known as vasomotor tone.

- The flow of a fluid through a vessel is determined by the pressure difference between the two ends of the vessel and the resistance to flow.

- Blood pressure (mmHg) is the force exerted on the wall of a blood vessel by its contained blood. The main parameter affecting BP is the relationship between cardiac output and peripheral resistance (BP = CO × PR).

- Contraction of the ventricles during systole ejects blood into the aorta and pulmonary artery and raises the arterial pressure. This is known as the systolic pressure. During diastole (relaxation) blood leaves the main arteries and BP falls to give the diastolic pressure. MAP (diastolic + one-third pulse pressure) is a useful guide to tissue perfusion.

- Neural, chemical and renal controls modify blood pressure by influencing cardiac output, peripheral resistance and/or blood volume. Blood pressure is highly variable both between individuals and within an individual. Physiological and genetic factors and a range of external influences can set blood pressure.

- In pregnancy, the maternal cardiovascular system changes to meet the demands of the fetus. Exchange of gases, nutrients and waste products between mother and fetus occurs via the uteroplacental circulation. The most important changes are increase in blood volume, increased cardiac output and reduced peripheral resistance.

- CO increases in the first and second trimesters of pregnancy. An initial rise in heart rate of 15 bpm occurs as early as 4 weeks, followed by a small increase in stroke volume.

- There is haemodilution of pregnancy and a fall in Hb level referred to as physiological anaemia. Little change is noted in the BP systolic reading, with a marked fall in the diastolic reading over the first two trimesters (lowest at mid-pregnancy) and rising in third trimester to non-pregnant levels.

- The rate of blood flow in the leg veins is much reduced, sometimes leading to varicosities in the leg veins and vulva as well as haemorrhoids in susceptible women. Gravitational oedema may occur.

- The increased circulation of pregnancy mainly targets the uterus. Renal blood flow rises in early pregnancy but this may fall towards the end of pregnancy. Blood flow to the skin, particularly that of the hands and feet, is increased. Mammary blood flow is probably increased.

- Control of cardiovascular system changes is partly hormonal and partly mechanical, as changes of growth and development of organs necessitate increased blood supply.

- The woman's physiological response to exercise includes changes in cardiac output, redistribution of blood, increased oxygen consumption and alterations in venous pooling.

References

Abbas, A.E., Lester, S.J., Connolly, H., 2005. Pregnancy and the cardiovascular system. Int. J. Cardiol. 98, 179.

Bamber, J. H., 2003. Aortacaval compression in pregnancy: the effect of changing the degree and direction of lateral tilt on maternal cardiac output. Anaes. Anal. 97, 256.

Blackburn, S.T., 2007. Maternal, Fetal and Neonatal Physiology: A Clinical Perspective, fourth edn. Elsevier Saunders, Missouri.

Bridges, E.J., Womble, E.J., Wallace, M., McCartney, J., 2003. Hemodynamic monitoring in high-risk obstetric patients. 1. Expected hemodynamic changes in pregnancy. Crit. Care Nurse 23, 53.

Cunningham, F.G., Levano, K., Bloom, S.I., et al., 2005. Maternal adaptations in pregnancy. In: Cunningham, F.G. (Ed.), Williams Obstetrics, twentysecond edn. McGraw-Hill Professional, New York.

de Swiet, M., 1998. The cardiovascular system. In: Chamberlain, G., Broughton Pipkin, F. (Eds.) Clinical Physiology in Obstetrics, third edn. Blackwell Science, Oxford.

Gilson, G.J., Samaan, S., Crawford, M.H., et al., 1997. Changes in hemodynamics, ventricular remodelling, and ventricular contractility during normal pregnancy: a longitudinal study. Obstet. Gynecol. 89 (6), 957–962.

Gordon, M.C., et al., 2007. Maternal physiology in pregnancy. In: Gabbe, S.G., Simpson, J.L., Niebyl, J.R. (Eds.) Obstetrics: Normal and Problem Pregnancies, fifth edn. Churchill Livingstone, Edinburgh.

Hartmann, S., Bung, P., 1999. Physical exercise during pregnancy: physiological considerations and recommendations. J. Perinat. Med. 27, 204.

Kramer, M.S., McDonald, S.W., 2006. Aerobic exercise for women during pregnancy. Cochrane Database Syst. Rev. (2) Update Software 2002, Oxford.

Marieb, E.N., Hoehn, K., 2008. Anatomy & Physiology, third edn. Pearson/Benjamin Cummings, New York.

Montague, S.E., Watson, R., Herbert, R.A. (Eds.). Physiology for Nursing Practice. third edn. Baillière Tindall, London.

O'Toole, M.L., 2003. Physiologic aspects of exercise in pregnancy. Clin. Obstet. Gynecol. 46, 379.

Rankin, J., 2002. Effects of Antenatal Exercise on Psychological Well-Being, Pregnancy and Birth Outcome. Whurr Publishers, London.

Monga, M., 2004. Maternal cardiovascular and renal adaptation to pregnancy. In: Creasy, R.K., Resnik, R., Iams, J.D. (Eds.) Maternal–Fetal Medicine: Principles and Practice, fifth edn. Saunders, Philadelphia.

Tsen, L.C., Gerard, W., Ostheimer, J., 2005. What's new in obstetric anaesthesia. Anaesthesiology 102, 672.

Warnes, C.A., 2004. Pregnancy and pulmonary hypertension. Int. J. Cardiol. 97, 11.

Annotated recommended reading

Blackburn, S.T., 2007. Maternal, Fetal and Neonatal Physiology: A Clinical Perspective, fourth edn. Elsevier Saunders, Missouri.
This textbook gives an in-depth review of studies relating to the adaptations to the cardiovascular system during pregnancy.

Marieb, E.N., Hoehn, K., 2008. Anatomy & Physiology, third edn. Pearson/Benjamin Cummings, New York.
This textbook presents a detailed overview of human anatomy and physiology. It is well illustrated with diagrams and pictures. Attention is given to the cardiovascular and haematological systems, homeostasis and the interrelationship with other body systems.

Chapter Eighteen

18

Respiration

CHAPTER CONTENTS

Introduction

Respiration is the process by which the body exchanges gases with the atmosphere in order to provide for the changing needs of cell metabolism. Oxygen (O_2) is taken from the atmosphere and transported around the body in the blood to the tissues. Carbon dioxide (CO_2), produced as metabolic waste by the cells, is returned to the lungs and excreted into the air. Efficient respiration depends on the interactions of respiratory, cardiovascular and central nervous system functions that alter the rate and depth of respiration as needed. An adult utilises about 250 ml of oxygen per minute and this can be dramatically increased in severe exercise.

Anatomy of the respiratory system

The respiratory system consists of the airways from the nasal passages to the pharynx and larynx as well as the bronchi, bronchioles and alveoli of the lungs (Fig. 18.1). The chest structures necessary for moving air in and out of the lungs are part of the system. It is usual to divide the respiratory system into the upper and lower airways at the level of the cricoid cartilage.

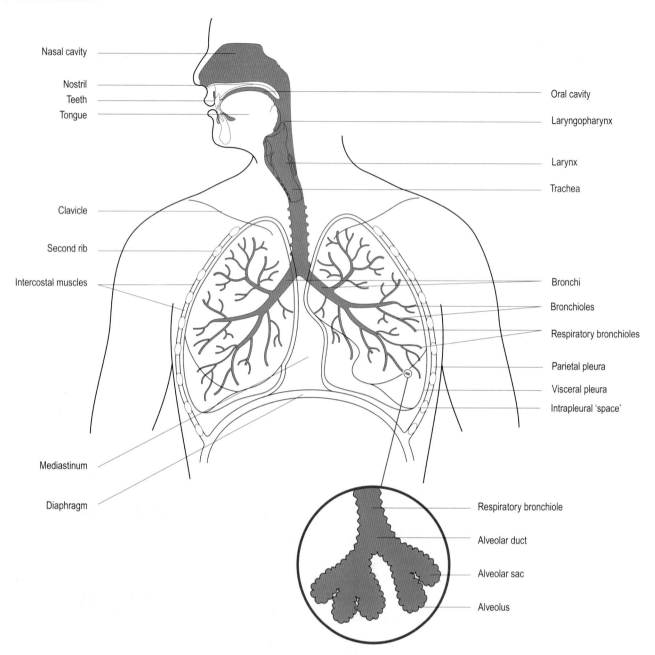

Figure 18.1 • Organisation of the respiratory system. (From Hinchliff S M, Montague S E 1990, with permission.)

The upper airways

The **nasal cavity** is a large, irregular-shaped cavity divided into two by a septum. Bony structures, called the **turbinates**, increase the surface area of the cavity and it is lined with ciliated epithelium which warms, filters and moistens the incoming air. The air now enters the upper pharynx through two internal nares.

The **pharynx** is a common passageway for water and food as well as air. It is a funnel-shaped tube extending from the internal nares to the level of the cricoid cartilage. The auditory or **Eustachian tubes** open into the upper pharynx and the mouth opens into the central portion or oropharynx. The tonsils and adenoids, which are organs of the lymphatic system, are found in the larynx. The oropharynx divides into the oesophagus, transporting food and water into the stomach, and the trachea, transporting air into the lungs.

The **larynx**, commonly called the voice box, is composed of pieces of cartilage connected by ligaments and moved by muscles. It is lined with mucous membrane continuous with the pharynx and trachea. In the larynx are the **vocal cords**, responsible for the production of sound, and between the vocal cords is the **glottis**,

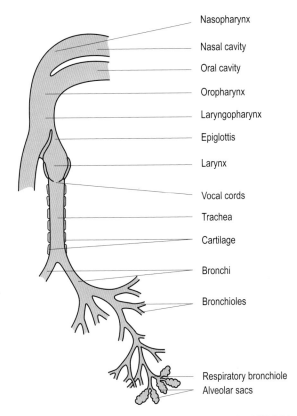

Nasopharynx

Nasal cavity

Oral cavity

Oropharynx

Laryngopharynx

Epiglottis

Larynx

Vocal cords

Trachea

Cartilage

Bronchi

Bronchioles

Respiratory bronchiole
Alveolar sacs

Figure 18.2 • Organisation of the airways. (From Hinchliff S M, Montague S E 1990, with permission.)

through which air passes. The **epiglottis** is a leaf-shaped piece of cartilage anchored to the thyroid cartilage. It moves up and down during swallowing to act as a cover for the glottis and prevent food and water from being inhaled into the larynx and lungs.

The lower respiratory tract

The lower part of the airway is also called the **bronchial tree** because of its resemblance to a trunk and branches (Fig. 18.2). The trachea is a cylindrical tube, 10–12 cm long, made up of 16–20 C-shaped cartilaginous rings joined together by fibrous and muscular tissue. This gives the trachea a firm structure to prevent collapse of the airway during inspiration. The posterior aspect of the cartilaginous rings is absent, facilitating the passage of food down the oesophagus, which lies immediately behind the trachea. The trachea extends from the larynx to the level of the fifth vertebra, where it divides into the two **primary bronchi**. The right primary bronchus is wider and shorter and more vertical than the left so that inhaled objects tend to enter the right lung rather than the left. The primary bronchi enter the lungs at the **hilum**, where the right bronchus goes on to divide into three: the right upper, middle and lower bronchi, to serve three lobes of the right lung. The left

primary bronchus divides into two: the left upper and lower bronchi, to serve the two lobes of the left lung.

The lower branches of the airway, known as bronchi, still have cartilage in their structure. After this they are known as **bronchioles** and have smooth muscle in their walls. The smooth muscle is able to respond to stimuli by causing dilatation or constriction of the lumen of the bronchioles. This function is mainly under the control of the autonomic nervous system, with sympathetic impulses causing bronchodilation and parasympathetic impulses causing bronchoconstriction. There are about 8–13 divisions from the trachea to the smallest bronchi and another 3–4 before the terminal bronchioles are reached. Each terminal bronchiole divides into about 50 respiratory bronchioles. About 200 sac-like **alveoli** are supplied with air by each respiratory bronchiole. Alveoli do not form part of the conducting zone of the respiratory system.

The thoracic cage

The thoracic cage forms the cavity and contains the two conical lungs and the heart. The organs are separated from each other by the mediastinum and its contents. Each lung is surrounded by a double-layered fluid-filled sac called the **pleura**, which also attaches them to the inner surface of the thorax. The inner, or visceral, pleura covers the outer surface of the lung and is reflected back to become the outer or parietal pleura which is attached to the inner surface of the thoracic cavity.

Physiology of the respiratory tract

The epithelial lining

The upper airway protects the alveolar tissues by warming, filtering and moistening the air. The structure of the epithelial lining is particularly good as a filter. It contains glands that secrete thick sticky mucus to trap particles and is ciliated to waft excess mucus and foreign particles towards the pharynx where they can be swallowed. The cilia beat about 600–1000 times per minute. Large numbers of phagocytic cells will engulf and destroy debris and bacteria trapped by the mucus.

Reflex mechanisms

Coughing is a forceful expiration reflex under the control of the respiratory centre in the medulla, which will expel irritant particles from the larynx. Air rushes out at a speed of 500 miles per hour! It is instigated by messages from a sensitive part of the airway at the bifurcation of the trachea, called the **carina**. **Sneezing** is a similar reflex, instigated by irritation of the nasal mucosa. The **swallowing reflex** is extremely important for respiration. Absence of this reflex, as is seen in unconscious or anaesthetised patients, may result in inhalation of particles of food or water into the larynx or lung. The airway may be obstructed or infection and pneumonia may occur.

Structure and function of the alveoli

The terminal bronchioles feed into respiratory bronchioles which branch into the alveolar ducts. These lead into alveolar sacs and the alveoli, where most of the gas exchange occurs (Fig. 18.3). The alveoli are expansions off the alveolar sacs, making the latter resemble bunches of grapes. Alveoli open into a common chamber called the **atrium** at the terminus of the alveolar duct. There are about 300 million alveoli in the lungs, providing an enormous area for gas exchange.

The alveolar wall (Fig. 18.4) consists of a single layer of flattened squamous epithelial cells called type I cells. The external surface of an alveolus has a few elastic fibres around the opening. There is a dense network of pulmonary capillaries surrounding each alveolus, providing a continuous encircling sheet of blood. Each capillary wall is also only one cell thick so that the interstitial space between the alveolus and its capillary network, forming the air–blood interface, is extremely thin (0.2 µm, compared with the 7 µm diameter of an average red blood cell). This interface is called the **respiratory membrane** and has blood flowing on one side and gas on the other. Gas exchange occurs by simple diffusion across the respiratory membrane and depends on the existence of pressure gradients between the lungs and the atmosphere. The total surface area of alveoli in contact with capillaries is roughly the size of a tennis court. This extensive area and the thinness of the barrier permit the rapid exchange of large quantities of oxygen and carbon dioxide for diffusion.

Surfactant

In addition to the type I cells forming the alveolar wall, the alveolar epithelium contains cuboidal type II alveolar cells which secrete pulmonary surfactant. This is a phospholipid that helps to keep the membrane moist and also maintains the patency of the alveolus. Macrophages called dust cells, part of the defence system of the body, are also present in the lumen of the alveoli, mopping up bacteria, dust and other inhaled particles. The alveolar surface is usually sterile. There

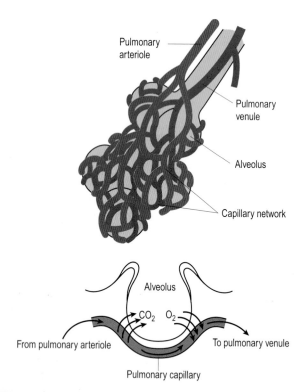

Figure 18.3 • Relationship between alveoli and blood vessels. Gas exchange can occur across the vast surface area provided by the dense network of capillaries. (From Hinchliff S M, Montague S E 1990, with permission.)

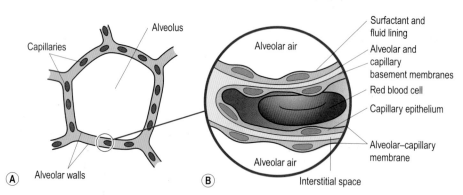

Figure 18.4 • (A) Cross-section through an alveolus. (B) Higher magnification showing histology of part of the alveolar–capillary membrane. The dense network of capillaries forms an almost continuous sheet of blood in the alveolar walls, providing a very efficient arrangement for gas exchange. (From Hinchliff S M, Montague S E 1990, with permission.)

are minute pores of Kohn present in the alveolar walls, allowing air flow between adjacent alveoli (**collateral ventilation**), which is useful if the terminal airways are blocked by disease.

Blood supply to the lungs

The lungs act to oxygenate the blood but they also need their own blood supply to maintain healthy tissue. The blood to be oxygenated reaches the lungs by branches of the pulmonary arteries, is re-oxygenated in the pulmonary capillary network surrounding the alveoli and returns to the heart via the pulmonary veins. The two left and one right bronchial arteries arising from the aorta provide the blood supplying the lung tissue with oxygen. Venous return is by both bronchial veins and the pulmonary veins.

Nerve supply to the respiratory muscles

The phrenic nerve to the diaphragm (originating in cervical nerves 3, 4 and 5) and the intercostal nerves to the intercostal muscles (originating in the thoracic nerves 1–12) innervate the respiratory muscles. This is why severance of the spine above C3 results in total respiratory paralysis but, below that, diaphragmatic breathing can occur although the intercostal muscles will be paralysed.

The physiology of pulmonary ventilation (breathing)

The major function of the respiratory system is to supply the body with oxygen and dispose of carbon dioxide. Four distinct events, collectively called respiration, must occur to perform this function:

1. **Pulmonary ventilation**—This process is called breathing and includes the movement of air in and out of the lungs.

2. **External respiration**—This involves the exchange of gases (oxygen loading and carbon dioxide unloading) between the pulmonary blood and alveoli.

3. **Respiratory gas transport**—Oxygen and carbon dioxide must be transported to and from the lungs and body tissues via the bloodstream.

4. **Internal respiration**—This involves the process of gas exchange between the blood and the tissue cells in the body.

There are two phases to breathing: **inspiration** or breathing in and **expiration** or breathing out. Mechanical factors and neural factors are involved in the control of respiratory rate. Atmospheric air contains about 21% oxygen and 79% nitrogen with traces of inert gases, carbon dioxide and water vapour. Alveolar air exchanges oxygen for carbon dioxide and water vapour. By the time alveolar air reaches the point of expiration it will be mixed with the atmospheric air in the dead space so that the content of expired air will be between the two extremes of atmospheric and alveolar air.

Mechanical factors

Under normal conditions and pressure gradients, oxygen passes from the alveolus into the blood and carbon dioxide from the blood into the alveolus. The movement of gases flowing from a high to a lower pressure down a gradient is said to occur by bulk flow. Air flows in and out of the lungs during breathing by bulk flow. Expansion of the thoracic cage, by contraction of the respiratory muscles during inspiration, increases lung volume and causes a temporary drop in the pressure in the alveoli. Atmospheric air flows in until pressure inside the lung is equal to the atmospheric pressure. Relaxation of the respiratory muscles causes expiration, by reducing the volume of the thoracic cage, creating a temporary rise in pressure within the lung to above atmospheric pressure.

Inspiration

The diaphragm, the most important muscle of inspiration, is a strong dome-shaped sheet of muscle separating the thoracic and abdominal cavities from each other. The diaphragm flattens when it contracts. This change in shape presses down the abdominal contents and lifts the rib cage, enlarging the thoracic cavity both from top to bottom and from front to back. Normally the external intercostal muscles, which are accessory muscles of respiration lying between the ribs, play little part in this expansion of the rib cage but do help to stabilise it. However, during any need for extra oxygen, such as in exercise and in upper airway obstruction, the upper intercostal muscles as well as other accessory muscles of respiration help to enlarge the rib cage and so enhance lung expansion.

Expiration

Under resting conditions, expiration is a passive process brought about by the relaxation and elastic recoil of the diaphragm and intercostal muscles at the end of inspiration. The elastic lung returns to its original volume as air is pushed out of the lung (the **functional residual capacity**), because the reduction in volume makes the alveolar pressure temporarily exceed atmospheric pressure. Active expiration may occur when the need for

222

gas exchange increases under certain conditions such as during exercise or constriction of the airways.

Pulmonary ventilation

Respiratory parameters

Respiratory volumes and respiratory capacities can be described and measured using a spirograph. The measurements below are given for the average healthy adult (Marieb & Hoehn 2008).

Respiratory volumes

- **Tidal volume** (TV) is the volume of air entering and leaving the lungs during a single breath. The tidal volume during normal quiet breathing averages 500 ml for both males and females.
- **Inspiratory reserve volume** (IRV) is the maximum amount of air that can be increased above the tidal volume value during the deepest inspiration. Volumes differ significantly by gender: males average 3200 ml and females average 1900 ml.
- **Expiratory reserve volume** (ERV) is the maximum amount of air that can be voluntarily expelled after a normal quiet respiratory cycle. This averages 1200 ml.
- **Residual volume** (RV) is the volume of air remaining in the lungs at the end of maximal active expiration and is typically 1200 ml in males and 1100 ml in females.

Respiratory capacities

- **Total lung capacity** (TLC) is the amount of air in the lungs at the end of a maximum inspiration. It includes TV + IRV + ERV + RV and averages 6100 ml in males and less in females (4200 ml) because of their smaller size.
- **Vital capacity** (VC) is total capacity minus RV and is typically 80% of TLC. This averages 4800 ml in males and 3100 ml in females.
- **Inspiratory capacity** (IC) is the maximum volume of air that can be inspired after a normal expiration. It is the sum of the tidal volume and the inspiratory reserve volume and averages 3600 ml for males and 2400 ml for females.
- **Functional residual capacity** (FRC) is the amount of air remaining in the lungs after a normal expiration. It is the sum of the expiratory reserve volume and the residual volume and averages 2200 ml in males and 1800 ml in females.

Minute volume

The total volume of air exchanged with the atmosphere in 1 min is called the **minute volume** or **pulmonary ventilation**. This volume depends on tidal volume and respiratory rate and varies considerably in different states of health and according to age. An average tidal volume in a resting adult is about 500 ml with a respiratory rate of 12 breaths per minute. Therefore pulmonary ventilation would be 6000 ml/min. Of this, about 150 ml of each breath is trapped in the **dead space** above the respiratory tissue and is breathed out with its composition unchanged.

Alveolar ventilation

The volume of fresh air entering the alveoli each minute is called the **alveolar ventilation**. The calculation from the parameters mentioned above is as follows:

$$\text{Respiratory rate} \times (\text{Tidal volume} - \text{Dead space}) = \text{Alveolar ventilation}$$

For example, for values given above:

$$12 \times (500 - 150) = 4200 \text{ ml/min}$$

Shallow rapid breathing is not as efficient as slower, deeper respiration because of the greater proportion of each breath wasted in the dead space.

Transport of gases around the body

Gas exchange in tissues

Gas exchange in the tissues occurs at the capillary level and the constant usage of oxygen and production of carbon dioxide by the cells creates the necessary pressure gradients, as discussed in Chapter 16. Oxygen is not very soluble in water and must therefore be carried around the blood in association with haemoglobin. Carbon dioxide is about 20 times more soluble than oxygen and readily dissolves in water to form carbonic acid. However, if all carbon dioxide was carried in solution then the acidity of the blood would be far too great to sustain life so a more complex mechanism is needed.

Transport of oxygen

About 99% of oxygen in the blood is bound to haemoglobin. There is a small quantity of oxygen dissolved in the blood, helping to determine the partial pressure of oxygen in the blood (Po_2) and maintains the pressure gradients, as the bound oxygen is not free to exert a pressure. The oxygen content of the blood is determined partly by the haemoglobin level but the hydrogen ion content of the blood also plays its part. As more oxygen is available, the Po_2 rises and haemoglobin will take it up. At a certain Po_2 when oxygen content is equal to oxygen capacity, the haemoglobin will be unable to take up any more oxygen and is said to be **fully** or **100% saturated**.

Partial pressure gradients and gas diffusion

The partial pressure gradient needed for the diffusion of oxygen is steep. For instance, the Po_2 of pulmonary blood is only 40 mmHg (5.3 kPa) whereas the Po_2 in the alveoli is 100 mmHg (13.3 kPa). Oxygen diffuses from the alveoli into the pulmonary capillary blood until there is equilibrium, with a Po_2 of 100 mmHg (13.3 kPa) on both sides of the respiratory membrane. Carbon dioxide moves in the opposite direction down a much less steep gradient from about 45 mmHg (6.1 kPa) to 40 mmHg (5.3 kPa) with equilibrium at 40 mmHg (5.3 kPa). Although the gradients are so different, both gases are exchanged equally well because carbon dioxide has solubility in plasma and alveolar fluid 20 times that of oxygen.

The oxygen dissociation curve

The oxygen–haemoglobin dissociation curve demonstrates the equilibrium between oxygen and haemoglobin (Fig. 18.5). The curve relates the partial pressure of oxygen to the percentage of haemoglobin that is saturated. There are two aspects of the curve that must be considered: its shape and position. The shape of the curve is sigmoid (S-shaped), indicating that at higher levels (less than 50 mmHg) the curve flattens and an increase in Po_2 produces little increase in saturation. The upper range is the Po_2 range in which oxygen binds to haemoglobin in the lungs. At low Po_2 levels the curve is steep and small changes in Po_2 result in large changes in haemoglobin saturation. In this range oxygen is released from haemoglobin and cellular activities occur. A small drop in Po_2 here allows a large amount of oxygen to be unloaded to the tissues.

Although each of the four haem groups in a haemoglobin molecule can take up a molecule of oxygen, they vary in their affinity. The first haem group in the molecule to take up oxygen does so with difficulty but also holds on to its oxygen tightly. This association changes the shape of the haemoglobin molecule so that the second and third haem molecules take up oxygen readily for a relatively small increase in Po_2 as oxygen saturation goes from 25% to 75%. This is shown on the graph as the steep part of the sigmoid curve. The fourth haem group takes up oxygen more slowly and only at high Po_2. The unloading of oxygen at the tissues is also efficient, with the unloading of one molecule facilitating the unloading of the next. The binding and dissociation of oxygen to haemoglobin is a typical reversible reaction.

Effects of the sigmoid curve on oxygen uptake

Physiological effects of the oxygen dissociation curve include the following aspects. First, oxygen diffuses into the blood at the alveoli and, by increasing the plasma Po_2, creates a pressure gradient so that oxygen can enter the red cell. Within the erythrocyte, the Po_2 rises more slowly; as the dissolved oxygen is rapidly bound to the haemoglobin molecules, so the pressure gradient is maintained. Loading to 90% saturation occurs rapidly at Po_2 of 60 mmHg (8 kPa). However, loading from 90% saturation to full saturation is slower and needs a higher erythrocyte Po_2 of 100 mmHg (13.3 kPa). Secondly, this flattened upper portion of the curve provides a safety factor in illness or at altitude as the blood leaving the lungs will still reach 90% saturation even when Po_2 remains moderate at 60 mmHg (8 kPa).

Effects of sigmoid curve on oxygen release

Blood enters the capillary circulation with a Po_2 of 100 mmHg (13.3 kPa) and is exposed to a tissue Po_2 of only 40 mmHg (5.3 kPa). This tissue pressure lies on the steep part of the oxygen dissociation curve so that up to 80% of the bound oxygen is readily released into the blood so that it can diffuse to the tissues. Below 10 mmHg (1.3 kPa) the affinity of haemoglobin for oxygen is increased so that the last molecule of oxygen associated with haemoglobin is lost with difficulty. However, this low level is very rarely reached. In working muscles, Po_2 of this low level may occur, but **myoglobin**, a special oxygen-carrying molecule, can extract all the oxygen.

Factors influencing the oxygen–haemoglobin dissociation curve

The position of the curve depends on the oxygen affinity for the haemoglobin molecules. The affinity of haemoglobin

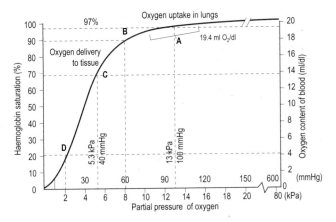

Figure 18.5 • The oxygen–haemoglobin dissociation curve. This applies when pH is 7.4, Pco_2 is 40 mmHg (5.3 kPa) and blood is at 37°C. The total blood oxygen content is shown, assuming a haemoglobin concentration of 15 g/dl blood (i.e. O_2 capacity of 20 ml/dl). (From Hinchliff S M, Montague S E 1990, with permission.)

for oxygen must be sufficient to oxygenate the blood during its movement through the pulmonary circulation. However, it must be weak enough to allow release of the oxygen to the tissues. Several factors can influence the affinity of haemoglobin for oxygen at any given P_{O_2}. These include factors that move the oxygen dissociation curve to the right or to the left. A shift to the right implies a lowered affinity and enhances oxygen unloading, while a shift to the left indicates that oxygen is more tightly bound to haemoglobin and unloading is inhibited.

Increase in carbon dioxide

An increase in carbon dioxide will reduce the ability of haemoglobin to bind oxygen. This reduced affinity for oxygen in the presence of increased carbon dioxide is called the **Bohr effect**. Blood entering the tissues with a P_{CO_2} of 46 mmHg (6.1 kPa) will release more of its oxygen than blood with a P_{CO_2} of 40 mmHg (5.3 kPa). This will shift the oxygen dissociation curve to the right.

Increase in hydrogen ions

The oxygen dissociation curve moves to the right when the blood becomes acidic. As acidity increases in the blood, as occurs with the addition of lactic acid to the extra carbon dioxide during anaerobic cell metabolism in exercise, oxygen release to the tissues is facilitated by the presence of extra hydrogen ions.

Increase in 2,3-diphosphoglycerate (2,3-DPG)

This substance is a product of red cell metabolism and binds reversibly to haemoglobin, reducing its affinity for oxygen. As the red cells reach the tissues 2,3-DPG is produced in more quantity and oxygen release is facilitated by moving the dissociation curve to the right.

Increase in temperature

Local elevation of temperature due to muscle cell metabolism in exercise or other actively metabolising cells will enhance the release of oxygen from the red cells. This moves the dissociation curve to the right.

The effects are reversed in the lung where the extra CO_2 is blown off and the local temperature is cooler. Haemoglobin therefore has a higher affinity for oxygen in the pulmonary capillaries, an appropriate effect!

Carbon monoxide

Carbon monoxide poisoning is a unique type of hypoxaemic hypoxia, and a leading cause of death from fire (Marieb & Hoehn 2008). Carbon monoxide (CO) and oxygen compete for the same binding site on haemoglobin but the affinity of haemoglobin for CO is 240 times greater than that of oxygen (Sherwood 2006). The product of haemoglobin with CO is carboxyhaemoglobin (HbCO). Even small amounts of CO will block the uptake of oxygen and shift the oxygen dissociation curve to the left. The amount of oxygen in the blood is reduced and the cells die from oxygen deprivation. CO is odourless, colourless and tasteless and is produced during the incomplete combustion of carbon products. If introduced into a small space it is lethal as the victim has no sense of breathlessness.

Transport of carbon dioxide

There are three ways in which carbon dioxide is carried around the blood:

1. 5% is carried in simple solution.

2. 5% is carried in combination with the globin rather than the haem part of haemoglobin as carbaminohaemoglobin.

3. 90% is transported as hydrogen carbonate (bicarbonate) ions.

Bicarbonate ions

As the cells metabolise they constantly produce CO_2 so that the P_{CO_2} of intracellular fluid is always greater than that of the blood in the tissue capillaries. This creates the pressure gradient for the removal of CO_2 from the tissues into the plasma. A small quantity will dissolve in the plasma to give carbonic acid. This is a reversible reaction:

$$CO_2 + H_2O \rightleftharpoons H_2CO_3 \qquad (18.1)$$

An enzyme called **carbonic anhydrase** can catalyse (speed up) this reaction. There is little of this enzyme in the plasma but the amount inside the red cell is much greater so that most of the CO_2 from the tissues diffuses through the plasma into the red cells. The rapid production of carbonic acid mops up the CO_2, keeping the red cell P_{CO_2} low. This ensures maintenance of the pressure gradient along which the CO_2 flows.

As is characteristic of acids, the carbonic acid in the red cell quickly ionises (dissociates) into hydrogen (H^+) and bicarbonate (HCO_3^-) ions, another reversible reaction:

$$CO_2 + H_2O \rightleftharpoons H_2CO_3 \rightleftharpoons H^+ + HCO_3^- \qquad (18.2)$$

The chloride shift

HCO_3^- ions can readily pass out of the red cell into the plasma, unlike the H^+ ions, so that the HCO_3^- ions, but not the H^+ ions, can pass down a concentration gradient into the plasma. HCO_3^- ions are much more soluble in blood than is CO_2. This movement out of the cell of HCO_3^- ions leaves the erythrocyte with a more positive electrical charge than the plasma and creates an electrical gradient down which chloride ions (Cl^-), the main plasma anion (**anions** are negatively charged ions and **cations** are positively charged ions), can diffuse into the red cell to restore electrical neutrality. This is known as the **chloride shift**.

Hydrogen ions, carbon dioxide and the acid–base balance

Most of the accumulated H^+ ions inside the red cell become bound to the haemoglobin, as reduced haemoglobin has an affinity for them. This action of haemoglobin acts as buffer, which neutralises the released H^+ ions to prevent any rise in acidity within the red cell. The increased affinity for the uptake of CO_2 and H^+ ions that follows the removal of oxygen is called the **Haldane effect**. The Bohr effect and the Haldane effect work together to facilitate O_2 release and the uptake of CO_2 and H^+ ions by the red cells at tissue level. During exercise, much larger amounts of CO_2 are produced by the tissues but the increase in alveolar ventilation and in cardiac output ensure that arterial Pco_2 remains constant between 37 mmHg (4.9 kPa) and 43 mmHg (5.7 kPa).

The reactions are reversed once the blood reaches the lungs because of the reversed pressure gradients caused by the presence of atmospheric air in the alveoli. Here, CO_2 leaves the red cell to enter the plasma and crosses into the alveoli, and the freed H^+ ions combine with HCO_3^- ions to form H_2CO_3, which then separates into CO_2 and H_2O (see Eqn 18.2), generating more CO_2 to diffuse out to the alveoli. This reaction is also catalysed by carbonic anhydrase.

As the HCO_3^- ions within the red cell are used up to generate CO_2, there is a shift inside the red cell to a positive electrical charge and plasma HCO_3^- ions and Cl^- ions now move back into the cell to restore electrical neutrality once more. This is a major pathway through which acid is removed from the body to maintain the acid–base balance: about 200 ml/min are removed from the tissues and eliminated from the lungs. Oxygen now crosses from the alveoli into the plasma and then to the red cell to bind to haemoglobin.

Because of the importance of fluid and electrolyte balance and the maintenance of pH, a full discussion of the role of the respiratory system in maintaining the pH is presented in Chapter 20.

Control of ventilation

Breathing, like the beating of the heart, must occur in a continuous rhythmic cycle in order to provide oxygen for the cells. The control of breathing is complex. The respiratory muscles, unlike cardiac muscle with its intrinsic pacemaker, are skeletal muscles and must receive nervous stimulation from the brain to make them contract. In normal circumstances respiration is an involuntary act. The control of rhythmic breathing originates in the respiratory centre in the medulla.

Medullary respiratory centres

The dorsal respiratory group

The pace-setting nucleus within the medulla oblongata is called the **inspiratory centre** or dorsal respiratory group (DRG). There is a second nucleus called the **expiratory centre** or ventral respiratory group but its function is not well understood. Two other centres that influence the respiratory centre (higher in the brainstem in the pons) are the **pneumotaxic centre**, which sends out inhibitory impulses to the DRG to prevent overinflation of the lungs, and the **apneustic centre**, which continuously stimulates the DRG to prolong inspiration. The pneumotaxic centre normally inhibits the apneustic centre. There is also a voluntary pathway of control by the cerebral cortex with descending pathways to the respiratory centre.

The respiratory cycle

Descending neurons from the respiratory centre terminate on the motor neurons controlling the respiratory muscles. As inspiration starts, there is a rapid increase in the number of nerve impulses from the DRG travelling along the phrenic and intercostal nerves to arrive at the respiratory muscles. The force of inspiration gradually increases and thoracic expansion occurs. At the end of inspiration the DRG becomes dormant and there is a sudden reduction in the number of impulses, resulting in relaxation of the respiratory muscles and passive elastic recoil of the thoracic cage and lungs. Inspiration lasts about 2 s and expiration about 3 s. This cycle is repeated about 12–18 times in a minute but the level of ventilation is continuously adapted to changes in bodily requirements or atmospheric conditions so that adequate oxygenation is maintained.

Factors influencing the rate and depth of breathing

Multiple factors are involved in the regulation of respiration. These include neural, mechanical and chemical events and are best summarised in a diagram (Fig. 18.6).

Voluntary control of breathing

Voluntary control of the rate and rhythm of respiration, such as hyperventilation or breath holding, is limited by the chemical stimuli that such efforts induce. Complex

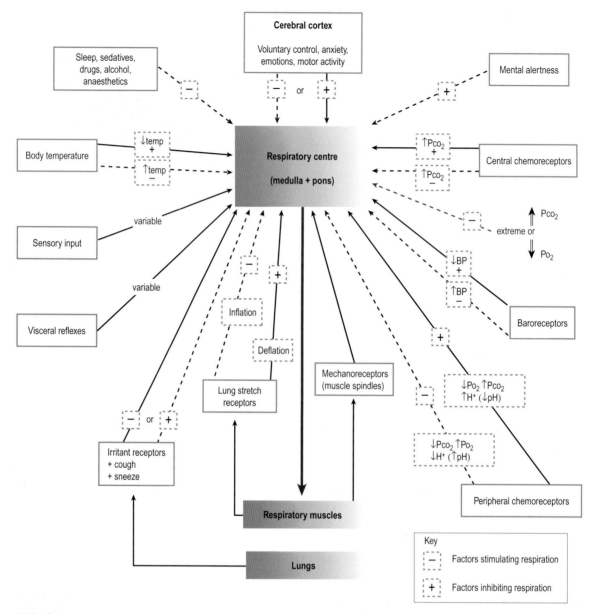

Figure 18.6 • Summary of factors controlling respiration. (From Hinchliff S M, Montague S E 1990, with permission.)

control of the respiratory system is necessary during speech and singing as well as playing a musical wind instrument. Response to emotional states with laughing and crying also change respiratory patterns. When nerve impulses are sent to the vocal cords, simultaneous impulses are sent to the respiratory centre to control the flow of air between the vocal cords. Mental states influence respiratory rhythm: mental alertness and wakefulness have a stimulating effect and sleep, sedatives, alcohol and some anaesthetics have an inhibitory effect.

Chemoreceptor effects

Both peripheral and central chemoreceptors are able to respond to small changes in arterial Po_2 and Pco_2 to

affect the rate and rhythm of respiration. **Peripheral chemoreceptors** are situated in the carotid bodies and other vascular structures around the aortic arch (Fig. 18.7). These receptors respond to chemical changes in the blood. They sense the levels of Po_2, Pco_2 and H^+ ions and relay the information to the respiratory centre.

The response to oxygen levels depends primarily on these peripheral chemoreceptors but the response to excessive levels of CO_2 (**hypercapnia**) depends on **central chemoreceptors** situated under the surface of the medulla. It is probable that with a rise in arterial Pco_2 carbon dioxide crosses the blood–brain barrier from the cerebral blood vessels into the cerebrospinal fluid (CSF). This bathes the central chemoreceptors. Once in the CSF, hydrogen ions are released (as in Eqn 18.2)

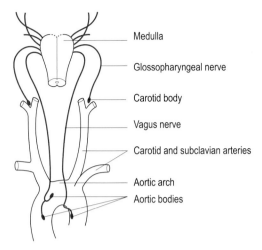

Figure 18.7 • Peripheral chemoreceptor system involved in the control of breathing. (From Hinchliff S M, Montague S E 1990, with permission.)

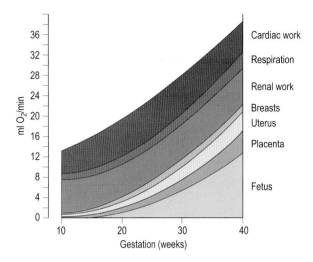

Figure 18.8 • Partition of the increased oxygen consumption in pregnancy among the organs concerned. (Reproduced with permission from de Swiet 1991.)

and these stimulate the central chemoreceptors, sending excitatory messages to the respiratory centre to increase the rate of respiration. A fall in Pco_2 will inhibit respiration.

The Hering–Breuer reflex

Stretch receptors are present in the visceral pleura and in the conducting passages in the lungs and are stimulated if the lungs are overinflated. Inhibitory impulses are sent by these receptors via the vagus nerve to the medullary inspiratory centre, resulting in the termination of inspiration so that expiration can occur. The stretch receptors quieten down as the lungs recoil so that inspiration can begin again. This is called the **inflation** or **Hering–Breuer** reflex.

Maternal adaptations to pregnancy

Pregnancy is associated with major changes in the respiratory system in lung volume and ventilation. The anatomical and functional changes during pregnancy are needed to meet the increased metabolic needs for oxygen of the maternal body and fetoplacental unit (Fig. 18.8). The changes occur very early due to hormonal and biochemical influences, even before the growing uterus impairs ventilation.

Upper respiratory tract changes

The mucosa of the nasopharynx becomes more hyperaemic and oedematous during pregnancy with hypersecretion of mucus due to the increase in circulating oestrogen. As a result there may be marked nasal stuffiness, the occurrence of epistaxis is more common, and

polyposis of the nose and nasal sinuses may develop in some women although these will regress postpartum (Gordon 2007).

Anatomical changes

The muscles and cartilage of the thorax relax, creating anatomical changes in the shape of the chest. These develop as pregnancy progresses and have implications for respiratory function (Fig. 18.9). The diaphragm becomes raised by a maximum of 4 cm and the transverse diameter of the chest is increased by 2 cm. The subcostal angle widens from the normal 68° to 103° in late pregnancy (Funai et al 2008). There is a change from abdominal to thoracic breathing, the main work of respiration being carried out by increased diaphragmatic movement during pregnancy. Some of these changes occur in advance of the increasing size of the uterus.

Biochemical changes

Maternal pulmonary ventilation increases by 40% during pregnancy, possibly because of a direct effect of progesterone on respiratory mechanisms in the brainstem (Johnson 2007).

Carbon dioxide

The tendency to overbreathe causes CO_2 to be washed out of the lungs so that the alveolar and arterial CO_2 concentration is lower than in the non-pregnant woman. This reduction in arterial Pco_2, from a norm of 35–40 mmHg (4.7–5.3 kPa) to a level of 30 mmHg (4 kPa), has been found in the luteal phase of each menstrual cycle before any embedding of a fertilised ovum is possible.

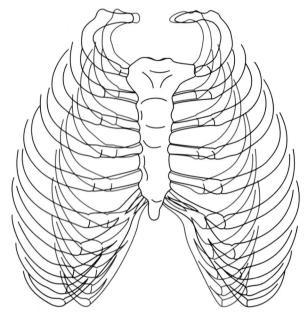

Figure 18.9 • The rib cage in pregnancy and the non-pregnancy state showing the increased subcostal angle, the increased transverse diameter and the raised diaphragm in pregnancy. (Reproduced with permission from de Swiet 1991.)

It is the result of progesterone, which is thought to stimulate the respiratory centres directly, causing an increased sensitivity to CO_2 with a lowered threshold (Blackburn 2007). Progesterone also causes an increase in carbonic anhydrase in the red cells, which in turn facilitates CO_2 transfer, tending to decrease P_{CO_2} even without the presence of a change in ventilation. The resulting mild respiratory alkalosis is essential to create the gas gradients for exchange across the placenta (Funai et al 2008).

Progesterone may also contribute to the decrease in airway resistance by relaxing the smooth muscles of the bronchioles (up to 50%). This will reduce the work of breathing and facilitate a greater airway flow in pregnancy. Prostaglandins may also influence the smooth muscle in the lung tissue, with $PGF_{2\alpha}$ acting as a bronchoconstrictor and PGE_1 and PGE_2 acting as bronchodilators (Blackburn 2007). Increases have been seen in PGFs throughout pregnancy and PGEs in the last trimester but their role is not clear.

Oxygen

The increased alveolar ventilation not only causes a decrease in P_{CO_2} but also raises P_{O_2}. However, this rise is only slight and has no significance on the oxygen–haemoglobin dissociation curve. During pregnancy, maternal O_2 consumption at rest and during exercise is increased compared with non-pregnant female proportionate to the growing tissue mass of pregnancy (Johnson 2007).

Respiratory parameters

The respiratory parameters discussed by Funai et al (2008) are summarised below.

Pregnancy causes less stress to the respiratory system than to the cardiovascular system. Therefore women with respiratory disease are less likely to show deterioration in their condition than those with cardiac disease. Over the years, findings from studies both support and refute an increase in vital capacity during pregnancy. The truth may be that some, but not all, pregnant women increase or decrease their vital capacity during pregnancy and the difference may be related to body build. Where there is probably an increase, this has taken place from mid-pregnancy and is of the order of 100–200 ml.

Recent studies agree that inspiratory capacity increases by about 300 ml and this occurs progressively throughout pregnancy. Expiratory reserve volume reduces by 200 ml progressively from early pregnancy. Tidal volume rises throughout pregnancy from the normal 500 ml to about 700 ml, an increase of 40%. Therefore ventilation increases during pregnancy by the woman deepening her respirations and not by breathing more frequently. Minute ventilation rises by 40% in parallel with tidal volume. Oxygen consumption increases by about 16% and alveolar ventilation is increased by 50%, resulting in a physiological change to overbreathing.

Postpartum changes

The changes in the respiratory system rapidly return to normal after delivery. This is initiated by the fall in progesterone levels following delivery of the placenta and the reduction in intra-abdominal pressure following delivery of the baby. A rise in P_{CO_2} is seen within 48 h of delivery. Overall, anatomical changes and ventilation parameters return to normal between 1 and 3 weeks following delivery (Blackburn 2007).

Clinical implications

Dyspnoea

As discussed above, the resting pregnant woman increases her ventilation, oxygen consumption and minute ventilation and there is a physiological change to overbreathing. The major influence leading to the overbreathing is central respiratory control but there are alterations in the lung volumes due to the anatomical changes mentioned above. The woman may be uncomfortable with dyspnoea and giddiness and mention or complain of 'shortness of breath'. This is not always related to exercise but is more likely to be present when sitting down rather than when walking about.

Smoking

Smoking remains one of the potentially preventable factors associated with adverse pregnancy and birth outcomes and for this reason it is an important public health issue in pregnancy (Enkin et al 2000). It is probably one of the most dangerous avoidable risks taken by people and it is essential that both men and women who are thinking about starting a family should stop smoking for the health and safety of mother and baby (Foresight 2006). Cigarette smoking during pregnancy is common and between 1 in 5 and 1 in 3 pregnant women in developed countries report smoking. There is strong evidence to suggest that cigarette smoking has harmful effects on the fetus in addition to the adverse health outcomes for the mother. The effects of smoking on human reproduction are discussed in Chapter 8, where the following list is addressed in detail.

Major reproductive effects of tobacco smoking on reproduction

- Male and female infertility.
- Very preterm birth.
- Low birth weight.
- Spontaneous abortions.
- Increased perinatal mortality (stillbirths + neonatal deaths in the 1st week).
- Fetal malformations.
- Reduced immunocompetence.

Main points

- The process of respiration enables the exchange of gases between the body and the atmosphere. Oxygen is taken from the atmosphere and transported around the body in the blood to the tissues. Carbon dioxide, produced as metabolic waste by the cells, is returned to the lungs and excreted into the air.
- The respiratory system consists of the airways from the nasal passages to the alveoli of the lungs which provide an enormous area for gas exchange. Pulmonary surfactant helps to keep the membrane moist and also acts to maintain the patency of the alveolus.
- Inspiration and expiration are the two phases of breathing. Mechanical and neural factors are involved in the control of respiration rate. Expiration is a passive process and active expiration may occur when the need for gas exchange increases.
- Respiratory parameters include tidal volume, inspiratory reserve volume, expiratory reserve volume and residual volume. Respiratory capacities include total lung capacity, vital capacity, inspiratory capacity and functional residual capacity.
- The relationship between haemoglobin saturation and Po_2 is called the oxygen dissociation curve. Several factors can influence the affinity of haemoglobin for oxygen. In situations where the oxygen dissociation curve moves to the right then this enhances the unloading of oxygen to the cells. In contrast, if the oxygen dissociation curve moves to the left then this inhibits oxygen transfer.

- The control of breathing involves the respiratory centre in the medulla and neural, mechanical and chemical events. Both peripheral and central chemoreceptors are able to respond to small changes in arterial Po_2 and Pco_2, affecting the rate and rhythm of respiration.
- In pregnancy, changes in the respiratory system are brought about by hormonal and biochemical influences as well as by the mechanical effect of the enlarging uterus.
- Respiratory function is affected by the mechanical changes of pregnancy. The diaphragm is pushed upwards and the transverse diameter of the chest increases. Breathing changes from abdominal to thoracic, with increased diaphragmatic movement.
- Inspiratory capacity increases progressively throughout pregnancy. Ventilation during pregnancy increases by the woman deepening her respirations and not by breathing more.
- The pregnant woman may be uncomfortable with dyspnoea and giddiness perceived as shortage of breath. This is more likely to occur when sitting down.
- Smoking is a preventable factor associated with adverse pregnancy and birth outcomes. Some adverse effects on reproduction include male and female infertility, premature birth, low birth weight and increased perinatal mortality. It is an important public health issue in pregnancy.

References

Blackburn, S.T., 2007. Maternal, Fetal and Neonatal Physiology: A clinical perspective, 4th edn. Elsevier Saunders, Missouri.

Enkin, M., Keirse, M.J.N.C., Neilson, J., et al., 2000. A Guide to Effective Care in Pregnancy, 3rd edn. Oxford University Press, Oxford.

Foresight 2006 The adverse effects of tobacco smoking on reproduction (literature review by Tuormaa T E 1995,

first published in Nutrition and Health). Foresight, AB Academic Publishers, Tacoma, Washington.

Funai, E.F., Gillen-Goldstein, J., Roque, H., 2008. Changes in the Respiratory Tract During Pregnancy. UpToDate Inc.

Gordon, M.C., et al., 2007. Maternal physiology in pregnancy. In: Gabbe, S.G., Simpson, J.L., Niebyl, J.R. (Eds.) Obstetrics: Normal and Problem

pregnancies, 5th edn. Churchill Livingstone, London.

Johnson, M.H., 2007. Essential Reproduction, 6th edn. Blackwell, Cambridge.

Marieb, E.N., Hoehn, K., 2008. Anatomy and Physiology, 3rd edn. Pearson Benjamin/Cummings, New York.

Sherwood, L., 2006. Human Physiology: From cells to systems, 6th edn. Brookes Cole, New York.

Annotated recommended reading

Foresight 2006 The Adverse Effects of Tobacco Smoking on Reproduction (literature review by Tuormaa T E 1995, first published in Nutrition and Health). Foresight, AB Academic Publishers, Tacoma, Washington.

This publication provides a detailed literature review of the adverse effects of smoking on reproduction.

Sherwood, L., 2006. Human Physiology: From Cells to Systems, 6th edn. Brookes Cole, New York.

This textbook provides an in-depth introduction to the respiratory system and is suitable for undergraduate students in health-related studies.

Website

UpToDate is an evidence-based, peer-reviewed information resource, available via the Web, desktop and PDA through many educational and professional institutions.

Chapter Nineteen

19

The renal tract

Introduction

The structure and function of the renal tract and how these change in pregnancy will be discussed within this chapter. Although the production of urine is also discussed, fluid and electrolyte balance and the regulation of acid–base balance are discussed in Chapter 20 in an attempt to integrate the roles of the respiratory and renal systems. This should be of value to the reader interested in the interactions between systems and may avoid turning backwards and forwards in the text to synthesise material. The role of renin and the angiotensin–aldosterone system and the control of blood pressure will be discussed in Chapter 20.

Kidney functions

The kidneys play a major role in maintenance of homeostasis within the internal environment by their regulation of the volume and composition of the body fluids. Each day the kidneys filter several litres of fluid from the bloodstream, ensuring that toxins, metabolic wastes and excess ions are excreted from the body in urine. Other than the excretory function, the roles of the kidney are:

- Regulation of the volume and chemical make-up of the blood.
- Maintenance of balance between water and salts, acids and bases.
- Production of the enzyme renin, which helps to regulate blood pressure, and production of the hormone erythropoietin, which stimulates red cell production in the bone marrow.
- Conversion of vitamin D to its active form.

Also part of the renal system are the two ureters, which convey urine to the urinary bladder where urine is stored until it is voided through the urethra.

Anatomy of the kidney

The kidneys are paired, compact organs situated on either side of the vertebral column between the 12th thoracic and the 3rd lumbar vertebrae. They are situated behind the peritoneum and are attached to the posterior abdominal wall by adipose tissue. An adult kidney is bean-shaped with a convex lateral surface and concave medial surface. A cleft in the medial surface is called the **hilum** and leads to a space within the kidney called the **renal sinus**. The hilum is the site of entry and exit of structures that include the ureters, renal blood vessels, lymphatics and nerves. Each kidney weighs about 150 g and measures 12 cm long, 6 cm wide and 3 cm thick. The adrenal gland sits on top of the kidney.

Structure

Three layers of supporting tissue surround each kidney:

1. The **renal capsule** is closest to the kidney and is fibrous and transparent. This is a strong barrier that prevents infections in nearby regions spreading to the kidneys.

2. The **adipose capsule** is a middle layer of fatty tissue that helps hold the kidney in place and protects it from trauma.

3. The **renal fascia** is the outermost covering and is made of dense fibrous connective tissue that surrounds both kidney and adrenal gland and anchors them to surrounding structures.

Beneath the capsule lie three distinct regions: the outer **cortex**, the **medulla** and the inner **renal pelvis** (Fig. 19.1). The cortex has a light granular appearance. The medulla is darker and reddish brown with cone-shaped masses of tissue called **medullary** or **renal pyramids**. The base of each pyramid is broad and faces the renal cortex while the pointed apex **(papilla)** projects into a minor calyx. Several minor calyces open into each of two or three major calyces, which then open into the renal pelvis. The pyramids have a striped appearance because they consist of bundles of microscopic tubules. The renal columns are extensions of cortical tissue that separate the pyramids. Each medullary pyramid and its cap of cortical tissue is known as a **lobe** of the kidney. There are usually between 8 and 18 lobes in a kidney.

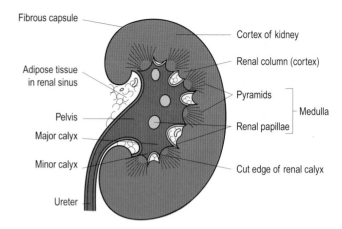

Figure 19.1 • Coronal section through a kidney. (From Hinchliff S M, Montague S E 1990, with permission.)

The renal pelvis

The renal pelvis is a flat funnel-shaped tube that is continuous with the ureter. The urine produced by the kidney flows continuously from the papillae into the calyces and down the ureter where it is then stored in the bladder. The walls of the calyces, pelvis and ureter contain smooth muscle, which contracts in peristaltic movements to propel urine towards the bladder.

Microscopic structure of the kidney

Each kidney contains over 1 million nephrons, which are the functional units of the kidney. Each nephron consists of a renal tubule and a tuft of blood vessel capillaries called the **glomerulus**. The end of the tubule, called a **Bowman's capsule**, is enlarged and invaginated to hold the glomerulus. The outer or parietal layer of the Bowman's capsule is composed of simple squamous epithelium and has a purely structural function. The inner or visceral layer that clings to the glomerulus is made up of branching epithelial cells called **podocytes** which form part of the filtration membrane. The branches of the podocytes end in **pedicles** or foot processes. The clefts between the pedicles form filtration slits or slit pores.

The capillary endothelium of the glomerulus is porous, which allows large quantities of solute-rich fluid to pass from the blood into the glomerular capsule. This fluid is called the **filtrate** and is processed by the renal tubules to form urine. A basement membrane divides the endothelium of the capillary from the epithelium lining the Bowman's capsule. The Bowman's capsule and its contained glomerulus are known as a **renal corpuscle** and are situated in the renal cortex. The structure comprising the capillary endothelium, basement membrane and podocytic epithelium constitutes the selective filtration barrier.

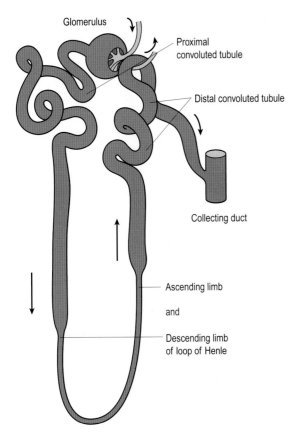

Figure 19.2 • Microanatomy of nephron. (From Hinchliff S M, Montague S E 1990, with permission.)

The remainder of the renal tubule is about 3 cm long and can be divided into four anatomically distinct regions: the proximal convoluted tubule, the loop of Henle, the distal convoluted tubule and the collecting duct (Fig. 19.2).

The **proximal convoluted tubule** extends about 16 mm through the cortex. This region of the tubule is lined by large columnar epithelial cells, which have a brush border of microvilli on their internal surface for solute reabsorption.

The **loop of Henle** has a descending limb and an ascending limb. The thin-walled descending limb extends from the proximal convoluted tubule, dips down into the medulla and makes a U turn, moving back into the cortex by the thick-walled ascending limb. In this loop the columnar cells are flatter and contain fewer microvilli on their luminal (side facing into the lumen) surfaces.

The **distal convoluted tubule**, continuous with the loop of Henle, is comparatively short (about 4–8 mm) and leads into the **collecting ducts**, which fuse together as they approach the renal pelvis to form papillary ducts. These ducts open at the tips of the medullary papillae to discharge their urine into the calyces and renal pelvis. The first part of the distal tubule folds back to bring it nearer to the afferent arteriole. This forms the juxtaglomerular apparatus (see below).

Cortical and juxtamedullary nephrons

About 85% of the nephrons are called **cortical nephrons** because they are situated in the cortex (except where their loops of Henle dip into the medulla). The remaining 15% of nephrons are different in structure and are called **juxtaglomerular nephrons**. They are located near the cortex–medullary junction and their loops of Henle are found deep in the medulla. Their thin segments are more extensive than those of the cortical nephrons. The juxtamedullary nephrons have long thin-walled looping capillaries, called the **vasa recta**, running parallel with their loops of Henle.

Capillary beds of the nephron

Every nephron is closely associated with two capillary beds which form the microvasculature of the nephron. These are the glomerulus and the peritubular capillary bed. The glomerulus is unlike any other capillary bed because it is fed and drained by arterioles. Glomeruli originate from an afferent arteriole arising from interlobular arteries that permeate the renal cortex and drain into efferent arterioles. The peritubular capillary bed consists of capillaries arising from the efferent arterioles draining the glomeruli. These capillaries cling closely to the renal tubules and empty into nearby venules. Just as the glomerular capillary bed is adapted for filtration, the peritubular bed is adapted for reabsorption. They are low-pressure porous capillaries. The additional vessels of the vasa recta play a part in reabsorption of salts.

The blood pressure within the glomerular capillary bed is very high for two reasons:

1. Arterioles are high-resistance vessels.

2. The afferent arteriole has a much larger diameter than the efferent arteriole.

This high pressure forces fluids and solutes out of the glomerular blood along its entire length into the Bowman's capsule. About 99% of this filtrate is reabsorbed into the blood in the peritubular capillary beds. As blood flows into the renal circulation, it encounters high resistance, first in the afferent and then in the efferent arterioles. Renal blood pressure declines from 95 mmHg in the renal arteries to 8 mmHg in the renal veins. The resistance of the afferent arterioles protects the kidney from large fluctuations in the systemic blood pressure. Resistance in the efferent arterioles maintains the high glomerular pressure and reduces the hydrostatic pressure in the peritubular arteries to facilitate reabsorption.

The juxtaglomerular apparatus

The juxtaglomerular apparatus is a region found in each nephron where the distal convoluted tubule lies against the afferent arteriole as it supplies the glomerulus (Fig. 19.3). Where the two parts of the nephron touch,

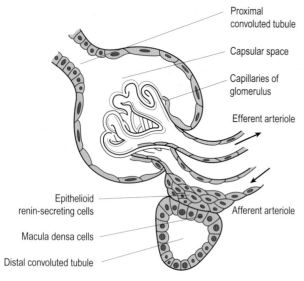

Proximal convoluted tubule

Capsular space

Capillaries of glomerulus

Efferent arteriole

Afferent arteriole

Epithelioid renin-secreting cells

Macula densa cells

Distal convoluted tubule

Figure 19.3 • The juxtaglomerular apparatus showing the macula densa. (Redrawn from Creager 1983.)

the cellular structures are modified. The afferent arteriolar wall contains juxtaglomerular cells. These are enlarged smooth muscle cells that contain granules filled with **renin**. They seem to be mechanoreceptors responding to the blood pressure in the afferent arterioles. The **macula densa** is a group of tall, closely packed distal tubule cells that act as chemoreceptors or osmoreceptors responding to sodium chloride concentration in the distal tubule. These two types of cell are important in the regulation of filtrate formation and systemic blood pressure.

Blood supply

About 25% of cardiac output is delivered each minute to the kidneys. This is a higher blood supply than to any other tissue. The two renal arteries arise high up on the abdominal aorta and enter the hilum, dividing in the renal tissue to form interlobar arteries between the pyramids. Arcuate arteries arise here and give rise to interlobular arteries, which branch to form the afferent arterioles supplying each glomerulus. Efferent arterioles emerge from the glomerulus and form a dense peritubular capillary network. Venous capillaries drain into interlobular, arcuate and interlobar veins and then into the renal veins. The renal veins drain into the inferior vena cava that lies to the right of the vertebral column. Therefore, the left renal vein must be twice as long as the right one.

Nerve supply

The kidneys are supplied by the autonomic nervous system. There is a rich supply of sympathetic fibres and a few parasympathetic fibres. These fibres supply the smooth muscle of the arterioles and the juxtaglomerular apparatus. Stimulation of these nerves causes vasoconstriction, a reduced renal blood flow, a reduced glomerular filtration rate (GFR) and the release of renin from the juxtaglomerular apparatus. The kidneys also have some sensory nerve fibres that allow the sensation of pain to be perceived. These fibres are stimulated by distension of the renal capsule in such situations as bleeding, inflammation or obstruction by renal calculi. Ischaemia may also cause pain.

Renal function

The production of urine

In an adult about 180 litres of plasma are filtered every day and 99% of the filtrate is reabsorbed by the nephrons. This results in the production of about 1.5 litres of urine per day. Fluid intake, diet and extrarenal fluid losses will affect the amount of urine produced (Sherwood 2006). Glomerular filtration is the first step in urine production. Prior to describing the physiology of glomerular filtration, some concepts to facilitate understanding will be briefly outlined.

Electrolytes

These substances are solutes that are electrically charged and dissociate into their constituent ions when placed in solution. Electrolytes are polarised into those carrying a positive charge (**cations**) and those carrying a negative charge (**anions**). They are located in both extracellular fluid (ECF) and intracellular fluid (ICF). In ECF, sodium is the cation (Na^+) and chloride is the main anion (Cl^-). In ICF, potassium is the cation (K^+) and protein the anion. Electrolytes are measured in milliequivalents per litre (mEq/L), which is the number of electrical charges per litre.

Diffusion

Diffusion is the movement of a solute molecule down a concentration gradient across a permeable membrane. This movement depends on the electrical potential across the membrane, the particle size, lipid solubility and water solubility.

Osmosis

Osmosis is the movement of **water** down a concentration gradient across a semipermeable membrane from a high water content to a lower one. The membrane must be more permeable to water than to the solutes and there must be a greater concentration of solutes in the destination solution for water to move easily. Osmosis is directly related to hydrostatic pressure and solute concentration but not to particle size. For example, in the plasma the protein albumin is smaller but more concentrated than the protein globulin; therefore albumin exerts the greater osmotic force for drawing fluid back from the ECF into the intravascular compartment.

Osmolality is the concentration of molecules per weight of water, measured in milliosmoles/kilogram. **Osmolarity** is the concentration of molecules in water, measured in millosmoles/litre of water. The two terms are often used interchangeably.

Hydrostatic pressure

Hydrostatic pressure is the mechanical force of water pushing against cell membranes. In the vascular system it is generated by the blood pressure. In the capillaries a hydrostatic pressure of 25 mmHg is sufficient to push water across the capillary membrane into the extracellular space. It is partly balanced by **osmotic pressure**. The excess water moves into the lymph system.

The amount of hydrostatic pressure needed to oppose the osmotic pressure of the solution depends on the type and thickness of the plasma membrane, size of the molecules, concentration of the molecules on the gradient and solubility of the molecules. An example would be the movement of water in the glomerulus of the kidney.

Tonicity is the effective osmolality of a solution. Solutions can be: **isotonic**, with the same concentration of particles as the body fluids; **hypotonic**, with less concentration of particles (will cause water to be pulled into the cells by osmosis); or **hypertonic**, with more concentration of particles (will cause water to be pulled out of the cells).

Oncotic pressure is the overall osmotic effect of the plasma proteins, sometimes called colloid osmotic pressure.

pH and acid–base balance

The pH is a measure of the **hydrogen ion concentration** [H^+]. It is the negative logarithm of the hydrogen ions in solution on a scale of 1–14. This means that from one pH unit to the next there is a 10-fold change in hydrogen ion concentration. It is negative because as hydrogen decreases, the pH value increases. Low pH values with more hydrogen ions result in an acid solution and high pH values with a low hydrogen ion concentration result in an alkaline solution. A pH of 7 is neutral and most body fluids, with the exception of acid gastric juices (pH 1–3) and urine (pH 5–6), are just alkaline with a pH between 7 and 8. Many pathological conditions disturb the acid–base balance.

Glomerular filtration

Filtration is a largely passive, non-selective process in which fluids and solutes are forced through a membrane (i.e. filtrate) by hydrostatic pressure (Marieb & Hoehn 2008). The passage of water and solutes across the filtration membrane of the glomerulus is similar to that in other capillary beds, moving down a pressure gradient. However, the glomerular filtration membrane is thousands of times more permeable to water and solutes and glomerular pressure is much higher than normal capillary blood pressure. There is a high net filtration pressure.

This results in 180 litres of filtrate per day compared to the 4 L/day formed by all other capillary beds combined. Unlike other capillary beds, where water and solutes move back into the capillary as the balance of hydrostatic pressure changes, movement is one way only, from the capillary into the glomerulus. The **glomerular filtration rate** (GFR) is the volume of plasma filtered through the glomeruli in 1 min and is normally 120 ml/min.

The filtration membrane of the glomerulus lies between the blood and the interior of the glomerular capsule. As described above, it is a porous membrane made up of three layers:

1. The fenestrated capillary endothelium.

2. The podocytic visceral membrane of the glomerular capsule.

3. The intervening basement membrane.

The membrane allows free passage of water, solutes and small protein molecules (less than 3 nm in diameter), but larger molecules such as blood cells and larger protein molecules are prevented from passing through by the capillary pores. The basement membrane may also act as a selective molecular sieve. It is made up of anionic (negatively charged) glycoproteins and therefore repels filtrate anions and prevents their passage; therefore the filtrate contains more cationic (positively charged) and uncharged molecules. The presence of the plasma proteins in the capillary provides the colloid osmotic pressure of the glomerular blood, limiting the loss of water to one-fifth of the plasma fluid.

Regulation of glomerular filtration

Intrinsic control by autoregulation

The kidney can control its own blood supply over a wide range of arterial blood pressure, from 80 to 180 mmHg. This intrinsic system is called **autoregulation** and

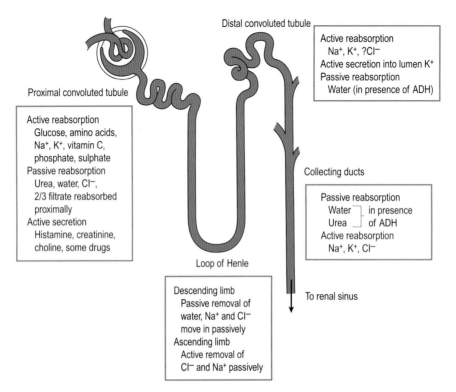

Distal convoluted tubule

Active reabsorption
  Na⁺, K⁺, ?Cl⁻
Active secretion into lumen K⁺
Passive reabsorption
  Water (in presence of ADH)

Proximal convoluted tubule

Active reabsorption
  Glucose, amino acids,
  Na⁺, K⁺, vitamin C,
  phosphate, sulphate
Passive reabsorption
  Urea, water, Cl⁻,
  2/3 filtrate reabsorbed
  proximally
Active secretion
  Histamine, creatinine,
  choline, some drugs

Collecting ducts

Passive reabsorption
  Water ⎤ in presence
  Urea ⎦ of ADH
Active reabsorption
  Na⁺, K⁺, Cl⁻

To renal sinus

Loop of Henle

Descending limb
  Passive removal of
  water, Na⁺ and Cl⁻
  move in passively
Ascending limb
  Active removal of
  Cl⁻ and Na⁺ passively

Figure 19.4 ● Regional specialisation in reabsorption and secretion in the nephron. Throughout the nephron, exchange of Na^+ for H^+, HCO_3 reabsorption and NH_2 secretion occur. (From Hinchliff S M, Montague S E 1990, with permission.)

depends on alterations in the diameter of the afferent and efferent arterioles in response to a systemic blood pressure change. Factors involved in autoregulation may include:

- The myogenic mechanism—the tendency of vascular smooth muscle to contract when stretched.
- A tubuloglomerular feedback mechanism directed by the macula densa cells and solute concentration.
- The renin–angiotensin mechanism and renal vasoconstriction (see below).
- Prostaglandin E_2 and renal vasodilation.

Extrinsic control by sympathetic nervous system stimulation

When the body is stressed, adrenaline (epinephrine) is released into the blood from the adrenal medulla. This causes strong constriction of the afferent arterioles and inhibits filtrate formation. Blood can be shunted to the brain and muscles at the expense of the kidneys. The juxtaglomerular cells are also stimulated to release renin, which activates angiotensin II to raise systemic blood pressure by generalised vasoconstriction. If there is a less intensive response, afferent and efferent arterioles are constricted to the same extent. This restricts blood flow out of the glomerulus as well as into it and GFR declines only slightly.

Tubular reabsorption and secretion

During the second stage of urine production, the filtrate is greatly modified as it moves along the tubule. Most reabsorption occurs in the proximal tubule where two-thirds of the filtrate is removed. Prior to this modification, filtrate is similar in every way to plasma, except it does not contain blood cells and large protein molecules. Figure 19.4 shows regional specialisation in reabsorption and secretion by the nephron.

Vital solutes such as glucose, amino acids and electrolytes are reabsorbed together with water. They pass from the lumen of the nephron, across the epithelial layer into the peritubular capillary network. A few substances are secreted into the filtrate from the peritubular capillaries. Mechanisms for reabsorption from the nephron may be active or passive.

Transport mechanisms in the nephron

Active transfer

Active transfer is the uphill movement of solutes against an unfavourable chemical or electrical gradient. Solutes move from a low to a high chemical concentration or electrical potential. Energy in the form of adenosine triphosphate (ATP) is used. Sodium is actively transported bound to a carrier protein. About 80% of energy is used in the transport of sodium ions. Substances actively reabsorbed include glucose, amino acids, lactate, vitamins and most ions. Many of these are cotransported bound to the sodium carrier complex (Martini & Nath 2009). There is a transport maximum depending on the number of carriers available in the renal tubule. When the maximum is exceeded any surplus substance will be excreted in the urine. This is what happens when people develop glycosuria.

Passive transfer

Passive transfer is the movement of non-electrolytes and ions across cell membranes according to the chemical or electrical gradients that prevail. Solutes could be said to move downhill from an area of high to low chemical concentration or electrical potential (see Ch. 2). No energy is directly used in passive transfer. Passive transfer includes diffusion, facilitated diffusion and osmosis.

Positively charged sodium ions are moved from the tubule to the peritubular capillaries and create an electrical gradient that favours the transfer of anions such as HCO_3^- and HCl^- so that electrical neutrality is restored in the plasma and filtrate. Sodium movement also establishes a strong osmotic gradient so that water moves from the lumen of the tubule into the peritubular capillaries. This movement of water out of the tubule increases the concentration of solutes in the filtrate and they begin to follow their concentration gradients out of the tubules. This movement of solutes after the solvent is called **solvent drag**.

Non-reabsorbed substances

Substances are not reabsorbed because:

- They lack carriers.
- They are not lipid-soluble and cannot diffuse through cell membranes.
- They are too large to pass through the plasma membrane pores in the tubular cells.

These substances include the end-products of protein and nucleic acid metabolism: urea, creatinine and uric acid. Urea is a small molecule and about 45% is reabsorbed, but creatinine is not reabsorbed at all; it is therefore a useful substance to measure when assessing GFR and glomerular function.

Tubular secretion

Tubular secretion is an important mechanism in clearing the blood of unwanted substances. Urine is therefore composed of both filtered and secreted substances. Secreted substances include hydrogen ions, ammonia and drug metabolites. Also secreted into the tubules are drugs such as penicillin and undesirable substances that might have been reabsorbed such as urea or excess potassium ions.

Regulation of urine concentration and volume

The role of the kidney in maintaining fluid and electrolyte balance and regulating pH is discussed in detail in Chapter 20. Briefly, an important function of the kidney is to keep the solute load of the body constant by regulating urine concentration and volume. This is accomplished by a function called the **countercurrent exchange**. The term countercurrent exchange means that something flows in opposite directions through adjacent channels. In this case, the loop of Henle and its adjacent blood vessels, the vasa recta, are involved.

The descending limb of the loop of Henle is quite impermeable to solutes and permeable to water. Water passes out of the filtrate into the interstitial fluid by osmosis along the course of the descending loop and the solute load becomes concentrated. The ascending limb of the loop of Henle is impermeable to water and actively transports sodium into the surrounding interstitial fluid. The concentration of solutes in the filtrate as it enters the ascending limb is very high. Sodium is pumped out of the lumen into the interstitial fluid. The urine becomes more dilute and becomes hypotonic with respect to plasma.

The two loops are close enough to influence each other's activity. Water diffusing out of the descending limb produces the salty filtrate that the ascending limb uses to raise the osmolarity of the medullary interstitial fluid. The more salt the ascending limb extrudes, the saltier the filtrate in the descending limb becomes. This positive feedback mechanism is referred to as a **countercurrent multiplier**.

The collecting tubules add to the osmolality of the renal medulla by allowing urea to leak out into the interstitial space.

The vasa recta are freely permeable to both water and salt and provide another countercurrent exchange to regulate the content of the interstitial fluid while still maintaining the gradient established by the loop of Henle. Blood moving down the descending limb of the vasa recta gains solutes and loses water while in the ascending limb the blood loses solutes and gains water.

Formation of concentrated urine

Because water follows the osmotic gradients established by salt concentration, sodium and water balance are interrelated. Water balance is mainly regulated by antidiuretic hormone (ADH) from the posterior pituitary

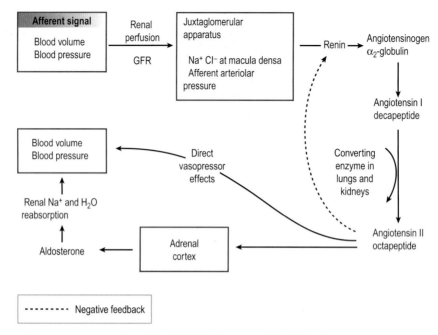

Figure 19.5 • The renin–aldosterone system. (From Hinchliff S M, Montague S E 1990, with permission.)

gland. The secretion of ADH is initiated by an increase in plasma osmolality, by a decrease in circulating blood volume and by a lowered blood pressure. If blood volume decreases, volume receptors (located in the right and left atria and thoracic vessels) and baroreceptors (located in the aorta, pulmonary arteries and carotid sinus) stimulate the release of ADH. The action of ADH is to increase the permeability of the renal tubular cells to water. Water absorption increases plasma volume and urine concentration is increased. This is called **facultative water reabsorption**. The amount of urine excreted is reduced and its concentration is increased.

The renin–angiotensin–aldosterone system

Sodium is regulated by aldosterone from the adrenal cortex. Sodium, along with its associated ions chloride and bicarbonate, regulates osmotic forces and therefore water balance. Sodium also works with potassium to maintain neurotransmission, regulate acid–base balance (via sodium bicarbonate) and participate in membrane reactions. The main anion in the ECF that neutralises the positive electrical charge of sodium is chloride. The transport of chloride is passive (following sodium) and concentrations of chloride vary inversely with concentrations of bicarbonate, which competes for sodium binding.

Concentrations of sodium are maintained within a narrow range of 136–145 mEq/L, primarily via renal tubular reabsorption. The average daily intake of sodium

is 6 g but the need is only 500 mg. If sodium is taken in excess a combination of hormonal (aldosterone), neural and renal mechanisms (via the renin–angiotensin system) work together to control the balance (Fig. 19.5). Renin is produced by the juxtaglomerular apparatus in the kidney and stimulates production of the inactive blood peptide angiotensin I. This is converted into the active angiotensin II, which acts as a hormone to stimulate the secretion of aldosterone and cause vasoconstriction.

Natriuretic hormone

The atria of the heart produce antinatriuretic hormone (ANH), which promotes urinary excretion of sodium by reducing tubular reabsorption. The excretion of sodium results in a diuresis. The hormone ANH is synthesised by the atrial myocytes and secreted into circulating blood by the coronary sinus. Increased right atrial pressure stimulates this hormone release. Increased circulating blood volume causes increased pressure on the atrial myocytes and the release of hormone seems to be directly related to the degree of mechanical load.

The lower urinary tract

The ureters

The structural changes occurring in the lower urinary tract are important and need to be taken into account by those involved in caring for pregnant women. The

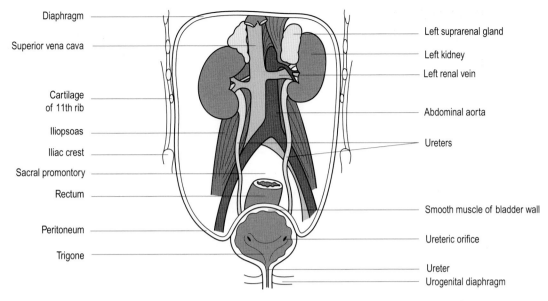

Figure 19.6 • Anatomy of the lower urinary tract. (From Hinchliff S M, Montague S E 1990, with permission.)

two ureters are hollow muscular tubes (Fig. 19.6). Urine that is secreted into the renal pelvis drains down through the ureters to be stored in the bladder. The muscle walls of the ureter undergo peristaltic movements to propel urine towards the bladder.

Structure

The walls of the ureters are composed of the following layers:

1. A lining layer of mucous membrane in longitudinal folds.

2. A fibrous tissue layer containing elastic fibres on which the epithelium rests.

3. A smooth muscle layer consisting of three sets of fibres – a weak inner layer of longitudinal fibres, a middle layer of circular fibres and an outer well-defined longitudinal layer.

4. A coat of fibrous connective tissue.

Situation and size

The ureters lie outside and behind the peritoneum throughout their length. They extend from the renal pelvis to the posterior wall of the urinary bladder, crossing the pelvic brim anterior to the sacroiliac joints. The ureters run through the pelvic fascia and pass through special tunnels in the cardinal ligaments. They enter the posterior bladder wall in front of the cervix and run at an oblique angle for about 20 mm, which prevents the back flow of urine. They open into the cavity of the bladder at the posterior lateral angles of the **trigone**. In an adult, the ureter is about 30 cm long and 3 mm in diameter.

Blood supply, lymphatic drainage and nerve supply to the ureters

Blood supply is from the common iliac, internal iliac, uterine and vesical arteries and drainage is by corresponding veins. Lymphatic drainage is to the internal, external and common iliac nodes. The nerve supply is via aortic, renal and hypogastric plexi.

The bladder

The bladder is a hollow, distensible muscular organ acting as a reservoir for the storage of urine. It is roughly pyramidal in shape when empty and lies in the pelvis. It has a posterior base or **trigone** (resting on the vagina) and an anterior apex. The bladder lies in the pelvis when empty. In a healthy adult the capacity of the bladder when full is normally 500 ml (300–700 ml). It then becomes globular and expands upwards and forwards into the abdomen when full.

The trigone of the bladder is triangular in shape and each side measures 2.5 cm. The two ureteric orifices are situated on either side of the base of the trigone and the apex is formed by the internal meatus of the urethra. This region may be called the **bladder neck**.

Structure

The bladder walls are formed of the following structures:

1. A lining of transitional epithelium resting on a layer of **areolar tissue**. The lining, except for the trigone, is thrown into folds or **rugae** to allow it to distend. Over the trigone the epithelium is firmly bound to the muscle.

2. Three coats of smooth muscle (inner longitudinal, middle circular and outer longitudinal) called the **detrusor muscle**. This contracts to expel urine during micturition. Around the internal meatus the circular muscle is thickened to form the **internal sphincter** of the bladder. This thickened muscle is in a state of sustained contraction except during micturition. There is a special arrangement of muscle fibres in the trigone. The fibres, which run between the ureteric openings, form a band known as the **interureteric ridge**. The muscle fibres running from each ureteric opening to the urethral orifice are also raised into ridges.

3. The upper surface of the bladder is covered by peritoneum reflected off the uterus to form the **uterovesical pouch**. Its remaining surfaces are covered by visceral pelvic fascia.

Ligaments

There are five ligaments attached to the bladder:

- A fibrous band called the **urachus** runs from the apex of the bladder to the umbilicus.
- Two **lateral ligaments** pass from the bladder to the side walls of the pelvis.
- Two **pubovesical ligaments** attach the bladder neck anteriorly to the pubic bones. They form part of the pubocervical ligaments of the uterus.

Relations

- Anterior: the pubic bones are separated from the bladder by a space filled with fatty tissue called the **cave of Retzius**.
- Posterior: the cervix and ureters.
- Lateral: the lateral ligaments of the bladder and the side walls of the pelvis.
- Superior: the body of the uterus and the intestines lying in the uterovesical pouch.
- Inferior: the upper half of the anterior vaginal wall and the levator ani muscles.

Blood supply, lymphatic drainage and nerve supply

Blood supply is from the superior and inferior vesical arteries and drainage is by corresponding veins. Lymphatic drainage is to the external iliac and obturator nodes. The nerve supply is via sympathetic and parasympathetic fibres of the autonomic system.

The urethra

In the female the urethra is a narrow tube about 4 cm long passing from the internal meatus of the bladder to the vestibule where it opens externally. It runs embedded in the lower half of the anterior vaginal wall. The internal sphincter surrounds it as it leaves the bladder. As it passes between the levator ani muscles it is enclosed by bands of striated muscle known as the **membranous sphincter** of the urethra, which is under voluntary control.

Structure

The walls of the urethra consist of the following layers:

1. The lumen is thrown into small longitudinal folds and is lined by transitional epithelium in the upper half and squamous epithelium in the lower half. It is normally closed.

2. A layer of vascular connective tissue.

3. An inner longitudinal layer of smooth muscle.

4. An outer circular layer of smooth muscle.

Several small crypts open into the urethra at its lowest point. The two largest are **Skene's ducts** and correspond to the prostate gland in the male.

Blood supply, lymphatic drainage and nerve supply

Blood supply is from the inferior vesical and pudendal arteries and drainage is by corresponding veins. Lymphatic drainage is to the internal iliac nodes. The nerve supply to the internal sphincter is from the sympathetic system and the voluntary control of the membranous sphincter is achieved via sympathetic and parasympathetic fibres of the autonomic system.

The physiology of micturition

Micturition requires the coordination of autonomic nerves and somatic nerves. Motor and sensory sympathetic and parasympathetic nerves pass to and from the bladder but the sympathetic fibres appear to play a minor role. When the bladder contains about 300 ml of urine, stretch receptors are stimulated and sensory parasympathetic nerves convey sensations of fullness to the basal ganglia, reticular formation and cortical centres of the brain. The need to pass urine is perceived but can be voluntarily postponed until a suitable time. There is a centre for the reflex control of micturition in the second to fourth sacral segments of the spinal cord. When the bladder contains 700 ml it may become impossible to avoid micturition.

Nerve impulses from the cerebral cortex increase parasympathetic activity and decrease sympathetic activity, causing relaxation of the internal sphincter and contraction of the detrusor muscle. The external sphincter is relaxed, intra-abdominal pressure is raised and expulsion of urine occurs. Cortical control of micturition is learned in infancy and usually achieved at about 2 years of age.

Maternal adaptations to pregnancy

During pregnancy the renal system undergoes a range of structural and functional changes with many of the structural changes persisting well into the postpartum period. It is important that practitioners understand these normal changes in order to be aware of the possible effects of pregnancy on women with renal disease, hypertension or following renal transplant.

The main changes of pregnancy are sodium retention and increased extracellular volume. Parameters used to assess normal renal function become altered and alterations in renal function may be difficult to assess.

The prenatal period

The maternal kidneys must act as the primary excretory organ for fetal waste besides dealing with the increased intravascular and extracellular volume and metabolic waste products. As in many of the widespread physiological adaptations to pregnancy, renal changes are related to the effects of progesterone on smooth muscle, pressure from the enlarging uterus and cardiovascular alterations such as increased cardiac output and increased blood volume (Blackburn 2007). A summary of the main changes in the renal tract is presented in Table 19.1.

Structural changes—the kidneys and ureters

Kidney size
Kidneys enlarge and the length may increase by 1.5 cm. This increase in size is mainly due to increased blood flow and vascular volume in addition to an increase in the interstitial space. Glomerular size increases but there is no change in the number of cells. Overall, the microscopic structure of the kidney is the same in the pregnant and non-pregnant woman.

Changes in the ureters
The most striking anatomical change is dilatation of the renal calyces, renal pelvis and ureters (Fig. 19.7). These changes are accompanied with alterations in haemodynamics, glomerular filtration and tubular performance. The dilatation of the renal calyces, renal pelvis and ureters begins in the first trimester and is maximal by the middle of the second trimester, when ureteric diameters may be as much as 2 cm (Gordon 2007). The

Table 19.1 The changes in the renal tract in pregnancy

Organ	Change
Renal calyces, renal pelvis, ureters	Dilatation, elongation, increased muscle tone, decreased peristalsis
Bladder	Mucosa becomes oedematous and hyperaemic, incompetence of vesicoureteric sphincter, displacement in late pregnancy Decreased bladder tone, bladder capacity increases to 1 litre
Renal blood flow	Increases 35–60%
Glomerular filtration rate	Increases 40–50%
Tubular function	Increased reabsorption of solutes Increased excretion of glucose, protein, amino acids, urea, uric acid, water-soluble vitamins, calcium, hydrogen ions, phosphorus Retention of sodium and water
Renin–angiotensin–aldosterone system	Increase in all components Resistance to pressor effects of angiotensin II

changes are mainly seen in that portion of the ureters above the pelvic brim and can be referred to as physiological hydroureter and hydronephrosis.

That portion of the ureters below the pelvic brim does not usually enlarge. This may be because the connective tissue surrounding the ureters hypertrophies and prevents the hormonally induced dilatation. The diameter of the lumen of the ureter increases, there is hypertrophy of the smooth muscle of the ureters, an increase in muscle tone and there is no decrease in peristalsis. The ureters elongate and become more tortuous in the latter half of pregnancy and are also displaced laterally by the growing uterus. The ureters may hold up to 25 times more urine and contain as much as 300 ml. The changes greatly increase the risk of urinary tract infection.

Physiological hydroureter
The cause of physiological hydroureter is not understood but the main factor may be the external compression of the ureters against the pelvic brim by the growing uterus. Growing blood vessels such as the iliac arteries and venous plexi may also add to the compression effect. Dilatation is more prominent in primigravidae

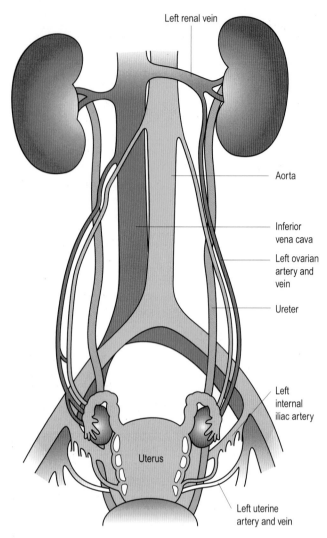

Figure 19.7 ● Obstruction of the right ureter at the pelvic brim by an enlarged ovarian vein. Note that the ovarian vein enters the vena cava by several trunks and that the pelvic portion of the ureter is normal. (From Hinchliff S M, Montague S E 1990, with permission.)

where the firmer abdominal wall does not permit the uterus to expand anteriorly. In 85% of women the right ureter is dilated more than the left, possibly because of dextrorotation of the growing uterus due to the presence of the sigmoid colon in the left quadrant of the pelvis. The increased flow of urine in pregnancy may result in a small amount of dilatation.

Structural changes—the bladder

Bladder capacity doubles by term to approximately 1000 ml (1 litre). Oestrogenic influences cause the trigone to become hyperplastic with hypertrophy of the bladder musculature (Blackburn 2007). The bladder mucosa becomes hyperaemic with an increase in size and tortuous route of blood vessels. The mucosa also becomes oedematous and is thus more vulnerable to trauma and infection. The decrease in bladder tone leads to incompetence of the vesicoureteric sphincters and there may be reflux of urine. This may be increased by the displacement of the bladder and of the terminal ureters.

Changes in renal physiology

Blood flow

There is a significant increase in renal blood flow in pregnancy. Blood flow increases by 35–60% by the end of the first trimester and then decreases slightly until the end of pregnancy. This is due to the increased blood volume and cardiac output as well as the decreased renal vascular resistance brought about by the relaxing effects of progesterone. There is vasodilation of the afferent and efferent glomerular capillaries.

Glomerular filtration

GFR increases 40–50% in pregnancy, with the increase beginning shortly after conception and peaking at 9–16 weeks before stabilising. The early second trimester level is maintained until term. Values for GFR may reach more than 150 ml/min. The volume of urine produced in 24 h is 25% higher during pregnancy. A greater proportion of renal blood flow is filtered and this increases the excretion of glucose, protein, amino acids, water-soluble vitamins and hydrogen ions.

No single cause has been identified for the increase in GFR in pregnancy. It is related to the increased renal blood flow. The decreased plasma oncotic pressure present because of the reduced concentration of plasma proteins due to haemodilution also increases GFR and there is involvement of hormones. Prolactin release from the pituitary gland has been found to induce changes in GFR in rats and is probably implicated in the human response to pregnancy. Prostaglandins may cause the renal vasodilation of pregnancy. Alterations in the renin–angiotensin–aldosterone system and in the role of antidiuretic hormone (see Ch. 20) accommodate the increase in blood plasma volume and thus add to renal blood flow.

Tubular function

Glucose

The rise in GFR increases the amount of fluid and solutes present within the tubules by 50–100%. Tubular reabsorption must increase to prevent the loss of sodium, chloride, glucose, potassium and water. However, tubular reabsorption rate and clearance may not accommodate the increased load and substances such as glucose and amino acids are excreted. Urinary glucose values may rise as much as 10-fold during pregnancy. There is a reduced ability of the tubules to reabsorb glucose in proportion to the amount in the filtrate (fractional reabsorption), possibly due to the changes in pregnancy steroid hormones (Baylis & Davison 1998). This leads to glycosuria commonly occurring in pregnancy. The changes are likely to be due to the increased plasma levels of oestrogen and progesterone and a similar effect is seen in some women taking the oral contraceptive pill.

Amino acids

Protein excretion increases during pregnancy and this can significantly vary on a day-to-day basis. Proteinuria is also more common during pregnancy with the extra excretion of amino acids. A value of 1+ on a protein labstick is not abnormal and protein excretion up to 300 mg/24 h can be accepted. Protein excretion does not correlate with the severity of renal disease and may not indicate progressive deterioration of the disease. However, proteinuria associated with hypertension is serious and associated with increased risk to the woman and her fetus.

The postnatal period

During the postnatal period, there is a rapid and sustained loss of sodium and a diuresis, especially within the first 5 postnatal days. The first postnatal day is associated with a marked glomerular hyperfiltration (+41%) with the GFR at 2 weeks postnatal remaining moderately elevated (+20%) above non-pregnant levels (Hladunewich et al 2004). A normal urine output for a woman during this time may be up to 3000 ml with voiding of 500–1000 ml at any one micturition. By the end of the 1st week urinary excretion of calcium, phosphate, vitamins, glucose and other solutes returns to normal but it may take up to 3 weeks to achieve normal fluid and electrolyte balance. Structural changes as described above may take up to 3 months to disappear although the structures will return to normal in 6–8 weeks in most women. This is important to remember when women who have had renal problems in pregnancy are assessed following delivery.

Main points

- The kidneys play a major role in maintenance of internal homeostasis by regulating the volume and composition of the body fluids. Kidneys regulate the volume and chemical make-up of the blood, maintain balance between water and electrolytes and produce renin and erythropoietin.
- The three distinct functional regions of the kidneys include the outer cortex, the medulla and the inner renal pelvis.
- Each kidney contains over 1 million nephrons (functioning units). There are two types of nephron: superficial cortical nephrons (85%) and juxtaglomerular nephrons (15%). About 25% of cardiac output is delivered to the kidneys each minute.
- Stimulation of the sympathetic and a few parasympathetic nerve fibres causes vasoconstriction, reduced renal blood flow, reduced glomerular filtration rate and the release of renin from the juxtaglomerular apparatus.
- In an adult about 180 litres of plasma are filtered every day and 99% of the filtrate is reabsorbed by the nephrons. As a result, 1.5 litres of urine is produced per day. Glomerular filtration is the first step in urine production.
- Filtration is a passive, non-selective process in which fluids and solutes are forced through a membrane by hydrostatic pressure. The glomerular filtration rate is the volume of plasma filtered through each glomeruli in 1 min (normally 120 ml/min). The presence of the plasma proteins (colloid osmotic pressure) limits the loss of water.

- An intrinsic system in the kidney controls blood supply over a wide range of arterial blood pressure. This autoregulation depends on alterations in the diameter of the afferent and efferent arterioles in response to a systemic blood pressure change. Extrinsic control is by sympathetic nervous system stimulation.
- During the second stage of urine production the filtrate is greatly modified as it moves along the tubule. Most reabsorption occurs in the proximal tubule where two-thirds of the filtrate is removed. Vital solutes such as glucose, amino acids and electrolytes are reabsorbed together with water.
- Transport across the nephron may be active or passive. Substances are not reabsorbed because they lack carriers, they are not lipid-soluble and cannot diffuse through cell membranes or they are too large. These include the end-products of protein and nucleic acid metabolism.
- Tubular secretion is an important mechanism in clearing the blood of unwanted substances. Urine is therefore composed of both filtered and secreted substances. Secreted substances include hydrogen ions, ammonia and drug metabolites.
- Water balance is mainly regulated by antidiuretic hormone. Sodium is regulated by aldosterone from the adrenal cortex. Renin is produced by the juxtaglomerular apparatus in the kidney and stimulates production of the inactive blood peptide angiotensin I. This is converted into the active angiotensin II, which acts as a hormone to stimulate the secretion of aldosterone and cause vasoconstriction.

- The two ureters drain the urine to the bladder for storage. The muscle walls propel urine through peristaltic movements. The bladder acts as a reservoir for urine and the normal capacity of the full bladder is 500 ml. The female urethra is about 4 cm long. Micturition requires the coordination of autonomic nerves and somatic nerves.

- The renal system undergoes structural and functional changes during pregnancy. Many of the structural changes are still present well into the postpartum period. The main changes are sodium retention and increased extracellular volume. Parameters used to assess normal renal function become altered and these alterations may be difficult to assess.

- Kidneys enlarge because of increased blood flow, and vascular volume and an increase in the interstitial space. That portion of the ureters below the pelvic brim does not usually enlarge because the connective tissue surrounding the ureters hypertrophies and prevents the hormonally induced dilatation. The ureters elongate, become more tortuous and are also displaced laterally by the growing uterus. The ureters may hold up to 25 times more urine.

- Bladder capacity doubles by term to 1000 ml. Under the influence of oestrogen, the trigone becomes hyperplastic with muscle hypertrophy. The bladder mucosa becomes hyperaemic with an increase in size and tortuous route of blood vessels. The mucosa also becomes oedematous and is thus more vulnerable to trauma and infection.

- There is a 60% increase in renal blood flow by the end of the first trimester, which then decreases slightly until the end of pregnancy. GFR increases 50% in pregnancy, the rise beginning soon after conception and peaking at 9–16 weeks.

- Urinary glucose values may rise as much as 10-fold during pregnancy. The tubules have a reduced ability to reabsorb glucose in proportion to the amount in the filtrate (fractional reabsorption) and glycosuria commonly occurs in pregnancy. Proteinuria is also more common during pregnancy with the extra excretion of amino acids.

- After birth there is a rapid and sustained loss of sodium and a diuresis, especially between the 2nd and 5th days, and it may take up to 3 weeks to achieve normal fluid and electrolyte balance. Structural changes may take up to 3 months to disappear although most women will return to normal in 6–8 weeks.

References

Baylis, C., Davison, J., 1998. The urinary system. In: Chamberlain, G., Broughton Pipkin, F. (Eds.), Clinical Physiology in Obstetrics, third edn. Blackwell Science, Oxford, p. 1.

Blackburn, S.T., 2007. Maternal, Fetal and Neonatal Physiology: A Clinical Perspective, fourth edn. Elsevier Saunders, St Louis MO.

Gordon, M.C., et al., 2007. Maternal physiology in pregnancy. In: Gabbe, S. G., Simpson, J.L., Niebyl, J.R. (Eds.), Obstetrics: Normal and Problem Pregnancies, fifth edn. Churchill Livingstone, London.

Hladunewich, M.A., Lafayette, G.C., Derby, K.L., et al., 2004. The dynamics of glomerular filtration in the puerperium. Am. J. Physiol.: Ren. Physiol. 286, F496–F503.

Marieb, E.N., Hoehn, K., 2008. Anatomy and Physiology, third edn. Pearson Benjamin/Cummings, New York.

Martini, F.H., Nath, J.L., 2009. Fundamentals of Anatomy & Physiology, eighth edn. Pearson Benjamin/Cummings, New York.

Sherwood, L., 2006. Human Physiology: From Cells to Systems, sixth edn. Brookes Cole, New York.

Annotated recommended reading

Blackburn, S.T., 2007. Maternal, Fetal and Neonatal Physiology: A Clinical Perspective, fourth edn. Elsevier Saunders, St Louis MO.
This textbook provides a detailed description of the major changes in the body systems during pregnancy and following childbirth.

Sherwood, L., 2006. Human Physiology: From Cells to Systems, sixth edn. Brookes Cole, New York.
This textbook provides an overview of the physiology of the body systems.

Chapter Twenty

20

Fluid, electrolyte and acid–base balance

Introduction

Cell function depends on the maintenance of a stable environment through the continuous supply of nutrients, removal of waste and homeostasis of the surrounding fluids. Therefore it is essential that the fluid, electrolyte, acid and base balances of the extracellular fluids be kept within a narrow range. For instance, changes in the composition of electrolytes can affect the electrical potentials of neurons and can move fluid from one compartment to another. Changes in pH can disrupt cellular enzyme systems. Cells also depend on a continuous supply of nutrients and the removal of metabolic wastes. Various organs are involved in coordinating this fluid balance and therefore the purpose of this chapter is to step outside of individual systems and examine the integration of systems in the control of this extremely important aspect of life. Understanding the basic information on biochemistry provided in Chapter 1 will be of benefit to the reader before proceeding with this chapter.

Fluid and electrolytes

Body water content

In an adult, water accounts for about 50% of the body mass although this ratio can vary depending on age, sex, body weight and relative amount of body fat (Marieb & Hoehn 2008). Infants contain approximately 73% of water because of their lower bone mass and body fat. Men contain more water than women because of the extra amount of female adipose tissue and their lower muscle mass. Body fat leads to a reduction in water content as fat is the least hydrated of all body tissues so that obese people contain less water proportionate to their body weight. Older people have less water as their fat content is increased and their muscle content is decreased. Also, as the kidney ages it is less able to concentrate urine so that more fluid is lost in urine. Other losses of body fluid can therefore be life threatening in the elderly. Table 20.1 provides a summary of the distribution of body fluid by weight in a 70 kg man.

Fluid compartments

There are three main **compartments** of the body where water can be found (Fig. 20.1). These are **intracellular fluid** (ICF), the fluid inside the cells, and **extracellular fluid** (ECF) which can be divided into **interstitial fluid**, the fluid between the cells, and **plasma**, the fluid inside the vascular system. Special types of ECF separate from interstitial fluid and plasma are lymph, transcellular fluid (secreted by cells), synovial, intestinal, cerebrospinal fluid, sweat, urine, pleural, peritoneal, pericardial and intraocular fluid (Martini & Nath 2009). These fluids are usually considered to be part of ECF because of the similarity in composition. The sum of all of the above is the **total body water** (TBW).

Composition of body fluids

Solutes: electrolytes and non-electrolytes

Water is the universal solvent and contains a variety of solutes. Broadly speaking, these can be divided into electrolytes and non-electrolytes. The **non-electrolytes**

Table 20.1 Distribution of body fluid by weight in a 70 kg man

Compartment	Body weight (%)	Volume (litres)
Intracellular fluid	40	28
Extracellular fluid—interstitial	15	11
Extracellular fluid—intravascular	5	3
Total body water	60	42

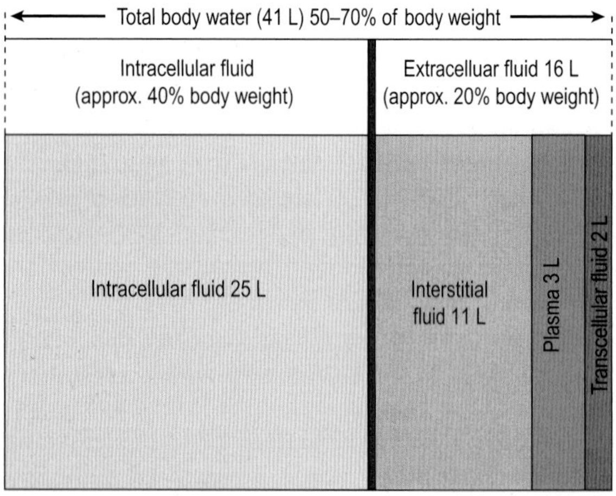

Figure 20.1 • Size of the major body fluid compartments. (From Hinchliff S M, Montague S E 1990, with permission.)

have bonds (usually covalent bonds) that prevent them dissociating into their component particles in solution and therefore do not carry electrical charges. These are mainly organic molecules such as glucose, lipids, creatinine and urea. **Electrolytes** are chemical compounds that do dissociate into ions in water. They are said to **ionise** and are charged particles capable of conducting an electric current. Electrolytes include inorganic salts, both inorganic and organic acids and bases and some proteins.

All dissolved solutes contribute to the osmotic activity of a fluid but electrolytes have the greatest osmotic power because each molecule can dissociate into at least two ions. An example is sodium chloride (NaCl):

$$NaCl \rightarrow Na^+ + Cl^- \qquad (20.1)$$

Electrolytes have the greatest ability to cause fluid shifts because water moves along osmotic gradients from areas of lesser osmolality to areas of greater osmolality.

Differences in composition between intracellular fluids and extracellular fluids

Each fluid compartment has its own pattern of electrolytes. Except for the high protein content of plasma, all extracellular compartments have a similar composition. Sodium is the most abundant ECF cation and chloride the major anion. In the ICF, potassium is the most abundant cation and the major anion is phosphate (HPO_4^{2-}). The balance in concentrations of sodium in ECF and potassium in ICF reflects the activity of the **sodium pump** (see Ch. 2).

Movement of fluid between compartments

Water movement between plasma and interstitial fluid

The distribution of water and the movement of nutrients and waste products between the plasma in the capillary and the interstitial space occur because of changes in hydrostatic pressure and osmotic forces between the arterial and venous ends of the capillary network. The capillary membrane is semipermeable and allows interchange of fluids and solutes between the intravascular and interstitial fluid (IF) compartments.

The movement of fluid back and forth across the capillary wall is called **net filtration** (Starling's hypothesis). The major forces of filtration are within the capillary. Net filtration is the balance between forces favouring filtration, such as capillary hydrostatic pressure (blood pressure) and interstitial oncotic pressure, and forces opposing filtration, such as plasma oncotic pressure. As the plasma flows from the arterial to the venous end of the capillary, blood pressure falls, reducing the hydrostatic pressure. Oncotic pressure remains constant. At the arterial end of the capillary, hydrostatic pressure exceeds oncotic pressure and fluid is forced out into the interstitial space. At the venous end of the capillary, oncotic pressure exceeds hydrostatic pressure and fluid is drawn back into the capillary (Sherwood 2006).

Water movement between ICF and ECF

This water movement between compartments is a function of osmosis. Water moves freely across cell membranes so that the osmolality of TBW is normally at equilibrium. The ICF balance is maintained by active transport of ions out of the cell and interstitial hydrostatic pressure. However, normally, the interstitial forces are negligible because only a very small amount of plasma protein crosses the capillary membrane so that the major forces of filtration are within the capillary. Movements of respiratory gases, nutrients and wastes are unidirectional.

Water balance

Water intake must balance water loss; Table 20.2 summarises the normal daily water balance in a healthy adult.

Regulation of water intake

Regulation of water intake is by the mechanism of thirst, which is poorly understood. A thirst centre in the hypothalamus responds to either a drop in plasma volume or an increase in plasma osmolarity. It is probable that the salivary glands, which obtain their fluid from the blood, produce less saliva and the resulting dry mouth makes us drink. Thirst is quenched as soon as we have taken on board the right amount of water, even before there has been time for it to affect blood volume.

Table 20.2 Normal daily water losses and gains

Intake	Amount	Output	Amount (ml)
Drinking	1400–1800	Urine	1400–1800
Water in food	700–1000	Faeces	100
Water of oxidation	300–400	Skin	300–500
		Lungs	600–800
Total	2400–3200		2400–3200

Regulation of water output

Water is lost from the body in ways that cannot be avoided. These are the **obligatory water losses** and explain why we cannot survive long without drinking. They include the insensible loss of water from the lungs and via the skin. Because of the large amount of perspiration lost daily, especially in a hot climate, humans are of necessity a riverine species. That is to say that most settlements before the advent of piped water were next to a river. Water in faeces must be added to the loss. There is an absolute minimum of 500 ml of urine per 24 h that the kidneys must excrete even when the urine is concentrated to its maximum level possible.

Disorders of water balance

Oedema

Oedema is the accumulation of fluid within the interstitial space. It is a problem of fluid distribution and does not necessarily indicate excess intake. Oedema may be accompanied by signs of dehydration if fluid becomes sequestered (locked) within a compartment. It may be caused by factors that increase fluid flow out of the plasma or hinder its return. There are four major contributors to oedema:

1. **Increased capillary hydrostatic pressure** may occur from venous obstruction such as in thrombophlebitis, hepatic obstruction, tight clothing or prolonged standing.
2. **Reduced plasma oncotic pressure** follows the loss of plasma proteins found in renal failure, diminished production of plasma proteins found in liver disease or protein malnutrition.
3. **Increased capillary membrane permeability** is usually associated with inflammatory or immune reactions. Burns, crush injuries, cancer and allergy also produce this effect.
4. If the **lymphatic system is blocked** by infection or inflammation or lymphatic cancer or has had to be surgically removed in areas to prevent the spread of cancer, proteins and fluids accumulate in the interstitial spaces causing localised lymphoedema.

Clinical manifestations

Oedema may be generalised or localised. It is associated with weight gain, swelling of the tissues and puffiness. Clothing may feel tight. Movement may be limited and blood flow may be restricted. Wounds tend to heal more slowly and the risk of pressure sores and wound infections is increased. The sequestered fluid is not available for metabolic processes and dehydration may occur, for instance following burns. Hypovolaemic shock may occur. Treatment is tailored to fit the individual case and could include elevation of affected limbs, support stockings, avoiding prolonged standing, reducing salt intake and the prescribing of diuretics.

Electrolyte balance

Electrolytes include salts, acids and bases. Salts are the main electrolytes and are involved in many physiological processes. The four main electrolytes are sodium, potassium, calcium and magnesium. Salts are obtained from the food we eat and also, to a lesser extent, in our drinking water. Small amounts of salts may be released during metabolism. An example would be the release of phosphate during the breakdown of nucleic acids.

A major problem for humans is the love of salty food. This may be an acquired taste but is equally as likely to have an innate factor because of the need to replenish salts lost in perspiration. Salts are lost from the body in faeces and urine as well as in perspiration, as mentioned above. If we are depleted of salt our perspiration will be more dilute but, even so, in hot weather a good deal of salt can be lost.

The role of sodium in fluid and electrolyte balance

Salts containing sodium account for at least 90% of solutes in the ECF. Regulating the balance between sodium intake and output is a major function of the kidneys. Sodium is the most abundant cation in the ECF and is the main cause of osmotic pressure. Sodium does not cross cell membranes very easily (Ch. 2) and is therefore ideal for controlling the ECF volume and water distribution in the body. Water follows salt so that a change in sodium content will be followed by a change in water content of a fluid compartment. Blood volume and blood pressure are linked to sodium balance and there is a hormonal regulatory effect by the hormone aldosterone; this is discussed more fully in Chapter 17.

Aldosterone

Aldosterone is produced by the cortical cells of the adrenal gland and its release is mediated by the production of renin by the juxtaglomerular apparatus of the kidney, as explained in Chapter 19. The renin–angiotensin–aldosterone system is also discussed fully in Chapter 19. In brief, renin catalyses a series of reactions leading to the activation of angiotensin II, which causes aldosterone release. Normally, without the influence of aldosterone, about 75% of the sodium in the renal filtrate is reabsorbed in the proximal tubules of the nephrons of the kidneys.

If aldosterone levels are high, most of the remaining sodium is reabsorbed in the distal tubules and collecting ducts. If the permeability of the tubules has been increased by antidiuretic hormone (ADH, also known as arginine vasopressin or AVP), water will passively follow the sodium. There will be sodium and water retention. When aldosterone release is inhibited, there will be little reabsorption of sodium beyond the proximal tubules. Urinary excretion of large amounts of sodium will always result in the excretion of large amounts of water. The effect of aldosterone is to allow large amounts of sodium-free water to be excreted in times of sodium depletion. Like all hormones, aldosterone has a slow effect, taking hours or days to alter fluid compartments.

Other influences on fluid and electrolyte balance discussed in other chapters are the cardiovascular system baroreceptors, the regulation of ADH and the influence of atrial natriuretic factor. Oestrogens and glucocorticoids also play a part in enhancing tubular reabsorption of sodium.

Regulation of potassium balance

Potassium (K^+) is the main cation in ICF and is necessary for normal neuromuscular functioning and other processes such as protein synthesis. Potassium is quite toxic, especially to heart muscle. Both hyperkalaemia (excess potassium) and hypokalaemia (potassium depletion) can cause abnormalities of cardiac rhythm and even cardiac arrest. Potassium also acts as a part of the buffer system which controls the pH of body fluids. Shifts of hydrogen ions (H^+) into and out of cells is compensated by shifts of potassium (K^+) in the opposite direction to maintain cation balance.

Potassium balance is similar to sodium balance as it is maintained by renal mechanisms. However, whereas sodium loss or retention is controlled to meet the specific needs of the body, potassium loss is constant. Most potassium is reabsorbed by the proximal tubule but about 10–15% is lost in the urine despite any need changes in the body.

Tubular cell secretion of potassium

The amount of potassium secreted into the lumen of the tubule can be changed. When potassium levels in the ECF are low, potassium leaves the cells. The kidneys then conserve potassium by reducing the amount secreted into the tubule. There are three factors which alter the rate and amount of potassium secretion: the intracellular potassium content of the tubule cells, aldosterone levels and the pH of the ECF.

Tubule cell potassium

If a high potassium load is taken on, there is an increase in potassium in the ECF and then in the ICF. This triggers the tubule cell to secrete potassium into the lumen of the proximal tubule of the nephron. A low potassium intake will have the reverse effect. Low ECF potassium levels result in low ICF potassium levels and the tubule cells reduce their secretion of potassium.

Aldosterone

Aldosterone helps to regulate potassium ions as well as sodium ions. To maintain electrolyte balance, there is a one-for-one exchange of Na^+ for K^+ in the collecting tubules of the kidney and for each Na^+ absorbed, a K^+ is secreted. Therefore, as plasma sodium levels rise, potassium levels fall. The adrenal cortex is also sensitive to high levels of potassium and will react by releasing aldosterone.

pH of ECF

The excretion of both K^+ and H^+ is linked to the reabsorption of sodium ions. They are cotransported with sodium and compete for places. If the pH of blood begins to fall, the secretion of H^+ increases and K^+ secretion falls.

Regulation of calcium balance

Almost all of the calcium content of the body, 99%, is found in the bones (Martini & Nath 2009). However, ionic calcium found in the ECF is extremely important for normal blood clotting, membrane permeability and secretory behaviour (Marieb & Hoehn 2008). Calcium is like potassium and sodium in having a large effect on neuromuscular excitability: hypocalcaemia increases excitability and leads to muscle tetany while hypercalcaemia inhibits muscle cells and neurons and may lead to cardiac arrhythmias.

Calcium is extremely well regulated and is balanced by the interaction of two hormones: parathyroid hormone (PTH) and calcitonin. PTH is released by the parathyroid glands situated on the posterior aspect of the thyroid gland. Calcitonin is produced by the parafollicular cells of the thyroid gland.

PTH acts to release calcium into the blood from the bones. It also stimulates the small intestine to absorb calcium by causing the kidneys to transform vitamin D into its active form. Activated vitamin D is necessary for the intestinal absorption of calcium. PTH increases calcium reabsorption by the kidneys, while at the same time there is a decrease in phosphate reabsorption. Declining plasma levels of calcium stimulate the release of parathyroid hormone.

Calcitonin encourages the deposition of calcium salts in bone tissue and inhibits bone reabsorption. Although it is an antagonist of PTH, its role in calcium homeostasis is small.

Regulation of magnesium balance

Magnesium is essential as an activator of coenzymes needed in carbohydrate and protein metabolism. It is also implicated in neuromuscular functioning. About 50% of the body's magnesium is in the skeleton and the remainder is found intracellularly in heart and skeletal muscle and in the liver. Although the mechanism of magnesium balance is not well understood, the renal tubules are probably involved.

Alterations in sodium, chloride and water balance

These alterations mainly involve changes in tonicity and can be classified as isotonic, hypertonic and hypotonic (Table 20.3).

Isotonic alterations

Depletion causes contraction of the ECF volume with weight loss, dry skin and mucous membranes, decreased urinary output and symptoms of hypovolaemia: rapid heart rate, flattened neck veins and normal or decreased blood pressure. **Excesses** are usually due to over-administration of intravenous fluids, hypersecretion of aldosterone or the effect of drugs such as cortisone. There will be weight gain and a decrease in haematocrit and plasma proteins. Neck veins distend and blood pressure increases. Increased capillary hydrostatic pressure results in tissue oedema. If the excess is severe enough pulmonary oedema and heart failure may be the consequence.

Hypertonic alterations

Hypertonicity may be due to excess sodium (**hypernatraemia**) or depleted water (**dehydration**). Hypernatraemia occurs when the serum sodium concentration exceeds

Table 20.3 Changes in tonicity

Tonicity	Mechanism
Isotonic (iso-osmolar) imbalance	Gain or loss of ECF results in a concentration equivalent to a 0.9% NaCl solution (normal saline) with no shrinkage or swelling of cells
Hypertonic (hyperosmolar) imbalance	An imbalance with an ECF concentration greater than 0.9% salt solution due either to water loss or solute gain. Cells shrink as fluid moves out of them into the ECF
Hypotonic (hypo-osmolar) imbalance	An imbalance with an ECF concentration of less than 0.9% salt solution due to either water gain or solute loss. Cells gain water from ECF and swell

147 mEq/L. This is rarely due to dietary excess. Causes include inappropriate use of hypertonic saline solution such as the administration of sodium bicarbonate to correct acidosis. Medical conditions leading to hypernatraemia include hyperaldosteronism and Cushing's syndrome with over-secretion of adrenocorticotrophic hormone (ACTH).

Dehydration occurs mainly in people who cannot take in water by themselves. Pathological causes include water loss in fever, respiratory infections, diabetes insipidus, diabetes mellitus, profuse sweating and diarrhoea. Clinical manifestations include thirst, dry skin and mucous membranes, elevated temperature, weight loss and concentrated urine except in patients who have diabetes insipidus. Isotonic salt-free solutions such as 5% dextrose can be given in both hypernatraemia and water loss until the plasma serum concentration returns to normal. Plain water cannot be given as it would increase intracellular fluid and cause cell lysis.

Hypotonic alterations

The most common causes are sodium deficit (**hyponatraemia**) and water excess (**water intoxication**). Hyponatraemia develops when plasma sodium concentration falls below 135 mEq/L. It is rarely caused by low intake and may be caused by vomiting, diarrhoea, gastrointestinal suctioning and burns. Hyperglycaemia increases ECF osmolality and pulls fluid from the plasma into the tissues.

Water excess may occur following over-intake in thirsty people (**dilutional hyponatraemia**). Pathological conditions include reduced urinary output in oliguric renal failure, congestive cardiac failure and cirrhosis of the liver. Clinical manifestations include neurological symptoms such as lethargy, confusion, apprehension, nausea, headache, convulsions and coma. If symptoms are severe small doses of hypertonic saline can be given with caution. With dilutional hyponatraemias, oedema may develop. Sodium and water balances are calculated and appropriate intravenous solutions are given. Restriction of fluid may be necessary in dilutional hyponatraemias. A summary of hypertonicity and hypotonicity is presented in Table 20.4.

Acid–base balance

Almost all biochemical reactions in the body are influenced by the pH of their fluid environment (Ch. 1). The acid–base balance of body fluids is crucial to many biochemical reactions. There is a slight difference in pH between fluid compartments. Arterial blood pH is normally 7.4, venous blood and interstitial fluid have a pH of 7.35 while inside the cell the pH is 7.0. The fall in pH

Table 20.4 Summary of hypertonicity and hypotonicity

Hypertonicity		
Sodium excess	Water normal	Hypervolaemia
Sodium normal	Water deficit	Hypernatraemia
Hypotonicity		
Sodium deficit	Water normal	Hypovolaemia
Sodium normal	Water deficit	Hypervolaemia

is due to the presence of acid metabolites. **Alkalosis** is present when arterial blood pH is over 7.45 and **acidosis** when arterial blood pH falls below 7.35 (Martini & Nath 2009). This could be said to be a misuse of the term, as even at pH of 7.0 a fluid is not acidic but neutral.

The structure of proteins, particularly enzymes, is affected by small changes in pH and significant alterations could disrupt metabolic processes and result in death. The pH scale may soon be replaced and the hydrogen ion concentration expressed in nanomoles per litre (nmol/L). The hydrogen ion content of arterial blood in these units is 40 nmol/L.

Chemical buffers tie up excess acids and bases as a temporary measure but cannot excrete them from the body. The lungs can dispose of carbonic acid by excreting carbon dioxide. However, it is the kidneys that dispose of the **metabolic** or **fixed acids** generated by cellular metabolism. These include phosphoric acid, uric acid and ketone bodies, the causes of **metabolic acidosis**. Also, only the kidneys have the power to regulate blood levels of alkaline substances. The kidneys are therefore the main regulators of acid–base status and act slowly and steadily to regulate the large acid–base imbalances that occur due to diet, metabolism or disease. Their most important mechanisms are the regulation of hydrogen ions (H^+) and the conservation or generation of bicarbonate ions.

The role of the kidney in acid–base balance

Regulation of hydrogen ion secretion

The tubule cells and the cells of the collecting ducts appear to be able to respond directly to the pH of the ECF. They then alter their H^+ secretion as needed to restore balance. The secreted ions are obtained from the dissociation of carbonic acid, H_2CO_3 (carbon dioxide + water), within the tubule cells, and for each H^+ ion secreted into the lumen one Na^+ ion is reabsorbed into the tubule cell from the filtrate. This maintains the electrochemical balance. The rate of H^+ secretion varies directly with CO_2 levels in the ECF. The kidneys can respond to alterations in blood pH because CO_2 levels in blood are directly associated with blood pH.

Conservation of filtered bicarbonate ions

Bicarbonate ions (HCO_3^-) are an important part of the carbonate buffer system. In order to maintain the **alkaline reserve** (available bicarbonate ions) to act in the buffer system (see below) the kidneys must replenish stores of HCO_3^- as necessary. The tubule cells are almost impermeable to bicarbonate ions and cannot re-absorb them from the filtrate. However, they can shunt bicarbonate ions generated within them into the peritubular blood. Dissociation of one molecule of carbonic acid inside the tubule cell releases one HCO_3^- ion and one H^+ ion.

There is a one-to-one exchange of bicarbonate ions depending on the numbers of H^+ ions secreted by the tubule cells. For each filtered HCO_3^- ion that is lost from the body, another one is generated from the dissociation of carbonic acid in the tubule cells. When large amounts of H^+ are secreted, equally large amounts of HCO_3^- enter the peritubular blood.

Respiratory regulation of hydrogen ions

Respiration and carbon dioxide transport have an important effect on the acid–base status (pH) of the body. The acidity of blood and body fluids is determined by hydrogen ion concentration, $[H^+]$; the hydrogen ions are the most highly reactive cations in the body. The intake and production of hydrogen ions varies according to the diet, energy output, disease and some drugs. To maintain homeostasis it is essential to both buffer these ions in body fluids and excrete them from the body via the lungs and kidneys.

These three mechanisms are brought into effect sequentially. Chemical buffers act within a fraction of a second and are the first line of defence against a change in pH. Respiratory rate is adjusted in 2–3 min. The kidneys are the most efficient regulator but it may take hours for the kidney to bring about a change in blood pH.

Excretion of hydrogen ions by the lungs

Any increase in P_{CO_2} and $[H^+]$ with a consequent fall in pH will be sensed by the central and peripheral chemoreceptors. Then there will be a rapid rise in alveolar ventilation, leading to a speeding up of the reaction:

$$H^+ + HCO_3^- \rightleftharpoons H_2CO_3 \rightleftharpoons CO_2 + H_2O \quad (20.2)$$

This leads to the rapid excretion of excess CO_2 and H^+ ions. The reverse situation will occur with any decrease in P_{CO_2} and $[H^+]$, with a consequent rise in pH leading to a decrease in respiratory effort. These two mechanisms form an efficient response to short-term chemical changes in blood. The kidneys play the main role in long-term control of pH and acid–base balance.

Chemical buffer systems

Buffers are systems that minimise changes in pH. Acids are proton donors releasing free H^+ ions into a solution. Bases are proton acceptors and mop up free H^+ ions from a solution. Chemical buffers minimise the changes in pH by binding to H^+ ions when there is a fall in pH, i.e. when the fluid is becoming more acidic, and releasing H^+ ions when pH rises, i.e. when the fluid is becoming more alkaline. There are three major buffer systems in the body which work together:

1. The bicarbonate buffer system.
2. The phosphate buffer system.
3. The protein buffer system.

The bicarbonate buffer system

In a solution, strong acids dissociate into their component molecules and release H^+ ions. In a similar manner strong alkalis dissociate to release hydroxyl (OH^-) ions. The bicarbonate buffer system is important in both ECF and ICF. It is a mixture of carbonic acid (H_2CO_3) and its salt, sodium bicarbonate ($NaHCO_3$), in the same solution. Carbonic acid is a weak acid that does not dissociate to release H^+ ions in neutral or acidic solutions. However, in a buffered solution in the presence of a stronger acid such as hydrochloric acid, bicarbonate ions of the salt will tie up the H^+ ions released by the stronger acid to form more carbonic acid:

$$HCl + NaHCO_3 \rightarrow H_2CO_3 + NaCl \quad (20.3)$$

In the same manner, if a strong base such as sodium hydroxide ($NaOH$) is added to a buffered solution, the weak base $NaHCO_3$ will not dissociate to release hydroxyl ions (OH^-) but the carbonic acid will be forced to dissociate and release H^+ ions to mop up the OH^- ions released by the strong alkali to form water (H_2O):

$$NaOH + H_2CO_3 \rightarrow NaHCO_3 + H_2O \quad (20.4)$$

In either Eqn. 20.3 or Eqn. 20.4 the result will be to drive the pH of the solution back to a biologically acceptable level. Potassium bicarbonate or magnesium bicarbonate acts as a buffer within cells where there is little sodium present. The bicarbonate ion concentration in ECF is normally about $25\,mEq/L$. The concentration of carbonic acid is about one-twentieth of the bicarbonate. It is freely available from cellular respiration and is subject to respiratory control.

The phosphate buffer system

The phosphate buffer system is almost identical to the bicarbonate buffer system with the control of H^+ ions occurring in a similar manner. Phosphate ions (HPO_4^-) replace bicarbonate ions in the equations. It is a very effective buffer in ICF and in urine, where phosphate concentrations are high.

The protein buffer system

Proteins in plasma and within the cells are the body's most plentiful and powerful source of buffers. In fact, at least three-quarters of buffering power of body fluid resides within the cells, and most of this reflects the buffering activity of intracellular proteins. Some amino acids have side groups called organic acid or **carboxyl groups** (COOH), which can release the H^+ ion if needed. Other amino acid side chains can accept hydrogen ions. An exposed NH_2 group can bind H^+ to form NH_3 or release it as needed. This type of molecule is said to be **amphoteric**. Haemoglobin in red cells is an excellent example of a protein that acts as an intracellular buffer.

Abnormalities of acid–base balance

- **Respiratory acidosis** develops when the respiratory system cannot eliminate all the CO_2 generated by peripheral tissues. It is caused by any condition that impairs lung ventilation and gas exchange: rapid shallow breathing, narcotic or barbiturate overdose.
- **Metabolic acidosis** has three major causes:
  - The most widespread cause is the production of a large number of fixed or organic acids resulting in the released H^+ ion overloading the carbonic acid–bicarbonate buffer system and reducing pH levels, e.g. during starvation, untreated diabetes mellitus, prolonged tissue hypoxia.
  - The less common cause is an impaired ability to excrete H^+ ions at the kidneys, e.g. glomerulonephritis.
  - Following severe bicarbonate loss, e.g. severe diarrhoea.
- **Respiratory alkalosis** develops when respiratory activity lowers plasma CO_2 to below normal levels, a condition called hypocapnia. It is always caused by hyperventilation whatever the triggering factor.
- **Metabolic alkalosis** occurs when HCO_3^- concentrations become elevated and is caused by vomiting of acid gastric contents, diuretics that cause salt loss, and severe constipation.

The effects of acidosis and alkalosis

Severe acidosis will depress the central nervous system and the person will go into a coma, shortly followed by death if not corrected. Alkalosis overexcites the central nervous system (CNS), resulting in muscle tetany, extreme nervousness and convulsions. Death may occur due to respiratory arrest.

Respiratory and renal compensation

If an acid–base imbalance occurs due to failure of either the lungs or kidneys, the other system will try to compensate. Changes in respiratory rate and rhythm are usually easy to observe. In metabolic acidosis the respiratory rate and depth are increased due to stimulation of the respiratory centres by high levels of H^+ ions. The respiratory system blows off as much carbon dioxide as it can to reduce blood pH. In respiratory acidosis the respiratory rate is normally depressed and is actually the cause of the acidosis. In metabolic alkalosis respiratory compensation involves slow, shallow breathing, which allows carbon dioxide to accumulate in the blood.

Maternal adaptations in childbearing

Pregnancy

In order to meet the needs of the fetus and her own metabolic changes, a woman's body retains fluids and electrolytes. Renal processes are modified and a new balance is achieved, especially in sodium and water homeostasis (Blackburn 2007). This adaptation is achieved by the antidiuretic hormone (ADH) and the renin–angiotensin–aldosterone system.

Sodium

The increase in glomerular filtration rate (GFR) brings about an increase of up to 50% in filtered sodium. Tubular reabsorption increases so that 99% of the filtered sodium is reabsorbed. Sodium retention is highest in the last 8 weeks of pregnancy when about 60% of the retained sodium is utilised by the fetus. The rest is distributed in maternal blood and ECF.

The maintenance of sodium retention during pregnancy is influenced by multiple factors. Besides ADH and the renin–angiotensin–aldosterone system, a decrease in plasma albumin, the vasodilatory effects of prostaglandins and the effects of the pregnancy hormones human placental lactogen (hPL) and oestrogen play their parts. Water accumulation is directly proportional to sodium retention.

Renin–angiotensin–aldosterone system

The increases in the components of the renin–angiotensin–aldosterone system and the decrease in response to the vasoconstrictor effects of angiotensin II are brought about by oestrogens, progesterone and prostaglandins and the alterations in sodium processing (Baylis & Davison 1998). Plasma renin activity increases by a factor of 4–10 times during the first trimester and remains elevated until delivery. Renin release is stimulated by oestrogens. Progesterone also has an effect by stimulating renal sodium loss, which causes the release of renin and aldosterone.

Angiotensinogen levels double by 8 weeks and increase 3–5 times by 20 weeks (Blackburn 2007). This is due to the effect of oestrogen on the liver, which manufactures the plasma protein. The plasma aldosterone level reaches a peak at 24 weeks of 2–5 times that in non-pregnant women. There is a second peak at 36 weeks when the aldosterone level can be 8–10 times that in the non-pregnant woman. Although angiotensin II rises during pregnancy, blood pressure actually decreases because of the decreased peripheral vascular resistance.

Water

Pregnant women accumulate about 7 L of fluid over the normal level to meet the needs of the fetus and their own altered metabolism. About 75% of the weight gain in pregnancy is due to the accumulation of fluid in the ECF. Interstitial fluid increases by about 1.5 L, beginning as early as 6 weeks and peaking at 30 weeks. This increase occurs despite decreases in plasma osmolality and colloid osmotic pressure, which would normally lower the fluid in the intravascular compartment. The vasodilation brought about by oestrogen and progesterone, which enables the vascular system to accommodate more blood volume, is probably a major cause as the increased volume is retained without stimulating the production of ADH. Thirst and urine output remain in balance.

Antidiuretic hormone

Early in pregnancy plasma osmolality decreases, in particular the decreased solute load. ADH secretion and its effect on reabsorption of water are similar in the pregnant and non-pregnant woman. During pregnancy the osmotic threshold is reset so that ADH release occurs at the lower plasma osmolality. As mentioned above, this allows the vascular tree to accommodate more fluid volume with a lower osmolarity due to the haemodilution of pregnancy. Human chorionic gonadotrophin (hCG) may be the main influence on osmoregulation in pregnancy. Circulating hCG levels decrease the thresholds for thirst and also the secretion of ADH.

Acid–base regulation

The plasma hydrogen ion concentration decreases by 2–4 mmol/L in early pregnancy and the change is sustained until term. This makes the blood slightly more alkaline with a pH change to 7.44 from a non-pregnant value of 7.4. Plasma bicarbonate concentration also decreases. This mild alkalaemia is thought to be respiratory in origin since women normally hyperventilate in pregnancy, reducing their arterial Pco_2 by about 25% (Johnson 2007). Renal bicarbonate reabsorption and H^+ excretion appear to be unchanged in pregnancy. The blood changes, especially the reduction in plasma CO_2 level, place the pregnant woman at a disadvantage if she develops significant metabolic acidosis such as in diabetic ketoacidosis or acute renal failure.

Potassium and calcium excretion

There is selective retention of potassium during pregnancy, most of which is utilised by the fetus. However, urinary calcium excretion increases. This may be to combat high levels of circulating 1,25-dihydroxyvitamin D (calcitriol), which increases the absorption of calcium in the intestines. Serum calcium levels are raised and renal calcium reabsorption is reduced.

The intrapartum period

During labour and delivery the renin–angiotensin–aldosterone systems of both mother and fetus are altered with an elevation of the components. It is possible that this mechanism may assist uteroplacental blood flow during labour (Blackburn 2007). The result is to cause fluid retention. Labouring women may suffer from water intoxication if given too much intravenous fluid, especially if it contains oxytocin (which has an antidiuretic effect). This may produce symptoms of agitation and delirium in a few women although most women will cope with over-enthusiastic fluid administration in labour (Millns 1991). Nutrition and fluid needs in labour are discussed in Chapter 37.

A decrease in GFR and sodium excretion and an increase in vasoconstriction complicate the use of general anaesthesia. If the woman is stressed, this effect may be increased. It is important to maintain accurate fluid balance recordings in labour and after a general anaesthetic.

The postnatal period

Renal blood flow and GFR usually return to normal by 6 weeks following delivery (Hladunewich et al 2004).

Urinary excretion of electrolytes and glucose returns to normal after 1–2 weeks. There is a diuresis with loss of sodium and water until prepregnancy levels are reached by 3 weeks.

Main points

- Cell function depends on the maintenance of a stable environment. The fluid, electrolyte, acid and base balances of ECF must be kept within a narrow range.
- In an adult, water accounts for about 50% of the body mass depending on the age, sex and weight of individuals. Water can be found in the ICF (fluid inside cells) and ECF (interstitial fluid and plasma). The sum of all of these is total body water.
- Water is the universal solvent and contains a variety of solutes, mainly divided into non-electrolytes and electrolytes. Non-electrolytes do not carry electrical charges and do not dissociate in solution. Electrolytes dissociate into ions in solution.
- Dissolved solutes all contribute to the osmotic activity of fluid but electrolytes have the greatest osmotic power because each molecule can dissociate into at least two ions. Electrolytes have the greatest ability to cause fluid shifts.
- The movement of water, nutrients and waste products across the capillary membrane is due to changes in hydrostatic pressure and osmotic forces between the arterial and venous ends of the capillary network. The movement of fluid across the capillary wall is called net filtration.
- Water intake must balance water loss. Regulation of water intake is by the mechanism of thirst. Water is lost via the lungs, skin, urine and faeces.
- Oedema is the accumulation of fluid within the interstitial space. Oedema may be generalised or localised and is associated with weight gain, swelling and puffiness.
- Electrolytes include salts, acids and bases. Salts are the main electrolytes and these are obtained through ingestion of food and also, to a lesser extent, in drinking water. Regulating the balance between sodium intake and output is a major function of the kidneys.
- Baroreceptors, ADH and atrial natriuretic factor influence fluid and electrolyte balance. Oestrogens and glucocorticoids also play a part in enhancing tubular reabsorption of sodium.
- Potassium is the main cation in ICF and is necessary for normal neuromuscular functioning and other processes such as protein synthesis. It also acts as a part of the buffer system to control the pH of body fluids. Potassium balance is maintained by renal mechanisms.
- Aldosterone helps to regulate potassium ions as well as sodium ions and as plasma sodium levels rise, potassium levels fall. If the pH of blood begins to fall then the secretion of H^+ ions increases and K^+ ions secretion falls.
- Ionic calcium found in the ECF is extremely important for normal blood clotting, membrane permeability and secretory behaviour. Calcium is extremely well regulated by the interaction of parathyroid hormone and calcitonin. Calcium has a large effect on neuromuscular excitability. Hypocalcaemia increases excitability, leading to muscle tetany, while hypercalcaemia may lead to cardiac arrhythmias.
- Almost all biochemical reactions in the body are influenced by the pH of their fluid environment. The structure of proteins, particularly enzymes, is affected by small changes in pH and significant alterations could disrupt metabolic processes and result in death.
- Chemical buffers neutralise excess acids and bases but cannot excrete them from the body. The lungs can dispose of carbonic acid by excreting carbon dioxide but the kidneys dispose of the metabolic acids or fixed acids generated by cellular metabolism. Bicarbonate ions are important for the carbonate buffer system.
- Respiration and carbon dioxide transport have an important effect on the acid–base status of the body. The hydrogen ion concentration $[H^+]$ determines the acidity of blood and body fluids. It is essential to buffer these ions to maintain homeostasis. Chemical buffers act in less than a second and are the first line of defence against a change in pH. There are three chemical buffer systems in the body which work together: the bicarbonate, the phosphate and the protein buffer systems.
- Respiratory acidosis is caused by any condition that impairs lung ventilation and gas exchange. Metabolic acidosis can be caused by severe diarrhoea, untreated diabetes mellitus, or starvation. Respiratory alkalosis is always caused by hyperventilation. Metabolic alkalosis can be caused by vomiting of acid gastric content, some diuretics or severe constipation.
- The pregnant woman's body retains fluids and electrolytes and renal processes are modified to achieve a new balance, especially in sodium and water. Changes are due to the ADH and the renin–angiotensin–aldosterone system. Pregnant women

accumulate about 7 L more water and about 75% of the weight gain due to the accumulation of ECF fluid.

- The plasma [H^+] decreases early in pregnancy and the change is sustained until term. This makes the blood slightly more alkaline. Plasma bicarbonate concentration also decreases. This mild alkalaemia may be respiratory in origin as pregnant women hyperventilate.

- There is selective retention of potassium during pregnancy, most of which is utilised by the fetus. However, urinary calcium excretion increases. Serum calcium levels are raised and renal calcium reabsorption is reduced.

- During labour and delivery the renin–angiotensin–aldosterone system of mother and fetus are altered with an increase in the components. This causes fluid retention. Labouring women may suffer from water intoxication if given too much intravenous fluid, especially if it contains oxytocin (antidiuretic effect).

- Urinary excretion of electrolytes and glucose returns to normal after 1–2 weeks. There is a diuresis with loss of sodium and water until prepregnancy levels are reached by 3 weeks.

References

Baylis, C., Davison, J., 1998. The urinary system. In: Chamberlain, G., Broughton Pipkin, F. (Eds.) Clinical Physiology in Obstetrics, third edn. Blackwell Science, Oxford.

Blackburn, S.T., 2007. Maternal, Fetal and Neonatal Physiology: A clinical perspective, fourth edn. Elsevier Saunders, St Louis MO.

Hladunewich, M.A., Lafayette, G.C., Derby, K.L., et al., 2004. The dynamics of glomerular filtration in the puerperium. Am. J. Physiol. Ren. Physiol. 286, F496–F503.

Johnson, M.H., 2007. Essential Reproduction, sixth edn. Blackwell, Cambridge.

Marieb, E.N., Hoehn, K., 2008. Anatomy & Physiology, third edn. Pearson/Benjamin Cummings, New York.

Martini, F.H., Nath, J.L., 2009. Fundamentals of Anatomy & Physiology, eighth edn. Pearson Benjamin/Cummings, New York.

Millns, J.P., 1991. Fluid balance in labour. Curr. Obstet. Gynaecol. 1, 35–40.

Sherwood, L., 2006. Human Physiology: From Cells to Systems, sixth edn. Blackwell Science, Oxford.

Annotated recommended reading

Blackburn, S.T., 2007. Maternal, Fetal and Neonatal Physiology: A Clinical Perspective, fourth edn. Elsevier Saunders, St Louis MO.

This textbook provides a detailed description of the major changes that occur in the body systems during pregnancy. There is an extensive review of the literature, extending from classical research studies to the more recent research findings.

Martini, F.H., Nath, J.L., 2009. Fundamentals of Anatomy & Physiology, eighth edn. Pearson Benjamin/Cummings, New York.

This textbook presents a detailed overview of the maintenance of fluid balance. Attention is given to the nature of the structure and function of body systems, their interrelationships and homeostasis.

Chapter Twenty-One

21

The gastrointestinal tract

Introduction

In general, the form in which we eat food is unsuitable for use by the body for growth, repair and energy production. A healthy digestive system is essential to maintaining life by converting the foods we eat into the raw materials necessary to build and fuel our body's cells. The organs of the digestive system can be divided into two main groups: alimentary canal (*aliment* = nourish) and the accessory digestive organs, which include teeth, tongue, salivary glands, liver, gall bladder and pancreas. The alimentary canal, also called the gastrointestinal tract, will be discussed in this chapter followed by significant changes in pregnancy. The accessory organs of salivary glands, liver, gall bladder and pancreas will be discussed fully in Chapter 22 and nutrition in Chapter 23.

Anatomy of the gastrointestinal tract

The adult gastrointestinal tract (GI tract) is a continuous, coiled, fibromuscular tube of variable diameter about 4.5 metres long, open to the external environment at both ends and extending from the mouth to the anus. It varies in structure and function throughout its length. The organs of the GI tract are the mouth, pharynx, oesophagus, stomach, small intestine and large intestine (Fig. 21.1). Readers are referred to a textbook such as Martini & Nath (2009) for detailed anatomy. A brief description is given below.

The basic structure of the gastrointestinal tract is the same throughout its course. From the oesophagus to the anal canal, the walls of every organ consist of the same four basic layers (Fig. 21.2):

1. The **mucosal layer** is innermost and lines the tube. This layer is very variable along the length of the tube depending on the required function. The lumen is lined with stratified epithelial cells from which mucus-secreting cells develop. The turnover rate for the epithelial cells is high because of the amount of frictional damage. The epithelial cells are supported by a sheet of connective tissue called the **lamina propria**, and beneath that is a thin layer of smooth muscle called the **muscularis mucosae**. The mucosal layer also contains patches of lymphoid tissue, which defend the tract against micro-organisms.

2. The **submucosa** consists of loose connective tissue that supports blood vessels, lymphatics and nerves. The nerve fibres are called the **submucosal** or **Meissner's plexus**.

3. The **muscularis layer** is formed of smooth involuntary muscle fibres, bound together in sheets called **fasciculi**. There are two sheets: an inner circular layer and an outer longitudinal layer. In the stomach there is an additional oblique layer. Between the two layers of muscle fibres is a network of nerve fibres called the **myenteric** or **Auerbach's plexus**. The muscle fibres respond rhythmically to stimulation by the autonomic nervous system and some hormones. They respond slowly and less forcefully than striated muscle fibres and their contractions are not as finely controlled.

4. The **adventitia** or **serosa** (visceral peritoneum) is the outermost protective layer and is formed of connective tissue and squamous, serous epithelium. It is continuous with the mesentery of the abdominal cavity and supports blood vessels and nerves.

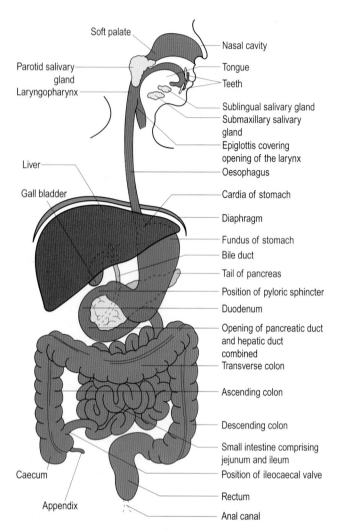

Figure 21.1 • Diagrammatic representation of the gastrointestinal tract. (From Hinchliff S M, Montague S E 1990, with permission.)

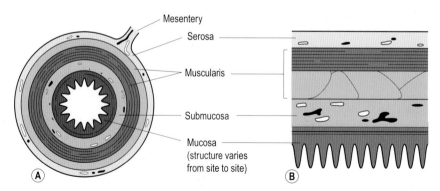

Figure 21.2 • Generalised structure of the gut wall. (A) Cross-section. (B) Longitudinal section. (From Hinchliff S M, Montague S E 1990, with permission.)

The peritoneum

Most of the digestive organs lie in the abdominopelvic cavity. All body cavities contain friction-reducing serous membranes and the peritoneum of the abdominopelvic cavity is the largest of these membranes. The visceral peritoneum covers the external surface of most of the digestive organs and is continuous with the parietal peritoneum that lines the walls of the abdominopelvic cavity. Between the two layers is the **peritoneal cavity** containing fluid secreted by the serous membranes.

The mesentery

Connecting the visceral and parietal layers of the peritoneum is a fused double layer of peritoneum called the mesentery. This supports the blood vessels, lymphatics and nerves to the digestive organs and helps support the organs. It also stores fat and is able to wall off areas of infection and inflammation to prevent the spread of peritonitis. Another fold of peritoneum, the **lesser omentum**, runs from the liver to the stomach. The **greater omentum** is a fold of peritoneum that hangs in front of the intestines and is reflected off the stomach. In most places the mesentery is attached to the posterior abdominal wall. The peritoneum surrounding the small intestine is like a fan with the small intestine attached to its outer edge.

Blood supply

Branches of the abdominal aorta serve the digestive organs and the special hepatic portal circulation. These include the hepatic, splenic and left gastric branches of the coeliac trunk supplying the liver, spleen and stomach and the superior and inferior mesenteric arteries supplying the small and large intestines. The hepatic portal circulation collects nutrient-rich venous blood from the digestive organs and takes it to the liver, as discussed in Chapter 22.

Control of the gastrointestinal tract

Autonomic nervous system

Nerve fibres from the autonomic nervous system (ANS) control the function of the gastrointestinal tract. The submucosal and myenteric nerve plexi are the local tracts. In the submucosal plexus, parasympathetic nerve fibres synapse with ganglion cells present in small clusters in the submucosal tissue. Postganglionic fibres, accompanied by some sympathetic fibres, leave the ganglion cells and send impulses to the glands and smooth muscle of the tract.

In the myenteric plexus parasympathetic nerve fibres synapse with ganglion cells which lie in large clusters between the circular and longitudinal fibres of the muscularis layer. Postganglionic fibres leave the ganglion cells and send impulses to the smooth muscle. Sympathetic fibres also supply this muscle. Both plexi run the length of the gut and receive both sympathetic and parasympathetic nerve fibres. The two plexi are connected and activity in one can affect the other. Stimulation at the upper end of the gastrointestinal tract can be transmitted to more distal parts; for instance, stimulation of gastric and intestinal enzyme secretion follows entry of food into the oesophagus.

Parasympathetic activity leads to an increase in both the motility and secretory functions of the tract and to relaxation of the gut sphincters. The vagus nerve, which is the 10th cranial nerve, is the source of parasympathetic supply to the oesophagus, stomach, pancreas, bile duct, small intestine and proximal colon. The parasympathetic supply to the distal colon is via the nervi erigentes from the sacral outflow.

Sympathetic activity leads to a decrease in blood supply to the gut with a decrease in secretions and in gut motility. There is contraction of the gut sphincters. As in other parts of the body, there are two types of catecholamine receptors in the gut: α and β_2 receptors. Note that β_1 receptors are present only in cardiac muscle. Stimulation of α receptors causes contraction of the smooth muscle of the gastrointestinal tract whereas stimulation of the β_2 receptors causes relaxation.

Regulatory chemicals

Two chemicals produced by the tract help in neural regulation. These are substance P and serotonin:

1. **Substance P**, a small peptide of only 11 amino acids, is found in high concentrations in the gut and may be a chemical mediator. It acts like a neurotransmitter and is referred to as a regulatory peptide or neuropeptide. It is involved in the conduction of pain impulses but brings about vasodilation and contraction of non-vascular smooth muscle.

2. **Serotonin** (5-hydroxytryptamine or 5-HT) is synthesised in the myenteric plexus and may also act as an interneuronal transmitter substance.

Functions of the gastrointestinal tract

The role of the gastrointestinal (alimentary) tract is to alter food so that it can be utilised by the body cells. Six processes can be described:

1. Ingestion.
2. Propulsion.
3. Mastication.
4. Mechanical and chemical digestion.
5. Absorption.
6. Elimination of non-usable residues as faeces.

Ingestion and mastication

These two processes take place in the mouth. Food is mixed with saliva, broken into small pieces by the teeth and propelled backwards into the oesophagus by the tongue. The tongue allows us to taste food. On its superior surface are numerous peg-like projections called **papillae**. These contain most of the 10000 taste buds, which allow differentiation between the four taste modalities: sweet, sour, salty and bitter (Marieb & Hoehn 2008). All taste buds have the potential for recognising the four tastes, although particular ones are associated with one taste. The four tastes result in different neural firing patterns, which are interpreted in the cerebral cortex. Taste is aided by the sense of smell, which sends impulses to the brain via the olfactory nerve. This is why any inflammation and hypersecretion of the nasal mucosa, which may occur in pregnancy, will result in a loss or alteration of taste.

Saliva

The salivary glands and the production of saliva are discussed more fully in Chapter 22. The three pairs of salivary glands—the parotid, submaxillary and sublingual glands—produce 1.5 L of saliva daily, consisting of 99% water and with a pH 6.75–7.0. Saliva contains the digestive enzyme α-**amylase** which acts upon cooked starch to convert polysaccharides into disaccharides. It facilitates the formation of a bolus of partly broken up food ready to swallow, once lubricated by salivary mucins. Saliva is produced in response to the cerebral perception of the thought, sight or smell of food or the presence of food in the mouth.

The ingested and masticated food is propelled down the oesophagus into the stomach for digestion of the food to continue. The process is called **deglutition**. The tongue contracts and presses the bolus of food against the hard palate in the roof of the mouth. It then arches backwards and the bolus of food is propelled into the oropharynx.

The stomach

Chemical breakdown of food by the secretion of enzymes begins in the stomach and is completed in the small intestine. The stomach is 25 cm long and lies in the left side of the abdominal cavity partly hidden by the diaphragm and liver. It is continuous with the oesophagus above and the duodenum below. When empty, it is J-shaped. Its mucosal layer has folds (**rugae**) which allow distension. The rugae are further folded, providing a large absorptive surface, and contain millions of deep **gastric pits** with microscopic gastric glands that produce gastric juice.

Functions of the stomach

- A reservoir for food.
- Production of the intrinsic factor.
- Gastric absorption.
- A churn to mix food.
- Secretion of mucus, hormones and gastric juice.

A reservoir for food

At rest the stomach's capacity is only 50 ml, but receptive relaxation of the stomach wall musculature can allow distension of up to 1.5 L. Under exceptional circumstances the stomach can hold 4 L of content. The pyloric sphincter prevents a too rapid transfer of food to the small intestine.

Production of the intrinsic factor

The intrinsic factor is a glycoprotein necessary for the absorption of **vitamin B_{12}** (cyanocobalamin) produced by the gastric parietal cells, which also produce gastric acid. Intrinsic factor binds to vitamin B_{12} in the terminal ileum of the small intestine to form a complex which appears to bind to receptors in the wall of the ileum and is transferred into the blood. Vitamin B_{12} is required for the maintenance of healthy myelin sheaths around the nerves and also for the formation of red blood cells in the bone marrow. Lack of vitamin B_{12} may lead to a megaloblastic anaemia. The resulting pernicious anaemia may lead to subacute combined degeneration of the spinal cord.

Gastric absorption

Food that has reached the stomach is only partly broken down there and many of the molecules are still too large to be absorbed. There are also no carrier systems present in the gastric mucosa. Water and some drugs such as aspirin (acetylsalicylic acid), which is a weak acid, can be absorbed from the stomach. Absorption of aspirin lowers intracellular pH and may cause damage, leading to gastric irritation and bleeding.

A churn to mix food

The stomach converts food to a thick soup consistency by mixing it with gastric secretions. This also dilutes

Table 21.1 Hormones that aid digestion

Hormone	Stimulus	Target organ	Effect
Gastrin	Presence of food in the stomach	Stomach	Increased gastric gland secretions, most effect on HCl production
		Small intestine	Causes contraction of intestinal muscle
		Ileocaecal valve	Relaxes valve
		Large intestine	Stimulates mass movements
Serotonin	Food in stomach	Stomach	Contraction of stomach musculature
Histamine	Food in stomach	Stomach	Release of HCl
Somatostatin	Food in stomach	Stomach	Inhibits gastric secretion, motility, emptying
	Sympathetic nerve stimulus	Pancreas	Inhibits secretion
		Small intestine	Inhibits GI blood flow and intestinal absorption
		Gall bladder	Inhibits contraction and bile release
Intestinal gastrin	Acidic/partly digested food in duodenum	Stomach	Stimulates gastric glands and motility
Secretin	Acidic or irritant chyme, partially digested fats and proteins	Stomach	Inhibits gastric secretion and motility during gastric phase
		Pancreas	Increases bicarbonate-rich pancreatic juice. Potentiates CCK action
		Liver	Increases bile output
Cholecystokinin (CCK)	Fatty chyme or partially digested proteins	Liver/pancreas	Potentiates secretin's action
		Gall bladder	Increases enzyme-rich output
		Sphincter of Oddi	Stimulates contraction with expulsion of bile. Relaxes to allow bile and pancreatic juice to enter duodenum
Gastric inhibitory peptide (GIP)	Fatty and/or glucose-containing chyme	Stomach	Inhibits gastric gland secretion and motility during gastric phase

the food and makes it compatible with the extracellular fluid in the duodenum. The semiliquid, formed by waves of peristalsis of the smooth muscle in the stomach wall, is called **chyme**.

Secretion of mucus

Mucus is produced by the cells in the necks of the deep gastric glands in both the cardiac and pyloric sphincters. It adheres to the gastric mucosa to protect the stomach from being digested by the proteolytic gastric enzyme **pepsin**. The layer of mucus that protects the mucosa must be 1mm thick.

Secretion of hormones

Enteroendocrine cells release a variety of hormones, which diffuse into blood capillaries and are returned to the GI tract to influence digestive system target organs. These include gastrin, serotonin, cholecystokinin, somatostatin and endorphins. Histamine, produced by circulating mast cells and basophils, increases gastric acid secretion by binding to histamine receptors (H_2 receptors) on the gastric parietal cells (Table 21.1).

Secretion of gastric juice

Two to three litres of gastric juice (a mixture of secretions from two types of cells present in the gastric pits but absent from the pylorus) is produced daily (Fig. 21.3). The gastric pit cells are:

1. Parietal or oxyntic cells, which secrete hydrochloric acid (HCl) and the intrinsic factor.
2. Chief or zygomen cells, which secrete the enzymes.

There are about 1000 million parietal cells in the gastric pits of an adult stomach. Hydrogen ions (H^+) are secreted into the lumen of the stomach against a concentration gradient, probably by an active pump mechanism in the cell membrane. Carbon dioxide (CO_2) diffuses into the parietal cells from arterial blood and combines with water to form H_2CO_3 (carbonic acid). Equal numbers of H^+ ions, formed by the dissociation of H_2CO_3 into H^+ and bicarbonate ions (HCO_3^-), and chloride ions (Cl^-) are secreted into the lumen of the gastric pits. They form HCl, which is then diluted by water. Histamine or the hormone gastrin stimulates the secretion of the HCl into the lumen of the stomach.

The functions of gastric acid are:

- Inactivation of salivary amylase.
- Bacteriostasis.

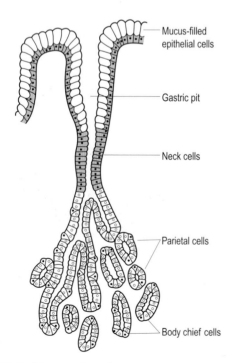

Figure 21.3 • Diagram of gastric pit. (From Hinchliff S M, Montague S E 1990, with permission.)

Labels: Mucus-filled epithelial cells; Gastric pit; Neck cells; Parietal cells; Body chief cells

- Alteration of the molecular structure of ingested proteins to tenderise them.
- Curdling of milk.
- Conversion of pepsinogen to pepsin.

Children produce an enzyme called **rennin** which acts on the milk protein casein and converts it into curds.

The chief cells produce a pepsinogen-rich secretion. When gastric pH is lower than 5.5, pepsinogen is converted into the active proteolytic enzyme pepsin by HCl, which converts proteins to polypeptides by breaking the bonds between specific amino acids. Once chyme leaves the stomach there is a change to an alkaline medium and pepsin's activity ceases.

Control of gastric juice secretion

There are both neural and hormonal aspects of control of gastric juice secretion.

Neural control

There are two phases in the neural control of gastric juice secretion although the two work interdependently. The **cephalic phase** is an anticipatory conditioned reflex to the sight, smell or thought of food. This phase is mediated by the vagus nerve, which stimulates both parietal and chief cells. The **gastric phase** is mediated by stretch receptors and chemoreceptors. Stretch receptors in the stomach wall respond to distension by food. Chemoreceptors respond to the presence of protein molecules within the stomach. Impulses from these two types of receptor are sent to the submucosal plexus where they synapse with parasympathetic neurons. Excitatory impulses are then dispatched to the parietal cells.

Hormonal control

Although the neural influences described above are important, hormonal influences, especially gastrin, contribute most to the gastric phase of secretion. Throughout, the gut regulatory hormones called **peptides** are active. Many of them are also found in the central nervous system and alternative names for them are neurohormones, neuropeptides or neurotransmitters. The term **gastrin** refers to a group of similar hormones produced by **G cells** in the lateral walls of the gastric glands in the antrum of the stomach. A small amount of gastrin is produced by the duodenal mucosa, sometimes referred to as a third or **intestinal phase** of gastric juice secretion. The production of gastrin is stimulated by food in the stomach, particularly by partially digested proteins and caffeine.

P cells throughout the gastrointestinal tract secrete **bombesin**, the gastrin-releasing peptide. Gastrin enters the gastric circulatory capillaries and the systemic circulation and when it reaches the stomach via the bloodstream gastrin has the following actions:

- Stimulates the production of gastric acid by the parietal cells by the release of histamine.
- Has a minor role in stimulating the production of pepsinogen by the chief cells.
- Stimulates the growth of the gastric and intestinal mucosa.
- Causes enhanced contraction of the cardiac sphincter to prevent gastric reflux.
- Stimulates the secretion of insulin and glucagon in the pancreas.

Control of gastric motility

Increase of gastric motility

Stomach contractions empty the stomach and also compress, knead and mix the food with gastric juice to produce chyme. Waves of peristalsis pass from the cardiac sphincter to the pylorus about three times a minute. The more liquid parts of chyme pass through the pylorus into the small intestine, while the more solid parts are sent back to the body of the stomach for further gastric mixing. The regulatory peptide **motilin**, produced by cells in the duodenum and jejunum in response to the entry of acid chyme, increases gastric motility.

Food remains in the stomach depending on its consistency and composition. Carbohydrates and liquids leave the stomach fastest followed by proteins and fats. The **enterogastric reflex** is initiated when the products of protein digestion, together with the acid, enter the duodenum, resulting in a slowing of gastric motility. Gastric emptying usually takes 4–5 h, during which the antrum, pylorus and duodenal cap contract in sequence. This is the gastric pump mechanism, which results in squirts of chyme entering the duodenum.

Inhibition of gastric motility

When glucose and fats enter the duodenum a regulatory peptide called **gastric inhibitory peptide** (GIP) is secreted by the **K cells** of the duodenal and jejunal mucosa. GIP, also known as glucose-dependent insulin-releasing peptide, decreases gastric secretion and motility and stimulates the secretion of insulin. **Vasoactive intestinal polypeptide** (VIP), produced in the D cells of the duodenum and colon, also inhibits gastric motility by acting as a smooth muscle relaxant. It also stimulates the intestinal secretion of electrolytes.

The small intestine

The structure of the small intestine

The small intestine is a long coiled tube about 3–3.5 m long that extends from the pyloric sphincter to the ileocaecal valve. Its diameter is only 2.5 cm. It is the body's main digestive organ, where food digestion is completed and absorption of nutrients and most of the water from the chyme takes place.

There are three sections of the small intestine:

1. The C-shaped duodenum lies mainly behind the peritoneum. It is about 25 cm long and surrounds the head of the pancreas.
2. The jejunum, 250 cm long, makes up about 40% of the remainder of the small intestine.
3. The ileum, 360 cm long, makes up the other 60%, joining the large intestine at the ileocaecal valve. The jejunum has thicker walls and is more vascular while the ileum has fewer folds in its lumen. Protective lymph nodes called **Peyer's patches** are present in the ileum.

The duodenum

Salivary amylase begins the digestion of cooked starch into maltose and dextrins. Pepsin begins the breakdown of proteins into polypeptides. There is no secretion of enzymes by the duodenum although it does secrete hormones. The duodenum receives the secretions of the pancreas and liver via the pancreatic duct and common bile duct (Fig. 21.4) after they join together at the

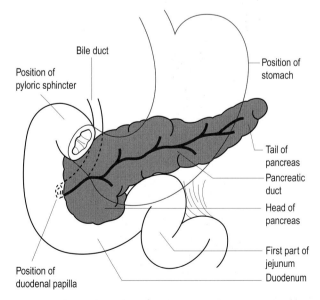

Figure 21.4 • The position of the pancreas. (From Hinchliff S M, Montague S E 1990, with permission.)

ampulla of Vater, at the sphincter of Oddi. These secretions are alkaline (pH of about 8) and produce a sharp change in pH from the acidity of the stomach to the alkalinity of the duodenum. Enzymes are pH-sensitive and function within a narrow range. The first few centimetres of the duodenum are called the **duodenal cap**. The tissue is protected from the acid chyme by a large number of mucus-secreting **Brunner's glands**.

Pancreatic extrinsic secretions

The exocrine function of the pancreas is achieved by secretions from **acinar cells** and plays a major role in digestion. The production of the enzymes is discussed more fully in Chapter 22. The enzymes are secreted into the pancreatic duct and the duodenum. The three proteolytic enzymes are:

1. **Trypsinogen**, which is in an inactive form to safeguard the gut from autodigestion.

2. **Trypsin**, which is formed from trypsinogen in a reaction catalysed by the enzyme enterokinase (enteropeptidase). Trypsin completes the breakdown of proteins to amino acids.

3. **Carboxypeptidase**, which acts on peptides.

Other enzymes are:

- Pancreatic amylase, which converts starch to maltose.
- Pancreatic lipase, which breaks down triglycerides to three fatty acids and glycerol.

- Ribonuclease (RNAase), which breaks down RNA.
- Deoxyribonuclease (DNAase), which acts on DNA to release free nucleotides.

Control of pancreatic juice secretion

The hormone **secretin** results in the secretion of the watery component, rich in bicarbonate but low in enzymes. Another hormone, **cholecystokinin** (CCK), causes the release of the enzymes. Stimulation of pancreatic juice secretion can be divided into a cephalic phase, with vagal control brought about by the sight, smell or thought of food or the presence of food in the mouth, and a gastric phase stimulated by the release of gastrin (Fig. 21.5).

CCK causes:

- Stimulation of enzyme-rich pancreatic secretion.
- Augmentation of the activity of secretin.
- Slowing of gastric emptying and inhibition of gastric secretion.
- Stimulation of the secretion of enterokinase.
- Stimulation of glucagon secretion.
- Stimulation of intestinal motility.
- Contraction of the gall bladder with the release of bile.

Bile

Bile is produced by the liver and stored in the gall bladder. It contains no digestive enzymes but emulsifies fats so that the fat-soluble vitamins and iron can

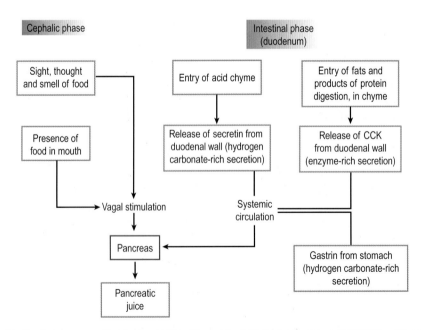

Figure 21.5 • Flow chart to illustrate pancreatic juice secretion. (From Hinchliff S M, Montague S E 1990, with permission.)

be absorbed. Its production, content and function are discussed more fully in Chapter 22. The control of bile secretion also involves neural and hormonal factors. CCK is the major controller, causing contraction of the gall bladder and relaxation of the sphincter of Oddi. Once the gall bladder is empty, further flow of bile into the duodenum occurs directly from the liver. Vagus nerve stimulation will bring about a similar action. About 97% of bile salts are reabsorbed into the portal circulation and returned to the liver.

Intestinal juice

The process of digestion is completed by juices secreted by the duodenum and jejunum. This juice is rich in mucus, some of which comes from the Brunner's glands in the proximal duodenum. **Lieberkühn glands** in the jejunum and ileum secrete most of the watery juice. The nutrients are absorbed into the circulating blood through small finger-like projections in the surface of the small intestine called **villi**, which are covered by a layer of mucus to prevent autodigestion.

Intestinal enzymes

These enzymes are produced by enterocytes in the villi and break down food particles into an absorbable form. They are probably released from shed enterocytes. Proteins are broken down into amino acids, while fats are in the form of fatty acids and glycerol.

Carbohydrates are broken down into monosaccharides: glucose, fructose and galactose. The enzymes are:

- Aminopeptidases: act on peptides.
- Dipeptidases: act on dipeptides.
- Maltase: converts maltose to glucose.
- Lactase: converts lactose to glucose and galactose.
- Sucrase: converts sucrose into glucose and fructose.

The villi

Visible folding of the mucosa and submucosa into **plicae circularis** (circular folds) increases the surface area of the small intestine. The addition of villi and microvilli increases the surface area to 600 times that of a simple tube of the same size, giving a surface area of 200 m^2 (Marieb & Hoehn 2008). Between the villi are small pits called the **crypts of Lieberkühn** where the mucus-secreting glands are situated. Villi have an external covering of simple columnar epithelium continuous with the crypts (Fig. 21.6) and a central lacteal containing lymph, which empties into the local lymphatic circulation. There is a capillary blood supply linked to both hepatic and portal veins.

Two other types of cell are associated with the villi: **goblet cells** that secrete mucus are situated mainly in the crypts while **enterocytes** are tall columnar cells involved in digestion and absorption. Enterocytes have many mitochondria to provide the energy for enzyme secretion and nutrient absorption. They have a high rate of mitosis and those at the tip of the villi are replaced every 30 h.

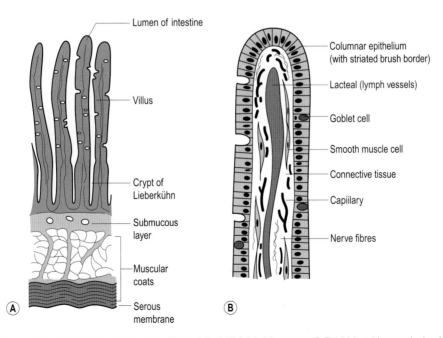

Figure 21.6 • (A) Villi in small intestine. (B) A single villus. (From Hinchliff S M, Montague S E 1990, with permission.)

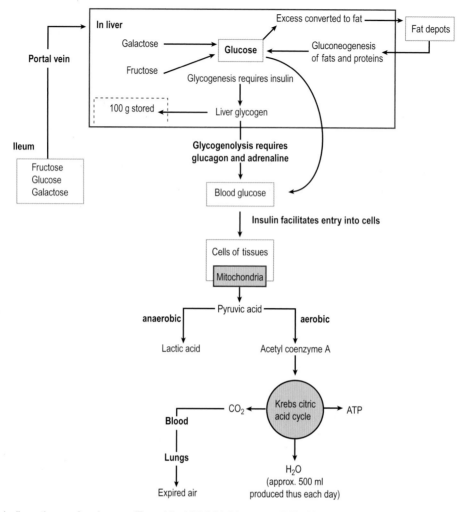

Figure 21.7 ● Metabolic pathways for glucose. (From Hinchliff S M, Montague S E 1990, with permission.)

A few smooth muscle cells are present in villi, contracting to assist lymph drainage in the central lacteals. Lymphocytes and plasma cells are situated at intervals between the enterocytes. The plasma cells secrete immunoglobulin A (IgA) to protect the gut from pathogens.

There are also cells in the intestinal wall secreting 5-hydroxytryptamine (5-HT), which may increase intestinal motility.

Absorption

Eight to nine litres of water and 1 kg of nutrients daily are absorbed across the gut wall. The transport of nutrients can be either active or passive. **Active transport** requires energy and is usually against a concentration gradient. Most such substances require carrier molecules, including vitamin B_{12}, iron, sodium ions, glucose, galactose and amino acids. Water follows passively along an osmotic gradient. **Passive transport** requires no

energy, depending on the direction of concentration and electrical gradients. It includes water, lipids, drugs and some electrolytes and vitamins. Some substances passively cross the gut wall membrane, with the help of carrier molecules, by **facilitated diffusion**.

Nutrients and minerals

Monosaccharides

About 500 g of monosaccharides are absorbed daily. Galactose and glucose pass into the villous capillaries and then to the hepatic portal vein. A high concentration of sodium ions on the surface of the enterocytes facilitates the active transport of these molecules. Glucose and sodium ions share the same carrier molecule. Sodium concentration in the enterocyte is low so that sodium moves into the cell along a concentration gradient accompanied by glucose. Fructose has a different carrier molecule and its transport is not influenced by sodium.

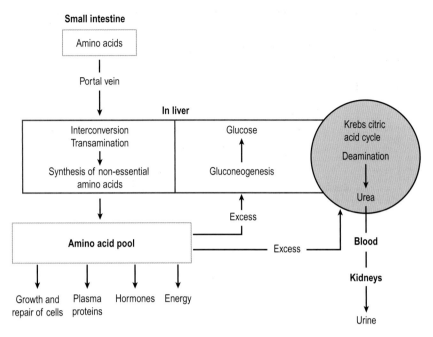

Figure 21.8 • Metabolic pathways for amino acids. (From Hinchliff S M, Montague S E 1990, with permission.)

Monosaccharides are transported to the liver where galactose and fructose are converted to glucose (Fig. 21.7). Some of the glucose is converted to glycogen (**glycogenesis**) under the influence of insulin. About 100 g of glucose are stored in the liver, sufficient to maintain blood glucose levels for 24 h. Some glycogen is stored in skeletal muscle to provide energy for muscle action. The liver converts any glucose that is surplus to the body's needs into adipose tissue.

Blood glucose is maintained normally at a level of 3.5–5.5 mmol/L. When the glucose level falls, liver glycogen is broken down (**glycogenolysis**) to release glucose. This occurs under the influence of glucagon and adrenaline (epinephrine). Once glycogen stores in the liver are depleted, the liver manufactures glucose from amino acids and glycerol (**gluconeogenesis**).

When circulating glucose arrives at the tissues, the cells take it up by facilitated diffusion, under the influence of insulin. In the mitochondria of the cells glucose is oxidised to form energy in the **Krebs** or **citric acid cycle**. The glucose is converted to pyruvic acid, which, in turn, is converted to acetyl coenzyme A, usually referred to as **acetyl CoA** in a process requiring oxygen, i.e. aerobic. Acetyl CoA enters the Krebs cycle to undergo changes mediated by enzymes. The process of oxidation forms the energy-storage molecule adenosine triphosphate (ATP), along with water and carbon dioxide. If there is insufficient oxygen to convert pyruvic acid to acetyl CoA, lactic acid is formed.

Amino acids

In an adult, approximately 200 g of amino acids are absorbed daily from the ileum, of which 50 g/day are needed to maintain nitrogen balance and to provide for tissue growth and repair. The mechanism for absorption of amino acids is not fully understood but may depend on whether the amino acid is acidic, basic or neutral. Sodium appears to facilitate the absorption of amino acids.

Amino acids cannot be stored by the body and are absorbed into the blood to enter a common circulating pool from which cells can remove them as necessary (Fig. 21.8). However, the liver can interconvert amino acids by utilising the eight essential amino acids to synthesise the non-essential amino acids. The process of **deamination** in the liver breaks down any excess amino acids. The nitrogen portion is converted into urea, which enters the blood and is excreted by the kidney.

Fats

About 80 g of fat is absorbed daily, mainly in the duodenum. The contents of the micelles are discharged onto the microvilli and enter the enterocytes by passive diffusion. Short-chain fatty acids enter the capillary network and travel in the hepatic portal vein as free fatty acids. Longer-chain fatty acids are resynthesised in the enterocyte to become triglycerides coated with a layer of lipoprotein, cholesterol and phospholipid. These complexes enter the central lacteals to form **chyle**, which enters the

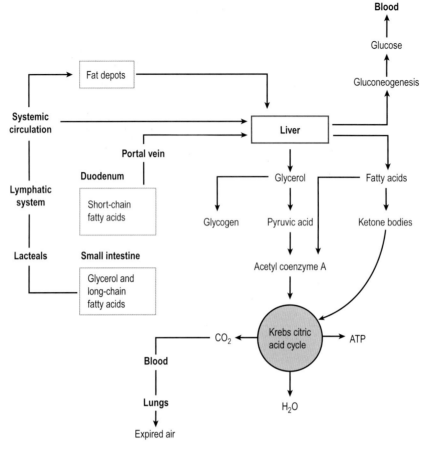

Figure 21.9 • Metabolic pathways for fats. (From Hinchliff S M, Montague S E 1990, with permission.)

lymphatic system and then the bloodstream. Faeces contain about 5% fat.

Bile salts, steroid hormones and cell membranes are formed from cholesterol. Cholesterol is found in the blood, mainly in combination with a protein carrier, as lipoproteins, of which there are three types:

1. High-density lipoproteins (HDLs).
2. Low-density lipoproteins (LDLs).
3. Very low-density lipoproteins (VLDLs).

Cholesterol (in the form of LDLs and VLDLs) is laid down in arterial walls as atheromatous plaques. A high ratio of HDLs to LDLs and VLDLs may offer protection against ischaemic heart disease. An increased ratio of HDLs to LDLs and VLDLs has been shown in vegetarians, in those whose fat intake is largely unsaturated and in those who take regular exercise. The ratio is reduced in those who smoke cigarettes.

Fat can be utilised by the body to form energy and any excess fat is stored as adipose tissue. When fat stores are needed for energy production they are mobilised under the influence of growth hormones or cortisol and taken to the liver where the triglycerides are broken down into free fatty acids and glycerol. The fatty acids

are converted to acetyl CoA in the presence of oxygen and glucose and these enter the Krebs citric acid cycle (Fig. 21.9). If glucose is not available, acetyl CoA metabolism is deranged and the ketone bodies acetoacetic acid and β-hydroxybutyric acid accumulate in the blood. These can be oxidised to release energy but metabolic acidosis will occur.

Sodium, potassium and water

About 2 L of fluid are ingested daily. A further 8–9 L of fluid are added to the gut during the production of digestive juices. Only 50–200 ml are lost in the faeces, the rest being absorbed from both the small and large intestine at a rate of 200–400 ml/min. The jejunum, ileum and colon actively reabsorb sodium ions, which are followed passively by chloride and water. Some potassium is actively secreted into the gut and reabsorbed from the ileum and colon along a concentration gradient.

Vitamins

The water-soluble vitamins, with the exception of vitamin B_{12} (absorbed as a complex with the intrinsic

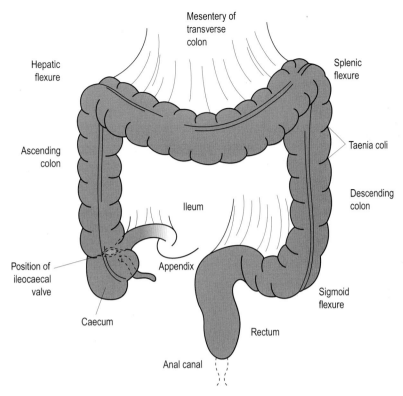

Figure 21.10 • The large intestine. (From Hinchliff S M, Montague S E 1990, with permission.)

factor in the terminal ileum), are passively absorbed with water. The fat-soluble vitamins, A, D, E and K, enter the enterocytes in the micelles. Bile and lipase are necessary for their absorption.

Most calcium is absorbed in the upper part of the small intestine under the influence of parathyroid hormone and calcitonin. The active process is facilitated by vitamin D.

Iron

In developed countries about 15–20 mg of iron is ingested daily, mostly as ferric salts, but only 5–10% is absorbed into the blood. There is a daily loss of 1 mg/day from desquamation of the skin and in the faeces. Women lose about 25 mg each month during menstruation. Iron is more readily absorbed in the ferrous form and the ferric form is reduced to the ferrous form by gastric juice and vitamin C.

Iron is actively absorbed in the upper part of the small intestine and is stored in the enterocytes when their cellular stores are low. The enterocytes discharge iron into the bloodstream when serum levels fall. Iron travels in the blood bound to **apoferritin**, which is known as **ferritin** when iron is bound to it. About 70% of iron in the body is in haemoglobin and 3% in myoglobin in muscle protein. The rest is stored in the liver as ferritin or as **haemosiderin**.

The large intestine

The adult large intestine is about 1.5 m long, consisting of the caecum, appendix, colon and rectum (Fig. 21.10). It has a diameter of 5–6 cm and can store large quantities of food residues. The large intestine has no villi and a much smaller internal surface than the small intestine. The colon differs from the generalised structure of the gastrointestinal tract as the longitudinal muscle bands are incomplete and the wall is gathered into three longitudinal bands, the **taeniae coli**. These bands are shorter than the remaining colon, so that the wall pouches outwards into **haustrations** (buckets) between the taeniae when the circular muscles contract. The filling and emptying of the haustrations help to mix the colonic contents. Patches of lymphoid tissue are scattered throughout the length of the large intestine, providing a protection against pathogens.

About 1 L of porridge-like chyme enters the large intestine daily through the ileocaecal valve. This valve, normally closed because of back pressure from the colon's contents, opens in response to peristaltic waves. The caecum relaxes and the ileocaecal valve opens, a reflex called the **gastrocolic reflex**. The colonic peristalsis that follows fills the rectum with faeces, resulting in the urge to defecate.

The **caecum**, a blind pouch between the ileocaecal valve and the colon, is about 7 cm long. This has no known function in humans although it is involved in cellulose digestion in herbivores. The **vermiform appendix**, a worm-like blind-ending sac projecting from the end of the caecum about the size of an adult's little finger, contains lymphoid tissue and enlarges in the presence of infection or inflammation (appendicitis). An enlarged appendix may rupture so that faecal material and bacteria enter the abdominal cavity, leading to peritonitis.

The colon

The large intestine is divided anatomically into three regions:

1. The **ascending colon**, about 15 cm long, commences at the caecum and extends upwards on the right of the abdominal cavity as far as the lower border of the liver.

2. The **transverse colon** begins at the hepatic flexure and traverses the abdominal cavity below the liver and stomach to the slightly higher splenic flexure.

3. The **descending colon**, about 25 cm long, descends along the left side of the abdominal cavity. The sigmoid (S-shaped) colon, about 40 cm long, is a continuation of the descending colon and empties into the rectum.

The large intestine has five functions:

1. Storage of unabsorbed food residues prior to defecation. About 70% of food residues are excreted within 72 h of ingestion, but the remainder may stay in the colon for 1 week. Non-absorbable dietary fibre gives bulk to the faeces.

2. Absorption of water, electrolytes and some vitamins. Sodium is actively reabsorbed into the hepatic portal vein, followed passively by water and chloride. The amount of water reabsorbed depends on how long the residue remains in the colon. In constipation the residue may stay in the colon for several days, resulting in removal of most of the water.

3. Synthesis of vitamin K and some B vitamins—thiamine, folic acid and riboflavin—by commensal colonic bacteria. Bacterial fermentation of food residues results in the formation of flatus, which consists of nitrogen, carbon dioxide, hydrogen, methane and hydrogen sulphide. Between 500 and 700 ml of flatus is produced daily depending on the type of food eaten; legumes lead to an increase in flatus production.

4. Secretion of mucus, which acts as a lubricant for elimination of faeces. The mucus contains bicarbonate, which gives the contents of the colon a pH of 7.5–8.0.

5. Secretion of potassium ions.

Movements of the colon

Contraction of the circular muscle fibres occurs about once every 30 min. This causes **segmentation**, a non-propulsive movement in the colon, which mixes the colonic contents and facilitates absorption. Peristalsis moves the faeces towards the rectum. Following meals, there is an increase in colonic activity due to the gastrocolic reflex. Associated with the gastrocolic reflex is **mass movement**, which propels the faeces towards the rectum. The haustrations in the mid-colon disappear and the tube becomes flattened and shortened by waves of rapid, powerful contractions, moving the colonic contents rapidly into the sigmoid colon.

The rectum

The rectum is a muscular tube about 15 cm long. It is capable of great distension but is usually empty until just before defecation. The sudden distension of the rectal walls brought about by filling of the rectum during mass movement brings about the urge to defecate. The rectum opens to the exterior by the anal canal, which has both internal and external sphincters.

The anal canal

The anal canal is about 3 cm long and begins where the rectum perforates the levator ani muscle of the pelvic floor. It has a sphincter at both ends. The **internal anal sphincter** is composed of smooth muscle fibres and is not under voluntary control. When nerve fibres from the sympathetic system are stimulated, the muscle fibres in the internal anal sphincter contract. Fibres from the parasympathetic system inhibit contractions and the sphincter relaxes. The **external anal sphincter** is made up of striated voluntary muscle and is supplied by fibres from the pudendal nerve. The sphincter is under conscious control from about 18 months of age. Damage to the sphincter or its nerve supply may occur in childbirth, resulting in incontinence of faeces.

The mucosa of the anal canal hangs in long ridges called **anal columns** and is made of stratified squamous epithelium. Mucus is secreted from the anal recesses between the columns, which aids in defecation. Two superficial venous plexi, the haemorrhoidal veins, are associated with the anal canal. These may become distended, resulting in varicosities or haemorrhoids.

Defecation

Afferent nerve impulses travel to the sacral spinal cord when faeces enter the rectum. Impulses then travel back from the spinal cord in a reflex arc to the terminal ileum and anal sphincter to allow defecation. The cerebral cortex receives nerve messages, which allow inhibition of the spinal reflex arc if it is not convenient to defecate. Defecation is usually assisted by voluntary effort, which raises intra-abdominal pressure. A deep breath is taken and is expired against a closed glottis. This is called **Valsalva's manoeuvre**. The levator ani muscles contract and the pressure in the rectum is raised to about 200 mmHg (26 kPa). The anal sphincters relax and the contents of the rectum are expelled. During straining there is a sharp rise in blood pressure followed by a sudden fall.

Faeces

About 100–150g of faeces are eliminated each day, consisting of 30–50g solids and 70–100g water. The solid portion consists mainly of cellulose, shed epithelial cells, bacteria, some salts and stercobilin, which gives it the brown colour. The characteristic odour of faeces is caused by bacterial breakdown of amines.

Maternal adaptations to pregnancy

The gastrointestinal and hepatic systems during pregnancy have dramatic anatomical and physiological alterations that are essential in supporting the nutritional demands of the mother and fetus. The related alterations are often accompanied by upsets of the gastrointestinal function, which are probably the commonest cause of complaint by pregnant women. These minor disorders are discussed in Chapter 30.

The mouth

Pregnant women usually find that they have an increased appetite, cravings or aversions for certain food, and pica, which is a craving for non-food substances. Specific changes in food consumption and food habits are strongly influenced by cultural and economical factors and may also change to meet the needs of the fetus. Progesterone is a known appetite stimulant and evidence for this is supported by changes in appetite, which closely follow the hormonal changes during the menstrual cycle. During pregnancy, alterations in the balance of oestrogen, progesterone, glucagon and insulin contribute to the changes in food intake.

The gums and teeth

The gums may become swollen and spongy and bleed easily. This results from oedema due to the effects of oestrogen on blood flow and the consistency of connective tissue. There is an increase in gingivitis and periodontal disease, caused by the oedema rather than by an increased presence of irritant particles of food. This is often more extreme with increased maternal age and parity and where there are pre-existing dental problems. About 5% of pregnant women will develop an **epulis** (pregnancy tumour), which is a friable growth or hyperplasia of the gum usually found on the palatal side of the maxillary gingiva (Laine 2002). It may bleed or interfere with chewing and will usually regress after delivery, although occasionally excision of the growth may be necessary.

Although dentists and women believe that pregnancy damages teeth, there is no evidence to suggest that demineralisation of teeth occurs from pregnancy. The calcium needs for the fetus are drawn from maternal stores (skeleton) and not from maternal teeth (Laine 2002). Changes in saliva and the nausea and vomiting of pregnancy may increase the risk of caries during pregnancy.

Saliva

Ptyalism or excess salivation may occur but there is no evidence to suggest that more saliva is actually produced. The problem is due to a reluctance of women to swallow because of the associated nausea. This is often a particular problem in Afro-Caribbean women. Ganglion-blocking drugs may be required if ptyalism becomes a major problem. There is uncertainty as to the changes in the pH of saliva. It is more likely that the pH drops and saliva becomes more acid in pregnancy.

The oesophagus

Heartburn affects about two-thirds of all women at some stage in pregnancy (Enkin et al 2000). It is probably due to reflux oesophagitis due to the effects of progesterone on the muscle tone of the cardiac sphincter between the oesophagus and stomach. The competence of the sphincter is impaired and regurgitation of gastric acid is more likely. This may not be the single cause as acid reflux has also been found to be present in 40% of people with no heartburn. There is an increased risk of **hiatus hernia** where there is displacement of the cardiac sphincter into the thorax. Displacement of the sphincter has probably a minor role to play in heartburn and the more likely factor to be considered is the strength of the sphincter (Hytten 1991).

The stomach

Acid secretion

The effect of pregnancy on gastric acid secretion is unclear (Blackburn 2007). Gastric acid secretions may remain unaffected whilst there is a tendency for secretions to decrease during pregnancy, beginning in the early weeks and becoming even less in late pregnancy. This may explain why a peptic ulcer is rarely detected in pregnancy and those women with an ulcer have a clear remission during pregnancy, with a return to the symptoms experienced by the third month after delivery (Scott & Abu-Hamda 2004).

Emptying time

Gastric muscle tone and motility are reduced during pregnancy due to the effect of progesterone (Blackburn 2007). However, low levels of circulating motilin have been found during pregnancy. This results in delay in emptying, which is probably due to the lower secretion rate of gastric juices. The digestion time for solid food is prolonged although watery food is digested and passed on to the small intestine with little delay. Drinks containing high levels of glucose such as those administered in glucose tolerance tests have a high osmotic effect and gastric emptying is delayed in hyperosmotic foods. The reduced activity of the gastric muscle may exaggerate the effect and result in nausea. During labour, reduced stomach motility leads to a delay in emptying and a risk of acid aspiration.

The small intestine

There is no increase in the absorption of food even though metabolism is anabolic during pregnancy. Any increased nutrition must come from increased intake and there is facilitated absorption of nutrients such as iron and calcium. The prepregnant levels of calcium absorption (20–25%) increase early in pregnancy, to a 50% absorption by mid-pregnancy, and thereafter remains stable (Kovacs 2001). Phosphate and magnesium absorption is assumed to follow calcium in terms of intestinal absorption. The transit time of food and waste products through the intestine is prolonged due to reduced mobility and a decrease in the tone of the intestinal musculature as a result on the action of progesterone on smooth muscle (Blackburn 2007).

The large intestine

The colon shares in the general relaxation of smooth muscle found throughout the body. Constipation is a common complaint during pregnancy and is made worse by the prolonged transit time of waste materials and the resulting increased absorption of water in the colon. Increased flatulence may also occur (Blackburn 2007).

Main points

- The gastrointestinal tract is a continuous, coiled, fibromuscular tube extending from the mouth to the anus. It consists of the mouth, pharynx, oesophagus, stomach, small intestine and large intestine.
- The function of the gastrointestinal tract is controlled by the autonomic nervous system (ANS). Parasympathetic activity leads to an increase in both the motility and secretory functions of the tract and to relaxation of the gut sphincters. Sympathetic activity leads to a decrease in blood supply to the gut with a decrease in secretions and in gut motility.
- The gastrointestinal tract processes the food to be used by the body cells. Six processes can be described: ingestion, propulsion, mastication, digestion, absorption and elimination.
- Digestion of food begins in the stomach and is completed in the small intestine. Saliva contains the digestive enzyme salivary amylase, which acts upon starch to convert polysaccharides into disaccharides.

- Gastric acid inactivates salivary amylase, alters the molecular structure of ingested proteins to tenderise them, curdles milk and converts pepsinogen to pepsin. Pepsin converts proteins to polypeptides. Once chyme leaves the stomach, there is a change to an alkaline medium and pepsin's activity ceases.
- Both neural and hormonal aspects are involved in the control of gastric juice secretion. The neural control has two phases: the cephalic phase mediated by the vagus nerve, and the gastric phase, mediated by stretch and chemoreceptors. Hormonal influences contribute most to the gastric phase of secretion.
- The three sections of the small intestine comprise the duodenum, the jejunum and the ileum. Digestion is completed and absorption of nutrients and most of the water takes place in the small intestine.
- Pancreatic digestive enzymes are secreted into the duodenum (pH 8). Pancreatic juice contains three proteolytic enzymes: trypsinogen, trypsin and carboxypeptidase. Bile emulsifies fats so that

fat-soluble vitamins and iron can be absorbed. Cholecystokinin (CCK) is the major controller of bile release, causing contraction of the gall bladder and relaxation of the sphincter of Oddi.

- Juices secreted in the duodenum and jejunum complete digestion. Basic nutrients are then absorbed into the circulating blood through intestinal villi.
- About 2 L of fluid are ingested daily. A further 8–9 L of fluid are added to the gut during the production of digestive juices. Only 50–200 ml are lost in the faeces, the rest being absorbed from both the small and large intestines.
- Most calcium is absorbed in the upper part of the small intestine under the influence of parathyroid hormone and calcitonin. The active process is facilitated by vitamin D.
- The large intestine is about 1.5 m long in an adult and consists of the caecum, appendix, colon and rectum. It can store large quantities of food residues. The gastrocolic reflex and colonic peristalsis fill the rectum with faeces, resulting in the urge to defecate.
- The colon absorbs most of the remaining water and electrolytes, synthesises vitamin K and some B vitamins, secretes mucus and acts as a lubricant for elimination of faeces. Sudden distension of the rectum results in the urge to defecate. The rectum opens to the exterior by the anal canal. About 100–150 g of faeces are eliminated each day.

- Pregnant women usually find that they have an increased appetite and food consumption, craving of certain foods and avoidance of others. Pica is a craving for non-food substances. The gums may become swollen and spongy in pregnancy and bleed easily.
- Gastric muscle tone and motility are reduced during pregnancy due to the effect of progesterone. The delay in emptying may also be due to the lower secretion of gastric juices, resulting in prolonged digestion time for solid food.
- Absorption of food does not increase even though the metabolism of pregnant women is anabolic. Any increased nutrition must come from increased intake. Iron and calcium appear to be absorbed more readily. Constipation is a common complaint as the colon shares in the general relaxation of smooth muscle found throughout the body.

References

Blackburn, S.T., 2007. Maternal, Fetal and Neonatal Physiology: A Clinical Perspective, fourth edn. Elsevier Saunders, St Louis MO.

Enkin, M., Keirse, M.J.N.C., Neilson, J., 2000. A Guide to Effective Care in Pregnancy, third edn. Oxford University Press, Oxford.

Hytten, F., 1991. The alimentary system. In: Hytten, F., Chamberlain, G. (Eds.), Clinical Physiology in Obstetrics, second edn. Blackwell Science, Oxford.

Kovacs, C.S., 2001. Calcium and bone metabolism in pregnancy and lactation. J. Clin. Endocrinol. Metab. 86 (6), 2344–2348.

Laine, M.A., 2002. Effect of pregnancy on peridontal and dental health. Acta Odontologica Scandinavica 60, 257.

Marieb, E.N., Hoehn, K., 2008. Anatomy and Physiology, third edn. Pearson Benjamin/Cummings, New York.

Martini, F.H., Nath, J.L., 2009. Fundamentals of Anatomy & Physiology, eighth ed. Pearson Benjamin/Cummings, New York.

Scott, L.D., Abu-Hamda, G., et al., 2004. Gastrointestinal disease in pregnancy. In: Creasy, R.K. (Ed.), Maternal–Fetal Medicine: Principles and Practice, fifth edn. Saunders, Philadelphia.

Annotated recommended reading

Blackburn, S.T., 2007. Maternal, Fetal and Neonatal Physiology: A Clinical Perspective, fourth edn. Elsevier Saunders, St Louis MO.
This text provides a detailed description of the major changes that occur in the body systems during pregnancy. There is an extensive review of the literature, extending from classical research studies to the more recent research findings.

Sherwood, L., 2006. Human Physiology: From Cells to Systems, sixth edn. Brookes Cole, New York.
This textbook provides in-depth information on the physiology of the gastrointestinal tract relevant for undergraduates in the health care profession.

Chapter Twenty-Two

The accessory digestive organs

22

Introduction

The alimentary system contains not only the gastrointestinal tract discussed in Chapter 21 but also the associated and accessory organs for digestion. It is an artificial division to separate out these accessory organs, as their function is integrated into the system. However, the sheer complexity of the physiology may be better understood by this format. This chapter discusses the contribution of the salivary glands, the pancreas and the liver to the process of digestion. The role of the liver in detoxification of drugs and ingested substances and the limitations to the protective role of the placenta are also discussed. Readers are referred to the selection of referenced textbooks if more detailed information is required.

The salivary glands

Three pairs of salivary glands produce the saliva that aids speech, chewing and swallowing. They are the parotid, submaxillary and sublingual glands. The **parotid glands** are the largest pair and are situated by the angle of the jaw. These glands produce a watery solution forming 25% of the daily saliva secretion. The **submaxillary glands** lie below the upper jaw and produce thicker saliva which forms 70% of the total daily output. The **sublingual glands** lie under the tongue on the floor of the mouth and produce only 5% of the daily output. Their solution is rich in glycoproteins, called mucins, which are primarily responsible for the lubricating action of saliva. Salivary glands produce 1–1.5 L of saliva each day. Saliva consists of 99.5% water and 0.5% solutes and has a pH value around 7.0.

The functions of saliva

- It cleanses the mouth. It contains lysozyme, which has an antiseptic action and the immunoglobulin IgA as a defence against micro-organisms.
- It provides oral comfort, reducing friction and allowing speech.
- It ensures that food is in solution so that the taste buds can recognise the contained chemicals.

- It facilitates the formation of a bolus of partly broken up food ready to swallow. The mucins present in saliva help to mould and lubricate the bolus.
- It contains a digestive enzyme, salivary or α-amylase (formerly know as ptyalin), which acts upon starch to convert polysaccharides into disaccharides.

Control of saliva production

The secretion of saliva is controlled primarily by parasympathetic supply from the facial (VII cranial) nerve and the glossopharyngeal (IX cranial) nerve. Normally, parasympathetic stimulation produces continuous moderate watery amounts of saliva while sympathetic activity produces a sparse viscid secretion and the dry mouth most of us experience during times of stress or following the administration of atropine or hyoscine, which block receptor sites for the neurotransmitter acetylcholine.

Saliva is produced as a conditioned reflex in response to the cerebral perception of the thought, sight or smell of food. The salivary nuclei are situated in the reticular formation in the floor of the fourth ventricle and, when stimulated by the thought, sight or smell of food, secretion of saliva occurs. The presence of food in the mouth will also lead to saliva production—an unconditioned reflex where the impulse created by the physical presence of the food in the mouth directly stimulates the salivary nuclei without the cerebral cortex being involved. The process of deglutition propels the food into the stomach and the next stage in the digestion of food can continue.

The pancreas

The pancreas is a gland lying just below the stomach that has both endocrine and exocrine functions. It is a soft friable pink gland, is 'tadpole'-shaped, with a head surrounded by the C-shaped loop of the duodenum and a tail which extends towards the right side of the abdomen. Most of the pancreas is retroperitoneal. Through the centre of the pancreas runs the **pancreatic duct**, which fuses with the common bile duct just before it enters the duodenum at the hepatopancreatic ampulla.

Exocrine functions of the pancreas

Within the pancreas are the acini, which are clusters of cells surrounding small ducts. These provide the exocrine function and play a major role in digestion. The cells form and store zygomen granules, consisting of a wide range of digestive enzymes that act on all nutrients. The enzymes are secreted into the pancreatic duct and then into the duodenum.

Pancreatic juice

The pancreatic enzymes were briefly mentioned in Chapter 21. About 1.5–2 L of pancreatic juice are secreted daily with a pH of 8–8.4. A mixture of two types of secretions are produced: a copious watery solution and a scanty solution rich in enzymes. The profuse watery solution contains the ions hydrogen carbonate (bicarbonate), sodium, potassium, calcium, magnesium, chloride, sulphate, phosphate and some albumin and globulin proteins. The enzyme-rich secretion contains the three proteolytic enzymes trypsinogen, trypsin and carboxypeptidase. Enzyme activity is summarised in Figure 22.1. Other enzymes are pancreatic amylase, pancreatic lipase, ribonuclease and deoxyribonuclease.

Control of pancreatic juice secretion

The hormones secretin and cholecystokinin (CCK) were mentioned in Chapter 21. Secretin is produced by the S cells in the duodenum and upper jejunum, when acid chyme enters the duodenum. This enters the venous systemic circulation and arrives back at the pancreas via the pancreatic artery. Its presence results in the secretion of the watery component, which is rich in bicarbonate but low in enzymes.

Cholecystokinin secreted by the columnar cells of the duodenum and jejunum in response to the presence of the products of protein and fat digestion, also circulates and returns to the pancreas via the pancreatic artery. Its presence causes the release of the enzyme-rich secretion. CCK has many important functions:

- Stimulation of the enzyme-rich pancreatic secretion.
- Augmentation of the activity of secretion.

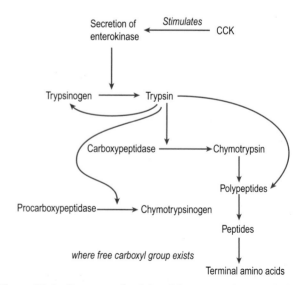

Figure 22.1 • Summary of activity of the pancreatic proteolytic enzymes. (From Hinchliff S M, Montague S E 1990, with permission.)

- The slowing of gastric emptying and inhibition of gastric secretion.
- Stimulation of the secretion of enterokinase.
- Stimulation of glucagon secretion.
- Stimulation of motility of the small intestine and colon.
- Contraction of the gall bladder with the release of bile.

Endocrine functions of the pancreas

Scattered among the acinar cells are approximately a million pancreatic islets (also called **islets of Langerhans**), which are tiny cell clusters that make up 1% of the pancreas and produce pancreatic hormones (Marieb & Hoehn 2008). There are two types of cells: the α cells synthesise glucagon, and a more numerous population of cells; the β cells, produce insulin. The normal human pancreas produces about 40 international units (IU) of insulin in 24h. The other cells produce somatostatin, which acts to suppress islet cell hormone production. A hormone called **amylin** appears to be an insulin antagonist.

Glucagon

Glucagon is a short polypeptide of 29 amino acids and a potent hyperglycaemic agent. One molecule of glucagon causes the release of 100 million molecules of glucose into the blood (Marieb & Hoehn 2008). Glucagon acts mainly in the liver to promote:

- Glycogenolysis (the breakdown of glycogen to glucose).
- Lipolysis.
- Gluconeogenesis (the formation of glucose from fatty acids and amino acids).

The liver releases the glucose into the bloodstream, raising the blood sugar level. There is a fall in serum amino acid levels as the liver then takes up amino acids to synthesise new glucose molecules.

Falling blood sugar levels stimulate secretion of glucagon from α cells. Increasing amino acid levels also stimulates glucagon release. Glucagon release is suppressed by increasing blood sugar levels and by somatostatin.

Insulin

Insulin is also a small polypeptide consisting of 51 amino acids. It begins as the middle part of a larger polypeptide chain called **proinsulin**. Enzymes cut amino acid bonds to release the functional hormone just before the insulin is secreted from the β cell. Insulin affects the metabolism of fat and protein as well as of glucose (Table 22.1).

Production of insulin

Insulin production is stimulated by glucose, amino acids and fatty acids in blood and hyperglycaemic agents such as glucagon, adrenaline (epinephrine), growth hormone, thyroxine and glucocorticoids. Insulin production is inhibited by somatostatin. Insulin binds firmly to a receptor site on the cell membrane. It appears to modify cellular activity without entering the cell. The presence of calcium is necessary for its functioning. A high-carbohydrate diet leads to increased sensitivity of tissues to insulin and this may be due to a rise in the number of insulin receptors in the cell walls.

The role of insulin at cellular level

Insulin assists the entry of glucose into muscle cells, connective tissue cells and white blood cells. It does not facilitate entry of glucose into liver, kidney and brain cells. Those cells have easy access to glucose regardless of insulin (Marieb & Hoehn 2008). Insulin counters any metabolic activity that would increase plasma glucose levels such as glycogenolysis and gluconeogenesis. These last effects are probably due to insulin inhibition of glucagon. Once glucose has entered the cells, insulin triggers enzyme activity which:

- Catalyses the oxidation of glucose to produce ATP.
- Joins glucose molecules together to form glycogen.
- Converts glucose to fat, particularly in adipose tissue.

These processes are considered in more detail in Chapter 23.

Table 22.1 The effects of insulin on foods

On glucose	On fat	On protein	On electrolytes
Stimulates glucose utilisation Stimulates glycogen synthesis Inhibits glycogen breakdown Inhibits gluconeogenesis	Stimulates fatty acid and triglyceride synthesis Inhibits triglyceride breakdown	Stimulates incorporation of amino acids into protein molecules	Stimulates the entry of potassium into cells

The liver and gall bladder

The liver, which is one of the accessory organs and is associated with the small intestine, is one of the body's most important organs. While it has many metabolic roles (see Ch. 23), its only digestive function is to secrete **bile**, which it stores in the gall bladder and discharges into the duodenum. Bile acts on fats to emulsify them; i.e. to break fat up into tiny particles so that it is more accessible to digestive enzymes.

Anatomy

The liver is a very large gland and weighs on average 1.4 kg. It is located in the abdominal cavity under the diaphragm, extending more to the right of the midline than the left, obscuring the stomach (Fig. 22.2). It lies totally protected by the rib cage (Fig. 22.3). The liver has four lobes (Fig. 22.4):

1. The right lobe, which is the largest.

2. The smaller left lobe.

3. The caudate lobe, which is the posterior lobe.

4. The quadrate lobe, which lies inferior to the left lobe.

The right lobe is the largest and is separated from the left lobe by a deep fissure. The right and left lobes are also separated by the **falciform ligament**, a cord of mesentery which suspends the liver from the diaphragm and the anterior abdominal wall. A fibrous remnant of the left umbilical vein, called the **ligamentum teres**, runs along the free edge of the falciform ligament. The superior aspect of the liver, or bare area, is fused to the

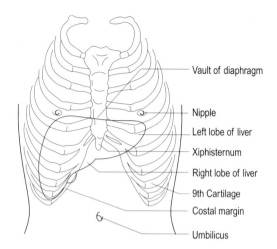

Figure 22.3 • The position of the liver in relation to the rib cage. (From Hinchliff S M, Montague S E 1990, with permission.)

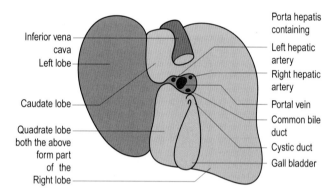

Figure 22.4 • The interior surface of the liver showing the position of the four lobes. (From Hinchliff S M, Montague S E 1990, with permission.)

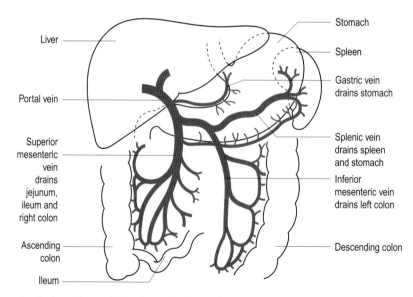

Figure 22.2 • The liver: anatomical position and blood supply. (From Hinchliff S M, Montague S E 1990, with permission.)

diaphragm while the remainder of the organ is enclosed in visceral peritoneum. The lesser omentum anchors the liver to the lesser curvature of the stomach.

Microscopic anatomy

The liver is composed of small units called liver lobules. Lobules are small hexagonal cylinders consisting of plates of **hepatocytes** (epithelial liver cells) (Fig. 22.5). The hepatocytes produce bile, process blood-borne nutrients and play an important role in detoxification (see below). The hepatocytes radiate outwards from a central vein running along the longitudinal axis of each lobule. At each of the six corners of a lobule is a **portal** triad (see Fig. 22.5). The three structures present in a triad are:

1. A branch of the hepatic artery, supplying arterial blood to the liver.

2. A branch of the hepatic portal vein, carrying nutrient-rich blood from the digestive tract.

3. A bile duct.

The hepatic artery and the hepatic portal vein enter the liver at the **porta hepatis**. Between the hepatocyte plates are enlarged capillaries called **sinusoids**. Blood percolates through the sinusoids from both the hepatic artery and the hepatic portal vein and is collected up into the central veins. Inside the sinusoids are the **Kupffer cells**, hepatic macrophages which remove debris such as worn-out blood cells and bacteria from the blood.

Digestive functions of the liver

The liver produces bile and also many enzymes that are able to detoxify the many noxious substances arriving at the organ via the bloodstream.

The production of bile

Bile produced by the hepatocytes flows into tiny channels called **bile canaliculi** and enters the bile duct branches in the portal triads. Collectively, the hepatocytes produce as much as 1000 ml (1 L) of bile daily, with more being produced if a fatty meal is taken. Blood and bile flow in opposite directions in the liver lobules (Fig. 22.6). The bile flows into the hepatic duct

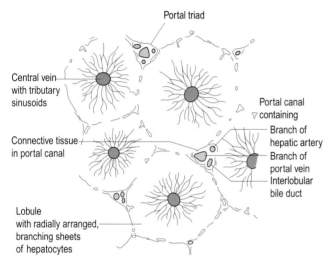

Figure 22.5 • The general features of the liver lobules at low magnification, showing the portal triad. (From Hinchliff S M, Montague S E 1990, with permission.)

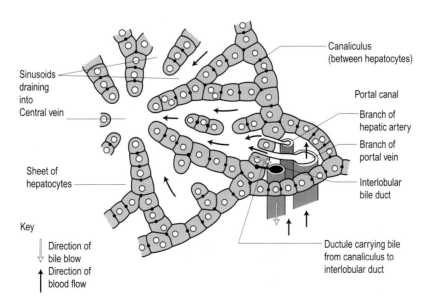

Figure 22.6 • The flow of blood and bile within the liver lobule. (From Hinchliff S M, Montague S E 1990, with permission.)

and, if needed by the digestive system, flows into the duodenum. If no bile is needed, the sphincter of Oddi is tightly closed and bile flows through the cystic duct to be stored in the gall bladder (Fig. 22.7).

The gall bladder is a thin-walled muscular bag about 10 cm long, situated in a fossa on the inferior surface of the right lobe of the liver. It stores secreted bile and concentrates it by absorbing water and ions. When empty, its walls are thrown into rugae to allow for distension. When the muscular wall contracts, bile is ejected into the cystic duct, leading to the common bile duct. It is covered with visceral peritoneum.

Bile contains no digestive enzymes and its chief role in digestion is to emulsify fats so that they and the fat-soluble vitamins and iron can be absorbed. Bile is a viscous fluid coloured greeny-yellow to brown. It contains 97% water, 0.7% bile salts, mucin and bicarbonate. Also present in bile are fatty acids, lecithin, inorganic salts, alkaline phosphatase and the excretory products of steroid-based hormones. Bile is alkaline with a pH of 7.8–8.0.

Bile salts

Bile salts are formed from the steroids cholic acid and deoxycholic acid, manufactured in the liver from cholesterol. In the liver, cholic acid is **conjugated** (joined together with the elimination of water) with the amino acids taurine and glycine to form taurocholic acid and glycocholic acid. The bile acids form salts with sodium and potassium, which are in solution in the bile.

The functions of the bile salts are to:

- Deodorise faeces.
- Activate lipase and proteolytic enzymes in the duodenum.
- Reduce the surface tension of fat droplets which helps to emulsify them.

Bile salts combine with lipids, lecithin and cholesterol to form micelles that are water-soluble and allow fat to be more easily absorbed. If bile salts are absent, about 25% of ingested fat will be lost in the stools. These stools will be bulky and have an offensive odour.

Bile pigments

Bile pigments make up 0.2% of the composition of bile. They are produced from the breakdown of red blood cells and are mainly bilirubin with a small amount of biliverdin. The pigments are taken to the liver bound to plasma albumin where they are conjugated with glucuronic acid in the presence of the enzyme glucuronic transferase. This forms the water-soluble bilirubin diglucuronide which enters bile to give it the golden colour. In the gut stercobilinogen is formed and, following conversion by bacterial action, is excreted as stercobilin. Some stercobilinogen is absorbed by the bloodstream and is then excreted as urobilinogen by the kidneys.

Control of bile secretion

As with other secretions into the gastrointestinal tract, the control of bile secretion involves neural and hormonal factors. CCK is the major controller, causing contraction of the gall bladder and relaxation of the sphincter of Oddi. Once the gall bladder has emptied its contents, further flow of bile into the duodenum occurs directly from the liver. Vagus nerve stimulation will bring about a similar action. About 97% of bile salts are reabsorbed into the portal circulation, following their passage through the intestine, and are returned to the liver; this is called the **enterohepatic circulation of bile salts**. The production of bile by the liver depends on the blood level of bile salts. High blood levels of bile salts stimulate the liver cells to secrete more bile.

Detoxification of ingested material

A second important function of the liver is the detoxification of ingested substances. Systems have evolved to protect humans from ingested poisons found especially in plants (see Ch. 8). This involves detoxification by enzyme systems and subsequent excretion of the by-products by the liver. Any alteration in liver or kidney function may reduce the ability of the body to handle harmful chemicals. Many drugs are simply purified naturally occurring chemicals and even those synthesised

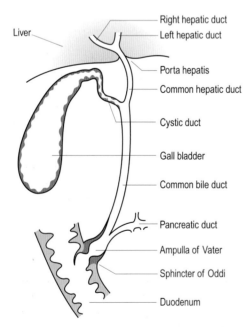

Figure 22.7 • The drainage of bile from the liver to the intestine (the biliary tract). (From Hinchliff S M, Montague S E 1990, with permission.)

Labels: Liver, Right hepatic duct, Left hepatic duct, Porta hepatis, Common hepatic duct, Cystic duct, Gall bladder, Common bile duct, Pancreatic duct, Ampulla of Vater, Sphincter of Oddi, Duodenum

in the laboratory will have similar chemical structures to naturally occurring substances.

The role of the liver in metabolism

The liver processes nearly every type of nutrient absorbed from the digestive tract. It also plays a major part in controlling plasma cholesterol levels. The hepatocytes carry out at least 500 metabolic functions. It would take a textbook devoted to the topic to begin to explore all of the functions of the liver. That is why the liver is such an important organ. Major metabolic roles include:

- Packaging fatty acids into forms that can be stored and transported.
- Synthesising plasma proteins.
- Synthesising non-essential amino acids.
- Converting ammonia, from the deamination of amino acids, to urea for excretion.
- Storing glucose as glycogen.
- Regulating blood sugar level by glycogenolysis and gluconeogenesis.
- Storing vitamins.
- Conserving iron from the breakdown of red blood cells.
- Detoxifying substances such as alcohol and drugs.

The absorption, distribution and fate of drugs

There are two main ways of describing drugs in the body:

1. **Pharmacokinetics**, which is concerned with the way the body handles drugs.
2. **Pharmacodynamics**, which is concerned with the effect drugs have on the body function (Rang et al 2007).

Drugs are often given to patients because of a need to support a failing system or organ. Examples are the administration of insulin when the pancreas is unable to make sufficient or no insulin of its own in diabetes mellitus, or the use of antibiotics to support the immune system in bacterial invasion. Drugs may also be used to control a function: for example, the administration of the contraceptive pill to control reproductive function. Drugs usually have the following attributes:

- They bind to protein targets.
- They exert chemical influences on one or more cellular components.
- They may affect one or more tissues.
- They may have agonist or antagonist effects.

The protein targets of drugs may be enzymes in metabolic reactions, carrier molecules on cell membranes, receptor molecules on cell membranes or ion channels in cell membranes (Rang et al 2007).

Drug disposition

Drug disposition is the process of drug molecule behaviour in the body. There are four stages:

1. Absorption from the site of administration.
2. Distribution within the body.
3. Metabolic alteration.
4. Excretion from the body.

Absorption

Absorption is the passage of a drug from the site of administration into the plasma. Except for some topical applications and some inhaled substances, most drugs must enter the plasma to travel to target tissues. Drugs are absorbed at different rates from sites and some may be unsuitable for some routes.

Distribution within the body (translocation)

There are two main phases in drug distribution. The first is **bulk flow transfer**, which is the transport of drugs around the body by the circulatory system. Some drugs may be transported freely in solution but many are carried around the blood attached to a carrier molecule such as plasma albumin. At cellular level **diffusional transfer** describes the carriage of drugs into the cells in a specific tissue. Diffusional transfer may be by:

- Diffusion through the lipid cell membrane.
- Diffusion through aqueous pores which traverse the lipid membrane.
- Combination with a carrier molecule to ferry the drug across the membrane.
- Pinocytosis to engulf the substance.

There is controversy as to whether aqueous pores exist; if they do, they are probably too small to allow entry of most molecules. Pinocytosis, where a piece of cell membrane surrounds the substance and draws it into the cell, concerns large biological molecules only.

Diffusion through the lipid membrane
This is one of the most important pharmacokinetic characteristics of a drug. Fat-soluble drugs diffuse across capillary walls and through cell membranes easily. Other determinants of diffusion include the pH of body fluids (acids and alkalis neutralise each other to precipitate a salt and water) and ionisation (drugs that are strongly

ionised are not lipid-soluble and may not be able to enter cells unaided).

Carrier mediation

Many drugs have specialised transport mechanisms to regulate entry and exit from cells. This usually involves a carrier molecule incorporated into the cell membrane. In facilitated diffusion, energy is not needed, but in active transport the cell must use energy. Some pharmaceutical effects are the result of interference with the function of carrier proteins.

Drug metabolism in the liver

Drugs pass through the liver several times while they are in the circulation. Metabolic alteration of drug molecules involves two kinds of biochemical reactions brought about by liver enzymes:

1. **Phase 1 reactions**, which may result in a more active or toxic metabolite of the drug, involve:

    a. Oxidation—adding oxygen or removing hydrogen.

    b. Reduction—adding hydrogen or removing oxygen.

    c. Hydrolysis—splitting of the molecule into separate parts by water.

2. **Phase 2 reactions** involve conjugation by liver enzymes, resulting in a water-soluble inactive product ready for excretion.

Excretion of drugs

Drugs are mainly excreted by the kidney but may also be excreted in expired air, perspiration, faeces and breast milk. In pregnancy, they may cross the placental barrier to the fetus. In the kidney there are three processes for excretion of drugs:

1. **Glomerular filtration**: if drugs are free in the plasma, i.e. not bound to plasma proteins and if their molecular weight is below 20 000.

2. **Active tubular secretion/reabsorption**: independent carrier systems are present in the cells of the proximal tubule for non-lipid-soluble drugs or ionised drugs (one for acids and one for bases).

3. **Passive diffusion across the tubular epithelium**: diffusion of lipid-soluble drugs occurs across the tubular and capillary cell membranes in the distal tubule and collecting tubule.

Drugs that are hydrophilic and poorly lipid-soluble such as antibiotics do not enter cells readily. They have a lower density volume and are readily excreted by the kidney. Lipid-soluble drugs are readily reabsorbed in the renal tubule and need breaking down to water-soluble by-products, usually in the liver, in order to be excreted.

Maternal adaptations to pregnancy

The pancreas

Although there is a slight decrease in serum amylase and lipase, this seems to have no significance. The alterations in glucose metabolism, due to increasing insulin resistance, are much more significant. This may be enough to precipitate diabetes mellitus in susceptible women. Glucose metabolism is discussed in Chapter 23 and diabetes in pregnancy in Chapter 35.

The gall bladder

The decrease in muscle tone and motility of the gall bladder during pregnancy is probably due to the effects of progesterone on smooth musculature. As a result, the volume is increased and the emptying rate is decreased. An increased fasting volume is probably due to decreased water absorption by the mucosa of the gall bladder. This change is due to reduced activity of the cell wall sodium pump, which is a function of the increased circulating oestrogens. Alterations in gall bladder tone lead to a retention of bile salts, leading to pruritus (Blackburn 2007). Pregnancy may predispose to gall stones but there is little empirical evidence to support this belief.

The liver

Liver size and liver blood flow appear to be unchanged and no histological changes have been seen in pregnancy (Reynolds 1998). However, as pregnancy progresses, the liver is displaced superiorly, posteriorly and anteriorly by the growing uterus. Although there is no change in blood flow to the liver there may be a reduction in the proportion of cardiac output to the liver of about 30% (Blackburn 2007).

There is an alteration in the production of plasma proteins, bilirubin, serum enzymes and serum lipids by the liver. Some changes arise from the presence of oestrogen and some from haemodilution. The changes reduce liver function and make normal testing of liver function less useful.

There may be a reversible disturbance of liver function in pregnancy in women who are otherwise healthy. A small proportion of women taking the contraceptive pill show the same effect. There will be jaundice, histologically dilated bile canaliculi and increased bile viscosity. Increased phagocytosis by the Kupffer cells, under the stimulus of oestrogen, has been seen in primate studies and may occur in humans. Storage and mobilisation of liver glycogen may occur more rapidly because of the 50% increase in glomerular filtration rate.

Pharmacokinetics and pregnancy

Health professionals who prescribe drugs must consider the likelihood of a woman being pregnant or lactating (Weiner & Buhimshi 2009). Drugs taken in early pregnancy may be teratogenic, a prime example being the tragedy of thalidomide in the 1960s (Reynolds 1998). Drugs given in late pregnancy may cause behavioural anomalies in children. Many women are unaware of the danger of taking over-the-counter drugs. Taking drugs in pregnancy may be essential for some women, and their life and the life of the fetus may be endangered if the drugs are discontinued even though the drugs may be involved in causing abnormalities in the fetus. A good example would be the use of Epanutin (phenytoin) in epilepsy, which may cause oral deformities.

Modification of pharmacokinetics

Ingestion

Many knowledgeable women will not comply with taking medicines in pregnancy. Nausea and vomiting may cause rejection of the drug.

Absorption

Most drugs are taken orally and are absorbed by the stomach and small intestine. Gastric motility is reduced throughout pregnancy and especially in labour. This slows down absorption of some drugs but may increase absorption of others. Most common drugs show little change from normal. Taking antacid preparations will lead to the absorption of some drugs being reduced.

Distribution

Increased extracellular fluid and body fat may alter the compartmental distribution of drugs. The fetus is considered to be a compartment and, although probably resistant to bolus doses, may be at risk in long-term drug therapy of some chemicals.

Protein binding

Many drugs circulate around the body bound to plasma proteins, especially albumin, which is reduced in pregnancy. There is an increase in some specific proteins such as transferrin and thyroid-binding hormone. Some drugs which bind to α_1 acid glycoprotein are more likely to cross the placenta.

Elimination

Drugs that act within the central nervous system or within cells are lipid-soluble. These cannot be effectively excreted without conjugation to water-soluble by-products in the liver. The kidney will excrete those drugs excreted by the renal tubules. The rule of the placenta as a barrier to drugs is discussed in Box 22.1.

BOX 22.1 THE PLACENTA AND FETUS

Almost all drug reactions carried out by the liver have been identified in placental tissue. To date, no studies have been carried out in vivo. This means we cannot trust the placenta to protect the fetus from the effect of drugs. The main trophoblastic layer in the placenta is a syncytium, covered by a continuous lipid membrane. This membrane acts in a similar way to the blood–brain barrier so that lipid substances of low molecular weight (below 1000) can readily diffuse across the membrane. Water-soluble molecules of up to 100 MW can also diffuse easily but charged ionic molecules cannot pass unless they are bound to a carrier protein (Weiner & Buhimschi 2009). Therefore drugs that affect the central nervous system will readily cross the placental barrier.

Other drugs such as barbiturates, non-steroidal anti-inflammatory agents, warfarin and anticonvulsants are weak acids while narcotics, local anaesthetics, beta blockers or beta stimulants are weak bases. These act as non-ionic substances and will cross the placental barrier slowly. Polar drugs such as the penicillins and cephalosporins are transferred so slowly that the fetus has no problem eliminating the drugs faster than they are transferred. Heparin is a large molecule and cannot cross the placenta. The fetus and neonate have a much reduced ability to handle drugs because of immaturity of liver enzyme systems.

Maternal elimination of polar non-lipid drugs is much faster during pregnancy, as the kidney excretes

(Continued)

 BOX 22.1 (CONTINUED)

them. This means that the dose requirements of some drugs, such as anticonvulsants, may rise during pregnancy. Some of these drugs cannot cross the placental barrier while others are excreted rapidly by the fetus and pose no problem. Some drugs such as anticonvulsants build up slowly in the fetus and may cause malformations. Maternal breakdown of lipid-soluble drugs is slower in pregnancy and these drugs readily cross the placenta into fetal tissues and may be excreted very slowly (Reynolds 1998).

Main points

- Salivary glands (three pairs) produce saliva, which aids speech, chewing and swallowing. Saliva contains lysozyme and immunoglobulin IgA as defence against micro-organisms. A digestive enzyme, salivary or α amylase, acts upon starch to convert polysaccharides into disaccharides.

- The secretion of saliva is controlled primarily by parasympathetic supply, producing continuous moderate amounts of watery saliva. Saliva is produced as a conditioned reflex in response to the perception of the thought, sight or smell of food.

- The pancreas has both endocrine and exocrine functions. The pancreas produces 1.5–2 L of alkaline pancreatic juice daily. Pancreatic juice secretion is divided into a cephalic phase in response to food stimuli and a gastric phase stimulated by the release of gastrin.

- About 1% of the pancreas consists of the islet of Langerhans cells. The α cells synthesise glucagon and the β cells produce insulin. The δ cells produce somatostatin, which acts to suppress islet cell hormone production.

- Glucagon acts in the liver to promote glycogenolysis, lipolysis and gluconeogenesis. Insulin stimulates glucose utilisation, glycogen synthesis, inhibition of glycogen breakdown and inhibition of gluconeogenesis. Insulin assists the entry of glucose into muscle, connective tissue and white blood cells.

- The liver is composed of lobules, consisting of plates of hepatocytes radiating outwards from a central vein. The hepatocytes produce bile, process blood-borne nutrients and play an important role in detoxification.

- Bile produced by the hepatocytes flows into tiny channels called bile canaliculi and enters the bile duct branches in the portal triads. If no bile is needed, the sphincter of Oddi is tightly closed and bile flows through the cystic duct to be stored in the gall bladder.

- Bile salts manufactured in the liver, from cholesterol, deodorise faeces, activate lipase and proteolytic enzymes in the duodenum and reduce the surface tension of fat droplets, which helps to emulsify them. Bile pigments are produced from the breakdown of red blood cells.

- The control of bile secretion involves neural and hormonal factors. CCK is the major controller, causing contraction of the gall bladder and relaxation of the sphincter of Oddi. High blood levels of bile salts stimulate the liver cells to secrete more bile.

- The liver detoxifies ingested substances by enzyme systems and excretes the by-products. The liver processes nearly every type of nutrient absorbed from the digestive tract.

- Pharmacokinetics is concerned with the way the body handles drugs. Pharmacodynamics is concerned with the effect drugs have on the body function. Drug disposition is the process of drug molecule behaviour in the body. There are four stages: absorption from the site of administration, distribution, metabolic alteration and excretion.

- Liver size and liver blood flow seem to be unchanged in pregnancy and no histological changes have been found. The growing uterus displaces the liver as pregnancy progresses.

- Increased extracellular fluid and body fat during pregnancy may alter the compartmental distribution of drugs. The fetus is considered to be a compartment and, although probably resistant to bolus doses, may be at risk in some long-term drug therapy. Many drugs circulate around the body bound to plasma proteins, especially albumin. Some drugs are likely to cross the placenta.

- Almost all drug reactions carried out by the liver have been identified in placental tissue. The fetus and neonate have a reduced ability to handle drugs because of immaturity of liver enzyme systems.

- Maternal elimination of polar non-lipid drugs is much faster during pregnancy, as the kidney excretes them. Maternal breakdown of lipid-soluble drugs is slower in pregnancy and these drugs readily cross the placenta into fetal tissues and may be excreted very slowly.

References

Blackburn, S.T., 2007. Maternal, Fetal and Neonatal Physiology: A Clinical Perspective, fourth edn. Elsevier Saunders, St Louis.

Marieb, E.N., Hoehn, K., 2008. Anatomy & Physiology, third edn. Pearson/Benjamin Cummings, New York.

Rang, H.P., Dale, M.M., Ritter, J.M. (Eds.), et al., 2007. Pharmacology, sixth edn. Churchill Livingstone, Edinburgh.

Reynolds, F., 1998. Pharmacokinetics. In: Chamberlain, G., Broughton, PipkinF. (Eds.) Clinical Physiology in Obstetrics, third edn. Blackwell Science, Oxford.

Weiner, C.P., Buhimschi, C., 2009. Drugs for Pregnant and Lactating Women, second edn. Elsevier Saunders, Philadelphia.

Annotated recommended reading

Marieb, E.N., Hoehn, K., 2008. Anatomy & Physiology, third edn. Pearson/Benjamin Cummings, New York.

This textbook presents a detailed overview of human anatomy and physiology related to the gastrointestinal tract and accessory organs. It is well illustrated with diagrams and pictures.

Rang, H.P., Dale, M.M., Ritter, J.M. (Eds.), et al., 2007. Pharmacology, sixth edn. Churchill Livingstone, Edinburgh.

This textbook presents a detailed overview of pharmacokinetics for information about drugs and how they affect the body and how the body handles drugs.

Chapter Twenty-Three

23

Nutrition and metabolism during pregnancy

CHAPTER CONTENTS

Introduction

A good nutritional status for a woman is essential for a healthy pregnancy outcome. Nutritional advice for pregnant women has recently changed from eating for two to more careful consideration of dietary quality as well as quantity on a need basis. Adequate energy and nutrient intake during pregnancy has significant impact on the well-being of the mother and her growing fetus, in both the short term and the long term. However, some health professionals do not feel confident enough to give nutritional advice to their clients. In this chapter, the principles of general nutrition as well as pregnancy-specific nutritional requirements and metabolic adaptation are discussed.

Nutrition

Nutrition is based on two fundamental areas of science: biochemistry and physiology. For practical purposes, this section will focus on a brief overview of basic nutrition physiology: general food groups, energy and nutrients and metabolism. Nutrients are utilised by the body for tissue growth, maintenance and repair. They can be divided into six categories: three major nutrients (macronutrients) are carbohydrates, lipids and proteins; and micronutrients including vitamins and minerals which are required in small amounts as well as water which is considered as a food because of its role as a solvent. Most foods provide a combination of nutrients, and water makes up 60% of the volume of food intake.

Food groups

There are four food groups which must be eaten in order to provide a balanced diet. The types and a general guide on the daily food choices are:

1. Grains, bread, cereal, rice and pasta 6–11 servings.
2. Fruits 2–4 servings, vegetables 3–5 servings.
3. Meat, poultry and fish 2–3 servings.
4. Dairy products, milk, cheese and yoghurt 2–3 servings.

Tiran (1997) adds a fifth group—fats and sugary foods. The five groups can be arranged in a pyramid, showing the quantities in relation to the health benefits of consumption (Fig. 23.1).

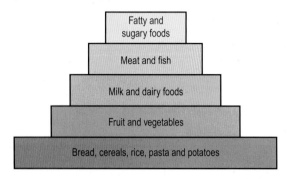

Figure 23.1 • The 'good food guide', showing the five main groups of food. (From Henderson C, Macdonald S 2004, with kind permission of Elsevier.)

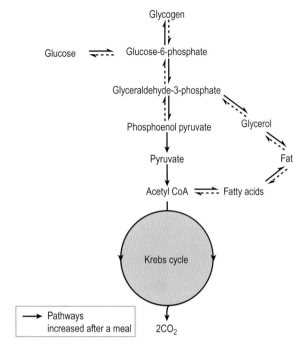

Figure 23.2 • A summary of glucose metabolism after a meal. (From Hinchliff S M, Montague S E 1990, with permission.)

Carbohydrates

Carbohydrate is the main source of energy in our food although the other macronutrients can also be metabolised to yield energy. According to their structure, there are three types of carbohydrates; their main food sources are explained below.

1. Monosaccharides (single sugars):
   a. Glucose, which is the ultimate example (corn syrup, processed foods).
   b. Fructose (fruits, honey).
   c. Galactose (milk).

2. Disaccharides (double sugars):
   a. Sucrose, which is made from glucose and fructose (sugar).
   b. Lactose, which is made from glucose and galactose (milk).
   c. Maltose, which is made from two glucoses (commercial malt product of starch breakdown, intermediate sweetener in food products).

3. Polysaccharides (multiple sugars or complex carbohydrates):
   a. Starch (grains, legumes, root vegetables).
   b. Glycogen (liver and muscle meats).
   c. Dietary fibre (whole grain, fruit and vegetables, seeds and nuts).

Carbohydrates play a fundamental role in the physiology of the body. Glucose, for example, is the ultimate common refined body fuel that is oxidised in cells to give energy; it is important to maintain a certain range in the blood of between 3.9 and 7.8 mmol/L to allow normal functioning. Cellulose is a form of plant carbohydrate (dietary fibre) that the human digestive system cannot process. It provides roughage to increase the bulk of faeces, thus facilitating defecation. Dietary fibres are also believed to have a role in the management of serum lipid and glucose levels; they are therefore helpful in prevention and management of chronic diseases such as diabetes and cardiovascular disease.

Carbohydrate metabolism

The Krebs (tricarboxylic acid or citric acid) cycle

When glucose in the circulating blood arrives at the tissues it is taken up by the cells by facilitated diffusion under the influence of insulin. Glucose is taken to the cells' mitochondria where it is oxidised to form energy via the Krebs cycle (Figs 23.2, 23.3). A series of reactions are involved when glucose, a 6-carbon molecule, is broken down into two 3-carbon molecules of pyruvic acid in a process called glycolysis.

Pyruvic acid is broken down further to a 2-carbon molecule called acetic acid and the released carbon atom forms carbon dioxide by combining with oxygen. The acetic acid now combines with coenzyme A (a derivative of a B complex vitamin, pantothenic acid) to form the enzyme acetyl coenzyme A (acetyl CoA). Acetyl CoA enters the Krebs cycle to undergo changes mediated by enzymes; ATP, water and carbon dioxide are formed in the process of oxidation.

The Krebs cycle consists of a series of eight separate biochemical reactions. This cycle of reactions is like one revolution of a wheel with acetyl CoA sitting at the top.

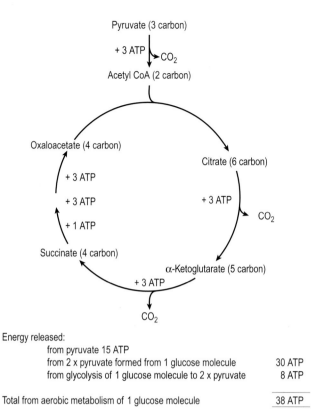

Pyruvate (3 carbon)

+ 3 ATP → CO_2

Acetyl CoA (2 carbon)

Oxaloacetate (4 carbon)

Citrate (6 carbon)

+ 3 ATP

+ 3 ATP

+ 3 ATP

+ 1 ATP

CO_2

Succinate (4 carbon)

α-Ketoglutarate (5 carbon)

+ 3 ATP

CO_2

Energy released:
from pyruvate 15 ATP
from 2 x pyruvate formed from 1 glucose molecule   30 ATP
from glycolysis of 1 glucose molecule to 2 x pyruvate   8 ATP

Total from aerobic metabolism of 1 glucose molecule   38 ATP

Figure 23.3 • A summary of the Krebs cycle. (From Hinchliff S M, Montague S E 1990, with permission.)

Each glucose molecule produces two pyruvic acid molecules and allows two turns of the cycle. Carbon dioxide produced when the excess carbon atoms unite with oxygen and surplus hydrogen atoms need to be disposed of. Two hydrogen carrier molecules, nicotinamide adenine dinucleotide (NAD) and flavin adenine dinucleotide (FAD), perform this function. The transfer of the hydrogen atoms converts the compounds into NADH and $FADH_2$, respectively.

ATP synthesis

Energy is stored in carbon–hydrogen bonds in food but cells cannot use energy in this form. They must convert it into the high-energy phosphate bonds of adenosine triphosphate (ATP) (Guyton & Hall 2006). ATP consists of adenosine with three phosphate groups attached. When a bond between adenosine (a nucleotide) and one of the phosphate groups is split, large amounts of energy are released and adenosine diphosphate plus an inorganic phosphate molecule (P_i) is formed. Some of the energy produced is in the form of heat and helps to maintain the temperature of the body. This can be written as:

Splitting by hydrolysis: ATP → ADP + Pi + energy

Cellular respiration

Aerobic cellular respiration

The main role of the Krebs cycle is to prepare the hydrogen acceptors for entry into the electron transport chain (respiratory chain) in the inner mitochondrial membrane. Electron transfer molecules are mostly brightly coloured protein-bound iron-containing pigments called cytochromes. These are arranged in a specific order which allows high-energy electrons to pass through a chain of reactions, resulting in a lowering of the energy levels at each step. At the end of this chain, the electrons are passed to the final electron acceptor, which is inspired oxygen.

The stepwise release of energy during the progression through the electron transport chain is used to pump protons into the intermembrane space. This creates an electrochemical proton gradient across the mitochondrial inner membrane which temporarily stores the energy. Protons flow back across the membrane through the enzyme ATP synthetase, providing the energy to attach a phosphate group to ADP to create a further 32 ATP molecules for each glucose molecule processed. The total production of ATP for one turn of the cycle is therefore 38 molecules. NAD and FAD are released to capture more hydrogen and begin the energy transfer again. This process, which uses oxygen and phosphate, is called oxidative phosphorylation or aerobic respiration (Marieb 2008).

Anaerobic cellular respiration

If there is no oxygen available, a few molecules of ATP are synthesised during glycolysis but the process cannot proceed further. Only two molecules of ATP are available for each glucose molecule. This is called substrate-level phosphorylation (Marieb 2008). The energy remains trapped in the molecules of pyruvic acid, and lactic acid is formed (anaerobic respiration). An oxygen debt arises and metabolic acidosis is created (Guyton & Hall 2006). When oxygen is available, the lactic acid is gradually converted to pyruvic acid and fed into the Krebs cycle.

Lipids

Lipid is the chemical name for fats and fat-related compounds. The most common source of lipids is in the form of triglycerides. Triglycerides are made up of fatty acids and glycerol. Fats provide the highest-density source of energy for the body. Carbohydrates can also be converted to fat and stored in the adipose tissue. Fat is essential for maintaining health; what is harmful is excess fat intake (more than 30% of the total calories).

Fatty acids, the common structural units of lipids, are also a refined fuel form which is preferred by some cells (e.g. heart muscle) over glucose.

Fatty acids consist of carbon, hydrogen and oxygen atoms. If a given fatty acid is filled with as much hydrogen as it can take, the fatty acid is saturated with hydrogen and the lipids containing them are called saturated fats. Saturated fats are mainly in animal fats such as meat and dairy products. Monounsaturated fats are fats containing fatty acids with one less hydrogen atom, creating one double bond between carbon atoms. The main sources of such fats are olive oils and canola oil, which is derived from the rape seed. Finally, lipids made mainly from unsaturated fatty acids with two or more places unfilled with hydrogen, creating double bonds, are called polyunsaturated. These are also from plant sources (Rodwell-Williams 1999).

Humans can synthesise saturated and monounsaturated fatty acids but there are some that the liver cannot make such as the n-3 and the n-6 families of long-chain polyunsaturated fatty acids (LC-PUFA). From this family, linolenic acid (LA) and α-linolenic (ALA) are essential fatty acids and must be included in the dietary intake. Arachidonic, eicosapentanoic and decosahexanoic acids (DHA) can all be synthesised from LA and ALA, but, if the supply of linoleic and α-linolenic acid is limited, they can become essential fatty acids. These fatty acids are found in vegetable oil and oily fish.

Body fat stores and functions

Body fat is mainly stored under the skin and around the abdominal organs. It is continually being interchanged with the fats circulating in the bloodstream and being metabolised for use as fuel. The dietary reference value for total fat intake is that 35% of energy should be provided by fat. Fats are essential for many of the body's functions:

- They are a source of energy.
- They are involved in the absorption of the fat-soluble vitamins.
- Triglycerides provide the major fuel for energy for hepatocytes and skeletal muscle.
- Phospholipids are a component of myelin sheaths that surround larger nerves and all cell membranes.
- Fatty deposits act as protective cushions for the vital organs such as eyes and kidneys.
- Fats provide an insulating layer under the skin.
- Prostaglandins are formed from linoleic acid; they play a role in smooth muscle contraction and inflammatory responses.
- Fats are part of the cell membrane structure.

- Fats are involved in cell metabolism; combinations of lipids and protein, called lipoproteins, carry lipids in the blood to cells.
- They are involved in nerve impulse transmission.

Lipid metabolism

The energy obtained from fat breakdown or lipolysis is twice that obtained from the metabolism of glucose or protein (4 kcal/g each), providing 9 kcal/g. Any excess fat is stored as adipose tissue in subcutaneous tissues and retroperitoneal tissue. When fat stores are needed for energy production, as in glucose shortage, they are mobilised from the stores under the influence of growth hormones or cortisol. They are taken to the liver where the triglycerides are broken down into free fatty acids and glycerol which are released into the blood.

Glycerol is converted to one of the intermediate products of glycolysis called glyceraldehyde phosphate and is thus assimilated into the energy-releasing process. Further oxidation of the fatty acids releases the 2-carbon acetic acid which is fused to coenzyme A to form acetyl CoA, which enters the Krebs cycle. Fatty acids cannot be used for gluconeogenesis (glucose synthesis) because they enter the cycle beyond the pyruvic acid stage when the changes are irreversible.

In the presence of oxygen and glucose, fatty acids are converted to acetyl CoA, which enters the Krebs cycle. If no glucose is available (e.g. in starvation, diabetes mellitus, some slimming diets or hyperemesis gravidarum) metabolism of a large amount of fat may occur, acetyl CoA accumulates and the liver converts the molecules to ketone bodies, i.e. acetoacetic acid and β-hydroxybutyric acid, which accumulate in the blood. These can be oxidised to release energy but metabolic acidosis will occur.

Cholesterol

Despite common perception, cholesterol is not a fat itself but is a fat-related compound vital in human metabolism. Cholesterol belongs to the steroid family and helps in production of vitamin D, formation of bile acids, digestion and absorption of fats, steroid hormones and cell membranes. Cholesterol is found in all animal foods, mainly in egg yolk and organ meats such as kidneys and liver. Even with no dietary intake of cholesterol, it is synthesised in the liver.

Bile salts, steroid hormones and cell membranes are formed from cholesterol. Cholesterol is found in the blood—mainly in combination with a protein carrier—as lipoproteins, of which there are three types:

1. High-density lipoproteins (HDLs);
2. Low-density lipoproteins (LDLs);
3. Very low-density lipoproteins (VLDLs).

It is also thought that cholesterol is laid down as atheromatous plaques in arterial walls in the form of LDLs and VLDLs. A high ratio of HDLs to LDLs and VLDLs may offer protection against ischaemic heart disease (Marieb 2008). The ratio of HDLs to LDLs and VLDLs has been shown to be increased in vegetarians, people whose fat intake is largely unsaturated and who take regular exercise and reduced in smokers.

Proteins

Animals (including humans) can synthesise protein from amino acids but are unable to synthesise amino acids de novo. Plants can synthesise amino acids from carbon dioxide, water and nitrogen. Therefore, human dietary sources of amino acids/proteins are plants or other animals. Amino acids can be converted to each other through a process in the liver called transamination. Those amino acids that the body either cannot make or cannot make in sufficient amount are called essential or semi-essential amino acids. The best source of essential amino acids is animal products.

Protein foods that have all the essential amino acids such as eggs, meat and human breast milk are said to have a high biological value. Protein foods from plant sources tend to have a lower biological value and should be eaten as a mixture, for their proteins complement each other, hence improving their biological values. Strict vegetarians can obtain adequate levels of essential amino acids by varying their diet carefully. For instance, cereals and legumes contain all the essential amino acids when taken together. Examples of such meals are West Indian rice and peas or the Middle Eastern meals of dishes including a mixture of peas and beans eaten with bread.

The functions of proteins

Proteins include important structural molecules such as muscle protein, collagen and elastin in connective tissue and keratin in skin. They produce new tissue and are therefore essential for growth, recovery from injury, pregnancy and lactation. Proteins also function as hormones, enzymes and transport molecules such as haemoglobin. Amino acids can be used to synthesise proteins or can be converted to glucose to provide energy. These uses depend on adequacy of calorie intake, nitrogen balance (balance between protein synthesis and protein breakdown) and the influence of hormones (anabolic hormones such as growth hormone and the sex hormones against the glucocorticoids produced in stress which enhance protein breakdown and the conversion of amino acids to glucose).

The amount of protein needed in the diet is influenced by age, size, metabolic rate and nitrogen balance.

The recommended daily intake (RDA) is 0.8 g/kg body weight in non-obese individuals. This is equivalent to 60 g of fish or meat and a glass of milk daily. Meat eaters in developed countries eat far in excess of the daily amount needed while some people in developing countries rarely eat meat.

Amino acids

At least 50 g a day is needed to maintain nitrogen balance and to provide for growth and repair of tissues. Amino acids cannot be stored by the body. However, the liver can interconvert amino acids by utilising the eight essential amino acids to synthesise the non-essential amino acids. Any excess amino acids are broken down by the liver by a process of deamination. The nitrogen portion is converted into urea, which enters the blood and is excreted by the kidney.

Proteins are needed by the body for the following functions:

- The formation of new cells.
- The manufacture of enzymes, hormones and antibodies.
- The transport molecules such as haemoglobin.
- Plasma proteins which act as buffers to maintain acid–base balance.
- The control of osmotic pressure between body fluid compartments.
- Amino acids can be used in gluconeogenesis once glucose stores are depleted.

Vitamins

Vitamins are needed in small amounts for growth and health (Marieb 2008). They mainly function as coenzymes to assist in the catalysis of chemical processes and metabolism in the body. The human body is unable to synthesise most vitamins with the exception of vitamin K and some of the B vitamins. Vitamins are distinguished usually according to their solubility in either fat or water. Some vitamins, such as vitamins A, D, E and K, are fat-soluble and are absorbed bound to digested lipids. The water-soluble vitamins, such as most of the B complex and vitamin C, are absorbed with water from the gastrointestinal tract. A normal varied diet should provide them all. Excessive intake can create as many health problems as insufficient intake. Details of the vitamins are given in Box 23.1.

Minerals, trace elements and water

Minerals and trace elements known as micronutrients are inorganic elements that are widely distributed in nature.

BOX 23.1 THE VITAMINS

Fat-soluble vitamins

Vitamin A

Vitamin A is available in two forms: β-carotene and the active form, retinol. β-Carotene is found in plant food (e.g. carrots and deep-green leafy vegetables such as broccoli and spinach), whereas retinol is from animal food sources such as fish liver oils, egg yolk, liver and fortified milk. Butter and commercial products such as margarine are fortified with vitamin A.

Deficiency

Vitamin A is shown to have an antioxidant capacity and may protect against the ageing process. Its absorption is impeded by alcohol, coffee and vitamin D deficiency. The early sign of vitamin A deficiency is a poor dark adaptation or night blindness. Severe deficiencies may lead to blindness, skin disorders, tooth decay and gastrointestinal disorders. Birth defects have occurred in women taking supplements or eating excessive amounts, such as found in liver. It is thought that retinol is a teratogenic agent (Ranjan 1991).

Vitamin D

Vitamin D (7-dehydrocholesterol) is a sterol hormone precursor ingested from animal products. The precursor obtained from plants is called ergosterol. Following ingestion these two substances are transported to the skin where 7-dehydrocholesterol is changed in the skin by the action of ultraviolet (UV) light to an intermediate product vitamin D_3 (cholecalciferol) and ergosterol is converted to vitamin D_2 (ergocalciferol). The most important is cholecalciferol, which is modified first by the liver and then by the kidneys to produce physiologically active vitamin D_3 (calcitriol, 1,25-dihydroxycholecalciferol). It is absorbed in the small intestine with the aid of bile. Vitamin D is stored in liver and skin and is stable to heat and light. Dark-skinned people or those who avoid dairy products may be prone to deficiency. The major source of vitamin D is that formed in the body as a result of ultraviolet irradiation of skin. Dietary sources of vitamin D are fish liver oils, egg/egg yolk, liver and fortified milk. Laxatives and antacids may inhibit gut absorption.

Deficiency

It activates absorption of calcium, promotes bone mineralisation and is involved in blood clotting. Deficiency causes poor mineralisation of bones and teeth such as rickets in children and osteomalacia in adults. There may be poor muscle tone, restlessness and irritability.

Vitamin E (tocopherol)

Vitamin E is chemically related to the sex hormones. It is an antioxidant that is unstable in oxygen. Vitamin E is found in vegetable oils, margarine, whole grains (wheat germ oil) and dark-green leafy vegetables. It is destroyed by food processing and its absorption is reduced by the contraceptive pill.

Deficiency

In vitamin E deficiency, cell membranes are more in danger of oxidation and breakdown. There is therefore more risk of haemolytic anaemia. Vitamin E is an antioxidant and may prevent against cancer. It may have a role in reproduction. In particular, its deficiency can occur in premature infants, as vitamin E stores are normally built up in the last month or two of fetal life. It may also cause neurological symptoms, as it is involved in myelin, the protective fat covering the long axons of nerve cells (Ch. 25). Deficiency may result in spontaneous abortion, preterm labour and stillbirth.

Vitamin K (coagulation vitamin)

There are different forms of vitamin K, including vitamin K_1 (phylloquinone), the dietary form found in green leaves, vegetables (and small amounts in fruit, meat, dairy products and cereal), and vitamin K_2 (menaquinone), which is mainly produced by intestinal bacteria. The approximate recommended dietary allowance (RDA) for men is 80 μg/day and 65 μg/day for women. No additional amount is advised for pregnancy or lactation. The vitamin is stored in the liver, is heat-resistant but is destroyed by acids, alkalis, light and oxidising agents.

Deficiency

Vitamin K has a role in blood clotting. In severe deficiency easy bruising and bleeding occur due to prolonged clotting time. Deficiency occurs as a result of anticoagulant or antibiotic therapy.

Water-soluble vitamins

Vitamin C (ascorbic acid)

Humans cannot synthesise vitamin C and must obtain it from food. It is rapidly destroyed by heat, light and alkalis so that food containing vitamin C should be cooked with minimum water for brief periods and kept covered. It is not stored in a single tissue, but is distributed throughout body tissues. Sufficient vitamin C is present in mother's milk (with a

BOX 23.1 (CONTINUED)

balanced diet) but very little exists in cow's milk so it is added to formula milk.

Vitamin C is found in fruits and vegetables, particularly in citrus fruits, strawberries, tomatoes and fresh potatoes. Some drugs such as aspirin, anticoagulants, antibiotics, diuretics, cortisone, the contraceptive pill and antidepressants may interfere with absorption. Other factors that interfere with absorption are pollution, industrial toxins, overcooking or poor food storage (Tiran 1997).

Deficiency

Vitamin C is an antioxidant and helps in maintenance of body tissues (e.g. collagen) and formation of haemoglobin. Its deficiency can cause poor resistance to bacterial infections, anaemia, bruising and haemorrhage, oedema, poor digestion and gum disease. Recent research appears to suggest that a very low intake of vitamin C may more than double the risk of women developing pre-eclampsia (Zhang et al 2002). Supplementation with antioxidants (vitamins C and E) was associated with a reduced incidence of pre-eclampsia (Alexander 2002).

Vitamin B_1 (thiamine)

B vitamins are mostly part of enzymes involved in the metabolism of carbohydrate, fat and proteins and in tissue building. They can be stored in small amounts (a continuous supply is necessary); excess is eliminated in urine. Vitamin B_1 is a fairly stable antioxidant but is destroyed by alkalis and high temperature. Its requirement depends on carbohydrate and energy intake. The RDA for adults is 0.5 mg/1000 kcal daily. It is not necessary to increase intake during pregnancy and lactation. Vitamin B_1 is found in lean meat, liver, eggs, whole grains, nuts, leafy green vegetables and legumes. Its absorption in the small intestine is reduced by alcohol, coffee, food additives and overcooking and it is lost in cooking water.

Deficiency

As it is involved in energy and glucose metabolism, deficiency of thiamine can affect the gastrointestinal (deficiency of hydrochloric acid), nervous, cardiovascular and musculoskeletal systems. Its deficiency causes the disease beri-beri (Sinhalese *I can't, I can't*) with pain, weakness, degeneration of muscles and inability to perform coordinated movements. The full disease is rarely seen in developed countries. The other disease due to thiamine deficiency is Wernicke–Korsakoff syndrome

which could occur in people with long-term vomiting or in alcoholics. Its symptoms include poor memory, confusion, apathy and ataxia.

Vitamin B_2 (riboflavin)

This vitamin contains the sugar ribose and is stable to heat but sensitive to light. Vitamin B_2 is found in lean meat, yeast, liver, eggs, whole grains, nuts, meats, legumes and mainly in milk.

Deficiency

Poor wound healing and cracks in lips, corner of mouth and tongue are typical signs of vitamin B_2 deficiency. Because of the sensitivity of riboflavin to light, attention should be given to premature infants who are getting phototherapy treatment for the symptoms of riboflavin deficiency. Its absorption will be reduced by the contraceptive pill and antibiotics.

Vitamin B_3 (niacin)

Niacin exists in two forms: nicotinic acid, which is easily converted to its amide form, and nicotinamide, which is a simple, stable organic compound. It is found in any protein food: meat, peanuts, dry beans and peas. It can easily be synthesised in the body from the amino acid tryptophan. Its absorption will be reduced by alcohol, coffee, antibiotics and antitubercular drugs.

Deficiency

Vitamin B_3 deficiency causes the disease pellagra with headache, weight loss, loss of appetite and, later, soreness and redness of the lips and tongue, vomiting and diarrhoea and skin ulceration. Neurological symptoms may also occur.

Vitamin B_6 (pyridoxine)

This vitamin is stable to heat and acids but destroyed by alkalis and light. The RDA standard is 2 mg/day for men and 1.6 mg/day for women, with additions for pregnancy and lactation. Vitamin B_6 is found in grains, seeds, meat, liver and kidney. Its absorption is reduced by antibiotics and antitubercular drugs.

Deficiency

Vitamin B_6 is important for the nervous system, amino acid formation, sulphur transfer, formation of niacin from tryptophan and formation of antibodies and haemoglobin. A dosage of vitamin B_6 of up to 100 mg/day is likely to be beneficial in treating premenstrual symptoms and premenstrual depression (Wyatt et al 1999). Deficiency of vitamin B_6 causes anaemia, convulsions, irritability, vomiting and

(Continued)

BOX 23.1 (CONTINUED)

abdominal pain in infants and dermatitis and depression in adults. It could be toxic in large amounts (up to 5 g/day).

Vitamin B$_{12}$ (cyanocobalamin)

This vitamin is complex and contains cobalt. It is stable to heat but inactivated by acids and alkalis. Vitamin B$_{12}$ is found mainly in meat, but milk, eggs, butter and cheese are also valuable sources. Some synthesis is done by human intestinal bacteria and it is found in some seaweeds. It is not found in any vegetable or fruit.

Deficiency

Vitamin B$_{12}$ is the intrinsic factor necessary for the transportation of iron across the intestinal membrane. It is stored in the liver, with stores sufficient to last 3–5 years in normal health. It is also involved in enzymes working in bone marrow in the formation of DNA. In its absence, erythrocytes do not divide. It is necessary for normal protein metabolism and production of myelin sheath around nerve cells. Vitamin B$_{12}$ deficiency causes pernicious anaemia and neurological symptoms. Vegans and vegetarians may have a diet deficient in vitamin B$_{12}$.

Folic acid

Folic acid is not a stable vitamin, so considerable losses occur in cooking. It is stored mainly in the liver. It is toxic in excessive amounts. Folic acid is widely distributed in food sources such as liver, yeast, eggs, whole grain, deep-green vegetables and nuts. It is also synthesised in the gut by enteric bacteria. Absorption is hindered by alcohol as well as drugs that are folic acid antagonists such as anticonvulsants, aspirin and sulphonamides.

Importance

Folic acid is essential for the formation of red blood cells. It is necessary for the health of the nervous system and for the development of the fetus.

Deficiency

Folic acid is essential for the formation of red blood cells. It is necessary for the health of the nervous system and for the development of the fetus. It is believed that perinatal supplementation of folic acid has a strong protective effect against neural tube defects (Lumley et al 2001; see also Ch. 15).

The mineral content of the human body is very similar to that of the Earth. There are seven minerals that the human body requires in greater amount: calcium, phosphorus, potassium, sulphur, sodium, chloride and magnesium. The remaining 18 elements, called trace elements, include iron, iodine and zinc and are no less important, but they occur in very small amounts, contributing 20–40% of the total inorganic elements in the body.

Iron (in haemoglobin) is discussed in Chapter 16, sodium and potassium in Chapter 20 and calcium and phosphorus (in bone) in Chapter 24. Generally, minerals and trace elements (4% of total body) function as structural and catalyst substances. These include regulation of fluid balance and acid–base balance, transmission of action along nerves and contraction of muscle fibres. They are also important as components of enzymes and hormones essential for energy metabolism and functioning of the immune system.

Regulation of food intake and energy balance

Energy is produced from oxidation of macronutrients in the body and is essential to maintain life. When there is

a balance between energy intake and energy output, the body weight remains stable. Obesity occurs when energy intake exceeds energy output. However, this is more complicated than a straightforward equation, as two people with the same energy intake may have totally different body type and size. Genetic as well as environmental factors are believed to have a role in causing obesity. There appear to be body mechanisms that control intake which enable most people to maintain a steady weight.

Nutritional states

There are two nutritional states: the absorptive state when nutrients are being eaten and absorbed by the digestive tract and the postabsorptive state when the gastrointestinal tract is empty and energy requirements are met by breakdown of body stores. The absorptive state lasts for about 4 h after a reasonable meal has been eaten. If three meals are eaten in the day there is a balance between the two states, each occupying about half of a 24-h period. Insulin directs the events of the absorptive state, mainly by its control of blood glucose levels.

The body can be maintained in the postabsorptive state for days or weeks in a famine or during illness as long as sufficient water is taken. Glucose is made available to cells via the bloodstream by glycogenolysis in the liver. Muscle glycogen cannot be broken down to glucose because it lacks the enzymes. It is partly oxidised to pyruvic acid or, in anaerobic conditions, to lactic acid. These substances enter the blood and are converted to glucose by the liver. The hormone glucagon is released when blood sugars become too low. Glucagon targets the liver and adipose tissue to enable glucose to be released into the blood.

Total energy expenditure

The total energy requirements in the body are to support three main energy uses: the basal metabolic rate (BMR) or resting metabolic rate (RMR), which are used interchangeably (BMR and RMR are slightly different in measurement but practically the same); the thermic effect of food; and variable amounts of physical activities.

Metabolic rate

BMR is the amount of energy required for the body's internal organs to maintain resting activities; it is measured after an overnight fast in a normal environmental temperature. In general, the younger the person, the higher the BMR, and males have a higher BMR than females because of the ratio of metabolically active muscle to the metabolically sluggish fatty tissue. Four main factors that positively influence BMR are lean body mass, growth, fever and disease condition as well as cold climate. BMR makes the largest contribution to total energy expenditure (about 60–70%).

The effect of food intake and body heat production

The ingestion of food stimulates metabolism and requires energy to meet the needs of the processes involved: digestion, absorption and transport of nutrients. This is called the thermic effect of food and comprises 10–15% of total energy expenditure.

Regulation of body temperature

The maintenance of body temperature depends on the balance between heat production and heat loss. The body temperature of humans is usually maintained within a range of 36.1–37.8°C independently of external environment or internal heat production. A rise in body temperature increases enzyme activity and most adults will have convulsions when their temperature reaches 41°C and die if their temperature exceeds 43°C. Temperature varies slightly depending on where in the body it is recorded. The body's core (organs within the body cavities) has the highest temperature and the shell (heat loss surface of the skin) has the lowest temperature. Rectal temperature is nearer the core than oral temperature. The hypothalamus (Ch. 26) is the major heat-regulating centre.

Body composition and body weight

In simple terms, body composition can be divided into two main compartments: lean mass and fat mass. Other more detailed models classify the body to three, four or five compartments (including lean, fat, water, mineral mass—bones and glycogen stores). In the concept of weight and health, the emphasis has been too much on the anthropometric side of measurements rather than body composition. However, what is important is the amount of excess fat and its distribution rather than just excess weight. Central obesity (accumulation of excess fat around the abdomen and upper body) is related to diseases such as diabetes and cardiovascular disease.

Maternal adaptation to pregnancy

Nutrition

Nutritional advice during pregnancy has had little supporting research-based evidence to date. However, available evidence (Tiran 1997) suggests that nutrition is an essential foundation for a happy and healthy mother and baby. There is a relationship between poor intake of essential nutrients and a higher-than-normal perinatal morbidity and mortality. Fetal growth may be compromised with an increase in preterm delivery and a decrease in weight for gestational age. The implications of low birth weight in the causation of adult diabetes mellitus and hypertension have been postulated (Barker 1992, 2003).

Specific requirements of pregnancy

During pregnancy, maternal weight increases significantly and includes the products of conception, increased water and excess uterine and breast tissue. There are additional nutritional requirements to meet both the increase in maternal tissue and fetal needs. Other factors that influence nutritional requirement during pregnancy include age, gravidity and parity as well as the time interval between pregnancies.

Energy

Factors influencing energy needs during pregnancy include metabolic cost, prepregnancy fat and weight, level of activity and the stage of pregnancy. The significant differences between the pattern of changes in BMR between women from developing and developed countries indicate that there may be some energy-sparing mechanism in process that causes variation in estimation of energy requirements during pregnancy.

The average total energy cost of pregnancy is estimated to be about 70 000 kcal for a woman with a pre-pregnancy weight of 60 kg and fat deposition of 2–2.4 kg during pregnancy. The UK dietary reference value (DRV) for extra energy requirement in pregnancy is 200 kcal/day, but only during the last trimester. This recommendation varies in different countries: e.g. 300 kcal/day during the second and third trimester in the USA. These are guidelines and the actual requirements depend on the individual basis: e.g. size, activity and original nutritional status of the woman.

Protein

The quality of protein intake depends on both the type and quantity of food eaten and the conditions under which it is eaten. For example, if the total energy supplied by the diet is so low that gluconeogenesis utilises amino acids to provide energy, the ability to construct new tissue will be reduced. The average pregnant woman in Britain will need an extra 6 g of dietary protein daily, a total of 51 g/day. However, Kramer (2000) concluded that there appeared to be no long-term benefits to the babies when mothers significantly increased their protein intake above normal. This is probably because most women in developed countries eat far more protein than is needed for health.

Carbohydrates and fats

There is little need to increase either glucose or fats for energy but the absorption of fat-soluble vitamins must be considered when advising women about diet in pregnancy. During pregnancy women should have adequate dietary intakes of essential fatty acids and their longer derivatives, omega-6 (mainly arachidonic acid) and omega-3s (mainly docosahexaenoic acid or DHA). Dietary fat intake in pregnancy and lactation, particularly long-chain fatty acids and DHA, are shown to play an important role in brain, cognitive and visual development of the growing baby (Koletzko et al 2007). In addition, the consumption of oils rich in LC-PUFA during pregnancy reduces the risk of premature birth (Koletzko et al 2008). Dietary fat intake for pregnant and lactating women is recommended to be the same as that required for the general population including an average intake of 200 mg DHA/day. This can be achieved by consuming one or two portions of oily fish (tuna, salmon and mackerel) per week. Caution should be applied by avoiding large predatory fish which are more likely to be contaminated with pollutants such as methylmercury.

Vitamins

In developed countries for healthy women with a balanced diet there is usually no need for vitamin supplementation. However, in women with restricted dietary intake or those having had gastrointestinal surgery, especially ileostomy, supplementation may be necessary. In particular it is important to remember the role of folic acid in the cause or prevention of neural tube defects (Wald & Bower 1995). There has been an effort to add folic acid to basic foods to ensure compliance with intake, especially prior to conception. Reference values for some of the vitamins are summarised below.

Vitamin A

The DRV for retinol during pregnancy is an extra 100 μg (Barker 2002). However, because of the teratogenic effects of retinol, the Department of Health and Social Security (DHSS 1990) recommends that the RDA should not be exceeded and that pregnant women should avoid liver and liver products.

Vitamin D

Routine supplementation of vitamin D in pregnancy is not recommended. Asian women in the UK, in particular those who are vegetarian, may be prone to vitamin D deficiency and need consideration.

Thiamine, riboflavin and folate

The need for thiamine increases by increased energy requirements. The increment for average riboflavin intake is 0.3 mg/day throughout pregnancy. The reference nutrient intake (RNI) for folic acid is 200 μg/day for adults and it should be increased during pregnancy (+100) and lactation (+60).

Vitamin C

To ensure sufficient maternal stores, an increment of 10 mg/day during the last trimester of pregnancy is recommended.

Calcium

The adult average requirement is 700 mg but no increment is established for pregnancy since calcium absorption increases and maternal stores meet the requirement. However, for teenage pregnant mothers, calcium-rich diets are particularly advisable since they have their own growth requirements to deal with as well.

Iron

The iron requirements are met by utilisation of maternal stores, cessation of menstrual losses and increased absorption. Therefore, no extra iron is required in a healthy woman with a balanced diet. Iron supplementation during pregnancy is discussed in Chapter 16.

Metabolism

The addition of a new endocrine organ (placenta) and increased endocrine activity have major influences on maternal metabolism to allow provision of nutrients for fetal growth. Human chorionic gonadotrophin (hCG), human placental lactogen (hPL), oestrogen and progesterone affect metabolism, some by antagonising insulin.

Plasma T_3 and T_4 (thyroxine) are increased, leading to a physiological state of hyperthyroidism (see Ch. 35). Maternal insulin plasma level is also increased to ensure availability of glucose for placental uptake. An increased state of maternal insulin resistance assists glucose availability for fetal utilisation. The changes in glucose tolerance and insulin levels during pregnancy make it a diabetogenic condition. Women who have predisposing factors may develop gestational diabetes (see Ch. 35).

The BMR rises during pregnancy, reflecting increased oxygen demands of the fetus, placenta and mother. Metabolism of carbohydrate, protein and fat alters, with a major shift in the fuel sources: fat becomes the maternal fuel, whereas glucose becomes the major fetal fuel. Approximately 50–70% of energy required daily by the fetus in the third trimester is derived from glucose, about 20% of it from amino acids and the remainder from fat (Worthington-Roberts & Rodwell-Williams 1996). Maternal metabolic adjustments occur in more than one way depending on the fetal size and therefore energy demand as well as maternal metabolic and nutritional status. For example, to meet the extra required energy in late pregnancy several changes may occur, including reduction in lipid synthesis and fat storage, alteration in physical activity and increase in food consumption (King 2000).

Carbohydrates

Blood glucose levels are generally between 10% and 20% lower than in the non-pregnant state. This decrease leads to lower insulin levels in the postabsorptive state and a tendency towards ketosis. As pregnancy progresses, there is less peripheral use of glucose by the mother because of increasing insulin antagonism (blockage of cellular uptake). Glucose therefore becomes more readily available to the fetus. Insulin resistance is thought to be due to a decrease in sensitivity of cell receptors, resulting from the effects of hPL, progesterone and cortisol. In response, the pancreatic β islet cells undergo hyperplasia and hypertrophy to produce increased insulin during meals. The results of changes in the above hormones are listed briefly below:

- Progesterone also helps to increase insulin secretion, decreases peripheral insulin usage and increases insulin levels after meals.
- Oestrogen increases the level of plasma cortisol, which is an insulin antagonist, stimulates β-cell hyperplasia and enhances peripheral glucose usage.
- Cortisol depletes hepatic glycogen stores through glycogenolysis and increases hepatic glucose production.
- The role of hPL is not very clear but it is biologically similar to growth hormone and it correlates with fetal and placental weight. It increases in the plasma as pregnancy progresses and is higher in multiple pregnancy. It antagonises insulin to increase glucose availability and increases the synthesis and availability of lipids which can be used as an alternative fuel to glucose.

Proteins

Pregnancy is an anabolic state with significant nitrogen retention, especially in late pregnancy. Protein metabolism is complex and changes gradually through pregnancy including reduction in nitrogen excretion to achieve nitrogen conservation for fetal growth. Serum amino acid and protein levels are decreased in pregnancy because of placental uptake, increased insulin levels and hepatic use of amino acids for gluconeogenesis. The 50% expansion of plasma volume as well as changes in hormone levels account for the reduction of biochemical substances such as plasma albumin and haemoglobin.

Lipids

Every aspect of lipid metabolism changes in pregnancy. During the first two trimesters, triglyceride synthesis and fat storage (lipogenesis) increase, mediated by the increase in insulin production and enhanced by progesterone. About 60% of fat storage occurs in the first 16 weeks of gestation (Forsum et al 1988). There is an overall store of 3.5 kg in normal pregnancy.

During the third trimester lipolysis increases further, probably due to the increase in hPL. There is accelerated ketogenesis in the liver due to increased oxidation of free fatty acids for conversion into energy. Fats are therefore acting as an alternative source of energy so that the mother can conserve glucose for the fetus. At the same time in the last trimester, when glucose transfer to the fetus is maximal, there is decreased lipogenesis in adipose tissue and the balance is tipped in the direction of lipolysis (Blackburn 2003). Blood cholesterol increases steadily as pregnancy progresses and stays stationary for the last few weeks before delivery. This is unrelated to diet.

Changes in the absorptive and postabsorptive states

During the absorptive state ingested nutrients are digested and absorbed by the gastrointestinal tract. The absorptive state in pregnancy is characterised by relative hyperinsulinaemia and hyperglycaemia due to reduced liver uptake. There is also hypertriglyceridaemia and increased lipogenesis due to the conversion of glucose to fat for storage.

In the postabsorptive or fasting state, energy has to be supplied from the body stores. Most of this comes from the catabolism of fat. Fat and protein synthesis are decreased and catabolism exceeds anabolism. The central nervous system has no alternative but to carry on using available glucose but other organs move to production of energy from lipids. Triglycerides are broken down and fed into the Krebs cycle with the production of ketone bodies. If these accumulate, ketoacidosis will occur. After an overnight fast, maternal plasma glucose falls significantly below that of a non-pregnant woman because of extra demand by the fetus and impaired gluconeogenesis. Gluconeogenesis and circulating free fatty acids are decreased. The reduced gluconeogenesis capacity preserves maternal muscle mass.

Maternal weight gain and body composition

The amount of weight gain may vary to a great extent among individual pregnant women. However, the average weight gain for most mothers is about 11–15 kg for a full-term pregnancy. About 35% of weight gain is accounted for by the weight of the fetus and placenta unit in developed countries, compared with 50% in less well-developed countries (Norgan 1992). Of the total weight gain, approximately 62% represents water, 30% fat and 8% protein. Fat distribution is not uniform and mostly accumulates in abdominal, subscapular and upper thigh areas (Forsum et al 1988).

A wide range, from weight loss to a weight gain of 30 kg, is reported during pregnancy. A greater incidence of poor outcome is associated with the extreme of this range. A higher risk of low birth weight is reported more in women with a low net weight gain during pregnancy. Maternal prepregnancy weight, socioeconomic status, genetic factors and pregnancy weight gain have all been shown to influence infant birth. High net weight gain during pregnancy is also problematic as it leads to complicated pregnancy, prolonged labour, retained weight after birth and increased birth weight. Most excess weight is lost within the first 3 months after birth. Factors that influence postpartum weight loss are maternal age, prepregnancy weight, mother's desired weight and length of lactation.

It is not advisable to encourage a strict diet for pregnant women in general (Enkin et al 2000). Nonetheless, a modest reduction in energy intake for some women seems most unlikely to have any adverse effect on the birth weight, yet it may prevent the problem of excessive fat gain by the woman. A study by Mathews et al (1999) showed that maternal nutrition (intake of macronutrients), at least in industrial countries, seems to have only a very small effect on the placental and infant birth weight.

Main points

- Many cells, especially in the liver, can convert one type of food molecule to another but there are about 50 essential nutrients that cannot be manufactured by the body cells and must be provided in the diet.
- Four food groups provide a balanced diet: grains; fruits and vegetables; meat and fish; and milk products.
- The best source of essential amino acids is animal products. The proteins found in legumes, nuts and cereals are nutritionally incomplete and are low in one or more of the essential amino acids. Vegetarians can obtain all the essential amino acids by varying their diet carefully.
- Vitamins may be fat-soluble or water-soluble. Their main role is to function as coenzymes to assist in the catalysis of chemical processes in the body. The human body is unable to synthesise most vitamins with the exception of vitamin K and some of the B vitamins.

- Body cells must convert ingested food into the high-energy phosphate bonds of ATP. When glucose arrives at the tissues it is taken up by the cells by facilitated diffusion under the influence of insulin. Glucose is taken to the mitochondria where it is oxidised to form energy in the Krebs cycle.
- Excess fat is stored as adipose tissue. When fat is needed for energy production it is mobilised from the stores under the influence of growth hormones or cortisol, taken to the liver and broken down into free fatty acids and glycerol which are released into the blood.
- Cholesterol, found in the blood in combination with a protein carrier such as lipoprotein, exists as three types: high-density lipoproteins (HDLs), low-density lipoproteins (LDLs) and very low-density lipoproteins (VLDLs). The ratio of HDLs to LDLs and VLDLs is increased in those whose fat intake is largely

- unsaturated and who take regular exercise and reduced in cigarette smokers.
- At least 50 g of protein per day is needed to maintain nitrogen balance and to provide for growth and repair of tissues.
- In pregnancy, increased nutrients are needed to supply the increase in maternal and fetal needs, although reducing energy expenditure without increased intake may be sufficient, depending on maternal stores. More protein is required but there is little need to increase glucose or fats. In women with restricted dietary intake or those with ileostomy, vitamin supplementation may be necessary. Folic acid deficiency is implicated in the cause of neural tube defects.
- As pregnancy progresses, there is less peripheral use of glucose by the mother because of increasing insulin antagonism. Glucose becomes more readily available to the fetus.
- There are decreased serum amino acid and protein levels in pregnancy because of placental uptake, increased insulin and gluconeogenesis. Nitrogen excretion is reduced to achieve nitrogen conservation for fetal growth.
- During the first two trimesters fat storage increases due to increased insulin production and progesterone. During the third trimester lipolysis increases. Fats act as an alternative source of energy to conserve glucose for the fetus.
- The central nervous system can only use available glucose but other organs move to production of energy from lipids. Triglycerides are broken down and fed into the Krebs cycle with the production of ketone bodies. If these accumulate, ketoacidosis will occur.
- A wide range of weight loss to a weight gain of 30 kg is reported during pregnancy. A greater incidence of poor outcome is associated with the extreme of this range.

References

Alexander, S., 2002. On the prevention of pre-eclampsia: nutritional factors back in the spotlight. Epidemiology 13 (4), 382–383.

Barker, D.J.P. (Ed.), 1992. Fetal and Infant Origins of Adult Disease. BMJ Books, London.

Barker, H.M., 2002. Nutrition and Dietetics for Health Care, tenth edn. Churchill Livingstone, Edinburgh.

Barker, D.J.P., 2003. The Best Start in Life. Century, London.

Blackburn, S.T., 2003. Maternal, Fetal and Neonatal Physiology, second edn. Saunders, Philadelphia.

DHSS, 1990. Vitamin A and pregnancy PL/C (90) 10 and 11. DHSS, London.

Enkin, M., Keirse, M.J.N.C., Renfrew, M., Neilson, J., 2000. A Guide to Effective Care in Pregnancy and Childbirth, third edn. Oxford University Press, Oxford.

Forsum, E., Sadurskis, A., Wager, J., 1988. Resting metabolic rate and body composition of healthy Swedish women during pregnancy and lactation. Am. J. Clin. Nutr. 47, 942–947.

Guyton, A.C., Hall, J.E., 2006. Textbook of Medical Physiology, eleventh edn. Elsevier Saunders, Philadelphia.

Henderson, C., Macdonald, S. (Eds.), 2004. Mayes' Midwifery: A Textbook for Midwives, thirteenth edn. Baillière Tindall, London.

King, J.C., 2000. Physiology of pregnancy and nutrient metabolism. Am. J. Clin. Nutr. 71 (5), 1218S–1225S.

Koletzko, B., Cetin, I., Brenna, J.T., 2007. Dietary fat intakes for pregnant and lactating women. Br. J. Nutr. 97, 873–877.

Koletzko, B., Lein, E., Agostoni, C., Bohles, H., et al., 2008. The roles of long-chain polyunsaturated fatty acids in pregnancy, lactation and infancy: review of current knowledge and consensus recommendations. J. Perinat. Med. 36, 5–14.

Kramer, M.S., 2000. Balanced protein/energy supplementation in pregnancy. Cochrane Database Syst. Rev. (1) Update Software 2003, Oxford.

Lumley, J., Watson, L., Watson, M., Bower, C., 2001. Periconceptual supplementation with folate and/or multivitamins for preventing neural tube defects. Cochrane Database Syst. Rev. (1) Update Software 2003, Oxford.

Marieb, E.N., 2008. Human Anatomy and Physiology, nineth edn. Benjamin/Cummings, New York.

Mathews, F., Yudkin, P., Neil, A., 1999. Influence of maternal nutrition on outcome of pregnancy: prospective cohort study. Br. Med. J. 319, 339–343.

Norgan, N.G., 1992. Maternal body composition: methods for measuring short term changes. J. Biosoc. Sci. 24, 367–377.

Ranjan, V., 1991. Vitamin A and birth defects. Prof. Care Mother Child 1 (1), 3–4.

Rodwell-Williams, S., 1999. Essentials of Nutrition and Diet Therapy, seventh edn. Mosby, St Louis.

Tiran, D., 1997. Maternal nutrition. In: Sweet, B.R., Tiran, D. (Eds.), Mayes Midwifery, twelfth edn. Baillière Tindall, London.

Wald, N.J., Bower, C., 1995. Folic acid and the prevention of neural tube defects. Br. Med. J. 310, 1019–1020.

Worthington-Roberts, B.S., Rodwell-Williams, S., 1996. Nutrition Throughout the Life Cycle, sixth edn. Mosby, St Louis.

Wyatt, K.M., Dimmock, P.W., Jones, P.W., O'Brian, P.M.S., 1999. Efficacy of vitamin B_6 in the treatment of premenstrual syndrome: systematic review. Br. Med. J. 318, 1371–1381.

Zhang, C., Williams, M.A., King, I.B., et al., 2002. Vitamin C and the risk of pre-eclampsia: results from dietary questionnaire and plasma assay. Epidemiology 13 (4), 409–416.

Annotated recommended reading

Barker, D.J.P., 2003. The Best Start in Life. Century, London.

This easy-to-read book develops Barker's theory on the effects of pregnancy on the fetus in causing disease in later life and is suitable for both practitioners and prospective parents.

Guyton, A.C., Hall, J.E., 2006. Textbook of Medical Physiology, eleventh edn. Elsevier Saunders, Philadelphia.

Chapters 67–72 give a detailed account of metabolism and this is an excellent book to own or borrow although it does not discuss pregnancy changes in any detail.

King, J.C., 2000. Physiology of pregnancy and nutrient metabolism. Am. J. Clin. Nutr. 71 (5), 1218S–1225S.

This paper gives an excellent overview of the topic of nutrition in pregnancy.

Soltani, H., Fraser, R.B., 2002. Pregnancy as a cause of obesity: myth or reality? RCM Midwives J. 5 (5), 193–195.

This paper is accessible and worth reading for both the content and conclusions and also to demonstrate the necessity for good research to be carried out by midwives.

Chapter Twenty-Four

The nature of bone—the female pelvis and fetal skull

Introduction

Successful childbearing depends on the relationship between the size and shape of the maternal pelvis and the fetal skull. The evolution of bipedalism (walking on two legs) and the large human brain have increased the risk to both mother and fetus. This chapter examines the general structure and function of bone and calcium and phosphorus metabolism. A detailed description of the pelvis and fetal skull follows.

The nature of bone: function and structure

Functions of bone

Bone is a highly vascular, constantly changing, hard mineralised connective tissue (Guyton & Hall 2006) which contains depositions of calcium and phosphorus. It performs important functions for the body:

- Support and protection of the soft organs.
- Movement by acting as anchorage for muscles and levers.
- Storage of fat.
- Large reservoir of calcium and phosphorus.
- Storage of smaller amounts of potassium, sulphur, magnesium and copper.
- Blood cell formation.

Structure of bone

Bone is a living matrix consisting of three basic components: an organic matrix of **collagen** known as **osteoid**, a cartilage-like material differing from cartilage in that calcium salts are readily deposited in it, a **mineral matrix** of calcium and phosphorus and **bone cells** which include **osteoblasts**, **osteoclasts** and **osteocytes**. Calcium (Ca^{2+}), the most common mineral in the body, and phosphorus are present in bone as crystals of **hydroxyapatite**, $(Ca_3(PO_4)_2)_3 \cdot Ca(OH)_2$, attached to collagen fibres. This results in the hardness of bone. Bone is continually being remodelled as osteoblasts deposit new bone and osteoclasts reabsorb it. Calcium and phosphorus are slowly exchanged between bone and extracellular fluid (ECF). Bone can be divided into **compact** (lamellar) bone and **spongy** (trabecular) bone (Guyton & Hall 2006).

Bone cells

- **Osteoblasts** are present on all bone surfaces in single layers next to the unmineralised osteoid of newly forming bone. They may be differentiated from haemopoietic stem cells. They are uniformly sized and linked together by cytoplasmic processes. Osteoblasts synthesise and secrete the constituents of the organic matrix and promote mineralisation.
- **Osteocytes** are derived from osteoblasts that have become trapped in lacunae. They maintain the bone matrix and if they die the surrounding matrix is absorbed.
- **Osteoclasts** reabsorb bone and are found on or near surfaces undergoing erosion. They may have developed separately to osteoblasts and derive from monocytes. They vary greatly in size and nuclear form and are very mobile. Osteoclasts contain both proteolytic enzymes and acids such as lactic acid and citric acid which remove both the organic and mineral matrix.

Compact bone

Compact bone forms the outer rim or cortex of all bones and consists of **osteons** or **Haversian systems**. There is a central Haversian canal oriented to the long axis of the bone. Running at right-angles to the long axis of the bone are secondary canals called perforating or **Volkmann's canals** which carry nerves, blood vessels and lymphatic vessels. Around the central canal are concentric hollow tubes of bone called **lamellae**. Each lamella has small concavities at its junctions with others called **lacunae** which contain the spider-shaped osteocytes. Hair-like canals called **canaliculi** connect the lacunae to each other and to the central canal, linking all the osteocytes in an osteon together. This facilitates exchange of nutrients and removal of waste products.

Spongy bone

Spongy bone contains far fewer Haversian systems and is made up of a lattice of **trabeculae** with red or fatty bone marrow filling the cavities (Figs 24.1, 24.2). Trabeculae are only a few cell layers thick and contain irregularly arranged lamellae and osteocytes connected by canaliculi. There are no osteons present. Nutrients arrive at the osteocytes by diffusing through narrow spaces between bony spicules. The tiny struts of bone are arranged to combat the stress placed on the bone during activity.

Periosteum and endosteum

Most bones have a tough outer covering of fibrous connective tissue, the **periosteum**, which does not cover the articular surfaces of joints. Periosteum transmits blood vessels and acts as an attachment surface for ligaments and muscles. It is supplied abundantly with nerve fibres. Beneath this is a layer of osteoblasts. Lining the marrow cavity is the **endosteum**, a layer of tissue containing the osteoblasts and osteoclasts.

Calcium and phosphorus metabolism

There are about 1000 g of calcium in an adult, of which the skeleton contains 99%, leaving only 10 g available for other cellular processes (Hinson et al 2007). The small amount of calcium found in body fluids and cells plays an important part in metabolic processes and is maintained within narrow limits. Phosphorus is also crucial to body function and the skeleton contains 85%. The normal plasma concentration of calcium is 2.10–2.70 mmol/L and of phosphate 0.70–1.40 mmol/L.

Functions of calcium

Calcium is an intracellular and extracellular ion with many functions. It is present in ECF in two forms: half is bound to the proteins albumin and globulin and half is in an ionised form (Ca^{2+}) which is important in many cell activities (Hinson et al 2007):

- Nerve and muscle function.
- Hormonal actions.
- Blood clotting.
- Cell motility.
- A secondary messenger between environmental stimulus and cell function by modulation of enzyme response when bound to the protein **calmodulin**.

Functions of phosphorus

Phosphorus in the form of phosphates plays a large role in cellular function:

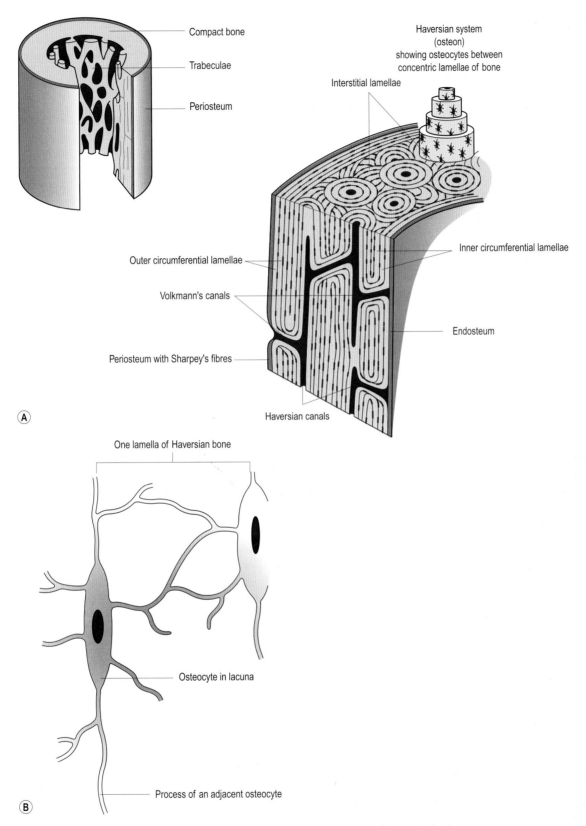

Figure 24.1 • Structure of compact bone. (From Hinchliff S M, Montague S E 1990, with permission.)

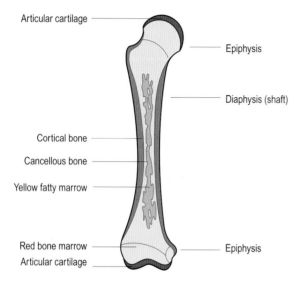

Figure 24.2 • Anatomical features of a long bone. (From Hinchliff S M, Montague S E 1990, with permission.)

- As a component of nucleic acids.
- By regulating energy storage as adenosine triphosphate (ATP).

Hormonal control of calcium and phosphorus metabolism

Regulation of calcium balance is closely associated with that of phosphate. There is continuous exchange of calcium between different sites (calcium pools) in the body. Three hormones control calcium and phosphorus metabolism by maintaining the concentration of calcium in ECF. These are **parathyroid hormone** (PTH), **vitamin D** and **calcitonin**. Plasma inorganic phosphate is more loosely controlled than calcium (Hinson et al 2007).

If there is no change in the amount of skeletal calcium, ECF calcium level depends on the balance between calcium absorption in the gut and its excretion in urine and faeces. About 50% of calcium in the blood passing through bone capillaries is exchanged in a single passage and about 300 mmol of calcium is involved in calcium exchange between blood and bone every day.

Parathyroid hormone

Four parathyroid glands which are embedded in the thyroid gland secrete parathyroid hormone (PTH). PTH increases the concentration of Ca^{2+} in blood and depresses plasma phosphate concentration by acting on bone and kidneys. PTH increases osteocyte reabsorption of bone with a rapid release of calcium and phosphorus into the blood. Calcium reabsorption in the kidney tubules is increased but the excretion of phosphate is increased. This results in a rise in plasma calcium and a

fall in plasma phosphate. PTH activity is directly related to serum calcium concentration. When plasma calcium level rises, PTH production falls, resulting in calcium deposition in bone, and vice versa.

Vitamin D

The D vitamins are steroid substances formed from **ergosterol** in plants and **7-dehydrocholesterol** in animals. Ultraviolet radiation modifies these to **ergocalciferol** (vitamin D_2) and **cholecalciferol** (vitamin D_3). Humans can either ingest vitamin D from plants and animals or manufacture it by the action of sunlight on skin to form cholecalciferol. Vitamin D has to be further metabolised by adding hydroxyl groups before it can become active. The liver first converts it to **25-hydroxycholecalciferol** and the kidney produces the active form **1,25-dihydroxycholecalciferol** (calcitriol) in response to PTH stimulation. Calcitriol is released into the circulation and transported to its target organs of intestine, bone and kidneys (Hinson et al Chew 2007).

Calcitonin

Calcitonin is secreted by the **parafollicular cells** (**clear** or **C cells**) of the thyroid gland. Its main effect is opposite to PTH, causing a fall in plasma calcium and phosphate concentrations. This hormone may play a part in skeletal growth in children but appears to have no role in adults other than in pregnant women. Calcitonin secretion is directly related to plasma calcium concentration.

The pelvic girdle

The pelvic girdle offers attachment for the lower limbs and for support of the pelvic and, to some extent, the abdominal organs. In an upright posture the pelvic girdle transmits the weight of the trunk to the legs, so the sacroiliac joints must be strong and stable. The size, shape and rigidity of the pelvic girdle is related directly to bipedal locomotion and the human pelvis compared to other primates is short, squat and basin-shaped (Trevathan et al 1999).

The mammalian spine is highly efficient for walking on four legs as the abdominal organs are suspended from a single horizontal arch (the backbone). This single arch is present in the human neonate but when babies sit up their spines develop a forward curve near the top. When babies stand their spines develop a second forward curve near the base. Both curves are essential for maintaining an upright posture.

The evolving changes in pelvic shape placed limits on the baby's head size, limiting human gestation length and resulting in an immature baby (Morgan 1990), a feature referred to as **altricial** (see Ch. 57). The gynaecoid pelvis is adapted for giving birth to a comparatively

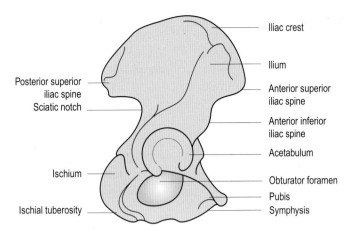

Figure 24.3 • The outer or lateral surface of the right innominate bone. (From Henderson C, Macdonald S 2004, with kind permission of Elsevier.)

large-headed baby but **mechanisms of labour** are necessary to facilitate descent of the head through the pelvis. These include passive alterations to fetal position and moulding of the fetal skull.

Pelvic bones

Although diagrams and text can illustrate features of the pelvis there is no substitute for handling a life-size model. Familiarity with the shape and size of the pelvis may enable life-saving decisions to be made. During vaginal examinations relevant pelvic features must be identified in vivo.

The pelvis is made up of four irregularly shaped bones: **two innominate bones** forming the lateral and anterior walls, and the **sacrum** and **coccyx** forming the posterior wall. Each innominate bone consists of three fused bones: the **ilium, ischium** and **pubis**. These were formed as cartilage in the fetus and their ossification centres begin to fuse at puberty and is completed about age 25. The description of these bones is mirrored to the left and right of the pelvis.

The ilium

The ilium has an upper flat plate of bone and forms part of the **acetabulum** below (Figs 24.3, 24.4). The external part of the plate of bone is curved and has a roughened surface for attachment of the **gluteal muscles** which form the buttocks. The inner surface forms the **iliac fossa** which is smooth and concave. The **iliacus muscle**, which forms a platform on which the abdominal organs rest, originates from this surface. The upper ridge of the ilium is called the **iliac crest** and is S-shaped. The muscles of the abdominal wall have attachments to this surface.

At the anterior end of the iliac crest is the **anterior superior iliac spine**, which can be identified under the skin. At the posterior end is the **posterior superior iliac spine**, marked externally by a dimple at the level of the

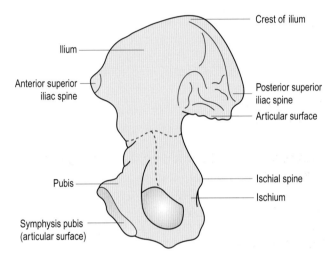

Figure 24.4 • The inner or medial surface of the right innominate bone. (From Henderson C, Macdonald S 2004, with kind permission of Elsevier.)

second sacral vertebra. Two **inferior iliac spines**, anterior and posterior, can be found below the superior spines. The lower margin of the ilium forms two-fifths of the acetabulum where it fuses with the ischium and pubis. Behind the acetabulum the ilium forms the **greater sciatic notch**, through which nerves from the sacral plexus pass. Above the greater sciatic notch is the area of the ilium which articulates with the sacrum at the **sacroiliac joint**.

The ischium

The ischium forms the lowest aspect of the innominate bone. The upper part forms two-fifths of the acetabulum, where it fuses with the ilium and pubis. Below the acetabulum, a thick buttress of bone called the **ischial tuberosity** takes the weight of the seated body. The **hamstring muscles** of the thigh arise from this bone. Passing upwards and inwards from the ischial tuberosity, a shaft of ischium meets the **inferior ramus of the pubic bone** to form the **pubic arch**.

The ischium also forms the lower border of the **obturator foramen**, a large opening in the lower part of the innominate bone below the acetabulum. On its internal surface, protruding from its posterior edge and about 5 cm above the tuberosity is the **ischial spine**, an important landmark to be found on virginal examination. The ischial spine separates the **greater sciatic notch** from the **lesser sciatic notch**.

The pubis

This square-shaped bone forms the anterior aspect of the innominate bone. The two pubic bones articulate medially to form a joint called the **symphysis pubis**. Laterally, the **superior ramus of the pubic bone** forms one-fifth of the acetabulum. The superior ramus also forms the upper boundary of the obturator foramen. The inferior ramus passes downwards and outwards to join the ischium and form the pubic arch. The upper surface of the pubis forms the **pubic crest** ending laterally in the **pubic tubercle**.

The sacrum

The sacrum is a shield-shaped mass of bone formed from five fused sacral vertebrae (Fig. 24.5). It articulates with the two innominate bones at the sacroiliac joints. The anterior surface is smooth and concave, both from above downwards and from side to side, forming the **hollow of the sacrum**. The first sacral vertebra overhangs the sacral hollow and the central point of this projection is called the **sacral promontory**. Through the centre of the bone, sacral and coccygeal nerves pass in the **sacral canal**.

Four pairs of **foramina** (openings) are present anteriorly between the five fused sacral vertebrae where sacral nerves exit to form the **sacral plexus**. Posteriorly, posterior branches of the sacral nerves pass through eight small foramina to supply the skin of the buttocks and the muscles of the lower back. On its upper surface a smooth oval area forms an articular surface for the fifth lumbar vertebra to form the **lumbosacral joint**. Lateral masses of bone on either side of the sacrum are called the **wings of the sacrum** or **sacral alae**.

The coccyx

This small triangular bone with its base uppermost is made of four fused coccygeal vertebrae. The first coccygeal vertebra articulates with the lower end of the sacrum to form the sacrococcygeal joint. The rudimentary vertebrae forming the rest of the coccyx are smooth on their inner surface and support the rectum. The external anal sphincter is attached to the lowest point.

Pelvic joints

There are four pelvic joints: one symphysis pubis, two sacroiliac and one sacrococcygeal joint:

- The **symphysis pubis** consists of an oval disc of fibrocartilage about 4 cm long lying between the two pubic bones. The joint is reinforced by ligaments crossing from one pubic bone to the other.
- The **sacroiliac joints** are synovial joints with a cavity filled with synovial fluid, a capsule formed of synovial membrane and tough external supporting ligaments. There are very strong posterior ligaments which transmit the weight of the trunk, head and arms to the legs. Movement of these joints is slight but increases in range during pregnancy when relaxin softens the ligaments.
- The **sacrococcygeal joint** lies between the sacrum and coccyx. There is sometimes a small synovial joint cavity present. Slight movement can occur backwards and this is increased greatly when the baby's head passes through the pelvis in labour.

Pelvic ligaments

Besides the ligaments supporting the pelvic joints, there are three other pairs of ligaments:

- The **sacrotuberous ligament** crosses from the posterior superior iliac spine and the lateral borders of the sacrum and coccyx to the ischial tuberosity. It bridges the greater and lesser sciatic notches.
- The **sacrospinous ligament** passes in front of the sacrotuberous ligament from the side of the sacrum and coccyx, crosses the greater sciatic notch and attaches to the ischial spine.
- The **inguinal ligament** (Poupart's ligament) runs from the anterior superior iliac spine to the pubic tubercle and forms the groin.

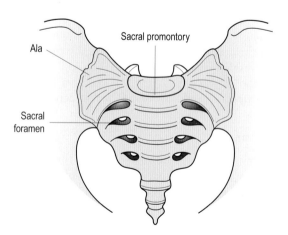

Ala

Sacral promontory

Sacral foramen

Figure 24.5 • The sacrum. (From Henderson C, Macdonald S 2004, with kind permission of Elsevier.)

Regions of the pelvis

There is a clear line of bone called the **pelvic brim** separating the upper flare of the iliac fossae which is the **false pelvis** from the basin-shaped part of the pelvis which is the **true pelvis**. The true pelvis has a cavity and outlet through which the fetus passes during birth.

The pelvic brim

Landmarks are identifiable on the pelvic brim (inlet) and important measurements are made between them. In the normal **gynaecoid (female) pelvis** the brim is oval in shape with the anteroposterior diameter reduced by the sacral promontory. Starting at the centre of the sacral promontory and tracing the brim round to the symphysis pubis, the landmarks are (Fig. 24.6):

- The sacral promontory.
- The sacral ala.
- The upper border of the sacroiliac joint.
- The ileopectineal line.
- The ileopectineal eminence.
- The inner upper border of the superior pubic ramus.
- The inner upper border of the body of the pubis.
- The inner upper border of the symphysis pubis.

If a piece of paper is placed across the landmarks, an imaginary flat surface is formed. This is called a **plane** and the concept is also applied to the cavity and outlet. The **pelvic diameters** are measured from landmarks across the planes.

The pelvic cavity

The cavity is that part of the pelvis between the brim and the outlet. It is a **curved canal** with a short anterior surface measuring 4.5 cm, formed by the inner aspect of the pubic bones and symphysis pubis and a longer posterior surface measuring 12 cm formed by the hollow of the sacrum. The lateral walls are formed from the greater sciatic notch, the inner surface of part of the ilium, the body of the ischium and the obturator foramen. The plane of the pelvic cavity is taken from the midpoint of the symphysis pubis anteriorly to the junction of the second and third sacral vertebrae posteriorly.

The pelvic outlet

Two pelvic outlets, the **anatomical** and the **obstetric outlets**, may be described. The anatomical outlet is traced from the lower border of the symphysis pubis along the pubic arch to the inner border of the ischial tuberosity and along the sacrotuberous ligament to the tip of the coccyx. It is of no value in labour as it is not a flat surface, just the lower border of the pelvis. It varies in size during labour because of the range of backwards tilting of the coccyx in different women. The obstetric outlet, which is the constricted lower portion of the true pelvis, is a more useful landmark and its structures are:

- The lower border of the symphysis pubis.
- A line passing along the pubis, obturator foramen and ischium to the ischial spine.
- The sacrospinous ligament.
- The lower border of the sacrum.

The plane of the outlet is an imaginary flat surface between these structures which is occupied by the muscles of the pelvic floor (Ch. 25).

Pelvic dimensions (diameters)

Measurements are taken of the planes of the brim, cavity and outlet, using the landmarks described above, in three directions: anteroposterior, oblique and transverse.

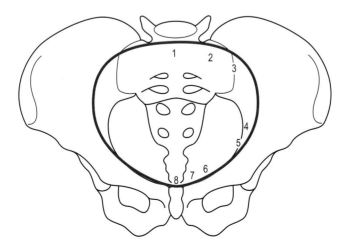

Figure 24.6 • The pelvic brim. 1, sacral promontory; 2, sacral ala; 3, sacroiliac joint; 4, ileopectineal line; 5, ileopectineal eminence; 6, superior pubic ramus; 7, body of pubic bone; 8, symphysis pubis. (From Henderson C, Macdonald S 2004, with kind permission of Elsevier.)

Table 24.1 gives the average measurements for a gynaecoid pelvis.

The brim

- The smallest diameter of the brim is the **anteroposterior diameter** which is measured from the upper part of the symphysis pubis to the sacral promontory. This is the **anatomical conjugate** which measures 12 cm. However, this is not available for accommodating the fetal head. If the measurement is taken from the inner border of the symphysis pubis to the sacral promontory the measurement is 11 cm; this is the **obstetric conjugate**. Both of these two measurements can be referred to as the **true conjugate**. The **diagonal conjugate**, measured during pelvic assessment, is taken from the lower border of the symphysis pubis to the sacral promontory and measures 13 cm. It is normally difficult to measure because its length exceeds the reach of most people. If the sacral promontory is reached, the obstetric conjugate is calculated by subtracting 2 cm.
- The two **oblique diameters** are taken from one sacroiliac joint to the opposite ileopectineal eminence. They are right and left after the corresponding sacroiliac joint. All the oblique diameters of the pelvis are 12 cm.
- The **transverse diameter** is taken between points on the ileopectineal lines that are further apart and measures 13 cm. The descending colon passes the left sacroiliac joint and may limit the space available for passage of the fetus.
- The **sacrocotyloid diameter** is a brim measurement taken from the sacral promontory to the ileopectineal eminence. It measures 9.5 cm and in an occipitoposterior presentation the fetal parietal eminences may become caught in this diameter, causing the head to extend.

The cavity

- The cavity is considered to be circular in diameter and the measurements taken through its plane are 12 cm.

The obstetric outlet

- The outlet is diamond-shaped with its longer diameter being anteroposterior. This is measured from the lower border of the symphysis pubis to the sacrococcygeal joint and is 13 cm.
- The oblique diameter has no fixed points but is between the obturator foramen and the opposite sacrospinous ligament. It is 12 cm.
- The transverse diameter is measured between the two ischial spines and is 11 cm.

Pelvic inclination

When a person stands up the pelvic basin is tilted with the plane of the brim forming an angle of 60° to the horizontal. If the reader stands facing and pressed up against a vertical surface, the two points touching that vertical surface are the pubic bones and the anterior superior iliac spines. The plane of the cavity forms an angle of 30° and that of the outlet 15° (Fig. 24.7).

Three other angles are important indicators of pelvic size all of which should measure at least 90°:

1. The subpubic angle of the pubic arch.
2. The sacral angle lying between the plane of the brim and the anterior surface of the first sacral vertebra.
3. The greater sciatic notch.

Axes of the pelvic canal

If imaginary lines are drawn at right-angles through the pelvic planes, axes can be created. If these lines are joined together a curve called the **curve of Carus** can be traced because each plane is at a different angle to the horizon. This unique feature of the human pelvis is the price paid for an upright posture as it makes delivery of the

Table 24.1 Pelvic measurements (gynaecoid pelvis)			
	Anteroposterior	**Oblique**	**Transverse**
Brim	11 cm	12 cm	13 cm
Cavity	12 cm	12 cm	12 cm
Outlet	13 cm	12 cm	11 cm

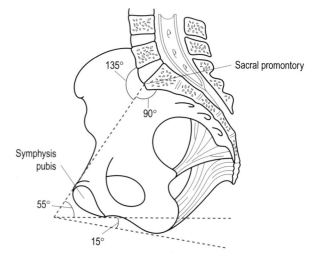

Figure 24.7 • The pelvis, showing the degrees of inclination. Inclination of the pelvic brim to the horizontal, 55°; inclination of the pelvic outlet to the horizontal, 15°; angle of pelvic inclination, 135°; inclination of the sacrum, 90°. (From Henderson C, Macdonald S 2004, with kind permission of Elsevier.)

fetus more difficult. Instead of an easy journey through a straight pelvic canal, the fetus must be moved passively by mechanisms to overcome the changing curves and diameters (Figs 24.8, 24.9).

Basic types of pelvis

There are four basic types of pelvis described according to the shape of the brim and other features (Fig. 24.10). These are gynaecoid, android, anthropoid and platypelloid. However, many pelves cannot be classified as easily as they contain features of different types. It is now considered that the size of the pelvis in relation to the fetus is more important than a slight abnormality of shape and there is a saying that 'the fetal head is the best pelvimeter'.

The gynaecoid pelvis

This ideal female pelvis which is associated with women of average height and shoe size 4 or over has:

- A rounded brim.
- Large forepelvis (that portion in front of the widest transverse diameter).
- A transverse diameter that bisects the anteroposterior diameter.
- Parallel side walls.
- A shallow cavity.
- Blunt ischial spines.
- A wide sciatic notch.
- A pubic angle of 90°.

The android pelvis

This pelvis has male features:

- A brim that is more heart-shaped.
- A narrow forepelvis.
- A widest transverse diameter set towards the back.
- Side walls which converge.
- A straight sacrum.

- A funnel-shaped cavity.
- Prominent ischial spines.
- Subpubic and greater sciatic notch angles of less than 90°.

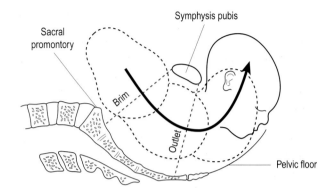

Figure 24.8 • The axis of the birth canal. (From Henderson C, Macdonald S 2004, with kind permission of Elsevier.)

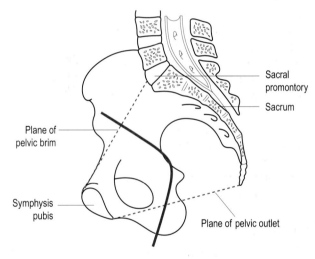

Figure 24.9 • The curve of the birth canal. (From Henderson C, Macdonald S 2004, with kind permission of Elsevier.)

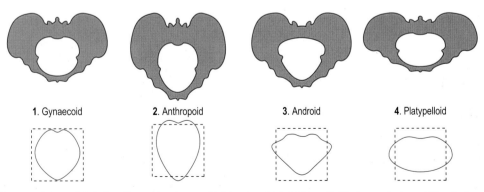

Figure 24.10 • Shapes of the pelvic brim. (From Henderson C, Macdonald S 2004, with kind permission of Elsevier.)

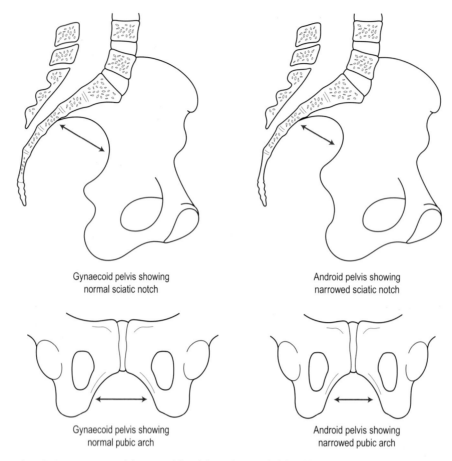

Gynaecoid pelvis showing
normal sciatic notch

Android pelvis showing
narrowed sciatic notch

Gynaecoid pelvis showing
normal pubic arch

Android pelvis showing
narrowed pubic arch

Figure 24.11 • Comparison between a normal (gynaecoid) pelvis and an android pelvis. An android pelvis has a narrower outlet because of the narrow sciatic notch and pubic arch. (From Henderson C, Macdonald S 2004, with kind permission of Elsevier.)

Women with this type of pelvis may be of short stature, heavily built and tend to be hirsute. There may be an occipitoposterior position of the fetal head at the commencement of labour and this is the least suitable pelvis for childbearing as it becomes narrower as the fetus descends (Fig. 24.11).

The anthropoid pelvis

This pelvis has an oval brim with the anteroposterior diameter greater than the transverse. This is found in other primates and anthropoid means ape-like. There is:

- Reduction in the transverse diameter but the pelvis tends to be large all over.
- The side walls diverge.
- The sacrum is long and deeply concave.
- There may be a sixth sacral vertebra present, especially in tall African women. This is called a **high assimilation pelvis**.
- The ischial spines are not prominent.

- The angle of the greater sciatic notch is wide.
- The subpubic angle may be normal or wide.

The fetus may present with the occiput anterior or posterior but the pelvis is so large that delivery occurs without rotation.

The platypelloid pelvis

This pelvis (Fig. 24.12) is flat with:

- A reduced anteroposterior diameter.
- A kidney-shaped brim.
- Side walls that diverge.
- A flat sacrum.
- A shallow cavity.
- Blunt ischial spines.
- The greater sciatic notch and subpubic angles are wide.

The fetal head may have difficulty negotiating the brim, a feature that will be discussed in the chapters on labour, but once through the brim there should be no further difficulty.

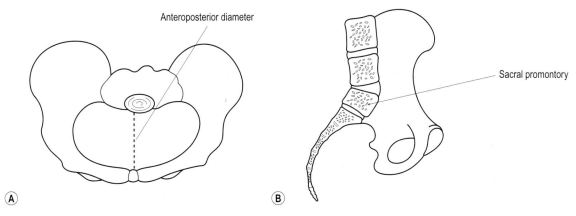

Figure 24.12 • A rachitic flat pelvis. (A) Reduced anteroposterior diameter; widened and irregular transverse diameter. (B) Sacral promontory pushed forwards and downwards; sacrum pushed backwards. (From Henderson C, Macdonald S 2004, with kind permission of Elsevier.)

Maternal physiological adaptations in pregnancy

Calcium and phosphorus metabolism in pregnancy

Calcium

Maternal calcium metabolism is altered during pregnancy to meet fetal needs for skeletal mineralisation, especially in the third trimester. Absorption and urinary excretion are increased. Maternal serum levels begin to fall shortly after fertilisation and reach their lowest at 30 weeks of pregnancy. These changes are reversible following delivery and cessation of lactation. Although bone mineral density falls during lactation, prolonged breastfeeding does not lead to permanent osteoporosis.

Fetal plasma calcium level exceeds that of the mother, suggesting that the mineral is actively transported across the placenta. Calcitonin and PTH cannot cross the placenta so the fetus must manufacture its own. The placenta can transfer vitamin D to the fetus and also synthesise vitamin D. During pregnancy maternal calcium, phosphorus and magnesium levels fall due to increased production of PTH, calcitonin and vitamin D. There may be an increase in calcium storage in preparation for lactation, but an increase in dietary calcium does not increase bone density. Any increase in bone calcium due to hPL is counterbalanced by oestrogen causing decreased reabsorption.

Diet

These changes are independent of calcium intake and supplements are unnecessary in countries where dietary intake is adequate. Supplementation may be needed in adolescents and where dietary insufficiency is suspected. The total extra calcium needed by term is about 25–30 g (Blackburn 2007). Some foods such as those containing excessive fats, phytates (found in some vegetables) and oxalates interfere with the absorption of calcium by forming calcium salts in the intestine. High sodium intake may also interfere with calcium absorption.

Vitamin D

Levels of active vitamin D (calcitriol) show a small rise by 10 weeks of pregnancy although staying within normal limits. They rise above normal in the last few weeks. However, there is little elevation in either intact PTH or calcitonin levels. Intestinal absorption of vitamin D is enhanced throughout pregnancy.

Diet

An increased intake of vitamin D is needed to ensure maternal and fetal needs for calcium are met and 400 IU/day is advised. Supplementation is advisable if dietary intake is poor or there is poor exposure to sunlight. Milk is an excellent source of calcium, phosphorus and vitamin D. Women who cannot drink milk should take cheese, yoghurt, sardines, whole grain foods or green leafy vegetables.

Phosphorus and magnesium

Serum inorganic phosphate and magnesium levels fall slightly until 30 weeks and return to non-pregnant levels by term. These changes are related to haemodilution.

Diet

Although phosphorus is essential during pregnancy, high intake levels limit calcium absorption while high plasma levels increase urinary excretion of calcium. Processed meats, snack foods and cola drinks all have high phosphorus but low calcium levels.

Clinical implications

Leg cramps

Pregnant women may suffer from intense, sudden cramping pain in the calf muscles, especially during the third trimester. These tend to occur in bed. Lowered serum ionised calcium and increased phosphates are thought to be responsible for the muscle spasm. Respiratory alkalosis may precipitate muscle spasm. Thrombophlebitis causing calf pain must be ruled out. Cramps may be prevented by reducing milk and processed food intake and performing stretching exercises before retiring. Jimenez (1994) suggested that taking calcium salts that are phosphate-free or taking the antacid aluminium hydroxide may prevent phosphorus absorption and correct the balance.

Restless leg syndrome

This disorder is seen in about 10–15% of pregnant women and usually occurs about 15 min after going to bed. There is a burning, twitching feeling in the lower leg and the more the wish to fidget is resisted, the worse the sensation becomes. The cause is unknown. Iron and folic acid deficiency have been implicated and replacement therapy has helped. Circulatory problems may be involved. Walking about and applying a cold compress help.

Backache in pregnancy

About 50% of pregnant women experience backache and it is more likely to be reported in very young women, women reporting back pain before pregnancy and multiparous women. Postural changes, overstretched abdominal muscles, strained back muscles and the effect of relaxin on the pelvic ligaments may contribute to backache. Other problems such as urinary tract infection should be ruled out before offering advice. Occasionally the woman may be in labour. More rarely, demineralisation of bone may cause back and hip pain (Davis 1996).

Relaxin

Relaxin is a small peptide which probably acts as a growth hormone affecting collagen. It appears to be a potent stimulator of uterine growth in pregnancy and is involved in the softening and effacement of the cervix and in the onset of labour. During pregnancy it helps to restrain uterine muscle contractibility.

With progesterone, relaxin causes relaxation of the ligaments and muscles, reaching its maximum effect in the last few weeks of pregnancy. Relaxation of the symphysis pubis and sacroiliac joints leads to instability of the pelvic girdle and relaxation of the sacrococcygeal joint allows extra backwards movement. These changes increase the pelvic diameters to facilitate birth. Some women develop a rolling gait and, as the developing weight and position of the uterus change the centre of gravity, the woman leans backwards to compensate, exaggerating the normal lumbar curve which leads to backache. Assessment of backache includes:

- Location and extent of pain.
- Onset and duration of pain.
- Nature and degree of pain.
- Any other symptoms.
- Relationship to activities.
- Self-treatment strategies.

In the absence of serious pathology localised heat or massage may help. The woman should rest and take analgesics. A supporting elasticated sacroiliac belt may help and a maternity girdle will support the uterus and relieve strain. Early advice on posture with exercise to strengthen the back muscles may be preventative. Shoes should have a heel of no more than 0.5–1.0 inch.

Rickets and osteomalacia

Malabsorption of calcium is caused by a deficiency in vitamin D due to a low intake. This is sometimes combined with low exposure to sunlight. The bones are poorly ossified and soft and become deformed. In childhood the condition is called **rickets** and in adults **osteomalacia**. Distortion of the pelvis may occur, leading to severe problems in childbirth, possibly requiring caesarean section. Low bone density is still more common in young South Asian women due to **hypovitaminosis D** (low vitamin D) (Roy et al 2007).

Spinal cord injury

Paraplegic or quadriplegic women can have a successful outcome to their pregnancy. Although there are dangers of urinary tract infections, constipation and pressure sores, these can be avoided. Uterine contractions in labour are mainly independent of neurological control and labour should progress normally. Pain may be perceived if the spinal lesion is below T10. Delivery of the baby may need to be assisted if the control of muscles used in active expulsion is lost.

The fetal skull

The shape and size of the human pelvis creates difficulties in the birthing process not found in other primates. This is further compounded by the large size of the fetal brain. At birth babies weigh about 3300 g of which 335 g is brain. The brain continues to grow at fetal rates for the next 20 months to reach 1000 g. Brain growth then slows down to reach adult size of 1400 g by age 8 years. A newborn gorilla weighs 2000 g of which only 225 g is brain, already half the adult size of 450 g after a gestation only 6 days shorter than the human pregnancy (Morgan 1994). Gorillas have very easy births! In humans evolutionary changes have developed to facilitate delivery:

- Birth when the fetus is very immature.
- Rapid brain growth after delivery.
- Flexion of the fetal head on its neck so that the narrowest diameters pass through the pelvis.
- Moulding of the skull bones to change the shape from ovoid to cylindrical.

Anatomy of the skull

The fetal skull is ovoid in shape and the bones can be divided into the vault, the face and the base. The vault extends from the orbital ridges to the base of the occiput and contains the brain which rests on the base of the skull. For the purposes of measurement and to describe the degree of flexion and extension in the different presentations, the fetal skull is divided into regions of face, brow, vertex and occiput (Fig. 24.13).

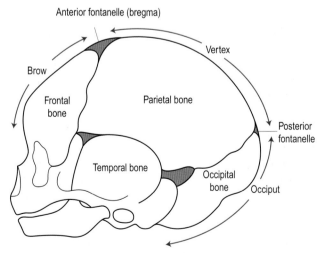

Figure 24.13 • The bones, fontanelles and regions of the fetal skull. (From Henderson C, Macdonald S 2004, with kind permission of Elsevier.)

- The **face** extends from the chin to the orbital ridges.
- The **brow** or **sinciput** is the area of the two frontal bones, extending from the orbital ridges to the anterior fontanelle.
- The **vertex** is bounded by the anterior fontanelle, the posterior fontanelle and the two parietal eminences.
- The **occiput** is the area over the occipital bone, extending from the posterior fontanelle to the nape of the neck.

The face and base of the skull are laid down in cartilage and are almost completely ossified by birth. The vault is composed of flat bones which develop from membrane. **Ossification centres** within the membrane lay down bone around them.

Bones: the vault

Five main bones make up the vault with two others helping to form the lateral walls – the squamous (flattened) portion of the temporal bones. Each bone is named for the portion of the brain lying beneath it:

- Two frontal bones whose ossification centres are indicated by the frontal bosses.
- Two parietal bones whose ossification centres are indicated by the parietal eminences.
- Two squamous portions of the temporal bones.
- One occipital bone whose ossification centre is indicated by the occipital protuberance.

Ossification is incomplete at birth and membranous sutures remain between the bones and membranous fontanelles where two or more sutures meet. These membranous areas facilitate moulding of the fetal skull during birth. They also provide landmarks that can be identified during vaginal examination (Fig. 24.14).

The sutures

- The **frontal** suture lies between the two frontal bones.
- The **sagittal** suture runs from the anterior to the posterior fontanelle, uniting the two parietal bones.
- The **lambdoidal** suture (it resembles the Greek letter lambda—λ) lies between the posterior edges of the parietal bones and the occipital bone.
- The **coronal** suture separates the posterior edges of the two frontal bones from the anterior edges of the two parietal bones.

The fontanelles

There are two main fontanelles:

- The **anterior** fontanelle or **bregma** is diamond-shaped and formed at the junction of four sutures: the frontal,

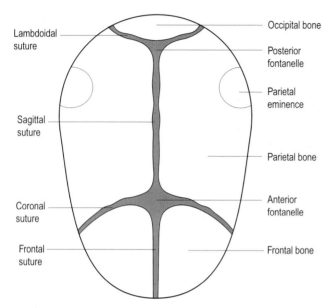

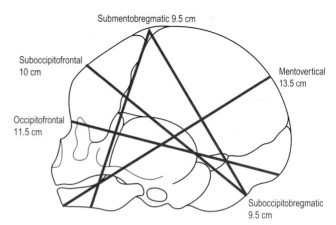

Figure 24.14 ● The fetal skull, showing the bones, fontanelles and sutures. (From Henderson C, Macdonald S 2004, with kind permission of Elsevier.)

Figure 24.15 ● The diameters of the fetal skull. (From Henderson C, Macdonald S 2004, with kind permission of Elsevier.)

parietal and two halves of the coronal sutures. It measures 2.5 cm across by 3 cm long and is not fully closed by ossification until 18 months of age.

- The **posterior** fontanelle or **lambda** is much smaller and triangular in shape and formed at the junction of three sutures: the sagittal suture and the two halves of the lambdoidal suture. It closes by the 6th week after birth.

Besides these two non-significant fontanelles there are four minor fontanelles on the side walls of the vault. There are two temporal fontanelles at the ends of the coronal suture and two mastoid fontanelles at the ends of the lambdoidal suture. These are not of any significance in childbearing.

Bones: the base

The fused bones of the base of the skull are perforated by the foramen magnum which allows passage of the spinal cord leading from the brain.

Diameters of the fetal skull

Measurements of the skull are used to assess its size in relation to the maternal pelvis. Longitudinal diameters are taken between key landmarks so that the diameters presenting at the pelvis in different degrees of flexion or extension can be estimated (Figs 24.15, 24.16):

1. **Suboccipitobregmatic** is measured from the nape of the neck to the centre of the anterior fontanelle. It is 9.5 cm and presents when the head is fully flexed.

2. **Suboccipitofrontal** is measured from the nape of the neck to the centre of the frontal suture. It is 10 cm and presents when the head is almost completely flexed.

3. **Occipitofrontal** is measured from the glabella (bridge of the nose) to the occipital protuberance. It is 11.5 cm and presents when the head is deflexed as in an occipitoposterior position.

4. **Mentovertical** is measured from the point of the chin to the highest point on the vertex. It is 13.5 cm and presents when the head is midway between flexion and extension in a brow presentation.

5. **Submentovertical** is measured from the junction of the chin with the neck to the highest point on the vertex. It is 11.5 cm and presents when the head is not fully extended in a face presentation.

6. **Submentobregmatic** is measured from the junction of the chin with the neck to the midpoint of the anterior fontanelle. It is 9.5 cm and presents when the head is fully extended in a face presentation.

Transverse diameters are also taken:

1. The **biparietal** is measured between the parietal eminences. It is 9.5 cm and is the widest transverse diameter.

2. The **bitemporal** is measured between the widest aspects of the coronal suture. It is 8 cm.

Circumferences of the skull are:

- **Suboccipitobregmatic**: 33 cm presents when the head is well flexed. The head engages, fits well onto the cervix and labour should progress easily.

- **Occipitofrontal**: 35 cm presents when the head is deflexed. Engagement is delayed, the membranes may rupture early and labour may be difficult.

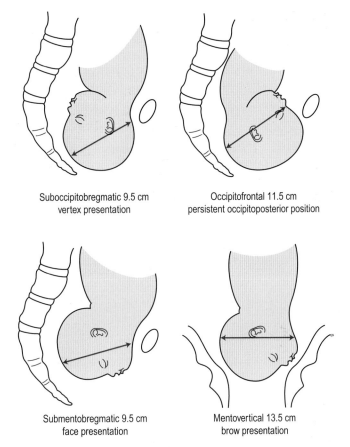

Suboccipitobregmatic 9.5 cm
vertex presentation

Occipitofrontal 11.5 cm
persistent occipitoposterior position

Submentobregmatic 9.5 cm
face presentation

Mentovertical 13.5 cm
brow presentation

Figure 24.16 • The diameters of the fetal skull in relation to the maternal pelvis. (From Henderson C, Macdonald S 2004, with kind permission of Elsevier.)

Table 24.2 Involvement of diameters of the fetal skull in moulding

Presentation	Diameters increased	Diameter decreased
Vertex	Suboccipitobregmatic Biparietal	Mentovertical
Brow	Mentovertical Biparietal	Suboccipitobregmatic
Face	Submentobregmatic Biparietal	Occipitofrontal
Occipitoposterior	Occipitofrontal Biparietal	Submentobregmatic

- **Mentovertical**: 39 cm presents when the head is midway between flexion and extension. The head cannot descend into the pelvis unless it completes extension and labour is obstructed.

Moulding

Moulding of the fetal skull results in a change in shape but not size of the vault brought about by the pressures of the pelvis and pelvic floor during labour. The diameters which are compressed reduce in size by at least 0.5 cm while those at right-angles to them are elongated (Table 24.2). Vertex and brow presentations affect the same diameters but in opposite ways as do face presentation and occipitoposterior position. The sutures and fontanelles allow overlap of the bones in a typical way:

- The frontal bones are pushed under the anterior edge of the parietal bones.
- The occipital bone is pushed under the posterior part of the parietal bones.
- The medial edge of the leading parietal bone is pushed under the other parietal bone.

Moulding is abnormal if it involves wrong diameters (Fig. 24.17), if it is too rapid or too extreme so that the brain is compressed, all with a risk of intracranial damage.

Caput succedaneum

During labour, especially after rupture of the membranes, the fetal head is pressed against the ring of the dilating cervix. In cephalic presentations venous return of the scalp circulation is impeded and oedema forms in the loose tissues. This is a **caput succedaneum** and varies in size with the length and difficulty of the delivery (Fig. 24.18). Caput forms on the leading parietal bone which is the left one when the occiput is to the right and vice versa.

It forms on the anterior part if the position is occipitoanterior and posteriorly if the position is occipitoposterior.

External features of the fetal skull

The fetal scalp consists of five layers. From the inside out these are:

1. The **pericranium** which covers the outer surface of the bones and is firmly attached to the edges of the bones. Bleeding may occur between the bone and the pericranium to form a swelling called a **cephalhaematoma**. The size of the haematoma is limited by the attachment of the pericranium to that of the bone over which it forms.

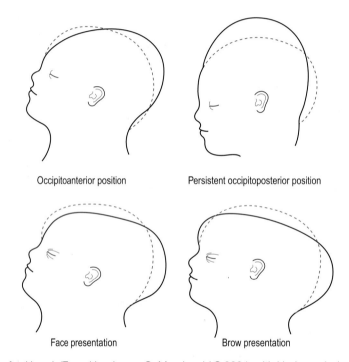

Occipitoanterior position

Persistent occipitoposterior position

Face presentation

Brow presentation

Figure 24.17 • Moulding of the fetal head. (From Henderson C, Macdonald S 2004, with kind permission of Elsevier.)

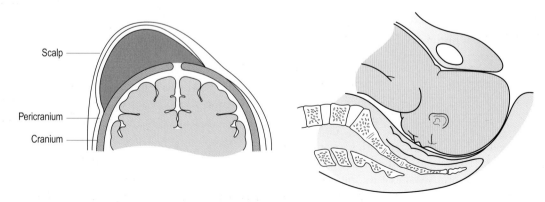

Scalp

Pericranium

Cranium

Figure 24.18 • Caput succedaneum. (From Henderson C, Macdonald S 2004, with kind permission of Elsevier.)

2. A loose layer of **areolar tissue** that permits limited movement of the scalp over the skull.

3. A layer of **tendon** known as the **galea** that is attached to the frontalis muscle anteriorly and the occipitalis muscle posteriorly.

4. A layer of **subcutaneous tis**sue containing blood vessels and hair follicles. This is the part of the scalp affected by the caput succedaneum (see Fig. 24.18).

5. The **skin**.

Internal structures of the fetal skull

The meninges

The brain is surrounded by three membranes; from the inside out these are:

1. The **pia mater** is very delicate and has many tiny blood vessels. It is closely applied to the surface of the brain.

2. The **arachnoid mater** forms a loose brain covering and is attached to the pia mater by thread-like extensions which cross the subarachnoid space which contains the cerebrospinal fluid. Knob-like extensions of the arachnoid are called **arachnoid villi** and protrude into the dura mater into the dual sinuses which carry venous blood.

3. The outer, tough **dura mater** which is a double-layered membrane lines the skull with its periosteal layer and is reflected back onto the surface of the brain as the meningeal layer. In places the dura extends inwards to form septa that anchor the brain to the skull and limit movement.

Sinuses and venous drainage

There are two main folds of the dura mater. The **falx cerebri** is a double fold forming a partition between the two cerebral hemispheres. It is attached to the skull following the line of the frontal and sagittal sutures from the root of the nose to the internal aspect of the occipital protuberance. Its lower edge is unattached and sickle-shaped.

The **tentorium cerebelli** lies horizontally, separating the cerebrum from the cerebellum. It is at right-angles to the falx cerebri and is horseshoe-shaped. Each side of the horseshoe is attached laterally to the sphenoid bone and along the inner surface of the petrous portion of the temporal bone. It meets the falx at the inner aspect of the occipital protuberance. The brainstem passes in front of this junction of the two folds of dura mater.

Venous drainage is by channels in the dural folds called sinuses (Fig. 24.19):

1. The **superior longitudinal sinus** (sagittal) runs along the upper border of the falx cerebri.

2. The **inferior longitudinal sinus** (sagittal) runs along the lower border of the falx cerebri.

3. The **straight sinus** is a continuation of the inferior longitudinal sinus which runs posteriorly to join the superior longitudinal sinus.

4. The **great vein of Galen** joins the straight sinus at the junction with the inferior longitudinal sinus.

5. From the confluence of sinuses, the **lateral sinuses** pass along the line of attachment of the tentorium cerebelli and emerge from the skull to become the internal **jugular veins** of the neck.

When moulding is abnormal these membranes and sinuses may be torn, especially at the junction of the two folds of dura. The tentorium is most likely to be damaged and bleeding involves the great vein of Galen, the straight sinus and the inferior longitudinal sinus.

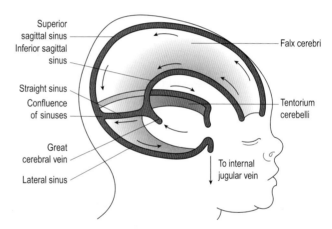

Figure 24.19 • Internal structures of the fetal skull. (From Henderson C, Macdonald S 2004, with kind permission of Elsevier.)

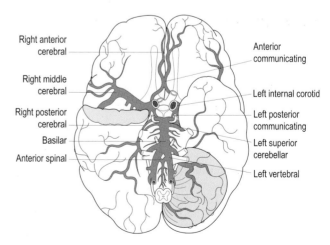

Figure 24.20 • Arterial blood supply to the brain including the circle of Willis.

Blood supply to the brain

The arterial blood supply is by two **internal carotid arteries** and **two vertebral arteries**. The internal carotid arteries give off pairs of **anterior, middle** and **posterior cerebral arteries**. Each vertebral artery gives off a branch which supplies the **cerebellum** and **medulla oblongata** before uniting with its partner to form the **basilar artery**. The basilar artery gives off two pairs of arteries to the cerebellum and upper brainstem before dividing into two terminal branches that link up with the ends of the internal carotid arteries. In 25% of people three cerebral arteries remain on both sides of the brain but in the majority of people the vertebral arteries take over from the posterior cerebral arteries. The intercommunicating arteries at the base of the brain are called the circle of Willis (Fig. 24.20).

Main points

- Bone is a connective tissue consisting of an organic matrix called osteoid, a mineral matrix of calcium and phosphorus and bone cells. Bone can be divided into compact bone and spongy bone.

- Most bones have a tough outer periosteum and a cavity lining of endosteum. Endosteum contains osteoblasts, osteoclasts and their precursor cells. Osteoblasts synthesise bone and promote mineralisation of the cortex. Osteoclasts contain enzymes that remove both organic and mineral matrix.

- The skeleton contains 99% of the calcium and 85% of the phosphorus present in the body. Three hormones control calcium and phosphorus metabolism: parathyroid hormone, vitamin D and calcitonin.

- The pelvic girdle provides attachment for the lower limbs and support for the abdominal organs. The shape, size and rigidity of the pelvic girdle and the curved spine are related to bipedal locomotion and maintaining an upright posture.

- The pelvis is made up of two innominate bones, one sacrum and one coccyx. Each innominate bone consists of three fused bones: the ilium, ischium and pubis.

- The four pelvic joints are the symphysis pubis, two sacroiliac joints and the sacrococcygeal joint. Ligaments support each joint and three other pairs are present: the sacrotuberous, sacrospinous and inguinal ligaments.

- The pelvic brim separates the upper flare of the iliac fossae known as the false pelvis above the brim from the basin-shaped true pelvis below the brim. The true pelvis forms the birth canal.

- Measurements are taken of the planes of the pelvic brim, cavity and outlet in three directions: anteroposterior, oblique and transverse.

- In the upright posture the pelvic basin is tilted in relation to the horizontal. Imaginary lines drawn at right-angles to the pelvic planes and joined together form the curve of Carus through which the fetus passes during birth. There are four basic pelvic types: gynaecoid, android, anthropoid and platypelloid.

- Maternal calcium metabolism alters to meet fetal needs for calcium and phosphorus for skeletal mineralisation. Serum calcium begins to fall soon after fertilisation and reaches its lowest level at about 39 weeks of pregnancy. Serum inorganic phosphate and magnesium levels fall slightly until 30 weeks and return to non-pregnant levels by term.

- Adequate calcium, phosphorus and vitamin D are essential in pregnancy. Foods which contain phytates and oxalates interfere with calcium absorption.

- Pregnancy problems related to calcium include leg cramps, restless leg syndrome and backache. Serious problems include rickets, osteomalacia and spinal cord injury.

- The bones of the fetal skull are divided into vault, face and base. The face and base are laid down in cartilage and are almost completely ossified by term. The vault is composed of flat bones which develop from membranes.

- The fetal skull is divided into regions of face, brow, vertex and occiput. Measurements of the skull are used to assess its size in relation to the maternal pelvis.

- Vault ossification is incomplete at birth so that membranous sutures and fontanelles remain between the bones. This allows the change in shape but not size, called moulding, to occur. Moulding is abnormal if it involves wrong diameters, is extreme or too rapid.

- The brain is surrounded by three meninges: the pia mater, the arachnoid mater and the dura mater. The dura mater covers the outer surface of the brain and dips down to form compartments. The two main folds are the falx cerebri and the tentorium cerebelli. Venous drainage is by sinuses lying in the dural folds.

- The arterial blood supply to the brain is from two internal carotid arteries and two vertebral arteries. The internal carotid arteries give off three pairs of anterior, middle and posterior cerebral arteries. The intercommunicating arteries at the base of the brain are known as the circle of Willis.

References

Blackburn, S.T., 2007. Maternal, Fetal and Neonatal Physiology: A Clinical Perspective, third edn. Saunders, Philadelphia.

Davis, D.C., 1996. The discomforts of pregnancy. JOGNN (Journal of Obstetric, Gynecologic & Neonatal Nursing) 25 (1), 73–80.

Guyton, A.C., Hall, J.E., 2006. Textbook of Medical Physiology, eleventh edn. Elsevier Saunders, Philadelphia.

Henderson, C., Macdonald, S. (Eds.), 2004. Mayes' Midwifery: A Textbook for Midwives, thirteenth edn. Baillière Tindall, London.

Hinson, J., Raven, P., Chew, S., 2007. The Endocrine System. Elsevier Churchill Livingstone.

Jimenez, S., 1994. If you can't get comfortable. Childbirth 11 (1), 37–40.

Morgan, E., 1990. The Scars of Evolution. Penguin Books, Harmondsworth.

Morgan, E., 1994. The Descent of the Child. Souvenir Press, London.

Roy, D.K., Berry, J.L., Pye, S.R., et al., 2007. Vitamin D status and bone mass in UK South Asian women. Bone 40 (1), 200–204.

Trevathan, W.R., 1999. Evolutionary obstetrics. In: Trevathan, W.R., Smith, E. O., McKenna, J.J. (Eds.), Evolutionary Medicine. Oxford University Press, New York.

Annotated recommended reading

Hinson, J., Raven, P., Chew, S., 2007. The Endocrine System. Elsevier Churchill Livingstone.

This endocrinology textbook is presented in a straightforward, easily readable manner. The content is of adequate depth for degree students but the text ensures that those with no previous knowledge can understand the principles.

Morgan, E., 1994. The Descent of the Child. Souvenir Press, London.

This book is written by a specialist in human evolution. She discusses why our babies are so small and helpless at birth compared with other species. There are also insights into family relationships.

Prentice, A., 2000. Maternal calcium metabolism and bone mineral status. Am. J. Clin. Nutr. 71 (Suppl), 13112S–13126S.

Prentice has collated what is currently known about calcium in pregnancy and lactation in a succinct manner. Although detailed, it is well set out and highly readable at the right level for midwifery students.

Roy, D.K., Berry, J.L., Pye, S.R., et al., 2007. Vitamin D status and bone mass in UK South Asian women. Bone 40 (1), 200–204.

This is a slightly technical paper but important in its discussion of an on-going medical phenomenon within a population in the UK.

Chapter Twenty-Five

25

Muscle—the pelvic floor and the uterus

Introduction

Muscle makes up almost half of the body's mass and is specialised tissue which generates forces and enables movement to occur. It has the ability to transform the chemical energy in adenosine triphosphate (ATP) into mechanical energy. This chapter will describe the nature of muscles and, for the purpose of this text, only the individual muscles of the pelvic floor and uterus will be described in detail.

Three basic muscle types can be identified on the basis of structure, contractile properties and control mechanisms: skeletal muscle, smooth muscle and cardiac muscle. Most skeletal muscle is attached to bone and is responsible for supporting and moving the skeleton. Smooth muscle is found in the walls of the hollow viscera of the gastrointestinal, genitourinary and respiratory tracts and the specialised cardiac muscle propels blood through the circulation. Although there are significant differences in these types of muscle, the force-generating mechanism is similar in all of them.

All muscle cells are elongated and therefore referred to as fibres and they all contain two kinds of protein filaments: **actin** and **myosin**. Muscles have **four functions**: they produce movement, maintain posture, stabilise joints and generate heat (Marieb & Hoehn 2008). They have **four properties**: excitability, which is the ability to receive and respond to a stimulus; contractility, or the ability to shorten when stimulated; extensibility, or the ability to be stretched or extended beyond its resting length; and elasticity, or the ability of muscle to recoil back to its resting length.

Skeletal muscle

Skeletal muscles, as the name implies, are attached to and cover the bony skeleton. The longest muscle fibres are found in skeletal muscle. One striking feature of the fibres is obvious bands or **striations**, hence the term **striated muscle**. Another term used for skeletal muscle is **voluntary** as this is the only muscle type under voluntary control. Skeletal muscle can contract rapidly

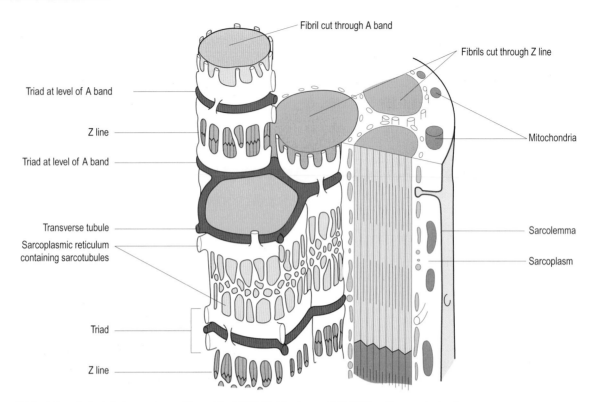

Figure 25.1 • Intracellular tubular systems. (From Hinchliff S M, Montague S E 1990, with permission.)

Labels (clockwise from top):
- Fibril cut through A band
- Fibrils cut through Z line
- Mitochondria
- Sarcolemma
- Sarcoplasm
- Z line
- Triad
- Sarcoplasmic reticulum containing sarcotubules
- Transverse tubule
- Triad at level of A band
- Z line
- Triad at level of A band

but tires easily and must be rested after short bursts of activity. Each skeletal muscle is a discrete organ made up of multiple muscle fibres. Other tissues found in the individual muscles include connective tissue, blood vessels and nerve fibres. Muscle fibres are gathered into functional units by a network of fibrous connective tissue. This connective tissue condenses into the **tendons** which form the muscular origins and insertions onto bone.

The activity of skeletal muscle depends on its rich blood supply and nerve supply. While the other muscle types can contract without nerve stimulation, each skeletal muscle fibre is supplied with a nerve ending. The blood supply is essential to deliver the large amounts of oxygen and nutrients and to remove equally large amounts of metabolic waste. The smaller blood vessels are long and winding, which permits the changes in muscle length to occur.

Microscopic anatomy of a skeletal muscle fibre

Skeletal muscle fibres are long cylindrical cells which taper at both ends. The plasma membrane is called the **sarcolemma** and there are multiple oval nuclei arranged just below the surface. Skeletal muscle fibres are huge. The fibre length is variable, ranging from a few millimetres (mm) in short muscles to lengths of 300 mm in longer muscles (1 ft in length). Their diameter ranges from 10 to 100 µm which is up to 10 times that of other body cells. The presence of multiple nuclei indicate that each muscle fibre is a **syncytium** (fusion of many cells) formed during embryonic development. The cytoplasm in muscle cells is called **sarcoplasm** and the endoplasmic reticulum is referred to as **sarcoplasmic reticulum**. The sarcoplasm contains large amounts of stored glycogen and a unique oxygen-binding protein called **myoglobin** similar to haemoglobin (Marieb & Hoehn 2008).

Myofibrils

Each muscle fibre contains a large number of rod-like **myofibrils** extending the full length of the cell and parallel to each other (Fig. 25.1). Myofibrils are densely packed and form 80% of the cellular content. Mitochondria, the energy-producing organelles, and other organelles are packed in between the myofibrils. Myofibrils are the contractile elements of the cell and each myofibril consists of smaller contractile units called **sarcomeres**. Several sarcomeres are arranged along each myofibril.

Myofibrils appear to be made of alternate dark or **A bands** and light or **I bands**, giving the characteristic striped appearance under the light microscope. The

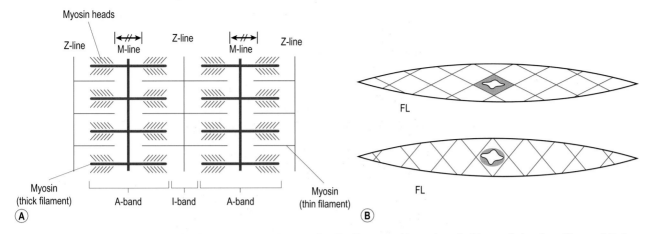

Figure 25.2 • Striated (A) and smooth (B) fibres. A, actin; M, myosin; FL, filaments. (Reproduced with permission from Huszar & Roberts 1982.)

bands are named according to how they refract (bend) polarised light (light waves with a definite direction): **A bands** (**anisotropic**) refers to their ability to refract light, depending on its angle; **I bands** (**isotropic**) refers to their ability to refract light, whatever its angle (Martini & Nath 2009).

The A band is interrupted in mid-section by the highly refractive **H zone** (**H** stands for *helle*, which means bright). Each H zone is bisected by a dark line called the **M line**. The I bands also have a midline interruption called the **Z line** (Figs 25.1, 25.2). A sarcomere is the region of a myofibril that extends from one Z line to the next. Brief explanations of these other features are as follows:

- The Z line is a network of interconnecting proteins that form a point of attachment for thin filaments.
- The H zone is only visible in relaxed muscle when the thick filaments are not overlapped by the thin filaments.
- The M line in the centre of the H zone appears darker because it is slightly thicker due to the presence of fine strands that connect adjacent thick filaments together.

The higher magnifying power of the electron microscope shows that the A bands are formed of thick **myosin** filaments (Fig. 25.3). The thin filaments are formed of three different proteins: **actin**, **troponin** and **tropomyosin**. These run the length of the I band, overlapping the thick filaments (Fig. 25.4). In an intact muscle fibre the bands are aligned horizontally across the width of the cell. Each myosin molecule has a rod-like tail (axis) and two globular heads (cross-bridges) that interact with special sites on the thin filaments. Each thick filament within a sarcomere contains about 200 myosin molecules.

The thin filaments are mainly composed of actin. Subunits called **globular** or **G actin** bear the active sites to which the **myosin cross-bridges** attach themselves

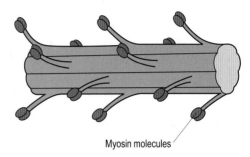

Figure 25.3 • Structure of a thick filament. (From Hinchliff S M, Montague S E 1990, with permission.)

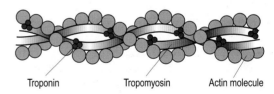

Figure 25.4 • Structure of a thin filament. (From Hinchliff S M, Montague S E 1990, with permission.)

during muscle contraction. The backbone of each actin molecule is formed by two strands of **fibrous** or **F actin** arranged in a helical structure. Regulatory proteins include tropomyosin, which spirals around the F actin to stiffen it. In resting muscle the orientation of the tropomyosin blocks the myosin-binding sites on the actin molecules. This prevents the formation of cross-bridges. Troponin actually consists of three polypeptides: one binds to actin, another to tropomyosin helping to position it on the actin, while the third binds calcium.

Intracellular tubular systems

The muscle cell is penetrated by two tubular systems (see Fig. 25.1), both ending near the A–I band junctions. One tubular system is called the **transverse** or

T system, extending from the cell exterior into the sarcoplasm where they branch and terminate. The other is the **internal system** formed by fine tubules called **sarcotubules** of the **sarcoplasmic reticulum**. These sarcotubules end in terminal sacs called the **terminal cysternae**. Both systems play a key role in muscle contraction. T tubules conduct electrical stimuli deep within the muscle cell to the sarcomeres. The sarcoplasmic reticulum regulates the calcium (Ca^{2+}) ions.

Muscle contraction

There are several theories of how muscle fibres contract but most evidence supports the **sliding filament theory**. The theory explains that during contraction the thin filaments slide past the thick ones, increasing the amount of overlap. This allows the thin filaments to penetrate more deeply into the central region of the A band. Overlapping is brought about by the crossbridges of the sarcomeres acting simultaneously as a ratchet to pull the thin filaments towards the centre of the sarcomeres. This results in shortening of the muscle cell. The myosin heads are said to 'walk up' the actin filaments step by step from one binding site to the next (Fig. 25.5). This requires the presence of calcium, which binds to the troponin to form a complex. In the absence of calcium ions, tropomyosin blocks access to the myosin-binding site of actin. When calcium binds to troponin, the positions of troponin and tropomyosin are altered on the thin filament and myosin then has access to its binding site on actin. Thus the configuration of tropomyosin is changed to move it away from the myosin-binding sites. As calcium is removed by the sarcoplasmic reticulum, the contraction comes to an end and the muscle cell relaxes.

Regulation of contraction

Skeletal muscles contract in response to nerve stimulation, which results in an **action potential** being sent along the sarcolemma. This electrical event results in a rise in intracellular calcium (Ca^{2+}) ion levels that triggers off the contraction. The axon of a **lower motor neuron** branches profusely as it enters the muscle and each mound-shaped unmyelinated axonal terminal forms a junction with a single muscle fibre, approximately in the middle of the cell. This is called a neuromuscular junction or **motor end plate** (Fig. 25.6). The plasma membrane of the axonal ending does not actually touch the muscle fibre; between them is a small fluid-filled extracellular space called the **synaptic cleft**.

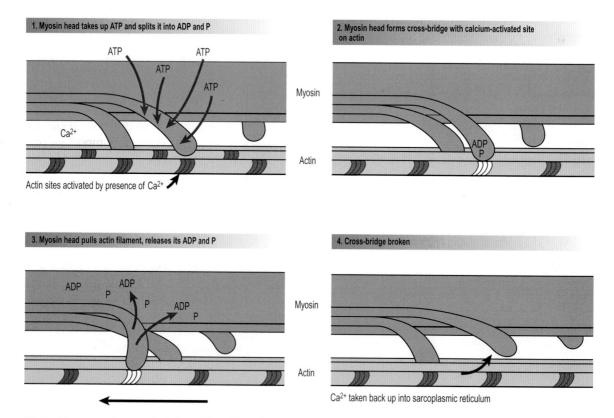

Figure 25.5 • Diagrammatic representation of the sliding-filament theory showing how the thick filaments of skeletal muscle move relative to one another as cross-bridges are formed and broken. (From Hinchliff S M, Montague S E 1990, with permission.)

The action potential must be transmitted across the space and this happens by the release of the neurotransmitter substance **acetylcholine (ACh)** from small membranous sacs in the axon terminal called **synaptic vesicles**.

When a nerve impulse reaches the end of an axon, **voltage-regulated calcium channels** open and calcium flows in from the extracellular fluid (ECF). The entry of the calcium causes some of the synaptic vesicles to fuse with the plasma membrane and release ACh into the synaptic cleft. This process is called **exocytosis**. ACh diffuses across the synaptic cleft and attaches itself to ACh receptors on the sarcolemma. All plasma membranes are polarised with a **voltage gradient** (membrane potential) across the membrane. The inside of the cell is negative. This attachment of ACh molecules opens chemically regulated ion gates. The positively charged sodium ion (Na^+) passes from its higher concentration in the ECF fluid down a gradient into the cell, leading to a slight decrease in the negative potential. This event, called **depolarisation**, allows a muscle cell action potential to be generated and to pass in all directions across the sarcolemma.

Repolarisation of the sarcolemma occurs following the wave of the muscle action potential when sodium channels close and potassium channels open. Potassium ions (K^+) rapidly diffuse out of the cell into the ECF down a gradient to restore the negativity inside the cell. The normal ionic balance of sodium and potassium is restored during the refractory period when the muscle cannot respond to stimuli. After the release of ACh and its binding to the ACh receptors, it is quickly destroyed by the enzyme **acetylcholinesterase**. This prevents the muscle contraction lasting longer than the stimulus requires.

Excitation–contraction coupling

This refers to the process whereby the generation of an action potential is followed by activation of the contractile machinery in the myofibrils. It involves the exposure of the binding sites on the actin to allow the formation of cross-bridges. Energy released from ATP is used to fuel the muscle contraction. As action potentials continue to arrive, the process is repeated many times, allowing sustained muscle contraction. Calcium ions are continuously released and taken up by troponin. This also requires energy from ATP. However, muscles store very little ATP and the supply is soon exhausted. If contraction is to continue, ATP must be regenerated (Martini & Nath 2009). This can occur in three ways:

1. By the interaction of ADP with creatine phosphate.
2. By aerobic respiration.
3. By lactic acid fermentation.

The pelvic floor

The bony pelvis provides protection to the pelvic organs while the **pelvic floor** holds them in position. The pelvic floor is primarily composed of soft tissues which fill the outlet of the pelvis. The most important of these is the strong funnel-shaped diaphragm of muscle attached to the pelvic walls. The posterior part of the diaphragm of muscles lies higher than the anterior. Through it pass the urethra, vagina and anal canal (Fig. 25.7).

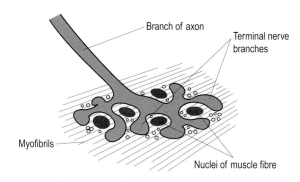

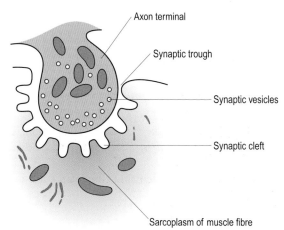

Figure 25.6 • The neuromuscular junction. (From Hinchliff S M, Montague S E 1990, with permission.)

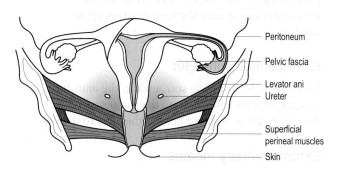

Figure 25.7 • The layers of the pelvic floor. (From Henderson C, Macdonald S 2004, with kind permission of Elsevier.)

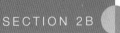
The pelvic floor consists of six layers of tissue. From the inside outwards:

1. Pelvic peritoneum.
2. Visceral layer of pelvic fascia thickened to form pelvic ligaments which support the uterus.
3. **Deep muscles** encased in fascia.
4. **Superficial muscles** encased in fascia.
5. Subcutaneous fat.
6. Skin.

Superficial muscles

These muscles lie external to the deep muscles and provide additional strength—a little like the webbing beneath the cushion on some chairs. They consist of:

- The transverse perinei.
- The bulbocavernosus.
- The ischiocavernosus.
- The external anal sphincter.
- The external urethral meatus, sometimes called the membranous sphincter of the urethra (Fig. 25.8).

The transverse perinei

One muscle arises from the inner surface of each **ischial tuberosity** of the pelvis and passes transversely to meet its fellow, inserting into the **perineal body**. Some fibres pass posteriorly to blend with the anal sphincter.

The bulbocavernosus

This arises in the centre of the perineum and fibres pass on either side of the vagina and urethra, encircling them both, to insert into the corpora cavernosa (body) of the clitoris just under the pubic arch. This muscle is responsible for erection of the clitoris and contraction of the vaginal walls.

The ischiocavernosus

A muscle runs from each ischial tuberosity along the pubic arch to the corpora cavernosa of the clitoris and fibres interweave with the membranous sphincter of the urethra.

External anal sphincter

This is a circle of muscle surrounding the anus formed by merging of muscle fibres from deep and superficial layers. The sphincter is attached behind the anus to the coccyx.

External urinary meatus

The membranous sphincter of the urethra is a weak and not too important muscle. It is composed of muscle

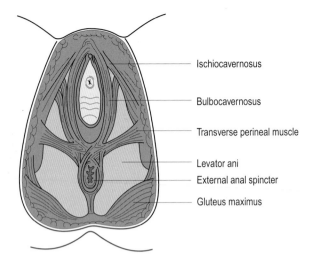

Figure 25.8 • The perineal muscles. (From Henderson C, Macdonald S 2004, with kind permission of Elsevier.)

fibres passing above and below the urethra and attached to the pubic bones. It is not a true sphincter since it is not circular, but it acts to close the urethra.

The superficial muscles do not form a continuous sheet and there are gaps filled with other tissues. Anteriorly is the **triangular ligament** bounded by the ischiocavernosus and the transverse perinei. It consists of two layers of fascia. Where the triangular ligaments stretch across the **pubic arch**, they help to support the bladder neck. Posteriorly, the gap is filled with fat and is bounded by the gluteus maximus muscle, the sacrotuberous ligament and the transverse perinei. This area is known as the **ischiorectal fossa**.

Deep pelvic floor muscles

The deep floor muscles are situated above the superficial muscles and are about 5 cm deep. Deep muscles called **levator ani** are by far the largest and most important muscles of the pelvic floor. The levator ani muscles raise or elevate the anus. They are collectively termed coccygeus muscles because they insert around the coccyx. Together with the fascia covering their surfaces, these muscles are referred to as the pelvic diaphragm. The arrangement of these muscle (pelvic diaphragm) gives the appearance of a funnel or sling suspended from its attachments on the pelvic wall (Fig. 25.9). These muscles are *vital* to the control of bladder and bowel function.

It is conventional to describe the levator ani in three pairs of deep muscles:

1. Pubococcygeus.
2. Iliococcygeus.
3. Ischiococcygeus.

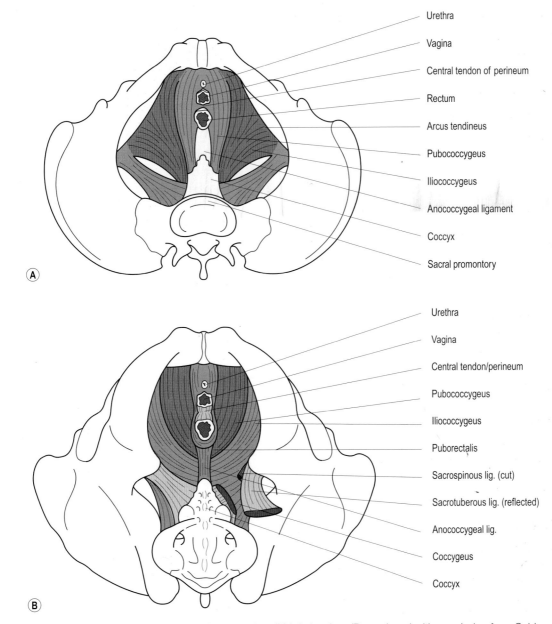

Figure 25.9 • Muscles of the pelvic diaphragm. (A) Superior view. (B) Inferior view. (Reproduced with permission from Gabbe et al 1991.)

The pubococcygeus

These are the most medial muscles. Fibres arise from the inner border of the body of the pubis and from the white line of fascia (arcus tendineus fasciae). They sweep posteriorly in three bands:

1. A central band of fibres surrounding the urethra.

2. Some fibres form a U-shaped loop around the vagina and insert into the lateral and posterior vaginal walls in the perineum.

3. Other fibres loop around the anus and insert into the lateral and posterior walls of the anal canal and the coccyx.

These muscles support and maintain the position of the pelvic viscera; resist increased intra-abdominal pressure during forced expiration, vomiting, coughing, urination and defecation; constrict the anus, urethra and vagina; and support the fetal head during childbirth. During childbirth the muscles may be injured as a result of a difficult childbirth or trauma during an episiotomy.

The iliococcygeus

These muscles arise from the inner border of the white line of fascia on the iliac bone and also from the ischial spines and run to the coccyx, some crossing over in the perineal body. They support and maintain position of the pelvic viscera; resist increased intra-abdominal pressure during forced expiration, vomiting, coughing, urination and defecation; and pull the coccyx anteriorly following defecation or childbirth. During childbirth the muscles may be injured as a result of a difficult childbirth or trauma during an episiotomy.

The ischiococcygeus

Fibres arise from each ischial spine and insert into the upper edge of the coccyx and lower border of the sacrum. These muscles help to stabilise the sacroiliac and sacrococcygeal joints of the pelvis and also flex the coccygeal joints.

Blood supply, lymphatic drainage and nerve supply

Blood supply

Arterial supply is by branches of the two internal iliac arteries and drainage is by corresponding veins.

Lymphatic drainage

Lymph drainage is widespread, both laterally and medially.

Nerve supply

The pelvic floor muscles are under voluntary control. The nerve supply is by branches of the pudendal nerve via the sacral plexus.

The **perineal body** is a wedge-shaped mass of muscular and fibrous tissue situated between the vaginal and anal canals. Both the superficial and deep pelvic floor muscles are involved in its structure. The wedge of tissue is pyramidal or triangular in shape; the apex is uppermost and is the central point of the pelvic floor. The perineal body measures approximately 4 cm in each direction.

Functions

Effective functioning is dependent on the integrity of the muscle fibres and maintenance of muscle tone. The pelvic floor has the following functions:

• Supports the weight of the abdominal and pelvic organs.
• Maintains intra-abdominal pressure.
• Allows voluntary control of defecation and micturition.
• Facilitates the movements of the fetus through the birth canal.
• Enables flexion of the sacrum and coccyx.

Clinical implications

Loss of integrity and trauma to the pelvic floor can often be associated with childbearing (Smith 2007). In the event of damage to the pelvic floor, the following reproductive anomalies may occur.

Uterovaginal prolapse

Prolapse of the pelvic organs with the possibility of urinary and faecal incontinence may cause women much anxiety, embarrassment and discomfort. Symptoms may occur with ageing due to loss of muscle tone and withdrawal of oestrogen, prolonged immobility due to muscle atrophy and congenital weakness of the muscles. However, the problems are most often related to childbearing and damage to the pelvic floor during childbirth may lead to long-term problems. This includes uterine prolapse, which is downward displacement of the uterus to varying degrees. It is now rare to see **procidentia**, which is total prolapse of the uterus outside the body.

Vaginal prolapse: anterior wall

A **cystocele** is a herniation of the bladder which may present with bladder irritation or a feeling of a lump in the vagina. This is often symptomless but, if large, may lead to collection of residual urine, infection and pyelonephritis. A **urethrocele** is a displacement of the urethra with loss of the acute angle between it and the bladder. This angle helps to maintain continence so the result may be urinary stress incontinence, which is the involuntary loss of small amounts of urine during coughing, sneezing or any other activity that increases intra-abdominal pressure.

Vaginal prolapse: posterior wall

A **rectocele** is a prolapse of the posterior middle vaginal wall, allowing herniation of the rectum. As in the cystocele, this may be symptomless unless very large, when faeces become lodged in the herniated sac. Defecation will be difficult unless digital pressure is applied on the vaginal side of the sac. An **enterocele** is a herniation higher in the vagina and on examination will not be palpable per vaginam.

Dyspareunia (painful sexual intercourse)

This may occur depending on the degree of prolapse (Reader 2007).

Treatment

Treatment of reproductive anomalies is usually by surgical repair. In a few women, such as those who refuse surgery or are too ill or frail, insertion of a ring pessary may be the treatment of choice.

Prevention of prolapse

A midwife can minimise the risk by careful practice:

- Attempt to avoid pushing until full dilatation of the cervix.
- Prevent delivery of the baby before full dilatation of the cervix.
- Ensure that the second stage is not prolonged without obvious progress.
- Avoid fundal pressure to deliver the placenta.
- Ensure careful repair of any perineal trauma.
- Ensure early ambulation of the woman.
- Encourage pelvic floor exercises in the puerperium.

Smooth muscle

Smooth muscle has two characteristics: it lacks the cross-striated banding pattern found in skeletal and cardiac fibres, and nerve supply is derived from the autonomic division of the nervous system rather than the somatic division. Hence, the muscle is described as smooth, **non-striated**, **involuntary** and is often referred to as **visceral muscle** (Martini & Nath 2009). Smooth muscle, like skeletal muscle, uses cross-bridge movements between actin and myosin filaments to generate force and calcium ions to control cross-bridge activity. However, there are differences between the two types of muscles in the organisation of the contractile filaments and in the excitation–contraction coupling process. There is also diversity within the range of smooth muscle types in respect of the mechanism of excitation–contraction coupling.

The contractions of smooth muscle are slow and sustained. The fibres of smooth muscle are small, spindle-shaped cells with a central nucleus. They have no striations and have a large surface area, allowing calcium ions to enter the cells easily. There are notably fewer myosin fibres than actin fibres in smooth muscle. The myosin heads are arranged along the length of the myosin fibre so that each myosin fibre is attached to many actin fibres.

The fibres are arranged in a spiral around the muscle cell and can change their lengths much more than skeletal muscle fibres can. The fibres are arranged in two (or more) sheets, usually at right-angles to each other. For instance, there are three layers in the body of the uterus: an outer, mainly longitudinal layer; an oblique middle layer; and an inner, mainly circular layer (Romanini 2008). Muscle fibres in the cervix are mainly circular with only a few longitudinal fibres.

There are no clear neuromuscular junctions in smooth muscle. The innervating fibres have bulbous varicosities and release their neurotransmitter substance directly onto many fibres. This allows a slow, **synchronised contraction** of the whole muscle sheet. Action potentials are transmitted from cell to cell until the whole muscle sheet is contracting. Some fibres act as **pacemaker cells** to set the contractile pace for the whole muscle sheet. It is thought that such fibres in the uterus are beneath the cornua so that the fundus dominates. Both the rate and intensity of smooth muscle contraction can be modified by neural and chemical stimuli.

Calcium triggers the onset of contractions and ATP provides the energy. Contraction in smooth muscle is slow, sustained and resistant to fatigue. Smooth muscle fibres take 30 times longer to contract and relax than skeletal muscle fibres. The same muscle tension can be maintained for long periods at less than 1% of the energy cost of skeletal muscle. In many parts of the body smooth muscle tone is maintained continuously with low energy expenditure and often by anaerobic ATP production.

Special features of smooth muscle include:

- Less vigorous contractile response to being stretched so that distension of a hollow organ can occur without provoking expulsive contractions.
- Ability to change more in length and create more tension than skeletal muscle.
- Ability to divide—hyperplasia.
- Secretion of the connective tissue proteins collagen and elastin.

Uterine muscle during pregnancy

Like most other smooth muscle the uterus is spontaneously contractile. When required, it has the ability to perform considerable muscular feats to expel its contents such as during menstruation and childbirth. At other times it is prevented from contracting and must remain quiescent to allow development and growth of the fetus and placenta during pregnancy. The uterus is unique among smooth muscular organs in that it undergoes profound, largely reversible, changes during pregnancy. In early pregnancy, muscle fibres become more compliant and growth of fibres is mainly due to hyperplasia. This occurs under the influence of oestrogen and independently of fetal growth. If the fetus embeds outside of the uterus (ectopic gestation), this early growth of the uterus would still occur.

The size of the non-pregnant uterus is 7.5 cm in length, 5 cm in width and 2.5 cm in depth but by term the uterus has grown to 20 cm long, 25 cm wide and 22.5 cm deep. There is 20-fold increase in weight of the uterus from 50 g to between 80 and 1200 g (Blackburn 2007). The main part of uterine growth during the second half of pregnancy is almost entirely due to hypertrophy (increase in size) in response to various stimuli. The growth of the fetus stretches the uterus and this acts as a powerful stimulator of growth-promoting synthesis of the contractile proteins of the myometrium. By 3–4 months the uterine wall has thickened from 10 to 25 mm but by term the wall has thinned to between 5 and 10 mm (Blackburn 2007). The lower part of the uterus, consisting of the isthmus, softens and elongates from its original 7 mm until about 10 weeks of pregnancy when it measures 25 mm. This is the beginning of differentiation of the lower uterine segment (Dunlop 1999).

Uterine shape and position: uterine growth

The uterus is expected to follow a predicted rate of growth during pregnancy. However, this is only a reliable indicator of gestational age in the first 20 weeks of pregnancy. Routine measurement of fundal height of the uterus is used to assess the growth of the fetus and the umbilicus and xiphisternum are useful landmarks for this purpose.

By 12 weeks the uterus has risen out of the pelvis and has become an abdominal organ. It is no longer anteverted and anteflexed. As it becomes upright, the uterus often inclines to and rotates to the right. This may be because the colon occupies the space in the left side of the pelvic cavity. This is known as **right obliquity of the uterus** and increases as pregnancy progresses. At this time the conceptus fills the uterine cavity and the isthmus opens out. The fundus of the uterus can be palpated abdominally just above the symphysis pubis.

As pregnancy progresses, the shape and position of the uterus change to accommodate the growing fetus. Following implantation, the embedded blastocyst does not require much space but the upper part of the uterus begins to enlarge due to the influence of oestrogen. The uterus becomes globular in shape until about 20 weeks and then pear-shaped or cylindrical until term. The fundus may be palpated at the level or just below the level of the umbilicus at 20 weeks and midway between the umbilicus and xiphisternum at 30 weeks. At this time the lower uterine segment (LUS) is identified but is not complete. By 36 weeks, the fundus reaches its maximum height at the xiphisternum. A reduction in fundal height may now occur as the presenting part of the fetus enters the pelvis. This is due to softening of the pelvic floor tissues together with good uterine tone and further formation of the LUS (Dunlop 1999). Lay people generally know this as 'lightening'.

Hormonal influences on the uterus in pregnancy

Oestrogen and progesterone, initially from the corpus luteum and then the placenta, are mainly the hormones responsible for influencing the uterus. Oestrogen promotes growth of muscle fibres and progesterone maintains the quiescence of the myometrium by possibly blocking the excitation and conduction mechanisms of the muscle cells. In particular, the interaction of these hormones has a growth-promoting effect and increases uterine muscle compliance. By term, each muscle fibre increases three-fold in diameter and 10-fold in length.

Actions of oestrogen and progesterone on target cells

The hormones probably enter the target cell by passive diffusion across the cell membrane and then bind to specific receptor proteins present in the cellular cytoplasm. The complex formed between the steroid and the receptor is transferred to the nucleus where gene function is regulated. The hormone estradiol stimulates RNA synthesis. The RNA is transferred to the cytoplasm where it is responsible for the synthesis of new protein. The role of progesterone is less well understood mainly due to the lack of thorough research. It may be responsible for increasing membrane resting potential in pregnancy so that muscle fibre contractions are less likely to occur.

The uterus at term

The uterus at term is generally described as having two main structural compartments: the upper uterine segment (UUS), formed of the body and fundus, and the lower uterine segment (LUS), formed of the isthmus and cervix. The uterus cannot simply be divided in this way as there is a gradual fall in the smooth muscle content from the fundus to the cervix. The muscle content of the cervix is estimated to be 10% and the functional significance of this cervical muscle is not understood. The physiological mechanisms regulating these functions are becoming clearer but there remains uncertainty about the pathophysiology, for example in incompetent cervix (Calder 2008).

The decidua

During pregnancy the endometrium becomes thicker, richer and more vascular in the upper part of the body of the uterus and the fundus, the normal site for implantation. It is now termed the decidua, because it is similar to the deciduous tree in that it sheds at the end of pregnancy. The decidua is thinner and less vascular in the lower pole of the uterus. The decidua provides a glycogen-rich environment for the blastocyst until the placenta is able to fulfil its functions. As the zygote embeds, the following changes occur in the endometrium due to increased progesterone production by the corpus luteum:

- Endometrium hypertrophies to become 6–8 mm thick.
- Stroma become more vascular and oedematous and the functional layer becomes organised into two distinct areas.
- Stroma cells enlarge and become more closely packed together to form the compact layer. They are now known as **decidual cells** and become polygonal in shape because of the pressure they exert on each other.
- Tubular glands become dilated and more tortuous in their deeper parts and the lumen becomes packed with secretion. This dilatation below the compact layer gives the stroma a cavernous spongy appearance and is known as the spongy or cavernous layer.
- The basal layer remains unchanged.

The myometrium

The myometrium forms the greater part of the uterine wall and the detailed arrangement of muscular tissue is highly effective, especially for evacuation of uterine contents. During pregnancy, the muscle fibres of the myometrium become more differentiated and organised in order to fulfil their roles in labour (Figs 25.10, 25.11). The myometrium is composed of at least three interdigitating muscle layers: an outer, a middle and an inner layer (Romanini 2008). Each layer performs a different function.

The middle layer forms the bulk of the organ and is composed of obliquely interdigitating strands of muscle fibres forming a network around blood vessels. It is involved with expulsion of the fetus and the control of bleeding after delivery of the placenta. The outer and inner layers contain both circular and longitudinal fibres and functional and structural studies indicate that these layers may be continuous (Garfield & Yallampalli 2008). The outer layer, with mainly longitudinal fibres, contracts and retracts during labour. The inner layer, with mainly circular fibres, is more evident around the cornua and lower uterine segment and cervix. It is involved in distension of the lower uterine segment and dilatation of the cervix during labour.

The muscle cells of the myometrium are grouped into bundles with thin sheets of connective tissue including collagen, elastic fibres, fibroblasts and mast cells between the bundles. The collagenous connective tissue probably serves two functions: a support for the

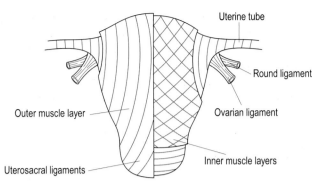

Figure 25.10 • The outer and inner layers of uterine muscle. (From Henderson C, Macdonald S 2004, with kind permission of Elsevier.)

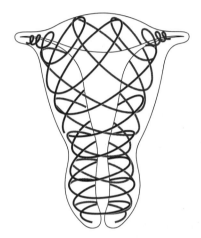

Figure 25.11 • The spiral arrangement of the uterine muscle fibres. (From Henderson C, Macdonald S 2004, with kind permission of Elsevier.)

muscle fibres and a transmission network for the tension developed by smooth muscle contraction. Around the bundles of smooth muscle cells are fibroblasts, blood and lymphatic vessels and nerve cells.

The perimetrium

This outer layer of peritoneum does not totally cover the uterus. It drapes over the bladder anteriorly to form a fold called the uterovesical pouch and posteriorly it drapes over the rectum to form the pouch of Douglas (Ramsay 2008). It forms the broad ligament, thus maintaining the anatomical position of the uterus. This loosely applied layer allows for unrestricted growth of the uterus during pregnancy.

Cervical changes

In line with the gradual build-up of uterine activity in pregnancy, changes take place in the cervix. Its function changes from a firm structure to an elastic tissue which can stretch to a diameter of 10 cm or more during labour and then almost return to its original state. During pregnancy the cervix increases in mass, water content and vascularity (Blackburn 2007). It remains 2.5 cm long throughout pregnancy until effacement begins. Early in pregnancy cervical softening occurs and some opening of the external os is detectable from 24 weeks and of the internal os in about one-third of primigravidae by 32 weeks (Steer & Johnson 1998). **Effacement** or shortening of the cervix and its gradual inclusion in the LUS occurs in the last few weeks of pregnancy. Tension exerted by the outer longitudinal muscle fibres of the fundus may contribute to the process of effacement (O'Lah 2006). These changes are seen only in the human cervix; the cervices of most other animals studied remain closed until the onset of parturition.

Dramatic changes need to occur in the cervix at time of delivery to allow uterine contractions to influence dilatation of the cervix. The changes involve degradation of the collagen content by enzymes such as collagenase and elastase. Changes also occur in the proteoglycans ground substance matrix which attracts water, and smooth muscle fibres which become more stretchable (Blackburn 2007). Oestrogen causes increased vascularity and the cervix appears purple when viewed through a speculum.

Myometrial contractions have little effect on the ripening of the cervix which usually occurs prior to the onset of labour. Hormonal control of cervical ripening may involve multiple changes in oestrogen, progesterone, relaxin and prostaglandins and seems to correlate well with a gradual rise in circulating oestrogens. PGE_2 and $PGF_{2\alpha}$ have a localised action on cervical softening that is independent of uterine activity and PGE_2 is used to improve the cervical state prior to induction of labour (Blackburn 2007). However, there is much variation in individual women in the changes in the cervix outlined above. Labour may begin in some women when the cervix is long, firm, uneffaced and undilated. In others, the cervix may be soft, effaced and partly dilated for some weeks prior to the onset of labour.

The cervix also acts as an efficient barrier to infection. Under the influence of progesterone the mucus secreted by the endocervical cells becomes thicker and more viscous. It forms a cervical plug called the **operculum** which prevents ascending infection.

Uterine blood flow

Increased vessel diameter and lowered resistance cause an increase in uterine blood flow during pregnancy. Prostacyclin (PGI_2) is produced by the pregnant and non-pregnant myometrium as well as by the placental blood vessels. This acts as a potent vasodilator to inhibit platelet aggregation and also to protect the vascular epithelium. It is therefore important in maintaining blood flow to the placenta and the uterus during labour. Unlike other prostaglandins, PGI_2 has little effect on uterine contractability.

Innervation of the human uterus

The uterus is innervated by sympathetic and parasympathetic fibres of the autonomic nervous system. In comparison to other smooth muscle cells, the uterus is poorly innervated with a low density of nerves to smooth muscle. The physiological result of the innervation of the uterus is unknown as labour will occur even if complete spinal transection is present. It is probable that central nervous system connections are not essential to the onset and progress of labour.

Sympathetic fibres

Preganglionic fibres leave the spinal cord and enter a chain of ganglia running alongside the spinal column from T1 to L5 vertebrae. In the ganglia they synapse with postganglionic fibres that synapse with the target organ. The uterus is unusual, as the preganglionic fibres leaving T10–T12 run directly to the uterus to synapse with the postganglionic fibres. Preganglionic fibres release acetylcholine into the synapse from their endings and postganglionic fibres release noradrenaline (norepinephrine) onto the target organ from their terminals.

There are two types of adrenergic receptors in target organs, alpha (α) receptors, which are normally excitatory, and beta (β) fibres, which are normally inhibitory. There are two types of beta receptors: beta-1 (β_1) and beta-2 (β_2). Beta-1 (β_1) receptors are cardiospecific and are excitatory, whereas beta-2 (β_2) receptors are present in the uterus and are inhibitory. Drugs such as salbutamol and ritodrine inhibit uterine contractions in preterm labour but will excite cardiac muscle, causing a rise in pulse rate, leading to increased cardiac output and blood pressure. The beta-blocking agent propranolol will enhance uterine activity.

Parasympathetic fibres

The parasympathetic innervation to the pelvis is through the sacral outflow from S2, 3 and 4. The preganglionic fibres end in or near the target organs and synapse with short postganglionic fibres. Acetylcholine is the neurotransmitter substance in both pre- and postganglionic fibres. The fibres innervating the uterus synapse in two nerve plexi on either side of the pouch of Douglas. These are the **paracervical plexi** (Lee–Frankenhäuser's plexi).

Changes in the vagina in pregnancy

Oestrogen produces changes in both the muscle layer and the epithelium. There is hypertrophy of the muscle layer and changes in the surrounding connective tissue allow the vagina to become more elastic, allowing it to distend during the second stage of labour. There is a marked desquamation of the superficial cells of the epithelium giving rise to an increased amount of normal vaginal discharge called **leucorrhoea** because of its white colour.

The epithelial cells also have an increased glycogen content and interaction with Döderlein's bacillus produces a more acid environment which adds to the protection against many micro-organisms. Unfortunately, this means an increased susceptibility to the organism *Candida albicans*, which causes moniliasis or thrush. There is increased vascularity and the vagina appears reddish purple in colour, a change in pregnancy referred to as **Jacquemenier's sign**. The increased vascularity of the pelvic organs gives rise to another sign of pregnancy called **Osiander's sign**, which is increased pulsation in the lateral vaginal fornices.

Uterine activity in pregnancy

As in skeletal muscle, myosin-containing thick filaments interact with the actin-containing thin filaments and the energy source is from ATP. There are no clear neuromuscular junctions in smooth muscle and innervating neurons release their neurotransmitter substance directly onto many fibres, resulting in a change in intracellular calcium concentration and allowing a slow, synchronised contraction of the whole muscle sheet. As pregnancy progresses, the timing and speed of the myometrial action potentials change and the muscle cells increase their content of contractile proteins, gap junctions, sarcoplasmic reticulum and mitochondria.

Calcium is a key ion in the contraction process and mainly comes from the ECF where its concentration is 10 000 times that of the myometrial cell. At rest the cell membrane does not allow calcium to enter the cell but after a contraction calcium enters the cell through ion channels. Action potentials are transmitted from cell to cell until the whole sheet is contracting. The uterus at term appears to have enhanced communication between cells and the action potential can spread across the entire uterus in only 2–3 s.

The role of pacemakers in uterine activity

Some fibres may act as pacemaker cells to set the contractile pace for the whole sheet. Specific pacemaker cells have not yet been identified. It was previously thought that fibres beneath the cornua of the uterus acted as pacemakers so that the fundus dominates.

Investigations no longer support this theory and although it is likely that cells near the cornua may initiate contractions it is now thought that any myometrial cell would have this property (Garfield & Yallampalli 2008). Both the rate and intensity of smooth muscle contraction can be modified by neural and chemical stimuli. Contraction in smooth muscle is slow, sustained and resistant to fatigue. The action potential is conducted from the cell membrane down the sarcoplasmic reticulum so that there is a rapid release of calcium deep in the cell.

In pregnancy, uterine activity gradually evolves, with activity being seen as early as 7 weeks with high frequency (about two contractions per minute) but very low intensity (about 1–1.5 kPa) (Steer & Johnson 1998). This pattern continues until about 20 weeks when uterine contractions increase in both frequency and amplitude until term. These tend to occur more rapidly in the last 6–8 weeks of pregnancy. This is thought to be facilitated by the development of gap junctions within the myometrium where the plasma membranes of adjacent cells are closely applied, which act as areas of low resistance so that conduction of electrical impulses can spread rapidly from one cell to another. They are important in the spread of action potentials and the development of the coordinated uterine activity that is seen in efficient labour.

Gap junctions

The appearance of gap junctions seems to depend on changes in the levels of oestrogen, progesterone and prostaglandins occurring in late pregnancy. The absence of gap junctions may be important for the maintenance of pregnancy and their appearance may be necessary to allow the development of effective uterine contractions in labour. Low-frequency but high-pressure Braxton Hicks' contractions are perceived by the mother. They may be as strong as labour contractions but are not painful and the cervix does not dilate.

Sensitivity to oxytocin and prostaglandins

Sensitivity to oxytocin is dependent on both gestational age and the level of spontaneous uterine activity. Up to about 30 weeks the uterus is very insensitive to oxytocin and it is necessary to give very high infusion rates of oxytocin in order to stimulate uterine activity (up to 128 mU/min). After 30 weeks the uterus will respond to much smaller concentrations of oxytocin of 8 mU/min and by 40 weeks as little as 4 mU/min will cause uterine activity similar to that seen in spontaneous labour. In contrast to this variable response, prostaglandins E_2 and $F_{2\alpha}$ will induce uterine contractions at any gestational age. Therefore, prostaglandins are probably the final mediator of uterine contractions.

Main points

- Muscle is specialised tissue with the ability to transform chemical energy to mechanical energy to produce force and enable movement to occur. All muscle cells are elongated and contain two kinds of protein filaments: actin and myosin.

- The three basic muscle types are skeletal muscle, smooth muscle and specialised cardiac muscle. The four functions of muscle are the production of movement, maintenance of posture, stabilisation of joints and the generation of heat. The four properties of muscle are excitability, contractility, extensibility and elasticity.

- Skeletal muscles are attached to and cover bones. Fibres have obvious bands or striations. Skeletal muscle contracts rapidly and tires easily. Activity depends upon a rich blood supply to deliver oxygen and nutrients and remove metabolic waste.

- The sliding filament theory of muscle action is commonly supported. Skeletal muscles contract in response to nerve stimulation, resulting in an action potential being sent along the sarcolemma. This electrical event results in the contraction.

- The pelvic floor is formed by the soft tissues (six layers) which fill the outlet of the pelvis. The most important tissue is the strong funnel-shaped diaphragm of skeletal muscle attached to the pelvic walls. Through it pass the urethra, vagina and anal canals.

- The superficial muscles lie external to the deep muscles and provide additional strength. The deep muscles called the levator ani are the major muscles of the pelvic floor. The deep muscles, because of their insertion, are also collectively known as the coccygeus muscles and are vital for bladder and bowel function.

- The perineal body is a wedge-shaped mass of muscular and fibrous tissue situated between the vaginal and anal canals. Superficial and deep pelvic floor muscles are both involved in its structure.

- Effective functioning of the pelvic floor depends on the integrity of the muscle fibres and maintenance of muscle tone. The pelvic floor supports the abdominal and pelvic organs, maintains intra-abdominal pressure, enables defecation and micturition, facilitates the fetus through the birth canal and enables flexion of the sacrum and coccyx.

- Prolapse of the pelvic organs with the possibility of urinary and faecal incontinence may cause physical and emotional discomfort for women. Treatment is usually by surgical repair. The risk of prolapse can be minimised by careful management of labour and careful repair of any perineal trauma.

- Smooth muscle is non-striated, involuntary and is referred to as visceral muscle. Contractions are slow and sustained. There are no clear neuromuscular junctions in smooth muscle. Innervating fibres release their neurotransmitter substance directly onto many fibres, allowing slow, synchronised contraction of the whole muscle sheet.

- Smooth muscle has special features which include a less vigorous contractile response to being stretched so that distension of a hollow organ can occur without provoking expulsive contractions; ability to divide and change more in length and width than skeletal muscle; and ability to secrete collagen and elastin (connective tissue proteins).

- Smooth muscle fibres in the uterus undergo hyperplasia in early pregnancy but the main part of uterine growth is due to hypertrophy. Uterine growth is a reliable indicator of fetal gestation in the first 20 weeks, becoming less reliable as pregnancy progresses.

- The uterus at term has two main structural compartments: the upper uterine segment formed of the body and fundus; and the lower uterine segment formed of the isthmus and cervix.

- During pregnancy the endometrium becomes thicker, richer and more vascular in the upper part of the body of the uterus and the fundus, the normal site for implantation. It is now called the decidua, which is thinner and less vascular in the lower pole of the uterus.

- The smooth muscle fibres of the myometrium are arranged in two (or more) sheets, usually at right-angles to each other. The body of the uterus has three muscle layers: an outer layer with mainly longitudinal fibres, a middle oblique layer and an inner layer with mainly circular fibres.

- Changes in the cervix include an increase in mass, water content and vascularity. Under the influence of progesterone, endocervical cell mucus thickens, becomes more viscous and forms the operculum which prevents ascending infection.

- Under the influence of oestrogen the muscle layer in the vagina hypertrophies and the surrounding connective tissue becomes more elastic, allowing distension during the second stage of labour. Increased desquamation of superficial epithelial cells leads to leucorrhoea.

- Contraction of uterine smooth muscle involves a slow, synchronised contraction of the whole muscle sheet. Some fibres may act as pacemaker cells. Sensitivity to oxytocin and prostaglandins depends on gestational age and the level of spontaneous uterine activity. Prostaglandins are probably the final mediator of uterine contractions.

References

Blackburn, S.T., 2007. Maternal, Fetal and Neonatal Physiology: A Clinical Perspective, fourth edn. Elsevier Saunders, Missouri.

Calder, A.A., 2008. The cervix during pregnancy. In: Chard, T., Grudzinskas, J.G. (Eds.), The Uterus, third edn. Cambridge Reviews in Human Reproduction. Cambridge University Press, Cambridge.

Dunlop, W., 1999. Normal pregnancy: physiology and endocrinology. In: Edmonds, D.K., Dewhurst, J. (Eds.), Textbook of Obstetrics and Gynaecology for Postgraduates, sixth edn. Blackwell Science, Oxford.

Garfield, R.E., Yallampalli, C., 2008. Structure and function of uterine muscle. In: Chard, T., Grudzinskas, J.G. (Eds.), The Uterus, third edn. Cambridge Reviews in Human Reproduction. Cambridge University Press, Cambridge.

Henderson, C., Macdonald, S. (Eds.), 2004. Mayes' Midwifery: A Textbook for Midwives, thirteenth edn. Baillière Tindall, London.

Marieb, E.N., Hoehn, K., 2008. Anatomy and Physiology, third edn. Pearson Benjamin/Cummings, New York.

Martini, F.H., Nath, J.L., 2009. Fundamentals of Anatomy and Physiology, eighth edn. Pearson Benjamin/Cummings, New York.

O'Lah, K., 2006. The cervix in pregnancy and labour. In: Studd, J., Lin Tan, S., Chervenak, F.A. (Eds.), Progress in Obstetrics and Gynaecology 17. Churchill Livingstone, Edinburgh.

Ramsay, E.M., 2008. Concepts of the uterus: a historical perspective. In: Chard, T., Grudzinskas, J.G. (Eds.), The Uterus, third edn. Cambridge Reviews in Human Reproduction. Cambridge University Press, Cambridge.

Reader, F., 2007. Sexual dysfunction. In: Edmonds, D.K., Dewhurst, J. (Eds.), Textbook of Obstetrics and Gynaecology for Postgraduates, seventh edn. Wiley-Blackwell, Oxford.

Romanini, C., 2008. Measurement of uterine contractions. In: Chard, T., Grudzinskas, J.G. (Eds.), The Uterus, third edn. Cambridge Reviews in Human Reproduction. Cambridge University Press, Cambridge.

Smith, A.R.B., 2007. Pelvic floor dysfunction: Uterovaginal prolapse. In: Edmonds, D.K., Dewhurst, J. (Eds.), Textbook of Obstetrics and Gynaecology for Postgraduates, seventh edn. Blackwell Science, Oxford.

Steer, P.J., Johnson, M.R., 1998. The genital system. In: Chamberlain, G., Broughton, Pipkin F. (Eds.) Clinical Physiology in Obstetrics, third edn. Blackwell Science, Oxford.

Annotated recommended reading

Chard, T., Grudzinskas, J.G. (Eds.), 2008. The Uterus, third edn. Cambridge Reviews in Human Reproduction. Cambridge University Press, Cambridge.

This text is at postgraduate level and provides a wide-ranging and authoritative account of the uterus and its physiological role in fertility, normal pregnancy and delivery.

Chapter Twenty-Six

The central nervous system

26

CHAPTER CONTENTS

Introduction

The ability to respond appropriately to environmental change depends on rapid communication achieved by the **nervous system** and the **endocrine system** (see Ch. 28). The nervous system communicates by the rapid transmission of **electrical signals**. The endocrine glands secrete **hormones** into the bloodstream which modify the working of target organs. Normal functioning of these systems is critical for maintaining **homeostasis** (the ability of a regulated system to maintain itself close to a fixed point).

The nervous system controls function of every body system, every thought, action and emotion. It is only possible to give a brief outline of this complex system and to elaborate on important functions such as pain perception. This chapter concentrates on the central nervous system; Chapter 27 considers the peripheral and autonomic nervous systems and neural integration.

Organisation of the nervous system

The **central nervous system** (CNS) consists of the **brain** and **spinal cord**. It has an integration function, receiving messages from and sending messages to all parts of the body via the **peripheral nervous system** (PNS). The **autonomic nervous system** (ANS) is that part of the PNS that innervates the smooth muscle and glands of the viscera and the cardiac muscle. It can be subdivided into the **sympathetic nervous system** and **parasympathetic nervous system**. Sensory organs such as eyes and ears feed environmental information back to the brain (Fitzgerald et al 2006).

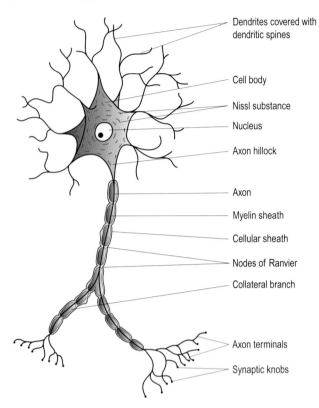

Dendrites covered with dendritic spines

Cell body

Nissl substance

Nucleus

Axon hillock

Axon

Myelin sheath

Cellular sheath

Nodes of Ranvier

Collateral branch

Axon terminals

Synaptic knobs

Figure 26.1 • Structure of a whole nerve fibre. (From Hinchliff S E, Watson R 1996, with permission.)

Neuroanatomy

Nervous tissue is made up of two cell types: the **neurons** (Fig. 26.1) and a group of cell types collectively known as **neuroglia**, the supportive connective tissue of the nervous system. The tissue is supplied by blood vessels.

Neurons

The structural units of the nervous system are the **neurons**. These specialised cells have the following characteristics (Marieb 2008):

- They have processes called axons and dendrites communicate with other cells.
- They conduct messages by nerve impulses from one body part to another.
- They are extremely long-lived but cannot undergo mitosis and divide.
- They have a very high metabolic rate needing continuous glucose and oxygen.
- They cannot survive more than a few minutes without oxygen.

Structure of neurons

The cell body

Each neuron has a cell body (**soma**) with a large spherical nucleus surrounded by granular cytoplasm and contains all the usual organelles except centrioles. **Neurotransmitters** (NTs) are synthesised in the soma. Most neuronal cell bodies are located in the central nervous system (CNS), where they are clustered together in groups called **nuclei**. The few neuronal cell bodies in the parasympathetic nervous system (PNS) are called **ganglia**.

Dendrites

Dendrites are short, diffusely branching extensions which receive messages from other cells at **synapses** by conducting electrical signals called **graded potentials** towards and into the cell body. Dendrites are the input part of the neuron and there may be hundreds clustering close to the cell body. They provide an enormous surface area for reception of signals from other cells.

Axons

Each neuron has only one axon arising from the **axon hillock** on the cell body. The axon is the same diameter along its length and some are over 1 metre long such as those travelling from the spine to the foot. Axons may give off branches called **axon collaterals** and usually have terminal branches ending in **synaptic knobs** or **boutons**. Axons contain **microtubules** and **microfilaments** that transport substances to the cell body (**anterograde**) and from the cell body (**retrograde**). They conduct messages to other cells by electrical nerve impulses and by neurotransmitters which excite or inhibit other neurons by attaching to receptors on their plasma membrane.

Myelin sheaths

Larger nerve fibres are covered in a white, fatty, segmented sheath called the **myelin sheath** which protects and insulates fibres and increases the rate of impulse transmission. Messages can be transmitted up to a 100 times more rapidly than in unmyelinated fibres (Fig. 26.2). Myelin sheaths in the PNS are formed by **Schwann cells** which wrap themselves around the axon. Schwann cell protoplasm is squeezed out of the cell to leave the axon wrapped in a multilayered membrane. The external portion is called the **neurolemma** or Schwann sheath. Adjacent Schwann cells along the axon do not touch and the gaps between them, which occur at regular intervals, are called the **nodes of Ranvier**. Axon collaterals can only emerge at these nodes.

The myelin sheaths of the CNS are produced by cells called **oligodendrocytes**. Myelinated fibres form the

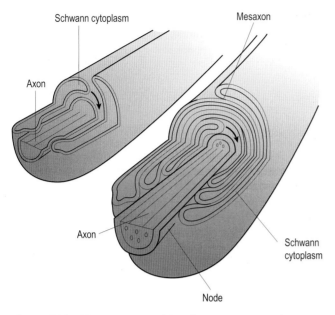

Figure 26.2 • Myelination in peripheral nervous system. Arrows indicate movement of flange of Schwann cytoplasm. (From Fitzgerald M T J 1996, with permission.)

white matter in the brain and spinal cord and the cell bodies form the grey matter. Cell bodies are outside the white matter in the brain and inside the white matter in the spinal cord.

Classification of neurons

Neurons may be classified structurally or functionally (Marieb 2008).

Structurally, neurons are grouped according to the number of processes extending from the cell body. There are three major groups:

1. **Multipolar neurons** are the most common type and have at least three processes, usually multiple dendrites and one axon. However, some do not have an axon.
2. **Bipolar neurons** have two processes—an axon and a dendrite. They are rare but are found in special sense organs such as the retina or in the olfactory mucosa.
3. **Unipolar neurons** have a single, very short process. They are found in the ganglia of the PNS where they act as sensory neurons.

Functional classification is into motor, sensory and association neurons.

- **Motor neurons** with cell bodies mainly in the CNS carry impulses to control effector organs such as the muscles or glands.
- **Sensory neurons** whose cell bodies are located in the sensory ganglia outside the CNS often have very long dendritic branches which gather impulses from the periphery such as the ends of the toes and fingers.
- **Association neurons**, often called interneurons, carry signals between motor and sensory neurons in complex networks.

Neuroglia

Neuroglial cells support and protect neurons, outnumbering them in a ratio of 5:1. As there are billions of neurons in the brain, the number of neuroglial cells is enormous. These cells are subdivided into four basic types (Fitzgerald et al 2006):

1. **Astrocytes** are star-shaped cells with long, fine processes arising from their bodies. They have one process against a neuron and other processes close to capillary walls.
2. **Oligodendrocytes** in the CNS and Schwann cells in the PNS are smaller than astrocytes and have fewer processes. They form myelin sheaths around nerve fibres.
3. **Ependyma** form a continuous layer of cells lining the ventricles of the brain and spinal cord central canal. They help to produce cerebrospinal fluid.
4. **Microglia** are small cells which are part of the immune system, acting as macrophages.

The structure of a nerve

The axons from single neurons are bound together to form **nerves** (Fig. 26.3). Nerves may contain **afferent fibres** (to the CNS), **efferent fibres** (from the CNS) or both when they are called **mixed nerves**. Each separate nerve fibre is embedded in a fibrous connective tissue sheath called the **endoneurium**. These are bound into groups by the **perineurium**, a connective tissue sheath and the complete nerve is surrounded by the **epineurium**. Each nerve has an arterial blood supply and venous drainage.

Neurophysiology

The nerve impulse

Both nerve fibres and muscle fibres are excitable tissues which conduct electrical signals. When a neuron is stimulated, an electrical impulse is sent along the axon (Fig. 26.4). Bodies are electrically neutral (positive and negative charges are equal). Potential electrical energy is called **voltage**, which is measured in volts (V) or millivolts (mV). The flow of electricity from one point to another

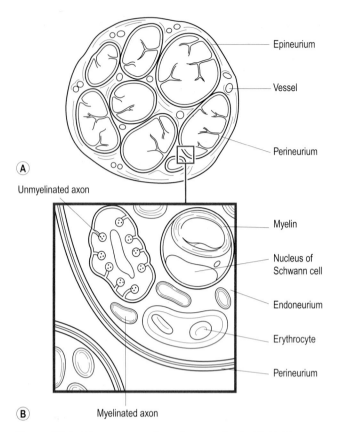

(A)

Unmyelinated axon

Epineurium

Vessel

Perineurium

Myelin

Nucleus of
Schwann cell

Endoneurium

Erythrocyte

Perineurium

(B)

Myelinated axon

Figure 26.3 • Transverse section of a nerve trunk. (A) Light microscopy. (B) Electron microscopy. (From Fitzgerald M T J 1996, with permission.)

is called a **current**. Substances that hinder the flow are said to provide **resistance**. Ions, which are electrically charged particles, provide the currents and usually flow through an aqueous solution across a plasma membrane. Plasma membranes are studded with proteinaceous ion channels.

Polarisation

When a membrane is resting, its potential is **polarised**, i.e. the inside has a different electrical potential from the interstitial fluid. The resting potential of neurons averages -70 mV. This is maintained by the distribution and relative contribution of negative and positive ions. Inside the cell the positive ion is potassium and the negative ion is protein. In the interstitial fluid the positive ion is sodium and the negative ion is chloride.

The role of sodium ions

When the cell is stimulated, sodium channels open in the membrane and sodium ions rush into the cell, changing the membrane potential to $+40$ mV. This is called **depolarisation**. The **action potential** is the sum of all negative and positive charges stimulating the cell and proceeds down the axon in a wave. Behind the wave the cell pumps three sodium ions out in exchange for two potassium ions. The membrane potential falls to -90 mV (hyperpolarisation) and then recovers.

The period of hyperpolarisation is called the **refractory period** during which the cell cannot generate an

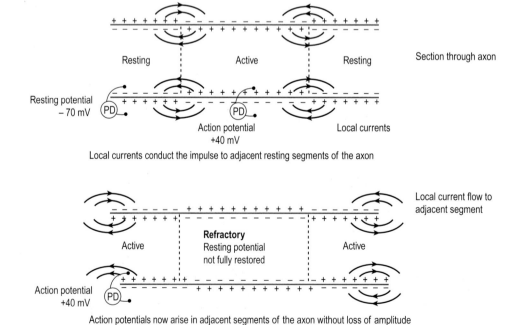

Resting   Active   Resting   Section through axon

Resting potential
-70 mV   PD   PD   Local currents

Action potential
$+40$ mV

Local currents conduct the impulse to adjacent resting segments of the axon

Local current flow to
adjacent segment

Refractory
Active   Resting potential   Active
not fully restored

Action potential
$+40$ mV   PD

Action potentials now arise in adjacent segments of the axon without loss of amplitude

Figure 26.4 • Propagation of an action potential along a nerve fibre. PD, potential difference. (From Hinchliff S E, Montague S E 1990, with permission.)

action potential. Depolarisation increases the chance of a nerve impulse being generated but hyperpolarisation decreases it. Firing of a neuron is an all-or-nothing phenomenon, occurring only if the potential reaches a threshold. Strong stimuli result in more impulses, not stronger impulses.

Saltatory conduction of the impulse

Nerve fibres can be classified according to the speed of conduction of the action potential. The larger the nerve, the more rapidly it conducts impulses. Myelinated nerves conduct impulses more rapidly than unmyelinated nerves. The myelin sheath increases electrical resistance of a nerve but it is leakier at the nodes of Ranvier. The electrical current flows smoothly along each section of the sheath between nodes of Ranvier and it is only necessary to generate an action potential at the nodes. The impulse seems to jump from node to node. This is called **saltatory conduction** (Fig. 26.5). In a non-myelinated nerve, new action potentials have to be generated across each adjacent section of the nerve membrane.

Classification of nerves by speed of conduction

Nerve fibres can be classified as follows:

- Group A fibres are myelinated and can conduct impulses at up to 120 metres per second (m/s). They are further subdivided into α, β, γ and δ (alpha, beta, gamma and delta) fibres.
- Group B fibres are myelinated. They are all preganglionic fibres of the autonomic nervous system.
- Group C fibres are non-myelinated and conduct impulses as slowly as 1 m/s.

The synapse

Synapses are junctions between the terminal bouton of the axon and its target tissue which may be a neuron cell body, a gland or a muscle (Fig. 26.6). Synapses enable transfer of information between one cell and another. They may be electrical or chemical (Fitzgerald et al 2006). The presynaptic neuron conducts impulses towards the synapse and the postsynaptic neuron transmits information away from the synapse.

Electrical synapses

These synapses are bridged junctions corresponding to gap junctions in other cells. Protein channels connect the cytoplasm of adjacent neurons, providing electrical pathways through which ions can flow from one neuron to another. Such neurons are electrically coupled and

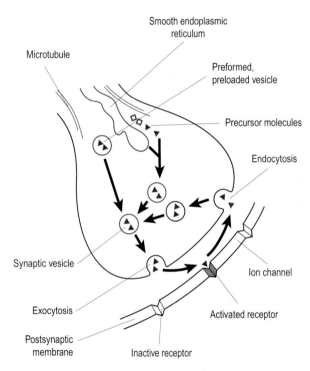

Figure 26.6 • Diagram to show origin and fate of synaptic vesicle and transmitter–receptor binding. (From Fitzgerald M T J 1996, with permission.)

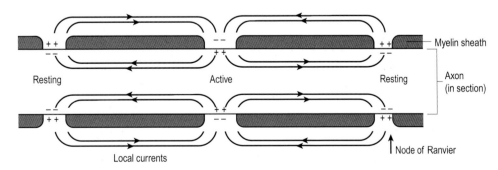

Figure 26.5 • Saltatory conduction in a myelinated nerve fibre. Local currents conduct the impulse from node to node. The action potential is regenerated at each node of Ranvier. (From Hinchliff S E, Montague S E 1990, with permission.)

communication between cells is extremely rapid. They synchronise interconnected neurons and are rare in the adult but much more common in the embryo, gradually being replaced by chemical synapses. They are responsible for stereotypical movements such as the jerky movements of the eyes. They remain abundant in some nervous tissues such as cardiac and smooth muscle.

Chemical synapses

Between the neuron and its target cell the synaptic cleft is a fluid-filled space into which NTs are released from the presynaptic membrane. These open and shut ion channels in the postsynaptic membrane. The electrical message of the action potential is conducted chemically across the gap. This is a reversible change and the NT is removed. Enzymes that degrade the NT are released into the synaptic cleft; the NT is taken up by the presynaptic membrane and then diffuses away from the synapse.

Neurotransmitters

Neurotransmitters (NTs) help neurons to communicate messages and regulate body activities and states (Marieb 2008). Over 100 different chemicals act as NTs and they are classified according to chemical structure. They are synthesised with the help of enzymes.

Acetylcholine

Acetylcholine (ACh) was the first NT to be identified. It is the NT released at neuromuscular junctions and is accessible for study. ACh is also found in the CNS.

ACh is synthesised and stored within synaptic vesicles in the presence of the enzyme **choline acetyltransferase**. Acetic acid is bound to coenzyme A to form **acetyl CoA**. This compound combines with choline and the coenzyme is released:

Choline acetyltransferase

$$Acetyl\ CoA + choline \rightarrow ACh + CoA$$

The released ACh binds to the postsynaptic membrane and is degraded to acetic acid and choline by the enzyme acetylcholinesterase (AChE). The released choline is captured by the presynaptic membrane and used to synthesise more ACh.

The biogenic amines

Biogenic amines include **catecholamines** such as **dopamine** and **noradrenaline** (norepinephrine) and **adrenaline** (epinephrine) and the **indolamines serotonin** (5-hydroxytryptamine, 5-HT) and **histamine**. Catecholamines are synthesised from the amino acid **tyrosine** in a common pathway. Neurons produce only the enzymes that control the steps for the NT they need. The common pathway is:

$$Tyrosine \rightarrow L\text{-}Dopa$$
$$\rightarrow Dopamine \rightarrow Noradrenaline \rightarrow Adrenaline$$

NTs are widely distributed in the brain and are involved in emotional behaviour and in regulation of the body clock. Catecholamines, especially noradrenaline, are released by some motor neurons of the ANS. Serotonin is synthesised from tyrosine by a different pathway. Histamine is synthesised from the amino acid histidine.

Amino acids

The most important amino acids involved in neurotransmission are **γ-aminobutyric acid (GABA)** and **glutamate**.

Peptides

The **neuropeptides** include any molecules with diverse effects. These include the **endorphins** and **encephalins** involved in pain perception (Ch. 38).

The brain

During the course of evolution there has been increasing elaboration of the brain, reaching its greatest complexity in humans. The average adult brain weighs 1500 g and is slightly heavier in men than in women. However, this extra size does not influence function. Although the brain is described as a single organ (Figs 26.7, 26.8), individual parts perform discrete functions. The brain can be subdivided into four main parts:

1. The cerebral hemispheres.
2. The diencephalon, comprising the thalamus and hypothalamus.
3. The brainstem comprising the midbrain, pons and medulla.
4. The cerebellum.

The cerebral hemispheres

The two **cerebral hemispheres** form 85% of the weight of the brain and sit like an umbrella over the **diencephalon** and **brainstem**. The neurons have their cell bodies outermost forming the **grey matter** or cortex and their fibres innermost forming the **white matter**. The cortex is thrown into elevated ridges called **gyri** which are separated by shallow grooves called **sulci**. This vastly increases the surface area of the cerebral cortex and most of it is hidden from view in the walls

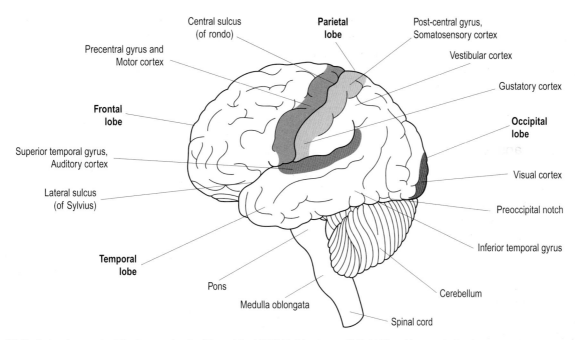

Figure 26.7 • Lateral aspect of the human brain. (From Hinchliff S E, Montague S E 1990, with permission.)

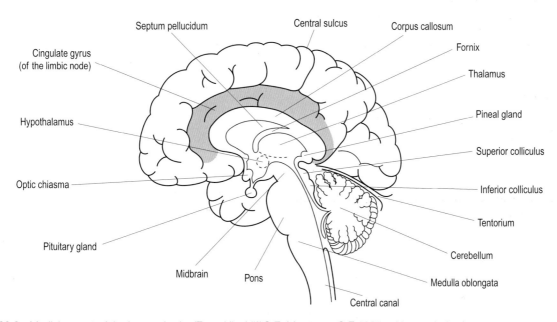

Figure 26.8 • Medial aspect of the human brain. (From Hinchliff S E, Montague S E 1990, with permission.)

of the sulci. The deepest grooves are called **fissures** and form important landmarks. There is a midline longitudinal fissure—the **midline sagittal fissure**—and **the transverse fissure** separates the cerebral hemispheres from the cerebellum.

Each hemisphere is divided into six main lobes. Four of these are the frontal, parietal, occipital and temporal lobes. The other two lobes are buried in the hemispheres and are the **insula**, revealed if the frontal and temporal lobes are eased apart and the **limbic lobe**,

which can be seen if the brain is divided along the mid-sagittal fissure.

The cerebral cortex

Structure

The cerebral cortex is also called the pallium (shell) and varies in thickness from 2 to 4 mm. It has a good blood supply via a dense capillary bed. The cortex contains about 50 billion neurons and is arranged in both a **laminar** (layered) and a **columnar** manner. There are three basic cell types: pyramidal cells, spiny stellate cells and smooth stellate cells. (There is an excellent chapter on the cerebral cortex in Fitzgerald et al 2006.)

- Pyramidal cells range in diameter from 20 to 30 µm in laminae II and III (see below) to 60 µm in lamina V. Very tall cells called **giant cells of Betz** situated in the motor cortex are 80–100 µm in diameter. All pyramidal cells are excitatory and use **glutamate** as their neurotransmitter.
- Spiny stellate cells have spiny dendrites and are mainly excitatory. They receive most of the afferent input from the thalamus and form glutamatergic synapses on pyramidal cells.
- Smooth stellate cells have non-spiny dendrites and are inhibitory. They receive collateral branches from pyramidal cells and form GABAergic synapses on other pyramidal cells.

The laminae

In the neocortex which forms 90% of the brain there are six well-organised laminae. These are:

1. The molecular layer contains the tips of the apical dendrites of pyramidal cells.
2. The outer granular layer contains small pyramidal and stellate cells.
3. The outer pyramidal layer contains medium-sized pyramidal cells and stellate cells.
4. The inner granular layer contains stellate cells receiving afferents from the thalami.
5. The inner pyramidal layer contains large pyramidal cells which project to the corpus striatum, brainstem and spinal cord.
6. The fusiform layer contains modified pyramidal cells which project to the thalamus.

Columnar organisation

The neurons have been found to be arranged functionally in columns of 50–100 µm in diameter. These columns only respond to very specific stimuli from very specific body areas. They are the functional units or modules of the cortex.

Function

The **cerebral cortex** enables conscious behaviour such as perception, communication, memory, understanding, appreciation and initiation of voluntary movements. It can be divided into three functional areas:

1. The **primary sensory area**, which receives stimuli from the periphery of the body.

2. The **primary motor area**, which sends out impulses to control the periphery.

3. The **association areas**.

Sensory areas are posterior and motor areas are anterior to the central sulcus. This same arrangement occurs in the spinal cord columns with sensory fibres posterior and motor areas anterior.

The association areas integrate diverse information to allow appropriate actions to be taken. These include the **prefrontal cortex** concerned with intellect, the **diffuse gnostic area** which contributes memory of sensation and emotional response and the two main **language areas**, Broca's and Wernicke's areas, usually in the left hemisphere.

Prefrontal cortex

The prefrontal cortex is concerned with higher mental functions such as abstract thinking, decision-making, social behaviour and anticipating the effects of actions. It has two-way connections with the cortex on the same side of the brain (**ipsilateral**), except the primary motor and sensory areas, the cortex on the opposite side of the brain (**contralateral**), the thalamus and the hypothalamus (Fitzgerald et al 2006).

Sensory cortex

Thalamic nerve fibres project to the sensory areas of the cerebral cortex. Nerves coming into the spinal cord from the body's periphery maintain **somatic organisation** so that a representation of the body is organised in the sensory cortex. The size of an area of sensory cortex given over to receiving input from the body depends on its innervation. This results in a peculiarly shaped **homunculus** represented upside down in the sensory cortex. Sensitive parts such as the tongue, lips, fingers and toes are represented as very large!

The control of movement

Motor cortex

Movement of the body by the skeletal muscles is controlled by input from the nervous system. Motor control can be divided into three neural systems:

1. The **pyramidal system**, a fast and usually direct descending pathway from the cortex.

2. The **extrapyramidal system** with multiple synapses involving many brain structures of which the basal ganglia are the most important.

3. The **cerebellum**.

The extrapyramidal system is very important and the intention to act is developed by the integration of widespread neural impulses. Efferent fibres from the motor cortex project to the **basal ganglia**, the **thalamus**, the **red nucleus**, the **lateral reticular formation** and the **spinal cord** in a topographically organised manner. The red nucleus lies between the substantia nigra and the aqueduct of Sylvius. It is oval-shaped and involved in the control of limb flexion.

The basal ganglia

The basal ganglia are the most important structure in the extrapyramidal system. They consist of large nuclei lying laterally to the thalamus. These are the **globus pallidus**, the **pars compacta** (including the **substantia nigra**) and the **striatum** (including the **caudate nucleus** and the **putamen**), which is the largest subcortical mass of cells in the brain. Motor activity is strongly influenced by the basal ganglia which constitute the main extrapyramidal control. Four circuits have been demonstrated (Fitzgerald et al 2006):

1. A motor loop concerned with learned movements.
2. A cognitive loop concerned with motor intentions.
3. A limbic loop concerned with the emotional aspects of movement.
4. An oculomotor loop concerned with voluntary saccades.

The cerebellum

This large brain structure lies beneath the occipital lobes and is separated from them by a fold of dura mater called the tentorium cerebelli. The **cerebellum** is bilaterally symmetrical, divided by a midline structure called the **vermis**. There are no interhemispheric nerve fibres so that messages are not relayed between the two halves. The cerebellum monitors the strength and execution of movements and therefore motor coordination using incoming sensory stimuli. Its function is entirely inhibitory and controlled by the NT GABA.

The limbic system

The **limbic system** consists of nuclei and fibres located on the medial aspect of each cerebral hemisphere. Its structures encircle the upper part of the brainstem (limbus means ring) and include the **cingulate gyrus**, the **parahippocampal gyrus**, the **hippocampus** and the **amygdala**, the **hypothalamus**, part of the **thalamus**, the **insula** and the **septum**. It is closely related to the **reticular formation**. Its function is concerned with emotional (affective) feelings. The limbic system interacts with higher brain centres and facilitates a close relationship between cognition and emotion. All the 'Trekkies' out there should wonder about Mr Spock's limbic system and the limitations of logic without emotions!

The cingulate gyrus

The cingulate gyrus involves part of the cortex and part of the limbic system. A bundle of fibres form a neural network interconnecting parts of the limbic lobe. The cingulate gyrus receives fibres from the parahippocampal gyrus, the temporal lobe, the thalamus and visual and tactile areas of the cortex. Its function is the emotional interpretation of pain and vision.

The hippocampus

The hippocampus is situated in the temporal lobe, has a complex three-dimensional trumpet shape and is called **Ammon's horn**. It communicates with the **neocortex**, the thalamus and other subcortical regions. Its functions include memory, learning, spatial awareness and cognitive mapping. In London taxi drivers their hippocampi were found to be enlarged significantly whilst they were 'doing the knowledge' (i.e. learning the routes).

The amygdala

The amygdalae (Greek for almond) are a group of paired nuclei in the temporal lobes. They are the focal point between incoming sensory systems and outgoing effector systems responsible for emotion and are linked to all sensory association areas of the cortex. They seem to be involved in the strength of emotion, especially in childhood and memories without hippocampal input may be laid down. Irrational states of fear such as phobias and anxiety states with no conscious recall of why the fear is felt are generated, including the physiological reactions of flight or fight (Fitzgerald et al 2006).

The hypothalamus

This structure is involved in homeostasis and survival. Despite its small size—it weighs only 4 g—the hypothalamus contains centres involved in the regulation of food intake, water intake, sleep–wake cycles, sexual behaviour and defence against attack. The hypothalamus controls the output of anterior pituitary hormones by producing releasing and inhibiting factors. It secretes the posterior pituitary hormones antidiuretic hormone and oxytocin directly.

The thalamus

The thalamus is the largest nuclear mass in the nervous system and consists of a pair of organs joined in the midline of the centre of the brain. It has been likened to a traffic conductor. The thalami contain multiple nuclei, each with a specific function. These include hearing, vision, memory, cognition, judgement and mood. There are multiple projections to the cortex and the structure is continuous with the reticular formation.

The insula

The insula lies deep within the brain. The **anterior insula** is a cortical centre for pain. The **posterior insula** is continuous with the **entorrhinal cortex** and the amygdala and may be involved in emotional response to pain. The **central region** is continuous with the frontoparietal and temporal cortex and may have a language rather than a limbic function (Fitzgerald et al 2006).

The septum

The connections of the septum lie central to the brain. Fibres are received from the amygdala, olfactory tract, hippocampus and brainstem. Fibres from the septum connect with the hypothalamus, brainstem and hippocampus. The septum controls sensations of pleasure and well-being and is also involved in memory.

The medulla oblongata and pons

The **medulla oblongata** is the conical-shaped lower part of the brainstem that blends into the spinal cord at the level of the **foramen magnum**. The central canal of the spinal cord broadens out in the medulla to form the **fourth ventricle**. The medulla functions as an **autonomic reflex centre**, maintaining homeostasis. Its nuclei include the **cardiac**, **vasomotor** and **respiratory centres** and nuclei that control vomiting, swallowing, coughing and sneezing.

The **pons** forms a bulbous structure between the medulla and midbrain and acts as part of the anterior wall of the **third ventricle**. It is a bridge of nerve fibres running between the spinal cord and higher brain centres. The transverse fibres of the pons belong to the giant **corticopontocerebellar pathway** which runs from one cerebral cortex to the contralateral cerebellar hemisphere.

The reticular formation

The reticular formation (RF) is an old part of the brain, sometimes called the **reptilian brain**. It is important in autonomic and reflex activities. It extends through the medulla, pons and midbrain and is closely related to the olfactory and limbic systems. Its neurons have long, branching dendrites and its fibres run in three columns: the main column or midline raphe, the medial nuclear group and the lateral nuclear group.

The part of the RF that makes multiple synapses throughout the brainstem is called the **reticular activating system (RAS)** which is involved in the level of consciousness, alertness and the sleep–wake cycle (Box 26.1). RF neurons maintain homeostasis by controlling the cardiac, vasomotor, respiratory, vomiting, swallowing, coughing and sneezing centres in the medulla.

The following summary of RS functions demonstrates its links to other brain centres (Fitzgerald et al 2006):

- Pattern generation and patterned cranial nerve activities.
- Posture and locomotion.
- Salivation and lacrimation.
- Bladder control.
- Involvement in circulation, respiration and blood pressure control.
- Conveys both somatic and visceral sensory information to the cerebellum.
- Sleeping and waking, attention, mood and arousal.

Protection of the brain

Nervous tissue is very delicate and neurons can be injured by even a slight pressure. Outwardly, the brain is protected by the bony skull and the **three meninges** (Ch. 24).

The ventricles

Four fluid-filled ventricles help to cushion and protect the brain (Fig. 26.9): the two **lateral ventricles** and the **third** and **fourth ventricles**. The ventricles are continuous with each other and with the central canal of the spinal cord via the aqueduct of Sylvius. The hollow chambers are filled with **cerebrospinal fluid** (CSF) and lined by ependymal cells. Three apertures in the wall of the fourth ventricle connect the ventricles to the fluid-filled subarachnoid space (Ch. 24) surrounding the brain.

Tufts of capillaries called **choroid plexi** hang from the roof of each ventricle and manufacture CSF, which moves freely though the ventricles and into the central canal of the spinal cord (Fig. 26.10). Most of the CSF enters the **subarachnoid space**, bathing the outer surface of the brain and spinal cord and returning to the blood via the **arachnoid** villi to the **dural sinuses**. An obstruction to the flow will result in CSF accumulating in the ventricles and putting pressure on the brain. In a neonate the skull bones are not fused and a collection of fluid in the ventricles causes skull enlargement (**hydrocephalus**).

The blood–brain barrier

The blood–brain barrier ensures that the brain's internal environment remains stable by providing a chemically optimum environment for neuronal function (Fitzgerald et al 2006). It selectively allows substances needed by the brain such as glucose, amino acids and some electrolytes to cross by facilitated diffusion while keeping toxic chemicals within the capillary network. In other body regions, extracellular concentrations of hormones, amino acids and other substances are in constant flux. If the brain was exposed to these variations, neurons would fire uncontrollably, as many of the substances act

BOX 26.1 THE SLEEP–WAKE CYCLE

Conscious awareness allows the nervous system to interact deliberately with the environment. The neural processes that underlie altered states of consciousness, even the sleep–wake cycle, are not well understood. Dark and light cycles (circadian rhythms) are known to play a role in the sleep-wake cycle. Waterhouse & Minors (1991) wrote that, left to it own devices, the body clock will complete its cycle in a period of about, but not exactly, 24 h. However, in our everyday life, environmental cues called **zeitgeibers** synchronise the clock with the 24 h solar cycle. Zeitgeibers include light, social activity and diet.

Sleep is a complex phenomenon defined as 'unconsciousness from which a person can be aroused by sensory or other stimuli' (Guyton & Hall 2006). The pattern of sleep has been studied by measuring the electrical activity of the brain by means of an electroencephalogram (ECG). Characteristic patterns in the electrical activity of cerebral cortical neurons accompany varying levels of consciousness.

Areas of the brain are involved in sleep, one of which is the raphe nuclei in the pons and medulla. Fibres from raphe cells spread locally in the brainstem reticular formation to the thalamus, hypothalamus and limbic system as well as the cortex. The NTs serotonin (stimulates waking) and acetylcholine (helps in sleep onset) as well as other substances may be involved in causing sleep.

Normal sleep consists of two types: slow-wave sleep and rapid eye movement (REM) sleep, also called paradoxical sleep or desynchronised sleep. In the normal waking state there are rapid, low-amplitude waves while the onset of sleep is accompanied by slow, high-amplitude waves due to the synchronisation of many neurons (slow-wave sleep). This lasts for about 90 min before being replaced by REM sleep when dreams occur. These two phases alternate several times during a normal night's sleep. In a phase of REM sleep which lasts 5–30 min several characteristics are seen (Guyton & Hall 2006):

- It is associated with active dreaming and active body muscle movements.
- The person is more difficult to arouse but they usually awake spontaneously from REM sleep.
- Muscle tone throughout the body is severely depressed indicating inhibition of spinal muscle control areas.
- Heart and respiratory rates become irregular when a person dreams.
- Despite inhibition of the peripheral muscles, irregular muscle movements occur.
- The brain is highly active and overall brain metabolism may be increased by as much as 20%. EEG brain waves are similar to those of wakefulness which is the source of the name paradoxical sleep.

Sleep may have two purposes: it may be restorative, a necessary part of replenishing energy and restoring tissues; or it may be protective to ensure safety for a daytime species relying on sight by limiting activity during darkness. REM sleep may allow the integration of the day's events into long-term memory, promoting learning, species-typical reprogramming or brain development.

---

as NTs, especially potassium. Blood-borne substances within the brain's capillaries are separated from the extracellular space and neurons by:

- A continuous endothelial capillary wall with tight junctions.
- A thick basal lamina surrounding the external face of the capillary.
- The bulbous feet of astrocytes clinging to the capillaries and signalling them to keep tight junctions.

The cranial nerves

Twelve pairs of cranial nerves are associated with the brain and pass through formina in the skull. The first two pairs originate from the forebrain and the rest are in the brainstem. The cranial nerves are:

- I: olfactory, concerned with the sense of smell.
- II: optic, concerned with vision.
- III: oculomotor, moves four of the external muscles of the eye.
- IV: trochlear, also innervates an extrinsic eye muscle.
- V: trigeminal, supplies facial sensory fibres and motor fibres for chewing muscles.
- VI: abducens, controls the extrinsic muscle that turns the eyeball laterally.
- VII: facial, innervates the muscles of facial expression.
- VIII: vestibulocochlear, the sensory nerve for hearing and balance.

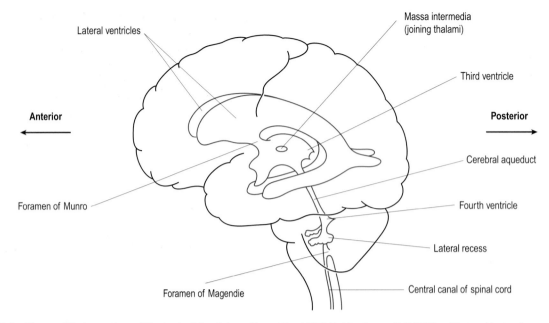

Lateral ventricles

Massa intermedia
(joining thalami)

Third ventricle

Anterior

Posterior

Cerebral aqueduct

Foramen of Munro

Fourth ventricle

Lateral recess

Central canal of spinal cord

Foramen of Magendie

Figure 26.9 • The ventricular system of the brain, lateral view. (From Hinchliff S E, Montague S E 1990, with permission.)

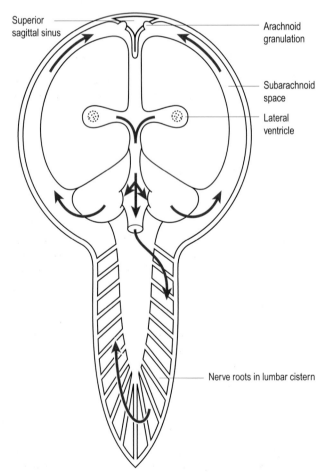

Superior
sagittal sinus

Arachnoid
granulation

Subarachnoid
space

Lateral
ventricle

Nerve roots in lumbar cistern

Figure 26.10 • Circulation of cerebrospinal fluid. (From Fitzgerald M T J 1996, with permission.)

- IX: glossopharyngeal, innervates the tongue and pharynx.
- X: vagus nerve, innervates thoracic and abdominal viscera.
- XI: accessory, helps the vagus nerve.
- XII: hypoglossal innervates the tongue moving muscle.

The spinal cord

Knowledge of spinal cord anatomy is important because of the use of epidural analgesia in childbirth (Ch. 38). The spinal cord is enclosed within the vertebral column and extends from the **foramen magnum** of the skull to the level of the first **lumbar vertebra**. It is about 48 cm long and 1.8 cm thick and carries ascending and descending nerve pathways (Fig. 26.11). There are spinal cord enlargements in the **cervical** and **lumbosacral regions** where the nerves supplying the limbs arise (Fitzgerald et al 2006).

Like the brain, the spinal cord is protected by bone, CSF and meninges. The dura mater is a single layer only and is unattached to the bony walls of the vertebral column. Between the bones and the dural sheath is the **epidural space** filled with fat and blood vessels. The subarachnoid space between the pia and arachnoid maters is filled with CSF. The dura and the arachnoid mater extend beyond the end of the spinal cord to the second sacral vertebra.

The spinal nerves

Thirty-one pairs of spinal nerves arise from the cord and leave the vertebral column by the **intervertebral foramina**

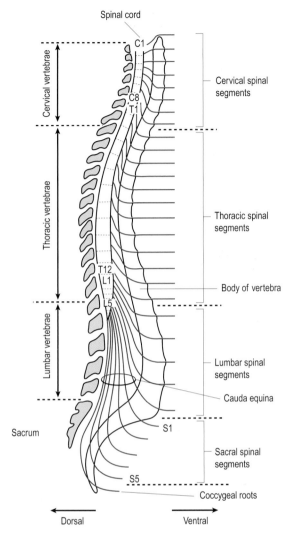

Figure 26.11 • The relationship between the spinal cord and the vertebral column. (From Hinchliff S E, Montague S E 1990, with permission.)

to target specific body areas (Fitzgerald et al 2006). Each segment of the segmented spinal cord is defined by a pair of spinal nerves. Each conducts sensory information from a specific body area called a **dermatome** (Fig. 26.12).

Inferiorly, the spinal cord ends in a cone-shaped structure, the **conus medullaris**, and nerve roots fan outwards and downwards to exit through relevant vertebrae. This collection of nerve roots is called the **cauda equinae** (horse's tail). A fibrous extension of the pia, the **filum terminale**, runs downwards to attach to the posterior surface of the coccyx.

A cross-section of the spinal cord

The grey matter and spinal roots

The grey matter of the cord consists of neuronal cell bodies, their unmyelinated processes and neuroglia. It is central to the white matter and looks like a letter H. There are two posterior or dorsal horns which contain interneurons and two anterior or ventral horns which house the cell bodies of somatic motor neurons (Fig. 26.13). The ventral roots of the spinal cord contain somatic motor neuron axons on their way to skeletal muscles. Afferent fibres of the peripheral sensory nerves form the dorsal roots of the spinal cord. Their cell bodies are in the dorsal root ganglion, an enlargement of the dorsal root. The dorsal and ventral roots are short and fuse to form the spinal nerves.

The white matter

The white matter of the spinal cord is composed of myelinated and unmyelinated nerve fibres running in three directions:

1. Ascending tracts of sensory inputs going to the higher centres.

2. Descending tracts of motor outputs coming from the brain.

3. Across from one side of the spinal cord to the other.

These will be discussed in detail in Chapter 27.

Adaptation to pregnancy

During pregnancy the following short list of changes can occur, mainly due to altered output from the endocrine system:

• Musculoskeletal discomforts.
• Sleep disturbances.
• Alterations in sensation.

The central nervous system

Pregnancy hormones affect the CNS but the phenomenon is not well understood. Women often report that their cognitive abilities diminish in pregnancy, with difficulty in concentration and poor memory being top of the list. Oatridge et al (2002) found that a woman's brain shrinks during pregnancy and returns to normal by 6 months following delivery. The amount of change seen was significantly more in pre-eclamptic women. The mechanism and physiological importance of these findings are not known as yet.

Sleep

Sleep patterns change during pregnancy and in the postpartum period. From about 25 weeks the pregnant woman experiences more REM sleep which decreases to non-pregnant levels by term. There is a corresponding

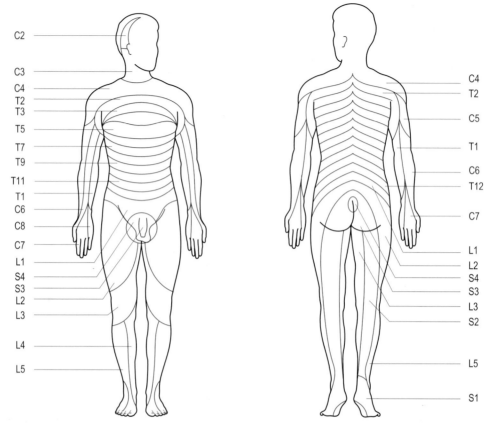

Figure 26.12 • Adult dermatome pattern. (From Fitzgerald M T J 1996, with permission.)

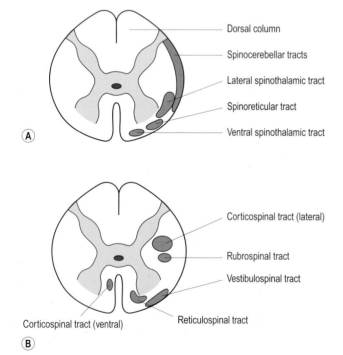

Figure 26.13 • Major nerve tracts of the spinal cord.
(A) Ascending nerve tracts. (B) Descending nerve tracts. (From Hinchliff S E, Montague S E 1990, with permission.)

decrease in slow-wave sleep which returns to normal immediately after delivery. During the first trimester sleep time and napping both increase but later night wakening occurs because of nocturia, dyspnoea, heartburn, nasal congestion, muscle aches and anxiety (Peterson 2008). In late pregnancy many factors contribute to poor sleep such as full bladder, muscle discomfort and anxiety.

Alterations in sensation

Changes in the ear, nose and larynx occur because of changes in fluid dynamics and vascular permeability. This is related to the increase in circulating oestrogen. Congestion and hyperaemia of the nasal mucosa causes nasal stuffiness and rhinorrhoea which may lead to nose bleeds or to loss of sleep. Laryngeal changes may result in voice changes or persistent cough.

The perceptions of smell and taste are closely related and a reduction in the sense of smell may lead to altered taste sensations and a change in food preference. There may also be nausea and food aversions, especially for foods that taste bitter. Profet (1992) believes these aversions are protective as bitter foods are often poisonous or teratogenic.

Main points

- The central nervous system receives messages from and sends messages via the peripheral nervous system to all parts of the body. It communicates by rapid transmission of electrical signals.
- The autonomic nervous system innervates smooth muscle and glands of the viscera and cardiac muscle. It is subdivided into the sympathetic and parasympathetic systems.
- Nervous tissue consists of neurons and the neuroglia which provide their support and protection. Neurons have axons and dendrites which communicate with other cells by nerve impulses and neurotransmitters.
- Large nerve fibres are covered in a myelin sheath which protects and insulates fibres and increases impulse transmission rate to up to 100 times more than unmyelinated fibres. Axons from single neurons are bound together to form nerves.
- Nerve electrical activity is maintained by the distribution and relative concentration of negative and positive ions. Neurotransmitters are released from the presynaptic membrane into the synaptic cleft.
- The brain weighs about 1500 g and can be subdivided into the cerebral hemispheres, the diencephalon (thalamus and hypothalamus), the brainstem (midbrain, pons and medulla oblongata) and the cerebellum.
- Each cerebral hemisphere is divided into frontal, parietal, occipital, temporal lobes, the insula and the limbic lobes. The cerebral cortex is divided into the primary sensory area, the primary motor area and the association areas.
- Nerves entering the spinal cord from the periphery maintain their somatotopic organisation so that the body is faithfully represented via the thalamus to the sensory cortex.
- The limbic system is concerned with emotional feelings and it links with higher brain centres forming a close relationship between cognition and emotion.
- The hypothalamus is involved in homeostasis and survival. It controls the output of anterior pituitary hormones by producing releasing and inhibiting factors but secretes posterior pituitary hormones directly.
- Functions of the thalamic nuclei include hearing, vision, memory, cognition, judgement and mood. The insula is involved in olfaction, taste and autonomic reflexes. The functions of the septum are sensations of pleasure and well-being and memory.
- The medulla oblongata maintains homeostasis. Its nuclei include the cardiac, vasomotor and respiratory centres and nuclei that control vomiting, swallowing, coughing and sneezing. The pons is a bridge formed of nerve fibres running between spinal cord and higher brain centres.
- The reticular formation is involved in the level of consciousness and alertness. Conscious awareness allows the nervous system to interact with the environment. Sleep may be restorative or it may ensure safety for a daytime species by limiting activity during darkness.
- The pia, arachnoid and dura mater protect the brain and spinal cord, protect blood vessels, enclose venous sinuses and contain CSF. Folds in the dura include the falx cerebri and the tentorium cerebelli.
- The four ventricles are filled with CSF and are continuous with each other and with the central canal of the spinal cord via the aqueduct of Sylvius. Their choroid plexi form the CSF.
- The blood–brain barrier ensures that the brain's internal environment remains stable. It is selective and substances needed by the brain cross over by facilitated diffusion whilst toxic chemicals are kept within the capillaries.
- Twelve pairs of cranial nerves pass through foramina in the skull. The first two pairs arise in the forebrain and the rest in the brainstem. All but the vagus nerve target structures in the head and neck.
- The spinal cord carries ascending and descending nerve pathways. The vertebral column is divided into segments and each segment conducts sensory information from a specific body part called a dermatome.
- Inferiorly the spinal cord ends in the conus medullaris and a collection of nerve roots called the cauda equina fan outwards and downwards to attach to the posterior surface of the coccyx.
- The grey matter of the spinal cord is central to its white matter and is H-shaped with two posterior horns and two anterior horns. The white matter is composed of nerve fibres running in three directions: ascending tracts, descending tracts and across from one side of the spinal cord to the other.
- Musculoskeletal discomforts, sleep disturbances and alterations in sensation such as smell and taste occur in pregnancy. Women report difficulty in concentration and poor memory. Research shows that the brain shrinks during pregnancy but returns to normal within 6 months postpartum. Congestion and hyperaemia of the nasal mucosa cause nasal stuffiness and rhinorrhoea which may lead to nose bleeds and sleep loss.

References

Fitzgerald, M.J., Gruener, G., Mtui, E., 2006. Clinical Neuroanatomy and Neuroscience, fifth edn. Elsevier, Saunders.

Guyton, A.C., Hall, J.E., 2006. Textbook of Medical Physiology, eleventh edn. Elsevier, Saunders.

Marieb, E.N., 2008. Essentials of Human Anatomy and Physiology, nineth edn. Benjamin/Cummings, New York.

Oatridge, A., Holdcroft, A., Saeed, N., et al., 2002. Change in brain size during and after pregnancy: study in healthy women and women with preeclampsia. Am. J. Neuroradiol. 23, 19–26.

Peterson, E.A., 2008. Pregnancy and Sleep: A Contradiction in Terms? EBSCO Publishing, Ipswich, MA.

Profet, M., 1992. Pregnancy sickness as adaptation: A deterrent to maternal ingestion of teratogens. In: Barkow, J., Cosmides, L., Tooby, J. (Eds.), The Adapted Mind: Evolutionary Psychology and the Generation of Culture. Oxford University Press, New York, pp. 327–365.

Waterhouse, J.M., Minors, D.S., 1991. Your Body Clock. Oxford Paperbacks.

Annotated recommended reading

Fitzgerald, M.J., Gruener, G., Mtui, E., 2007. Clinical Neuroanatomy and Neuroscience, fifth edn. Elsevier, Saunders.

This is a very well laid out and detailed but easy-to-read textbook on the human nervous system. The format is full of interesting diagrams and the headings make the book content easy to find and follow.

Marieb, E.N., 2008. Essentials of Human Anatomy and Physiology, nineth edn. Benjamin/Cummings, New York.

This is still, in my opinion, one of the best general anatomy and physiology textbooks for the student of nursing and midwifery. Although not applied to reproduction in any depth, it has extremely succinct and easy-to-follow explanations on the anatomy and physiology of the nervous system.

Oatridge, A., Holdcroft, A., Saeed, N., et al., 2002. Change in brain size during and after pregnancy: Study in healthy women and women with preeclampsia. Am. J. Neuroradiol. 23, 19–26.

This concise but well-researched article concerning this interesting physiological phenomenon is worth obtaining for the information about a poorly understood occurrence.

Chapter Twenty-Seven

27

The peripheral and autonomic nervous systems

CHAPTER CONTENTS

The peripheral nervous system

Introduction

The **peripheral nervous system** (PNS) detects changes in the body's external or internal environments. Sensory receptors code them into nerve impulses and pass the information back to the central nervous system (CNS) so that appropriate action can occur. Some messages are not passed to the brain; they influence reflex actions at the level of the spinal cord or brainstem. The PNS includes all the neural structures outside the brain and spinal cord (i.e. sensory receptors), peripheral nerves and associated ganglia and efferent motor endings (Marieb 2008). For ease of understanding of **nerve pathways** to the brain, the spinal cord columns are placed in this chapter.

Ascending sensory tracts

Categories of sensation

There are two kinds of sensation (Fig. 27.1): **conscious** sensations perceived at the level of the cortex and **non-conscious** sensations that are not. Conscious sensation can be divided into **exteroception** and **proprioception**. Exteroception involves messages from the outside world perceived in the cerebral cortex. Sensations may originate in body surface receptors or in telereceptors of the special senses such as vision or hearing. **Proprioceptors** in the locomotor system and the inner ear labyrinth inform the brain of the position when stationary (**position sense**) and during movement (**kinaesthetic sense**).

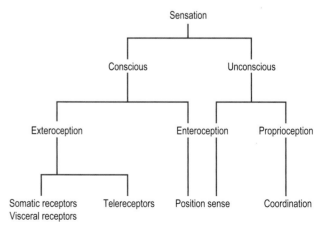

Figure 27.1 • Categories of sensation.

Non-conscious sensation can also be divided into two kinds: non-conscious proprioception, which affects the cerebellum, involving messages essential for smooth muscle coordination received through spinocerebellar pathways and the brainstem, and enteroception which refers to non-conscious signals from visceral reflexes (Fitzgerald et al 2006).

Somatic sensory perception

Two major pathways are involved in somatic perception sensations: the **posterior column–medial lemniscal pathway** and the **spinothalamic pathway** (Fig. 27.2). There are common features:

- They contain first-order, second-order and third-order sensory neurons.
- The cell bodies of the first-order neurons are in the posterior root ganglia.
- The cell bodies of the second-order neurons are on the same side of the CNS grey matter as the first-order neurons.
- Second-order axons cross the midline to ascend and terminate in the thalamus.

- Third-order neurons project to the somatosensory cortex.
- Both pathways are somatotopic, representing the body parts in an orderly fashion up to the sensory cortex.
- Both pathways can be modulated, either by inhibition or stimulation by other neurons.

The posterior column–medial lemniscal pathway

The first-order nerve fibres enter the dorsal columns of the spinal cord without synapsing. They are usually large **A fibres** with conduction velocities of about 70 metres per second (m/s). As nerve fibres from higher levels in the cord are added, they take up lateral positions so that the higher the level of origin is, the more lateral the position of the fibre in the column. The fibres of second-order neurons at the level of the brainstem cross the midline to be projected to the thalamus. Crossing over is why one side of the brain controls the opposite (contralateral) side of the body. Cells in the sensory relay nucleus of the thalamus are third-order neurons and project their fibres to the **somatosensory cortex**.

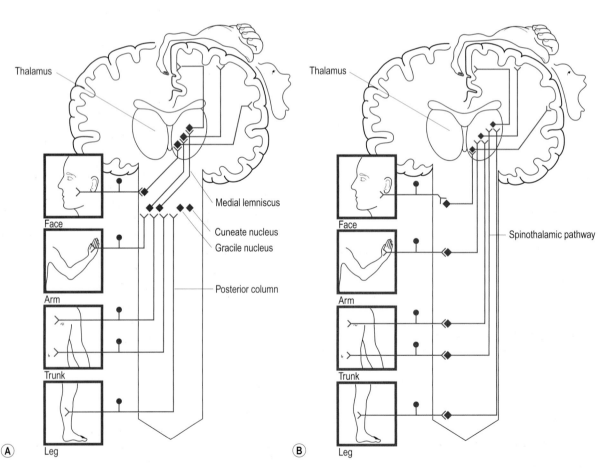

Figure 27.2 • Basic plans of (A) posterior column–medial lemniscal pathway, (B) spinothalamic pathway. (From Fitzgerald M J T 1996, with permission.)

The chief functions of this pathway are conscious proprioception and discriminatory touch. These provide the parietal lobe with an instantaneous body image of our position both at rest and when moving. Disturbances of this pathway cause demyelinating diseases such as multiple sclerosis.

The spinothalamic tract

The **dorsal root fibres** of this pathway tend to be the smaller **A-δ** or unmyelinated **C fibres** with slow conduction velocity. The dorsal root fibres enter the spinal cord and may ascend or descend a few segments before synapsing with cells of the dorsal horn in the **substantia gelatinosa**. The dorsal horn second-order fibres ascend or descend a few segments before crossing over the midline to ascend in the spinothalamic tract. These fibres terminate on thalamic third-order neurons whose fibres synapse on cells of the sensory cortex. The role of this pathway is the perception of heat, cold and touch on the opposite side of the body. The role of the substantia gelatinosa in the gate control theory of pain perception is discussed in Chapter 38.

Somatosensory receptors

Sensory receptors are mostly adapted nerve fibre endings that respond to environmental changes. Sensory afferent nerves arising from the body are grouped together as the somatosensory system and include sensation from the skin, muscles, joints and viscera. The special senses are associated with organs in the head and include vision, hearing, balance, taste and smell; they are not discussed in this book but a useful source is Marieb (2008).

Types of somatosensory receptors

- **Mechanoreceptors** respond to touch, pressure, vibrations and stretch.
- **Thermoreceptors** respond to temperature change.
- **Photoreceptors** respond to light.
- **Chemoreceptors** respond to smell, taste and changes in blood chemistry.
- **Nociceptors** respond to damage by causing pain (see Ch. 38).

Descending motor pathways

The descending tracts carry efferent messages from the brain down the spinal cord and are divided into four main pathways:

1. **Corticospinal** (pyramidal).
2. **Reticulospinal** (extrapyramidal).
3. **Vestibulospinal**.
4. **Tectospinal**.

The corticospinal tract

The corticospinal tract (Fig. 27.3) is the major motor pathway involved with voluntary movement. It contains about 1 million nerve fibres, more than 60% of which originate in the primary motor cortex. The tract descends through the internal capsule to the brainstem. It continues through the pons to the medulla oblongata where about 80% of the fibres **decussate** (cross over to the other side of the body). The fibres, which are arranged **somatotopically** (Fig. 27.4), synapse with interneurons or directly with anterior horn neurons.

The reticulospinal tract

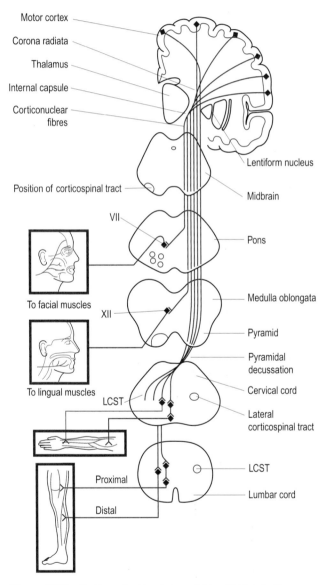

Figure 27.3 • Corticospinal tract viewed from the front. At spinal cord level, only the lateral corticospinal tract is shown. LCST, lateral corticospinal tract; VII, nucleus of facial nerve; XII, hypoglossal nucleus. (From Fitzgerald M J T 1996, with permission.)

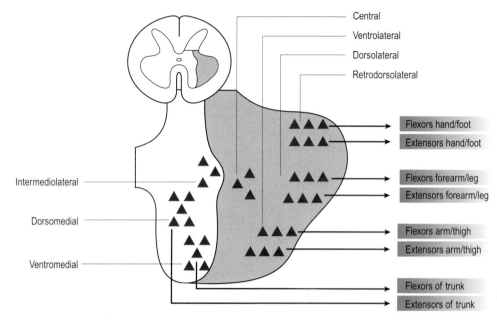

Figure 27.4 • Cell columns in the anterior grey horn of the spinal cord: somatotopic organisation. (From Fitzgerald M J T 1996, with permission.)

The reticulospinal tract is partially crossed and originates in the reticular formation of the pons and medulla. It is involved in two kinds of motor behaviour: locomotion, where it controls bilateral rhythmicity (try moving the arm and leg of the same side together when walking), and postural control.

The vestibulospinal tract

The vestibulospinal tract is an uncrossed paired pathway originating in the vestibular nucleus of the medulla oblongata. It maintains balance when the head is tilted to one side.

The tectospinal tract

The tectospinal tract is a crossed pathway descending from the tectum of the midbrain to the medial part of the anterior horn at cervical and upper thoracic levels. In reptiles it orients the head and trunk towards visual or auditory stimuli and may have a similar function in humans.

Upper and lower motor neurons

The neurons of the motor cortex are called the pyramidal cells because of the shape of their bodies. They are referred to as the upper motor neurons. The anterior horn neurons whose axons leave the cord to innervate skeletal muscles are called the lower motor neurons. Damage to upper motor neurons causes floppy paralysis with loss of tendon reflexes. Damage to lower motor neurons causes weakness and wasting of muscles. Motor neuron disease

is characterised by progressive degeneration of both upper and lower motor neurons (Fitzgerald et al 2006).

Reflex activity

A reflex is a rapid, predictable, unlearned, involuntary response to a stimulus. Some reflex activity is protective, such as rapid removal of the body from a noxious stimulus such as heat. Other reflexes which control visceral activities occur without any awareness of change. Some reflexes are learned, such as driving a car. Many reflexes can be modified by learning and conscious effort.

The reflex arc

Reflexes occur over specific neural paths called **reflex arcs** (Fig. 27.5) which have five main components:

1. The receptor at the site where the stimulus occurs.

2. The sensory neuron which takes the message to the CNS.

3. The integration centre within the CNS which may be a single synapse or may involve a chain of interneurons.

4. The motor neuron which conducts efferent impulses from the integration centre to an effector organ.

5. The effector which may be a gland or muscle fibre and acts to complete the reflex action. Reflexes may be somatic or autonomic. Somatic reflexes can be tested to confirm normal neural function.

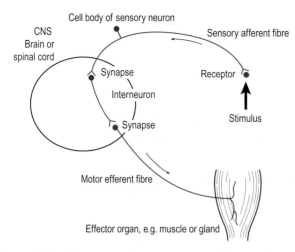

Figure 27.5 • The component structures of a reflex arc. (From Hinchliff S M, Montague S E 1990, with permission.)

Spinal reflexes

Many spinal reflexes occur with little or no brain input:

- Stretch and deep tendon reflexes, where the messages from the proprioceptors in the muscles and joints are transmitted to the cerebellum and cerebral cortex. These allow normal muscle tone and activity to be maintained.
- The flexor reflex, which causes automatic withdrawal from a painful stimulus.
- The crossed extensor reflex consists of an ipsilateral withdrawal reflex and a contralateral extensor reflex. These are important in maintaining balance.
- Superficial reflexes can be elicited by gentle stroking of the body. The best known are the plantar reflex with incurling of the toes in response to stroking the sole of the foot. Babinski's reflex with extension of the toes occurs in infants less than 1 year old. The abdominal reflex occurs when the skin on one side of the trunk is stroked.

The autonomic nervous system

The **autonomic** (self-regulating) system or ANS is responsible for maintaining the stability of the body's internal environment. ANS motor neurons innervate smooth muscle, cardiac muscle and glands, making adjustments to alter function in response to messages from the viscera sent to the CNS. Systemic changes brought about by the ANS include making adjustments to:

- Shunting of blood to needy areas.
- Heart rate.
- Blood pressure.
- Respiratory rate.
- Body temperature.
- Stomach secretions.

The role of the two divisions

There are differences between the somatic and autonomic nervous systems in their pathways and neurotransmitters (NTs). The ANS is divided into two arms: the sympathetic system (Fig. 27.6), which prepares the body for emergency action, and the parasympathetic system (Fig. 27.7), which counterbalances the sympathetic system and has a calming effect, allowing general body maintenance and the conservation of energy to occur. There is usually a dynamic interaction between the two systems maximising homeostasis.

The sympathetic nervous system

The sympathetic nervous system is so called because it acts in sympathy with the emotions. It is sometimes referred to as the 'fight or flight' system and is activated if we are excited or in a threatening situation. The heart and respiratory rates increase, the skin is cold and sweaty and the eye pupils dilate. Visceral blood vessels are constricted and digestion ceases. Blood is shunted to the heart and skeletal muscles and the liver releases glucose into the blood to provide cells with energy.

The parasympathetic nervous system

The parasympathetic division is active when the systems are unstressed. It has been called the 'resting and digesting' system and is active during digestion of food and elimination of waste. Blood pressure, heart and respiratory rates are low. The skin is warm as the skeletal muscles do not need extra blood supply. The eye pupils are constricted and the lenses adjusted for close vision.

Anatomy of the ANS

The motor unit of the ANS is a two-neuron chain:

- The first neuron is the **preganglionic neuron**. Its cell body is found in the brain or spinal column.
- The first neuron synapses with the second motor neuron or **postganglionic neuron** which has its cell body in the autonomic ganglion outside the CNS. The postganglionic neuron extends to the target tissue.

Preganglionic neurons are thin and lightly myelinated while postganglionic neurons are even thinner and unmyelinated. Both types of fibre may run with somatic nerves in spinal or cranial nerves.

Differences between the two divisions

- Parasympathetic fibres emerge from the brain and sacral spinal cord (craniosacral division) while sympathetic

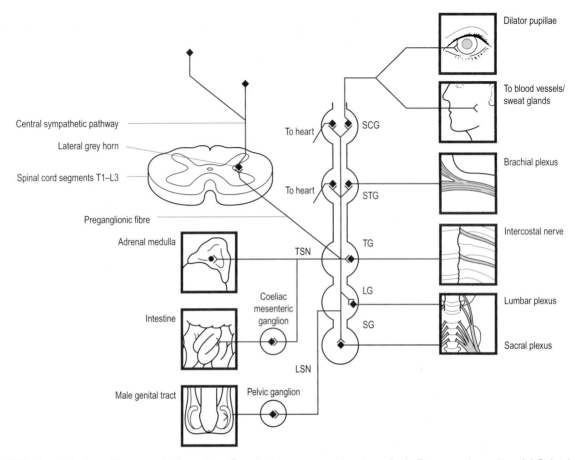

Figure 27.6 • General plan of the sympathetic system. Ganglionic neurons and postganglionic fibres are shown in red. LG, lumbar ganglia; LSN, lumbar splanchnic nerve; SCG, superior cervical ganglion; SG, sacral ganglia; STG, stellate ganglion; TG, thoracic ganglia; TSN, thoracic splanchnic nerve. (From Fitzgerald M J T 1996, with permission.)

fibres originate in the thoracolumbar region of the spinal cord.

- The parasympathetic division has long preganglionic fibres and short postganglionic fibres. The sympathetic division has short preganglionic fibres and long postganglionic fibres.
- Parasympathetic ganglia are located in terminal ganglia within or close to the target organs. Sympathetic ganglia lie close to the spinal cord.

Sympathetic division

The sympathetic division is more complex because it innervates more organs. Sympathetic activity tends to inhibit the activity of visceral organs, some body wall structures such as sweat glands and the smooth muscles, such as the hair-raising muscles (erector pili). All arteries and veins are innervated by sympathetic fibres.

Preganglionic fibres

Preganglionic fibres arise from cell bodies of neurons in the **thoracolumbar division** of the spinal cord segments T1–L2. The presence of these preganglionic sympathetic neurons produces the lateral horns (visceral motor horns of the spinal cord). The fibres leave the cord via the ventral root and pass through a myelinated white ramus communicans to enter the appropriate paravertebral (chain) ganglion which forms part of the sympathetic chain. Two sympathetic chains flank the spinal column. The fibres arising from the thoracolumbar region innervate 23 pairs of **ganglia** running from neck to pelvis:

- 3 cervical.
- 11 thoracic.
- 4 lumbar.
- 4 sacral.
- 1 coccygeal.

A preganglionic fibre reaching a paravertebral ganglion may:

- Synapse with postganglionic neuron in the same ganglion.
- Ascend or descend within the sympathetic chain to synapse in another ganglion.

Fibres from T5–L2 pass through the ganglion and emerge as preganglionic **splanchnic nerves** (Fitzgerald et al 2006).

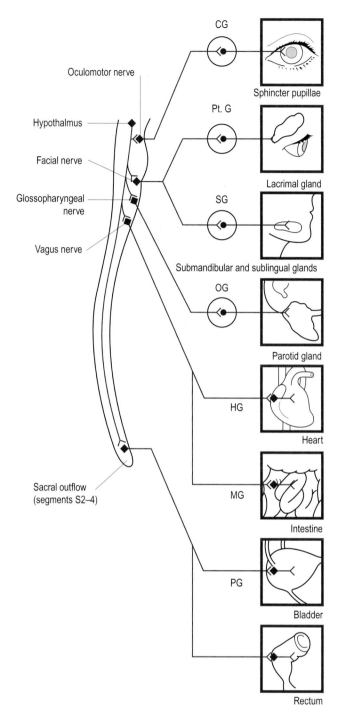

Table 27.1 Segmental sympathetic supply to the organs

Organ	Spinal cord segment
Head and neck + heart	T1–T5
Bronchi and lungs	T2–T4
Upper limb	T2–T5
Oesophagus	T5–T6
Stomach, spleen, pancreas	T6–T10
Liver	T7–T9
Small intestine	T9–T10
Kidney and reproductive organs	T10–L1
Lower limb	T10–L2
Large intestine, bladder, ureters	T11–L2

Figure 27.7 • General plan of the parasympathetic system. Ganglionic neurons and postganglionic fibres are shown in red. CG, ciliary ganglion; HG, heart ganglia; MG, myenteric ganglia; OG, otic ganglion; PG, pterygopalatine ganglion; SG, submandibular ganglia nerve. (From Fitzgerald M J T 1996, with permission.)

these, postganglionic fibres fan out to reach their target organs (Table 27.1).

Postganglionic fibres

From the synapse, postganglionic axons join the spinal nerves by non-myelinated branches called the **grey rami communicantes**. They are then distributed to sweat glands and smooth muscle of the hair roots and blood vessels. Some postganglionic fibres travelling in the thoracic splanchnic nerves synapse with the adrenal medullary cells and are stimulated to produce adrenaline (epinephrine) and noradrenaline (norepinephrine).

Parasympathetic division

The cranial outflow

Cranial parasympathetic preganglionic fibres run in several cranial nerves:

- Oculomotor nerve parasympathetic fibres innervate smooth muscle within the eye causing the pupils to constrict and the lenses to shorten and thicken for near vision.
- Facial nerve parasympathetic fibres stimulate large glands in the head: the lacrimal and nasal glands and the submandibular and sublingual salivary glands.
- Glossopharyngeal parasympathetic fibres activate the parotid salivary glands.
- Vagus nerve parasympathetic activity accounts for 90% of preganglionic nerve activity. Axons synapse on intramural (within walls) ganglia of target organs. Thoracic organs are the heart, lungs and oesophagus. Abdominal organs are the liver, stomach, small intestine, kidneys, pancreas and the proximal half of the large intestine.

The splanchnic nerves—thoracic, lumbar and sacral—contribute to **nerve plexi** such as the aortic abdominal plexus, the coeliac plexus, the superior and inferior mesenteric plexi and the hypogastric plexus. From

387

The sacral outflow

The sacral outflow arises from neurons in the lateral grey matter of sacral spinal cord segments S2–S4. Their axons run in the ventral roots of the spinal cord and branch off to form the splanchnic nerves which contribute to the inferior and hypogastric ganglia. Most postganglionic fibres synapse in intramural ganglia in the distal half of the large intestine, the urinary bladder, the ureters and the reproductive organs.

Visceral sensory neurons

Although the ANS is considered to be a motor system, there are **visceral pain afferents** in autonomic nerves which travel with somatic pain fibres. Visceral pain is caused by mechanisms such as inflammation, smooth muscle spasm, ischaemia and distension. It is usually vague and deep-seated and often accompanied by sweating and nausea. As it increases in severity, the pain perception is referred to the somatic structures innervated from the same embryonic segmental level (dermatome). Labour pains are referred to the sacral area of the back.

Physiology of the ANS

The terminal neurotransmitter (NT) differs between sympathetic and parasympathetic nerves. NTs are molecules which help neurons communicate messages and regulate body activities and states (Marieb 2008). The major NTs of the ANS are acetylcholine (ACh) and noradrenaline (norepinephrine).

ACh is released by all preganglionic axons and by the postganglionic axons of the parasympathetic system. ACh-releasing fibres are called **cholinergic fibres**. Most sympathetic postganglionic fibres release noradrenaline and are called **adrenergic fibres**. The exceptions to the rule are sympathetic postganglionic fibres innervating sweat glands, some skeletal muscle blood vessels and the external genitalia which release ACh. ACh and noradrenaline do not consistently produce excitation or inhibition on their target tissues. The response of visceral effectors depends on the type of receptor to which the NTs attach; there are at least two receptors for both NTs.

Cholinergic receptors

The two types of ACh-binding receptors are given names associated with the drugs that bind to them, mimicking their effects. They are **nicotinic receptors** to which nicotine binds, and **muscarinic receptors** (muscarine is a mushroom poison).

Site of nicotinic receptors

- Motor end plates of skeletal muscle cells (somatic targets).
- All postganglionic neurons, both sympathetic and parasympathetic.
- The hormone-producing cells of the adrenal medulla.

The effect of ACh binding to nicotinic receptors is always excitatory.

Site of muscarinic receptors

- All cells stimulated by postganglionic cholinergic fibres targeted by the parasympathetic system.
- A few sympathetic targets such as the sweat glands and some blood vessels of skeletal muscles.

The effect of ACh binding to muscarinic receptors may be excitatory or inhibitory depending on the target organ.

Adrenergic receptors

There are two major classes of adrenergic receptors: alpha (α) and beta (β). In general, adrenaline binding to α receptors is excitatory whilst binding to β receptors is inhibitory. There are medically important exceptions. Binding of adrenaline to β receptors of cardiac muscle induces vigorous activity in the heart. This is due to both α and β receptors having subclasses: α_1 and α_2, β_1 and β_2 (Marieb 2008).

Interactions of the autonomic divisions

Most visceral organs receive innervation from both sympathetic and parasympathetic fibres, i.e. dual innervation. If both divisions are partially active as is normal, a dynamic antagonism is present that allows precise control of visceral activity. Antagonistic effects are more easily seen on the activity of the heart, respiration and gastrointestinal organs, i.e. fight or flight versus rest and digest modes.

Sympathetic and parasympathetic tone

The vascular system is innervated by sympathetic fibres which control blood pressure, even at rest. The partial constriction of blood vessels maintaining vasomotor tone is under sympathetic control. If blood flow needs increasing, sympathetic impulses increase, vessels constrict and blood pressure rises. If bloods pressure needs decreasing, impulses decrease, smooth muscle relaxes and the vessels dilate. However, the heart, along with the gastrointestinal tract and urinary tract, is dominated by parasympathetic effects. The smooth muscles of these organs exhibit parasympathetic tone. The sympathetic division overrides this parasympathetic tone during stress.

Effects unique to the sympathetic division

Some physiological functions are not under parasympathetic influences and are controlled by the sympathetic division. These include:

- Control of the adrenal medulla.
- The sweat glands.
- The erector pili muscles.
- The production of rennin by the kidney.
- Thermoregulatory response to heat.
- Mobilisation of glucose and fats for fuel.

Control of autonomic functioning

Several levels in the CNS contribute to the regulation of the ANS. These include controls in the brainstem which can be modified by the hypothalamus and cerebral cortex.

Brainstem controls

Most sensory impulses that cause autonomic reflexes arrive in the brainstem via afferents from the vagus nerve. Centres in the medulla that are influenced include the cardiac, vasomotor and respiratory centres and those controlling gastrointestinal activities. Control of micturition and defecation are reflexes that can be overcome by conscious control.

Hypothalamic controls

Signals from the hypothalamus can affect the autonomic centres in the brainstem mentioned above. It coordinates heart activity, blood pressure, body temperature, water balance, endocrine activity, emotional states such as rage or pleasure and biological drives such as hunger and thirst. It can influence and be influenced by the higher cortical centres. The hypothalamus is the main integration centre for the ANS and the brainstem can be thought of as a relay station. Medial and anterior hypothalamic regions direct parasympathetic activities while the posterior and lateral areas direct sympathetic functions.

Cortical controls

Signals from the cerebrum can influence the activities of most of the brainstem autonomic control centres (Guyton & Hall 2006). The research area includes meditation, biofeedback, neuropsychoimmunity and psychosomatic illness (Sapolsky 2004).

Adaptation to pregnancy

Changes in the functioning of the peripheral and autonomic nervous systems are related to changes in the endocrine system during pregnancy. The relevant neurohormonal reflexes such as lactation will be discussed in the relevant chapters. The role of the sympathetic system in the stress response is important for understanding uterine muscle activity and cervical dilatation in labour.

Main points

- The peripheral nervous system passes information about changes in the external and internal environment back to the central nervous system so that appropriate action can be taken. Sensory afferent nerves include sensation from the skin, muscles, joints and viscera.
- First-order nerve fibres enter the dorsal columns somatotopically and cross the midline to synapse with second-order neurons at the level of the medulla. Thalamic third-order fibres project an accurate representation to the sensory cerebral cortex.
- Dorsal root fibres of the spinothalamic tract ascend or descend a few segments before crossing over the midline to ascend in the spinothalamic tract and terminate on third-order neurons in the thalamus. Axons from these third-order fibres terminate in the sensory cortex.
- Descending tracts carry efferent messages from the brain down the spinal cord. The pyramidal cells of the motor cortex are the upper motor neurons. The

- anterior horn neuron axons which leave the cord to innervate skeletal muscles are the lower motor neurons.
- Reflexes occur over reflex arcs and may be somatic or autonomic. Many spinal reflexes occur with little or no brain input.
- The ANS maintains stability of the body's internal environment. Its motor neurons innervate smooth muscle, cardiac muscle and glands, making functional adjustments in response to visceral messages sent to the CNS.
- The ANS is divided into the sympathetic nervous system, which prepares the body for emergency action, and the parasympathetic system, which has a calming effect. The dynamic interaction between the two divisions is aimed at maximising homeostasis.
- Sympathetic activity tends to inhibit the activity of visceral organs. Sympathetic fibres innervate sweat glands, smooth muscle fibres such as the erector pili and all blood vessels.

- Visceral pain afferents in autonomic nerves respond to ischaemia, distension, smooth muscle spasm and inflammation and travel along the same pathways as somatic nerve fibres.
- The NTs of the ANS are acetylcholine and noradrenaline. ACh is released by all preganglionic axons and by parasympathetic postganglionic axons. Most sympathetic postganglionic fibres are adrenergic. Most visceral organs are innervated by both sympathetic and parasympathetic fibres.
- The partial constriction of blood vessels to maintain vasomotor tone is controlled by the sympathetic division. The heart, gastrointestinal tract and urinary tract are dominated by parasympathetic impulses.
- Several layers in the CNS contribute to regulation of the ANS. These include brainstem, hypothalamus and cerebral cortex.

References

Fitzgerald, M.J., Gruener, G., Mtui, E., 2006. Clinical Neuroanatomy and Neuroscience, fifth edn. Elsevier Saunders.

Guyton, A.C., Hall, J.E., 2006. Textbook of Medical Physiology, eleventh edn. Elsevier Saunders.

Marieb, E.N., 2008. Essentials of Human Anatomy and Physiology, nineth edn. Benjamin/Cummings, New York.

Sapolsky, R.M., 2004. Why Zebras Don't Get Ulcers. Saint Martin's Press Inc.

Annotated recommended reading

Fitzgerald, M.J., Gruener, G., Mtui, E., 2006. Clinical Neuroanatomy and Neuroscience, fifth edn. Elsevier Saunders.

This is a very well laid out and easy-to-read textbook on the human nervous system. The format is full of interesting diagrams and the headings make the book content easy to find and follow.

Marieb, E.N., 2005. Essentials of Human Anatomy and Physiology, eighth edn. Benjamin/Cummings, New York.

This is still, in my opinion, one of the best general anatomy and physiology textbooks for the student. Although not applied to reproduction in any depth, it has extremely succinct and easy to follow explanations on the anatomy and physiology of the nervous system.

Sapolsky, R.M., 2004. Why Zebras Don't Get Ulcers. Saint Martin's Press Inc.

This small paperback covers the topic of mind–body interactions in an easily read manner. It acts as an excellent introduction to the topic and covers sleep, addiction, the impact of spirituality on managing stress and much more. It is well researched and is also full of humour and practical advice.

Chapter Twenty-Eight

28

The endocrine system

CHAPTER CONTENTS

Introduction

The nervous system (Chs 26 and 27) is the rapid controller of the body whereas the endocrine system provides a much slower control. By coordinating the body's internal physiology and modifying cell function, the endocrine system helps it to adapt to external environmental changes (Hinson et al 2007). The nervous system and the endocrine system are closely related with the hypothalamus providing a major link between them. Each gland will be discussed in turn.

The hypothalamus

The **hypothalamus** controls the function of the **endocrine glands** and has wider links with parts of the nervous system. The hypothalamus is therefore a **neuroendocrine** organ, producing both releasing and inhibiting hormones to influence the production of anterior pituitary gland hormones. Endocrine glands include the thyroid, parathyroid, adrenal and pineal glands.

Other organs produce hormones, including the pancreas (Ch. 22), ovaries (Ch. 4), testes (Ch. 5) and placenta (Ch. 12). Functions of endocrine glands include reproduction, growth and development, mobilisation of body defences against stress, maintenance of fluid and electrolyte balance, blood nutrient content, regulation of cell metabolism and energy balance. Tissue responses to hormones may take only a few seconds or may take days.

Hormones

Hormones are regulatory molecules synthesised in specialist cells which may be collected into distinct endocrine glands or found as single cells within organs, e.g. the gastrointestinal tract. Hormone-secreting glands are arranged in cords and branching networks to maximise contact between cells and the capillaries that receive their secretions directly. Exocrine glands pass their products through ducts into a body cavity or onto the surface of the skin.

Hormones affect tissues by binding to specific receptors on the surface of target cells. Some hormones act locally and are secreted into the extracellular fluid without entering the bloodstream. They affect adjacent cells of a different type (**paracrine**) or on the same cell type (**autocrine**) (Guyton & Hall 2006).

Types of hormones

Hormones are classified into three groups: those derived from the amino acid tyrosine; polypeptide and protein hormones; and steroid hormones. Most are polypeptides (Guyton & Hall 2006).

Tyrosine-derived hormones

Hormones derived from tyrosine include **adrenaline** (epinephrine), **noradrenaline** (norepinephrine), **dopamine** and the thyroid hormones **thyroxine** and **tri-iodothyronine**.

Protein and polypeptide hormones

These hormones include **parathyroid hormone**, **oxytocin**, **vasopressin**, **insulin**, the anterior pituitary gland glycoprotein hormones such as gonadotrophins, follicle-stimulating hormone and luteinising hormone and gastrointestinal hormones such as **secretin** and **gastrin**.

Steroid hormones

Steroids, which are derived from **cholesterol**, include cortisol and aldosterone from the adrenal cortex and the sex hormones testosterone, progesterone and oestrogen.

Target cells

Hormones circulate to nearly all tissues but can only influence cells with specific receptors in their plasma membranes. Some only influence a few tissues; for example, **adrenocorticotrophic hormone** can only influence certain adrenal cortical cells. Others such as thyroxine are essential for the metabolism of all cells.

Water-soluble hormones such as peptides and catecholamines are dissolved in plasma and transported to their target cells diffusing out of the capillaries to reach their targets. Thyroxine and the steroid hormones are bound to specific plasma carrier proteins and are inactive until they dissociate from their carriers.

Metabolic clearance rate is millilitres of plasma cleared of a hormone per minute (ml/min). This may be achieved by:

- Metabolic destruction by the tissues.
- Binding with the tissues.
- Excretion in bile by the liver.
- Excretion in urine by the kidneys.

Most peptide hormones and catecholamines are water-soluble and are degraded by enzymes in the blood to be excreted by the kidneys and liver. The actions of some hormones are short-lived, developing their full action within a few seconds. Hormones bound to plasma proteins may stay in the blood for hours or even days. Some such as thyroxine and growth hormone may require months to achieve their full effects. Cellular activity depends on blood levels of the hormone, the number of cell-surface receptors and the affinity of the receptor for the hormone. Hormone receptors are large proteins and there are thousands of receptors on a cell, each specific for a single hormone. Different types of hormone receptors are located:

1. In or on the surface of the cell membrane, mainly for protein, peptide and catecholamine hormones.

2. In the cell cytoplasm, mainly for steroid hormones.

3. In the cell nucleus, mainly for thyroxine.

Cell-surface receptors

There are two major groups of cell-surface receptors: **single-transmembrane domain receptors**, a pathway utilised by hormones such as insulin and prolactin; and **G-protein coupled receptors** (seven-transmembrane domain receptors), so called because the receptor structure crosses the lipid bilayer of the plasma membrane seven times (Hinson et al 2007).

Cytoplasm receptors

Most amino acid-based hormones cannot penetrate cell membranes and have to utilise intracellular second messengers such as cyclic AMP. Others involve a different second messenger: calcium, which either acts directly by altering the activity of specific enzymes or indirectly by binding to an intracellular protein **calmodulin**.

Nuclear receptors

Steroid and thyroid hormones bind to protein members of a superfamily of **intracellular receptors**. They are lipid-soluble and diffuse across plasma membranes to gain access to intracellular receptors in the cytosol or nucleus. Responses to steroid and thyroid hormones are sluggish compared with hormones which act via cell-surface receptor/second messenger systems.

The mechanisms of hormone action

Hormones increase or decrease cellular activity by producing one or more of the following (Marieb 2008):

1. Changes in cell membrane permeability and/or electrical potential.

2. Enzyme synthesis, activation or deactivation.

3. Induction of secretory activity.

4. Stimulation of mitotic cell division.

Regulators of receptors

Target cells may make more receptors in response to high levels of hormones, this is up-regulation, or respond to high hormone levels by losing receptors, down-regulation. Hormones may also influence receptors responsive to other hormones. The presence of progesterone causes a loss of oestrogen receptors but oestrogen causes an increase in progesterone receptors, causing the cells to have an enhanced ability to respond to progesterone.

Control of hormone release

The synthesis and release of hormones depends on inhibition by negative feedback. Hormone secretion is triggered by a stimulus and blood levels rise until they reach the required level when further hormone release is inhibited. This maintains blood levels within a narrow range. Stimuli can be hormonal, humeral or neural:

- Hormonal stimulus: hypothalamic releasing and inhibiting hormones regulate the pituitary gland hormones, some of which in their turn induce other glands to secrete their hormones.
- Humeral stimulus: changing blood levels of ions and nutrients; for example, the production of parathyroid hormone is prompted by decreasing blood calcium levels.
- Neural stimuli: for example, the release of catecholamines by the sympathetic nervous system in response to stress.

The pituitary gland

The pituitary gland or **hypophysis** is a small ovoid gland weighing 500 mg and situated in the **sella turcica** of the sphenoid bone. It has a stalk called the **infundibulum**, which connects it to the hypothalamus, and two lobes:

- The posterior lobe (**neurohypophysis**) consists of nerve fibres and neuroglia and is a downwards growth of the hypothalamus. It does not manufacture hormones but stores hypothalamic hormones, releasing them as necessary.
- The anterior lobe (**adenohypophysis**) is composed of glandular tissue and manufactures and releases its own hormones.

The gland has a rich blood supply derived from the internal carotid artery via superior and inferior hypophyseal branches. Venous drainage is into the dural venous sinuses. The gland is susceptible to blood loss, particularly in pregnancy.

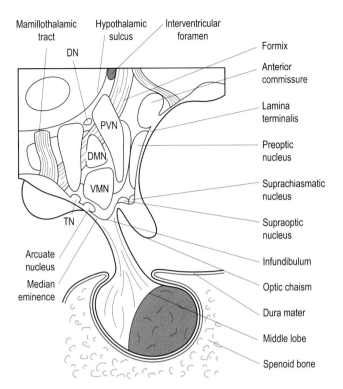

Figure 28.1 • Hypothalamic nuclei and hypophysis, viewed from the right side. DN, dorsal nuclei; DMN, dorsomedial nucleus; MB, mamillary body; PN, posterior nucleus; PVN, periventricular nucleus; TN, tuberomamillary nucleus; VMN, ventromedial nucleus. (From Fitzgerald M J T 1996, with permission.)

Table 28.1 Actions of hypothalamic neurohormones

Name	Major function(s)
Thyrotrophin-releasing hormone (TRH)	Stimulates release of thyroid-stimulating hormone (TSH) and prolactin (PRL)
Gonadotrophin-releasing hormone (GnRH)	Stimulates release of luteinising hormone (LH) and follicle-stimulating hormone (FSH)
Growth hormone-releasing hormone (GHRH)	Stimulates release of growth hormone (GH)
Growth hormone-release inhibiting hormone (somatostatin, SMS)	Inhibits release of GH, gastrin, vasoactive intestinal peptide (VIP), glucagons, insulin, TSH and PRL
Corticotropin-releasing hormone (CRH)	Stimulates release of adrenocorticotrophic hormone (ACTH)
Dopamine (DA)	Inhibits release of PRL

The pituitary–hypothalamic axis

A nerve bundle called the hypothalamic–hypophyseal tract runs through the infundibulum (Fig. 28.1). The tract neurons are situated in two groups of nuclei in the hypothalamus:

1. Oxytocin is secreted from the hypothalamic paraventricular nuclei and antidiuretic hormone from the supraoptic nuclei. These hormones are transported along axons to their terminals on the posterior pituitary lobe.

2. The hypothalamic–hypophyseal nuclei are responsible for anterior pituitary function. There is no direct neural connection between the adenohypophysis and the hypothalamus. The vascular hypophyseal portal system carries hypothalamic releasing and inhibiting hormones to the anterior pituitary lobe.

Regulation of function

A number of hypothalamic neurohormones regulate anterior pituitary function. They have short half-lives in the circulation and act rapidly on specific anterior pituitary cells (Table 28.1).

Anterior pituitary hormones

The anterior lobe of the pituitary is called the 'master endocrine gland' because of its control of other glands. There are six anterior pituitary hormones, four of which regulate the hormonal functioning of other glands:

1. Thyroid-stimulating hormone (TSH).

2. Adrenocorticotrophic hormone (ACTH).

3. Follicle-stimulating hormone (FSH).

4. Luteinising hormone (LH).

The other two hormones influence non-endocrine targets:

5. Growth-hormone (GH).

6. Prolactin (PRL).

All these hormones use the second messenger system.

Growth hormone

GH stimulates cells to grow and divide. It promotes growth of bone, soft tissue and viscera. Indirectly it promotes clonal expansion of newly differentiated cells mediated by **insulin-like growth factors** (IGF-1 and IGF-2). The amount secreted daily declines with age and GH has a diurnal cycle, with the highest levels occurring during sleep. It is anabolic and stimulates protein synthesis, facilitates the use of fats for fuel and conserves glucose.

Two hypothalamic hormones with antagonistic effects regulate production of GH: GH-releasing hormone and GH-inhibiting hormone (somatostatin). Hypersecretion of GH in childhood results in **gigantism** and the person may reach a height of 2.4m (8ft). After cessation of longitudinal growth, enlargement of bony areas of the hands, feet and face occurs (**acromegaly**). Hyposecretion of GH in children leads to **pituitary dwarfism**. Body proportions are normal but the maximum height is 1.2m (4ft).

Prolactin

PRL is similar to GH. The only known effect is the stimulation of breast milk production (Ch. 54). PRL is regulated by the negative control of dopamine (DA) in men and non-lactating women.

Prolactin levels are influenced by the effect of oestrogen on the breast. The release of PRL just before menstruation accounts for premenstrual breast swelling and tenderness but no milk is produced. Hypersecretion of PRL causes inappropriate lactation (**galactorrhoea**) and is seen in both sexes, mostly due to an anterior pituitary gland tumour. Women will have amenorrhoea and men may become impotent.

Posterior pituitary hormones

Oxytocin

Oxytocin is a strong stimulator of uterine action and is important in childbirth. Oxytocin is released during the final stage of labour due to the stretching of the lower genital tract, a phenomenon known as Ferguson's reflex. It is also secreted after birth as a response to suckling.

Antidiuretic hormone

Antidiuretic hormone (ADH) inhibits urine formation by influencing the renal tubules to reabsorb more water. Less urine is produced and blood volume rises. Hypothalamic osmoreceptors monitor the solute concentration in blood and, if too much is detected, they send excitatory messages to the ADH-secreting neurons in the hypothalamus. ADH release is also stimulated by pain, low blood pressure and drugs such as nicotine, morphine and barbiturates. In a large blood loss enormous amounts of ADH are released, causing vasoconstriction and a rise in blood pressure. ADH is therefore sometimes called vasopressin.

Alcohol ingestion inhibits ADH production causing a diuresis. This accounts for the thirst and dry mouth! Drinking large amounts of water will also suppress ADH release. Diabetes insipidus is a rare disorder resulting in inadequate release of ADH. There is excessive urination and thirst and it can be life-threatening if the individual cannot drink enough. ADH production is similar in pregnant and non-pregnant women but the osmoreceptors are reset to accommodate the extra blood volume of pregnancy.

Anterior pituitary changes during pregnancy

The pituitary gland changes in pregnancy. In non-pregnant women it is about 20% heavier than in men. During pregnancy its weight increases by 30% in first pregnancies and 50% in subsequent pregnancies, almost entirely due to an increase in the number of prolactin-secreting cells (**lactotrophs**). The enhanced blood supply makes the pituitary gland more vulnerable to vasospasm which may lead to **Sheehan's syndrome** (Box 28.1). The number of GH-producing cells falls, probably due to the presence of human placental lactogen. GH returns to normal within a few weeks of delivery.

During pregnancy the fetoplacental hormones greatly influence the pituitary gland and the secretion of FSH and LH are inhibited, possibly due to hCG release. Pregnancy hyperprolactinaemia also contributes to the fall in gonadotrophic secretion. Anterior pituitary hormone production changes in the puerperium to accommodate lactation.

The thyroid gland

The thyroid gland lies in the neck in front of the trachea and below the larynx. It has two lateral lobes joined by a medial isthmus. It is the largest endocrine gland, weighing 10–20g in an adult and is well supplied with blood via superior and inferior thyroid arteries. It concentrates **iodine** from the bloodstream to synthesise hormones.

The internal structure of the thyroid gland consists of hollow spherical structures called **follicles**, lined by cuboidal epithelial cells which produce **thyroglobulin**, a glycoprotein. The follicles store an amber-coloured sticky material called **colloid** which consists of thyroglobulin molecules attached to iodine. This produces two thyroid hormones: **thyroxine** or T_4, and **tri-iodothyronine** or T_3. Another group of cells, the **parafollicular cells**, produce the hormone calcitonin.

Thyroid hormones

Thyroxine is the major hormone and more is secreted than tri-iodothyronine. The structure of the two hormones is similar, each consisting of two linked tyrosine molecules. Thyroxine binds four iodine atoms (hence T_4) and tri-iodothyronine binds three iodine atoms (hence T_3). Although both T_3 and T_4 bind to tissues, T_3 is 10 times more active. Most of the T_3 is formed in target tissues by removal of an iodine group from T_4. Iodine atoms attached to a tyrosine molecule make **iodotyrosine**.

If two iodine atoms are attached to a tyrosine molecule, **di-iodotyrosine** (DIT) is produced. The attachment of one iodine atom to a tyrosine produces **mono-iodotyrosine** (MIT). A coupling of DIT with DIT within the thyroglobulin molecule forms T_4 while DIT plus MIT forms T_3. Enzymes split the hormones off the thyroglobulin molecule.

Secretion of thyroid hormones

In the adult about 1 mg/week of dietary iodine is required for the manufacture of the thyroid hormones

BOX 28.1 SHEEHAN'S SYNDROME

The increase in size of the anterior pituitary gland in pregnancy necessitates an increased oxygen supply carried by an increased circulation. The unique blood supply to the pituitary gland makes it vulnerable to a reduction in arterial blood supply if there is vasospasm of the superior hypophyseal artery. This leads to swelling and necrosis of the gland (Sheehan & Stanfield 1961). Because the posterior pituitary gland has a separate blood supply, Sheehan's syndrome does not affect it. The symptoms are caused by loss of the anterior pituitary hormones. The earliest sign is failure to lactate due to prolactin deficiency, followed by amenorrhoea due to loss of the gonadotrophic hormones.

Sheehan's syndrome or anterior pituitary necrosis is a condition associated with a sudden decrease in blood volume or a localised bleed disrupting the hypophyseal portal system. Although rare it is most commonly associated with severe and prolonged obstetric shock, usually following haemorrhage during labour (Hinson et al 2007). The activity of the thyroid and adrenal glands gradually diminishes and the woman becomes lethargic and feels cold. Her hair and skin become coarser and she suffers loss of libido. Her genitalia and breasts atrophy. Adequate and prompt treatment of obstetric shock will prevent the syndrome from developing. If the diagnosis is not made the woman may die. Treatment is by total hormone replacement.

(Guyton & Hall 2006). Transfer of iodide from blood to follicular cells occurs against a steep iodide concentration gradient (Hinson et al 2007). The hormones circulate round the body bound to **thyroid-binding globulin** (TBG). Less than 1% of the hormones is free in the blood and it is this that stimulates tissues. The hormones are broken down by the tissues and some iodine is returned to the thyroid for reuse whilst some is excreted. Regulation of thyroid hormone secretion is by a negative feedback loop from T_3 so that blood levels are maintained within a narrow limit. Hypothalamic TRH influences the secretion of TSH from the anterior pituitary gland (Fig. 28.2).

Functions of thyroid hormones

Thyroid hormones affect most cells except the tissues of the brain, spleen, testes, uterus and the thyroid gland itself. They are essential for maintenance of normal metabolism by increasing **basal metabolic rate**. Thyroid

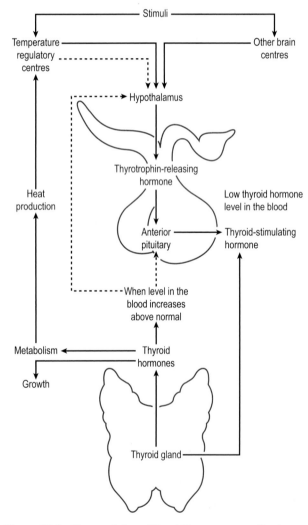

Figure 28.2 • The regulation of thyroid hormone secretion by negative feedback loop.

hormone binds to nucleic acid proteins which can bind to specific DNA sequences. The hormone–receptor complex directly induces transcription of the genes responsive to thyroid hormones. Abnormalities of thyroid function are discussed in Chapter 35.

Changes in the thyroid gland during pregnancy

Secretion of TSH is reduced in the first trimester, returning to normal for the remainder of pregnancy. Thyroid function remains normal during pregnancy although some women exhibit some signs associated with an overactive thyroid gland, including thyroid hyperplasia or goitre. During pregnancy a balance is achieved by alterations in the metabolism of iodine. Renal iodide clearance doubles, plasma inorganic iodide falls and thyroid clearance of iodide trebles. The absolute uptake of iodine remains within normal limits. From 12 weeks there is an increase in plasma TBG and free thyroxine and the ability of TBG to bind doubles. Basal metabolic rate increases by 25% from 4 months (ACOG 2001). The changes revert to normal in the puerperium but may take 12 weeks.

The above alterations have been linked with nausea and vomiting in early pregnancy, especially with hyperemesis gravidarum (Vitoratos et al 2000). Maternal immunological reactiveness also seems to be involved (Leylek et al 1999). Human chorionic gonadotrophin (hCG) is similar in structure to TSH. When hCG peaks in pregnancy it is matched by a corresponding fall in TSH. hCG levels are high in hyperemesis and there is an increase in T_4 and T_3. Thyroid function reverts to normal for pregnancy when vomiting stops (Hershman 2004).

The adrenal glands

The two pyramid-shaped glands each weigh about 4 g and are situated on the superior poles of the kidneys. The inner medulla is derived from the neural crest and is functionally part of the sympathetic nervous system. It is composed of **chromaffin cells** which give it a reddish-brown colour. The outer cortex forms 80–90% of each gland and is derived from embryonic mesoderm similar to the ovary and testis. It is yellow due to its high lipid content.

Adrenal blood supply

The adrenal gland blood supply is derived from a circle of arteries arising from the superior, middle and inferior adrenal arteries. These give off three types of artery: capsular vessels, cortical vessels and medullary vessels. The medulla has a double blood supply: one derived from medullary arterioles and one derived from cortical capillaries. The latter is similar to a portal system and ensures that blood arriving in the medulla is rich in the corticoid hormones necessary for the production of adrenaline (epinephrine). Medullary venules empty blood into the central vein. The central vein of the right adrenal gland empties into the inferior vena cave while the left venous drainage is into the left renal vein.

The adrenal cortex

The cortex consists of large, lipid-filled cells arranged in three concentric regions. These synthesise corticosteroids from cholesterol:

1. The outer **zona glomerulosa** produces mineralocorticoids.

2. The middle zona fasciculata makes up 5–10% of the cortex and secretes glucocorticoids.

3. The inner **zona reticularis** forms about 75% of the cortex and produces glucocorticoids and small amounts of the sex hormones or gonadocorticoids.

The mineralocorticoids

Mineralocorticoids regulate the amount of water and electrolytes in extracellular fluid by affecting sodium and potassium concentrations. **Aldosterone** is the most common and most important mineralocorticoid. It regulates sodium balance by stimulating kidney tubule reabsorption of sodium ions from urine and returning them to the blood. Aldosterone also helps sodium reabsorption from perspiration, saliva or gastric juice. Potassium, hydrogen, bicarbonate and chloride ions are coupled to sodium regulation and water follows sodium passively.

Four mechanisms help to regulate the secretion of aldosterone (Fig. 28.3):

1. The renin–angiotensin mechanism.

2. Rising potassium and low levels of sodium in blood.

3. Release of atrial natriuretic factor by the heart as blood pressure rises.

4. Decreasing blood volume and blood pressure causes the hypothalamus to release corticotrophin-releasing factor (CRH) which steps up ACTH production. This leads to increases in aldosterone production.

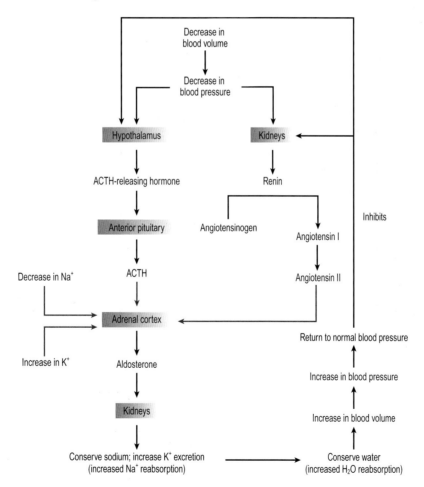

Figure 28.3 • The regulation of aldosterone secretion. (From Montague S E, Watson R, Herbert R A 2005, with kind permission of Elsevier.)

The glucocorticoids

Glucocorticoids include **cortisol** (hydrocortisone), **cortisone** and **corticosterone**. Only cortisol is secreted in significant amounts in humans. The control of glucocorticoid secretion is by feedback mechanism (Fig. 28.4). CHR from the hypothalamus causes ACTH release by the anterior pituitary gland which causes the release of cortisol.

Cortisol affects the metabolism of most cells by converting the intermittent intake of food to a steady level of plasma glucose by stimulating **gluconeogenesis**, the mobilisation of fatty acids and the breakdown of proteins.

Other functions of cortisol include:

- Reducing inflammation following injury.
- Enhancing the vasoconstrictive effects of noradrenaline.
- Increasing blood pressure and circulatory efficiency.
- Maintenance of fluid balance by preventing the shift of water into tissue cells.

In severe stress, whether physiological or psychological, the output of glucocorticoids rises dramatically to help the body though the crisis.

Gonadocorticoids

The main gonadocorticoids secreted are the androgens with small amounts of oestrogen and progesterone. In adult women, adrenal androgens are thought to be responsible for libido. Adrenal oestrogens may replace ovarian oestrogens after the menopause.

The role of the fetal cortex

In the term fetus the adrenal gland is 20 times larger in relation to other organs than in an adult. It regresses after birth to reach normal proportions by 1 year. The fetal cortex appears to produce mainly **dehydroepiandosterone sulphate** (DHEAS) which is the substrate for placental oestrogen synthesis. The fetal adrenals cannot synthesise glucocorticoids. These may be obtained from the mother or made by the placenta for:

- Surfactant production.
- Development of the hypothalamic–pituitary axis.
- Changes in placental structure and amniotic fluid composition during development.
- Initiation of fetal endocrine change in the fetus and mother that is responsible for the onset of labour.
- The development of liver enzymes.
- Induction of thymic gland reduction.

The adrenal medulla

The chromaffin cells produce the hormones adrenaline (epinephrine) and noradrenaline (norepinephrine), known collectively as the **catecholamines**. About 80% of production is adrenaline. Sympathetic nerve endings stimulate the adrenal medulla to produce the fight or flight response. Adrenaline stimulates the heart and metabolic activity while noradrenaline affects peripheral vasoconstriction and blood pressure. Catecholamines produce short-term responses. During short-term stress the main effects of the sympathetic nervous system are a rise in blood sugar levels and constriction of blood vessels. The heart beats faster, blood pressure rises and blood is diverted to the brain and skeletal muscles.

Changes in the adrenal gland during pregnancy

Cortical function

ACTH plasma concentrations rise progressively during pregnancy associated with a doubling of plasma cortisol, but still remain in the range for non-pregnant women. Normally, a rise in plasma cortisol would suppress ACTH production but the feedback mechanism appears to change during pregnancy. The placenta may contribute to the increase in ACTH. The myometrium and decidua convert cortisone to cortisol, resulting in a local cortisol concentration of nine times normal. This may contribute to immunological protection of the fetus.

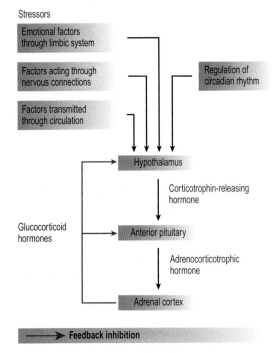

Figure 28.4 • The regulation of glucocorticoid secretion.

Cortisol

There is a steady rise in plasma cortisol due to a doubling of cortisol-binding globulin (also called transcortin). Free plasma cortisol is increased with loss of diurnal variation so that there is a greater maternal tissue exposure to it, especially in late pregnancy. The cushingoid appearance of pregnancy with striae gravidarum, impaired carbohydrate tolerance and hypertension may be due to the excess cortisol. There is increased cortisol production in labour, probably due to stress.

Aldosterone

There is an increase in renin substrate due to higher oestrogen level. Excretion of sodium and chloride is increased in response to the presence of progesterone.

Alterations in the renin–angiotensin mechanisms lead to increased aldosterone production which enhances the reabsorption of sodium to maintain balance.

The pineal gland

The minute pineal gland hangs from the floor of the third ventricle. Neural connections between the retina and the pineal gland allow a light-regulated diurnal secretion of the hormone melatonin from its pinealocytes. This is highest during the night and lowest about noon. In animals melatonin controls reproduction so that lengthening periods of light affect gonadal size and mating behaviour. In humans melatonin causes the hypothalamus to inhibit gonadotrophin-releasing hormone. It also causes daily variations in temperature, sleep and appetite.

Main points

- The hypothalamus controls the function of the endocrine glands and has wider links with parts of the nervous system. It is a neuroendocrine organ producing releasing and inhibiting hormones to influence the production of anterior pituitary hormones.
- The pituitary gland controls hormone production from the other endocrine glands and single cells within organs such as the gastrointestinal tract. Hormones are classified into three groups: those derived from tyrosine; polypeptide and protein hormones; and steroid hormones. Most are polypeptides.
- Hormones can only influence cells with specific receptors. Some hormones only influence a few tissues. ACTH can only influence certain adrenal cortical cells. Others such as thyroxine are essential for all cellular metabolism.
- Cellular activity depends on the blood levels of its hormone, the number of target cell receptors and the receptor affinity for the hormone. Target cells may up-regulate or down-regulate receptors in response to the hormone level.
- The pituitary gland has a stalk called the infundibulum which connects it to the pituitary gland, and two lobes. The posterior lobe is derived from a downwards growth of the hypothalamus. It stores hypothalamic hormones, releasing them as necessary. The anterior lobe is glandular and manufactures and releases its own hormones.
- Fetoplacental hormones greatly influence the pituitary gland inhibiting the secretion of FSH and LH. Hyperprolactinaemia also contributes to the fall in gonadotrophin secretion. Hormone production by the anterior pituitary changes in the puerperium to accommodate lactation.

- ACTH plasma concentrations rise during pregnancy associated with a doubling of plasma cortisol. The placenta may contribute to the increase in ACTH. A local uterine cortisol concentration of nine times normal may contribute to fetal immunological protection.
- During pregnancy the size of the pituitary gland increases due to more prolactin-secreting cells. The enhanced blood supply makes the pituitary gland vulnerable to vasospasm with a risk of Sheehan's syndrome.
- Antidiuretic hormone production is similar in pregnant and non-pregnant women but osmoreceptors are reset to accommodate the extra blood volume of pregnancy.
- The thyroid gland has two lateral lobes joined by a medial isthmus and is well supplied with blood. It synthesises the hormones thyroxine or T_4 and tri-iodothyronine or T_3. Its parafollicular cells produce the hormone calcitonin.
- Thyroid hormones affect most cells except the brain, spleen, testes, uterus and the thyroid gland itself and are essential for maintenance of normal metabolic functions by causing an increased basal metabolic rate.
- Thyroid function remains normal during pregnancy although some women exhibit some of the signs associated with an overactive thyroid gland, including goitre. Basal metabolic rate increases by 25% from 4 months.
- In the adrenal cortex large lipid-filled cells synthesise corticosteroids from cholesterol: the outer zona glomerulosa produces mineralocorticoids; the middle zona fasciculata secretes glucocorticoids; the inner zona reticularis produces glucocorticoids and small amounts of the sex hormones.

- Aldosterone regulates sodium balance by stimulating reabsorption of sodium ions from urine in the renal tubules and returning them to the blood.
- Cortisol affects cellular metabolism by converting the intermittent intake of food to a steady level of plasma glucose. It reduces inflammation, enhances the vasoconstrictive effects of noradrenaline, increases blood pressure and circulatory efficiency and maintains fluid balance by preventing the shift of water into cells.
- In severe stress the output of glucocorticoids rises dramatically to help the body through the crisis.
- The fetal adrenal cortex produces DHEAS, the substrate for placental oestrogen synthesis. The fetal adrenals cannot synthesise glucocorticoids, which may be obtained from the mother or made by the placenta.
- Sympathetic nerve endings stimulate the adrenal medulla to produce the fight or flight response. Adrenaline stimulates the heart and metabolic activity while noradrenaline affects peripheral vasoconstriction and blood pressure.
- There is a steady rise in plasma cortisol and free plasma cortisol is increased with loss of diurnal variation so that there is a greater exposure to it of maternal tissues, especially in late pregnancy.
- The cushingoid appearance of pregnancy with striae gravidarum, impaired carbohydrate tolerance and hypertension may be due to the excess cortisol. There is increased cortisol production in labour, probably due to stress.
- There is an increase in renin substrate due to a rise in circulating oestrogen. Excretion of sodium and chloride is increased in response to the presence of progesterone. Alterations in the renin–angiotensin mechanisms lead to increased aldosterone production which enhances the reabsorption of sodium.
- The pineal gland secretes melatonin. In humans melatonin causes the hypothalamus to inhibit gonadotrophin-releasing hormone. It also causes daily variations in temperature, sleep and appetite.

References

ACOG (American College of Obstetricians and Gynecologists), 2001. Thyroid diseases in pregnancy. Pract. Bull. (32) Obstetrics and Gynecology 98(5): 879–888.

Guyton, A.C., Hall, J.E., 2006. Textbook of Medical Physiology, eleventh edn. Elsevier Saunders, Philadelphia.

Hershman, J.M., 2004. Physiological and pathological aspects of the effect of human chorionic gonadotrophin on the thyroid. Best Pract. Res.: Clin. Endocrinol. Metab. 18 (2), 249–265.

Hinson, J., Raven, P., Chew, S., 2007. The Endocrine System: Basic Science and Clinical Conditions. Elsevier Churchill Livingstone, Philadelphia.

Leylek, A., Toyaski, M., Arselcan, T., Dokmetas, S., 1999. Immunologic and biochemical factors in hyperemesis gravidarum with or without hyperthyroxaemia. Gynecol. Obstet. Investig. 47, 299–334.

Marieb, E.N., 2008. Essentials of Human Anatomy and Physiology, ninth edn. Benjamin/Cummings, New York.

Montague, S.E., Watson, R., Herbert, R.A. (Eds.), 2005. Physiology for Nursing Practice, third edn. Baillière Tindall, London.

Sheehan, H.L., Stanfield, P., 1961. The pathogenesis of postpartum necrosis of the anterior lobe of the pituitary gland. Acta Endocrinol. 37, 479.

Vitoratos, N., Salamalekis, E., Kassanos, D., et al., 2000. Hyperemesis gravidarum: its relation ship to maternal immune response and thyroid function. Prenat. Med. 5, 363–367.

Annotated recommended reading

Guyton, A.C., Hall, J.E., 2006. Textbook of Medical Physiology, eleventh edn. Elsevier Saunders, Philadelphia.

This large hardback book is very detailed but very easy to understand. The use of language is straightforward and the explanations are logically presented. There is detail on every system of the body.

Hershman, J.M., 2004. Physiological and pathological aspects of the effect of human chorionic gonadotrophin on the thyroid. Best Pract. Res.: Clin. Endocrinol. Metab. 18 (2), 249–265.

This learned paper is full of information and gives excellent insight into how one system can influence another, including pregnancy and hyperemesis gravidarum.

Hinson, J., Raven, P., Chew, S., 2007. The Endocrine System: Basic Science and Clinical Conditions. Elsevier Churchill Livingstone, Philadelphia.

This textbook is one of a series on systems of the body by Elsevier Churchill Livingstone. Although it is not referenced within the text it is well laid out and clinically very informative. There are very helpful question and answer sections to each chapter.

Chapter Twenty-Nine

The immune system

CHAPTER CONTENTS

Introduction

The immune system protects us from environmental factors such as micro-organisms, irritants and abnormal cells. Pathogens such as viruses, bacteria and fungi constantly invade the body, both on its surface and internally (Male

et al 2006). Larger organisms such as worms are parasitic, obtaining their food from our metabolic processes (Kendall 2007). Many micro-organisms cannot harm us if we are well but may cause death if the immune system is defective.

In developed countries, infection accounts for less than 2% of deaths. However, there are developing problems such as resistant strains of bacteria such as meticillin-resistant *Staphylococcus aureus* (MRSA) and *Clostridium difficile* (C-diff.). Also, global travel makes the transfer of deadly organisms such as the so-called bird flu more rapid.

Divisions of the immune system

The immune system recognises pathogens and mounts an immune response to eliminate them. Because there are many pathogens a wide variety of immune responses is needed and there are three lines of defence. The first two, **surface barriers** and the **inflammatory response**, are non-specific (**innate**) and the third is a specific response (**acquired, adaptive**) to a particular foreign protein. Innate immunity immediately protects the body from a range of substances whilst acquired immunity acts against a particular invader but must be primed by its presence and takes time to develop. The two categories of immune response are interdependent and work together to either destroy the invader or reduce its harmful effects (Fig. 29.1).

Cells of the immune system

Immune responses are mediate by a variety of cells and the soluble molecules they secrete. Leucocytes (white blood cells, WBCs) are protective against bacteria, viruses,

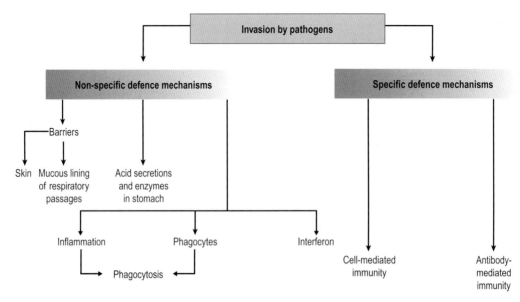

Figure 29.1 • Summary of specific and non-specific defence mechanisms. Non-specific mechanisms prevent entry of many pathogens and act rapidly to destroy those that manage to cross the barriers. Specific defence mechanisms take longer to mobilise but they are highly effective in destroying invaders. (From Montague S E, Watson R, Herbert R A 2005, with kind permission of Elsevier.)

parasites, toxins and tumour cells. There are normally about 4000–11 000 per cubic mm ($4–11 \times 10^9$/L). Most leucocytes are in the tissues and there is a wide variation in the blood count as cells enter and leave the circulation from hour to hour. All leucocytes are produced in the bone marrow from **haemopoietic stem cells** (Male et al 2006).

Types of leucocyte

Several types of leucocyte are distinguished by their shape, appearance and function. **Granulocytes** (polymorphonuclear leucocytes) have granules in their cytoplasm which contain substances that fight infection. They are 10–14 μm in diameter and have a lobed nucleus. They are divided into three groups by the size of their granules: **neutrophils**, **eosinophils** and **basophils**. All are **phagocytic**, engulfing and destroying foreign proteins. **Agranulocytes**, which include **lymphocytes** and **monocytes**, do not contain granules. **Natural killer cells** (NK cells) are a specialised type of large, granular lymphocyte.

Granulocytes

1. Neutrophils contain granules that stain violet because they take up both acidic red dyes and basic blue dyes. They account for more than 50% of granulocytes and have the most lobular nuclei. Neutrophils migrate to inflammation sites. They are short-lived cells that engulf foreign material such as bacteria, destroy it and die.

2. Eosinophils have large granules that stain red with acidic dyes. They make up 1–4% of leucocytes.

They attack parasitic worms by surrounding them and releasing granular enzymes onto the parasite's surface to digest it from the outside. Eosinophils also deal with allergy by destroying antigen–antibody complexes.

3. Basophils have large granules that take up a basic dye and stain blue-black. They account for only 0.5% of white cells. Their granules contain histamine, an inflammatory substance that acts as a vasodilator and draws other white cells to an inflammation site. Mast cells are similar to basophils and are present in connective tissue. Both cell types release histamine when they bind to immunoglobulin E.

The production of granulocytes

The process of **granulopoeisis** takes about 14 days but is considerably reduced if cells are needed. There is progressive condensation and lobulation of the nucleus, loss of organelles and development of granules in the cytoplasm. Within 7 h of reaching the circulation, half of the granulocytes will have migrated into tissue and will not return. They survive about 5 days and are eliminated in faeces and respiratory secretions and form pus at infection sites. For every granulocyte in blood there are 50 in bone marrow.

Natural killer (NK) cells are present in blood and lymph and account for 15% of blood lymphocytes. Unlike other lymphocytes which only react to specific virus-infected or tumour cells, **NK cells** react against cells which do not express major **histocompatibility complex (MHC) class 1 molecules** (see below), an important factor in the immunology of pregnancy.

Agranulocytes

Lymphocytes are round cells with large round nuclei and are the second most common type of leucocyte. Large numbers exist in the body, mostly in **lymphoid tissue**. They recirculate between blood and lymph and are subdivided into small and large lymphocytes. There are two types of lymphocytes: **T** and **B lymphocytes**. Some lymphocytes leave the bone marrow and migrate to the **thymus gland** where they will become T cells. They are selected so that they will not attack **self-antigens** present on the surface of an individual's cells. B cells were first identified in the **bursa of Fabricius**, a pocket of lymphoid tissue associated with the digestive tract in birds. T cells are involved in cell-mediated immunity and account for 80% of the lymphocytes found in blood. B cells are involved in humoral immunity and produce antibodies.

Monocytes are large cells produced in the bone marrow from **myeloid progenitors**. Mature cells spend about 30h in the blood and then migrate to the tissues where they develop into phagocytic **macrophages** (giant eaters). Macrophages regulate the immune response by presenting antigens to activate B and T cells.

Non-specific responses

These can be divided into surface barriers, such as skin and mucous membranes, and cellular and chemical defences.

Surface barriers include:

- A thickly keratinised unbroken skin.
- Intact mucous membranes lining the organs.
- Acidic secretions, such as in the vagina, gastric juices and urine.
- Sticky mucus to trap organisms.
- Ciliated cells that sweep particles towards the outside.
- Lysozyme, an enzyme that destroys bacteria, in saliva and tears.

Phagocytes

If the intact surfaces are breached, cellular and chemical non-specific mechanisms are triggered. In most cases, phagocytic cells (Fig. 29.2) are involved. These are amoeba-like and travel through tissue spaces in search of invading organisms or other debris to engulf and destroy.

Macrophages are the main phagocytic cells but neutrophils become phagocytic if an infection is present. Macrophages are long-lived but neutrophils are destroyed during phagocytosis. Both cells destroy microbes by producing **free radicals**. Neutrophils also produce antibiotic-like chemicals called **defensins. Complement proteins** and antibodies coat foreign proteins and provide binding sites for phagocyte attachment, a process called **opsonisation**.

Inflammation

Inflammation is a localised response when there is a tissue injury due to trauma or invasion by micro-organisms. The inflammatory response prevents the spread of damaging substances to nearby tissues, disposes of cell debris and pathogens and allows repair to begin. There are **four cardinal signs** of inflammation: heat, redness, swelling and pain. Depending on the site and type of tissue damage, chemicals are released into the extracellular fluid by injured cells, phagocytes, lymphocytes, mast cells and blood proteins. Four major plasma enzyme systems are involved in the control of inflammation (Male et al 2006):

1. The clotting system.
2. The fibrinolytic system.
3. The kinin system.
4. The complement system.

The most important molecules are **histamine, kinins, prostaglandins, complement** and **lymphokines**. They induce vasodilation of localised small blood vessels, causing heat and redness. Capillary wall permeability increases, allowing a fluid exudate containing clotting factors and antibodies to seep into the tissue spaces and cause oedema and swelling. Clotting proteins form a **fibrin mesh** which limits the spread of harmful agents and acts as scaffolding for tissue repair. Pain results from pressure on local nerve endings, release of bacterial toxins, lack of cellular nutrition and the effects of prostaglandins and kinins. Loss of function may occur, forcing the person to rest the injured part to aid healing.

The damaged area is first invaded by phagocytes. Rapid release of neutrophils by the bone marrow is caused by **leucocyte-inducing factors** so that four times as many neutrophils may be in the blood stream after a few hours. These cells are attracted to the injury site by chemicals called **chemotactic agents**. At the site they

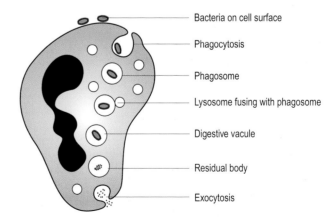

Figure 29.2 Diagram of a neutrophil undergoing phagocytosis. (From Montague S E, Watson R, Herbert R A 2005, with kind permission of Elsevier.)

Labels:
- Bacteria on cell surface
- Phagocytosis
- Phagosome
- Lysosome fusing with phagosome
- Digestive vacule
- Residual body
- Exocytosis

cling on to capillary walls (**margination** or **pavementing**) and squeeze through capillary walls (**diapedesis**) to the site where they devour bacteria, toxins and dead tissue. Monocytes now enter the tissue, swell and mature into macrophages.

If the infection is severe, pus—a mixture of dead neutrophils, living and dead pathogens and damaged tissue cells—is produced. If this becomes walled off by collagen fibres, an abscess forms. Some bacteria like the tuberculosis bacillus are resistant to digestion by macrophages because of their waxy outer coat and remain alive inside the macrophage. Infectious **granulomas** develop which have a central core of infected macrophages surrounded by uninfected macrophages and an outer fibrous capsule. The person only becomes ill if his resistance to infection is reduced when the bacteria may break out and cause disease.

Fever

Fever is an elevation of the body temperature in response to chemicals called **pyrogens** such as the **interleukins**. High fevers are dangerous because they inactivate enzymes and disrupt cellular metabolic processes but mild to moderate fevers are helpful in stimulating the immune system (Kendall 2007) and speeding up both metabolic rate of tissue and defensive actions to aid repair. Antibacterial responses include the sequestering of zinc and iron in the liver and spleen to prevent their use as nutrients by bacteria.

Complement

Complement is a system of about 30 antimicrobial plasma proteins constituting about 10% of total plasma proteins. They normally circulate in the blood in an inactive state. In evolutionary terms they are very old and developed long before the adaptive immune system (Male et al 2006). Their functions are:

- Control of inflammatory reactions.
- Chemotaxis.
- Clearance of immune complexes.
- Cellular inactivation.
- Antimicrobial defence.
- Development of antibody responses.

Important complement proteins are **C1–C9**. Activation of the complement system releases chemical mediators that increase most parts of the inflammatory response and enhance the specific immune system. Complement can be activated by three pathways, which activate C3, causing it to split into two fragments, C3a and C3b:

1. The **classical pathway** (Fig. 29.3) is activated by the formation of antigen–antibody complexes.

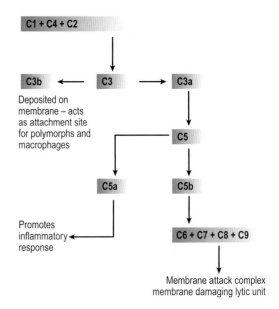

Figure 29.3 • Simplified complement pathway. (From Montague S E, Watson R, Herbert R A 2005, with kind permission of Elsevier.)

2. The **lectin pathway** is similar but activated by bacterial carbohydrates.

3. The evolutionary older alternative pathway provides non-specific immunity and is triggered by the presence of microbial pathogens.

An orderly **cascade** of complement protein activation occurs and C3b binds to the target cell's surface, resulting in the insertion of a group of complement proteins called the **membrane attack complex** (MAC) into the bacterial cell wall, punching a hole and allowing solutes to leak from the cell which destroys it (Male et al 2006).

Specific defence: the immune system

Tissues of the lymphatic system

The lymphatic system consists of two parts: a network of lymphatic vessels and lymphoid organs and tissues throughout the body. The organs and tissues are divided into **primary lymphoid organs** such as the bone marrow and thymus gland where B and T cells mature and the **peripheral lymphoid system** where they spend most of their active lives (Fig. 29.4). The peripheral lymphoid system includes encapsulated organs such as the spleen, tonsils and lymph nodes. Uncapsulated lymphoid tissue is found associated with mucosal surfaces in the gut, lungs and urogenital tract.

Lymph nodes

The immune response takes place in the lymphatic system. The kidney-shaped **lymph nodes** (Fig. 29.5)

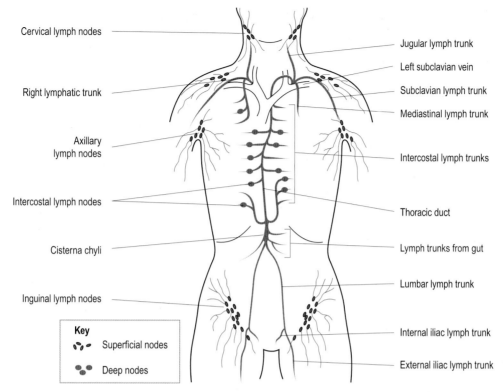

Cervical lymph nodes

Right lymphatic trunk

Axillary
lymph nodes

Intercostal lymph nodes

Cisterna chyli

Inguinal lymph nodes

Jugular lymph trunk

Left subclavian vein

Subclavian lymph trunk

Mediastinal lymph trunk

Intercostal lymph trunks

Thoracic duct

Lymph trunks from gut

Lumbar lymph trunk

Internal iliac lymph trunk

External iliac lymph trunk

Key

Superficial nodes

Deep nodes

Figure 29.4•General arrangement of the lymphatic system. (From Montague S E, Watson R, Herbert R A 2005, with kind permission of Elsevier.)

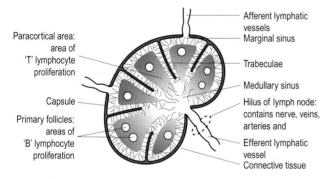

Paracortical area:
area of
'T' lymphocyte
proliferation

Capsule

Primary follicles:
areas of
'B' lymphocyte
proliferation

Afferent lymphatic
vessels
Marginal sinus

Trabeculae

Medullary sinus

Hilus of lymph node:
contains nerve, veins,
arteries and

Efferent lymphatic
vessel
Connective tissue

Figure 29.5•Section through a lymph gland. (From Montague S E, Watson R, Herbert R A 2005, with kind permission of Elsevier.)

are about 2–10 mm in diameter and filter lymph. They consist of a radial network of fibres in which lymphocytes are embedded. The inner medulla contains macrophages, T cells, B cells and plasma cells. B cells are concentrated in primary and secondary follicles in the cortex. Cells at the centre of a follicle divide while those at the periphery produce antibodies. T cells are found in the paracortical area.

Macrophages tend to be fixed in lymphoid organs, whereas lymphocytes also circulate throughout the body. Lymph capillaries pick up pathogens and other foreign protein. Immune cells in lymph nodes are protective locally; for instance those in the tonsils combat organisms that invade the nasal and oral cavities.

The spleen

The **spleen** is the largest lymphoid organ and is located on the left side of the body below the diaphragm. It is about 18 cm × 8 cm in size and weighs about 200 g. It is composed of venous sinuses and reticular connective tissue forming the **red pulp** where removal of ageing and defective red cells, cellular debris and micro-organisms takes place. There are areas of reticular fibres with attached lymphocytes called the **white pulp**, which provides sites for lymphocyte proliferation. The spleen stores the products from broken-down red cells and platelets.

The thymus gland

This bilobed gland, found in the mediastinum of the thorax, is more active during childhood. It is organised into lobules separated by connective tissue. Within each lobule, the lymphoid cells (**thymocytes**) are arranged in an outer cortex and inner medulla. The cortex contains immature cells and the medulla contains densely packed, more mature cells. During adolescence it decreases in size and atrophies. The thymus is involved in the differentiation of T lymphocytes. Embryonic stem cells migrate from bone marrow to thymus, where they mature and differentiate.

Lymphatic vessels

An extensive network of lymphatic vessels connects tissues to lymphoid organs. Lymphatic capillaries are like blood capillaries but their cell wall endothelium does not lie on a basement membrane. They join up to make larger vessels which contain smooth muscle in their walls and have one-way valves. The flow of lymph is ensured by skeletal muscle contraction and negative intrathoracic pressure. Unlike veins, lymphatic vessels contract rhythmically to help lymph flow.

Lymph

Lymph originates as plasma which leaks from blood capillaries. It transports water and small molecules and contains proteins which enter the lymph capillary lumen along its length between endothelial cells. Dietary fat is absorbed as triglycerides from the small intestinal villi. Lymph enters lymph nodes by afferent vessels and leaves via an efferent vessel.

Up to 4 L of lymph accumulates over 24 h and is returned to the blood into the large neck veins via the thoracic duct, which arises anterior to the second lumbar vertebra as an enlarged sac called the cisterna chyli. It drains the lower limbs, digestive system, the left arm and left side of the thorax, neck and head. The smaller right lymphatic duct accepts lymph from the right arm and right side of the thorax, neck and head.

The immune response

There are three important aspects of the immune response:

1. It is antigen-specific—directed against particular pathogens or foreign substances.

2. It is systemic—not restricted to the initial site of infection.

3. It has memory—once it recognises an antigen it responds by producing antibodies to subsequent invasions by the same molecule.

Immunity can be divided into two types. **Humoral immunity** or **antibody-mediated immunity** is provided by the presence of antibodies in body fluids (humors). **Cellular immunity** or **cell-mediated immunity** is when lymphocytes attack an invader directly (Fig. 29.6). Three cell types are involved in the immune response:

1. B lymphocytes produce antibodies and are responsible for humoral-mediated immunity.

2. T lymphocytes are involved in cell-mediated immunity.

3. Macrophages support the two sets of lymphocytes.

The humoral immune response

Recognition of a foreign antigen (non-self molecule) is the basis for specific adaptive immunity (Male et al

2006). Two different types of molecule are involved: antibodies (immunoglobulins, Igs) and T cell antigen receptors. The first encounter between an invading antigen and an immunocompetent lymphocyte involves the activation of a B cell and the collaboration of T cells. Foreign antigens are molecules such as proteins, nucleic acids, lipids and large polysaccharides. A small area on the antigen called an **epitope** is recognised by a small area on a B lymphocyte cell membrane receptor called the **antigen-binding site**.

Pollen grains and micro-organisms are the strongest antigens. Small molecules such as peptides, nucleotides and hormones are not immunogenic but may form complexes with the body's proteins to cause allergies. These are **haptens** and include drugs, detergents, plant products and industrial pollutants. The immune system responds by producing antibodies.

Clonal selection

The binding of the antigen and the lymphocyte stimulates the B cell to divide rapidly, forming a clone of identical cells that recognise that antigen. As the response is so specific, a huge variety of lymphocytes are available to recognise the enormous number of antigens a person encounters throughout life and produce antibodies (see Box 29.1). This specific response is called clonal selection.

Most clone cells differentiate into **antibody-forming cells** (AFCs or **plasma cells**), which secrete antibodies at about 2000 per second for 5 days before the cell dies. Antibodies circulate in blood and lymph where they bind to antigens and present them to phagocytes for destruction. This primary immune response occurs the first time the body meets the antigen. There is a lag of about 3–6 days as B cells proliferate and form AFCs. Plasma antibody levels reach a peak at 10 days.

Immunological memory

Those clone cells that do not differentiate into plasma cells become long-lived **memory cells**, able to respond with a rapid humoral response if the antigen is encountered again. This secondary immune response is faster, more prolonged and more effective. A new clone of plasma cells is produced within hours and peak levels reached within 2 days.

Antibodies

Antibodies, also called **immunoglobulins** (Igs), are a group of glycoproteins present in blood and tissue fluid (Fig. 29.7). Some are present on the surface of B cells, where they act as receptors for specific antigens. Others, secreted by the activated B cell and the cloned AFCs following an encounter with a specific antigen, are

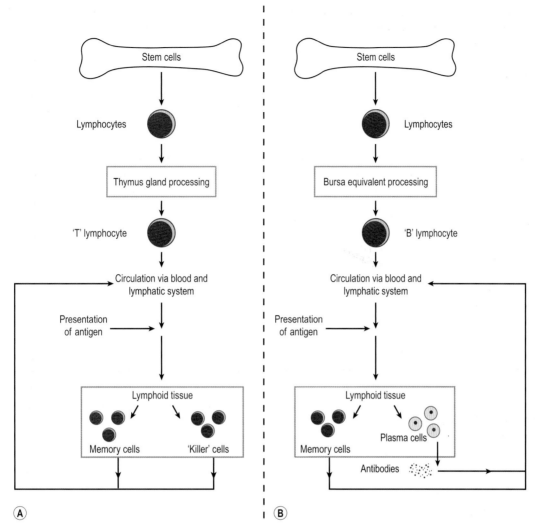

Figure 29.6 • Summary of the development of (A) the cell-mediated immune system and (B) the humoral immune system. Diagram to summarise the formation and protective function of the humoral immune system. (From Montague S E, Watson R, Herbert R A 2005, with kind permission of Elsevier.)

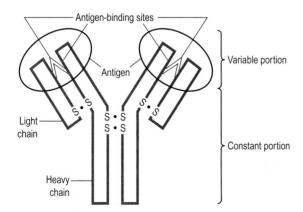

Figure 29.7 • Structure of a typical IgG antibody showing it to be composed of two heavy polypeptide chains and two light polypeptide chains. The antigen binds at two different sites on the variable portions of the chains. (From Guyton & Hall 2006, with kind permission of Elsevier.)

free in the blood and lymph. People come into contact with a large number of antigens and need a tremendous antibody diversity to combat them (see Box 29.1).

Antibody classes

The five classes of Ig are given Greek alphabet names. They are:

1. Gamma (γ)—IgG is produced in large quantities during the secondary response; it diffuses through blood vessel walls and is the major class of antibody found in tissue fluids. IgG activates the classical complement pathway. It crosses the placenta to confer passive immunity to the fetus and is found in colostrum and breast milk.

2. Alpha (α)—IgA protects the body's exposed surfaces against bacteria and fungi. It is found

407

BOX 29.1 GENERATION OF ANTIBODY DIVERSITY

The following facts help to explain antibody diversity:

- A small number of immunoglobulin genes are recombined in individual B cells so that each mature B cell contains a unique antibody molecule.
- The genes are found on different chromosomes so that antibody chains are made separately and recombined within the cell.

The basic structure of the five types of antibody consists of four polypeptide chains linked by disulphide bonds. There are two identical **heavy chains** and two identical **light chains** about half as long. The heavy chains are structurally distinct for each antibody class and are hinged about half way along their length. There are two types of light chain: λ (lambda) and κ (kappa). The chains form a Y-shaped molecule.

Each of the four chains is made up of different regions joined together. Each has a **variable** or V region, which differs between antibodies and forms the binding site at one end, and a much larger **constant** or C region. Between the V and C regions of light chains is the **joining** or J region. In heavy chains an additional region between the J and V sections is called the **diversity** or D region. These multiple regions increase the number of antibodies available to counteract antigens (Fig. 29.8). When the light and heavy chains with all their variable sites are combined, millions of antibody configurations are possible (Guyton & Hall 2006).

Some antibodies may have as many as 10 heavy and 10 light chains and therefore 10 antibody binding sites. When the antibody is highly specific there are so many binding sites that antigen–antibody attraction is strong. The two molecules are held together by hydrogen bonding, hydrophobic bonding, ionic attractions and van der Waals forces (see Ch. 1).

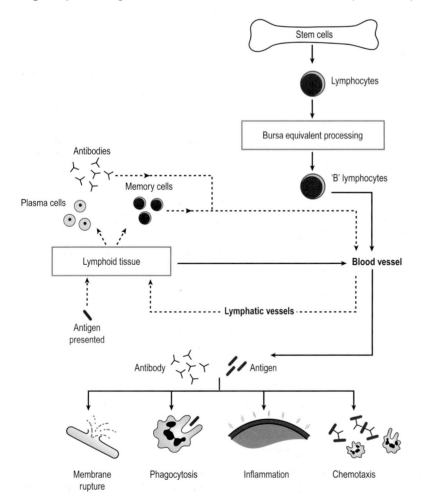

Figure 29.8●Diagram to summarise the formation and protective function of the humoral immune system. (From Montague S E, Watson R, Herbert R A 2005, with kind permission of Elsevier.)

in organ-lining mucous membrane secretions and in watery secretions such as tears, saliva and perspiration.

3. Mu (μ)—IgM is a large antibody found mainly in serum. It is the first and most abundant antibody secreted during the primary response. It binds to multiple antigens, causing them to agglutinate so that they are recognised by phagocytes. IgM is a potent trigger of the classical complement pathway.

4. Delta (δ)—IgD is mainly found attached to B cells and may be involved in their differentiation.

5. Epsilon (ε)—IgE precipitates inflammatory reactions around parasites. It is mainly bound to the surface of basophils and mast cells in skin, lungs and mucous membranes. IgE is implicated in allergy and hypersensitivity reactions.

Antibody functioning

Antibodies do not destroy antigens directly but inactivate them and tag them for other parts of the immune system to destroy by forming **antigen–antibody complexes**. Destruction is accomplished by mechanisms including complement fixation, neutralisation, agglutination and precipitation. The first two of these are most important:

- **Complement fixation** is the main protection against cellular agents such as bacteria. When antibodies bind to a target cell, their shape changes to expose complement-binding sites on their constant regions. This triggers the complement cascade.

- **Neutralisation** is when antibodies block specific sites on viruses or chemicals secreted by bacteria (exotoxins). This prevents them from binding to cells. Phagocytes destroy the resulting complexes.

- **Agglutination** of cell-bound antigens occurs because antibodies have more than one binding site and molecules have more than one antigenic site. Large lattices are formed by cross-linkage of immune complexes.

- **Precipitation** is a similar mechanism whereby soluble molecules are cross-linked into large complexes that settle out of solution. The large complexes formed by agglutination or precipitation are engulfed by phagocytes.

Cell-mediated immune response

T lymphocytes

T lymphocytes form the basis for cellular immunity. There are two major groups of T cells: **cytotoxic T cells (T_C or killer cells)** and T_H cells or **helper T cells** (Fig. 29.9). All T cells have glycoproteins on their cell surfaces. These are the **CD4** and **CD8 surface receptor molecules** (CD means cluster of differentiation).

Generally, T_H cells have CD4 proteins and are known as T4 cells; T_C cells have CD8 molecules on their cell surfaces and are known as T8 cells. Both CD4 and CD8 cells can suppress immune responses (Male et al 2006).

A further group of T lymphocytes has been identified but they are not well understood. These are **suppressor T cells** (T_S). They are capable of suppressing both CD4 and CD8 cells and their role may be to limit the ability of the immune system to attack its own tissues, a process called immune tolerance. T_S cells are classified with T_H cells as regulatory T cells. It is believed that during the processing of T cells by the thymus and bone marrow most of the clones that would damage a person's own tissues are destroyed before they can enter and colonise the tissues (Guyton & Hall 2006).

The T cell antigen receptor

T cells are also distinguished by the type of T cell antigen receptor (TCR) on their cell surface. The TCR recognises antigen fragments which are bound and presented by specialist antigen-presenting molecules. They do not recognise free antigen, that is the antibody's role. The most important of these molecules are the **class I** and **class II** molecules of the **major histocompatibility complex** (MHC). TCRs and antibodies are structurally related and both reproduce by cloning.

T cell differentiation: the MHC

For T cells to be selected and cloned there must be a double recognition of **antiself** (the antigen) and **self**. Every cell has surface proteins that identify it as self-coded for by the MHC, a very large gene complex. This provides the basis of human uniqueness as the genes can be combined in millions of ways. Only identical twins have identical MHC proteins, making tissue transplants difficult.

There are two main classes of MHC protein important in T cell activation: MHC class I and MHC class II (Engelhard 1994). MHC I proteins are present on most body cells to enable self-recognition, but MHC II proteins are found only on the surfaces of mature B cells, macrophages and some T cells. MHC cells are shaped like a hammock so that antigenic fragments to be displayed sit inside them, forming a self–antiself complex. T_H and T_C cells prefer different classes of MHC protein, a phenomenon called MHC restriction.

- T_H cells bind only to complexes that include MHC II proteins on the surfaces of macrophages.
- T_C cells are activated by complexes that include MHC I proteins on any cell.

Immunologic surveillance

T cells crawl over other cells searching for antigens, a process called **immunologic surveillance**. When the T cell

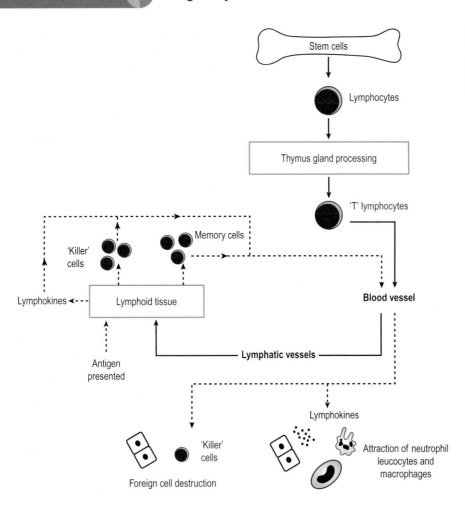

Figure 29.9 • Diagram to summarise the formation and protective function of the cell-mediated immune system. (From Montague S E, Watson R, Herbert R A 2005, with kind permission of Elsevier.)

is activated by binding to the self–antiself complex it enlarges and forms a clone. Some, as with B cells, are left as memory cells. T_C cells act mainly against virus-infected cells but can kill cells invaded by some bacteria such as the tubercle bacillus. T_H cells stimulate the proliferation of other B and T cells by releasing a **lymphokine** called **interleukin II.** Some T cells release lymphokines that inhibit the activated B and T cells, ensuring that the immune response is brought to an end after the successful destruction of an antigen. Most T cell activity consists of T_C cells attacking cells infected by micro-organisms or cancerous cells. They will also attack transplanted tissue.

The immune system cells release chemicals called cytokines (from cells) to stimulate each other. These soluble glycoproteins fall into different categories: e.g. they are called lymphokines when released from lymphocytes. Lymphokines enhance immune system cellular activity.

Cytokines

The principal sets of cytokines are (Male et al 2006):

* **Interferons** (IFNs) limit the spread of viral infections. They are produced by certain T cells early in a viral infection and may be the first line of resistance.

They diffuse to nearby cells and stimulate them to produce proteins that inhibit viral replication. Alpha (α) interferons are produced by most white cells and gamma (γ) interferons are produced by lymphocytes. NK cells produce gamma interferons which can activate macrophages.

* **Interleukins** (ILs) are a large group; 22 have so far been found. They are produced mainly by T cells and mainly direct other immune system cells to divide and differentiate.
* **Colony-stimulating factors** (CSFs) are primarily involved in directing the division and differentiation of bone marrow stem cells.
* **Chemokines** are chemotactic cytokines which direct cell movement around the body: e.g. movement of immune cells out of the blood and into the tissues.
* **Tumour necrosis factors** (TNFs) mediate inflammation and cytotoxic reactions.

The brain's immune system

White cells secrete substances capable of killing neurons but these are prevented from entering the brain by the blood–brain barrier unless blood vessels are damaged. Microglia can become phagocytic and are the cells that HIV attacks in the brain; their activation is implicated in AIDS dementia.

Physiological changes in pregnancy

During pregnancy the immune system undergoes minor alterations in both primary and secondary defence mechanisms. The fetus is antigenically unique and it is a mystery why it is not rejected as foreign tissue. The changes may help to protect the fetus but also increase the severity of autoimmune diseases (Blackburn 2007).

White cell count

The total white cell count rises early in pregnancy, mainly due to an increase in neutrophils. It is probably caused by circulating oestrogen. A peak is reached at 30 weeks and a plateau maintained until delivery. There is a further rise in labour and the count returns to normal by the 6th postnatal day. There is a slight rise in eosinophils in ratio to the increased white cell count but a sharp fall occurs during labour. They are absent at delivery but return to normal by the 3rd postnatal day. Basophil and monocyte counts appear to remain unchanged.

Cell-mediated immunity

Although the lymphocyte count remains unchanged in pregnancy, there is a change in cell-mediated immunity. T_H cells decline in relation to T_C cells able to suppress the immune response, possibly due to pregnancy hormones. However, these changes are insufficient to prevent fetal rejection and other mechanisms must be present. It is likely that both maternal and fetoplacental mechanisms prevent fetal rejection.

Immunology of the fetoplacental unit

The fetoplacental unit is an **allograft** (foreign tissue from the same species) with different MHC cell surface receptors. Paternal antigens are expressed on fetal cells as early as the 8-cell stage. If the skin of a newborn baby is grafted onto the mother she rejects it as foreign. In fact there is an immunological rejection response to the fetus seen in the blood of pregnant women (Johnson 2007). Alternative explanations have been explored.

Local inhibition of the immune response

There may be local immune regulation in the uterus due to high levels of circulating pregnancy hormones such as progesterone, corticosteroids and/or human chorionic gonadotrophin (hCG). Also local metabolism of the amino acid tryptophan might reduce maternal immunological response but the mechanism is not understood. Helper T cells are low in relation to suppressor T cells in the decidua and may not recognise the antigens on the invading trophoblast cells. NK cells may moderate local immune response by producing cytokines to create a local balance between placental invasion and maternal resistance (Johnson 2007).

Protective immunological barrier

The fetus, including its blood, is separated from the mother by the fetal membranes. The trophoblast at the fetal–maternal interface may be important in protecting the fetus from the maternal immune system by preventing maternal immune cells and antibodies from entering the fetal circulation. However, some trophoblastic cells break away and enter the maternal circulation via the spiral arteries and provoke antibody formation.

Neither the villous cytotrophoblast nor the syncytiotrophoblast express class I or class II MHC antigens. However, the trophoblast cells that invade the spiral arteries express other MHC molecules, namely human leucocyte antigens HLA-C and HLA-G. This may confer fetal resistance to destruction by NK cells by inhibiting cytokine production.

The fetal immune response

Although the placental barrier (or filter as it is not perfect) is effective against most cells and antibodies, IgG crosses to the fetus to protect it against any infectious diseases she has suffered and made antibodies against. Other antibodies such as rhesus may cross the placental barrier. The rhesus antigen exists as a cell surface antigen and is never found as a free molecule. As red blood cells are too large to cross the placental barrier, there is no possibility of raising fetal antibodies unless maternal red cells escape into the fetal circulation, usually at delivery.

However, other fetal cell surface antigens such as the ABO system and major MHC molecules are naturally present as soluble molecules in fetal blood or tissue fluid. The fetal immune system may be able to destroy such proteins. If any maternal immune cells or antibodies cross the placental barrier they are likely to be mopped up by free fetal antigens before they can damage fetal tissues.

411

In summary

Fetal protection from maternal immune response may depend on (Johnson 2007):

- An antigenically unique trophoblast giving local depression of immune reactivity.
- Special populations of NK cells in the decidua recognising specific HLAs and regulating invasion and maternal immune resistance.
- A complete barrier to transmission of immune cells or antibodies from mother to fetus.
- Fetal antigens mopping up any aggressive immune cells or antibodies before they can cause extensive damage to fetal tissues.

The immunology of breast milk

Colostrum and breast milk during the 1st week following delivery contain enormous quantities of immunoglobulin capable of reacting against many microorganisms. Bacteria that may cause gastroenteritis in the neonate are especially protected against. A discussion on the anti-infective benefits of breastfeeding is found in Chapter 54.

Clinical implications

Active and passive humoral immunity

Active immunity

Immunity to infectious diseases is naturally acquired when B cells produce antibodies against a bacterium or virus during an infection. However, the symptoms of the disease may cause serious illness or death. Edward Jenner noticed that people who caught cowpox were unaffected by smallpox. In 1796 he inoculated James Phipps with liquid from a pustule on the hand of a milkmaid who had cowpox. He then inoculated him with pus from a smallpox sufferer and James did not develop the disease.

This technique is now used on a massive scale: protection against infectious diseases by raising antibodies. The word vaccine derives from this experiment (the Latin word for cow is *vacca*). Most vaccines contain dead or attenuated (weakened) pathogens which challenge the immune system without producing symptoms.

Passive immunity

Just as active immunity can be naturally or artificially acquired, so can passive immunity. Antibodies are not produced by the immune system but obtained from another source. Protection against a disease is limited to the natural lifespan of the acquired antibody, at most 2–3 weeks. Naturally occurring passive immunity is acquired by the fetus through transfer of maternal IgG across the placenta and by the breastfed baby in breast milk. Injection of immune serum such as gamma-globulin can be offered passive immunity to a person needing short-term protection from a pathogen they have been in contact with such as hepatitis virus.

Autoimmune disorders

There may be improvement, deterioration or no change in the status of **autoimmune disorders** during pregnancy. Both T cells and autoantigens (self cells) are needed to allow production of **autoantibodies**. The resulting immune complexes activate the complement system and mediate phagocytosis and an inflammatory response (Male et al 2006).

Pregnancy changes in the immune system are exactly opposite to the above events so that women with an autoimmune disorder should experience relief from symptoms. Most women with **rheumatoid arthritis** improve during pregnancy.

However, women with **systemic lupus erythematosus** (SLE), particularly those with renal involvement, may have an exacerbation of their condition, affecting the fetus and neonate adversely. SLE is also associated with an increase in abortion and stillbirth (Andrade et al 2008).

Maternal antibodies and the fetus

The fetus of a woman with autoimmune disease may develop transient autoimmune symptoms. In **Grave's disease** a thyroid-stimulating immunoglobulin crosses the placenta and may cause neonatal hyperthyroidism. **Myasthenia gravis** is associated with an antibody against ACh receptors, resulting in profound muscle weakness. These antibodies can cross the placenta to produce transient myasthenia gravis in about 15% of their neonates.

A drug effect on immunity

Between 1940 and 1970 the drug **diethylstilbestrol** was given to 1.5 million women in the USA to prevent miscarriages. Many of their daughters developed vaginal **clear cell carcinoma** as teenagers and had increased incidences of infertility, fetal anomalies, ectopic pregnancies, miscarriages, stillbirths and premature deliveries. They have also a higher risk of autoimmune disorders. Researchers believe these have a common factor: alterations in their T-cell-mediated immunity (Burke et al 2001).

Main points

- The immune system cells and molecules protect us from environmental factors such as micro-organisms, irritants and abnormal cells by destroying them or rendering them harmless.

- There are two branches of the immune system: non-specific and specific immunity. Non-specific immunity includes surface barriers such as skin and mucous membranes and some cellular and chemical defences, usually involving phagocytic cells.

- The lymphatic system consists of primary lymphoid organs where B cells and T cells differentiate and mature, and the peripheral lymphoid system which includes encapsulated organs and unencapsulated lymphoid tissue.

- Specific immunity is divided into humoral and cellular immunity or cell-mediated immunity. B lymphocytes, T lymphocytes and macrophages are the main immune cells.

- B lymphocytes secrete antibodies. Macrophages present antigens to T cells for recognition and secrete substances that activate them. T cells secrete chemicals that activate macrophages. The immune response targets non-self antigens. Small molecules that are not immunogenic can link up with body proteins to form haptens which may trigger allergies.

- The binding of an antigen and lymphocyte stimulates formation of a clone of cells which recognise that antigen. Most clone cells differentiate into plasma cells which secrete antibodies for 5 days and die. A few become memory cells able to mount a secondary response if the antigen is encountered later.

- Five classes of antibody each have a specific function: IgG, IgA, IgM, IgD and IgE. Mechanisms that destroy antigen-bearing molecules include complement fixation, neutralisation, agglutination and precipitation.

- There are two types of T cell: T_C and T_H cells. T_H cells have CD4 proteins and T_C cells have CD8 molecules on their surfaces. Both types of cell suppress immune responses.

- Class I and class II MHC molecules on cell surfaces define self. MHC proteins are present on most body cells but MHC II proteins are found only on cell surfaces of mature B cells, macrophages and some T cells.

- T_H cells bind only to complexes which include MHC II proteins on macrophage surfaces. T_C cells are activated by complexes which include MHC I proteins on any cell.

- The immune system cells release cytokines to stimulate each other. T_C cells act mainly against virus-infected cells but also attack cancerous cells or transplanted tissue. T_H cells stimulate the proliferation of other T and B cells by releasing interleukin II.

- HIV attacks microglia in the brain and causes AIDS dementia.

- In pregnancy the immune system undergoes minor alterations to both primary and secondary defence mechanisms. Total white cell count increases, mainly due to an increase in neutrophils. Though protecting the fetus, the changes may influence the progress of autoimmune diseases.

- T_H cells decline in relation to T_C cells which may suppress the immune response but these changes are insufficient to explain fetal protection from maternal immune responses.

- There may be immune regulation in the uterus. Decidual T cells are low in number and may not recognise antigens on invading trophoblastic cells. High local levels of pregnancy hormones and high metabolism of tryptophan may moderate local immune response.

- The trophoblast may prevent most maternal immune cells and antibodies except IgG from entering the fetal circulation. Most MHC receptors are down-graded in trophoblastic cells. This may confer resistance to destruction by maternal NK cells.

- Most fetal cell surface antigens (except the rhesus factor) such as the ABO system and major MHC molecules are present in fetal blood and tissue fluids. Any maternal antibodies crossing the placental barrier may be mopped up by these free antigens.

- Colostrum and breast milk in the first week contain high levels of immunoglobulins capable of reacting against many micro-organisms, particularly those that cause gastroenteritis.

- Active immunity to infectious diseases can be acquired during an infection. Vaccines can challenge the immune system to produce specific antibodies.

- Passive immunity is acquired by the fetus by placental transfer of maternal IgG and by breast-fed babies via antibodies in breast milk.

- There may be improvement, deterioration or no change in the status of autoimmune disorders during pregnancy. Both T cells and autoantigens are needed to allow production of autoantibodies.

References

Andrade, R., Sanchez, M.L., Alarćon, G.S., Fessier, B.J., et al., 2008. Adverse pregnancy outcomes in women with systemic lupus erythromatosus from a multiethnic US cohort: LUMINA (LVI). Clin. Exp. Rheumatol. 26 (2), 268–274.

Blackburn, S.T., 2007. Maternal, Fetal & Neonatal Physiology: A Clinical Perspective, third edn. Saunders, Philadelphia.

Burke, L., Segall-Blank, M., Lorenzo, C., et al., 2001. Altered immune response in adult women exposed to diethylstilbestrol in utero. Am. J. Obstet. Gynecol. 185, 78–81.

Engelhard, V.H., 1994. How cells process antigens. Sci. Am. August, 44–51.

Guyton, A.C., Hall, J.E., 2006. Textbook of Medical Physiology, eleventh edn. Elsevier Saunders, Philadelphia.

Johnson, M.H., 2007. Essential Reproduction, sixth edn. Blackwell Publishing, Oxford.

Kendall, M.D., 2007. Dying to Live: How Our Bodies Fight Disease. Cambridge University Press, Cambridge.

Male, D., Brostoff, J., Roth, D., Roitt, I., 2006. Immunology, seventh edn. Mosby, St Louis.

Montague, S.E., Watson, R., Herbert, R. A. (Eds.), 2005. Physiology for Nursing Practice, third ed. Baillière Tindall, London.

Annotated recommended reading

Johnson, M.H., 2007. Essential Reproduction, sixth edn. Blackwell Publishing, Oxford.

This up-to-date textbook places human reproduction in a wider context and represents an integrated approach to the subject. Where appropriate, descriptions and discussions centre on the human reproductive system. Chapter 12 includes a clear discussion about the non-rejection of the fetus by the maternal immune system.

Kendall, M.D., 2007. Dying to Live: How Our Bodies Fight Disease. Cambridge University Press, Cambridge.

This popular science book presents the many levels of complexity of this subject in a manner that reduces the complexity without losing content. It is very readable and informative.

Male, D., Brostoff, J., Roth, D., Roitt, I., 2006. Immunology, seventh edn. Mosby, St Louis.

The first half of this book covers basic immunity whilst the second half is geared to clinical application of concepts. The plentiful use of paragraph headings ensures that concepts are well explained. There is on-line access to help available.

Section **2C**

Pregnancy—The Problems

SECTION CONTENTS

Although pregnancy is a normal physiological function, some women may develop illnesses independent of their pregnancy. Some minor health problems are caused by the pregnancy but are not life-threatening; these are discussed in Chapter 30. Long-term health problems such as diabetes mellitus are influenced greatly by the pregnancy, and perhaps the most widespread danger to pregnant women, pregnancy itself, may precipitate a hypertensive condition in up to 10% of women. Chapters 31–35 discuss pathological states relevant to the pregnant woman. Chapter 31 examines the possible causes and management of bleeding in pregnancy. Chapters 32–35 utilise a systems approach and each disorder is discussed in depth with its management in terms of diagnosis and treatment.

Chapter Thirty

Minor disorders of pregnancy

Introduction

During pregnancy women suffer inconvenient but not life-threatening symptoms referred to collectively as the minor disorders of pregnancy. It should also be considered that a minor disorder may suddenly become a much more serious illness. For these two reasons, it is essential for the midwife or doctor caring for women to pay attention to these symptoms and to offer safe and sensible advice on their alleviation.

Maintenance of pregnancy

Maternal physiological recognition of pregnancy begins with the presence of the blastocyst in the uterine cavity. The development of the embryo and placentation are described in Chapters 9–12. The corpus luteum normally regresses after about 14 days if a fertilised ovum does not reach the uterus. The maintenance of the **corpus luteum of pregnancy** has been ascribed to the production of **human chorionic gonadotrophin** (hCG) by the cells of the **syncytiotrophoblast** as they invade the endometrium. This is secreted into maternal blood and taken to the ovary where it augments the action of **luteinising hormone** from the anterior pituitary gland to continue production of **progesterone** from the corpus luteum. The role of the corpus luteum is to maintain the pregnancy by secreting steroid hormones, mainly progesterone, until the placenta can take over the major role about 4–5 weeks after the last menstrual period (Johnson 2007). The corpus luteum continues to secrete progesterone but this only plays a minimal role in later pregnancy.

The hormone hCG can be identified in the blood 6–7 days post fertilisation and before the first missed period; its excretion in the urine forms the basis of the widely available and highly efficient immunological pregnancy tests. There is no ovulation, and endocrine production is changed to maintain the pregnancy.

Another mechanism important in maintaining early pregnancy is the suppression of **prostaglandin** concentrations in decidual tissue. In the menstrual cycle these play a role in **luteolysis**, the breakdown of the corpus luteum. Prostaglandin concentrations in early pregnancy are lower than those measured in the endometrium during the menstrual cycle. It is possible that prostaglandin production is reduced by a substance which inhibits the biosynthesis of arachidonic acid, their precursor substance. The hormone **relaxin**, a small polypeptide, seems to be produced by the corpus luteum in early and late pregnancy. It inhibits myometrial activity and may play a role in the maintenance of early pregnancy (Fig. 30.1) (Johnson 2007). Other important factors include **inhibin**, **interferon**, **cytokines** and **growth factors** which assist in the early development of the conceptus (Coad & Dunstall 2001).

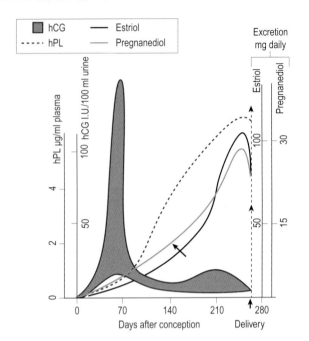

Figure 30.1 • Changes in hormone levels during pregnancy. hCG, human chorionic gonadotrophin; hPL, human placental lactogen. (From Hinchliff S M, Montague S E 1990, with permission.)

Minor disorders of pregnancy

The minor disorders occur because of physiological adaptation of the woman's body to pregnancy, in particular the effect of progesterone and other hormones on the smooth muscle and connective tissue.

The digestive system

Nausea and vomiting

This troublesome complaint begins early in pregnancy at the 4th week and persists until about the 12th week in most sufferers; a few continue to have symptoms until the 16th week. Although commonly referred to as morning sickness, many women feel nauseous but may not vomit. Others will vomit at any time of day. In a prospective study of 160 women, 80% found nausea lasted all day, and sickness occurred in 1.8% (Lacroix et al 2000). The duration of these symptoms in 90% of women lasted 22 weeks. Nausea and vomiting for approximately two-thirds of women is an expected and normal feature of pregnancy (Flaxman & Sherman 2000, Furneaux & Langley-Evans 2001). A few women will develop severe vomiting known as **hyperemesis gravidarum**, which is life-threatening to the woman; this is discussed in Chapter 34.

The aetiology of nausea and vomiting is not fully understood. It may be that a combination of physical and emotional factors is involved (Chou et al 2003, Furneaux & Langley-Evans 2001). However, this period

of time is close to the peak presence of hCG, which may be a trigger. Oestrogen and progesterone may also be involved. Andersson et al (2004) found an association between depression and increased nausea and vomiting.

Flaxman & Sherman (2000) reviewed the literature and mentioned other facts:

• Peak sickness occurred at 6–18 weeks, the period of embryonic organogenesis—increasing hormone levels.
• Women who experience sickness are less likely to miscarry.
• Aversions to some foods may be protective.

Huxley (2000) suggested that the nausea and vomiting stimulated placental growth by dividing nutrient factors from the mother to the benefit of the growing embryo. Alterations in thyroid function have been suggested as a cause (Mori et al 1988). The severity of morning sickness has been correlated with the increased amount of free thyroxine (T_4), and decreased thyroid-stimulating hormone (TSH). There is a link between altered thyroid gland function and nausea and excessive vomiting in pregnancy (Asakura et al 2000).

Perhaps morning sickness is **adaptive** in an evolutionary sense and nausea and food aversions minimise fetal exposure to toxins during the period of **organogenesis**. Women are inclined to eat bland food without strong odours and flavours. This avoids the ingestion of spicy plant toxins and foods produced by bacterial and fungal decomposition.

There have been anxieties about the safety of **antiemetic drugs**. Non-pharmacological measures are best used and are usually sufficient to combat pregnancy nausea. Light snacks instead of large meals and carbohydrate snacks at bedtime and before rising can prevent the hypoglycaemia that appears to be the cause (Lindsay 2004, McParlin et al 2008). The avoidance of iron supplements is advisable. Ginger capsules and ginger root tea have been found to combat nausea and vomiting in some diseases but Marcus et al (2005) warn that the safety of this substance taken in quantity has not been established (Vutyavanich et al 2001). If vomiting persists or becomes severe, a medical practitioner should be consulted. The use of pressure bands has been found to be beneficial to some women (Sook et al 2007, Steele et al 2001).

Heartburn

Heartburn (**reflux oesophagitis**) is a burning sensation felt behind the sternum caused by reflux of acid gastric contents into the oesophagus. It is most problematic after 30 weeks of pregnancy, increasing in intensity until term and disappearing after delivery. Some 30–70% of women at some time in their pregnancy complain of heartburn, with 25% of those complaining of symptoms daily in the latter half of pregnancy (Blackburn 2007).

The main cause is the relaxing effect of progesterone on the smooth muscle of the cardiac sphincter between stomach and oesophagus. In the non-pregnant woman, sphincter tone increases in response to raised intragastric pressure to prevent reflux. This ability is greatly diminished in pregnancy as peristaltic activity is slowed and gastric emptying time is lengthened. Pressure from the growing uterus increases the intragastric pressure and flattening of the diaphragm distorts the shape of the stomach and decreases the angle at the gastrojejunal junction (Girling 2000).

The anatomical changes may cause the sphincter to become incompetent, causing a **temporary hiatus hernia** (Coad & Dunstall 2001). Reflux can be prevented by avoiding bending over when doing housework such as cleaning the bath, particularly with a full stomach. Sleeping in a more upright position by using additional pillows helps at night. A balanced diet, not spicy, with small regular meals, is recommended. Antacids may be taken after meals and at bedtime under medical supervision (Lloyd 2000).

Ptyalism

This disorder, which is more common in women with an Afro-Caribbean background, is excess salivation and is the equivalent of morning sickness. In some cases the woman must continuously wipe saliva from her mouth. It is referred to as 'spitting' and is a sign of pregnancy, particularly in the West Indies. If severe, it may lead to loss of fluids and electrolytes and dehydration. Similar advice as for morning sickness may help. It may also accompany heartburn (Girling 2000).

Pica

This is the medical term for the ingestion of non-nutritive substances such as coal, washing starch, soap, toothpaste. There is a belief that the craving occurs because of a need of the fetus for certain minerals but this has not been substantiated by research. Hormones and metabolic changes have also been implicated. In a survey of 10 000 women only 14 respondents had experienced such cravings (Mikkelsen 2007).

Constipation

Constipation is a common and troublesome disorder of pregnancy and may lead to the development of haemorrhoids, which in turn may increase constipation because of a fear of pain. The increased production of progesterone in pregnancy causes relaxation and reduced peristalsis in the smooth muscle of the digestive tract. This increases the transit time of food through the gut and a greater time for water to be absorbed in the large intestine. A dryer bulkier stool is then more difficult to defecate. The gut is also displaced upwards and outwards by the growing uterus. Faulty diet and disregarding the need to defecate add to the problem. In a survey to investigate diet habits and activity in the three trimesters it was found that women who were constipated ate more and drank less water, and physical activity did not seem to affect constipation in this sample (Derbyshire et al 2006).

Oral iron therapy is also implicated by some women. Advice should be given to pregnant women as soon as they have had their pregnancy confirmed to avoid the situation if possible. It is necessary to ensure that they have an adequate fluid intake, maintain regular bowel habits and take in enough roughage in the form of fruits, vegetables and grains. Also live yoghurt is a natural laxative because of its **bifidus** content. Exercise is also useful. A stool softener or mild laxative can be useful as an adjunct to the above advice (Girling 2000).

Skin

Anterior pituitary production of **melanocyte-stimulating hormone** is increased by the progesterone and oestrogen levels of pregnancy. This increases skin pigmentation in pregnancy, which may lead to a condition called **chloasma** or 'pregnancy mask', typically found on the face. **Palmar erythema** may be seen, due to increased circulation and the palms may feel hot (Frederique et al 2006). The skin changes very common to all are the **striae gravidarum** of pregnancy due to the rupturing of small amounts of tissue under the skin caused through stretching of the skin layers. Although pink in pregnancy, as the skin returns to normal and after time the striae become mauve and less noticeable. Pruritus or itching of the skin is not a problem in itself but of great nuisance to the woman. It only becomes a problem when the liver enzymes are raised and **cholestasis of pregnancy** is suspected (Coggins 2002).

The cardiovascular system

Fainting

The effect of progesterone on smooth muscle increases the incidence of fainting in pregnancy. Although the increase in circulating blood volume partly compensates, there is decreased vascular resistance. This alters the blood pressure and the venous return, permitting the pooling of blood in the lower extremities. Standing erect for long periods and the increased vasodilatation by being too warm may precipitate a faint. Later in pregnancy **supine hypotension** can be a problem; it is caused by the gravid uterus pressing on the inferior vena cava, preventing venous return to the heart and thus reducing cardiac output. It is easily prevented or reversed by avoiding the total supine position or turning the woman quickly onto her side if she begins to feel faint.

Varicosities

Varicosities occur as an outcome of the relaxing effect of progesterone on the smooth muscle of the walls of the veins. This is commonly found in the lower limbs as circulation becomes sluggish and the veins dilate, reducing valvular efficiency. The situation is exacerbated by pressure from the growing uterus, causing pelvic congestion and poor venous return and weight gain in the woman. **Varicose veins** may also occur in the anus as haemorrhoids and in the vulva (Turner 2001). Varicose veins of the leg can be made more bearable with the use of support tights applied in the morning and gentle walking to maintain circulation. Where possible, women should sit with their legs elevated and uncrossed (Carr 2006).

Haemorrhoids occur as an outcome of the relaxing effect of progesterone on the veins of the anus, the reduction of venous return by the growing uterus and the incidence of constipation. They can be helped by the prevention and treatment of constipation. If needed, topical applications can be suggested and medical advice sought. As the haemorrhoids often disappear after delivery and because of the alteration in venous tone, surgery would not be performed in pregnancy.

Vulval varicosities, while rare, are very painful. A sanitary pad or sometimes a panty girdle may give support. Lying down will help to prevent congestion in the area. Care must be taken during delivery as there is a risk of haemorrhage from the distended veins, especially if cut through during an episiotomy (Turner 2001).

The musculoskeletal system

Backache

At least 50% of women may experience backache in pregnancy. It is essential to differentiate the cause of back pain so that appropriate treatment can be obtained. Some contributing factors are postural changes resulting in lumbar lordosis with overstretched abdominal muscles and strained back muscles (Borg-Stein et al 2005). Also, the relaxing effect of progesterone and relaxin on the pelvic ligaments allows movement of the symphysis pubis and lumbosacral joints. Symphysis pubic dysfunction (Bick 2004, Wellock & Crichton 2007) can be exceedingly painful and limit mobility. Relaxin may make the intervertebral joints unstable as they try to support the increased weight of pregnancy. Once the more worrying causes of backache are excluded, the woman is advised on back care to minimise pain. The following advice may be helpful:

- **Sitting**—She should choose a comfortable chair which supports both back and thighs when sitting. She should sit well back and it may be necessary to place a small cushion behind the lumbar spine.
- **Standing**—It is advised that standing tall with tummy and buttocks tucked in and weight evenly distributed on both legs with a flat shoe would be of benefit to prevent backache.
- **Lying**—Lying in the lateral position is preferable to supine with a good supportive mattress. Care should be taken when changing from lying down to sitting up to avoid strain on back and abdominal muscles. When getting off the examination couch, rolling on to the side and allowing the legs to fall over the side of the couch will place less strain on the back. The arms should be used to push up into a sitting position.
- **Work**—Lifting or dragging heavy objects should be avoided and women should discuss the best position for managing their work both in business and at home.

The nervous system

Carpal tunnel syndrome

Women who develop **carpal tunnel syndrome** (CTS) complain of numbness and tingling, often called pins and needles, in their fingers and hands. This is most likely to be present in the morning but can occur at any time of day. The cause is fluid retention of pregnancy and swelling of connective tissue which compresses the median nerve as it runs through the carpal tunnel in the wrist. It may be necessary for the woman to wear a splint at night and elevate the hand, to prevent fluid collecting in the night. Occasionally, the doctor may prescribe diuretics. A multicentre study found that many women suffered from CTS in pregnancy and half of these women will still be having symptoms post pregnancy (Pazzaglia et al 2005).

Fatigue and emotional changes

Ninety-seven per cent of women experience fatigue in the first trimester of pregnancy. The early weeks of pregnancy are a time of physiological and psychological change which will inevitably affect women's feelings about themselves. Sleep patterns change during the menstrual cycle so it would be anticipated that this would happen in pregnancy. This change is related to oestrogen levels (Ozaja et al 2005). Fatigue has been associated with depression and nausea and causes an inability to carry out mental and physical tasks. Sleep may be disturbed by urinary frequency, leg cramps, breathing problems and vomiting, therefore midwives need to be aware of sleep problems which can be helped by a rest during the day. This is easier said than done with women working and caring for young children but it has been associated with a greater risk of pre-eclampsia and preterm birth (Bialiobok & Monga 2000).

The genitourinary system

Frequency of micturition

Urinary frequency affects women most in the first and third trimesters of pregnancy, mainly because of pressure on the bladder by the growing uterus. During the second trimester the uterus is displaced upwards over the pelvic brim and the incidence of frequency is lower.

The increased reabsorption of sodium and water increases the need to pass urine through the night (**nocturia**). During the day excess water is trapped in the lower extremities because of venous stasis. When the woman lies down at night, pressure on the large veins is reduced and there is increased cardiac return, cardiac output and renal blood flow with a subsequent increase in urinary output, particularly in the left lateral position. There is an increased risk of urinary tract infection because of progesterone's effect on ureteric smooth muscle. This may cause **urinary reflux** or **stasis** (Turner 2000).

Small lifestyle changes can reduce nocturia:

- Restrict fluids in the evening by increasing the fluid intake earlier in the day.

- Limit the intake of natural diuretics such as caffeine.
- Lie down in the left lateral recumbent position during the evening to encourage a diuresis.

Leucorrhoea

There is an increase in white, non-irritant vaginal discharge in pregnancy. Once the possibility of vaginal moniliasis or trichomonal infection has been excluded, simple personal hygiene will ensure comfort for the woman. Wearing cotton pants and avoiding tights will also increase comfort.

Conclusion

Midwives play an important role in the management of minor disorders of pregnancy. Women often discuss their discomforts with the midwife, who can reassure women that their problem is not health-threatening and offer simple advice to minimise the particular problem. Occasionally, a more serious condition may be present and midwives should be vigilant about seeking medical advice in such cases.

Main points

- Maternal physiological recognition of pregnancy begins with the presence of the blastocyst in the uterine cavity. There is no ovulation and the endocrine production is changed to maintain the pregnancy. The corpus luteum continues to secrete progesterone until term.

- A minor disorder of pregnancy may suddenly become a much more serious illness. Minor disorders include breast tenderness, morning sickness, increased urinary frequency, leg cramps, carpal tunnel syndrome, increased fatigue, fainting/dizziness, constipation, heartburn, dyspnoea, varicose veins, haemorrhoids, ankle oedema, vaginal discharge, skin changes, backache, ligament pain, headache, stuffy nose, bleeding gums, mood swings, changing body image, depression, increased sensitivity, indecisiveness and alterations in libido.

- Midwives play an important role in the management of minor disorders of pregnancy. Women often discuss their discomforts with the midwife, who can reassure women that their problem is not health-threatening and offer simple advice to minimise the particular problem.

- Occasionally a more serious condition may be present and midwives should be vigilant about seeking medical advice in such cases.

References

Andersson, L., Sundstrom-Poromaa, I., Wulff, M., Astrom, M., Bixo, M., 2004. Implications of antenatal depression and anxiety for obstetric outcome. Obstet. Gynecol. 104, 467–476.

Asakura, H., Watanabe, S., Sekiguchi, A., Power, G.G., Araki, T., 2000. Severity of hyperemesis gravidarum correlates with serum levels of T3. Arch. Gynecol. Obstet. 264 (2), 57–62.

Bialiobok, K., Monga, M., 2000. Fatigue and work in pregnancy. Curr. Opin. Obstet. Gynecol. 12 (6), 497–500.

Bick, D., 2004. Content and organization of postnatal care, Ch. 41. In: Henderson, C., Macdonald, S. (Eds.) Mayes Midwifery: A Textbook for Midwives. Baillière Tindall, London.

Blackburn, S.T., 2007. Maternal, Fetal and Neonatal Physiology, third edn. W B Saunders, Philadelphia.

Borg-Stein, J., Dugan, S., Gruber, J., 2005. Musculoskeletal aspects of pregnancy. Am. J. Phys. Med. Rehabil. 84 (3), 180–192.

Carr, S., 2006. Current management of varicose veins. Clin. Obstet. Gynecol. 49 (2), 414–426.

Chou, F.H., Lin, L.L., Cooney, A., Waller, L., Riggs, M., 2003. Psychological factors related to nausea and vomiting and fatigue in early pregnancy. J. Nurs. Sch. 35 (2), 119–125.

Coad, J., Dunstall, M., 2001. Anatomy and Physiology for Midwives. Mosby, St Louis.

Coggins, J., 2002. Early pregnancy care. Pract. Midwife 5 (9), 14–17.

Derbyshire, E., Davies, J., Vassilikki, C., Dettmar, P., 2006. Diet, physical inactivity and prevalence of constipation throughout and after pregnancy. Matern. Child Health 2 (3), 127–134.

Flaxman, S.M., Sherman, P.W., 2000. Morning sickness: a mechanism for protecting mother and embryo. Q. Rev. Biol. 75 (2), 113–148.

Frederique, H., Quatresooz, P., Valverde-Lopez, J., Pierard, G., 2006. Blood vessel changes during pregnancy: a review. Am. J. Clin. Dermatol. 7 (1), 65–69.

Furneaux, E.C., Langley-Evans, A.J., 2001. Nausea and vomiting of pregnancy. Obstet. Gynecol. Surv. 56, 775–782.

Girling, J.C., 2000. Physical adaptation to pregnancy. In: Page, L. (Ed.), The New Midwifery. Churchill Livingstone, Edinburgh.

Huxley, R.R., 2000. Nausea and vomiting in early pregnancy: its role in placental development. Obstet. Gynecol. 95 (5), 779–782.

Johnson, M.H., 2007. Essential Reproduction, 6th edn. Blackwell Science, Oxford.

Lacroix, R., Eason, E., Melzack, R., 2000. Nausea and vomiting during pregnancy: a prospective study of its frequency, intensity and pattern changes. Am. J. Obstet. Gynecol. 182 (4), 931–937.

Lindsay, P., 2004. Nausea and vomiting, Ch 43. In: Henderson, C., Macdonald, S. (Eds.) Mayes' Midwifery: A Textbook for Midwives. Baillière Tindall, NY.

Lloyd, N., 2000. How to cope with heartburn during pregnancy. Br. J. Midwifery 8 (4), 254.

McParlin, C., Graham, R.H., Robson, S.C., 2008. Caring for women with nausea and vomiting in pregnancy: new approaches. Br. J. Midwifery 16 (5), 280–285.

Marcus, D.M., Snodgrass, W., 2005. Do no harm: avoidance of herbal medicines. Obstet. Gynecol. 105, 1119–1122.

Mikkelsen, B.T., Andersen, A.M.N., Olsen, S.F., 2007. Pica in pregnancy in a privileged population: myth or reality. Obstet. Gynecol. Surv. 62 (2), 94–95.

Mori, M., Amino, N., Tamaki, H., et al., 1988. Morning sickness and thyroid function in normal pregnancy. Obstet. Gynaecol. 72 (3 Part 1), 355–359.

Ozaja, A., Arber, S., Hislop, J., Kerkhofs, M., Kopp, C., et al., 2005. Women's sleep in health and disease. J. Psychiatr. Res. 39 (1), 55–76.

Pazzaglia, C., Caliandro, P., Aprile, I., Mondelli, M., Foschini, M., et al., 2005. Multicentre study of carpal tunnel syndrome and pregnancy incidence and natural course. Acta Neurochir. Suppl. 92, 35–39.

Sook, H. S., Young, S., Sunhee, S. 2007. Effect of Nei-Guan point (P6) acupressure on ketonuria levels, nausea and vomiting in women with hyperemesis gravidarum. Available on line: <http://ovidsp.uk.ovid.com/spb/ovidweb.cgi> (accessed 14.04.08.).

Steele, N.M., French, J., Gatherer-Boyles, J., 2001. Effect of acupressure by sea-bands on nausea and vomiting of pregnancy. J. Gynaecol. Neonatal Nurs. 30 (1), 61–70.

Turner, A., 2000. How to manage urinary tract infection in pregnancy. Br. J. Midwifery 8 (12), 777.

Turner, A., 2001. Varicose veins during pregnancy. Br. J. Midwifery 9 (7), 464.

Vutyavanich, T., Kraisarin, T., Ruangsri, R.A., 2001. Ginger for nausea and vomiting in pregnancy: randomised, double masked, placebo-controlled trial. Obstet. Gynecol. 97 (4), 577–582.

Wellock, V.K., Crichton, M.A., 2007. Symphysis pubis dysfunction: women's experiences of care. Br. J. Midwifery 15 (8), 494–499.

Annotated recommended reading

Coggins, J., 2002. Early pregnancy care. Pract. Midwife 5 (9), 14–17.

This is the second of two articles covering all aspects of antenatal care with application to the physiological and psychological changes women experience.

Girling, J.C., 2000. Physiological adaptation to pregnancy. In: Page, L. (Ed.), The New Midwifery. Churchill Livingstone, Edinburgh.

This chapter covers adaptation to pregnancy, including the minor ailments women complain of. It is well set out and easy to read.

McParlin, C., Graham, R.H., Robson, S.C., 2008. Caring for women with nausea and vomiting in pregnancy: new approaches. Br. J. Midwifery 16 (5), 280–285.

A good guide for midwives, discussing pathophysiology and key interventions.

Smith, C., Crowther, C., Beilby, J., 2002. Acupuncture to treat nausea and vomiting in early pregnancy: a randomised controlled trial. Birth 29 (1), 1.

This is a report of a trial in Australia to help women with vomiting in pregnancy.

Chapter Thirty-One

31

Bleeding in pregnancy

Bleeding in early pregnancy

Bleeding from the genital tract during pregnancy is abnormal and a doctor should see all women who report bleeding, irrespective of the amount. Bleeding prior to the 24th week of pregnancy may be caused by implantation bleeding, abortion, ectopic pregnancy, trophoblastic disease and lesions of the cervix or vagina. Research by Weiss et al (2004) compared 16 506 women, some of whom did not bleed and others who had light or heavy bleeding. Women with light bleeding were more likely to develop pre-eclampsia, have a preterm birth or placental abruption. The women with heavy bleeding were more likely to lose their pregnancy before 24 weeks. The conclusions were that the severity of bleeding was a risk factor for adverse pregnancy outcome.

Implantation bleeding

Normal implantation is thought to occur in three stages (Potdar & Konje 2005):

* Apposition: the blastocyst sits adjacent to the endometrium—an unstable situation.
* Stable adhesion: increased activation of the syncytiotrophoblast with the endometrium.
* Invasion.

As the syncytiotrophoblast cells erode the maternal endometrium during embedding, a small amount of bleeding may occur at about 6–7 days (Norwitz et al 2001). By 10 days the blastocyst is completely covered by the decidua; this is just before the next menstrual period is due. Women may think this is a normal but short menstruation. Implantation is a complex interaction between the blastocyst and the endometrium and 'various adhesion molecules' (Potdar & Konje 2005). At this early stage women often do not know they are pregnant. If the blastocyst does not implant, then menstruation begins, although a little late, and the conceptus is lost with menstrual debris.

Abortion

Spontaneous abortion is the complete loss of the products of conception prior to the 24th week of pregnancy; 10–15% of diagnosed pregnancies are lost before 20 weeks (Potgar & Konje 2005). However, most of them are lost before implantation and only a quarter of them are clinically recognized as abortions. The aetiology of abortion is shown in Table 31.1.

About 80% of all abortions will occur before 12 weeks gestation; the rest will occur between 13 and 24 weeks and are referred to as late abortions. The majority

Table 31.1 Aetiology of abortion

Cause	Percentage of total
Genetic abnormalities: mainly chromosomal abnormalities arising during meiosis of ovum or sperm	50–60
Endocrine abnormalities: progesterone deficiency, thyroid deficiency, diabetes, increased androgens, elevated luteinising hormone as in polycystic ovary	10–15
Chorioamniotic separations: there may be bleeding beneath the chorion or between the amnion and chorion	5–10
Incompetent cervix: usually the result of cervical trauma	8–15
Infections: usually ascending, but occasionally due to systemic microbial infections such as rubella, listeria, toxoplasmosis, chlamydia	3–5
Abnormal placentation: failure of the trophoblastic invasion of the spiral arteries, linked to raised blood pressure	5–15
Immunological abnormalities: may be the cause of repeated spontaneous abortions and have recognisable serum antibodies	3–5
Uterine anatomic abnormalities: caused mainly by failure of the Müllerian ducts to unite in the embryonic stage resulting in septate uterus; a fibroid uterus may also cause abortion	1–3
Unknown reasons	<5

of early abortions are due to anembryonic pregnancies or blighted ova suggestive of genetic faults, while those with a formed fetus suggest the possibility of many causes and occur after 13 weeks. Fifty per cent of conceptions are lost before the next menstruation, 30% soon after the missed cycle and 65–90% of these losses are recognised as chromosomally abnormal (Lockwood 2000). This may be linked to older women and pregnancy loss. The incidence of loss is higher in IVF pregnancies probably due to the underlying causes of infertility in the first place (Mukhopadhaya & Arulkumaran 2007).

Classification of abortion (Fig. 31.1)

Threatened abortion

In threatened abortion, painful or painless bleeding occurs, the cervical os is closed and ultrasound will define a live fetus when conservative treatment such as bed rest is advised. The outcome may be resolution and continuance of the pregnancy or proceed to an inevitable abortion.

Inevitable abortion

A diagnosis of inevitable abortion is made on the fact that the cervical canal is open; ultrasound will define if the fetus is alive. Blood loss may be heavy and cause maternal collapse with increasing abdominal pain. The uterus may spontaneously evacuate its contents or surgical or medical removal with **mifepristone** (RU4B6) may be necessary to remove retained products. Expectant management is sometimes an alternative to operative measures for removing retained products of conception. Ultrasound measures endometrial thickness and the presence of a gestational sac. If left to nature, most women will lose the retained products naturally. This management requires regular follow-up as an outpatient and access to the clinic by phone (Cahill 2001, Luise et al 2002).

Missed abortion

This is now termed early fetal demise (Cahill 2001). A blood-stained or brown loss may be evident, the woman may or may not still feel pregnant and the signs of pregnancy may disappear. Low levels of human chorionic gonadotrophin (hCG) may be found, in which case the conceptus has died or ultrasound confirms fetal death. A suction curette or oral mifepristone may be used. If the uterus is larger than 13 weeks, a combination of vaginal prostaglandins and intravenous Syntocinon (oxytocin) may be prescribed. Although the uterus would eventually expel the mole, there is a risk of disseminated intravascular coagulation because of the toxins produced by a dead fetus.

Recurrent miscarriage (abortion)

Recurrent abortion is the term used for three or more consecutive abortions. Only 0.4% of women suffer in this way but they have a 55% increased risk of having a fourth miscarriage (Eblen et al 2000). In some women the cause is unknown but there is a specific group of women who suffer from **antiphospholipid antibodies (Hughes syndrome)**, some 10–16% who will continually abort. In other words, the mother produces antibodies against the fetus. These antibodies also affect clotting factors and the process of abortion is thought to involve the activation of clotting mechanisms on the endothelial decidual cell surface (Singh 2001).

Induced abortion (therapeutic)

Therapeutic abortions have been available in the UK since 1967 but there are other countries where the procedure is illegal. The lack of an abortion law leads to the risk of women seeking illegal abortions, often carried out in unfavourable conditions by unskilled practitioners.

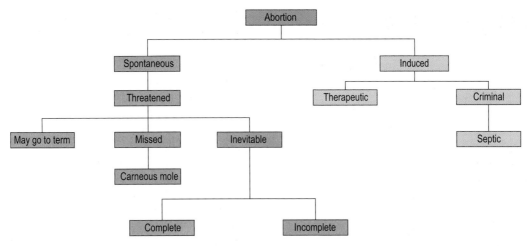

Figure 31.1 • The classification of abortion. (From Henderson C, Macdonald S 2004, with kind permission of Elsevier.)

In the past this often resulted in a septic abortion, which occurred because of infection, and the woman suffered from **septicaemia**, **endotoxic shock** and **disseminated intravascular coagulation**. Infection leads to the development of adhesions, and infertility. Fatalities were common. As for long-term health problems, there seems to be no connection between induced abortion and later early pregnancy loss or the incidence of ectopic pregnancy, but the risk of preterm birth and placenta praevia in subsequent pregnancies is increased (Thorp et al 2003).

It should be considered that, if a woman is pregnant and the pregnancy is unwanted, then she may choose the route to abort the baby. Other women abort because of fetal abnormality and this in itself is difficult for the woman and her partner. Some women are treated as outpatients using mifepristone or prostaglandins followed by a suction evacuation under a general anaesthetic if deemed necessary.

Gestational trophoblastic tumours

Chorionic tumours deriving from the placenta include **hydatidiform mole** (partial or complete), **placental site tumours** and **choriocarcinoma** with varying degrees of the diseased tissue spreading and causing malignancy. Placental site tumours are rare and generally treated with hysterectomy followed by chemotherapy (Hassadia et al 2005, Trommel et al 2005).

Hydatidiform mole

Hydatidiform mole is a benign neoplastic disease, an abnormal growth of the trophoblast where the chorionic villi proliferate, become avascular and are filled with fluid. The mole looks like a bunch of grapes, often filling the uterus, which clinically palpates large

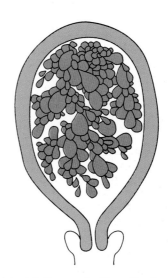

Figure 31.2 • A hydatidiform mole. (From Henderson C, Macdonald S 2004, with kind permission of Elsevier.)

for dates (Fig. 31.2). Complete and partial moles have abnormal sets of chromosomes (Fig. 31.3); a complete mole will have a 46XX where all chromosomes are of paternal origin. The ovum has no nucleus but has been fertilised by one spermatozoon. A partial mole where a fetus may be present is usually triploid, either 69XXX or 69XXY where two spermatozoa have fertilized one ovum (Blackburn 2007, Trommel 2005).

Aetiology

There are wide variations in incidence: 2:1000 in Japan; 1:1000 in Europe and North America; and 1:1945 in Ireland. It is suggested that diet and socioeconomic factors may play a role, particularly the lack of carotene and animal fats (Berkowitz & Goldstein 1996). Women over 35, and who have had a previous mole, have an increased risk of a complete mole.

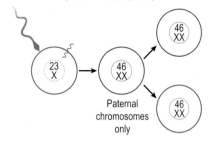

Paternal chromosomal origin of a complete hydatiform mole (46XX)

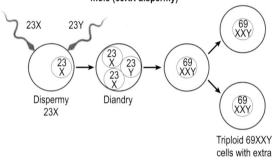

Triploid chromosomal origin of a partial mole (69XX dispermy)

Figure 31.3 • Genetic origins of complete and partial hydatidiform moles.

Signs and symptoms

Signs and symptoms

- Intermittent vaginal bleeding with increasing bleeding as the mole is aborted.
- Early onset of pre-eclampsia.
- The uterus is large for dates and no fetal parts will be palpated in a complete mole.
- There may be mild signs of thyrotoxicosis and hyperemesis gravidarum due to the action of hCG, which is similar to thyroid-stimulating hormone (TSH) (Misra et al 2002).
- Diagnosis is confirmed by ultrasound scan, which will show a snowstorm effect of multiple vesicles.
- Urinary or serum hCG is very high, exceeding that of a multiple pregnancy.

Management

Complete emptying of the uterus by suction and then curettage to eliminate all diseased tissue is essential. The molar tissue always expresses the RhD factor; therefore Rh-negative women require rhesus immunoglobulin following evacuation (Berkowitz & Goldstein 1996). Follow-up at one of the three centres in the UK for the measurement of hCG until hCG levels are normal (urine hCG 0–24 IU/L; serum hCG 0–4 IU/L) will be routine. Follow-up will continue for life with an incidence of recurrence of a molar pregnancy being

1:75 (http://www.Hmole-chorio.org.uk, accessed June 2008). Hormonal contraception should be avoided, as it increases the chance of developing malignant disease.

Choriocarcinoma and placental site tumours

The diagnosis of a choriocarcinoma is the presence of a persistently raised level of hCG (>2000 IU/L). A tumour consisting of placental tissue and haemorrhage debris and the spread to lung and brains is typical. Other symptoms such as haemorrhage and rising levels of hCG are also diagnostic. The tumour is very invasive and treatment must be commenced immediately following diagnosis. Placental site tumours can be difficult to diagnose, with hCG levels less elevated but not markedly as in choriocarcinoma; irregular bleeding may be a first sign.

Treatment

Choriocarcinoma in all its presentations responds very well to **chemotherapy**. To assist in the treatment process a scoring system is used: women scoring 0–8 are low risk and are administered methotrexate and folinic acid; those scoring above 8 receive etoposide, methotrexate, cyclophosphamide and vincristine (McNeish et al 2002). The problem of toxicity is as for every use of cytotoxic drugs with malaise, stomatitis, pharyngitis, diarrhoea, leucopenia and alopecia occurring. Follow-up treatment will continue for life with some women opting for hysterectomy.

Ectopic pregnancy

An ectopic pregnancy occurs when the fertilised ovum implants outside the uterine cavity, commonly diagnosed between 6 and 10 weeks (Murray et al 2005). In 95% of cases the site of implantation is the uterine tube. More rarely, the implantation site may be the ovary, the cervical canal or the abdominal cavity. Ectopic pregnancy is a serious condition and is a major cause of maternal death. Reasons for death have been stated as, in the main, missed diagnosis in primary care and accident and emergency. The Royal College of Obstetricians and Gynaecologists (RCOG 2002) recommend the use of the urinary hCG dipstick test to ascertain pregnancy to prevent missed diagnosis. The use of vaginal ultrasound also aids diagnosis and may prevent the drastic operative measures of salpingectomy (Farquhar 2003, Levine 2007).

Tubal pregnancy

There is a rise in the incidence of tubal pregnancies due to the increase in sexually transmitted diseases, in particular by *Chlamydia trachomatis* (Tay et al 2000). Any condition that delays the transport of the zygote along

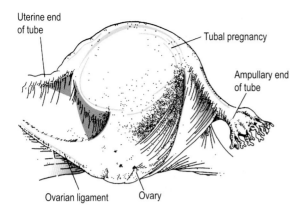

Figure 31.4 • Tubal pregnancy. (From Henderson C, Macdonald S 2004, with kind permission of Elsevier.)

the uterine tube may lead to a tubal pregnancy (Fig. 31.4). This may be due to malformation of the tubes but is more likely due to tubal scarring and the loss of cilia due to pelvic infection.

Risk factors

Risk factors for tubal pregnancy include (Tay et al 2000):

- An older woman.
- Women of low gravidity or parity.
- Previous tubal pregnancy.
- Tubal surgery.
- Salpingitis.
- Intrauterine contraceptive device.
- Hormonal stimulation of ovulation.
- In vitro fertilisation and embryo transplant.
- Tubal endometriosis.
- Pelvic inflammatory disease (PID).
- Pelvic or abdominal surgery.
- Progestogen-only pill (interferes with the action of the cilia).

Pathophysiology

Implantation may occur in various sites along the genital tract (Table 31.2).

Table 31.2 Sites of ectopic implantation

Position	Percentage occurrence
The fimbriated part of the tube	17
The ampulla	55
The isthmus	25
The ovary	0.5
The abdominal cavity	0.1

The outcome varies depending on where in the tube implantation occurs, the ability of the tube to distend and the size of blood vessels eroded. If the pregnancy occurs in the fimbriated end or the ampulla, the conceptus may continue to grow until 10 weeks. The gestation sac may be expelled into the abdominal cavity as a tubal abortion (Fig. 31.5). Blood clot may be organised around the separated sac to form a tubal mole, which may remain in the uterine tube or be expelled from the fimbriated end as a tubal abortion. Tubal rupture (Fig. 31.6) may lead to devastating haemorrhage. The most severe haemorrhage occurs if the zygote implants at the level of the isthmus where the mucosa is thinner and the blood vessels larger. Tubal rupture is likely to occur between the 5th and 7th weeks of pregnancy.

Diagnosis

The condition may be subacute or acute with signs of shock and collapse. The condition is serious and should always be suspected in women of childbearing age, especially if there is a history of amenorrhoea or previous salpingitis. The likely signs and presenting history of ectopic pregnancy are given in Table 31.3 (Tay et al 2000).

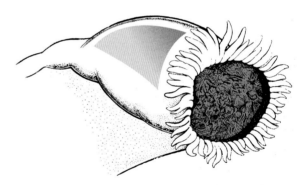

Figure 31.5 • Tubal abortion. (From Henderson C, Macdonald S 2004, with kind permission of Elsevier.)

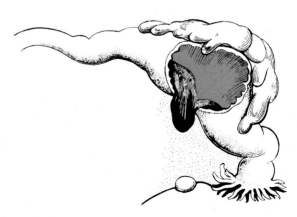

Figure 31.6 • Rupture of the uterine tube. (From Henderson C, Macdonald S 2004, with kind permission of Elsevier.)

Table 31.3 Signs and presenting history of ectopic pregnancy

Sign	Percentage occurrence
Abdominal pain	97
Abdominal tenderness	91
Vaginal bleeding	79
Adnexal tenderness	54
History of infertility	15
Use of intrauterine device	14
Previous ectopic pregnancy	11

Delay in diagnosis may be fatal as the clinical picture is similar to PID or threatened abortion:

- The woman will give a history of early pregnancy signs.
- The uterus will have enlarged but feel soft.
- Abdominal pain may occur as the tube distends and uterine bleeding may be present as the endometrium begins to degenerate.
- The abdomen is tender and may be distended.
- Shoulder tip pain may be due to referred pain.
- The woman may appear pale, complain of nausea and collapse.
- Severe pain may be felt during pelvic examination, especially if the cervix is moved.
- A mass may be felt in the adnexi on one or other side of the uterus.
- Hormonal assay will find progesterone levels to be low and hCG levels may be low or falling (Farquhar 2003).
- Ultrasound scanning may show fluid in the pelvic cavity, a mass in the pelvic cavity and absence of an intrauterine pregnancy (Levine 2007).

Management
Although an acute emergency when rupture of the tube and bleeding occurs, surgery is indicated and salpingectomy is performed, ectopic pregnancy can be treated expectantly, particularly with early ultrasound diagnosis. The ectopic resolves naturally in 88% of patients if the hCG titre is <1000 IU/L (Tay et al 2000). The use of systemic methotrexate in women who have not ruptured and are haemodynamically stable has been beneficial; however, it is not without side-effects.

Prognosis
About 40% of women may never become pregnant following an ectopic pregnancy. About 75% of these women avoid pregnancy voluntarily and 25% are infertile. The risk of a second ectopic pregnancy is 10% compared with only 0.4% in other women.

Bleeding from associated conditions

The following conditions may cause bleeding at any time in pregnancy but are not caused by the pregnancy.

Cervical polyps

Cervical polyps are benign growths which are bright red, fleshy and attached by a pedicle. They usually originate in the cervical canal and can be seen on speculum examination. Polyps may have been present before the onset of pregnancy but bleed during pregnancy because of the increased blood supply.

Cervical erosion

Cervical erosion (**eversion, ectropion**) forms when the columnar epithelium lining the cervical canal proliferates because of the influence of the pregnancy hormones. Columnar epithelium secretes mucin and the woman may complain of profuse vaginal discharge. This may be blood-stained because of rupture of capillaries, especially following sexual intercourse. The epithelium should recede after delivery but, if it persists, treatment by diathermy or cryosurgery can be given (Hefner 2001).

Carcinoma of the cervix

Carcinoma of the cervix if diagnosed early is a very treatable condition; the fact that 50% of women diagnosed have never had a Papanicolaou test (pap test) and 10% more have not had one in 5 years shows that regular testing works (Tiffen & Mahon 2006). If diagnosed in pregnancy treatment may depend on the stage of pregnancy and the severity of the findings. Prospective parents have a difficult choice to make and must be guided to make an informed decision. **Cellular dysplasia** (abnormal growth of cells) and **nuclear dyskaryosis** (abnormal chromosomes) are associated with human papillomavirus (HPV) infection types 6, 16 and 18, and between 10% and 30% of women have been affected by age 30. HPV is transmissible and is a cause of genital warts. About 60% of the partners of women with HPV infection of the cervix have penile infection. HPV virus acts with a co-agent to cause carcinoma of the cervix. Clinical findings may show **cervical intraepithelial neoplasia** (CIN invasive carcinoma of the cervix) (Tiffen & Mahon 2006).

Cervical intraepithelial neoplasia (CIN)

Cervical cytology may show normal cells, mild, moderate or severe dysplasia or carcinoma in situ. When carried out in the antenatal period, 1 in 200 mothers have abnormal cell changes. If these are consistent with CIN, a repeat Papanicolaou smear is taken and the cervix is assessed by **colposcopy**. A small cervical biopsy may be carried out. If the tissue is precancerous, treatment can be deferred until after delivery (Cancer Research UK 2008, Hefner 2001, Tiffen & Mahon 2006).

Invasive carcinoma of the cervix

Invasive carcinoma of the cervix occurs in about 1 in 5000 women of childbearing age. It is an aggressive cancer and may progress rapidly. The cervix feels hard and nodular and bleeds when touched. Decisions about treatment should be discussed with each woman and will depend on the degree of invasion and the duration of pregnancy.

Vaginitis

Occasionally the use of vaginal deodorants may lead to inflammation and bleeding from the vaginal epithelium. Infections by organisms such as *Candida albicans* or *Trichomonas vaginalis* are more likely causes of vaginitis, which may be accompanied by slight bleeding. Following culture of the organism, the correct antibiotic should be given.

Antepartum haemorrhage

Antepartum haemorrhage is bleeding after the 24th week of pregnancy and before the birth of the baby and is always a serious complication. Bleeding from a placenta implanted wholly or partly in the lower uterine segment is termed **placenta praevia**; bleeding from a normally sited placenta is a **placental abruption**. **Intrapartum haemorrhage** occurs during labour and may be life-threatening for both mother and baby necessitating emergency measures to deliver the baby.

Placenta praevia

Normally, the chorionic villi surround the whole embryo but later degenerate under the decidua capsularis to form the chorion laeve. The fetus grows to fill the uterine cavity and the decidua capsularis fuses with the decidua vera by about 4 months. If the chorionic villi near the lower pole of the uterus fail to degenerate as the decidua capsularis fuses with the decidua vera, the area will become part of the placenta, encroaching on the lower uterine segment (Blackburn 2007).

The incidence of placenta praevia ranges between 0.5% and 1% at term, rising to 2% in grand multiparity (Enkin et al 2000). Although a low-lying placenta may be detected on routine ultrasound scanning in early pregnancy, it may be detected in as many as 25% of pregnancies in the second trimester. Growth of the lower segment in later pregnancy appears to remove the placental site away from the internal os. In the later weeks of pregnancy sheering stresses may detach the placenta from the uterine wall, resulting in haemorrhage.

Classification of placenta praevia

The standard classification of placenta praevia has been defined as types I–IV as shown in Figure 31.7. In practice this cannot always be as easily defined and the RCOG (2005) suggests that a more useful one is major praevia covering the os and minor praevia within the area but not covering the os. The use of ultrasound has improved the diagnosis and allows prognosis of outcome (Bhide & Thilaganathan 2004). If the placenta is low lying at the 20–24-week scan then a transvaginal ultrasound should define the exact position of the placenta and is safe for these women (RCOG 2005). At 32 weeks if no symptoms such as blood loss have occurred, a follow-up scan would define placental position and subsequent management (NICE 2008).

Vaginal examination is an extremely dangerous procedure in placenta praevia and must never be carried out unless in theatre with the ability to perform an immediate caesarean section.

Aetiology of placenta praevia

The evidence suggests that the placenta is low-lying because of defects in the uterine endometrium and musculature. Women with previous caesarean sections, terminations, intrauterine surgery with increasing parity, uterine infections, those who smoke and are older are all at risk of placenta praevia. Multifetal pregnancies are at risk of the placenta being large and covering a greater area of the uterus and thus covering the os (Oyelese & Smulian 2006).

The clinical ability to diagnose a low-lying placenta is not so important if scanning is carried out as a routine measure; however, women book late, miss antenatal visits and may miss the important scans (RCOG 2005).

On palpation the following may be found:

- Malpresentation of the fetus.
- Non-engagement of the presenting part.
- The presence of a loud maternal pulse that originates in the placental bed below the umbilicus.

Blood loss

In 98% of cases painless fresh recurrent vaginal bleeding occurs after 24 weeks due to stretching of the lower uterine segment and detachment of the placenta,

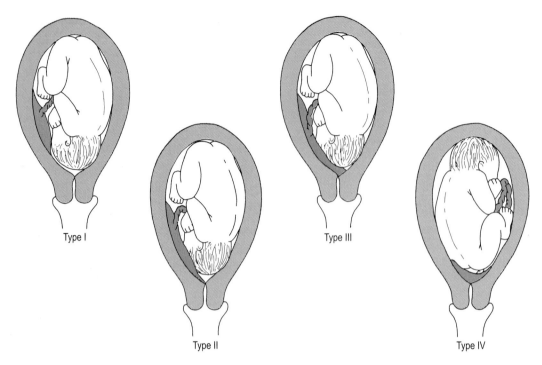

Figure 31.7 • Placenta praevia types I–IV. (From Henderson C, Macdonald S 2004, with kind permission of Elsevier.)

although it may occur earlier. Blood loss usually stops after a few hours and is rarely dangerous. Subsequent episodes of bleeding due to increased development of the lower uterine segment and further detachment of the placenta tend to become worse and a blood transfusion may be required. Torrential maternal haemorrhage may occur at any time, especially if labour commences and the cervix begins to dilate. The fetus may be compromised if maternal bleeding is severe enough to reduce the uterine blood supply. The placenta may be torn and fetal bleeding occurs. Massive haemorrhage will require an emergency caesarean section performed by an experienced obstetric consultant as suggested under the guidelines of the enquiries into maternal deaths (Hall 2004).

Management

Management may be conservative or active. Any woman bleeding in her own home should be transferred to hospital by ambulance. Vital signs should be assessed and intravenous fluids used to stabilise the condition. The amount of blood lost should be estimated.

General examination

- There may be a history of spotting or small blood losses.
- Observations of maternal pulse and blood pressure should correspond with the amount of blood loss and the degree of shock.
- Temperature should be normal.

Abdominal examination

- The uterus should feel soft and should not be tender.
- The size will correspond to the period of gestation.
- There may be a malpresentation, an unstable lie and a high presenting part.
- Usually the fetus is in good condition with a fetal heart of normal rate and rhythm.

Blood is taken for cross-matching and at least 2 units placed on standby. Full blood count and Kleihauer estimation is needed if the woman is rhesus negative. An intravenous infusion of Hartmann's solution is commenced if bleeding is persistent. Blood loss is estimated. The woman remains on bed rest until the bleeding ceases. **On no account should a vaginal examination be performed.**

Conservative management

If bleeding is slight to moderate and occurs before the 38th week of pregnancy and both maternal and fetal conditions are satisfactory, conservative treatment is commenced. The aim is to maintain the pregnancy until 38 weeks to avoid preterm delivery of an immature fetus.

Ultrasound examination is used to identify the placental site and, if this is found to be normal, the woman is allowed home. If placenta praevia is diagnosed the woman will be advised to remain in hospital to reduce any risk of severe bleeding in the absence of immediate medical help. Fetal growth will be monitored and any women who are rhesus negative will receive anti-D γ-globulin after each episode of bleeding (RCOG 2005).

However, Love & Wallace (1996) reviewed the outcome of 58 pregnancies complicated by placenta praevia in Edinburgh. Of these women, 42 (72%) had one or more episodes of bleeding. Repeated episodes of bleeding did not affect the outcome of pregnancy. Both diagnosis and delivery occurred earlier in the women who bled and delivery by caesarean section was more common in the women who were bleeding. Only three women required emergency delivery because of bleeding. These authors concluded that, as the clinical outcome of placenta praevia is so variable in both women who have no bleeding and those who bleed, outpatient management is safe and appropriate.

Delivery

If no serious haemorrhage occurs, the fetus is delivered at 38 weeks. Placental localisation is clarified by ultrasound. If the fetal head is below the rim of the placenta then vaginal delivery is permitted. Enkin et al (2000) list the hazards of vaginal delivery as:

- Profuse maternal haemorrhage.
- Malpresentation.
- Cord accidents.
- Placental separation.
- Fetal haemorrhage.
- Dystocia if the placenta is situated posteriorly.

Active management

This is more likely to be needed in the last 2 weeks of pregnancy. If bleeding is severe or continuous or there is deterioration in maternal or fetal condition or if labour has commenced, the woman's condition is stabilised and an emergency caesarean section is carried out. Blood must be cross-matched but it may be necessary to give the woman a transfusion of O-negative blood in a dire emergency. Surgery can be complicated if the placenta underlies the site of normal surgical incision. Even if the fetus has died, caesarean section will be needed to stop the haemorrhage and stabilise the woman.

Third stage

The lack of oblique fibres in the lower uterine segment may fail to control bleeding and postpartum haemorrhage may occur. **Placenta accreta** is often associated with placenta praevia as the thin decidua over the lower uterine segment increases the likelihood of myometrial invasion. It has also been noticed that, as the caesarean section rate rises, so does the incidence of placenta accreta (Oyelese & Smulian 2006, Usta et al 2005). Hysterectomy may be required to control haemorrhage and to save life.

Placental abruption (abruptio placentae)

Placental abruption (accidental haemorrhage) is bleeding due to the separation of a normally situated placenta and occurs in about 1% of pregnancies (Oyelese & Ananth 2006) (Fig. 31.8). It may occur at any stage in pregnancy or labour and bleeding occurs into the decidua basalis beneath the placenta. A haematoma is formed which separates the placenta from the maternal vascular system and the fetus is deprived of oxygen and nutrients. If 50% of the placenta is involved fetal loss is likely (Oyelese & Ananth 2006). Most maternal complications arise from hypovolaemia and collapse of the systems (Yerby 2002). The haemorrhage may be secondary to degenerative changes in the arteries supplying the intervillous spaces (Blackburn 2007).

Risk factors

In the majority of cases bleeding is slight and no cause may be found. The following risk factors are associated with this serious complication of pregnancy:

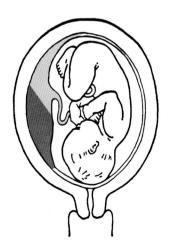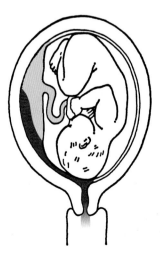

Figure 31.8 • Abruptio placentae. (From Henderson C, Macdonald S 2004, with kind permission of Elsevier.)

- **Hypertensive states**—essential hypertension or pre-eclampsia is present in 50% of severe cases (Hladky et al 2002).
- Sudden decompression of the uterus, as when membranes rupture in **polyhydramnios** (Hladky et al 2002, Oyelese & Ananth 2006).
- Preterm, pre-labour rupture of the membranes (Major et al 1995).
- Previous history of placental abruption, increasing parity (Hladky et al 2002, Oyelese & Ananth 2006).
- Trauma, as in a fall or road traffic accident, or domestic violence.
- Smoking (Andres 1996, Hladky et al 2002).
- Illegal drug abuse, such as cocaine (Hladky et al 2002).

Blood loss

Blood loss comes from the maternal venous sinuses and may be revealed, partly revealed or concealed (Fig. 31.9). The blood is darker than that seen in placenta praevia, because of the time taken to appear out of the vagina. Some experts believe that the magnitude of placental separation is determined at the outset and that no further separation occurs. Others believe that abruption causes progressive placental separation:

- **Revealed bleeding** occurs when the site of placental detachment is at the margin. The blood escapes between the membranes and decidua and is seen at the vulva. The condition of the woman is directly related to the observed blood loss.
- **Partially revealed bleeding** occurs when some of the blood remains in the uterus. The bleeding may exceed that which is visibly lost and the degree of shock may be greater than expected.

- **Concealed bleeding** occurs when the site of detachment is near to the centre of the site of placental attachment. Blood cannot escape and a large retroplacental clot forms. Extravasated blood may also infiltrate the full-thickness myometrium, a condition known as **Couvelaire uterus**. Under direct observation, the uterus would appear bruised and oedematous. There may be no vaginal blood loss but pain and shock are usually severe (Sundle 2002).

As shown in Table 31.4, depending on the amount of placental separation and blood lost, either revealed or concealed, placental abruption may be mild, moderate or severe (Lindsay 2004):

Table 31.4 The main features of bleeding in abruptio placentae

	Mild	**Moderate**	**Severe**
Blood loss	Slight	More than 1000 ml	More than 2000 ml
Uterus on abdominal examination	Soft, not tender	Firm and tender	Hard (woody) and tender; backache if the placenta is posterior
Pain	None or mild	Quite severe	Severe
Shock	No sign	Tachycardia, hypotension	Extreme shock
Fetus	Fetal heart normal	Signs of fetal distress	Fetal heart absent

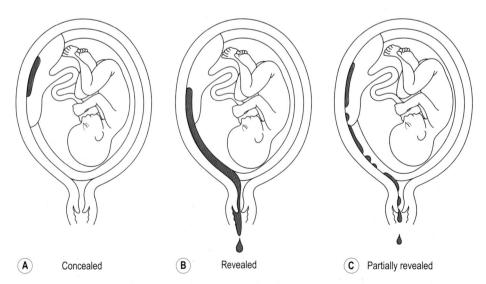

(A) Concealed   (B) Revealed   (C) Partially revealed

Figure 31.9 • Types of abruptio placentae. (A) Concealed. (B) Revealed. (C) Partially revealed. (From Henderson C, Macdonald S 2004, with kind permission of Elsevier.)

- Mild includes situations where the mother and fetus are not compromised in any way. Ultrasound will define where the placenta lies. Observation of the blood loss and fetal well-being will continue in hospital until bleeding stops. Discharge home will occur if before 37 weeks.

- Moderate blood loss may be greater than 1000 ml and the fetus may be alive. Immediate caesarean section may be necessary if the fetus is distressed. The mother may show signs of hypovolaemia and require stabilisation with intravenous fluids. The uterus may be tender and the mother in pain. Clotting screens should be undertaken. If the fetus is dead, a vaginal delivery could be possible if the mother is stable.

- Severe separation of the placenta is life-threatening for the mother, the fetus is nearly always dead, and blood loss may be in the region of 2000 ml or more. The uterus will be hard and woody and blood loss may not be totally revealed, giving a false impression of less blood loss. The maternal condition is poor with severe shock and pain. Complications which may arise from this are coagulation defects, kidney failure and Sheehan's syndrome. Most maternal deaths occur in this latter group of women and it is important to monitor cardiovascular and renal status closely to ensure a good maternal outcome. If the fetus is alive, the maternal condition should be stabilised and caesarean section performed.

The amount of bleeding per vaginam is no guide to the degree of placental separation.

Management of placental abruption

When bleeding is slight and there is no effect on maternal or fetal condition, it may be difficult to differentiate the cause of bleeding, especially if there is no sign of hypertension. Because of the risk of placenta praevia, the woman is treated as if that condition is present until it is excluded by ultrasound scan. If the placenta is localised in the upper uterine segment, the bleeding stops and the condition of mother and fetus is satisfactory, the woman may go home.

Moderate or severe placental abruption is usually easy to diagnose and is an obstetric emergency. The woman is resuscitated if necessary and an intravenous infusion commenced. Morphine 15–20 mg may be ordered to relieve pain and shock and the woman is then transferred to hospital. The aim is to restore blood loss and deliver the baby as quickly as possible to avoid complications such as renal failure and blood clotting defects.

Blood is taken for grouping and cross-matching and it is wise to have at least 6 units standing by. Full blood count with urea and electrolytes, clotting studies and fibrin degradation products should be routine. Central venous pressure is monitored to avoid under- or over-transfusion and the woman's blood pressure, pulse and respiratory rate are monitored frequently. A Foley urinary catheter is inserted to observe urinary output and allow urine to be tested.

The only way to stop the bleeding is to empty the uterus. Vaginal delivery may be achieved if the fetus has died or is in a good enough condition to allow time for induction. The membranes are ruptured and an oxytocic infusion is commenced. Caesarean section will be carried out if the fetus is alive but in poor condition. Postpartum haemorrhage is likely due to the poor ability of the uterine muscle to contract when it is infiltrated by blood; intravenous Syntocinon (oxytocin) infusion may be continued for some hours following delivery.

Blood coagulation disorders

Damage to tissue causes the release of **thromboplastins** from the cells. In normal circumstances thromboplastin activates the clotting mechanism and **fibrinogen** is converted to **fibrin**, forming a clot to seal any broken blood vessels. This clot is later dispersed by **plasmin**, releasing **fibrin degradation products**. The tissue damage in placental abruption is so severe that there is a massive release of thromboplastin into the circulation. Widespread clotting occurs within the vascular tree, a condition called disseminated intravascular coagulation (DIC). At the same time, the anticlotting mechanisms are affected and shut down, preventing dissolution of the clots. The **microthrombi** produced occlude small blood vessels, which results in ischaemic damage in organs (Lindsay 2004). The damaged tissue then releases more thromboplastins and a vicious circle commences.

- Damage to the kidney results in reduced urinary output and may result in **anuria**.
- The liver may be damaged, leading to **jaundice**.
- Damage to the lungs may result in **dyspnoea** and **cyanosis**.
- Brain involvement may result in **convulsions** or **coma**.
- The retina may be affected and cause **blindness**.
- If the pituitary gland is damaged, **Sheehan's syndrome** may occur.

Platelets and clotting factors are depleted and no further coagulation can occur. Spontaneous bleeding begins from puncture wound sites, mucous membranes, petechiae develop in the skin and there will be uncontrollable uterine bleeding. Transfusions of fresh frozen plasma, packed cells and platelets will be needed.

Specific tests for coagulation failure are:

- Partial thromboplastin time (normal = 60–90 s).
- Prothrombin time (normal = 11–16 s).
- Thrombin time (normal = 10–15 s).
- Fibrinogen levels (normal = 150–400 mg/dl).
- Fibrin degradation products.
- Whole blood film and platelet count.

Other complications

The complications of acute renal failure, Sheehan's syndrome, postpartum haemorrhage, infection, anaemia and mental disturbances are discussed in relevant chapters. Women who have had a placental abruption have a higher risk of complications such as spontaneous abortion or repeated abruption in later pregnancies.

Vasa praevia

Vasa praevia is an unusual cause of bleeding in pregnancy where the blood lost is fetal. It is associated with **velamentous insertion** of the umbilical cord where one of the fetal vessels crosses the membranes between the presenting part of the fetus and the internal os of the uterus. The vessel may be torn when the membranes rupture and fetal bleeding may be severe. There is a high incidence of perinatal mortality with this condition and the incidence is said to be 1:2500 (Oyelese et al 1999). Diagnosis has been possible since transvaginal ultrasound and Doppler ultrasound have been available. The condition can also be diagnosed by feeling a pulsating vessel on vaginal examination.

If the condition is suspected during a vaginal examination, the membranes are left intact and the fetus delivered by emergency caesarean section. If the woman is in the second stage of labour, rapid delivery is made by forceps. Any sudden vaginal bleeding accompanied by fetal distress following rupture of the membranes should alert the practitioner and the blood should be tested for fetal cells. Although this sounds sensible, in reality there may be no time and the fetus should be immediately delivered. A blood transfusion may be needed to restore the baby's blood volume. A much higher incidence of velamentous cord insertion following IVF pregnancies has been noted (Schachter et al 2002).

Main points

- Any bleeding from the genital tract during pregnancy is abnormal and all women who bleed should be seen by a doctor. The causes of bleeding prior to the 24th week of pregnancy are implantation bleeding, abortion, ectopic pregnancy, cervical lesions, vaginitis and bleeding from trophoblastic disease. Spontaneous abortion is a common serious cause of bleeding in early pregnancy.

- Inevitable abortion is accompanied by cervical dilatation. The bleeding is severe with increasing abdominal pain and may result in maternal collapse. The uterus may spontaneously evacuate its contents or it may be necessary to surgically evacuate the uterus. In women who have recurrent abortions, investigations to ascertain the cause are made in order to plan treatment.

- Abortions may be induced in unwanted pregnancies. Sepsis may follow any type of abortion, when the term septic abortion is used. This is a serious condition and is potentially fatal. Antibiotics are commenced before surgical intervention.

- Hydatidiform mole is an abnormal growth of the trophoblast. The uterus must be emptied by suction curettage. Following the emergency treatment, follow-up will be continued for life to ensure that there is no progression to choriocarcinoma. Between 5% and 10% of women may go on to develop choriocarcinoma, which responds well to chemotherapy.

- In 95% of cases of ectopic pregnancy the implantation site is the uterine tube. Ectopic pregnancy may be subacute with most of the signs but without the shock and collapse that is present with the classical acute picture with sudden collapse.

- Tubal rupture is an obstetric emergency; bleeding is heavy and can only be stopped surgically.

- Cervical polyps, vaginitis, cervical erosion and carcinoma of the cervix may cause associated bleeding and require treatment in pregnancy.

- The two main types of antepartum haemorrhage are placenta praevia and placental abruption. Placenta praevia causes bleeding from an abnormally sited placenta. In units where early ultrasound scanning is routine, at-risk women will be identified. If the placenta is still low-lying at 30 weeks, placenta praevia should be diagnosed and subsequent care modified. In 98% of cases, painless fresh recurrent vaginal bleeding occurs.

- Risk factors for placental abruption include hypertensive states, sudden decompression of the uterus, preterm pre-labour rupture of the membranes, previous history of placental abruption, trauma, smoking and abuse of cocaine. The bleeding is from maternal venous sinuses and may be revealed, partly revealed or concealed.

- Moderate or severe placental abruption is an obstetric emergency. The aim is to restore blood loss and deliver the baby as quickly as possible to avoid renal failure and blood clotting defects. The only way to stop the bleeding is to empty the uterus.

- Vasa praevia is associated with a velamentous insertion of the umbilical cord where one of the fetal vessels crosses the membranes between the presenting part of the fetus and the internal os of the uterus. The vessel may be torn when the membranes rupture and fetal bleeding may be severe. There is a high incidence of perinatal mortality with this condition.

References

Andres, R.L., 1996. The association of cigarette smoking with placenta praevia and abruptio placentae. Semin. Perinatol. 20 (2), 154–159.

Berkowitz, R., Goldstein, D., 1996. Chorionic tumours. N. Engl. J. Med. 355 (23), 1740–1748.

Bhide, A., Thilaganathan, B., 2004. Recent advances in management of placenta praevia. Curr. Opin. Obstet. Gynecol. 16 (6), 447–451.

Blackburn, S.T., 2007. Maternal, Fetal and Neonatal Physiology: A Clinical Perspective, third edn. W B Saunders, Philadelphia.

Cahill, D.J., 2001. Managing spontaneous first trimester miscarriage: we don't yet know the optimal treatment. Br. Med. J. 322 (7298), 1315–1316.

Cancer Research UK, 2008. Pregnancy and abnormal cervical cells. <http://www.cancerhelp.org.uk/hrlp/default.asp?page=2768> (accessed June 2008).

Eblen, A., Gercel-Taylor, C., Shields, L., et al., 2000. Alterations in humoral responses associated with recurrent pregnancy loss. Fertil. Steril. 73 (2), 305–313.

Enkin, M., Keirse, M.J., Neilson, J., et al., 2000. A Guide to Effective Care in Pregnancy and Childbirth. Oxford University Press, Oxford.

Farquhar, C., 2003. Ectopic pregnancy. Lancet 366 (9485), 583–591.

Hall, G.M., 2004. Haemorrhage. In: Lewis, G., Drife, J. (Eds.), Why Mothers Die, 2000–2002. The Sixth Report of the Confidential Enquiries into Maternal Death in the United Kingdom. RCOG, London, pp. 86–93.

Hassadia, A., Gillespie, A., Tidy, J., Everard, J., Wells, M., et al., 2005. Placental site trophoblastic tumour: clinical features and management. Gynecol. Oncol. 99 (3), 603–607.

Hefner, L., 2001. Human Reproduction at a Glance. Blackwell Science, Oxford.

Hladky, K., Yankowitz, J., Hanson, W., 2002. Placental abruption. Obstet. Gynecol. Surv. 57 (5), 299–305.

Levine, D., 2007. Ectopic pregnancy. Radiology 245, 385–397.

Lindsay, P., 2004. Bleeding in pregnancy, Ch. 44. In: Henderson, C., Macdonald, S. (Eds.), Mayes's Midwifery: A Textbook for Midwives, thirteenth edn. Baillière Tindall.

Lockwood, C., 2000. Prediction of pregnancy loss. Lancet 355 (9212), 1292–1293.

Love, C.D.B., Wallace, E.M., 1996. Pregnancies complicated by placenta praevia: what is appropriate management? Br. J. Obstet.Gynaecol. 103 (9), 864–867.

Luise, C., Jermy, K., Collins, W., 2002. Expectant management of incomplete spontaneous first trimester miscarriage: outcome according to initial ultrasound criteria and value of follow-up visits. Ultrasound Obstet. Gynaecol. 19 (6), 580–582.

McNeish, I., Strickland, S., Holden, L., et al., 2002. Low risk persistent gestational trophoblastic disease: outcome after initial treatment with low dose methotrexate and folinic acid from 1992–2000. J. Clin. Oncol. 20 (7), 1838–1844.

Major, C.A., de Vaciana, M., Lewis, D.F., et al., 1995. Preterm premature rupture of the membranes and abruptio placentae: is there an association between these pregnancy complications? Am. J. Obstet. Gynecol. 172 (2, part 1), 672–676.

Misra, M., Levitsky, L., Lee, M., 2002. Transient hyperthyroidism in an adolescent with hydatidiform mole. J. Paediatr. 140 (3), 362–366.

Mukhopadhaya, N., Arulkumaran, S., 2007. Reproductive outcomes after in-vitro fertilization. Curr. Opin.Obstet. Gynecol. 19 (2), 113–119.

Murray, H., Baakdah, H., Bardell, T., Tulandi, T., 2005. Diagnosis and treatment of ectopic pregnancy. CMAJ 173 (8).

NICE. Antenatal CareMarch 2008. Quick Ref. Guide 26 Website: <http://www.nice.org.uk> (accessed June 2008).

Norwitz, E.R., Schust, D., Fisher, S.J., 2001. Mechanisms of disease: implantation and survival of early pregnancy. N. Engl. J. Med. 345 (19), 1400–1408.

Oyelese, Y., Ananth, C.V., 2006. Placental abruption. Obstet. Gynecol. 108, 1005–1016.

Oyelese, Y., Smulian, J., 2006. Placenta praevia, placenta accreta and vasa praevia. Obstet. Gynecol. 107, 927–941.

Oyelese, K., Turner, M., Lees, C., Campbell, S., 1999. Vasa praevia: an avoidable obstetric tragedy. Obstet. Gynecol. Surv. 54 (2), 138–145.

Potdar, N., Konje, J.C., 2005. The endocrinological basis of recurrent miscarriage. Curr. Opin. Obstet. Gynecol. 17 (4), 424–428.

RCOG, 2002. Why Mothers Die, 1997–1999. Royal College of Obstetricians and Gynaecologists, London.

RCOG, 2005. Placenta praevia and placenta accreta: diagnosis and management. Green Top Guide (27) revised.

Schachter, M., Tovbin, Y., Arieli, S., et al., 2002. In vitro fertilization is a risk factor for vasa praevia. Fertil. Steril. 78 (3), 642–643.

Singh, A., 2001. Immunopathogenesis of the antiphospholipid antibody syndrome, an update. Curr. Opin. Nephrol. Hypertens. 10 (3), 355–358.

Sundle, H., 2002. Antepartum haemorrhage. In: Boyle, M. (Ed.), Emergencies Around Childbirth. Radcliffe Medical Press, Abingdon.

Tay, J., Moore, J., Walker, J., 2000. Ectopic pregnancy. Br. Med. J. 320, 916–919.

Thorp, J., Hartmann, K., Shadigian, E., 2003. Long-term physical and psychological health consequences of induced abortion: review of the evidence. Obstet. Gynecol. Surv. 58 (1), 67–79.

Tiffen, J., Mahon, S., 2006. Cervical cancer: what should we tell women about screening? Clin. J. Oncol. Nurs. 10 (4), 527–531.

Trommel, N.E., Sweep, F.C., Schijf, P.T., Massuger, L.F., Thomas, C.M., 2005. Diagnosis of hydatidiform mole and persistent trophoblastic disease: diagnostic accuracy of total human chorionic gonadotrophin (hCG), free hCG and β-subunits, and their ratios. Eur. J. Endocrinol. 153 (4), 565–575.

Usta, I., Hobeika, E., Abu Musa, A., Gabriel, G., Nassar, A., 2005. Placenta previa-accreta: risk factors and complications. Am. J. Obstet. Gynecol. 193 (3), 1045–1049.

Weiss, J., Malone, F., Vidaver, J., Ball, R., Nyberg, D., et al., 2004. Threatened abortion a risk factor for poor pregnancy outcome: a population- based screening study. Am. J. Obstet. Gynecol. 190 (3), 745–750.

Yerby M. In: Boyle, M. (Ed.), 2002. Emergencies Around Childbirth. Radcliffe Medical Press, Abingdon. Ch. 2.

Annotated recommended reading

Long, L., 2000. Antepartum haemorrhage. Pract. Midwife 3 (5), 32–35.

This article provides a sound base for students learning about antepartum haemorrhage.

Norwitz, E.R., Schust, D.J., Fisher, S.J., 2001. Mechanisms of disease: implantation and survival of early pregnancy. N. Engl. J. Med. 345 (19), 1400–1408.

This is a review paper that covers normal implantation, maintenance of early pregnancy and implications for infertility and loss of pregnancy.

Sundle, H., 2002. Antepartum haemorrhage. In: Boyle, M. (Ed.), Emergencies Around Childbirth. Radcliffe Medical Press, Abingdon, Oxfordshire.

This excellent chapter covers all aspects of antepartum haemorrhage, is worth reading and has some good references.

Website. <http://www.hmole-chorio.org.uk>.

This website is clearly set out and is full of very readable information on trophoblastic disease and hydatidiform mole.

Chapter Thirty-Two

32

Cardiac and hypertensive disorders

Introduction

Heart disease in pregnancy is a serious medical condition; there were 44 indirect deaths in 2000–2002 (Drife 2005). This has risen since the last Confidential Enquiry due to deaths from cardiomyopathy and myocardial infarction; these are both acquired problems and this may in part be due to women being older when becoming pregnant. However, there are younger women also embarking on a pregnancy who have undergone corrective surgery from heart disease in childhood where in the past they would not have survived heart surgery (Clarke & Butt 2005). This has implications within the maternity service for those women of childbearing years. The most dangerous cardiac lesions are those that involve pulmonary hypertension such as **primary pulmonary hypertension** and **Eisenmenger's syndrome,** and **Marfan's syndrome,** an autosomal dominant disorder of connective tissue which may result in aortic dilatation and rupture late in pregnancy or in labour.

Rheumatic heart disease is still fairly common despite the reduction in rheumatic fever in the British population. The most common lesion is **rheumatic mitral stenosis** with the most common complication being **pulmonary oedema** occurring in late pregnancy or immediately after delivery. It is important to consider that, although the indigenous population may have a changing pattern of heart disease, we see many immigrants who may have not been diagnosed with a condition.

Cardiac disorders in pregnancy

The incidence of heart disease in the pregnant population is about 1% (Lupton et al 2002). It is important to understand the physiological adaptation of the heart and circulation in pregnancy in order to understand the detrimental effects in pregnancy on the health of a woman with diagnosed heart disease. The changes in the cardiovascular system begin early, reach their maximum at about 30 weeks and are maintained until term. They include:

- An increase in cardiac output by 50%.
- An increase in blood volume up to 50%.

- A heart rate increase of 10–20 beats/min (bpm).
- A decrease in total peripheral resistance.
- A lowering of blood pressure in the first and second trimesters with a rise at 34 weeks, myocardial hypertrophy and heart chamber enlargement in the third trimester.

The changes in cardiac output in normal pregnancy without pre-existing cardiac problems may produce signs and symptoms of cardiac disease: for example, dyspnoea, orthopnoea, breathlessness on exertion, oedema and occasional palpitations (Lupton et al 2002). Heart sounds may change and confuse diagnosis (Prasad & Ventura 2001).

Risk factors

In some women the adaptive changes may exceed the ability of the heart to function, and **congestive cardiac failure** with pulmonary oedema may occur. More rarely, sudden death may be the outcome. There are times during pregnancy when **cardiac decompensation** is higher:

- At 12 and 32 weeks when the **haemodynamic changes** are increasing towards their maximum, with the most critical time between 28 and 32 weeks.
- The second dangerous period is during labour and delivery. During labour every uterine contraction injects blood from the uteroplacental circulation into the maternal bloodstream, which temporarily increases the cardiac output by 15–20%. The continuous demand on the heart may precipitate heart failure. Pushing during the second stage of labour increases the risk further by reducing venous return. Intravenous fluids should be accurately calculated, as overperfusion will be increased by the sudden injection of 300–500 ml of blood into the maternal circulation at delivery of the placenta. Congestive heart failure is frequent at this time (Lupton et al 2002).
- Finally, 4–5 days following delivery is a danger period, with thrombus formation and pulmonary embolism being a problem as blood constituents rapidly return to normal levels.

Main types of cardiac disorder

Rheumatic heart disease

The main effect of this disease is to cause valvular lesions. Mitral and aortic incompetence may be improved during pregnancy because of the lower pressure within the arterial tree. However, there is a risk of **endocarditis**. Mitral stenosis requires an increase in left atrial pressure to push blood into the left ventricle and will require an even greater effort in pregnancy. Women with mitral stenosis may develop increasing breathlessness.

The heart rate increases which decreases diastolic filling time and there is a rise in left atrial pressure which causes pulmonary oedema, hence the breathlessness (Lupton et al 2002).

To prevent pulmonary oedema **diuretics** should be given with β**-blockers** to aid diastolic filling (Prasad & Ventura 2001, Ray et al 2004, Sawhney et al 2003). **Anticoagulation** is important: warfarin crosses the placenta and causes embryopathy; heparin is safe for the fetus but the mother may develop thrombocytopenia and it affects bone density. Low-molecular-weight heparin may be used and is safer for the mother but may cause bleeding in the fetus (RCOG 2007, Uebing et al 2006). Most regimens use heparin for the first trimester, changing to warfarin until 2 weeks before the due date, when heparin is recommenced. This prevents the warfarin affecting fetal blood clotting time. Prophylactic antibiotics should be routine for operative or normal delivery to prevent infective endocarditis (Uebing et al 2006).

Congenital heart disease

A review of the literature by Drentham et al (2007) looking at 2491 pregnancies found that 11% exhibited cardiac complications, with a high incidence of preterm birth and consequent mortality and recurrence of heart defects in the babies was high.

Categorisation of congenital heart disease

- **Septal defects**: atrial septal defect (ASD), ventricular septal defect (VSD), patent ductus arteriosus (PDA), Eisenmenger's syndrome (Ammash & Warns 2001).
- **Obstruction defects**: pulmonary stenosis, aortic stenosis, coarctation of the aorta (Brickner et al 2000a).
- **Cyanotic defects**: tetralogy of Fallot, transposition of great vessels (American Heart Association 2002, Brickner et al 2000b).

Some of the defects mentioned above will not be problematic in pregnancy if the woman has been treated in childhood. There is a need to prevent infective endocarditis; thus, antibiotics in labour are necessary, as even though defects are repaired, some impairment may be present following the surgery. Women with prosthetic valve replacement are at risk of **thromboembolism** and should be anticoagulated (RCOG 2007, Uebing et al 2006).

Eisenmenger's syndrome

Eisenmenger's syndrome is an end-stage syndrome with pulmonary hypertension and has a high risk of maternal mortality (between 30% and 50%), and termination of pregnancy may be suggested (Lupton et al 2002). The syndrome is a result of various congenital heart defects: VSD, ASD, PDA, AVSD, or single ventricle. This causes systemic to pulmonary shunts—when the pulmonary pressures reach systemic pressures the shunt is reversed to a right to left shunt (American Heart Association 2002, Dumitresco & Walsh 2006). Cyanosis may be marked. During the third trimester, at birth and for 2 weeks post-natally the woman is at greatest risk of death and should be observed in hospital for at least 2 weeks post delivery.

Pregnancy adaptation causes the right-to-left shunt to increase cyanosis and creates back-pressure on the pulmonary circulation. Intrauterine growth restriction is seen in 30% of cases because of poor cardiac output and thus low oxygen levels in the circulation (Dumitresco & Walsh 2006). There is a high incidence of abortion and preterm birth (Siu & Colman 2001). During labour, haemodynamic monitoring should take place; vaginal delivery is preferable to caesarean section, with a shortened second stage.

Marfan's syndrome

Marfan's syndrome is an inherited condition involving connective tissue which causes skeletal, eye and heart abnormalities. High oestrogen levels present in pregnancy affect the structure of the aorta, where spontaneous rupture may take place, particularly in labour, where pressures within the vascular system may be variable (American Heart Association 2002, Blackburn 2003). Again, termination of the pregnancy may be advised, but, if there has been no pre-existing heart disease, pregnancy should not pose a problem.

Assessment of mothers with heart disease

Heart disease can present itself in pregnancy for the first time, or as an ongoing problem. Assessment is made jointly by the cardiologist and obstetrician so that counselling and decision making can be considered. If a termination of pregnancy is suggested, this should take place in the first trimester as, after 16 weeks continuing with the pregnancy, it may be the safer option. To assess client condition in heart diseases the following system has been widely used.

New York Heart Association classification

It is traditional to use the New York Heart Association classification (Ray et al 2004) to describe the severity of heart disease and how it affects daily activity. In practice this has little predictive value of the effect of pregnancy on the disease process.

- Class 1: no symptoms during ordinary physical activity.
- Class 2: ordinary physical activity, some fatigue, palpitations, dyspnoea.
- Class 3: symptoms during less than normal physical activity.

- Class 4: symptoms at rest, activity increased symptoms and discomfort.

If the woman is classified higher than class 2 it would indicate a poorer outcome in pregnancy. An increased risk to the fetus would be maternal smoking, prescribed anticoagulants and maternal age under 20 and over 35 (Uebing et al 2006).

Management of women with heart disease

The major maternal complications and the treatments aimed at avoiding them are:

- Endocarditis: routine antibiotics.
- Thromboemboli: anticoagulation.
- Cyanosis: rest, hospital admission.
- Arrhythmias: β-blockers, digoxin.
- Heart failure: hospital admission, dietary restriction of salt, diuretics.
- Urinary tract infection: antibiotics.
- Respiratory infection: antibiotics.
- Hypertension.
- Anaemia.

Care should be directed towards prevention of complications rather than treating them. An assessment of risk can be made during pregnancy, by using electrocardiography (ECG), echocardiography and maternal function in everyday circumstances. Counselling is important, especially if the woman is high risk. Assessment of the heart lesion is important, by examining ventricular function, pulmonary pressure, persistence of shunts and valvular obstruction (Siu & Colman 2001, Uebing et al 2006).

Specific aspects of care

Intrapartum care

Labour should take place in a unit with full resuscitation facilities and an intensive care unit. The cardiologist, obstetrician and anaesthetist should collaborate. If possible, labour should be spontaneous in onset with a vaginal delivery. The use of intravenous fluids could increase circulating blood volume, which may result in pulmonary oedema, so accurate fluid balance is essential. Blood should be cross-matched and oxygen and adult resuscitation equipment available. The heart should be monitored by ECG and pulse oximetry with accurate blood pressure recording. During active labour, the left lateral position is advantageous to assist venous return and prevent aortocaval compression.

Pain relief

Epidural is the best form of pain relief to assist women in labour, as it helps relaxation (Siu & Colman 2001).

Second stage

This stage should be kept short and without exertion; if delay occurs, forceps or vacuum extraction should be performed.

Third stage

To prevent blood loss a continuous Syntocinon (oxytocin) infusion should be used instead of intramuscular Syntocinon for the third stage. When the uterus empties and contracts, approximately 500 ml of blood is returned to the central circulation.

Postnatal care

The risk of cardiac failure with pulmonary oedema is greatest in the early puerperium. Signs include tachycardia, cyanosis, oedema and distension of the liver. If pulmonary oedema occurs, acute dyspnoea with frothy sputum and haemoptysis may occur. In most units the woman will be admitted to a high dependency unit to stabilise her condition (RCOG 2007).

Hypertension in pregnancy

Terminology

Raised blood pressure in pregnancy can be termed essential hypertension if it exists before pregnancy and is >140/90 mmHg; these women may develop pre-eclampsia (Pridjian & Puschett 2002a). Pregnancy-induced hypertension (PIH) is a condition specific to pregnancy and mainly occurs after the 20th week of gestation in some 5–10% of pregnancies (Hayman & Myers 2003, Magee et al 1999). The earlier the occurrence the greater the problems, and pre-eclampsia with raised blood pressure, proteinuria of >500 mg/L/24 h and multiorgan involvement may develop (Broughton Pipkin 1995). This has a 15–20% maternal mortality rate in developed countries (Sibai et al 2005). Eclampsia (convulsions) is caused by brain oedema, and where multiple organs are affected disseminated intravascular coagulation (DIC) defects may occur. Convulsions can occur postnatally for the first time (Zhang et al 1997) and the incidence is approximately 1:2000 pregnancies. HELLP syndrome (Nutt 1997, Sibai 2004a) is an acronym for Haemolytic anaemia, Elevated Liver enzymes and Low Platelet count. This may occur on its own or as part of pre-eclampsia.

Classification

It is generally accepted that hypertension in pregnancy may be defined as a diastolic pressure of greater than 90 mmHg. Davey & MacGillivray (1986) gave a clear definition:

The occurrence of a blood pressure of 140/90 mmHg on at least two occasions 4 hours apart after the 20th week of pregnancy. The woman is normotensive before this time.

If proteinuria of 500 mg/L or more is present, the condition is described as pre-eclampsia. **Severe pre-eclampsia** depends on the rise in blood pressure and the clinical or laboratory results (Chari et al 1995, Morley 2004). All or some of the following symptoms may be present:

- Blood pressure >160 mmHg systolic and >110 mmHg diastolic.
- Proteinuria >5.0 g in 24 h.
- Haemolytic anaemia, elevated liver enzymes, platelet count <100 000/ml.
- Headache.
- Epigastric pain.

Incidence

Pre-eclampsia is mainly a disorder affecting primigravidae. However, PIH may occur in a multiparous woman in a first pregnancy by another partner and who has a raised body mass index, a long pregnancy interval (>10 years) and is older than 40 (Duckitt & Harrington 2005). There is also evidence that women in a prolonged sexual relationship develop an immune response to sperm and are therefore immunologically protected in later pregnancies (Morley 2004, Ness & Grainger 2008). There is a genetic predisposition to this disease, women being more likely to develop the disorder if their mothers or sisters did (Zhang et al 1997). Multiple pregnancies and women who experience a hydatidiform mole may develop symptoms of PIH before 20 weeks due to hyperplacentation. Women who were hypertensive before pregnancy may develop pre-eclampsia superimposed on the existing condition and women who had pre-eclampsia in a previous pregnancy are more likely to have an occurrence.

A major problem is that PIH can really only be diagnosed in retrospect by a post-delivery return to normal blood pressure (Hearnshaw 1996). There is also difficulty in predicting which woman is likely to progress to a more serious condition. Severe pre-eclampsia can rapidly fulminate to eclampsia before blood pressure or proteinuria reach levels of concern (Zhang et al

1997). Blood pressure returns to normal within weeks. It is believed that there is no long-term link between hypertension in pregnancy and later onset of essential hypertension, although this may occur. Proteinuria may persist for longer than the hypertension and may indicate underlying renal disease.

Pathogenesis

The cause of PIH is still not completely understood and it has been described as a disease of theories. It is difficult to use animal models as there is no comparable process with which to make analogies. Pre-eclampsia is associated with an increase in the inflammatory response, poor placentation and poor placental blood flow to the fetus. Lockwood et al (2008) found high levels of interleukin-6, an inflammatory cytokine, in the plasma of pre-eclamptic women.

In normal pregnancy the spiral arterial walls are invaded by trophoblast and are transformed into large tortuous channels that carry large amounts of blood to the intervillous space. This occurs by 22 weeks, leading to a fall in peripheral resistance. In PIH this does not occur and the spiral arteries may only dilate to 40% of a normal pregnancy (Ghidini et al 1998, Morley 2004).

In women with pre-eclampsia there is inadequate invasion of the spiral arterioles by trophoblastic cells so that a decreased uteroplacental perfusion occurs (Fisher 2004). The symptoms of PIH are a maternal response to poor placentation and an attempt to prevent poor oxygenation of the fetus. Maternal compensatory mechanisms may break down, causing the woman symptoms such as DIC. This disruption of normal placentation may lead to altered endothelial cell function throughout the body, causing generalised vasoconstriction (Morley 2004).

In normal pregnancy, the renin–angiotensin–aldosterone system increases in activity, maintaining salt and water balance. In PIH this system is depleted (Pridjian & Puschett 2002b). Vasomotor tone depends on the relative influences of prostacyclin (a vasodilator) and thromboxane (a vasoconstrictor), which are substances from the prostaglandin family found in all tissues. In normal pregnancy there is an increase in substances that cause vasodilatation, including nitric oxide, which is a potent relaxing factor within the endothelium (Pridjian & Puschett 2002b, Zhang et al 1997).

The reduced volume of trophoblast in the spiral arterioles leads to an under-production of prostacyclin and a relative over-production of thromboxane, which encourages vasospasm of the spiral arteries. The damaged endothelium of the spiral arteries undergoes acute atherosclerosis (thickening of the vessel walls), thus narrowing the lumen. This causes a rise in blood pressure to overcome the increased resistance.

Proteinuria is a serious sign in pre-eclampsia, resulting from a swelling of the kidney glomeruli partly due to the raised blood pressure causing leakage of protein through enlarged capillaries (Morley 2004). Uric acid clearance is reduced and plasma urates rise, indicating kidney involvement showing impaired tubular function. The cardiac index (the ratio of cardiac output to body surface area) is reduced by 22% in established pre-eclampsia while systemic vascular resistance is raised (Broughton Pipkin 1995). This raised systemic resistance is not due to the action of the sympathetic nervous system. It is associated with vasoconstriction, a reduced plasma volume and haemoconcentration, and oedema usually develops. The reduced plasma volume is associated with intrauterine growth restriction (Ghidini et al 1998, Johnson et al 2002).

Oxidative stress

Oxidative stress causes **atherosclerosis**, resulting in endothelial cell damage causing clotting defects and microthombi which may be the link in causing pre-eclampsia. There is also a link between oxidative stress and early-onset cardiac disease (Stephens et al 1996). Oxidative stress produces circulating free oxygen radicals as a metabolic by-product. This influences **lipid peroxidation** and damages proteins, nucleic acids and the endothelium. Prostaglandin production is affected, disturbing the balance between thromboxanes and prostacyclins and thus diminishing the vasodilatory effect that pregnancy requires (Broughton Pipkin 1995). Excess **free radicals** affect the endothelium, causing vasoconstriction and platelet aggregation and initiating clotting mechanisms (Chappell et al 1999). Vitamins E and C, which work in tandem, are naturally occurring antioxidant substances that were found to be low in pre-eclamptic women. Supplementation of these substances has not been found to be beneficial (Spinnato et al 2007).

Outcomes

This multisystem disorder eventually affects the kidneys, the liver and the placental bed. The kidney changes are only distinguishable from acute **glomerulonephritis** by electron microscopy. Narrowing of the capillary lumen by vasospasm is worsened by the deposition of **fibrinous material** between the endothelial cells and the basement membrane as the disease progresses. In glomerulonephritis the narrowing is caused by swelling of the basement membrane. The same fibrinous deposits have been found in the liver of patients with pre-eclampsia. **Intracapsular haemorrhages** and necrosis occur, and oedema of the liver cells may produce

epigastric pain and impairment in liver function, showing diagnostically as raised liver enzymes.

The vessels supplying the placental bed may become constricted and the reduction in uterine blood flow along with placental vascular lesions may result in placental abruption. The reduced maternal capillary blood flow in the placental villi may result in the placental tissue becoming ischaemic. These changes have grave implications for fetal growth and survival. The release of thromboplastin into the maternal circulation results in DIC. The brain becomes oedematous with the development of headache and visual disturbances. As blood pressure continues to rise, fitting may occur. Thrombosis and necrosis of the cerebral blood vessel walls may result in a **cerebrovascular accident**. Seven deaths were reported in the maternal mortality report 1997–9 (Lewis 2001).

Eclampsia

The incidence of eclampsia is 2.7 per 10 000 births in the UK (Knight 2007) and has significantly fallen since the trials into the use of magnesium sulphate in the 1990s. Symptoms often include headaches, visual disturbance, nausea, vomiting, convulsions and coma (Cipolla 2007). A population-based study by Knight (2007) showed that 38% of the study population had raised blood pressure and proteinuria prior to their first fit; 56% of the women were admitted to an intensive care unit, indicating the seriousness of the condition. There were eight stillborns and five babies died postnatally. The underlying pathophysiology is a complicated process, but is due to changes in pressure within the blood–brain barrier as a complication of the vascular changes within the circulatory system causing oedema in the brain (Cipolla 2007).

Prediction

To be of use a test must be non-invasive to mother and fetus, be easy to perform and have a high predictive value. Endothelial cell numbers (CEC) are raised in pre-eclampsia; Grundmann et al (2008) are researching the use of CECs as markers in the blood to predict pre-eclampsia, but this has not been used in clinical practice. Research is ongoing in this area. Those involved in antenatal care should assess risk for pre-eclampsia at the booking visit, preferably before 10 weeks, and must be vigilant in detecting early signs and symptoms to prevent severe pre-eclampsia and eclampsia developing (NICE 2008). Research has shown that women have a greater risk of cardiovascular disease if they have pre-eclampsia early in a first pregnancy, showing symptoms of 'endothelial damage, abnormal lipids and insulin resistance' some years later (Roberts & Gammill 2005).

HELLP syndrome

There is uncertainty about whether the HELLP syndrome is a serious complication of pre-eclampsia or a process in itself. Women may present with malaise, nausea, vomiting and epigastric pain, typically before term. They may have normal blood pressure and no proteinuria. If these symptoms, which imitate gastric flu, are present, women may be sent home to recover but the practitioner should think again and take blood specimens for platelets, liver enzymes and await results before sending them home (Nutt 1997).

The resultant pathophysiology may be present alone or together with pre-eclampsia. The severe decrease in platelets alters clotting mechanisms and the haemolysis damages the internal strata of the blood vessels. The multisystem involvement causes kidney failure, hepatic failure and neurological problems in the form of multiple emboli which block capillaries. The placenta is involved and abruptio placentae may occur with the death of the fetus. The HELLP syndrome is a serious condition and delivery is essential to prevent the above complications. Criteria for diagnosis are perhaps a selection of abnormalities and not always all of them (Sibai 2004a).

Management of hypertensive conditions

Rest and observation

Women with mild PIH can rest at home but, if the disease is moderate to severe or worsening with proteinuria, hospitalisation is recommended. The mother is admitted to hospital where bed rest may be encouraged but this has never been found to be positively beneficial to the management of PIH (Enkin et al 2000). However, admission to hospital allows greater surveillance of maternal and fetal conditions.

A prime method of observing women antenatally is the assessment of blood pressure and urinalysis with estimation of maternal and fetal well-being. When proteinuria is present, hospital admission is generally advised once urinary tract infection is eliminated. Plasma urate concentrations are the only useful biochemical indicator of deterioration and severe disease is present if platelet counts begin to fall. Assessment of urinary output may be useful. As the blood pressure rises, visual disturbances, headache and epigastric pain may be experienced by the woman; these signs need investigating and acting on.

The measurement of blood pressure must be accurate and consistent (Bothamley & Boyle 2008). Doctors and midwives should be guided by the research into the taking and recording of blood pressure and the machines used for its measurement (Shennan 2005,

Shennan & Shennan 1996). Errors are created by observer technique or bias, the sphygmomanometer and the stethoscope and the client's anxiety and fear (white coat hypertension).

Good practice pointers for measurement of blood pressure

- Sit client up, with machine level with heart (if using mercury manometers).
- Always record on the same arm and use a correctly sized cuff.
- Automated blood pressure machines can under-record the pressure.
- Let cuff down slowly; read to the nearest 2 mmHg; do not round up or down.
- Korotkoff sound V should be recorded and the disappearance of the sound; if this is 0, then Korotkoff IV may be used; both should be noted on records.
- If measurement is raised, allow a rest before retaking; record findings of both observations.

Fetal observations

Fetal observations will include twice-daily cardiotocograph recordings, serial ultrasonic assessments of growth and Doppler measurements of blood velocity in placental bed and umbilical arteries. Any signs of impending eclampsia may necessitate rapid delivery, regardless of the gestational period, to save the mother's life.

Delivery

The only treatment for pre-eclampsia is delivery of the baby. A decision to deliver the baby will depend partly on how effective the treatment is considered to be, which depends on interpretation of the observations. The mode of delivery similarly depends on the risks to mother and baby, and delivery, whether by induction of labour, depending on cervical ripeness, or by caesarean section, depends on the condition of the mother and maturity of the fetus (Vidaeff et al 2005).

Control of blood pressure

There are alternative therapies for attempts to prevent complications and in some situations to control high blood pressure. **Methyldopa**, which affects noradrenaline (norepinephrine) synthesis (Rang et al 2007), reduces systemic peripheral resistance without changing heart rate or cardiac output (Chari et al 1995). It has been used safely for many years, particularly for women with essential hypertension, who may have been prescribed **angiotensin-converting enzyme** (ACE) inhibitors pre-pregnancy; these are contraindicated in

pregnancy. The aim is to maintain blood pressure below 90–100 mmHg diastolic to improve fetal outcome; too low a level would compromise placental blood flow (Tomlinson 2003).

Labetalol, a β-adrenoreceptor antagonist, may be given orally or parentally. Its effects can be seen in 2–5 min and it initiates a fall in blood pressure almost immediately. Maternal side effects such as headache or shaking could be mistaken for impending fitting. Labetalol does not pass through the placenta or decrease cardiac output.

Nifedepine, a calcium channel blocker affecting cell membranes and cardiac muscle, is absorbed by the gut and is only used orally. **Nicardipine** is its parenteral equivalent. Similar side effects may be seen in the mother as labetalol. It does not pass through the placenta but may have effects on labour as it is a tocholytic (Tomlinson 2003). Calcium channel blockers may be more effective than other hypotensive drugs but this is not conclusive (Abalos et al 2007).

Hydralazine directly relaxes arterial smooth muscle, resulting in increased heart rate and contractility with decreased placental blood flow and consequent fetal distress (Chari et al 1995, Tomlinson 2003), but it may cause maternal hypotension. Hydralazine should not be given to women with a pulse rate above 100 bpm as it causes a tachycardia. Research by Zu et al (2006) found that hydralazine increased the production of interleukin-10, an anti-inflammatory, thus having a dual effect on the maternal system.

Anticonvulsive therapy

Magnesium sulphate has been widely used in the USA for the last three decades to control the convulsive state (Belfort et al 2006). There is overwhelming evidence in favour of magnesium sulphate (Duley et al 2003, Sibai 2004b). Magnesium sulphate is toxic, thus monitoring blood levels and reflexes to test nervous system involvement is crucial. Long-term use could cause respiratory depression in both mother and fetus (BNF 2007). Calcium gluconate should be available in case toxicity is evident (Garovic 2000).

Diuretics are contraindicated in pre-eclampsia as they can aggravate plasma volume and balance of fluids. There is a place for them in women with chronic hypertension pre-pregnancy and hypertension in renal and heart failure, although they may adversely affect electrolyte imbalance (Garovic 2000).

Prevention

Aspirin prevents platelet aggregation by inhibiting thromboxane production. The multicentre Collaborative Low-dose Aspirin Study trial (CLASP Collaborative

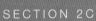
Group 1994) set out to show that, used prophylactically, it would prevent pre-eclampsia. In this study, the use of low-dose aspirin (60–150 mg) was not proven to be beneficial. However, in the follow-up studies by Duley et al (2001) and Askie et al (2007), which reviewed 60 000 women, there was a significant reduction in preterm birth and risk from pre-eclampsia. There was some benefit from starting aspirin early, before 12–16 weeks, and it was concluded that there is a small-to-moderate benefit in its use.

Main points

- There is a changing pattern of heart disease, with increasing numbers of women surviving congenital heart disease and an increase in coronary artery disease. The woman may already be aware of her heart disease and may have sought preconception advice. There will be a higher incidence of a heart defect in the baby if there is a family history of congenital heart defect.

- The main effects of rheumatic heart disease are to cause valvular lesions. Mitral stenosis requires an increase in left atrial pressure to push blood into the left ventricle and will require a greater effort in pregnancy.

- It is traditional to use the New York Heart Association classification to describe the severity of heart disease but in practice this has little predictive value of the effect of pregnancy on the disease process.

- Labour should take place in a unit with full resuscitation facilities and an intensive care unit. It should be spontaneous in onset, with a vaginal delivery where possible. The use of intravenous fluids increases circulating blood volume, which may result in pulmonary oedema, and an epidural reduces the risk. To prevent infective endocarditis antibiotic prophylaxis may be necessary in labour. Anticoagulants could avoid the risk of developing thromboemboli.

- The second stage should be kept short and without exertion. Elective forceps delivery and avoiding the supine position should be advocated.

- Hypertension which develops for the first time in the second half of pregnancy and is caused by the pregnancy is common. Pre-eclampsia is associated with proteinuria and may lead to eclampsia. It is a multisystem disorder, which may result in maternal and fetal morbidity and mortality.

- Pre-eclampsia is mainly a disease of primigravidae but may occur in a multiparous woman in a first pregnancy by a new partner.

- In pre-eclampsia there is inadequate invasion of the spiral arterioles by trophoblastic cells and decreased uteroplacental perfusion occurs. Associated with vasoconstriction is a reduced plasma volume and haemoconcentration and oedema usually develop. There are two common features of pre-eclampsia—vasoconstriction and DIC—leading to changes in the kidney, liver and placental bed.

- The aim of care is to prolong the pregnancy until the fetus is mature enough to survive. Antihypertensive drugs are useful at protecting the woman's circulation against the risk of cerebrovascular accident but have no effect on the disease or on fetal growth.

- Maternal observations include urinalysis for protein, fluid balance, presence of oedema, blood pressure and abdominal examination for pain and tenderness. Plasma urate concentrations are useful biochemical indicators of kidney function and severe disease is present if platelet counts fall.

- Deciding when to deliver the baby depends partly on how effective the treatment is considered to be, which will depend on the interpretation of the observations. The timing can be a fine line drawn between maternal condition and fetal maturity. The mode of delivery similarly depends on the risks to mother and baby.

- In a few women severe pre-eclampsia may affect the liver and be complicated by the HELLP syndrome. Immediate delivery will resolve the abnormal blood picture but there may be a need to give platelets or packed red cells to lessen the risk of haemorrhage. The long-term prognosis is that the blood pressure returns to normal within weeks.

References

Abalos, E., Duley, L., Steyn, D.W., Henderson-Smart, D.J., 2007. Antihypertensive drug therapy for mild to moderate hypertension during pregnancy. Cochrane. Database. Syst. Rev. 24 (1), CD002252.

American Heart Association. 2002 Congenital cardiovascular disease. <http://www.americanheart.org>

Ammash, N., Warnes, C., 2001. Ventricular septal defect in adults. Ann. Intern. Med. 35 (9), 812–824.

Askie, L.M., Duley, L., Henderson-Smart, D.J., Stewart, L.A. on behalf of the PARIS Collaborative Group, 2007. Anti-platelet agents for pre-eclampsia: a meta-analysis of individual patient data. Obstet. Gynecol. Surv. 62 (11), 697–699.

Belfort, M.A., Clark, S.L., Sibai, B., 2006. Cerebral hemodynamics in pre-eclampsia: cerebral perfusion and the rationale for an alternative to magnesium sulphate. Obstet. Gynecol. Surv. 61 (10), 656–665.

Blackburn, S.T., 2003. Maternal, Fetal and Neonatal Physiology: A clinical perspective, third edn. W B Saunders, Philadelphia.

BNF (British National Formulary), 2007. Magnes. sulphate March, 508.

Bothamley, J., Boyle, M., 2008. How to measure blood pressure. Midwives February/March, 29.

Brickner, E., Hillis, D., Lange, A., 2000a. Medical progress: congenital heart disease in adults (Part 1). N. Engl. J. Med. 342 (4), 256–263.

Brickner, E., Hillis, D., Lange, A., 2000b. Medical progress: congenital heart disease in adults (Part 2). N. Engl. J. Med. 342 (5), 334–342.

Broughton Pipkin, F., 1995. The hypertensive disorders of pregnancy. Br. Med. J. 311, 609–613.

Chappell, L., Seed, P., Briley, A., et al., 1999. Effects of anti-oxidants on the occurrence of pre-eclampsia in women at increased risk: a randomised trial. Lancet 354 (9181), 810–815.

Chari, R., Friedman, S., Sibai, B., 1995. Antihypertensive therapy during pregnancy. Matern. Med. Rev. 7, 71–75.

Cipolla, M.J., 2007. Cerebrovascular function in pregnancy and eclampsia. Hypertension 50, 14–24.

Clarke, J., Butt, M., 2005. Maternal collapse. Curr. Opin. Obstet. Gynecol. 17 (2), 157–160.

CLASP Collaborative Group, 1994. Collaborative low-dose aspirin study in pregnancy. Lancet 343 (8898), 619–629.

Davey, D., MacGillivray, I., 1986. The classification of the hypertensive disorders of pregnancy. Clin. Exp. Hypertens. B5, 97–133.

Drentham, W., Pieper, P., Roos-Hesselink, J., et al., 2007. Outcome of pregnancy in women with congenital heart disease. J. Am. Coll. Cardiol. 49, 2303–2311.

Drife, J., 2005. Why mothers die. J. R. Coll. Physicians Edinb. 35, 332–336 http://www.rcpe.ac.uk/publications/articles/journal_35_4/why%20mothers%20die.pdf.

Duckitt, K., Harrington, D., 2005. Risk factors for pre-eclampsia at antenatal booking: systematic review of controlled studies. BMJ 330 (7491), 565–567.

Duley, L. for the Eclampsia Trial Collaborative Group, 1995. Which anticonvulsant for women with eclampsia? Evidence from the Collaborative Eclampsia Trial. Lancet 345, 1455–1463.

Duley, L., Henderson-Smart, D., Knight, M., King, J., 2001. Antiplatelet drugs for the prevention of pre-eclampsia and its consequences: systematic review. Br. Med. J. 322 (7782), 329–333.

Duley, L., Gulmezoglu, A. M., Henderson-Smart, D. J., 2003. Anticonvulsants for women with pre-eclampsia. Cochrane Review. Cochrane Library, Issue, 2, Update Software, Oxford.

Dumitresco, A., Walsh, K.P., 2006. Eisenmenger's syndrome. Br. J. Cardiol. 13 (6), 419–424.

Enkin, M., Keirse, M., Neilson, J., et al., 2000. A Guide to Effective Care in Pregnancy and Childbirth, 3rd edn. Oxford University Press, Oxford.

Fisher, S. J. (2004). The placental problem: Linking abnormal cytotrophoblast differentiation to the maternal symptoms of pre-eclampsia. Reproductive Biology and Endocrinology 2:53. Online access: <http://www.rbej.com/content/2/1/53> (accessed 10.07.08).

Garovic, V., 2000. Hypertension in pregnancy: diagnosis and treatment. Mayo Clin. Proc. 75 (10), 1017–1076.

Ghidini, A., Salfia, C.M., Pijnenborg, R., 1998. Lesions of the placental bed and placenta in relation to pre-eclampsia. Contemp. Rev. Obstet. Gynaecol. June, 85–90.

Grundmann, M., Woywodt, A., Kirsch, T., Hollwitz, B., Oehler, K., et al., 2008. Circulating endothelial cells: a marker of vascular damage in patients with pre-eclampsia. Am. J. Obstet. Gynecol. 198 (3), 317.

Hayman, R., Myers, J., 2003. Definition and classification, Chapter 1. In: Baker, P., Kingdom, J., Kingdom, J.C. (Eds.) Pre-Eclampsia: Current Perspectives on Management. Informa Healthcare, Parthanon Publishing, Nashville.

Hearnshaw, A., 1996. The trouble with terminology. APEC Newsletter 11 (Spring), 17.

Johnson, M.R., Anim-Nyame, N., Johnson, P., Sooranna, S.R., Steer, P.J., 2002. Does epithelial cell activation occur with intrauterine growth restriction? Br. J. Obstet. Gynaecol. 109 (7), 836–839.

Knight, M., 2007. Eclampsia in the United Kingdom. Br. J. Obstet. Gynaecol. 114 (9), 1072–1078.

Lewis G, (ed.), 2001, Why mothers die. Fifth Report of Confidential Enquiries into Maternal Deaths in the United Kingdom 1997–99. Royal College of Obstetricians and Gynaecologists Press, London.

Lockwood, C.J., Yen, C.F., Basar, M., Kayisli, U.A., Martel, M., et al., 2008. Pre-eclampsia related inflammatory cytokines regulate interleukin-6 expression in human decidual cells. Am. J. Pathol. 172 (6), 1571–1579.

Lupton, M., Oteng-Ntim, E., Gubby, A., Steer, P., 2002. Cardiac disease in pregnancy. Curr. Opin. Obstet. Gynecol. 14 (2), 137–143.

Magee, L., Ornstein, M.P., von Dadelszen, P., 1999. Management of hypertension in pregnancy. Br. Med. J. 318, 1332–1336.

Morley, A., 2004. Pre-eclampsia: pathophysiology and its management. Br. J. Midwifery 12 (1), 30–37.

Ness, R.B., Grainger, D.A., 2008. Male reproductive hormones and reproductive outcomes. Am. J. Obstet. Gynecol. 198 (6), 620–624.

NICE. Antenatal care: routine care for the healthy pregnant woman, 2008. Guideline 62 Website: http://www.nice.org.uk; accessed July 2008.

Nutt, J., 1997. HELLP syndrome. Br. J. Midwifery 15 (1), 8–11.

Prasad, A., Ventura, H., 2001. Valvular heart disease and pregnancy. Postgrad. Med. 110 (2) online http://www.postgraduatemed.com/issues/2001/08/prasad.htm.

Pridjian, G., Puschett, J., 2002a. Pre-eclampsia, part 1, clinical and pathophysiological considerations. Obstet. Gynaecol. Surv. 57 (9), 598–618.

Pridjian, G., Puschett, J., 2002b. Pre-eclampsia, part 2, experimental and genetic considerations. Obstet. Gynaecol. Surv. 57 (9), 619–640.

Rang, H.P., Dale, M.M., Ritter, J.M., 2007. Pharmacology, 6th edn. Churchill Livingstone, Edinburgh.

Ray, P., Murphy, G.J., Shutt, L.E., 2004. Recognition and management of maternal cardiac disease in pregnancy. Br. J. Anaesth. 93 (3), 428–439.

RCOG 2007 Heart Disease and Pregnancy—Study Group Statement. <http://www.rcog.org.uk/index.asp?pageID=2236> (accessed 06.08).

Roberts, J.M., Gammill, H., 2005. Pre-eclampsia and cardiovascular disease in later life. Lancet 366 (9490), 961–962.

Sawhney, H., Aggarwal, N., Suri, V., et al., 2003. Maternal and perinatal outcomes in rheumatic heart disease. Int. J. Gynaecol. Obstet. 80 (1), 9–14.

Shennan A. 2005. How to reduce errors in blood pressure measurement. Online: <www.apec.org.uk/documents/elearning/bpmeasurement.htm> (accessed 10.07.08).

Shennan, C., Shennan, A., 1996. Blood pressure in pregnancy: the need for accurate measurement. Br. J. Midwifery 4 (2), 102–108.

Sibai, B.M., 2004a. Diagnosis, controversies, and management of the syndrome of hemolysis, elevated liver enzymes, and low platelet count. Obstet. Gynecol. 103, 981–991.

Sibai, B.M., 2004b. Magnesium sulphate prophylaxis in pre-eclampsia: lessons learned from recent trials. Am. J. Obstet. Gynecol. 190 (6), 1520–1526.

Sibai, B., Dekker, G., Kupferminic, M., 2005. Pre-eclampsia. Lancet 365 (9461), 789–799.

Siu, S., Colman, J., 2001. Heart disease in pregnancy. Heart 85 (6), 710–715.

Spinnato, J.A., Freire, S., Pinto, E., Silva, J.L., Cunha Rudge, M.V., et al., 2007. Antioxidant therapy to prevent pre-eclampsia: a randomised controlled trial. Obstet. Gynecol. 110 (6), 1311–1318.

Stephens, N., Parsons, A., Schofield, P., et al., 1996. Randomised controlled trial of vitamin E in patients with coronary artery disease: Cambridge Heart Antioxidant Study (CHAOS). Lancet 347, 781–786.

Tomlinson, J., 2003. Labour ward management of severe pre-eclampsia. Ch. 12. In: Baker, P., Kingdom, J., Kingdom, J.C. (Eds.) Pre-eclampsia: Current Perspectives on Management. Informa Healthcare, Parthanon Publishing, Nashville.

Uebing, A., Steer, P.J., Yentis, S.M., Gatzoulis, M.A., 2006. Pregnancy and congenital heart disease. Br. Med. J. 332 (7538), 401–406.

Vidaeff, A., Carroll, M., Ramin, S., 2005. Acute hypertensive emergencies in pregnancy. Crit. Care Med. 33 (10 Suppl), S307–S312.

Zhang, J., Zeisler, J., Hatch, M., Berkowitz, G., 1997. Epidemiology of pregnancy-induced hypertension. Epidemiol. Rev. 19 (2), 218–232.

Zu, B., Makris, A., Thornton, C., Ogle, R., Horvath, J., Hennessy, A., 2006. Antihypertensive drugs clonidine, hydralazine, and furosemide regulate the production of cytokines by the placenta and peripheral blood mononuclear cells in normal pregnancy. J. Hypertens. 24 (5), 915–922.

Annotated recommended reading

American Heart Association, 2002. Congenital cardiovascular disease. <http://www.americanheart.org>.

Within this site is a clearly written account of congenital heart defects; also there are many links to other pertinent sites about heart disease.

Oakley, C., Warnes, C. (Eds.), 2007. Heart Disease in Pregnancy. Blackwell Publishing, London.

This edited textbook gives a detailed account of all aspects of heart disease in pregnancy.

Sibai, B.M., 2004. Diagnosis, controversies, and management of the syndrome of hemolysis, elevated liver enzymes, and low platelet count. Obstet. Gynecol. 103, 981–991.

This paper gives the reader a depth of understanding of HELLP syndrome. It includes classification, pathophysiology, assessment of maternal health and treatment.

Sibai, B., Dekker, G., Kupferminic, M., 2005. Pre-eclampsia. Lancet 365 (9461), 789–799.

This paper is a must read as it is an overview of hypertension in pregnancy with clear physiological explanations of this puzzling disorder.

Zhang, J., Zeisler, J., Hatch, M., Berkowitz, G., 1997. Epidemiology of pregnancy-induced hypertension. Epidemiol. Rev. 19 (2), 218–232.

This paper defines pregnancy-induced hypertension. It contains a depth of physiology which clarifies many aspects of the cause of hypertension in pregnancy.

Chapter Thirty-Three

Anaemia and clotting disorders

Anaemia

Worldwide, the effects of anaemia and clotting disorders on maternal and fetal morbidity and mortality are enormous. This chapter examines these two clinical problems in detail. Anaemia is reduction in the oxygen-carrying capacity of the blood, which may be due to a reduced number of red blood cells, a low concentration of haemoglobin (Hb) or a combination of both (Bewley 2004). The effects of anaemia involve both mother and fetus. The mother may develop symptoms such as dyspnoea, fainting fatigue, tachycardia and palpitations. She may have reduced resistance to infection and her life may be threatened by antepartum or postpartum haemorrhage.

The fetus may suffer intrauterine hypoxia and growth restriction although it is difficult to separate the effects of anaemia from other factors such as social class, smoking and maternal age. Godfrey et al (1991) found that large placental weight with a reduction in fetal weight was associated with iron-deficiency anaemia. This correlated the change in placental/fetal weight ratio with a risk of hypertension in later life (Godfrey & Barker 1995).

Recognition and incidence of anaemia

The World Health Organization (WHO 2008) set criteria for diagnosis of anaemia in pregnancy as a haemoglobin (Hb) of <11g/dl, but because of increased understanding of the physiological changes in pregnancy many doctors only investigate women with an Hb of ≤10.0g/dl (Bewley 2004). The incidence is high in developing countries and is associated with helminth infections, poor nutrition and malaria (Walraven 2008). The WHO state that the prevalence of anaemia in pregnancy in developing countries is between 35% and 75%; however, in developed countries this is lower, at 18%.

Types of anaemia include:

- Iron-deficiency anaemia (IDA).
- Folic acid deficiency.
- Hereditary haemoglobinopathies, sickle cell anaemias and the thalassaemias.
- Anaemia due to blood loss.

Iron-deficiency anaemia

Pathology

Iron is essential for the bioavailability of oxygen to cells. Diminished iron levels are due to poor intake of available dietary iron (Conrad 2008). It is absorbed by the small intestine more readily in pregnancy (Milman 2006). Iron-deficiency anaemia (IDA) is a common pathology of pregnancy, but may be asymptomatic and difficult to diagnose. The physiological changes of blood plasma volume expansion make it appear that haemoglobin is lower. In pregnancy there is a greater demand for iron for haemoglobin synthesis, and demands increase to 7.5 mg/day by the end of pregnancy (Milman 2006). If haemoglobin is low, there is a poor red cell uptake of oxygen and poor oxygen delivery to the placental bed and fetus. The fetus obtains its iron from transferrin in the maternal blood across the placental–maternal interface, usually after 30 weeks of pregnancy. In the earlier weeks maternal iron consumption increases and should meet the later demands, but if iron stores as ferritin are low the demand may not be met. To ascertain those women at risk of IDA, the midwife's booking interview should highlight the following (Coggins 2001, Conrad 2008):

- Reduced food intake or malabsorption of iron or protein.
- Blood loss from previous heavy menses.
- Iron deprivation from previous pregnancies or short pregnancy gap.
- Multiple pregnancy.
- Chronic urinary tract infection (low iron status affects immunity).
- Previous antepartum or postpartum haemorrhage.
- Women from low social groups.

In a multicultural society such as Britain the likelihood of the **inherited haemoglobinopathies** should be considered as well as the effects of nutrition and infection on iron status.

Investigations

Identification of IDA involves screening, blood counts, history taking and investigations. Screening all pregnant women for haemoglobin (Hb) concentration regularly indicates the presence of anaemia but will not identify the cause. However, normal non-pregnant reference values may not consider the haemodilution of pregnancy and there may be a danger of overdiagnosing asymptomatic women with low Hb. Women who are identified as having a low Hb should be questioned about nutritional habits, gastrointestinal upset, and excessive menstrual bleeding prior to pregnancy.

IDA is a **microcytic anaemia** with a fall in mean cell volume (MCV), and a fall in **serum ferritin** (iron stores) before a fall in Hb. A fall in Hb is a late sign when iron stores have already been depleted. A urine sample should be obtained to exclude urinary tract infection as ferritin levels may be artificially high when an infection is present (Breymann 2005). Coggins (2001) outlined the parameters considered when making a diagnosis of IDA (Table 33.1).

Table 33.1 Blood tests used to diagnose iron-deficiency anaemia (IDA)

Blood test	Normal reference range	Validity in diagnosis
Haemoglobin	11–15 g/dl (pregnant)	Lacks specificity, affected by haemodilution and smoking
Mean cell volume (MCV)	75–99 fl (femtolitres)	Raised in pregnancy, decreased in IDA
Reticulocyte count	25–75 × 10^9/L	Increased by pregnancy, decreased by IDA
Serum ferritin	15–300 μg/L	Signifies iron stores, early indication of iron deficiency
Total iron-binding capacity	45–72 μmol/L	Non-specific in pregnancy, raised by pregnancy, false positive if infection present
Serum iron	13–27 μmol/L	Decreased by pregnancy, diurnal rhythm, non-specific in pregnancy

Management

An oral iron preparation is usually given once IDA has been diagnosed. Absorption is maximised if taken with orange juice (Coggins 2001). The daily amount of iron needed to treat IDA is 60–120 mg in divided doses. Oral ferrous salts are more absorbable than ferric salts but all iron preparations tend to have side-effects such as nausea, vomiting and constipation, although in a randomised double blind study of 404 women in four groups it was found that this was not true (Milman et al 2006). In most units in the UK, women are only given iron preparations if IDA has been diagnosed. Iron can be given by intramuscular injection or intravenous infusion if necessary (BNF 2007):

- Intramuscular iron is given in the form of **iron sorbitol** 50 mg/ml. The dose is 1.5 mg/kg body weight and it can be given daily or weekly. A deep intramuscular injection should be given to avoid staining the skin and fat necrosis.
- Intravenous iron is given as a total dose iron infusion in the form of **iron dextran** 50 mg/ml. It is given slowly in normal saline and the dose depends on body weight and the degree of iron deficiency. Anaphylactic shock is a major side-effect and intravenous iron should only be given if absolutely necessary.
- Blood transfusion may be an option (RCOG 2007). Further investigations should take place if treatment is not effective (BNF 2007).

The treatment for IDA has been reviewed by Cuervo & Mahomed (2003) who looked at 53 trials. Evidence about the effects of iron therapy in pregnancy was inconclusive as there was a shortage of quality trials. Intravenous iron was associated with an increased risk of venous thrombosis. The debate continues as to whether or not to routinely supplement with iron. As the babies of iron-depleted mothers may be adversely affected by their mother's low iron status supplementation would perhaps be beneficial (Müngen 2003).

Folic acid deficiency anaemia

Incidence

Folic acid is necessary for red cell proliferation and DNA synthesis, and in pregnancy demands are high as the fetus develops and grows (Blackburn 2007). Deficiency may occur in pregnancy in the undernourished, in multiple pregnancy, those on anticoagulants or anticonvulsants, heavy drinkers or smokers causing a megaloblastic anaemia (Bewley 2004). Positive diagnosis cannot be made without a bone marrow biopsy. Demands for folate (naturally occurring) and folic acid (synthesised) are high in pregnancy and many women will have low reserves to call on as the fetus grows (Tsunenobu & Picciano 2006). Synthesised folic acid is more readily acquired by the body systems than folate; hence supplementation may be required and is more successful in raising levels in pregnancy.

Investigations

The red cells are macrocytic (larger) and may be misshapen, fewer in number and the Hb level is low. Plasma folate and red cell folate can be estimated. There may be a low platelet count and white cell count. Serum folic acid is lower than $4\,\mu g/ml$ (Bewley 2004).

Management

The anaemia usually responds to folic acid supplementation of 5–15 mg folic acid daily. Prevention of anaemia by administration of prophylactic folic acid 300–500 µg daily can be given to those:

- With malabsorption syndrome.
- With haemoglobinopathies (see below).
- Who are on anticonvulsant therapy.
- With a multiple pregnancy.

Folate deficiency is involved in the causation of neural tube defects (Box 33.1).

Haemoglobinopathies

Two of the most common diseases are the recessively inherited **sickle cell disease** and **thalassaemias** which affect haemoglobin synthesis. In utero, the fetus is not affected as it carries fetal haemoglobin (HbF) which has a greater affinity to oxygen, but soon after birth the switch between fetal and adult haemoglobin (HbA) begins (Bailey & Gwinnutt 2008). As the ratio of HbF to HbA changes, the symptoms of inherited disease become evident (Stephen & Cunningham 1998).

The globin chains

The gene for the α-globin chain family is located on chromosome 16 and for the β-globin chain family on chromosome 11. The α-globin chain is 141 amino acids long and the β-globin chain is 146 amino acids long. All haemoglobin variants have a tetrameric structure with four protein chains in association with four haem molecules. The four protein chains in normal haemoglobin take up a particular shape which allows maximum uptake, delivery and release of oxygen into the tissues.

Inherited genes produce abnormal proteins that cannot carry out their function efficiently resulting in ill-health with anaemia, hypoxia, tissue damage and haemolysis (Fig. 33.1). There are three forms of inherited haemoglobinopathies:

- Structural Hb variants, in which there is a fault in either the α-globin chain or the β-globin chain.
- The thalassaemias, in which there is reduced production of either the α-globin chain or the β-globin chain.
- Failure to switch from the production of HbF to HbA, which is clinically insignificant, although in some instances helps the sufferer because oxygen is absorbed more easily by HbF (Weatherall 1997b).

Sickle cell disease

Sickle cell disease (SCD) is the most common of the structural haemoglobin defects (Weatherall 1997a) (Table 33.2). A single amino acid substitution of **valine** for **glutamic acid** results in a haemoglobin molecule that is less soluble. When oxygen is low, the molecules form long, linear stacks that distort the red cells into a sickle shape. The inheritance of one gene from each parent (homozygous genotype for HbSS) makes the individual sickle cell-positive. Those who inherit one gene (heterozygote) have the **sickle cell trait** (HbAS) and usually do not display signs of the disease. They do, however, have some protection against the organism *Plasmodium falciparum*, the cause of a severe form of malaria. The malarial parasite enters the red blood cell and makes it sickle. This cell and its parasite are destroyed by the spleen, protecting the individual from malaria (Frenette & Atweh 2007).

Heterozygote parents have a 50% chance of producing an infant affected by SCD (Sickle Cell Society 2008).

33.1 NEURAL TUBE DEFECTS IN THE FETUS AND FOLATE DEFICIENCY

Neural tube defects (NTDs) include conditions such as anencephaly and **spina bifida** with or without a **meningocele**, most of which occur from failure of closure of the caudal neuropore between 22 and 30 days of pregnancy. This leaves the spinal cord unprotected by the spinal column. α-Fetoprotein (AFP) is a fetal protein found in small amounts in maternal serum in normal pregnancies. Any open fetal defect leads to the leaking of AFP into the amniotic fluid, with higher levels than usual entering maternal serum. Higher levels of AFP occur if the gestational age is over-assessed or if more than one fetus is present.

The routine use of ultrasound at booking, then a further anomaly scan, identifies most of these defects so the parents can make a choice between continuing the pregnancy or termination (Devane & Devane 2000). The cause may involve both genetic and environmental triggers. A dietary factor was suspected for a long time and **folic acid** was implicated as early as 1964 (Wald 1991).

The Medical Research Council (MRC) Vitamin Study Group (1991) undertook a multicentred, double-blind, randomised trial across 33 centres in seven countries to see if supplementation with folic acid or a mixture of seven other vitamins around the time of conception could prevent NTDs. The findings were that folic acid supplements prevented three-quarters of the cases of NTD recurrence.

Folic acid is used in the metabolic chain to provide the chemical bases of three of the essential **DNA components**: guanine, adenine and thymine. Vitamin B_{12} is necessary to form an enzyme in the metabolic pathway of folate. Women who are epileptic tend to have more congenital abnormalities, in part due to the antiepileptic medication altering the absorption of folate (Steegers-Theunissen 1995).

Following the findings of the above study the Department of Health (1992) recommended the use of 4 mg of folic acid 3 months prior to conception continued until the early months of pregnancy. However, those women at risk, under-nourished, of low economic status and those with unplanned pregnancies would be unlikely to supplement diet with folic acid (Eichholzer 2006). Some foods such as cereals are fortified in the UK; however, fortification in USA and Canada of flour and cereals since 1998 has proven the benefits with no evidence of risk. Despite the RCOG recommendations to fortify bread flour in the UK this has not yet been agreed (Food Standards Agency 2008, RCOG 2008).

Diagnosis may be made in the first trimester of pregnancy by chorionic villus sampling. Molecular technology in the future may be able to diagnose SCD with a few fetal cells from maternal blood (Frenette & Atweh 2007).

Incidence

The incidence of SCD varies from country to country and is about 1 in 4 in parts of Africa and 1 in 10 of the black population of the USA and UK. It is estimated that 50 000 Americans have SCD. Amongst African-Americans 1:375 have HbSS, 1:832 have HbSC and 1:1667 have Hb β-thalassaemia (Sickle Cell Society 2008). Heterozygote incidence ranges from 0.9% in Europe to 13.3% in Africa. The incidence of SCD in the UK is 1 in 2400 live births and is the 'fastest growing genetic disorder' (Sickle Cell Society 2008). Other variants of the disease are being found and crossing racial and ethnic groups so it is no longer appropriate to assume that a particular group will have SCD. Routine screening is already taking place both antenatally and in the newborn (Anglin 2007a, Zack-Williams 2007).

Pathophysiology

Deoxygenation is the most common cause of **sickling**; HbSS reacts by creating non-pliable intracellular fibres which pull the cells into a banana shape or holly leaf shape. These block capillaries, creating the pain of a sickle cell crisis (Bailey & Gwinnutt 2008). Decreased plasma volume, hypothermia, infection and acidosis also precipitate sickling. This will occur with minor degrees of oxygen shortage in people with sickle cell disease, but lack of oxygen has to be severe to cause sickling in people with sickle cell trait.

Vascular occlusion occurs anywhere, but especially in the kidney and brain. In pregnancy the placental bed may be affected. Pain is severe and death of tissues may occur within affected organs. Sickled cells are haemolysed in the spleen, resulting in anaemia. Sickling is not permanent and most of the red cells regain their normal shape after reoxygenation and rehydration. The extent and clinical manifestations of sickling will depend on the percentage of haemoglobin that is HbS. This is why it is rare for a heterozygous person to suffer much sickling (McCance & Huether 2002).

Pregnancy outcomes

In general, women with sickle cell trait have uncomplicated pregnancies, whereas sickle cell-positive women may have complications. A US study compared HbSS and HbSC women with a group of women with normal haemoglobin. The HbSS and HbSC women were at

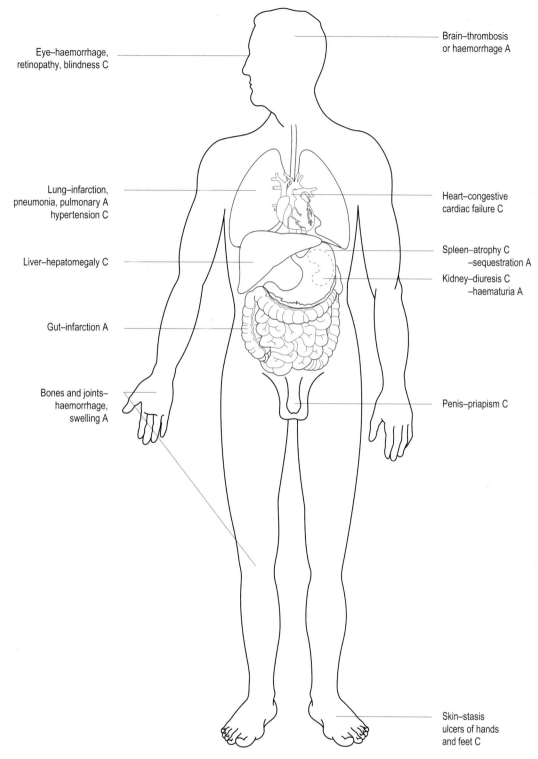

Eye–haemorrhage,
retinopathy, blindness C

Brain–thrombosis
or haemorrhage A

Lung–infarction,
pneumonia, pulmonary A
hypertension C

Heart–congestive
cardiac failure C

Liver–hepatomegaly C

Spleen–atrophy C
      –sequestration A

Kidney–diuresis C
      –haematuria A

Gut–infarction A

Bones and joints–
haemorrhage,
swelling A

Penis–priapism C

Skin–stasis
ulcers of hands
and feet C

Figure 33.1 • Major clinical manifestations of sickle cell anaemia. A, acute; C, chronic.

increased risk of fetal growth restriction, antenatal admissions, preterm labour and postpartum infections, although women with HbSS had more complications (Sun et al 2001). An English study of 81 pregnancies in several centres observed that there were 46.2% sickling crises in the antenatal period and 7.7% postnatal sickling episodes. These women were more likely to have anaemia, proteinuric hypertension and low-birth-weight babies. Prophylactic blood transfusion was used to prevent problems but there was no significance in

Table 33.2 Common variants of haemoglobin in sickle cell disease

Haemoglobin	Disease
HbSS	Homozygous sickle cell disease (sickle cell anaemia)
HbSC	Heterozygous sickle cell disease (sickle cell C disease), mild anaemia, and fewer crises, risk of retinal damage and thromboembolic problems in pregnancy
HbCC	Homozygous CC disease (not a sickling disorder)
HbS β-thalassaemia	Sickle β-thalassaemia, generally produces sickle Hb
HbAS	Sickle cell trait, generally no problems

preventing complications when compared with the untransfused women (Sickle Cell Society 2008).

Principles of treatment in pregnancy

- Anaemia may be prevented by prophylactic use of folic acid and iron.
- Blood transfusion may be necessary if Hb is extremely low.
- Avoidance of infection.
- Avoidance of cold and stress.
- In labour keep hydrated and prevent acidosis by intravenous therapy; use prophylactic antibiotics; oxygen may be necessary; this will prevent crisis.
- If crisis occurs, give pain relief; this may be the first sign of sickling.

Anyone with sickle cell disease needs specialised care by both the haematologist and the obstetrician with back-up from laboratory and a sickle cell centre (Bewley 2004). Treatment may include a blood transfusion every 6 weeks to maintain a high proportion of normal haemoglobin or it may be necessary to carry out an exchange transfusion (Boyle 2002).

Thalassaemia

Incidence

The incidence of the thalassaemias is high among Cypriots in which the carrier state is 15–20%. In Thailand, β-thalassaemia is common and children suffer severe ill-health due to the interactions of different thalassaemias. α-Thalassaemia causes severe health problems in parts of China, Cambodia and Vietnam. In the UK, each new wave of immigration may lead to increased incidence of inherited disorders and screening is essential (Anglin 2007b).

Pathophysiology

Thalassaemia is caused by a reduced rate of synthesis of either α-globin chains or β-globin chains. The heterozygote (**thalassaemia minor**) with one normal haemoglobin gene is generally asymptomatic but with reduced haemoglobin levels. The red cells are thin, and misshapen and short-lived (Bewley 2004). The homozygous condition (**thalassaemia major**) is life-threatening and if untreated leads to death in childhood. Homozygotes have severe anaemia which requires regular blood transfusions, but not replacement iron as stores are overloaded due to rapid breakdown of the short-lived red cells.

The thalassaemias can be categorised as (UK Thalassaemia Society 2008):

1. α^+-Thalassaemia with low production of α-globin chains due to one defective gene.

2. α^0-Thalassaemia, where neither gene is producing α-globin chains. Tetramers of β-chains and δ-chains are produced. β_4 (HbH) and δ_4 (Hb Bart's) are formed but the absence of α-globin chains means that oxygen cannot be released and the condition is incompatible with life.

3. β^+-Thalassaemia intermedia with low production of β-globin chains, due to one defective gene.

4. β-Thalassaemia major, where neither gene is producing β-globin chains. There is production of HbF and α-globin chains. The affected red cells are destroyed by the immune system, leading to ineffective erythropoiesis.

Clinical signs and symptoms

β-Thalassaemia is much more common than α-thalassaemia and in the carrier state leads to mild **microcytic hypochromic anaemia** and hyperplasia of bone marrow due to increased haemopoiesis. Haemolysis of immature erythrocytes may cause a slight rise in serum iron. The spleen may be enlarged because of the increased haemolysis.

Homozygotes have severe anaemia and HbF levels are always raised. Bone growth may be stunted in young children due to the hyperplasia. Regular blood transfusions shut off the bone marrow overgrowth. The accumulation of iron may result in death from damage to heart muscle, liver and pancreas. Blood transfusions can increase the life span by up to 20 years (UK Thalassaemia Society 2008). People who inherit the α-thalassaemia trait are usually symptom-free with a milder anaemia than seen in β-thalassaemia trait. However, homozygous α-thalassaemia leads to intrauterine congestive cardiac failure and **hydrops fetalis** with intrauterine death (Letsky 1995, UK Thalassaemia Society 2008).

Treatment

Heterozygotes seldom need treatment but the treatment for homozygous β-thalassaemia is only partially successful. It involves:

* Blood transfusions to top up the haemoglobin and haematocrit levels.
* Iron chelation therapy with an agent such as desferrioxamine to allow the excess iron to be excreted from the body (BNF 2007).
* Splenectomy to reduce the amount of haemolysis.
* Monitoring of hepatic iron and ferritin levels, which is essential.

Care in pregnancy

Anyone with thalassaemia trait is likely to develop anaemia that is similar to iron deficiency with microcytic cells. However, iron deficiency is not usually a problem as the reduced number of red cells and mild haemolysis ensure that iron is available; folic acid supplementation is advised.

Girls with homozygous β-thalassaemia die in childhood but treatment increases the likelihood of them living long enough to become pregnant. They need care, shared between the haematologist and obstetrician, preferably in a specialised centre (Bewley 2004).

Optimizing care in childhood will prevent infertility, as the pituitary and hypothalamus are prone to damage because of high iron levels. There are risks for the mother with an increase in cardiac disease and pre-existing diabetes. The fetus is more likely to inherit Hb disorders, with an increase of birth anomalies, pre-term birth and growth restriction.

Glucose-6-phosphate dehydrogenase deficiency

Glucose-6-phosphate dehydrogenase (G6PD) deficiency is the most common X-linked enzyme deficiency found in people of African, Asian and Mediterranean origin. It is more common in males, only manifesting itself when both X chromosomes are affected. The enzyme protects the haemoglobin molecules from oxidation and certain drugs precipitate haemolytic crises, such as antimalarial preparations, sulphonamides, some antibiotics such as nitrofurantoin, nalidixic acid, chloramphenicol and hydralazine (BNF 2007, Carter & Gross 2008). A gene frequency of 11% has been found in the American Black male population (McCance & Huether 2002). Neonates who inherit the gene may have prolonged jaundice.

Thromboembolism and pregnancy

Thrombosis in childbearing women is serious because of its association with deep vein thrombosis and pulmonary embolism, which remains the most common cause of maternal death, 30 direct deaths in 2000–2002 being recorded, mainly in those women with predisposing factors such as obesity and thrombophilia (Drife 2005). Thromboembolic diseases are much more likely to occur in the puerperium as the diuresis which occurs in the first 24h following delivery changes the blood viscosity. This becomes significant now that the rate of operative deliveries is rising. Thrombosis can be divided clinically into superficial **thrombophlebitis** and **deep vein thrombosis** (DVT).

Superficial thrombophlebitis

The superficial veins of the legs are affected. The vein is tender and may be reddened and hard. It is usually a varicose vein that is affected and there is no risk of pulmonary embolism unless there is a concomitant deep vein thrombosis. Women who are at risk tend to be older, overweight and of high parity. The use of supportive tights and TEDS (thromboembolic deterrent stockings) assists in the treatment of this condition. The woman should elevate her legs when resting but there is no need to restrict movement and anticoagulant therapy is not necessary.

Deep vein thrombosis

The deep veins of the calf, thigh or pelvis are usually affected, particularly on the left side. If there is no accompanying inflammation (**phlebitis**) and the blood clot (thrombus) does not obstruct the blood vessel, there may be no clinical signs. If the clot is friable and pieces become detached from the vessel wall, they will travel around the circulation (**embolus**), through the heart and into the pulmonary circulation, leading to a **pulmonary embolism**. This may be fatal, but recovery could be complete (Bewley & Bradshaw 2001).

Factors associated with pregnancy predisposing women to thromboembolism

* Caesarean section.
* Age over 30 years; high parity.
* Weight over 80kg.
* Family history or personal history of DVT.
* Thrombophilias; deficiency of antithrombin, protein C and protein S; antiphospholipid syndrome; factor V Leiden mutations.
* Smoking.
* Immobility, from paralysis or medical problems; admission to intensive care.
* Reduced plasma volume as in dehydration or pre-eclampsia.

Pathogenesis

During physiological adaptation to pregnancy some clotting factors are altered to prevent detrimental blood loss at delivery: von Willebrand factor, factors X, VIII and V and fibrinogen are increased. There is impaired fibrinolysis and the placenta produces plasminogen 1 and 2 activator inhibitors which prevent clotting at the placental bed (Brenner 2004). In a 30-year population study, it was found that women appeared to be more vulnerable in the postnatal period and although the incidence of pulmonary embolism had increased DVT had not (Heit et al 2006). The triad of factors described by Virchow of hypercoagulability, vascular damage and venous stasis which predispose to thrombosis exist in pregnancy (Auter 1996).

Prevention of thrombosis

Exercise encourages the return of blood to the heart and helps to prevent stasis. Any treatment which immobilises women increases their risk of DVT, whether antenatally, intrapartum or postnatally. High-risk women with previous thrombosis may be given prophylactic treatment antenatally and postnatally with low-molecular-weight heparin (LMWH). Oral warfarin may be prescribed to continue for 6 weeks following birth and is safe to use in breastfeeding, as is heparin (RCOG 1995). Some women could be treated with low-dose aspirin as a preventative measure (De Swiet 1999). The side-effects of heparin and warfarin include osteoporosis and embryopathy, respectively. A systematic review of LMWH for prevention and treatment of DVT found it to be effective (Greer & Nelson-Piercy 2005).

Diagnosis

DVT is most common in the first few days after delivery. The woman may complain of pain or discomfort in the leg, which is increased when the foot is dorsiflexed (**Homan's sign**). The affected leg may be swollen and measures 2–3 cm more than the unaffected leg, more common on the left. There may be a slight rise in systemic temperature. Diagnosis on clinical signs alone is difficult and there may be up to 50% error in diagnosing DVT of the lower extremity. Diagnosis is made by **Doppler** ultrasound. In 80% of pregnant women the thrombosis starts in the iliac and femoral veins and can be diagnosed by non-invasive methods such as ultrasound (Bothamley 2002, RCOG 2001). Blood estimation of **D-dimers** (fibrin degradation products) may be made but results are inaccurate antenatally and of no value postnatally.

Treatment

Intravenous heparin will be commenced and may be followed by oral warfarin, especially if the woman has delivered her baby. The danger of haemorrhage and haematoma formation should be kept in mind. The effects of warfarin can be monitored by serial estimation of blood prothrombin time.

Pulmonary embolism

Diagnosis and treatment

Chest pain, dyspnoea, cyanosis and hypotension are suggestive of pulmonary embolism and require action immediately. Oxygen may be given with intravenous (IV) heparin. The woman's physiological response depends on the size of the clot or clots. If she collapses and has a cardiac arrest a major embolic event has taken place and is life-threatening. Resuscitation should continue as this may disperse the clot and IV heparin given (Bothamley 2002, de Swiet 1995). Subsequent treatment should centre on positive diagnosis and immediate dissolution of the clot with streptokinase, urokinase or plasminogen activator. Anticoagulation over several months is necessary (Bothamley 2002).

Consumptive coagulopathies during pregnancy

Disseminated intravascular coagulation

Disseminated intravascular coagulation (DIC) is always secondary to some other occurrence: for example, abruptio placentae, postpartum haemorrhage, pre-eclampsia, a dead fetus or sepsis. Local activation of the clotting system releases thromboplastin into the circulation, leading to intravascular formation of fibrin. **Microthrombi** are released into the circulation, occlude blood vessels and may lead to **multiple organ failure** (Levi et al 2005). Consumption and reduction of clotting factors and platelets lead to severe bleeding. **Fibrinolysis** stimulated by DIC results in the formation of **fibrin degradation products** (FDPs). These interfere with the formation of firm fibrin clots and a vicious circle is established increasing the blood loss. FDPs are also thought to interfere with myometrial contraction and cardiac function (Letsky 1995).

Diagnosis

Clinical condition and laboratory tests will accurately diagnose DIC, such as the observation of the loss of blood from an IV site or the nose or the presence of **haematuria** (Crafter 2002). In laboratory tests (Levi et al 2005), the following tests will all deviate from normal:

- Platelet count.
- Clotting times (in series).
- Levels of antithrombin III.
- Fibrin degradation products.

Treatment

The replacement of blood cells and clotting factors is a priority, but treating the underlying disorder may in itself resolve DIC. A transfusion of fresh frozen plasma or plasma substitutes such as dextran and platelet concentrates will assist in preventing bleeding. Whole blood is not usually given but stored blood components are given separately (Letsky 1995).

Idiopathic thrombocytopenia

Idiopathic thrombocytopenia (ITP) is a disorder that is characterised by an autoimmune destruction of maternal and fetal platelets. Typical sufferers are women aged between 18 and 40 years; it is usually asymptomatic, but sufferers may report that they bruise easily and bleed excessively. Normal platelet levels are $150\,000–400\,000\,mm^3$. There may be an increased rate of miscarriage. Incidence is low in pregnancy (1:1000 to 1:10000) and may be associated with pre-eclampsia or HELLP syndrome.

Maternal platelets fall in pregnancy but ITP would be suspected if the count is $<5000\,mm^3$; the condition is diagnosed following a full blood count. In pregnancy, the aim is to maintain a platelet level $>100\,000\,mm^3$ by administering corticosteroids. It is important that the anaesthetist is happy with the level of platelets prior to epidural administration. Intravenous γ-globulin may be used to suppress **antiplatelet antibodies**. **Neonatal thrombocytopenia** is due to transplacental passage of antiplatelet antibodies, which may cause neonatal haemorrhage (Cines & Bussel 2005, Parnas et al 2006).

Main points

- Iron-deficiency anaemia (IDA), folic acid deficiency, hereditary haemoglobinopathies and anaemia due to blood loss are associated with pregnancy. Anaemia is reduction in the oxygen-carrying capacity of the blood, which may be due to a reduced number of red blood cells, a low concentration of haemoglobin (Hb) or a combination of both.
- Folic acid deficiency or vitamin B_{12} deficiency in pregnancy can lead to megaloblastic anaemia. Folic acid deficiency responds to folic acid supplementation.
- The Department of Health (1992) recommended the use of 4 mg of folic acid 3 months prior to conception, continued until the early months of pregnancy to prevent neural tube defects (NTDs).
- Sickle cell disease is the most common of the structural haemoglobin variants. A single amino acid substitution of **valine** for **glutamic acid** results in a haemoglobin molecule that is less soluble.
- In sickle cell disease, when oxygen availability is low, the red cells are distorted into a sickle shape and cannot pass through the capillaries. Vascular occlusion occurs, especially in the kidney and brain.
- Fetal blood can be tested for abnormal haemoglobin genes by cordocentesis. Chorionic villus sampling may also be used for DNA analysis. Cord blood may be taken at birth for screening purposes.
- β-Thalassaemia is much more common than α-thalassaemia and in the carrier state leads to mild microcytic hypochromic anaemia and hyperplasia of bone marrow. Homozygous people have severe anaemia and death from cardiac failure, which is common in untreated people. Blood transfusions can increase the life span by up to 20 years.
- Pregnant women with homozygous β-thalassaemia need specialised care shared between the haematologist and obstetrician. Treatment may include repeated blood transfusions and folic acid supplementation. Prenatal diagnosis and genetic counselling should be available to couples susceptible to having an affected child.
- Glucose-6-phosphate dehydrogenase (G6PD) deficiency is a rare X-linked enzyme deficiency. It affects women of African, Asian and Mediterranean origin. Certain drugs precipitate haemolytic crises. Neonates may have prolonged jaundice if they carry this gene.
- Thrombosis in childbearing women is serious because of its association with deep vein thrombosis (DVT) and pulmonary embolism (PE), which remains the most common cause of maternal death.
- In DVT the deep veins of the calf, thigh or pelvis are affected. If the clot is friable and pieces become detached from the vessel wall, they will travel around the circulation (**embolus**), through the heart and into the pulmonary circulation, leading to a **pulmonary embolism**. Women with an inherited thrombophilia are at increased risk of developing a DVT in pregnancy.
- Exercise encourages the return of blood to the heart and helps to prevent stasis. Any treatment which immobilises women will increase their risk of DVT.
- Massive release of thromboplastin into the circulation leads to intravascular formation of microthrombi with consumption of clotting factors and platelets and severe bleeding leading to organ failure. Fibrinolysis is stimulated by DIC. Replacement of blood cells and clotting factors is a priority.
- Idiopathic thrombocytopenia (ITP) is an autoimmune disease with destruction of platelets. It is usually asymptomatic but there may be easy bruising and excessive bleeding from the gastrointestinal and urinary tracts. Intracranial haemorrhage may be a complication.

References

Anglin, S., 2007a. Sickle cell and thalassaemia: screening for all. Pract. Midwife 10 (4), 22–24.

Anglin, S., 2007b. Sickle cell and thalassaemia screening early care. Pract. Midwife 10 (9), 22–25.

Auter, R., 1996. Deep Vein Thrombosis: The silent killer. Quay Books, Dinton.

Bailey, K., Gwinnutt, C., 2008. The physiology of red blood cells and haemoglobin variants. Website: <http://www.frca.co.uk/printriendly.aspx?articleid=100796/>.

Bewley, C., 2004. Medical disorders in pregnancy, Ch. 46. In: Henderson, C., Macdonald, S. (Eds.), Mayes Midwifery: A Textbook for Midwives. Baillière Tindall, Edinburgh, p. 793.

Bewley, C., Bradshaw, C., 2001. Thromboembolic disorders during pregnancy, birth and the puerperium. MIDIRS Midwifery Dig. 11 (11), 56–59.

Blackburn, S.T., 2007. Haematological and Homeostatic Systems, third edn. W B Saunders, Philadelphia Ch. 5.

BNF (British National Formulary), 2007. Nutr. Blood 4, 480, 487, 489.

Bothamley, J., 2002. Thromboembolism in pregnancy, Ch. 3. In: Boyle, M. (Ed.), Emergencies Around Childbirth. Radcliffe Medical Press, Oxford.

Boyle, M., 2002. Other causes of potential maternal collapse. In: Boyle, M. (Ed.), Emergencies Around Childbirth. Radcliffe Medical Press, Oxford.

Brenner, B., 2004. Haemostatic changes in pregnancy. Thrombosis Research 114 (5–6), 409–414.

Breymann, C., 2005. Iron deficiency anaemia in pregnancy: modern aspects of diagnosis and therapy. Eur. J. Obstet. Gynecol. Reprod. Biol. 123, S3–S13.

Carter, S. M., Gross, S. J., 2008. Glucose-6-phosphate dehydrogenase deficiency. <http://emedicine.medscape.com/article200390-overview/>.

Cines, D., Bussel, J., 2005. How I treat idiopathic thrombocytopenia purpura (ITP). Blood 106 (7), 2244–2251.

Coggins, J., 2001. Iron deficiency anaemia: a complication of pregnancy or a foregone conclusion? MIDIRS Midwifery Dig. 11 (4), 469–474.

Conrad, M.E., 2008. Iron deficiency anaemia. Website: <http://www.emedicine.com/med/topic118.htm/>.

Crafter, H., 2002. Intrapartum and primary postpartum haemorrhage. In: Boyle, M. (Ed.), Emergencies Around Childbirth. Radcliffe Medical Press, Oxford.

Cuervo, L., Mahomed, K., 2003. Treatments for iron deficiency anaemia in pregnancy. Cochrane Database Syst. Rev. (1) Update Software, Oxford.

Department of Health, 1992. Report from an Expert Maternity Group: Folic acid and the prevention of neural tube defects. Health Publications Unit, Lancashire.

De Swiet, M., 1995. Thromboembolism. In: de Swiet, M. (Ed.), Medical Disorders in Obstetric Practice, third edn. Blackwell Science, Oxford.

De Swiet, M., 1999. Thromboembolic disease. In: James, D., Steer, P., Weiner, C., Gonik, B. (Eds.) High Risk Pregnancy. W B Saunders, London.

Devane, D., Devane, M., 2000. Termination for fetal defects? The debate must go on. Br. J. Midwifery 8 (8), 475–479.

Drife, J., 2005. Why Mothers Die. Online: <http://rcpe.ac.uk/publications/articles/journal_35_4/why%20mothers%20die.pdf/>.

Eichholzer, M., Tonz, O., Zimmermann, R., 2006. Folic acid: a public health challenge. Lancet 367 (9519), 1352–1361.

Food Standards Agency, 2008 Folic acid fortification. Website: <http://food.gov.uk/healthiereating/folicfortification/>; accessed July 2008.

Frenette, P., Atweh, G., 2007. Sickle cell disease: old discoveries, new concepts, and future promise. J. Clin. Invest. 117 (4), 850–858.

Godfrey, K., Barker, J., 1995. Maternal nutrition in relation to fetal and placental growth. Eur. J. Obstet. Gynecol. Reprod. Biol. 61, 15–22.

Godfrey, K.M., Redman, C.W.G., Barker, D.J.P., et al., 1991. The effect of maternal anaemia and iron deficiency on the ratio of fetal weight to placental weight. Br. J. Obstet. Gynaecol. 98, 886–891.

Greer, I., Nelson-Piercy, C., 2005. Low molecular weight heparin for the thromboprophylaxis and treatment of venous thromboembolism in pregnancy: a systematic review of the safety and efficacy. Blood 106 (2), 401–407.

Heit, J., Kobbervig, C., James, A., Petterson, T., Bailey, K., Melton, L., 2006. Trends in the incidence of venous thromboembolism during pregnancy or postpartum: a 30 year population-based study. Obstet. Gynecol. Surv. 61 (4), 220–221.

Letsky, E., 1995. Blood volume, haematinics and anaemia. In: de Swiet, M. (Ed.), Medical Disorders in Obstetric Practice, third edn. Blackwell Science, Oxford.

Levi, M., 2005. Disseminated intravascular coagulation. What's new? Crit. Care Clin. Haematol. Issues Crit. Illn. 21 (3), 449–467.

McCance, K.L., Huether, S.E., 2002. Pathophysiology: The Biologic Basis for Disease in Adults and Children, fourth edn. Mosby Year Book, Chicago.

Milman, N., 2006. Iron and pregnancy a delicate balance. Ann. Haematol. 85 (9), 559–565.

Milman, N., Byg, K.E., Bergholt, T., Eriksen, L., 2006. Side effects of oral iron prophylaxis in pregnancy—myth or reality? Acta Haematol. 115 (1–2), 53–57.

MRC Vitamin Study Group, 1991. Prevention of neural tube defects. Lancet 238, 131–137.

Müngen, E., 2003. Iron supplementation in pregnancy. J. Perinat. Med. 31 (5), 420–426.

Parnas, M., Shiner, E., Shoham-Vardi, E., Burstein, T., Yermiahu, I., et al., 2006. Moderate to severe thrombocytopenia during pregnancy. Eur. J. Obstet. Gynecol. Reprod. Biol. 128 (1–2), 163–168.

RCOG, 1995. Report of the RCOG Working Party on Prophylaxis Against Thromboembolism in Gynaecology and Obstetrics. Royal College of Obstetricians and Gynaecologists Press, London.

RCOG, 2001. Thromboembolic Disease in Pregnancy and the Puerperium: Acute Management. Guideline 28. Royal College of Obstetricians and Gynaecologists Press, London.

RCOG, 2007. Green Top Guideline, Number 47. Royal College of Obstetricians and Gynaecologists Press, London.

RCOG, 2008. Periconceptual folic acid and food fortification in the prevention of neural tube defects. Website: <http://www.rcog.org.uk/index.asp?pageID=541/>; accessed July 2008.

Sickle Cell Society, 2008. Standards for the Clinical Care of Adults with Sickle Cell Disease in the UK. <http://www.sicklecellsociety.org/pdf/CareBook.pdf/>.

Steegers-Theunissen, R., 1995. Folate metabolism and neural tube defects: a review. Eur. J. Obstet. Gynecol. Reprod. Biol. 61, 39–48.

Stephen, J., Cunningham, J., 1998. Understanding fetal haemoglobin gene expression: a step towards effective HbF reactivation in haemoglobinopathies. Br. J. Haematol. 102, 415–422.

Sun, P., Wilburn, W., Raynor, B., Jamieson, D., 2001. Sickle cell disease in pregnancy: twenty years of experience at Grady Memorial Hospital, Atlanta, Georgia. Am. J. Obstet. Gynecol. 184 (6), 1127–1130.

Tsunenobu, T., Picciano, M.F., 2006. Folate and human reproduction. Am. J. Clin. Nutr. 83 (5), 993–1016 Online: <http://www.Ajon.org/cgi/content/full/83/5/993#top/>; accessed August 2008.

UK Thalassaemia Society, 2008. Standards for the Clinical Care of Children and Adults with Thalassaemia in the UK (2005). <www.ukts.org/>, accessed August 2008.

Wald, N., 1991. Prevention of neural tube defects: results of the Medical Research Council Vitamin Study. Report of the MRC Vitamin Study Research Group. Lancet 338 (8760), 131–137.

Walraven, G., 2008. Treatments for iron deficiency anaemia in pregnancy. The WHO Reproductive Library on line: <http://www.who.int.rhl./pregnancy_childbirth/medical/anaemia/gw/>.

Weatherall, D., 1997a. Fortnightly review: the thalassaemias. Br. Med. J. 314 (7095), 1675–1678.

Weatherall, D., 1997b. ABC of clinical haematology: the hereditary anaemias. Br. Med. J. 314 (7079), 492–496.

WHO, 2008. Treatments for iron-deficiency anaemia in pregnancy. World Health Organization, Geneva. <www.who.int/rhl/pregnancy_childbirth/medical/anaemia/gw/>; accessed July 2008.

Zack-Williams, D., 2007. Sickle cell anaemia in pregnancy and the neonates: ethical issues. Br. J. Midwifery 15 (4), 205–209.

Annotated recommended reading

Frenette, P., Atweh, G., 2007. Sickle cell disease: old discoveries, new concepts, and future promise. J. Clin. Invest. 117 (4), 850–858.

A very readable text with excellent pathophysiology, and advances in treatment and diagnosis.

Godfrey, K., Barker, J., 1995. Maternal nutrition in relation to fetal and placental growth. Eur. J. Obstet. Gynecol. Reprod. Biol. 61, 15–22.

This paper provides a basis for the understanding of the Barker hypothesis.

Levi, M., 2005. Disseminated intravascular coagulation. What's new? Crit. Care Clin. Haematol. Issu. Crit. Illn. 21 (3), 449–467.

This paper is well worth reading. It provides an in-depth account of DIC and its management.

Tsunenobu, T., Picciano, M.F., 2006. Folate and human reproduction. Am. J. Clin. Nutr. 83 (5), 993–1016 Online: <http://www.ajon.org/cgi/content/full/83/5/993#top/>; accessed August 2008.

A very detailed account of folate in pregnancy with excellent historical background to folic acid supplementation; slightly heavy reading for the student but well worth it for the information acquired.

Chapter Thirty-Four

34

Respiratory, renal, gastrointestinal and neurological problems

Respiratory tract problems

Asthma

Asthma is the most common respiratory problem found in pregnancy, with an incidence of between 0.4% and 1.3% (Liu et al 2001), although de Swiet (1995) quoted 5%. Asthma is an inflammatory disease with **hyper-responsiveness** of the airways characterised by constriction of the smooth muscle in the bronchioles, hypersecretion of mucus and mucosal oedema (McCance & Huether 2002). The work of breathing is increased and excessive negative intrapleural pressures can increase the demands on the right ventricle. There is a rise in pulmonary arterial pressure and a decrease in arterial systolic pressure and pulse pressure.

Aetiology

Asthma is a complex disorder, involving biochemical, autonomic nervous system, immunological, endocrine and psychological factors which differ from person to person. Airway inflammation is present even when the person is symptom-free. There is a familial incidence and environmental factors such as dust, pollens, moulds, animal dandruff and foods interact with inherited factors to cause **bronchospasm**. About half of sufferers develop asthma in childhood and another third before age 40. Complete remission is quite common in children but less so in adults, in whom symptomatic episodes tend to occur more frequently (Liu et al 2001).

Pathophysiology

Respiratory rate is not changed by pregnancy; progesterone increases hyperventilation by term. The effects of the gravid uterus on the diaphragm cause a decrease in expiratory and residual volumes and this may cause some problems for the woman who is pregnant and asthmatic (Blackburn 2007). **Bronchoconstriction** occurs after exposure to an allergen and causes immunoglobulin E (IgE) antigen to bind to mast cell surface receptors. These release inflammatory substances such as **histamine**, **bradykinin**, **prostaglandins** and **thromboxane** A_2 and **chemotactic factors** which attract eosinophils, neutrophils, T lymphocytes and platelets. Eosinophils produce a protein that stops epithelial cell cilia from beating, disrupts mucosal integrity and causes damage and sloughing of epithelial cells.

Asthma in pregnancy

During pregnancy some asthmatic women improve, some deteriorate and some experience no change in lung function. It is difficult to predict events, so close monitoring and ensuring compliance with treatment is essential. Pregnancy is a state of slight immunosuppression so the asthmatic may be slightly more prone to chest infections, depending on the season; it is less likely in the summer months (Ie et al 2002). Women with asthma may have more complications in pregnancy such as preterm birth and small-for-gestational-age babies particularly if asthma attacks increase, typically in the second trimester, and if there is non-compliance with medication (Murphy et al 2006). Other researchers suggest there are few complications but more caesarean sections in the moderate to severe asthmatic (Dombrowski et al 2004).

Treatment considerations

Asthma requires long-term administration of **bronchodilators** and **anti-inflammatory agents** and the effect of these on early fetal development must be considered. Women sometimes decrease their medication for fear of harming their babies to the detriment of treating their asthma. They must be encouraged to recognise the early symptoms of an attack to avoid hypoxia. Up to 15% of pregnant asthmatic women require hospitalisation for **status asthmaticus** or recurrent asthmatic episodes (Blackburn 2007). Anxiety exacerbates asthma attacks but sedative drugs are contraindicated, as these may cause respiratory depression.

Normal inhalation medications may continue, with regular examination of peak flow levels (Beckmann 2006). **Aminophylline** is safe in pregnancy and may be used in acute-to-severe asthma attacks to aid breathing, and **oral steroids** may be used to treat repeated asthma attacks. Medications in labour that cause vasoconstriction such as prostaglandin $F_{2\alpha}$ and ergometrine should not be used. Syntocinon (oxytocin) should be used for the third stage of labour (de Swiet 1995).

Tuberculosis

The prevalence of **pulmonary tuberculosis** (TB) in some areas of London exceeds 50 per 100 000. It is a global health problem (Watson & Moss 2001, WHO 2008) and 50% of UK cases were born overseas. In a survey of asylum seekers screened at Heathrow Airport in 1995–99 the incidence was 241 per 100 000, with high rates from the Indian subcontinent and sub-Saharan Africa (Callister et al 2002).

Improvements in urban conditions during the 19th century decreased the incidence of TB. However, with the increase of travel and immigration, the incidence rose between 1986 and 1993, particularly in the more deprived areas of London. A retrospective review of incidence in pregnancy in one area in London showed that all women came from ethnic minority groups and 88% had only been in the country 2 years (Kothari et al 2006). The white population cases declined, with an increase in the ethnic groups, particularly black African and Chinese. Co-infection with the **human immunodeficiency virus** (HIV) occurred in 3.3% of the TB-infected population (Rose et al 2001).

Aetiology

The disease is caused by the bacillus *Mycobacterium tuberculosis*, a soil-living organism pathogenic to some animals such as cattle. It infects far more people than it causes to be ill and infected people have a 10% lifetime risk of developing TB. It may manifest as **pulmonary** or **extrapulmonary** TB. Pulmonary TB with infected sputum is more contagious. The causative organism is a slow-growing bacterium with a waxy outer coat that protects it from immune system attack. The body responds by forming **fibrinous tubercles** to contain the microbe. The bacillus can lie dormant for years (latent TB) inside macrophages; 10% of these people will develop active TB (Bothamley 2006).

TB exploits the vulnerable, with poverty, overcrowding, institutionalisation, the presence of other disease and immune suppression leading to an increase in active disease. It is highly contagious and all contacts with tuberculosis should be followed up and vaccinated (Joint Tuberculosis Committee of the British Thoracic Society 2000).

Signs and symptoms

Pregnancy increases the demands on the body systems, but general tiredness of pregnancy may be overlooked as a normal occurrence until other factors accumulate such as country of origin, length of time in the UK, co-existing infection such as HIV (Bothamley 2006). There is a rare possibility of transplacental fetal infection (Ormerod 2001). The woman's poor health may affect fetal growth adversely.

Symptoms of active TB can include: (Bothamley 2006):

- Night fever.
- Poor appetite.
- Weight loss.
- Tiredness.
- Persistent productive cough.
- Haemoptysis.

Management of tuberculosis

A chest physician should be involved in the woman's care. If there are clinical signs of TB or the woman has been in contact with active TB, a chest X-ray is performed with adequate protection of the fetus. Sputum specimens and pleural effusions may be cultured to confirm the presence of the bacillus. If the sputum contains the organism, the woman may need to be admitted to hospital but drug therapy is usually carried out at home. After 2 weeks of therapy there is no risk of infection to others (BNF 2007a).

Tuberculin skin tests are performed in the USA on those who have been at risk of TB and the family is investigated. The sole manufacturer of tuberculin in the UK has recently put in its data sheet that tuberculin testing should not be carried out in pregnancy but does not supply any data to support this recommendation. This has not been backed up by the Vaccination and Immunisation Committee (Ormerod 2001). However, BCG vaccination should not be performed in pregnancy as it is a live vaccine.

Treatment

A combination of drugs is used if diagnosis is made in pregnancy; the drugs that have been shown to be safe for the fetus are rifampicin, isoniazid, pyrazinamide and ethambutol (Bothamley 2001). This regimen should be adhered to in order to treat tuberculosis satisfactorily and breastfeeding can continue as normal (BNF 2007a). Liver function should be monitored as 'drug induced hepatitis may be more common in pregnancy' (Bothamley 2006). Intramuscular streptomycin is contraindicated in pregnancy because of the incidence of hearing loss in those neonates exposed to it in utero and is rarely used in the UK (BNF 2007a).

The baby

If the mother is on effective treatment and has negative sputum, there is no reason for the baby to be isolated from her. Staff will be protected by vaccination, which is a prerequisite before employment. If treatment commenced late in pregnancy and sputum is still positive, the baby will need prophylactic isoniazid and a **tuberculin test** should be performed at 6 weeks. If the mother has a multiple drug-resistant strain of TB, the infant will need to be separated from her. The mother would also need to be isolated and staff should use dust/mist/fume masks. TB drugs cross into breast milk but there is no contraindication to breastfeeding, except where the neonate is separated from its mother (Ormerod 2001).

Vaccination: BCG

The bacillus Calmette-Guérin (BCG), a live attenuated strain developed from cattle TB, is given by injection into the skin to stimulate an immune response. In babies, care must be taken to inject intradermally to prevent abscess formation. The vaccine is effective in the prevention of tuberculosis in children but of variable value when given to adults. It can reduce the incidence of pulmonary tuberculosis by up to 80% and minimises the risk of complications.

The effectiveness of BCG programmes remains controversial. In the USA, vaccination is thought to create difficulties in interpreting the results of any future use of the tuberculin test performed to establish whether a person is infected with TB. In the UK, BCG vaccination has been discontinued in children aged 10–14 years. Adults who have contact with someone suffering from active pulmonary tuberculosis should be tuberculin tested and given BCG if the test is negative. Babies in contact with active TB should be vaccinated without having a tuberculin test as their immune systems may be too immature to show a response. In the UK it is recommended that all immigrants from countries with a high incidence of TB are tested and BCG vaccination given to those with a negative result and that all babies born to recent immigrants are vaccinated (BNF 2007a). All neonates born in an area of high TB incidence and neonates of health care workers are offered BCG soon after birth (Joint Tuberculosis Committee 2000, Bothamley 2006).

Contraindications

Harmful effects of BCG are rare. However, ulcers and abscess formation may occur at the site of the vaccination, sometimes with swollen lymph glands and inflammation of the underlying bone. Healing of such an ulcer may be slow and result in a **keloid scar**. The vaccine should not be given to people who have leukaemia, cancer or acute illness (including TB) or to patients taking corticosteroids or immunosuppressant drugs. It is also contraindicated in those who are HIV-positive (Joint Tuberculosis Committee 2000).

Renal disorders

Acute pyelonephritis

Pregnant women are more susceptible to renal tract infections than other women and there is an incidence of unsuspected asymptomatic bacteriuria in 4–10% of them; if this is not diagnosed and treated, about 25% develop pyelonephritis. Ascending infection caused by perineal bacteria is the most common route and the most common causative organisms are Gram-negative bacilli such as *Escherichia coli*, *Klebsiella pneumoniae* and *Proteus mirabilis* with *Escherichia coli* present in at least 80% of cases. Some strains of *E. coli* have fimbriae that bind to specific receptors on the surface of epithelial cells, increasing their selection of the urinary tract and their virulence (Lindsay 2000).

Screening for asymptomatic bacteriuria

Women who have had previous episodes of asymptomatic bacteriuria or urinary tract infection should have a midstream specimen of urine cultured. If the presence of a specific bacterium exceeds 10^5 organisms/ml of urine (100 000 organisms/ml) asymptomatic bacteriuria is diagnosed. Appropriate antibiotics should be successful in treating the condition (Lindsay 2000).

Clinical implications of acute pyelonephritis

Fetal risks

* Intrauterine growth restriction, even with asymptomatic bacteriuria alone.
* Preterm labour is more common.
* There may be an associated risk of congenital abnormality.

Maternal risks

* Endotoxic shock.
* Chronic renal infection.
* Renal failure.

Signs and symptoms

Acute pyelonephritis occurs in 1–2% of pregnancies, usually in the second and third trimesters. It begins with the onset of malaise, fatigue, chills and back pain located in the upper lumbar region, accompanied by muscle guarding. The pain follows the path of the ureters and may radiate round to the suprapubic area. Some women complain of nausea, vomiting and uterine contractions. Affected women may have a temperature as high as 40°C with a corresponding increase in pulse rate. There may be dehydration and frequency of micturition with scalding on voiding. The urine appears cloudy and even bloodstained and on urinalysis red blood cells, leucocytes and casts may be present as well as bacteria (Bewley 2004).

Management

It is essential to treat acute pyelonephritis immediately to avoid serious side-effects. The woman may need to be admitted to hospital and the following treatment instigated:

* A midstream specimen of urine should be sent to the laboratory for culture and sensitivity tests.
* A blood specimen (for full blood count and electrolytes) is taken if the woman is obviously very ill.
* Intravenous fluids may be required to correct any dehydration.
* Antibiotic therapy should be commenced, intravenously if women are nauseated. Oral medication

may be commenced after 48 h. *E. coli* is becoming increasingly resistant to **ampicillin** and a combination of antibiotics may be prescribed until the sensitivity reports are returned.

* Pain relief may be necessary and an antiemetic to counteract nausea.
* Renal function should be assessed both during the acute illness and as a follow-up.
* Maternal observations of temperature, pulse and blood pressure should be recorded at least 4-hourly.
* Tachycardia and hypotension may indicate the development of endotoxic shock.
* Fetal observations are as important as maternal and the early onset of labour should be recognised.

Most women will respond to the combination of rehydration and antibiotics. In cases of persistent problems, there may be an abnormality of the renal tract and such women should be referred appropriately (Bewley 2004).

Acute renal failure

Diagnosis

The onset of acute renal failure (ARF) has occurred if the urine output falls below 400 ml in 24 h or to less than 20 ml/h. There is a reduced glomerular filtration rate (GFR) and a rise in blood urea and creatinine. Acute renal failure usually results from a severe deficit in cortical renal blood flow that results in ischaemia to the kidneys. Pregnancy conditions associated with ARF are shown in Table 34.1 (Thorsen & Poole 2002).

If cortical hypoperfusion is allowed to persist, **acute tubular necrosis** or **cortical necrosis** may follow. Renal cortical necrosis is a severe form of ARF that usually results from large, sudden blood loss or vascular collapse such as in severe pre-eclampsia or haemorrhage. There is sudden

Table 34.1 Pregnancy conditions associated with acute renal failure

Prerenal hypoperfusion	Hypotension and coagulopathy	Urinary tract obstruction
Haemorrhage	Abruptio placentae	Polyhydramnios
Spontaneous abortion	Pre-eclampsia	Damage to ureters
Hyperemesis gravidarum	Incompatible blood transfusion	Pelvic haematoma
Adrenocortical failure	Drug reaction Acute fatty liver of pregnancy Sepsis	Calculus or clot in ureter

onset of oliguria (less than 400 ml in 24 h) or anuria and a rise in serum creatinine (Thorsen & Poole 2002). Immediate treatment of ARF prevents necrosis occurring.

In a study of 72 pre-eclamptic women with renal failure, median gestation was 32 weeks and perinatal mortality was 38%. Twelve women had previous renal disease and only seven women required short-term dialysis. In the long term there was no need for dialysis or transplantation (Drakeley et al 2002). Those women with renal impairment had HELLP syndrome or abruptio placenta.

Management

The aims are to re-establish urinary output and treat the underlying condition. Blood is taken for estimation of urea, electrolytes and plasma proteins. Haematocrit and blood osmolality findings indicate the degree of dehydration. Blood culture and liver function tests help to identify a cause. Urine is tested for culture and sensitivity of organisms, protein estimation, specific gravity and osmolality. Maternal and fetal condition is monitored closely with assessment of fetal growth and delivery gauged to both maternal and fetal condition (Gammill & Jeyabalan 2005, Thorsen & Poole 2002).

Re-establishing kidney function: principles of treatment

Treatment is guided by laboratory tests of kidney function and blood biochemistry results and includes:

- Control of bleeding, stabilisation of raised blood pressure or sepsis.
- Intravascular volume expansion with packed red cells, fresh frozen plasma and crystalloid solutions, guided by intake and output measurement. Insertion of a Foley's catheter for accurate documentation of fluid out.
- Restrict fluid intake to the volume of fluid lost in the previous 24 h plus 500 ml to replace insensible fluid loss. If the woman is pyrexial, an extra 200 ml may be added.
- Dialysis if there is cardiovascular overload, **hyperkalaemia**, electrolyte imbalances, metabolic acidosis or **uraemia**.
- Diet should be low in potassium and chloride; 1500 calorie, protein-free, fat/carbohydrate diet (Thorsen & Poole 2002).

Chronic renal disease

A successful pregnancy for women with chronic renal disease depends on the degree of renal impairment. Physiologically the kidney GFR and renal plasma flow increase in pregnancy by approximately 50%; if this does not occur the woman's future health may be jeopardised even if the pregnancy were successful. Pregnancy increases the possibility of significant renal function loss

and women should be counselled regarding this before embarking on a pregnancy; those with serum creatinine levels >180 mol/L come into this category (Davison 2001). Women with chronic renal impairment presenting with poorly controlled hypertension, proteinuria, oedema and poor kidney function may not have successful pregnancies. They are prone to delivering preterm and producing 'small-for-dates' babies.

Pathophysiologically oedema is present because of loss of protein in the urine and electrolytes become imbalanced because kidney excretion of urine is low. Blood acid–base balance is compromised. Erythropoietin and red cell production are decreased and anaemia occurs. Renal tissue damage causes decreased blood supply which results in the production of excess renin which in turn increases blood pressure (Bewley 2004).

A history of prior kidney problems or associated medical conditions is common, causing kidney function to deteriorate (Bewley 2004). These include:

- Glomerulonephritis.
- Chronic pyelonephritis.
- Renal calculi.
- Polycystic kidney disease.
- Nephrotic syndrome >3 g/day, a serum albumin of <3 g/dl plus oedema.
- Diabetic nephropathy.
- Systemic lupus erythematosus.

Antenatal care and prognosis

The mother

Antenatal care should take place with a multidisciplinary team in a referral centre with specific facilities available if kidney failure does occur and dialysis necessary. Outcome is dependent on the degree of hypertension and kidney function and optimum care should prevent deterioration in the mother and the delivery of a healthy infant. Early recognition of urinary tract infection is essential.

The fetus

Regular antenatal visits will observe fetal growth and delivery will be dependent on fetal well-being. Fetal distress occurs both antenatally and in labour in pregnancies complicated by intrauterine growth restriction, and fetal mortality may occur because of poor placental blood flow, abruptio placentae or hypoxia.

Pregnancy following renal transplant

A renal transplant will immediately improve the woman's health, and it is estimated that 1:50 will become pregnant after transplantation. The outcomes of these pregnancies are variable: 30% fail before the second trimester, some will miscarry and some will have a therapeutic termination; 95% will succeed beyond the first trimester (Davison 2001). Outcome will vary but, the lower the dose of steroids, the better the function of the allograft and the longer the time since transplantation the better the outcome. Women with renal transplants tolerate pregnancy well but it is important to continue **immunosuppressive medication**. Most women are prescribed azathioprine as an immunosuppressor and prednisolone to prevent rejection of the transplanted kidney (Armenti et al 2002). There have been no reports of congenital malformations due to these drugs. Cyclosporine, a more potent immunosuppressant agent, has been linked to fetal growth restriction (Alston et al 2001). These women are more prone to infections because of these drugs, which may increase problems for the fetus. The more common complications are preterm labour, small-for-dates infant and pre-eclampsia, and two follow-up studies agreed that pregnancy was not a contraindication after transplant surgery in stable women (Kashanizadeh et al 2007, Keitel et al 2004).

Gastrointestinal problems

Vomiting in pregnancy

Slight nausea and vomiting may affect up to 80% of women in the first trimester (Ch. 30). Causes and management of moderate to severe vomiting are discussed below.

Causes of vomiting

Pregnant women may suffer from diseases causing vomiting not associated with pregnancy. These disorders, such as gastric ulceration or infection, must be ruled out before accepting that moderate to severe vomiting is due to the pregnancy alone. Vomiting is a reflex which occurs because of stimulation of two centres in the brain (Rang et al 2007). These are the **vomiting centre (VC)** in the medulla and the **chemoreceptor trigger zone (CTZ)**.

The VC controls smooth muscle movements in the stomach wall and the related skeletal muscle of the respiratory and abdominal muscles. The CTZ lies outside the blood–brain barrier and responds to circulating chemical stimuli from ingested drugs and endogenous toxins produced in uraemia and radiation sickness. This centre also produces motion sickness. Stimuli arising in the CTZ are passed to the VC, which then activates the relevant respiratory and gastrointestinal muscles, resulting in vomiting. Vomiting can be triggered by the factors outlined in Table 34.2.

Table 34.2 Causes of vomiting in pregnant women

Non-pregnancy causes	Causes due to pregnancy
Stimulation of the sensory nerve endings in the stomach and duodenum and of the vagal sensory endings in the pharynx	High levels of pregnancy hormones, such as hCG or oestrogen, with multiple pregnancy and hydatidiform mole (trophoblastic disease)
Some stimuli to the heart and viscera, such as distension, damage or infection of the uterus, renal pelvis or bladder	Physiological changes in the gastrointestinal tract in pregnancy, resulting in decreased motility and in increased gastric reflux
Drugs or endogenous toxins produced as a result of radiation damage, infection or disease	Transient hyperthyroidism, causing high levels of hCG, stimulating thyroid secretion
Disturbance of the vestibular apparatus, as in motion sickness	Metabolic changes, including carbohydrate deficiency and alteration in lipid pathways
Raised intracranial pressure, migraine, cerebral tumour	Pre-eclampsia, HELLP syndrome
Nauseating smells, sights or thoughts	Renal tract infections
Endocrine factors such as increased oestrogen	Torsion of an ovarian cyst
A fall in blood pressure and reduced circulation to the brain (vasovagal events)	Genetic incompatibility between mother and fetus
Viral gastroenteritis	Psychological factors
Hepatitis, acute liver failure	
Gall bladder disease	

Hyperemesis gravidarum

Hyperemesis gravidarum (HG) is a severe condition that results in excessive vomiting throughout the day and continues on most occasions until birth. Dehydration and metabolic imbalance may lead to maternal death if not treated actively (Verberg et al 2005). HG usually begins in the first trimester and is continuous, severe and often associated with excessive salivation. The incidence is about 0.3–2% (Moran & Taylor 2002). It is associated with multiple pregnancies and hydatidiform mole and these conditions should be suspected if the uterus appears large for dates.

Numerous studies have tried to clarify the aetiology of HG, ranging from high levels of hCG and increasing levels of oestrogen and progesterone to the slowing of gastrointestinal peristalsis, which increases gastric reflux (Low 1996). Hyperthyroidism may be caused by high levels of hCG; this is similar in structure to thyroid-stimulating hormone (TSH) and increases thyroid function (Verberg et al 2005). When the two conditions occur together, women may present with vomiting, weight loss and increased thyroid activity which requires treatment to prevent adverse outcomes in pregnancy.

Signs and symptoms

Nausea and vomiting are continuous throughout the day, little food or fluids are ingested and signs of dehydration are present. There is marked **oliguria** with dark urine of high specific gravity which may contain **ketones**, bile, protein and glucose. Electrolyte disturbances include **hyponatraemia** and **hypochloraemia** as sodium and chloride ions are lost in the vomit. The woman's breath smells offensive, she loses weight and her condition will deteriorate rapidly without treatment. The pulse will be rapid and the blood pressure reduced. Anaemia may occur because of the disruption in vitamin B_{12}, folic acid and vitamin C absorption. Fatigue is evident and relationships are strained; work patterns may be totally disrupted (Farrell 2008).

Complications

- Liver and renal damage, resulting in jaundice (Hay 2008).
- Vitamin B_1 (thiamine) deficiency, resulting in neuropathy such as **polyneuritis**.
- Rarely, **Wernicke's encephalopathy** may occur, signalled by confusion ataxia, impairment of short-term memory, leading to coma (Togay-Isikay et al 2001).
- **Hyperthermia** may occur due to disturbance of temperature control. The condition responds well to treatment with thiamine.

Management

The woman is usually admitted to hospital for investigations and rehydration. The cause of vomiting may not be found. An **antiemetic** will be given and fluids and electrolytes replaced by intravenous infusion of a solution such as Hartmann's. Vitamin B_{12}, thiamine, vitamin C, folic acid and iron will be needed to prevent complications (Farrell 2008).

General observation of the woman's condition should be monitored. Strict fluid balance should be maintained until rehydrated. There is usually a rapid response to treatment and oral fluids may be recommended when vomiting has ceased for 24 h. Solid food should be then introduced gradually. Moran & Taylor (2002) found that weight loss of more than 5% of prepregnancy weight in women with HG was effectively treated with 10 mg of prednisolone three times a day. This shortened the stay in hospital and stopped vomiting. This treatment was gradually decreased and discontinued at 20 weeks of gestation.

Appendicitis in pregnancy

The appendix is gradually displaced upwards by the growing uterus so that typical signs of appendicitis may not be present. In early pregnancy appendicitis may be difficult to differentiate from threatened abortion; however, there will be no bleeding. Later in pregnancy the pain may be mistaken for urinary tract infection, abruptio placentae or the onset of labour. A scan will confirm the diagnosis. The appendix must be removed to save life and prevent peritonitis (Eryilmaz et al 2002).

The abdominal incision is made on **McBurney's point** although the appendix is slightly higher. In 94% of a small sample of 23 gravid women, the appendix was located through the normal incision point (Popkin et al 2002). **Laparoscopic surgery** is gaining favour and has been used in pregnancy to remove ovaries and the appendix. Evidence suggests that this is safe in pregnancy but more research is needed (Fatum & Rojansky 2001). There is a small risk of spontaneous abortion or preterm onset of labour but this has to be balanced against the need for surgery.

Pregnancy in women with a stoma

An ileostomy or colostomy for urinary or alimentary diversion should not affect the course of pregnancy. About 75% of women with stomas will have a normal vaginal delivery. The use of urinary diversion with an ileocaecal reservoir is now common treatment for congenital disorders, neurogenic disease or trauma and some women may require caesarean delivery in these circumstances. Problems that may need careful management include:

- Changes in shape and position of the stoma as the uterus enlarges.
- Leaking from the stoma as the opening changes shape.
- Hormonal changes that alter skin secretions, leading to reduced adhesiveness of the appliance.
- Reduced absorption of nutrients—for example, vitamin B_{12} and folic acid—which may lead to anaemia.
- Increased risk of gastrointestinal obstruction; the consequent abdominal pain is difficult to distinguish from appendicitis (Stables 1995, Takahashi et al 2007).

Obstetric cholestasis

Cholestasis is a last trimester problem with the development of pruritus, particularly of the hands and feet, abnormally high transaminase levels and elevated bile acids in women with no evidence of liver inflammation. Jaundice is not common, <10% (Kingham et al 2006). The incidence in the UK is 0.5–1%; in Chile and Bolivia it is 5–15% and in Scandinavia 1–2% (Pusl & Beuers 2007). Obstetric cholestasis may disappear postnatally but may reoccur when contraception or hormone replacement therapy is commenced or when the woman is pregnant again. It is thought to be caused in the susceptible by raised oestrogen levels and may be an autoimmune response to pregnancy; there is a strong familial link (Kingham et al 2006). There is a high incidence of stillbirth if left untreated. The recommended treatment is ursodeoxycholic acid, which may assist in reducing the bile acid pool and serum bile acids (Arrese & Reyes 2006).

Neurological disorders

Epilepsy

Epilepsy is a general term for a group of conditions that cause **seizures**. It occurs in approximately 1% of the population, a third of which are women who may become pregnant. There is a brief alteration in brain function with a high-frequency discharge that can involve motor, sensory, autonomic or psychic clinical features accompanied by an alteration in the level of consciousness (Adab & Chadwick 2006). Seizures may be provoked by hypoglycaemia, lack of sleep, raised temperature, emotional or physical stress, drinking large amounts of water, constipation, drugs, hyperventilation, strobe lights, loud noises, some music and being startled.

Classification of seizures

- **Generalised seizures** involve neurons bilaterally, often without a focal onset and usually originating from a subcortical or deeper brain focus. Consciousness is always impaired or lost. Other terms used to describe seizures are absence, myoclonic, akinetic and clonic-tonic often termed grand mal and petit mal epilepsy (Clarke 2007).
- **Partial seizures (focal)** such as temporal lobe epilepsy and **Jacksonian epilepsy** often have a local onset and usually originate from cortical brain tissue. Consciousness is maintained if the seizure is limited to one cerebral hemisphere, but voluntary loss of muscular control occurs in the affected part of the body. **Temporal lobe epilepsy** is often characterised

by continuous inappropriate rubbing of hands, or combing the hair (Rang et al 2007).

- In **status epilepticus** more seizures follow the first before consciousness is fully regained and the person is in the **postictal state** (a state following a seizure) when the next seizure begins. Cerebral hypoxia means that this state is a medical emergency and failure to treat adequately may result in deterioration in mental health and death. Impairment of the conscious state may lead to the aspiration of the stomach contents.

Pathophysiology of seizures

The abnormal discharge of electricity may rapidly spread throughout the brain to involve the cortex, basal ganglia, thalamus and brainstem, leading to a tonic phase with generalised muscle contraction and increased muscle tone. Respiration may stop, and involuntary urination or defecation may occur. This is followed by a clonic phase as inhibitory neurons begin to interrupt the seizure discharge, leading to an intermittent contract/relax pattern of muscle action. The clonic bursts gradually become more infrequent and the seizure ends. Immediately prior to the onset of a seizure there may be an aura which may involve a visual disturbance or sensing a peculiar smell (Rang et al 2007).

Treatment of epilepsy

Investigation into the background of seizures should be established in order to offer treatment. If no cause is found, which is common, antiepileptic medication, either as monotherapy or combination therapy, will be commenced. Drugs used in treatment are known to interact adversely, thus affecting the efficiency of the drug if used in combination therapy. Some drugs in use are:

- Valproate (Epilim).
- Phenytoin (Epanutin).
- Phenobarbital.
- Carbamazepine, oxcarbazepine and others.

Epilepsy in pregnancy

Epilepsy affects 1 in 200 of all pregnant women (Clarke 2007, Shorvon 2002). Many pregnancies are unplanned in women with epilepsy; antiepileptic drugs may increase the breakdown of oestrogens, rendering contraceptives less efficient. There may be an increase or decrease in seizures but there is no change for most women. The more severe the disorder, the greater the effect on pregnancy; however, 90% of pregnancies have a successful outcome.

Preconception advice is important but women who are epileptic perceive a lack of information and support in outpatient departments, particularly advice for pregnancy (Shorvon 2002). Preconception folic acid 4 mg daily is recommended to prevent neural tube defects when trying to conceive. The changing metabolism of pregnancy alters the effect of medication and there will be a need to increase the dose or change medication if it causes teratogenicity. In trials it has been shown that epileptic women have more birth defects, not because they are epileptic but because of their medication (Adab & Chadwick 2006). There is a 2–3-fold increased risk of deformity in these newborns. Specific abnormalities have been linked to specific drugs (Clarke 2007, Shorvon 2002):

- Sodium valproate: neural tube and skeletal defects, particularly in higher doses (Battino & Tomson 2007).
- Carbamazepine: neural tube and cardiac anomalies.
- Phenytoin: orofacial clefts, cardiac anomalies and digital defects.

Other problems associated with anticonvulsant drugs are anaemia, because of folate antagonism, and vitamin D deficiency. Seizures occurring during pregnancy may cause fetal hypoxia and therefore a risk to fetal well-being, even more so if status epilepticus occurs (Adab & Chadwick 2006).

Fetus to neonate

Anticonvulsant drugs cross the placenta and decrease the production of vitamin K, which may lead to **haemorrhagic disease of the newborn**. Vitamin K should be administered to mothers from 36 weeks' gestation (Shorvon 2002) and to all infants post delivery (NICE 2004). During pregnancy it may be advisable to divide the dose of medication evenly through the day to prevent high fetal dosage. Blood medication levels should be assessed monthly. If the baby is formula-fed it may have withdrawal symptoms from maternal medication at approximately 1 week, in the form of irritability, excessive crying and continuous hunger. Some babies may remain sleepy and difficult to feed. All the drugs are excreted in breast milk but as long as the dosage is not high there is no contraindication to breastfeeding (Adab & Chadwick 2006, BNF 2007b).

Main points

- Asthma is the commonest respiratory problem found in pregnancy. Close monitoring and ensuring compliance with treatment ensure mother and fetus remain well.
- Women with asthma may have more complications in pregnancy such as preterm birth and small-for-gestational-age babies particularly if asthma attacks increase. Women may decrease their medication for fear of harming their babies to the detriment of treatment.
- TB in some parts of London exceeds 50 per 100 000 and 50% of TB cases in the UK were born overseas. The bacillus lies dormant for years but lowered resistance activates it and the host becomes sick. TB exploits the vulnerable, with poverty, overcrowding, institutionalisation, the presence of other disease and immunosuppression leading to an increase in active disease.
- The signs of pulmonary tuberculosis include general malaise, anorexia, weight loss, low-grade fever and night sweats. Pulmonary-specific symptoms include productive cough with purulent sputum and haemoptysis. Rest and drug therapy form the basis for treatment.
- There is a worldwide epidemic of multiple drug-resistant TB and many strains may resist up to seven different antibiotics. Vaccination is effective in the prevention of tuberculosis in children but of variable value in adults.
- Pregnant women are more susceptible to renal tract infections than other women. There is an incidence of unsuspected asymptomatic bacteriuria in 4–10% of pregnant women which if not diagnosed and treated results in about 25% of them developing pyelonephritis.
- The onset of acute renal failure is diagnosed if the urine output falls below 400 ml in 24 h or less than 20 ml/h. The incidence is about 1 in 10 000 pregnancies.
- Pregnancy is rare when the kidneys are functioning with less than 50% efficiency. Women with chronic renal impairment may appear to have pre-eclampsia, from which it needs distinguishing. Hypertension is the most common and serious complication.
- Maternal mortality may occur because of cerebral haemorrhage, abruptio placentae or acute renal failure. Fetal mortality may occur because of poor placental blood flow, abruptio placentae or fetal hypoxia. If kidney function diminishes, renal and peritoneal dialysis are both possible and there is a 50% fetal survival rate.
- Following kidney transplantation, fertility returns and pregnancy is likely. If kidney function is adequate and there is no hypertension, women with renal transplants tolerate pregnancy well. Common complications are preterm labour and pre-eclampsia.
- Hyperemesis gravidarum is a severe condition that results in excessive vomiting throughout the day and continues on most occasions until birth. Dehydration and metabolic imbalance may lead to maternal death if not treated actively. The cause of vomiting should be identified, an antiemetic should be given and fluids

and electrolytes replaced by intravenous infusion. Vitamins B$_{12}$ and C, folic acid and iron will be needed to correct anaemia.

- In early pregnancy appendicitis may be difficult to differentiate from threatened abortion. Later in pregnancy the pain may be mistaken for urinary tract infection, abruptio placentae or the onset of labour. Careful consideration of the patient's symptoms should allow a correct diagnosis.

- An ileostomy or colostomy for urinary or alimentary diversion should not affect the course of pregnancy. About 75% of women with stomas will have a normal vaginal delivery.

- Cholestasis is a last trimester problem with the development of pruritus particularly of hands and feet, abnormal liver enzymes and jaundice.

- Epilepsy occurs in approximately 1% of the population and affects 1 in 200 pregnant women.

Many pregnancies are unplanned in women with epilepsy, possibly because anti-epileptic drugs increase the breakdown of oestrogens, rendering contraceptives less efficient. Preconception folic acid 4 mg daily will prevent neural tube defects. When pregnancy is confirmed, advice about type and dosage of anti-epileptic medication is important. Epileptic women have more birth defects because of their medication.

- Anticonvulsants cross the placenta and decrease the production of vitamin K, which may lead to haemorrhagic disease of the newborn. Vitamin K should be administered to mothers from 36 weeks' gestation and to all infants post delivery. Following birth, babies who are formula-fed may have withdrawal symptoms from maternal medication. As long as the maternal drug dosage is not high there is no contraindication to breastfeeding.

References

Adab, N., Chadwick, D., 2006. Management of women with epilepsy during pregnancy. Obstet. Gynaecol. 8 (1), 20–25.

Alston, P.K., Kuller, J.A., MacMahon, M.J., 2001. Pregnancy in transplant recipients. Obstet. Gynaecol. Surv. 56 (5), 289–295.

Arrese, M., Reyes, H., 2006. Intrahepatic cholestasis of pregnancy: a past and present riddle. Ann. Hepatol. 5 (3), 202–205.

Armenti, V.T., Moritz, M.J., Cardonick, E.H., Davison, J.M., 2002. Immunosuppression in pregnancy: choices for infant and maternal health. Drugs 62 (16), 2361–2375.

Battino, D., Tomson, T., 2007. Management of epilepsy during pregnancy. Drugs 67 (18), 2727–2746.

Beckmann, C.A., 2006. The impact of pregnancy on peak flow values in women with asthma. Br. J. Midwifery 14 (2), 62–66.

Bewley, C., 2004. Medical disorders in pregnancy, Ch. 46. In: Henderson, C., Macdonald, S. (Eds.), Mayes's Midwifery: A Textbook for Midwives. Baillière Tindall, Edinburgh.

Blackburn, S.T., 2007. Maternal, Fetal and Neonatal Physiology: A Clinical Perspective, third edn. W B Saunders, Philadelphia.

BNF, 2007a. BCG vaccines. Br. Nat. Formul. March (53), 632.

BNF, 2007b. Antiepileptics. Br. Nat. Formul. March (53) 4.8:241.

Bothamley, G., 2001. Drug treatment for tuberculosis during pregnancy: safety considerations. Drug Saf. 24, 553–565.

Bothamley, J., 2006. Tuberculosis in pregnancy: the role for midwives in diagnosis and treatment. Br. J. Midwifery 14 (4), 182–185.

Callister, M.E.J., Barringer, J., Thanbalasingam, G., Gair, R., Davidson, R., 2002. Pulmonary tuberculosis among asylum seekers screened at Heathrow Airport, London 1995–9. Thorax 57, 152–156.

Clarke, S.D., 2007. Epilepsy in pregnancy. Br. J. Midwifery 15 (12), 740–745.

Davison, J., 2001. Renal disorders in pregnancy. Curr. Opin. Obstet. Gynecol. 13 (2), 109–114.

De Swiet, M., 1995. Diseases of the respiratory system. In: de Swiet, M. (Ed.), Medical Disorders in Obstetric Practice, third edn. Blackwell Science, Oxford.

Dombrowski, M., et al., 2004. Asthma during pregnancy. Obstet. Gynecol. 103, 5–12.

Drakeley, A.J., Le Roux, P.A., Anthony, J., et al., 2002. Acute renal failure complicating severe pre-eclampsia requiring admission to an obstetric unit. Am. J. Obstet. Gynecol. 186 (2), 253–256.

Eryilmaz, R., Sahin, M., Bas, G., Alimoglu, O., Kaya, B., 2002. Acute appendicitis during pregnancy. Dig. Surg. 19 (1), 40–44.

Farrell, N., 2008. Hyperemesis gravidarum: how midwives can help. Pract. Midwife 11 (7), 12–14.

Fatum, M., Rojansky, N., 2001. Laparoscopic surgery during pregnancy. Obstet. Gynecol. Surv. 56 (1), 50–59.

Gammill, H.S., Jeyabalan, A., 2005. Acute renal failure in pregnancy. Crit. Care Medicine 33 (Suppl. 10), S372–S384.

Hay, J.E., 2008. Liver disease in pregnancy. Hepatology 47 (3), 1067–1076.

Ie, S., Rubio, E.R., Alper, B., Szerlip, H.M., 2002. Respiratory complications of pregnancy. Obstet. & Gynecol. Surv. 57 (1), 39–46.

Joint Tuberculosis Committee of the British Thoracic Society, 2000. Control and prevention of tuberculosis in the UK. Code of Practice 2000. Thorax 55 (11), 887–901.

Kashanizadeh, N., Nemati, E., Shrifi-Bonab, M., Moghani-Lankarani, M., Gazizadeh, S., et al., 2007. Impact of pregnancy on the outcome of kidney transplant ion. Transplant. Proc. 39 (4), 1136–1138.

Keitel, E., Bruno, R.M., Duarte, M., Santos, A.F., Bittar, A.E., et al., 2004. Pregnancy outcome after renal transplantation. Transplant. Proc. 36 (4), 870–871.

Kingham, J., Adams, D., Hayden, G., 2006. Liver disease in pregnancy. Clin. Med. 6 (1), 34–40.

Kothari, A., Mahadevan, N., Girling, J., 2006. Tuberculosis and pregnancy. Results of a study in a high prevalence area in London, European. J. Obstet., Gynaecol. Reprod. Biol. 126 (1), 48–55.

Lindsay, N.E., 2000. Asymptomatic bacteriuria: important or not? N. Engl. J. Med. 343 (34), 1037–1039.

Liu, S.M.B., Wen, Shi.Wu., Demissie, K., et al., 2001. Maternal asthma and pregnancy outcome: a retrospective cohort study. Am. J. Obstet. Gynecol. 184 (2), 90–96.

Low, K.G., 1996. Nausea and vomiting in pregnancy: a review of the research. J. Gen. Cul. Health 1 (3), 151–172.

McCance, K.L., Huether, S.E., 2002. Pathophysiology: The biologic basis for disease in adults and children, fourth edn. Mosby, St Louis.

Moran, P., Taylor, R., 2002. Management of hyperemesis gravidarum: the importance of weight loss as a criterion for steroid therapy. Qld. J. Med. 95 (3), 153–158.

Murphy, V.E., Clifton, V.L., Gibson, P.G., 2006. Asthma exacerbations during pregnancy: incidence and association with adverse outcomes. Thorax 61, 169–176.

NICE, 2004, The Epilepsies: The diagnosis and treatment of epilepsies in adults and children in primary and secondary care. Clinical Guideline 20, London. <www.nice.org.uk./nicemedia/pdf/CGO2Oadultsquickrefguide.pdf> (accessed 09.08).

Ormerod, P., 2001. Tuberculosis in pregnancy and the puerperium. Thorax 56, 494–499.

Popkin, C.A., Lopez, P.P., Cohn, S.M., et al., 2002. The incision of choice for pregnant women with appendicitis is through McBurney's point. Am. J. Surg. 183 (1), 20–22.

Pusl, T., Beuers, U., 2007. Intrahepatic cholestasis of pregnancy. Orphanet. J. Rare Dis. 29, 2–26.

Rang, H.P., Dale, M.M., Ritter, J.M., 2007. Pharmacology, sixth edn. Churchill Livingstone, Edinburgh.

Rose, A.M.C., Watson, J.M., Graham, C., et al., 2001. Tuberculosis at the end of the 20th century in England and Wales: results of a national survey. Thorax 156, 170–173.

Shorvon, S., 2002. Antiepileptic drug therapy during pregnancy: the neurologist's perspective. J. Med. Genet. 39 (4), 248–250.

Stables, D., 1995. Mother and child nursing: stomas and pregnancy. In: Heath, H.B.M. (Ed.), Potter and Perry's Foundations in Nursing Theory and Practice. Mosby, St Louis.

Takahashi, K., Funayama, Y., Fukushima, K., Shibata, C., Ogawa, H., et al., 2007. Pregnancy and delivery in patients with enterostomy due to anorectal complications from Crohn's disease. Int. J. Colorectal. Dis. 22 (3), 313–318.

Thorsen, M.S., Poole, H., 2002. Renal disease in pregnancy. J. Perinatal Neonatal Nurs. 15 (4), 13–26.

Togay-Isikay, C., Yigit, A., Mutluer, N., 2001. Wernicke's encephalopathy due to hyperemesis gravidarum: an under-recognised condition. Aust. N. Z. J. Obstet. Gynaecol. 41 (4), 453–456.

Verberg, M.F.G., Gillott, D.J., Al-Fardan, N., Grudzinskas, J.G., 2005. Hyperemesis gravidarum: a review. Hum. Reprod. Update 11 (5), 527–539.

Watson, J.M., Moss, F., 2001. TB in Leicester: out of control, or just one of those things? (Editorial). Br. Med. J. 322, 1133–1134.

WHO, 2008. Tuberculosis. World Health Organization. Website: <http://www.who.int/topics/tuberculosis/en>. (accessed 09.08).

Annotated recommended reading

Bothamley, J., 2006. Tuberculosis in pregnancy: the role for midwives in diagnosis and treatment. Br. J. Midwifery 14 (4), 182–185.

This article gives an overview of tuberculosis from the midwifery perspective.

Davison, J., 2001. Renal disorders in pregnancy. Curr. Opin. Obstet. Gynecol. 13 (2), 109–114.

This is a good review of renal disease.

Farrell, N., 2008. Hyperemesis gravidarum: how midwives can help. Pract. Midwife 11 (7), 12–14.

This paper is written from a midwifery perspective—a good overview.

Joint Tuberculosis Committee of the British Thoracic Society, 2000. Control and prevention of tuberculosis in the UK, Code of Practice 2000. Thorax 55 (11), 887–901.

This comprehensive guide to the control of tuberculosis in the UK includes management guidelines for health care workers in relation to open TB infection.

Kingham, J., Adams, D., Hayden, G., 2006. Liver disease in pregnancy. Clin. Med. 6 (1), 34–40.

This is a clearly written article about most liver diseases found in pregnancy.

Shorvon, S., 2002. Antiepileptic drug therapy during pregnancy: the neurologist's perspective. J. Med. Genet. 39 (4), 248–250.

The article is easy to understand and gives the main points about epilepsy and pregnancy.

Chapter Thirty-Five

Diabetes mellitus and other metabolic disorders in pregnancy

Introduction

Pregnancy in some endocrine disorders is rare and management is sometimes based on limited observation and clinical judgement rather than on evidence-based criteria (Hague 2001). However, **diabetes mellitus** is by far the most common of these diseases and much progress has been made in its management. Normal metabolism is discussed in Chapter 23 and readers may wish to remind themselves of normal carbohydrate utilisation.

Diabetes mellitus

Diabetes mellitus is a group of disorders characterised by **impaired carbohydrate utilisation** caused by an absolute or relative deficiency of **insulin production** by the endocrine pancreas. A total of 180 000 000 people worldwide have diabetes and this figure will double by 2030 (WHO 2008). The changes in uncontrolled diabetes are a rise in blood glucose (normal range 3–5 mmol/L) and increases in glycogen breakdown (gluconeogenesis), fatty acid oxidation, ketone production and urea formation. There is also a reduced production of glycogen, lipid and protein in cells of tissue such as muscle and adipose tissue that are normally dependent on insulin (Brook & Marshall 2001).

Pathophysiology

The inability of the tissues to receive enough glucose results in inhibition of **glycolytic enzymes** and activation of the enzymes involved in **gluconeogenesis** (Bewley 2004). This results in more blood glucose than can be utilised. Excessive glucose passes into the renal filtrate and **glycosuria** occurs. Glucose is osmotically active and pulls water after it, resulting in **polyuria** and **dehydration. Thirst** increases to try to maintain adequate body fluids (Brook & Marshall 2001).

The body tries to mobilise energy from fats and proteins. Urea, produced as a by-product of amino acid metabolism, is excreted in the urine. Fatty acid release always results in ketogenesis but in the diabetic person excess ketones are produced and excreted in the urine, and on the breath. The ketones in the blood cause metabolic acidosis and lowering of pH (Bewley 2004, Brook & Marshall 2001). The buffer systems attempt to correct this and become exhausted. Other metabolic processes are disturbed and all body systems are affected. If untreated, acidosis leads to shock, coma and death (Tortora & Grabowski 2000).

Diabetes mellitus in pregnancy

Diabetes mellitus in pregnancy includes type 1 or **insulin-dependent diabetes** (IDDM). Recently, more pregnant women were found to have type 2 or **non-insulin-dependent diabetes** (NIDDM) (Feig & Palda 2002). **Gestational diabetes** (GDM) is diagnosed if diabetes develops for the first time in pregnancy.

Aetiology

Type 1 diabetes mellitus (IDDM)

This is rare before 9 months and peaks at 12 years of age and there is an almost total lack of insulin production. Hyperglycaemia, polyuria and ketosis are present at onset and insulin treatment is necessary. There are differences between populations both within and between countries. IDDM accounts for about 10% of diabetes in the developed countries. It is thought to be more prevalent amongst white people than amongst non-white people and the incidence is highest in Finland and lowest in Japan. There is a seasonal variation in the onset of IDDM, with more new cases in the northern hemisphere being reported in autumn and winter.

The Coxsackie virus B4 (CB4) may be implicated in the onset of type 1 diabetes (Saunders 2002). This common childhood infection causes a high fever, sore throat and headache which lasts for about 3 days. The CB4 virus may destroy pancreatic islet cells and trigger an autoimmune response in genetically susceptible children. There is a long period of subclinical diabetes as β cells are progressively destroyed and islet cell antibodies have been found years before the onset of clinical signs. There is evidence that α-cell function is impaired, leading to excess **glucagon**, which exacerbates hyperglycaemia. Autoantibodies have been found in most people with juvenile-onset diabetes.

Type 1 diabetes mellitus is subdivided into two distinct types. **IDDM type 1A** develops in childhood and is thought to be due to a genetic–environment interaction. There is a link with the human leucocyte antigen HLA-DR4. The predisposing gene is carried on chromosome 6. About 12% of newly diagnosed diabetics of this type have a first-degree relative with the disease. **IDDM type 1B** tends to occur later in life, between the ages of 30 and 50 years, and is probably an autoimmune disorder linked to HLA-DR3 (Anastassios 2008).

Type 2 diabetes mellitus (NIDDM)

This is four times as common as IDDM and its incidence is increasing globally (WHO 2008). The onset is usually in later life in obese people. NIDDM occurs in pregnancy more frequently as women delay conception (Hague 2001). It varies with ethnicity, suggesting a genetic–environment interaction (Feig & Palda 2002). A form of NIDDM called **maturity-onset diabetes of the young** (MODY) is caused by an autosomal dominant gene. Sufferers are usually of normal weight and under 25 years of age.

Amyloid deposits associated with islet cell destruction are seen in about 25% of cases, usually correlating with the person's age and severity of disease. The ratio of α to β cells is normal and there is no reduction of insulin in the blood, but in obese people insulin has a decreased ability to influence cellular uptake of glucose. This is perhaps due to increased circulating free fatty acids, although reaction of other substances has also been proposed (Anastassios 2008). There is increased **insulin resistance** because of decreased numbers of **cellular insulin receptors**.

The incidence of NIDDM in pregnancy is difficult to assess as some women taking insulin may have type 2 diabetes, especially in susceptible populations such as East-Asian women. Many women may be undiagnosed prior to pregnancy. Pregnant women with type 2 diabetes are likely to be obese and to suffer hypertension and hyperlipidaemia. Screening women before pregnancy or early in the first trimester of pregnancy might help to differentiate between women with NIDDM and those with gestational diabetes (Feig & Palda 2002) but the dangers are the same.

Gestational diabetes mellitus (GDM)

Women with impaired glucose tolerance may develop diabetes in stressful situations. In pregnancy this is called gestational diabetes; these women may well go on to develop type 2 diabetes in later life, particularly if obese (Metzger et al 2007). GDM occurs in 2% of all pregnancies, mostly in the third trimester. Following delivery, glucose metabolism may return to normal.

Population differences in the incidence of GDM

Studies have been conducted into the incidence of gestational diabetes between different ethnic groups. There was found to be an increased risk in women of lower socioeconomic class, older women, obese women and those with infertility (Modder 2006). In Great Britain, 49% of women are from 'black, Asian and other minority groups'; 9% are type 1 diabetic (Modder 2006).

Shelley-Jones et al (1993) in Australia compared the physiology of 15 women with normal glucose tolerance,

16 Caucasian women with GDM and 19 Asian-born women with GDM. They found that:

- Caucasian women, unlike the Asian women, were obese compared to the control group of women.
- Both groups of women with GDM had a similar abnormal insulin response to a glucose load.
- Fasting serum triglycerides were increased in all women with GDM. Asian women had significantly lower serum cholesterol levels than the Caucasian women, with or without GDM.

They concluded that it is difficult to know whether the differences in obesity and serum cholesterol 'reflect a dietary difference or a major difference in lipid metabolism'.

Glucose tolerance test

The **glucose tolerance test** (GTT) can be used to confirm the presence of diabetes. Fasting blood and urine specimens are taken, then a 75 g glucose drink is given. Venous blood samples are then taken at intervals. Normally, blood glucose rises but returns to normal (3–5 mmol/L) within 2 h. The following abnormalities occur in glucose impairment (Porterfield & White 2007):

- A fasting plasma glucose >7 mmol/L.
- A blood glucose level >10 mmol/L after 2 h.
- If the 2 h blood glucose level is between 7 and 10 mmol/L, glucose tolerance is impaired.

General pathological effects of diabetes mellitus

The metabolic changes and physiological effects of diabetes mellitus are profound (Fig. 35.1). Seventy years ago young diabetics usually died within 2 years of onset. The identification of insulin by Banting and Best led to survival, but the acute and long-term effects of diabetes mellitus became apparent. Deaths from **cardiovascular disease** and **renal disease** are much more common than in the general population. Acute complications include **hypoglycaemia** and **diabetic ketoacidosis**. Pregnant women who have had IDDM for more than 10 years are significantly more at risk of associated cardiovascular, ophthalmic, renal and neuropathic problems, and in general diabetic women are at risk of a poor pregnancy outcome, particularly if diabetic control has been less than ideal (Hague 2001, Stenhouse 2007).

Hypoglycaemia

Hypoglycaemia occurs in 90% of IDDM sufferers and is also known as **insulin shock** or **insulin reaction**. Diabetic patients aim to prevent hypoglycaemia by diet and insulin administration. The balance of insulin versus available glucose becomes unbalanced and blood levels of glucose fall, brain cells are depleted of nutrients and loss of consciousness results in coma (Porterfield & White 2007, Tortora & Grabowski 2000).

Symptoms and treatment

Hypoglycaemia causes the secretion of glucagon, adrenaline (epinephrine) and growth hormone which in turn causes tachycardia, palpitations, tremors, pallor and anxiety. Other symptoms include headaches, dizziness, irritability, confusion, visual disturbances, hunger and convulsions. Coma will occur if not treated with oral or intravenous glucose (Porterfield & White 2007, Tortora & Grabowski 2000).

Diabetic ketoacidosis

Glucose is not available for cell metabolism because there is a deficit of insulin, thus the body breaks down fatty acids causing **ketoacidosis**. It is a serious condition because, as fatty particles are mobilised round the transport system, fatty deposits are left behind in the blood vessels causing atherosclerosis with consequent cardiovascular problems. There is an increase in hormones such as catecholamines, glucagon, cortisol and growth hormone antagonising the effect of insulin. Liver glucose production increases and peripheral glucose usage decreases. The most likely precipitating causes are interruption of insulin administration, infection and trauma (Porterfield & White 2007, Tortora & Grabowski 2000).

Symptoms and treatment

Polyuria, polydipsia and dehydration will occur because of **osmotic diuresis**. Coma is rare. Sodium, magnesium and phosphorus deficits may occur but the most severe electrolyte disturbance is potassium deficiency. Hyperventilation may occur to compensate for the acidosis with postural dizziness, anorexia, nausea and abdominal pain. Both glucose and ketones will be present in the urine. There may be a smell of acetone on the breath. Treatment will aim to decrease blood glucose levels by continual administration of low-dose insulin and maintaining normal electrolyte levels.

Long-term complications

- Diabetic neuropathy with sensory deficits.
- Microvascular disease with thickening of capillary basement membrane appears to be directly linked to the duration of the disease and blood glucose levels. Retinopathy causes blood vessel changes, leading to loss of sight. Nephropathy may result in end-stage renal disease.
- Atherosclerosis appears at a younger age and progresses more rapidly in the diabetic, leading to hypertension, coronary artery disease and stroke. This is unrelated to the severity of diabetes and may occur with only

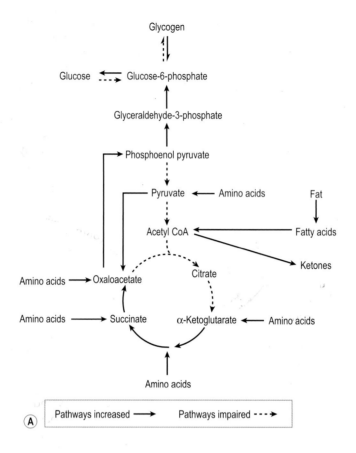

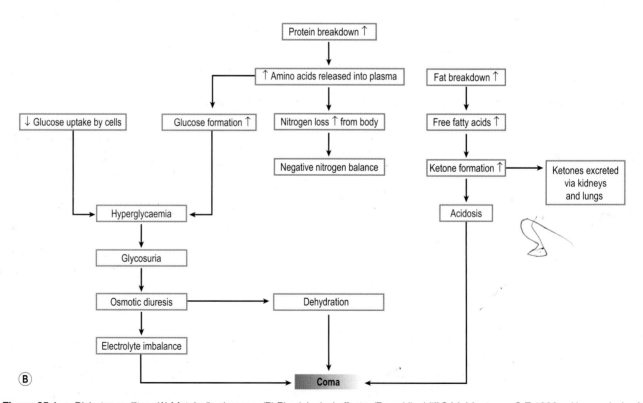

Figure 35.1 • Diabetes mellitus. (A) Metabolic changes. (B) Physiological effects. (From Hinchliff S M, Montague S E 1990, with permission.)

impaired glucose tolerance. Peripheral vascular disease, leading to gangrene and amputation, may result due to the abnormal level of glucose in the tissues.

- Infection is more common as pathogens utilise the increased tissue glucose to multiply and the function of phagocytic white cells is impaired.
- Pre-eclampsia will develop in about 13% of pregnant women (Evers et al 2004, Porterfield & White 2007).

Effects of diabetes on pregnancy

Pregnancy changes glucose metabolism creating a **diabetogenic effect**. Women with carbohydrate intolerance may not show signs or symptoms of diabetes, but there is a significant increase in fetal and maternal morbidity (Modder 2006). A comparison was made between women who tested negative on one glucose loading test and those with one positive result. There were 14 036 women in the study and those with an elevated glucose level were more inclined to have babies weighing >4000 g, have a caesarean section, pre-eclampsia and admission of the baby to a neonatal unit (McLaughlin et al 2006). Diabetes becomes more difficult to control in pregnancy although immediately after delivery women return to their pre-pregnancy needs.

Fetal problems

These include:

- The incidence of fetal malformations is higher in women with poor diabetic control as is first trimester abortions. Congenital anomalies of the nervous, cardiovascular, renal and skeletal systems may occur but are difficult to diagnose on ultrasound (Galindo et al 2006).
- **Fetal macrosomia** (i.e. birth weight >4500 g or >95th centile) is increasingly correlated with maternal obesity due to poor diabetic control in the second and third trimesters. This is not a simple relationship between blood glucose levels and fetal size, as both protein and triglyceride metabolisms have been implicated in excessive fetal growth (Clausen et al 2005, Ehrenberg et al 2004).
- Polyhydramnios.
- Traumatic delivery due to macrosomia (Jevitt 2008).
- Stillbirth.
- Neonatal asphyxia and respiratory distress syndrome.
- Hyperviscosity syndrome.

Effect of pregnancy on the diabetes

Pregnancy with additional fetal requirements places large demands on maternal metabolism, particularly in the last trimester. This changes to allow more efficient storage of nutrients while minimising catabolism of protein stores. There is progressive insulin resistance caused by oestrogens and progestins decreasing insulin efficiency. Normally, the β cells increase the amount of insulin they release in the presence of insulin resistance but glucose metabolism in diabetic pregnant women becomes unstable and more insulin will be needed to achieve metabolic control (Porterfield & White 2007).

Diabetic nephropathy

This is present in 5% of pregnant women with diabetes and increases perinatal risk and the incidence of pre-eclampsia. There is evidence to suggest that angiotensin-converting enzyme inhibitors are teratogenic; these drugs may have been taken pre-pregnancy to aid kidney function and as a hypotensive (BNF 2007, Landon 2007). Although in non-pregnant women a protein-restricted diet to aid kidney function would be commenced, this is generally avoided in pregnancy because of fetal nutritional needs.

Diabetic retinopathy

Pregnancy may temporarily increase the progression of retinopathy (Kaaja & Loukovaara 2007). It has been associated with poor control of blood glucose and blood pressure, albuminuria and poor perinatal outcome (Lauszus et al 2000). Ophthalmologic examination and evaluation should be carried out at regular intervals and the Valsalva manoeuvre avoided in labour to prevent possible retinal haemorrhage. Pregnant women who have proliferative retinopathy with neovascularisation (new blood vessel growth) risk loss of vision; this can be treated by laser photocoagulation.

Care in pregnancy

Preconception advice

Pregnancy should be discussed with the diabetic woman prior to conception (Hague 2001). Adequate blood glucose control prior to conception helps to reduce fetal loss due to early abortion, congenital abnormalities, fetal macrosomia, polyhydramnios and stillbirth. Research has shown that diabetic women whose blood sugar is well controlled around conception and during pregnancy have outcomes approaching the incidence of the non-diabetic population (Sacks 2006). Folic acid 5 mg daily should be taken preconceptually and blood glucose levels monitored (Modder 2006, Stenhouse 2007).

Management during pregnancy

Health professionals should collaborate with the diabetic woman in her care during pregnancy. The involvement of the **diabetic team**, the obstetrician and the midwife is essential. The woman should be booked for care and delivery in a consultant unit with neonatal facilities and is usually seen at least every 2 weeks (Hague 2001).

Diabetic control

The management of diabetes before and during pregnancy requires control of blood sugar and prevention of ketosis. Hypoglycaemia may be a particular problem in the first trimester particularly where excessive vomiting occurs. Dietary intake and insulin dosage should be monitored with blood glucose levels by self-assessment at home. Self-monitoring of ketoacidosis should also take place and if positive the woman should be admitted for stabilisation with IV insulin (NICE 2008). Ketoacidosis may present in pregnancy with normal glucose levels and is an emergency situation as the fetus has a greatly increased mortality rate (Wallace & Matthews 2004). Pregnancy alters the renal threshold for glucose, and therefore urinary glucose levels are unhelpful.

Glycaemic control

NICE (2008) targets for plasma glucose levels are 3.5–5.9 mmol/L in the fasting state and <7.8 mmol/L after a meal. They suggest that, to monitor hypoglycaemia, plasma levels should be taken before bedtime as well. Women must be told about the risk of nausea and vomiting likely to occur in the first trimester and how glucose metabolism is changed by the presence of the fetus. The added awareness will assist them in reporting abnormalities to their doctor. The effect of the pregnancy on lifestyle, including the implications of maintaining a demanding job and the possible need for medical leave, should be discussed.

Glycosylated haemoglobin

Glycosylated haemoglobin (HbA_{1c}) is a type of adult haemoglobin in which glucose is attached to part of the β-globin chain in the red cell and shows levels of blood glucose in the past 2 months. Pre-conceptually these levels of glucose can be used to obtain the optimum time for conception (Pearson et al 2007). They are increased in diabetes and indicate that blood glucose control has been inadequate. The optimum level set by NICE (2008) is <7% of the total (0.08 SI units) and should only be used in the first trimester.

Insulin

This is necessary for all women with type 1 diabetes and occasionally those with type 2 diabetes or gestational diabetes where diet control is insufficient. Better control can be obtained by tailoring the insulin regimen to the individual woman to avoid hypoglycaemia (Hague 2001). The regimen may be a combination of soluble, long- and short-acting insulins. Rapid-action insulin (insulin aspart, insulin lispro) may have advantages against soluble insulin (NICE 2008). Continuous insulin pump therapy may be necessary in the unstable diabetic (NICE 2008).

Oral hypoglycaemic agents

These are safe to use in pregnant women who are non-insulin-dependent, but the BNF (2007) suggests that metformin and glibenclamide should be discontinued in favour of insulin. Homco et al (2004) report that in a randomized controlled trial no glibenclamide was found in cord blood of infants in the trial group (Homco & Reece 2006). Recent meta-analysis of metformin in the first trimester showed no increase in major fetal abnormalities but there is a need for larger trials in this area (Gilbert et al 2006).

Diet

Dietary advice during pregnancy aims to achieve good diabetes control with optimum nutrition for both mother and baby. An ideal dietary composition would be 55% carbohydrate, 20% protein and 25% fats, with polysaturated fats no more than 10%. Foods with a low glycaemic index and small frequent meals are recommended and it is an ideal time to educate the woman in good diet which will help her and her family (Reader 2007). Ethnic differences in dietary habits should be discussed where necessary.

Monitoring the fetus

Ongoing fetal well-being should be monitored closely using the methods discussed in Chapter 13. Although fetal macrosomia is the main problem, the babies of women with renal disease or superimposed pre-eclampsia may suffer from intrauterine growth restriction.

Delivery

Women with uncomplicated diabetes and no obstetric problems may be delivered vaginally after 38 weeks. Women with unstable diabetes, complications or obstetric problems may be delivered earlier by caesarean section to avoid the possibility of intrauterine death. Following induced or spontaneous onset of labour, a continuous dextrose infusion and variable insulin infusion according to hourly blood glucose is maintained. Blood glucose levels should be maintained at 4–7 mmol/L (NICE 2008). Care is under a consultant endocrinologist and obstetrician. Immediately following delivery, insulin requirements usually revert back to pre-pregnancy needs (Bewley 2004).

Care in the puerperium

Control of diabetes

Insulin requirements fall and restabilisation is necessary. Women with type 2 diabetes or gestational diabetes can usually cease taking insulin and commence oral therapy if needed, which is safe for the infant (NICE 2008).

Infection prevention

It is important to avoid infection in all postpartum women, but diabetic women are especially at risk. Data suggest that breast infection is higher in diabetic women, so care must be taken to control blood glucose level and to inspect the breasts for early signs (Whittaker 2001).

Breastfeeding

Breastfeeding is possible but it is necessary to remember that lactating women have a higher energy turnover and this means diet and insulin dosage need to be monitored carefully. Diabetic women gain the same benefits as all mothers who breastfeed, including protection against premenopausal breast and ovarian cancer (Chilvers 1993) and osteoporotic hip fractures in later life (Cumming & Klineberg 1993). Today women with diabetes of all types choose to breastfeed their babies as frequently as non-diabetic women (Whittaker 2001).

Contraceptive advice

This must be discussed. The oral contraceptive pill can be taken but may mimic pregnancy, increasing the need for insulin. Intrauterine contraceptive devices may lead to infection and are not recommended for most diabetic women. A barrier method may be used by women wishing to add to their family. It is an ideal time to discuss future pregnancy and preconceptual care prior to getting pregnant again (Kjos 2007).

Type 2 diabetes (NIDDM) and gestational diabetes

Gestational diabetes developing for the first time in pregnancy may be due to the diabetogenic effect of pregnancy or a familial disposition to diabetes. It occurs in 3–5% of women (Ben-Haroush et al 2004). However, if women have not been screened before pregnancy or during the early part of the first trimester, it is difficult to differentiate this from pre-pregnancy-onset NIDDM. Gestational diabetes is associated with an increased risk of perinatal morbidity and mortality. There are usually no symptoms and diagnosis depends on abnormal blood glucose results, usually following a GTT.

Antenatal screening for GDM

This has been suggested for all pregnant women at 24–28 weeks' gestation; it is cost-effective considering that the diagnosis of GDM prevents poor pregnancy outcome and prevents long-term health problems when diagnosed. Women in certain groups do go on to develop NIDDM. Tests used include a 50 g oral glucose challenge test (OGCT) and a 100 g and 75 g oral glucose tolerance test (OGTT); positive results from an OGTT would be indicative of GDM (Ben-Haroush et al 2004).

The diagnostic value of the OGCT has been put into question (Montagnana et al 2008). NICE (2008) suggest that further research is needed to clarify the efficacy of testing all pregnant women and to assess the criteria from these tests in order to diagnose GDM.

Indicative clinical findings

Obstetricians may use clinical findings from history taking or from the present pregnancy to order tests for diagnosing the presence of GDM (Ben-Haroush et al 2004). These may include:

- A history of diabetes in close relatives.
- Chronic hypertension.
- Recurrent urogenital infections.
- Age over 30 years.
- Poor reproductive history (three or more spontaneous abortions).
- A previous baby weighing more than 4000 g.
- A previous unexplained perinatal death.
- A previous baby with unexplained congenital malformations.
- History of GDM in a previous pregnancy.
- Obesity.
- Glycosuria on two occasions at antenatal visit.
- The presence of polyhydramnios.

Complications of GDM

Macrosomia is twice as frequent, leading to a greater incidence of forceps delivery, caesarean section and shoulder dystocia which may result in injury to the mother or baby (Jevitt et al 2008). Postnatally, women should be counselled about ways to minimise the risk of developing NIDDM later in life. They should be reminded to maintain normal body weight, to exercise regularly, to have annual blood glucose tests and to receive early care if they become pregnant again (Ben-Haroush et al 2004).

Management of GDM

Once diagnosed, treatment should aim to control blood glucose, carry out additional fetal surveillance and decrease the incidence of macrosomia. Dietary control is usually sufficient in GDM but occasionally insulin injections will be necessary. The need for insulin should disappear after delivery (King 2006).

The baby of a diabetic mother

If there has been poor control of the diabetes mellitus the baby may be large, weighing over the 90th centile, and plethoric (Fig. 35.2). With the good control usually achieved in current practice, babies are more likely to be of a weight appropriate for gestational age (Bewley

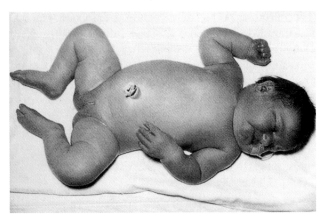

Figure 35.2 • A large-for-gestational-age baby from a diabetic mother. (From Kelnar C, Harvey D, Simpson C 1995, with permission.)

2004). Despite being 4000 g or more these babies may be physiologically immature and have problems similar to those of a preterm baby, including respiratory distress syndrome (see Ch. 51). Congenital defects are also related to the control of the diabetes around the time of conception. Birth injuries such as Erb's palsy may occur if the baby is large (see Ch. 53).

High maternal blood glucose levels in utero encourage the fetal pancreas to produce more insulin. This hyperinsulinaemia continues after birth, creating neonatal hypoglycaemia which will require stabilising, perhaps by intravenous glucose. Careful monitoring of neonatal blood glucose and early feeding should help to prevent severe side-effects. The baby will have high-fat deposits created by the hyperinsulinaemia which is a potent growth hormone. **Polycythaemia with hyperbilirubinaemia** may result from inadequate transfer of nutrients via the placenta which may hypertrophy in the diabetic with unstable glucose levels. The polycythaemia is a result of the fetus needing to increase oxygen levels thus producing more red cells to do so. Consequently there is hyperbilirubinaemia postnatally. The baby tends to be lethargic at first but development then proceeds normally (Blackburn 2007, Coad & Dunstall 2005).

Abnormalities of thyroid function

Overactivity and underactivity of the thyroid gland can produce serious illness.

Hyperthyroidism (thyrotoxicosis) in pregnancy

Thyrotoxicosis occurs in about 0.2% of pregnancies and **Graves' disease** (Fig. 35.3) accounts for 95% of cases (Lao 2005). **Thyroid-stimulating immunoglobulins** (TSIgs)

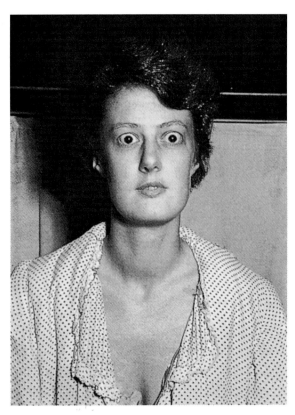

Figure 35.3 • A person with Graves' disease. (From Hinchliff S M, Montague S E 1990, with permission.)

(antibodies) activate **follicular cell TSH receptors**, leading to increased production of **thyroid hormones**. Signs include raised basal metabolic rate (BMR), excessive perspiration, weight loss despite good calorific intake, a rapid irregular heart beat, palpitations, hypertension and nervousness. **Exophthalmos** (protrusion of the eyeballs, see Fig. 35.3) may occur. Pre-pregnancy treatment may have been by surgical removal of the thyroid gland or radioactive iodine to destroy the most active thyroid cells.

Rarer conditions causing hyperthyroidism include **autonomous thyroid nodules. Biochemical thyrotoxicosis** may occur in women who develop hyperemesis gravidarum (Turner 2007) because of the similarity between thyrotrophin (TSH) and human chorionic gonadotrophin (hCG) (Lao 2005, Vitoratos et al 2000). In pregnancy the thyroid increases in size without increased hormone levels; it may also become more nodular, making diagnosis of thyroid problems difficult (Lao 2005). However, failure to gain weight despite a good appetite, a rapid sleeping pulse and lid lag are suspicious. Thyroxine (T_4) assays will be higher than normal in pregnancy.

Severe hyperthyroidism is associated with infertility but conception may occur if treatment has been successful or if the disease is mild (Bewley 2004). In mild hyperthyroidism, improvements may occur in pregnancy due to increased thyroxine-binding globulin, which can offset the excess of thyroid hormones. Women with Graves' disease may also experience improvement due to altered immune system functioning, and drug dosages can often be reduced (Hague 2001).

Management

Inadequately managed thyrotoxicosis is associated with severe pre-eclampsia and maternal heart failure (Lao 2005). Pregnant women with hyperthyroidism need more calories to compensate for the higher metabolic rate. Fluid loss may occur if there is diarrhoea. If antithyroid drugs are used, their effects must be monitored to avoid too high levels of drug. The drugs commonly used are **propylthiouracil** (PTU) or **carbimazole** (CBZ). PTU is the drug of choice in pregnancy and the puerperium. Failure to control the disease may necessitate a **partial thyroidectomy** if the disease is difficult to control or the woman has a large goitre (Hague 2001).

Thyroid storm

A **thyroid storm** is characterised by an extreme **hypermetabolic state**. It is a rare complication, occurring in 1% of hyperthyroid pregnancies, usually due to a stressful delivery or infection (Lao 2005). The woman develops hyperthermia, tachycardia, cardiac decompensation and mental disorientation. This carries a high rate of maternal morbidity and mortality and therefore treatment should take place in a unit with intensive care facilities (Hague 2001).

Effect of maternal treatments on the fetus

If hyperthyroidism is poorly controlled, intrauterine growth restriction, preterm labour and perinatal death may occur. No teratogenic effects have been reported for PTU or CMZ and perinatal mortality can be reduced by medical management of the mother (Hague 2001). Preterm labour should not be treated with β agonists such as salbutamol because of the risk of tachycardia. Calcium channel blockers such as nifedipine can be used instead.

Fetal hypothyroidism

Thionamide treatment of Graves' disease can suppress fetal and neonatal thyroid function (Lao 2005). There is a risk of 1:100 of fetal hypothyroidism as the drugs may cross the placenta and block the synthesis of thyroid hormones by the fetus so the lowest possible doses should be given.

Fetal hyperthyroidism

Women with Graves' disease who have been treated by **surgical** or **radioiodine ablation** of the thyroid, with or without thyroxine treatment, may have raised titres of thyroid-stimulating immunoglobulins (TSIg). Their fetuses may develop uncontrolled hyperthyroidism with

a heart rate above 160 beats/min. These women should be given thyroxine, which does not cross the placenta, to maintain their normal thyroid function and thionamides to treat the fetus, using its heart rate as a guide (Hague 2001). In pregnancies where there is placental transfer of **long-acting thyroid stimulator** from mother to fetus, fetal hyperthyroidism may result. The baby's thyroid function will return to normal within 3 weeks (Lao 2005).

Hypothyroidism in pregnancy

It may be due to **autoimmune thyroiditis (Hashimoto's disease)**, viral thyroiditis or congenital absence of the thyroid gland and affects only 1% of pregnancies (Bewley 2004, Hague 2001, Lao 2005). There may be a defect in the thyroid gland or in the control pathway of thyrotrophin-releasing hormone (TRH) or thyroid-stimulating hormone (TSH) release. In dietary iodine deficiency, the thyroid gland hypertrophies and a goitre occurs. The enlarged gland is stimulated by increasing amounts of TSH but produces unusable colloid. This used to be common in inland areas such as Derbyshire (hence **Derbyshire neck**).

Other causes of hypothyroidism in pregnancy are those secondary to immune disorders or following destruction of thyroid tissue either surgically or with radioactive iodine. Women with type 1 diabetes mellitus have a 5–8% incidence of hypothyroid disease and a 25% risk of developing postpartum thyroid dysfunction (Lao 2005).

Symptoms include a low basal metabolic rate, feeling cold, constipation, thick, dry skin, puffy eyes, oedema, lethargy and mental sluggishness. Untreated hypothyroidism is often associated with infertility because TRH stimulation induces **hyperprolactinaemia**, which prevents ovulation (Hague 2001). Confirmation is by measurement of tri-iodothyronine (T_3) and T_4 levels. Treatment is by thyroxine medication, and assessment of thyroid function once in each trimester is usually sufficient (Hague 2001). As long as the fetus is not exposed to iodine deficiency or teratogenic drugs, development should be normal. Complications of increased fetal loss and prolonged pregnancy may occur (Lao 2005).

Adrenal disorders in pregnancy

Adrenal disorders in pregnancy are uncommon and most women will have had their disorder diagnosed and treated before pregnancy (Hague 2001).

Addison's disease

Addison's disease is caused by inadequate secretion of the adrenal cortical hormones with deficiency of both glucocorticoids and mineralocorticoids. Symptoms include falling plasma sodium and glucose levels, a rise in serum potassium levels, **skin hyperpigmentation** and weight loss. Severe dehydration and hypotension are common. The main cause is **autoimmune destruction** of the adrenal cortex and it often occurs combined with other autoimmune endocrine disorders such as Graves' disease. In pregnancy, the condition is treated by replacement therapy of 20–30 mg/day of oral hydrocortisone (Hague 2001). In an acute episode, **intravenous hydrocortisone** is necessary.

Cushing's syndrome

Cushing's syndrome is rare in pregnancy because it is usually associated with amenorrhoea and anovulation (Hague 2001). It is caused by excessive levels of corticosteroids. The cause is often pituitary or adrenal carcinoma. Some normal pregnancy features mimic Cushing's syndrome but, unless other signs such as a moon face, hirsutism, acne and proximal myopathy are present, it is unlikely that true Cushing's syndrome is present. In the rare cases seen, fetal loss has been 25% and preterm delivery occurred in up to 50%.

Congenital adrenal hyperplasia

Congenital adrenal hyperplasia (CAH) is a group of conditions with a block in the biosynthesis of **cortisol**

(Brook & Marshall 2001). Women who remain undiagnosed tend to be infertile and few pregnancies occur (Hague 2001). Girls treated with hormones in childhood and adolescence may have clitoral and vaginal scarring, making vaginal delivery traumatic. The masculinisation of the pelvis causes **cephalopelvic disproportion**. Women with late-onset CAH usually have **polycystic ovary syndrome** and require adrenal suppression with glucocorticoids to allow ovulation to occur (Hague 2001) (see Ch. 7). Any women who have been given prolonged steroid therapy should be given hydrocortisone during labour or at the time of caesarean section to avoid a hypoadrenal crisis.

Phaeochromocytoma

A phaeochromocytoma is a tumour of the adrenal medulla and is rare in pregnancy. It may be misdiagnosed as pre-eclampsia or essential hypertension as blood pressure rises and proteinuria is present. Symptoms include intermittent or sustained hypertension, postural hypotension, sweating, palpitations and tachycardia, anxiety, nausea and vomiting. The tumour and symptoms are treated medically until the fetus is viable when surgical removal of the tumour is carried out.

Main points

- Diabetes mellitus is characterised by impaired carbohydrate metabolism and utilisation caused by an absolute or relative deficiency of insulin production. In pregnancy, abnormal carbohydrate metabolism occurs in women with IDDM, NIDDM or GDM. After delivery, glucose metabolism may return to normal. Gestational diabetes is likely to recur in subsequent pregnancies.

- The Coxsackie virus B4 may destroy pancreatic islet cells and trigger an autoimmune response in genetically susceptible children.

- Type 1 diabetes mellitus is subdivided into two types: type 1A begins in childhood and may be due to destruction of the β cells in the pancreas; type 1B occurs between the ages of 30 and 50 and may be an autoimmune disorder.

- Type 2 diabetes occurs mainly in obese people after the age of 40. MODY affects younger individuals, usually of normal weight. The incidence of NIDDM in pregnancy is difficult to assess, but may be confirmed by an OGTT.

- Long-term effects of diabetes mellitus include deaths from cardiovascular and renal disease. Chronic conditions include: diabetic neuropathy; microvascular disease, leading to retinopathy and nephropathy; and

atherosclerosis, leading to coronary artery disease and stroke. Peripheral vascular disease, leading to gangrene and amputation, may occur. Infection is more common.

- Acute complications include hypoglycaemia and diabetic ketoacidosis. The aim is to prevent hypoglycaemia. Emergency treatment is to provide glucose. Treatment of diabetic ketoacidosis is to decrease blood glucose levels by continual administration of low-dose insulin.

- Diabetes is difficult to control in pregnancy although immediately after delivery women return to their pre-pregnancy needs. Most women with carbohydrate intolerance show no signs or symptoms but there is a significant increase in fetal and maternal morbidity. Pre-eclampsia will develop in about 13% of pregnant women.

- Fetal problems include first trimester abortions, congenital abnormalities, macrosomia, polyhydramnios, traumatic delivery, stillbirth, neonatal asphyxia, respiratory distress syndrome and hyperviscosity syndrome.

- The management of diabetes requires control of blood glucose and prevention of ketosis. Adequate blood glucose control prior to conception helps to reduce

- fetal loss but, if control is too extreme, hypoglycaemia may endanger the mother and cause fetal intrauterine growth restriction. The diet and insulin dosage should be monitored by blood glucose levels.
- The need for insulin increases during pregnancy. Specific oral hypoglycaemic agents in pregnancies of women who are non-insulin-dependent are safe to use.
- Fetal complications include macrosomia with an increased incidence of shoulder dystocia, forceps delivery and caesarean section. Women with unstable diabetes, complications or obstetric problems may be delivered earlier by caesarean section to avoid intrauterine death.
- Women from India, the Middle East and Oriental women have a higher risk of developing gestational diabetes. There is an increased risk in women of lower socioeconomic class, older women, obese women and those with infertility.
- In the puerperium, insulin requirements fall and restabilisation is necessary. Women who breastfeed may take oral hypoglycaemic agents. Breast infection is higher in diabetic women.
- The oral contraceptive pill may mimic pregnancy, increasing the need for insulin. Intrauterine contraceptive devices may lead to infection and are not recommended for most diabetic women.
- If there has been poor diabetic control, the baby may be large and plethoric and birth injuries may occur. The baby may be physiologically immature and have problems similar to those of a preterm baby.
- High maternal blood glucose levels in utero encourage the fetal pancreas to produce more insulin. This hyperinsulinaemia continues after birth, creating neonatal hypoglycaemia which will require stabilising, perhaps by intravenous glucose. Other neonatal problems are skin infections and polycythaemia with hyperbilirubinaemia.
- Graves' disease accounts for 95% of cases of hyperthyroidism seen in about 0.2% of pregnancies. Thyrotoxicosis may be difficult to diagnose if it arises for the first time in pregnancy. Failure to gain weight despite a good appetite, a rapid sleeping pulse and lid lag should raise the possibility.
- Improvements may occur in pregnancy. If antithyroid drugs are used, their effects must be monitored carefully to avoid too high levels of drug treatment. A partial thyroidectomy may be necessary if there is failure to control the disease or the woman has a large goitre.
- Inadequately managed thyrotoxicosis is associated with severe pre-eclampsia and maternal heart failure. A thyroid storm with high maternal morbidity and mortality rate may occur if there is stress. Thionamide treatment of Graves' disease can suppress fetal and neonatal thyroid function, causing a transient hypothyroidism in the neonate.
- Neonatal hyperthyroidism may occur in women who have been treated by surgical or radioiodine ablation of the thyroid. These women should be treated with thyroxine to maintain their normal thyroid function and thionamides to treat the baby using its heart rate as a guide. The baby's thyroid function will return to normal within 3 weeks.
- Maternal hypothyroidism may be due to Hashimoto's disease, viral thyroiditis or congenital absence of the thyroid gland. It may result from a defect in the thyroid gland or in the control pathway of TRH or TSH release. Dietary iodine deficiency may be a cause. Hypothyroidism in pregnancy may be secondary to immune disorders or follow destruction of thyroid tissue. Treatment is by thyroxine medication.
- Addison's disease is mainly caused by autoimmune destruction of the adrenal glands. In pregnancy it is treated by oral hydrocortisone 20–30 mg/day. In an acute episode, intravenous hydrocortisone is necessary.
- Women with congenital adrenal hyperplasia who remain undiagnosed tend to be hirsute and infertile. Girls treated with hormones in childhood and adolescence have a fertility rate of 64%. Masculinisation of the pelvis causes cephalopelvic disproportion and can be a serious problem.
- The symptoms of phaeochromocytoma, which include hypertension, postural hypotension, sweating, palpitations and tachycardia, anxiety, nausea and vomiting, are treated medically until the fetus is viable, when surgical removal of the tumour is carried out.

References

Anastassiosis, G.P., 2008. Diabetes Mellitus: Diagnosis and Pathophysiology. Tuftsopencourseware Tufts University <http://ocw.tufts.edu/Content/14/lecturenotes/265878/>.

Ben-Haroush, A., Yogev, Y., Hod, M., 2004. Epidemiology of gestational diabetes mellitus and its association with type 2 diabetes. Diabet. Med. 21 (2), 103–113.

Bewley, C., 2004. Medical conditions complicating pregnancy, Ch. 46. In: Henderson, C., Macdonald, S. (Eds.), Mayes Midwifery, thirteenth edn. Baillière Tindall, London, p. 793.

Blackburn, S.T., 2007. Maternal, Fetal and Neonatal Physiology, third edn. W B Saunders, Philadelphia, Ch. 13.

BNF (British National Formulary), 2007. March 53. Angiotensin-converting enzyme inhibitors, p. 99; Treatment of diabetic nephropathy and neuropathy, p. 369.

Brook, C.G.D., Marshall, N.J., 2001. Essential Endocrinology, fourth edn. Blackwell Science, Oxford.

Chilvers, C., 1993. Breast-feeding and risk of breast cancer in young women, United Kingdom case control study group. BMJ 507, 17–20.

Clausen, T., Burski, T.K., Øyen, N., Godang, K., Bollerslev, J., Henriksen, T., 2005. Maternal anthropometric and metabolic factors in the first half of pregnancy and risk of neonatal macrosomia in term pregnancies. A prospective study. Eur. J. Endocrinol. 153 (6), 887–894.

Coad, J., Dunstall, M., 2005. Anatomy and Physiology for Midwives, second edn. Elsevier Mosby, Edinburgh, Ch. 9.

Cumming, R., Klineberg, R., 1993. Breast-feeding and other reproductive factors and the risk of hip fractures in elderly women. Int. J. Epidemiol. 22 (4), 684–691.

Ehrenberg, H., Mercer, B., Catalano, P., 2004. The influence of obesity and diabetes on the prevalence of macrosomia. Am. J. Obstet. Gynecol. 191 (3), 964–968.

Evers, I.M., de Valk, H.W., Visser, G.H.A., 2004. Risk of complications of pregnancy in women with type 1 diabetes: nationwide prospective study in The Netherlands. BMJ 328, 915.

Feig, D.S., Palda, A., 2002. Type 2 diabetes in pregnancy: a growing concern. Lancet 359, 1690–1692.

Galindo, A., Burguillo, A.G., Azriel, S., Fuente, P., de, L., 2006. Outcome of fetuses in women with pregestational diabetes mellitus. J. Perinat. Med. 34 (4), 323–331.

Gilbert, C., Valois, M., Koren, G., 2006. Pregnancy outcome after first trimester exposure to metformin: a meta-analysis. Fertil. Steril. 86 (3), 658–663.

Hague, W.M., 2001. Endocrine disease (including diabetes). Best Practice & Research Clin. Obstet. Gynaecol. 15 (6), 877–889.

Homco, C.J., Reece, E.A., 2006. Insulins and hypoglycaemic agents in pregnancy. J. Matern. Fetal Neonatal Med. 19 (11), 679–686.

Homco, C.J., Sivan, E., Reece, A.E., 2004. Is there a role for oral antihyperglycaemics in gestational diabetes and type 2 diabetes during pregnancy? Treat. Endocrinol. 3 (3), 133–139.

Jevitt, C., Morse, S., O'Donnell, Y.S., 2008. Shoulder dystocia: nursing prevention and post-trauma care. J. Perinat. Neonatal Nurs. 22 (1), 14–20.

Kaaja, R., Loukovaara, S., 2007. Progression of retinopathy in type 1 diabetic women during pregnancy. Curr. Diabetes Rev. 3 (2), 85–93.

King, J.C., 2006. Maternal obesity, metabolism, and pregnancy outcome. Annu. Rev. Nutr. 26, 271–291.

Kjos, S.L., 2007. After pregnancy complicated by diabetes: postpartum care and education. Obstet. Gynecol. Clin. North Am. 34 (2), 335–349.

Lao, T.T., 2005. Thyroid disorders in pregnancy. Curr. Opin. Obstet. Gynecol. 17 (2), 123–127.

Landon, M.B., 2007. Diabetic nephropathy and pregnancy. Clin. Obstet. Gynecol. 50 (4), 998–1006.

Lauszus, F., Klebe, J.G., Bek, T., 2000. Diabetic retinopathy in pregnancy during tight metabolic control. Acta Obstet. Gynecol. Scand. 79, 367–370.

McLaughlin, G., Cheng, Y., Caughey, A., 2006. Women with one elevated 3-hour glucose tolerance test value: are they at risk for adverse perinatal outcome? Am. J. Obstet. Gynecol. 194 (5), e16–e19.

Metzger, B.E., Buchanan, T.A., Coustan, D.R., de Leiva, A., Dunger, D.B., et al., 2007. Summary and Recommendations of the Fifth International Workshop–Conference on Gestational Diabetes Mellitus. Diabetes Care 30, S250–S251. Online: <http://care.diabetesjournals.org/cgi/content/full/30/Supplement_2/S251/>.

Modder, J., 2006. CEMACH report on pregnancy risk in women with diabetes. Br. J. Midwifery 14 (1), 44–45.

Montagnana, M., Lippi, G., Targher, G., Fava, C., Guidi, G.C., 2008. Glucose challenge test does not predict gestational diabetes. Intern. Med. 47 (13), 1171–1174.

NICE, 2008. Diabetes in Pregnancy. NICE Guideline No. 63. Website: <www.nice.org.uk/>.

Pearson, D.W., Kernaghan, D., Lee, R., Penney, G.C. Scottish Diabetes in Pregnancy Study Group, 2007. The relationship between pre-pregnancy care and early pregnancy loss, major congenital anomaly or perinatal death in type 1 diabetes mellitus. Br. J. Obstet. Gynaecol. 114 (1), 104–107.

Porterfield, S.P., White, B.A., 2007. Endocrine pancreas, diabetes mellitus, Ch. 5. In: Endocrine Physiology, third edn. Mosby, St Louis.

Reader, D.M., 2007. Medical nutrition therapy and lifestyle interventions. Diabetes Care 30 (Suppl), S188–S193.

Sacks, D.A., 2006. Pre-conception care for diabetic women: background, barriers, and strategies for effective implementation. Curr. Diabetes Rev. 2 (2), 147–161.

Saunders, R., 2002. Casualties of war. Balance (Diabetes UK) 189, 42–44.

Shelley-Jones, D.C., Wein, P., Nolan, C., Beischer, N.A., 1993. Why do Asian-born women have a higher incidence of gestational diabetes? An analysis of racial differences in body habitus, lipid metabolism and the serum insulin response to an oral glucose load. Aust. N. Z. J. Obstet. Gynaecol. 33 (2), 114–118.

Stenhouse, E., 2007. Diabetes: monitoring and managing. Midwives 10 (11), 520–521.

Tortora, G.J., Grabowski, S.R., 2000. Principles of Anatomy and Physiology. Wiley, New York.

Turner, M., 2007. Hyperemesis gravidarum: providing woman-centered care. Br. J. Midwifery 15 (9), 540–541.

Vitoratos, N., Salamalekis, D., Kassanos, D., et al., 2000. Hyperemesis gravidarum: its relationship to maternal immune response and thyroid function. Prenat. Neonatal Med. 5, 363–367.

Wallace, T.M., Matthews, D.R., 2004. Recent advances in monitoring the management of diabetic ketoacidosis. QJM 97 (12), 773–780. Online: http://qjmed.oxfordjournals.org/cgi/content/full/97/12/773; accessed September 2008.

Whittaker, K.M., 2001. Breast-feeding and the diabetic mother. Br. J. Midwifery 9 (8), 484–488.

WHO, 2008. Diabetic Fact Sheet No. 312. Website: <http://www.who.int/mediacentre/factsheets/fs312/en/index.html/>.

Annotated recommended reading

Hague, W.M., 2001. Endocrine disease (including diabetes). Best Practice & Research Clin. Obstet. Gynaecol. 15 (6), 877–889.

This paper gives an excellent overview of all the endocrine disorders, including diabetes mellitus, their effects on pregnancy and their current management.

Lao, T.T., 2005. Thyroid disorders in pregnancy. Curr. Opin. Obstet. Gynecol. 17 (2), 123–127.

A good review of thyroid disease in pregnancy.

Metzger, B.E., Buchanan, T.A., Coustan, D.R., de Leiva, A., Dunger, D.B., et al., 2007. Summary and Recommendations of the Fifth International Workshop–Conference on Gestational Diabetes Mellitus. Diabetes Care 30, S251–S250. Online: <http://care.diabetesjournals.org/cgi/content/full/30/Supplement_2/S251/>.

A report on the 5th International Workshop–Conference on Gestational Diabetes, includes discussion into pathophysiology and diagnosis of GDM and implications for future research.

Turner, M., 2007. Hyperemesis gravidarum: providing woman-centered care. Br. J. Midwifery 15 (9), 540–541.

This is a good paper, discussing all aspects of hyperemesis.

Section **3A**

Labour—Normal

SECTION CONTENTS

Perhaps the most challenging aspect of childbearing is the birth. Midwives within the UK are privileged to be the major carer during this short but intensively meaningful time in the life of a woman and her family. There is no denial of the importance in relation to the social and psychological aspects of this major life event, but these chapters concentrate on the management of labour that arises from a deep knowledge of physiology. Chapter 36 examines what is currently known about the causes of the onset of labour. Currently there is a rise in the number of babies delivered by caesarean section, with a decline in spontaneous vertex birth. If a return to more normal birth is to be achieved it is imperative that midwives understand the progress and management of normal labour. Therefore, there is a chapter dedicated to each of the so-called three stages of labour, although the authors recognise that labour is a continuum. Chapter 37 discusses the physiology and management of the first stage of labour; Chapter 38 is dedicated to the important topic of pain relief in labour. Chapters 39 and 40 discuss the second and third stages of labour, respectively.

Chapter Thirty-Six

36

The onset of labour

CHAPTER CONTENTS

Introduction

The main issues about providing care for women in labour are how to meet the social, psychological and spiritual needs and how to provide physiological safety for the woman and her baby. A major problem for anyone courageous enough to research the field of human behaviour, especially in physiological terms, is to place such behaviour in the context of cultural influences.

A great number of textbooks devoted to the social meaning of pregnancy and labour are worth reading for anyone considering how the management of childbearing is influenced by major changes and beliefs of society.

The purpose of this chapter is to examine the physiological concepts associated with normal uncomplicated labour so that the reader can make informed decisions on the management of labour based on current concepts and theories.

Timing of the onset of labour

Normal labour occurs between 37 and 42 weeks gestation (Johnson 2007). However, in humans the timing of the onset of labour is less precise than in many other species, with the mean timing being 39.6 weeks with a range of 3 weeks on either side of the mean. The timing may be related to fetal brain activity via **adrenocorticotrophic hormone** (ACTH) and the pituitary–adrenal axis. Progesterone is then metabolised to oestrogen, which gradually increases the sensitivity of the uterus to prostaglandins and oxytocin produced by both the fetoplacental unit and maternal tissues. Large numbers of research projects into the onset of labour in cattle, sheep and humans have found that, when there is an abnormality of the fetal hypothalamus and pituitary area of the brain, extreme prolongation of pregnancy may occur (Johnson 2007, Steer & Johnson 1998).

Two major physiological changes are necessary for the expulsion of the fetus to proceed smoothly. First, the cervix must go through a structural change called softening or ripening which changes its role from support to birth canal. Secondly, myometrial tone must change to allow coordinated contractions of the body of the myometrium (assisted later in labour by contractions of striated muscles in the abdominal wall) to increase uterine pressure (Johnson 2007).

The aetiology of labour is complex and at present is not fully understood and therefore there are numerous hypotheses and theories. Consequently, an outline only of key areas of discussion is given. If the sequence of events leading to the onset of labour were fully understood it might be easier to prevent the onset of preterm labour and the devastating fetal loss and morbidity resulting from extreme immaturity. There is good evidence for a central role for **prostaglandins** in the initiation of labour (Karim 1966) but the composition and biosynthesis of prostaglandins by the various tissues remains unclear (see below).

The role of the fetal endocrine system

There is evidence to support the concept that the fetus is largely responsible for triggering the onset of labour. However, there is still uncertainty about the role of the fetal hypothalamus–pituitary–adrenal axis in the initiation of labour in humans. It has become apparent that the extrapolation of experimental findings from one species to another is not reliable, as events may differ between species. In sheep, parturition is initiated by a surge of cortisol secreted by the fetal adrenal cortex. This acts on placental enzymes to convert progesterone to oestrogen (Coad & Dunstall 2005). The rapid change in steroid balance stimulates the release of prostaglandins from both the placenta and the myometrium. There is increased sensitivity of the myometrium to form oxytocin receptors which are sensitive to the hormone oxytocin, and there is a reduction of the hormone progesterone, which has maintained uterine quiescence, therefore uterine contractions are produced which are powerful enough to expel the fetus (Marieb 2009).

The adrenal cortex

Johnson (2007) has summarised the research findings and suggests it is unlikely that increased production of cortisol plays a major part, as labour begins in the congenital absence of the fetal adrenals. Cortisol levels measured in the umbilical cord blood after delivery are difficult to assess, as they may increase because of the stress of labour rather than be responsible for initiating labour. Scalp blood cortisol measurements made in early labour showed no difference in spontaneous or induced labour, although there was a rise in fetal plasma cortisol as labour progressed. There is no dramatic rise in total cortisol level in fetal circulation prior to the onset of labour.

The administration of corticosteroids such as **betamethasone** to women in late pregnancy results in a fall in maternal circulating oestrogen levels but there is little effect on the placental progesterone synthesis or the duration of pregnancy. In the human placenta, although **glucocorticoids** do not induce the fall in progesterone and rise in oestrogen leading to labour, they are involved in the maturation of the fetus, in particular the fetal lung, allowing survival of a fetus born 6 weeks early.

In sheep, cortisol produces both organ maturity and the onset of labour and a lamb born even 1 week or 2 weeks early may be too immature to survive.

One hormone that may be implicated in fetal control of the onset of labour is **dehydroepiandrosterone sulphate** (DHAS), which is the major precursor of placental estradiol and estrone synthesis. The human fetal adrenal gland is relatively large at birth with a fetal zone occupying 80% of the cortex and being responsible for the size. The function of the adrenal cortex is different in the fetus from the adult and the fetal zone atrophies after birth. It has been found that human chorionic gonadotrophin (hCG) is a major stimulator of the fetal zone during pregnancy and ACTH can also stimulate the production of DHAS.

The fetal posterior pituitary gland

Higher concentrations of the posterior pituitary hormones vasopressin and oxytocin have been found in the umbilical circulation than in the maternal circulation. Although the source of this fetal oxytocin is not clear, the levels are higher in fetal arterial blood than venous blood, which suggests fetal origin. It is possible that as much as 1–3 mU/min of oxytocin is transferred from fetus to mother, which is enough to promote uterine activity at term. An argument against the fetal role is that labour almost always follows fetal death in utero, depending on the gestational age of the fetus. Possibly the release of prostaglandins is more important and the mechanism of release differs when the fetus is dead, being provoked by the massive fall in progesterone level that accompanies fetal death.

The role of the placenta

Progesterone

It is now over 35 years since Csapo put forward a hypothesis that labour is initiated by the withdrawal of the progesterone block on myometrial activity. It has been difficult to prove or disprove this hypothesis (Steer & Johnson 1998). All attempts to use progesterone to prolong labour, postpone preterm labour or to prevent early abortion have been unsuccessful. Measurement of progesterone levels in the peripheral blood of women has not shown any withdrawal of progesterone at the end of pregnancy. However, this may not be significant if the progesterone acts locally and it may be an alteration in the binding of progesterone that is important rather than the level.

Oestrogens

Placental production of **oestrogens** rises as pregnancy progresses and DHAS of both maternal and fetal origin contributes to the placental production of oestrogens, most importantly of estradiol. However, women do go into labour without a rise in the concentration of estradiol and there is no dramatic rise in the levels of estradiol just prior to the onset of labour. It is probable that estradiol facilitates rather than causes the onset of labour. As yet, there is no clear evidence that changing concentrations of oestrogens and progesterone alter at the onset of labour. However, these changes in balance between the two steroid hormones facilitate increasing myometrial activity.

Fetal membranes

Steroid hormones

The fetal membranes are known to have a relatively high concentration of progesterone. Both the chorion laeve and the amnion have been shown to contain enzymes that can reduce the level of progesterone and also both chorion and amnion contain a protein which increases towards the end of pregnancy and that can bind progesterone. These two mechanisms would produce a local progesterone withdrawal effect. However, the membranes are avascular and any substance produced by them must travel by diffusion.

Prostaglandins

The amnion and chorion are both involved in the production of **prostaglandins**. Karim (1966) first suggested that prostaglandins play a role in the initiation of labour. It is still unclear whether prostaglandins initiate labour or maintain it. Findings from earlier studies have been unusable because of prostaglandin production by tissue trauma during sample collection. Making measurements of prostaglandins is extremely difficult as storage or temperature can affect the findings. Drugs such as aspirin act as **prostaglandin inhibitors**, preventing the first step in the metabolism of **arachidonic acid**. The fetal membranes contain significant amounts of arachidonic acid and research indicates that the membranes are significantly involved in the synthesis of prostaglandins, but once again there seems to be no significant change at the onset of labour.

Maternal influences

The decidua

The decidua within the endometrium is also implicated in the production of prostaglandins. Evidence suggests that the decidua is a major source of prostaglandins during labour. In the 1970s Gustavii studied the role of the decidua in controlling the onset of labour (Steer & Johnson 1998). Gustavii (1977) proposed that the decidual cells have lysosomes which contain **phospholipase A$_2$**, an enzyme necessary for the synthesis of prostaglandins. These lysosomes are fragile and degenerate under the influence of oestrogen in late pregnancy when progesterone levels fall and oestrogen levels rise. Steer & Johnson (1998) find this hypothesis useful in the explanation of the onset of labour at term.

Work carried out by Keirse and his colleagues in the 1970s showed that the primary prostaglandins present were PGE$_2$ and PGF$_{2\alpha}$. The precursor of the two prostaglandins is an essential fatty acid called arachidonic acid which is derived from glycerophospholipids and involves several stages of conversion by enzymes. Both these prostaglandins and other PGEs are known to stimulate myometrial contractions (Johnson 2007). Production rates of prostaglandins in decidual cells may be 30 times greater in labour than at elective caesarean section.

The endocrine system

The ovaries are not necessary for the initiation of labour and it seems that maternal oxytocin from the pituitary gland plays little part in the initiation of labour. The maternal adrenal glands do not seem to play any part in labour.

Neurohormonal control

James Ferguson, a Canadian physiologist, discovered that if the cervix is stretched it increases the production of oxytocin and subsequently increased uterine activity (Banting Research Foundation 2003). The **Ferguson reflex**, as it is termed today, is a neurohormonal reflex (Fig. 36.1) arising from the genital tract, which may be involved in the release of both oxytocin and prostaglandin in labour (Johnson 2007). The release of oxytocin could lead to increasing prostaglandin production as it does in some animal species. If this were so, then administration of epidural analgesia should block the spinal part of the reflex and oxytocin release, resulting in prolongation of the first stage of labour. Since there is no evidence to suggest this happens, prostaglandin release in human labour probably does not involve oxytocin release.

Control of cervical changes in labour

It is absolutely necessary that uterine contractions are coordinated with cervical dilatation. The increasing pressure placed on the cervix by the presenting part during active labour is said to aid dilatation of the cervix by the mechanism of Ferguson's reflex described above. Uterine contractions alone cannot bring about cervical softening and cervical dilatation. Changes in the collagen content of the cervix must occur and evidence is that it is the hormone estradiol that brings about the change. Prostaglandins also play a part in the ripening of the cervix and are often used prior to the induction of labour if the cervix is unfavourable.

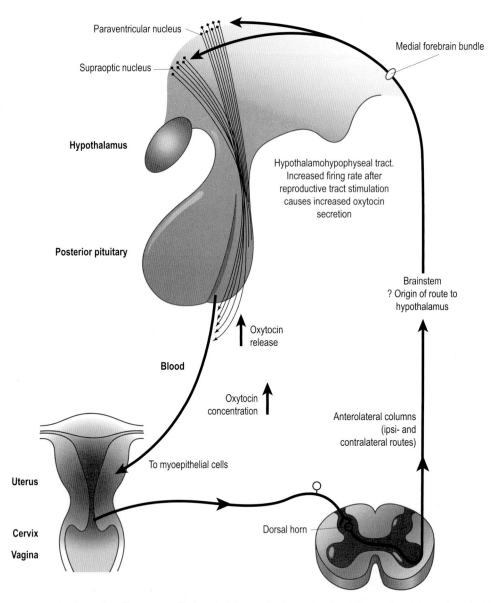

Paraventricular nucleus

Supraoptic nucleus

Medial forebrain bundle

Hypothalamus

Hypothalamohypophyseal tract.
Increased firing rate after
reproductive tract stimulation
causes increased oxytocin
secretion

Posterior pituitary

Brainstem
? Origin of route to
hypothalamus

Oxytocin
release

Blood

Oxytocin
concentration

Anterolateral columns
(ipsi- and
contralateral routes)

To myoepithelial cells

Uterus

Dorsal horn

Cervix

Vagina

Figure 36.1 • The neuroendocrine reflex (Ferguson reflex) underlying oxytocin synthesis and secretion. (Reproduced with permission from Johnson & Everitt 1995.)

Definitions of labour

The previous section considered the role of the myometrium, decidua, fetus, placenta and membranes in the initiation of labour and the maintenance of contractions resulting in progress. This progress must be achieved without compromising maternal or fetal safety. The key concepts associated with labour are defined below:

- Labour is the process by which the fetus, placenta and membranes are expelled through the birth canal.
- Normal labour is spontaneous in onset at term, with the fetus presenting by the vertex, and is completed within 18 h with no complications arising.

- Although labour is ultimately a continual process for the ease of education it can be subdivided into three stages:

  1. **Stage 1** begins with the onset of regular rhythmic contractions and is complete when the cervix is fully dilated. This stage can be further subdivided into the latent, active and transitional stages.

  2. **Stage 2** begins when the cervix is fully dilated and ends with complete expulsion of the fetus.

  3. **Stage 3** begins following expulsion of the fetus and ends when the placenta and membranes are expelled and control of any bleeding.

Each of these three stages of labour will be explored in more depth in Chapters 37, 39 and 40.

The causes of onset of labour have been discussed above and the timing is important as it allows decisions to be made about the progress and ongoing management of labour, yet it is difficult to establish with accuracy. The concept of pre-labour relates to the changes that occur in the last few weeks of pregnancy (Gibb 1988). It is often difficult to decide when the transition from the painless uterine contractions of pre-labour develop into true labour. The length of labour is variable and may be affected by parity, birth interval, psychological state, presentation and position, pelvic shape and size and the type of uterine contractions.

Maternal physiological adaptation in labour

The physiological changes in labour are examined separately from the process of labour so that sufficient depth can be achieved.

Cardiovascular system

There are profound changes in the cardiovascular system due to the effect of uterine contractions. The woman's emotional response to labour may affect the cardiovascular system, especially in primigravidae. The first stage of labour is associated with a progressive rise in cardiac output as each contraction adds 300–500 ml of blood to the circulating blood volume; thus during pregnancy the cardiac output rises by about 50% (Blackburn 2007). These changes are limited by epidural analgesia or supine position and by alleviation of pain and anxiety. Epidural analgesia appears to prevent the progressive increases in cardiac output while supine positioning lowers the cardiac output, decreases stroke volume but causes a compensatory increase in heart rate.

Pain, anxiety and apprehension may add to this effect, causing an increase in systolic and diastolic blood pressure and heart rate by increasing sympathetic tone. Blood pressure begins to rise 5 s before the contraction begins and returns to its baseline after the contraction has ended. During the first stage of labour there may be a rise in blood pressure of 35 mmHg systolic and it may rise even higher in the second stage. The diastolic pressure can rise 25 mmHg in the first stage of labour and up to 55 mmHg in the second stage. There is only a small change in peripheral vascular resistance in labour so the increase is probably due to the transient rise in cardiac output during the contraction.

Following the delivery of the fetus, placenta and membranes, there may be cardiovascular instability because of dramatic haematological changes. The changes occur because of blood loss at delivery and compensatory mechanisms. Within 10 min of the delivery, cardiac parameters fall to pre-labour levels and may then take up to 4 weeks to return to pre-pregnancy levels.

Haematological system

There are changes in the haematological system and haemostasis to ensure that blood loss is kept to a minimum and tolerated. Haemoglobin levels tend to increase slightly in labour because of haemoconcentration. This is related to an increase in erythropoiesis (formation of red blood cells) due to stress, muscular activity and dehydration. White blood cell (WBC) count increases during labour and immediately postpartum and may reach levels of 25–30×10^9/L. This is mainly due to an increase in neutrophils and is a probable response to stress.

The hypercoagulable state that is present in pregnancy is further magnified in labour (Coad & Dunstall 2005). There is a transitory increase in the activity of the coagulation system during and immediately after placental separation so that clot formation in the torn blood vessels is maximised and blood loss from haemorrhage minimised. However, it also increases the risk of disseminated intravascular coagulation and thrombosis (Coad & Dunstall 2005). The placenta and decidua are rich in thromboplastin and release of this factor during separation activates coagulation via the extrinsic system.

There is also a decrease in fibrinolytic activity, enhancing clot formation at the placental site. The placental site is rapidly covered by a fibrin mesh which utilises about 5–10% of the circulating fibrinogen. Levels of fibrin/fibrinogen degradation products rise after delivery, increasing the risk of coagulation disorders in the immediate postpartum period.

Respiratory system

Maternal acidosis

There is an increase in the work of the uterine and other muscles during labour and therefore a greater need for oxygen. Alterations in ventilation and acid–base status occur. If the contractions are occurring too frequently, there will be a decrease in the oxygenation of the myometrium with resulting metabolic acidosis. In the presence of strong, frequent uterine contractions, ischaemia and the resulting tissue hypoxia will occur with an increase in P_{CO_2} because of the change to anaerobic metabolism leading to a fall in pH (maternal acidosis). The ischaemia will increase the pain experienced during contractions.

In the second stage of labour pain will lead to an increase in respiratory rate and tidal volume (Coad & Dunstall 2005). Maternal P_{CO_2} may rise during pushing and also due to the use of voluntary muscles during bearing down. Fetal P_{CO_2} will rise if the mother is acidotic because the build-up of maternal P_{CO_2} will prevent placental transfer to the mother of fetal P_{CO_2}. This will lead to significant fetal acidosis and distress.

Maternal alkalosis

In some women there is a tendency to hyperventilation, leading to respiratory alkalosis. This appears to be mainly caused by pain. Anxiety, drugs, breath-holding, panic and excessive use of breathing exercises learned in the antenatal period will also add to the likelihood of hyperventilation. The end result will be a fall in P_{CO_2} and a level of 25 mmHg can commonly occur. Blackburn (2007) reports that levels as low as 17 mmHg have been seen in women during painful contractions. The woman may complain of tingling of the fingers and toes and dizziness due to overbreathing. She should be encouraged to change her respiratory rate, to lower it if necessary, to breathe when breath-holding is inappropriate and to deep breathe if oxygen is needed, such as between contractions.

Renal system

The renin–angiotensin systems of mother and fetus are altered during labour and delivery. There is an increase in maternal and fetal renin and angiotensin which may be important in reducing uteroplacental blood flow following delivery. The changes in pregnancy outlined in Section 2 of the book affect fluid and electrolyte status so that administration of intravenous fluids and their electrolytic content must be carefully monitored to avoid water intoxication. Also, it is important to remember that oxytocin has an antidiuretic effect so that oxytocin infusion during labour reduces water excretion.

Gastrointestinal system

Gastric emptying

Evidence suggests that gastric motility is decreased and gastric emptying is mildly delayed during labour (Blackburn 2007), with or without epidural analgesia. Factors dramatically increasing this delayed gastric emptying include:

- Fear and pain.
- The administration of opioid drugs.
- Intake of food during labour that contains high levels of fibre and fat.

There is also an increase in gastric acidity and relaxation of the cardiac sphincter leading to oesophageal reflux, thereby increasing the risk of aspiration pneumonitis (commonly known as **Mendelson's syndrome**) should a woman require general anaesthesia (Liu 2003). Nutrition and hydration in labour and the prevention of acid aspiration are discussed in the section on clinical implications below.

Metabolism

Generally, prior to labour, women have a degree of respiratory alkalosis and metabolic acidosis and a reduced ability to utilise glucose so that the main source of glucose for the fetus is met. Provision of glucose (gluconeogenesis) from the metabolism of body fat (lipolysis) occurs, causing an increase in plasma ketones throughout pregnancy. Labour has an effect on maternal metabolism and plasma electrolytes and these changes may affect the fetus.

The vigorous contractions of the uterus throughout labour require energy, and glucose is the main substrate for this. Most women have little reserve for aerobic metabolism and glucose stores are quickly used up, especially with the modern tendency to restrict oral intake in labour. The energy cost of active labour is estimated to be between 700 and 1100 calories/h. Compensatory lipolysis occurs to meet the body's energy requirements, resulting in the production of ketones which, in excess, may depress fetal pH and interfere with myometrial activity (Liu 2003). Anaerobic metabolism causes the accumulation of lactate (see Krebs cycle) and this produces a small drop in maternal plasma pH to about 7.34, a reduction in base excess to -5 mEq/L and a fall in P_{CO_2}.

Clinical implications

Recognition of the onset of labour

Women themselves usually recognise that labour has begun, especially if they have received antenatal education about what to expect. The woman may notice a **show**, although this may occur following a vaginal examination in the antenatal clinic. A 'show' is when the operculum plug and blood from the shearing of the cervical vessels become dislodged when the cervix dilates (Coad & Dunstall 2005). **Contractions** which are regular, rhythmic and increase in **length**, **strength** and **frequency** occur but the woman may only be aware of backache with hardening of her uterus. When the presenting part of the fetus is not well applied to the cervix, the membranes may rupture and the woman has a sudden gush of fluid. This must be reported to the midwife immediately as there is a small risk of cord prolapse, although this is very rare. Sometimes women find it hard to distinguish the trickle of amniotic fluid from urine and might seek guidance from the midwife.

Initial examination of the woman

Although this is a book on physiology, it is important to realise that the social and psychological background and approach to care may interfere with the process of labour. This interaction between the mind and body will be discussed in Chapter 57. For now, it is necessary to remember that the approach taken at this initial meeting of the woman and her midwife may influence not only her perception of labour but also her physical progress towards delivery. While it is desirable to provide a meaningful experience for the woman, it is of paramount importance that the physical safety of mother and fetus are ensured. Good history taking and risk assessment is a crucial part of the initial examination of the woman (Lewis 2007, NHS Quality Improvement Scotland 2004). This is the aspect of care that follows below.

The history

When a woman telephones her midwife, information may be obtained allowing the decision to be made either to visit at home, especially if there is to be a home birth, or admit to hospital. If there are no complications and the woman is in early labour, it will be beneficial for her to remain in her own surroundings for the time being. The history of the woman's health, any previous pregnancies and this pregnancy up to the onset of labour should be carefully scrutinised (NICE 2007) for any indications that complications might occur. **True labour** can be recognised by the midwife from what is termed **spurious** or **false** labour by the nature of the contractions and the state of the cervix. In true labour, contractions will show a pattern of increase in length, strength and frequency and the cervix will dilate progressively.

General examination

The general condition of the woman is important and her appearance may indicate aspects of her well-being to the midwife. Her general stance and gait may indicate pain or even imminent delivery. The midwife should look for any abnormality in skin colour such as flushing, pallor or cyanosis which may indicate underlying problems. Her behaviour may indicate how well she is coping with contractions and whether she is anxious or afraid. Observations of temperature, pulse rate and blood pressure, signs of oedema and urinalysis should be taken and recorded (NICE 2007).

Abnormal findings may indicate a problem with the general health of the woman or be associated with an abnormality of labour. If the temperature and pulse rate are elevated, it is necessary to find the cause. Infection may be present and care must be taken to avoid passing this on to other women and their babies. A rise in blood pressure should be reported to the obstetrician. The presence of slight oedema of the feet and ankles may be normal, depending on the time of day, but pretibial oedema or puffiness of the fingers or face, especially if there is a raised blood pressure, may indicate the presence of pregnancy-induced hypertension (PIH). Urine is tested for protein, which may indicate that the woman has had a show or that her membranes have ruptured, both easily confirmed, but may also indicate PIH or urinary tract infection. Glucose and ketones are also tested for and are considered in the light of the woman's past medical history, when she last ate and how her labour is progressing. Assessment of fetal well-being is also conducted and is explored in more depth in Chapter 37.

Assessing progress in labour

When as much detail as possible about the progress of labour prior to admission has been ascertained, the woman is examined to confirm details given verbally and to establish a baseline on which to judge further progress. An abdominal examination is made and this may be followed by a vaginal examination. Vaginal examination in low-risk women is only necessary if it adds further information to the decision making process of the woman's care as it can ultimately cause more distress and discomfort (NICE 2007). The health professional should use their clinical judgement along with a fully informed decision from the woman prior to conducting a vaginal examination. Progress can be considered as a function of descent of the presenting part through the pelvis and dilatation of the cervix. The presence of one in the absence of the other suggests lack of progress and is a cause for concern if this persists. These factors will be discussed in Chapter 37.

Main points

- In humans the timing of the onset of labour is less precise than in many other species and may be related to fetal brain activity via ACTH and the pituitary–adrenal axis. Progesterone is metabolised to oestrogen, which gradually increases the sensitivity of the uterus to prostaglandins and oxytocin produced by both the fetoplacental unit and maternal tissues.

- In humans prostaglandins and oxytocin are implicated in the cervicouterine changes at parturition. Prostaglandins appear to play a central role in the initiation of labour but their composition and biosynthesis by various tissues remains unclear.

- Dehydroepiandrosterone sulphate (DHAS), the major precursor of placental estradiol and estrone synthesis, may be implicated in fetal control of the onset of labour. Higher concentrations of the posterior pituitary hormones vasopressin and oxytocin have been found in the umbilical circulation than in the maternal circulation. The source of this fetal oxytocin is not clear but the levels are higher in fetal arterial blood than in venous blood, which suggests a fetal origin.

- One argument against the fetal role is that labour almost always follows fetal death in utero, depending on the gestational age of the fetus. Possibly the release of prostaglandins is more important, being provoked by the massive fall in progesterone level that accompanies fetal death.

- Placental production of oestrogens rises as pregnancy progresses but women go into labour without a rise in the concentration of estradiol and there is no dramatic rise just prior to the onset of labour. There is no clear evidence to suggest that concentrations of oestrogens and progesterone alter at the onset of labour, but changes in balance between them facilitate increasing myometrial activity.

- Fetal membranes have a relatively high concentration of progesterone. Both the chorion and amnion contain enzymes that can reduce the level of progesterone and both chorion and amnion contain a protein which increases towards the end of pregnancy and which can bind progesterone. The debate continues as to whether prostaglandins initiate labour or maintain it.

- Uterine contractions are coordinated with cervical dilatation. The increasing pressure placed on the cervix by the presenting part during active labour is said to aid dilatation of the cervix by the mechanism of the Ferguson reflex, which may be involved in the release of both oxytocin and prostaglandin in labour. Prostaglandin release in labour seems not to involve oxytocin release.

- Uterine contractions alone cannot bring about cervical softening and cervical dilatation. Changes in the collagen content of the cervix must occur and evidence is that it is the hormone estradiol that brings about the change. Prostaglandins also play a part in the ripening of the cervix.

- Normal labour is spontaneous in onset at term with the fetus presenting by the vertex and is completed within 18 h with no complications arising. Factors affecting the length of labour include parity, birth interval, psychological state, presentation and position, pelvic shape and size and the type of uterine contractions.

- There are profound changes in the cardiovascular system due to the effect of uterine contractions. The woman's emotional response to labour may affect the cardiovascular system, especially in primigravidae. Pain, anxiety and uterine contractions may cause an increase in blood pressures and heart rate. Within 10 min of delivery, cardiac parameters fall to pre-labour levels and may take up to 4 weeks to return to pre-pregnancy levels.

- Vital signs, blood pressure, signs of oedema and urinalysis findings should be recorded for baseline levels. Abnormal findings may indicate a problem with the general health of the woman or be associated with an abnormality of labour.

References

Banting Research Foundation, 2003. Available: http://www.utoronto.ca/bantresf/HallofFame/Ferguson.html/ (accessed 8.6.08).

Blackburn, S.T., 2007. Maternal, Fetal and Neonatal Physiology: A Clinical Perspective, fourth edn. Elsevier Saunders, St Louis.

Coad, J., Dunstall, M., 2005. Anatomy and Physiology for Midwives, second edn. Elsevier Churchill Livingstone, London.

Gibb, D., 1988. A Practical Guide to Labour Management. Blackwell Science, Oxford.

Gustavii, B., 1977. Human decidual and uterine contractility. In: Chamberlain, G., Broughton Pipkin, F. (Eds.), Clinical Physiology in Obstetrics, third edn. Blackwell Science, Oxford.

Johnson, M.H., 2007. Essential Reproduction, sixth edn. Blackwell, Cambridge.

Karim, S.M.M., 1966. Identification of prostaglandins in human amniotic fluid.

J. Obstet. Gynaecol. Br. Commonw. 73, 903.

Lewis, G. (Ed.), 2007. Saving Mothers Lives: The Seventh Report of the Confidential Enquiries into Maternal and Child Health 2003–2005. RCOG, London.

Liu, D.T.Y., 2003. Labour Ward Manual, third edn. Churchill Livingstone, Edinburgh.

Marieb, E.N., 2009. Essentials of Human Anatomy and Physiology, ninth edn.

Pearson Benjamin Cummings, San Francisco.

NHS Quality Improvement Scotland (NHS QIS), 2004. Maternal History Taking. Best Practice Statement, NHS QIS, Edinburgh.

NICE (National Institute for Health and Clinical Excellence), , 2007. Intrapartum Care: Care of Healthy Women and Their Babies during Childbirth Guideline No. 55. NICE, London, http://www.nice.org.uk.

Steer, P.J., Johnson, M.R., 1998. The genital system. In: Chamberlain, G., Broughton Pipkin, F. (Eds.), Clinical Physiology in Obstetrics, third edn. Blackwell Science, Oxford.

Annotated recommended reading

Blackburn, S.T., 2007. Maternal, Fetal and Neonatal Physiology: A Clinical Perspective, fourth edn. Elsevier Saunders, St Louis.

This book covers physiological changes that occur throughout the perinatal period, with the emphasis on the mother, fetus and the neonate and the relationship between them. It provides an in-depth study of the major body systems.

Johnson, M.H., 2007. Essential Reproduction, sixth edn. Blackwell, Cambridge.

This text provides a detailed account of parturition and the fetus and its preparation for birth.

Chapter Thirty-Seven

37

The first stage of labour

Introduction

It is essential to understand the physiology of any system or process to inform observations and care. One problem of caring for women in labour is to define the acceptable parameters for progress and maternal and fetal responses so that women view the experience as being satisfactory while safety is assured. In the past these parameters were arbitrarily decided by empirical methods but, more appropriately, research is being increasingly utilised. Practitioners have a duty to women to ensure that they read widely, develop a discerning mind and deliver evidence-based practice.

Physiology of the first stage of labour

Uterine activity in labour

In early labour, contractions may be 15–20 min apart and are fairly weak, lasting for about 30 s. These may not be recognised as labour pains by the woman for a while. In established labour, the uterus contracts 3–4 times every 10 min, and in advanced labour each contraction may last 50–60 s and is powerful. Contractions can be measured in mmHg (millimetres of mercury) by the pressure they exert on the amniotic fluid. This is called the **intrauterine hydrostatic pressure**. The resting pressure exerted by the muscular myometrium is about 5 mmHg. In pregnancy, the intensity of uterine contractions may reach 30 mmHg and up to 60–80 mmHg in labour.

Several concepts are described in relation to uterine activity in labour. The spread of each contraction across the uterine muscle is thought to begin in the fundus near the cornua, spreading outwards and downwards, remaining most intense in the fundus and being weakest in the lower uterine segment, a phenomenon known as **fundal dominance**. The spread of myometrial electrical activity to its maximum takes about 1 min and the same time is taken for the wave of contraction to pass off. This allows progressive dilatation of the cervix and, as the upper segment thickens and shortens, the fetus is propelled down the birth canal. During contractions, the upper and lower poles of the uterus act in harmony, with contraction and retraction of the upper **pole**, and dilatation of the lower pole to allow expulsion of the fetus. This is known as **polarity**.

Uterine muscle in labour has the unique property of **contraction** and **retraction** (Fig. 37.1). Following each contraction, the muscle fibres do not completely relax but retain some of the shortening of contraction. This is called **retraction** and leads to the progressive shortening and thickening of the upper uterine segment (UUS) and the diminishing of the uterine cavity to accommodate the descending fetus. A physiological ridge forms between the UUS and the lower uterine segment (LUS), known as a **retraction ring** (see Ch. 44 for the abnormal **Bandl's ring** which is an exaggerated pathological retraction ring that develops in obstructed labour and becomes visible above the symphysis pubis).

Effacement or 'taking up' of the cervix is the term used to describe the gradual mergence of the cervix into the LUS. In primigravidae, this process is sometimes complete before the onset of labour and before dilatation of the external cervical os occurs (Fig. 37.2A). In multigravidae, a perceptible cervical canal remains until labour is well established, a finding midwives refer to as a 'multip's os'. During labour there is **dilatation** of the external os until it is large enough for the widest diameter of the presenting part to pass through (Fig. 37.2B). In a fetus at term presenting by the vertex, the diameter of the cervix would normally have to reach 10 cm but this would be less in a fetus with a smaller head. As the cervix begins to dilate, the operculum or mucous plug formed in pregnancy is lost around the time of the commencement of labour and the woman will notice a

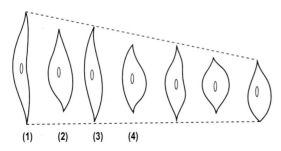

Figure 37.1 • Retraction of the uterine muscle fibres. (1) Relaxed. (2) Contracted. (3) Relaxed but retracted. (4) Contracted but shorter and thicker than those in (2). (From Henderson C, Macdonald S 2004, with kind permission of Elsevier.)

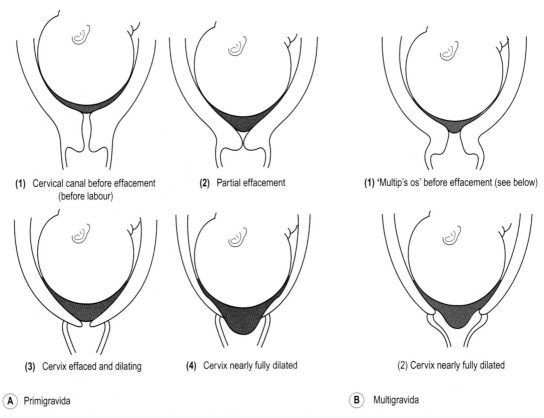

(1) Cervical canal before effacement (before labour)

(2) Partial effacement

(1) 'Multip's os' before effacement (see below)

(3) Cervix effaced and dilating

(4) Cervix nearly fully dilated

(2) Cervix nearly fully dilated

(A) Primigravida

(B) Multigravida

Figure 37.2 • (A) Effacement and dilatation of the cervix in a primigravida. (B) Effacement and dilatation of the cervix in a multigravida.

mucoid discharge, which may be blood-stained. This is termed the **show**. The blood originates from ruptured capillaries when the lining of the cervix is stretched or where the chorion has become detached from the dilating cervix.

Mechanical factors

Besides uterine action, there are mechanical forces that aid dilatation of the cervix. As the lower uterine segment is stretched, the chorion is detached from it. In normal labour the increased intrauterine pressure during contractions forces a well-flexed head snugly against the cervix, trapping a small amount of amniotic fluid in front of the head separate from the rest of the fluid surrounding the body of the fetus. This small sac of fluid is known as the **forewaters** and the rest of the fluid as the **hindwaters**. The forewaters bulge through the cervix, becoming more tense during contractions (Fig. 37.2A-4/B-2). This separation of the forewaters from the larger volume of the hindwaters keeps the membranes intact during the first stage of labour, providing a barrier against ascending infection.

When the membranes remain intact, the pressure of each contraction is exerted on the fluid and, as fluid is not compressible, pressure is equalised throughout the uterus. This is known as **general fluid pressure** (Fig. 37.3). If the membranes are ruptured and amniotic fluid is reduced, contraction pressure is applied directly to the fetus. The placenta is compressed between the uterine wall and the fetus, which further reduces the oxygen supply to the fetus. Therefore, there are two good reasons for maintaining intact membranes: to reduce the risk of infection and to maintain a good oxygen supply to the fetus. In a systematic review of 14 studies (4893 women) exploring amniotomy in labour, Smyth et al (2007) did not find any evidence of a statistical difference in length of first stage of labour, maternal satisfaction with childbirth experience or low Apgar score of <7 at 5 min. However, amniotomy was associated with an increased risk of delivery by caesarean section compared to women in the control group. The physiological moment for the membranes to rupture is when the cervix is fully dilated and no longer able to support the forewaters and the force of the uterine contractions reaches maximum. The evidence remains clear that routine amniotomy during the first stage of labour can never be justified as standard care in normal low-risk women (NICE 2007, Smyth et al 2007).

During each contraction, the force of the fundal contraction is transmitted to the upper pole of the fetus, down the long axis of the fetal spine, causing increasing flexion of the head. This ensures that the smallest possible circumference, which is the circular vertex, is applied to the circular cervical os. This is known as **fetal axis pressure** (Fig. 37.4).

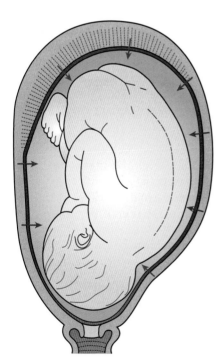

Figure 37.3 • General fluid pressure. (From Fraser & Cooper 2009, with kind permission of Elsevier.)

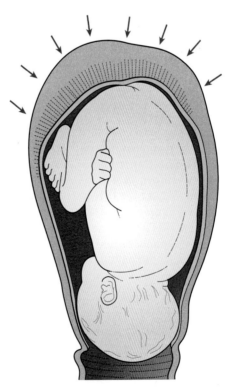

Figure 37.4 • Fetal axis pressure. (From Fraser and & Cooper 2009, with kind permission of Elsevier.)

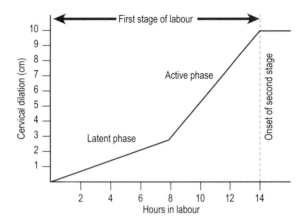

Figure 37.5 • A cervicograph. (From Henderson C, Macdonald S 2004, with kind permission of Elsevier.)

Phases of the first stage of labour

The present understanding of labour is based on the work of Emanuel A Friedman. He developed the graphic representation of labour by plotting cervical dilatation and descent of the presenting part against time. In normal labour, the rate of dilatation of the cervix follows a sigmoid-shaped curve. There are three distinct parts:

1. An initial part where there is little progress in cervical dilatation, which Friedman called the **latent phase**.

2. A part of the curve where there is rapid progress in dilatation, called the **active phase**.

3. A part of the curve where dilatation slows, called the **deceleration phase** (also termed the **transitional phase**).

The latent phase, which lasts until cervical dilatation is about 3–4 cm, can take 6–8 h in a primigravida. The active phase occurs with rapid dilatation of the cervix at about 1 cm/h in a primigravida and 1.5 cm/h in a multigravida. The length of established first stage of labour varies between women. First labours last on average 8 h and are unlikely to last over 18 h. Second and subsequent labours last on average 5 h and are unlikely to last over 12 h (NICE 2007). Plotting the rate of cervical dilatation has been commonly carried out in labour (a **cervicograph**), an average duration is indicated in Figure 37.5.

Individualised care

Childbearing experience for women encompasses both a biological and a social event. The midwife should carefully consider these aspects when planning care with the labouring woman. This should include the following:

- Assess the woman's needs and expectations, using a clear risk-assessment strategy.

- Plan care accordingly to meet the specific needs and expectations.
- Carry out the plan.
- Evaluate the effect of the care and modify it if necessary.

The physiological aspects of care in labour include assessing progress, positioning of the woman, nutrition and hydration and monitoring the condition of woman and fetus.

Assessing progress in the first stage of labour

When as much detail as possible has been ascertained about the progress of labour prior to admission, the woman is examined to confirm details given verbally and to establish a baseline on which to judge further progress. An abdominal examination is made and this may be followed by a vaginal examination. Progress can be considered as a function of descent of the presenting part through the pelvis and dilatation of the cervix. The presence of one in the absence of the other may suggest lack of progress and is a cause for concern.

Abdominal examination in labour

Most of the aims of abdominal examination, considered by Viccars (2003) in the context of antenatal care, apply equally well to labour. These are to assess fetal size and well-being, to diagnose the location of fetal parts—in particular, lie, presentation, position and engagement—and to detect any deviation from normal. Abdominal examination should always be carried out prior to performing a vaginal examination (if required) and repeated abdominal examinations can be used to assess descent of the presenting part.

Inspection

The size and shape of the uterus can be of value in ensuring that there is a normal longitudinal lie. The uterus will appear ovoid in shape. In the rare instance of a transverse lie, the uterus may appear to be low and broad. If there is a saucer-shaped depression below the umbilicus, the fetus may be lying in an occipitoposterior position. Fetal movements may be seen and can help in the diagnosis of position.

Palpation

The following terms are used to describe fetal palpation:

- **Lie**: The relationship of the long axis of the fetus and the long axis of the uterus. It may be longitudinal, oblique or transverse.

- **Presentation**: That part of the fetus which lies at the pelvic brim or in the lower pole of the uterus. This is usually cephalic but other possible presentations include breech, face, brow and shoulder.
- **Attitude**: The relationship of the fetal head and limbs to its body. It may be fully flexed, deflexed or partially or completely extended.
- **Denominator**: Identifies the name of the part of the presentation used when referring to fetal position in relation to the pelvis. Each presentation has a different denominator: occiput for cephalic presentation; sacrum for breech presentation; and mentum for face presentation.
- **Position**: The relationship of the denominator to six key points on the maternal pelvic brim. These points are right and left anterior, right and left lateral, and right and left posterior. However, a further two points could be direct anterior and direct posterior.
- **Engagement of the fetal head**: This occurs when the widest presenting transverse diameter has passed through the brim of the pelvis, i.e. biparietal diameter of 9.5 cm in cephalic presentation.

Practitioners often get the terms 'presentation' and 'presenting part' confused. The presenting part refers to that part of the fetus that lies over the cervical os during labour and on which the caput succudaneum may form (e.g. in a cephalic presentation); the presenting part would be the posterior part of the anterior parietal bone (Downe 2003).

Fundal palpation (Fig. 37.6A) (taking into account the overall size of the uterus) allows a judgement of the gestational age to be made (Fig. 37.7). It is also a necessary part of determining the lie of the fetus (Fig. 37.8).

Lateral palpation (Fig. 37.6B) is used to locate the fetal back to determine position. The length and frequency of contractions should be noted by palpation rather than by the reaction of the woman. The hardness of the abdomen may give a good indication of the strength of the contractions.

Pelvic palpation (Fig. 37.6C) using both hands identifies the presenting part (Fig. 37.9) and the amount of flexion (Fig. 37.10), and engagement of the head can be assessed by estimating the amount of head still present above the pelvic brim. If the head is engaged, it will be possible to feel less than half the fetal head above the pelvic brim and the head will not be mobile. It may not be possible to palpate the occiput if the head is deeply engaged (Fig. 37.11). Engagement is a good sign and indicates that the bony pelvis is adequate for the passage of the fetus and a vaginal delivery should follow. Stuart (2003) summarises descent of the head by abdominal assessment, which can be described in fifths of the head felt above the pelvic brim. Determination of the level of the fetal head by abdominal palpation excludes the variability due to caput and moulding and that produced by a different depth of pelvis.

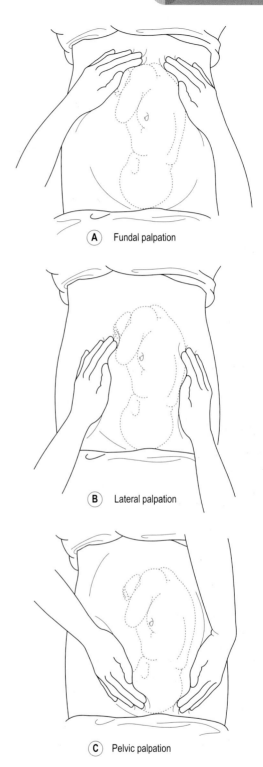

(A) Fundal palpation

(B) Lateral palpation

(C) Pelvic palpation

Figure 37.6 • Types of palpation per abdomen. (A) Fundal, (B) Lateral, (C) Pelvic. (From Henderson C, Macdonald S 2004, with kind permission of Elsevier.)

Auscultation

Listening to the fetal heart is an important part of any abdominal examination as it enables the practitioner to make an assessment of fetal well-being. The point of maximum intensity is located by considering the position of the fetus (Fig. 37.12). As labour progresses and descent takes place, the point of maximum intensity will change. Therefore the position of the Pinard's stethoscope on the abdomen will also change to ensure the best possible clarity of the fetal heartbeat in assessing, rate, rhythm and frequency. Continuous monitoring of the fetal heart may be necessary where there is doubt about fetal well-being.

Vaginal examination in labour

Vaginal examination has been routine practice for generations to assess progress in labour. The rationale for why vaginal examination is required in a low-risk situation is still unclear, with evidence to support it being unnecessary and a traumatic experience for women (NICE 2007). With good physiological knowledge of labour, healthcare professionals can use their skills in deciphering progress rather than using intervention. The purple line which creeps up the 'natal cleft' (cleavage between the buttocks) can be used as a measure of cervical dilatation (Byrne & Edmonds 1990). Hobbs (2003) proposes that this non-intervention method would be a useful tool

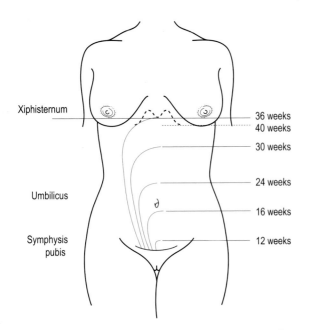

Figure 37.7 • The height of the fundus at different stages of pregnancy. (From Henderson C, Macdonald S 2004, with kind permission of Elsevier.)

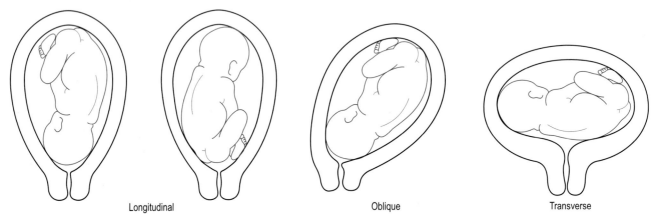

Longitudinal   Oblique   Transverse

Figure 37.8 • The lie of the fetus. (From Henderson C, Macdonald S 2004, with kind permission of Elsevier.)

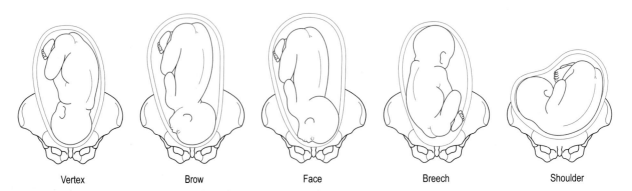

Vertex   Brow   Face   Breech   Shoulder

Figure 37.9 • The presentation of the fetus. (From Henderson C, Macdonald S 2004, with kind permission of Elsevier.)

to adopt in low-risk situations. At the start of labour the 'purple-red line' begins at the anal margin and gradually creeps up the anal cleft (much like mercury in a thermometer) as cervical dilatation occurs. Vaginal examinations in low-risk women are only necessary if they add further information to the decision-making process of the women's care as these examinations can ultimately cause more distress and discomfort (NICE 2007). Health professionals should use their clinical judgement along with a fully informed decision from the woman prior to conducting a vaginal examination. Low-risk

women with a strong history of pre-labour spontaneous rupture of membranes should not be offered a speculum examination routinely, but if there is any uncertainty then a speculum examination should be offered. However, if no uterine contractions are present then a digital vaginal examination should be avoided (NICE 2007).

It is acknowledged that vaginal examinations are not always required in labour. The following rationale for conducting a vaginal examination in labour are suggested:

• To make a positive identification of presentation.
• To determine whether the head is engaged if there is doubt.
• To ascertain whether the forewaters have ruptured or to rupture them artificially.
• To exclude cord prolapse if the forewaters rupture and the presenting part is high.
• To assess progress or delay in labour.
• To confirm full dilatation of the cervix.
• In multiple pregnancy, after the birth of the first baby, to confirm the lie and presentation of the second fetus and to rupture the second amniotic sac.

There is a way in which such a list, while comprehensive, does not do justice to the value of a well-performed

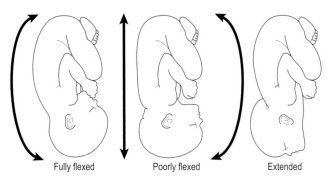

Fully flexed   Poorly flexed   Extended

Figure 37.10 • The attitude of the fetus. (From Henderson C, Macdonald S 2004, with kind permission of Elsevier.)

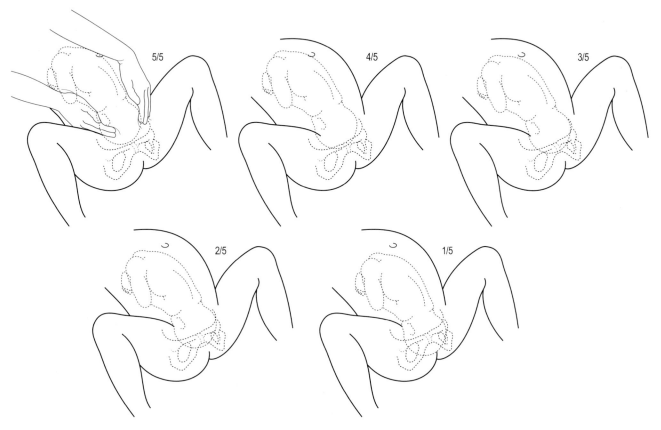

Figure 37.11 • Examination per abdomen to determine the descent of the fetal head in fifths. (From Henderson C, Macdonald S 2004, with kind permission of Elsevier.)

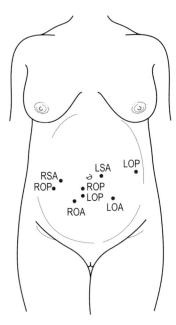

Figure 37.12 • The approximate points of the fetal heart sounds in vertex and breech presentations. ROA, right occipitoanterior; ROP, right occipitoposterior; LOA, left occipitoanterior; LOP, left occipitoposterior; RSA, right sacroanterior; RSP, right sacroposterior; LSA, left sacroanterior; LSP, left sacroposterior.

and carefully timed vaginal examination. Firstly, it is the combination of abdominal and vaginal findings that enables a clear picture of the progress in labour to be made; secondly, continuous careful observation of the woman will enable the avoidance of unnecessary vaginal examinations. Lai & Levy (2005) inform us that although women accept the need for vaginal examination they also wish to be treated with dignity and respect by the examiner and that it is also important to have the findings communicated to them.

In any clinical examination it is sensible to use the same order of findings each time. This ensures that there is less chance of missing an important feature. It is also important to continue with the examination until satisfied in all aspects, as it is essential to keep the number of vaginal examinations to a minimum to minimise the risk of infection and distress to the woman. The practitioner should adhere to local policies and procedures with regard to aseptic or non-aseptic technique as in some instances if the woman has intact membranes it is a clean procedure; however, if the membranes are ruptured full aseptic technique should be used to prevent the risk of infection to both woman and fetus.

The concept of a 'quick VE' is both futile and dangerous and should not be conducted! Contraindications to vaginal examinations are (Bowen & Taylor 2005):

- Bleeding per vaginum.
- Placenta praevia.
- Preterm rupture of membranes, preterm labour.

Findings

The following order is suggested for the performance and recording of a vaginal examination.

External genitalia

Prior to inserting fingers into the vagina, the external genitalia should be inspected as some findings may influence the course and management of labour. The labia should be examined for any varicosities or warts and the presence of oedema. The perineum should be inspected for scarring which could indicate a previous tear or episiotomy and, in some cultures, female circumcision. Signs of vaginal discharge or bleeding and, if the membranes have ruptured, the colour and quantity of any amniotic fluid should be recorded. Any offensive odour should be reported as this is likely to indicate the presence of infection.

Condition of the vagina

The normal vagina in labour should feel warm and moist. It is very rare but not impossible that the implications of a prolonged labour with obstruction would be seen. Women who have been cared for in pregnancy and have sought care early in their labour should never present with a hot and dry vagina. A cystocele and/or rectocele may be present in a multiparous woman. A loaded rectum can be easily felt through the posterior vaginal wall.

Condition of the cervix

The cervix is palpated for length, consistency and dilatation to diagnose the length of the cervical canal and the degree of effacement. The position of the cervix relative to the fetal presenting part is noted: if it is in the normal central position or in early labour can be very posterior. A long closed cervix may indicate early stages of labour or that labour has not begun. The cervix in labour should feel soft and elastic and will usually be applied closely to the presenting part. A primigravidae cervix has been described as the consistency of the nose, whereas the parous cervix has been described as the consistency of the lips.

Assessing the dilatation of the cervical os

The two examining fingers are gently inserted into the vagina and the cervical os is located. The fingers are then inserted into the os and parted gently to assess the diameter of cervical os dilatation in centimetres. This should be done gently to minimise discomfort to the woman. The cervix should be palpated in every direction, by a circular movement of the examining fingers to ensure a complete circle or that no lip of cervix remains; in particular, when assessing full cervical dilatation. Intact membranes can be felt through the dilating os.

They feel a little like clingfilm and become tense during a contraction. If the membranes are absent, the slightly rougher fetal scalp can be felt.

Level or station of the presenting part

The level of the presenting part is judged in relation to the ischial spines so that descent of the fetus through the pelvis can be monitored. The distance above or below the ischial spines is estimated in centimetres above or below the ischial spines (Fig. 37.13). If there is a caput succedaneum, care must be taken to establish the level of the bony skull above the swelling.

The presentation

In 96% of cases this will be vertex and easily confirmed. Only rarely will it be difficult to confirm presentation on vaginal examination and this usually indicates a very abnormal labour or even more rarely a fetal abnormality such as an encephalocele which may have slipped through the vaginal os and feel too soft to be a head.

Position

Landmarks such as sutures and fontanelles on the fetal skull can be felt to diagnose or confirm the position of the presenting part (Fig. 37.14). The most commonly identified landmark is the sagittal suture as it is found in a vertex presentation (Fig. 37.15). It is identifiable by moulding that occurs with the leading anterior parietal bone overriding the posterior parietal bone and is usually in one or other of the oblique diameters. The

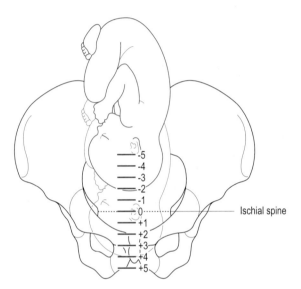

Figure 37.13 • The stations of the head. Descent in relation to the maternal ischial spines is expressed in centimetres. (From Henderson C, Macdonald S 2004, with kind permission of Elsevier.)

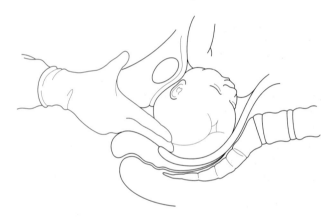

Figure 37.15 • Identifying the sagittal suture and fontanelles during examination per vaginam. (From Henderson C, Macdonald S 2004, with kind permission of Elsevier.)

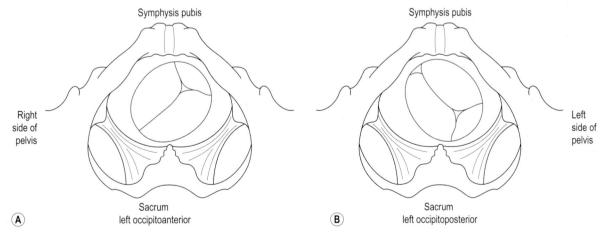

Figure 37.14 • Identifying the position of the fetus. (A) Left occipitoanterior: the sagittal suture is in the right oblique diameter of the pelvis. (B) Left occipitoposterior: the sagittal suture is in the left oblique diameter of the pelvis. (From Henderson C, Macdonald S 2004, with kind permission of Elsevier.)

posterior fontanelle can be identified because of its small size and the three sutures that leave it. The anterior fontanelle is larger, diamond-shaped and has four sutures leaving it.

Moulding of the fetal skull

Moulding is described in Chapter 24. The most important aspect is to make a judgement on whether the amount of moulding is normal or excessive, suggesting disproportion between the fetal skull and the bony pelvis.

Pelvic capacity

An estimation of pelvic size has probably been made antenatally but the practitioner responsible for the safe conduct of the delivery should make her own estimation of the pelvic outlet by assessing the ischial spines and the angle of the subpubic arch. Prominent ischial spines often accompany a pubic arch that is less than 90° and the features suggest an android pelvis.

Fetal heart rate

An assessment of the fetal heart should always be made after the vaginal examination is completed, especially if the membranes are ruptured, to ensure that the examination has had no adverse effect on the fetus.

Maternal position in the first stage of labour

Mobility and positions for labour and delivery have been an area of interest for a number of years. Where appropriate, most labouring women are encouraged to move about in labour and adopt the position they find to be most comfortable while still maintaining safety (Hughes 2003). Women remaining mobile in labour (Fig. 37.16) have shown this to be a core attribute of physiological labour (Gould 2000). As well as adding to the discussion on placental perfusion, it is proposed that there is better alignment between the descending presenting part and the pelvic brim so that engagement of the presenting part is facilitated and, in occipitoposterior presentation, rotation of the occiput to the anterior may be helped.

Labour normally begins with the fetal head in **asynclitism**. This means that the head is tilted so that one of the parietal bones enters the pelvis first. This tilting facilitates passage of the fetal head through the pelvic inlet. Once through the inlet, the head shifts to **synclitism** so that the vertex presents as the head descends further through the pelvis. Encouraging women with firm abdominal muscles to adopt forward leaning positions can promote the fetal head to adopt more favourable

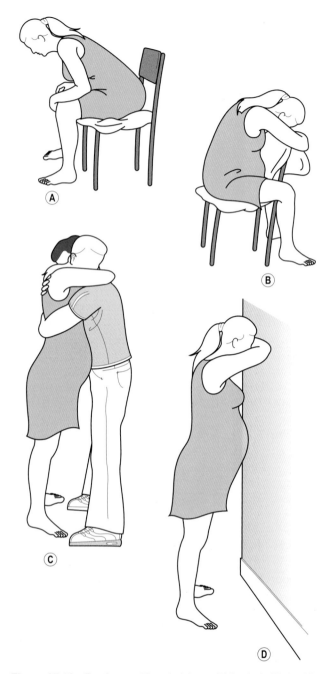

Figure 37.16 • Resting positions in labour. (A) In chair. (B) Astride chair. (C) Supported by partner. (D) Leaning. (Illustrations courtesy of Jim Morrin 1993.)

positions (Simkin & Ancheta 2005). The forces of gravity may also lead to better application of the presenting part to the cervix, promoting the Ferguson reflex. The strength and length of uterine contractions are increased, leading to a more rapid dilatation of the cervix; the supine position should be avoided as it can compromise uterine blood flow (Enkin et al 2000). Women who remain ambulant and adopt an upright posture during labour report a greater level of maternal satisfaction, perceive less pain and backache and often request delivery in an upright position for a subsequent labour (Enkin et al 2000, Walsh 2000).

Immersion in water

Immersion of the body in warm water has been in use for decades and is acceptable to many women. Although its main use is for relaxation and pain relief it may also shorten the labour and decrease the need for augmentation. The warmth of the water relaxes the muscles and enhances a state of mental relaxation, with women reporting a greater sense of satisfaction (Nikodem 2002) and a greater sense of control over their labour (Hall & Holloway 1998). There may be a decrease in the release of the stress hormones such as catecholamines, resulting in better uterine perfusion and more efficient contractions (Schorn et al 1993). The woman feels weightless, can support her body in whatever position she prefers and is helped to cope with the discomfort of contractions. However, there may be problems such as unrealistic expectations, restricted choice of analgesia, restriction of mobility, increase in perineal trauma, postpartum haemorrhage, infection to both the woman and the baby and severe blood loss of the neonate due to rupture of the umbilical cord (de Graaf et al 1999). Emergency interventions may be delayed if there is difficulty in getting the woman out of the water. Overall, the reports on the safety aspects for woman and baby have been reassuring (Gilbert & Tookey 1999, Otigbah et al 2000). Cluett et al (2002) conducted a systematic review of the use of water in labour and highlighted that both the woman's perceptions of pain and requirement for pharmacological analgesia are less for women in labour, but they did explain that there were limitations to the quality of the evidence obtained. They did not find any evidence to support poorer outcomes for babies or longer labours although the reviewers did stress that further evidence is required to support birthing in water.

Nutrition and hydration in labour

Nutrition

The nutritional needs of labouring women are poorly understood. The process of labour uses energy and the body stores fat in pregnancy to use as fuel in longer labours (Odent 1998). If insufficient carbohydrate is available, then body fat will be utilised with the release of ketones and the development of ketoacidosis. Prior to admission, women can be advised to take carbohydrate foods such as toast, cereal and plain biscuits. The

main problem with food intake in normal labour is the possible need for the administration of a general anaesthetic. Coupled with the delayed emptying of the stomach and the relative inefficiency of the cardiac sphincter brought about by the influence of progesterone is a risk of inhalation of acid gastric reflux, resulting in **inhalational pneumonitis** (Mendelson's syndrome).

Practices for eating and drinking in labour vary considerably across the world and within the UK (McCormick & Champion 2002). Fasting in labour has been a feature of management since the relationship between anaesthesia and Mendelson's syndrome was established more than 40 years ago. In a review of the literature, Sleutal & Golden (1998) noted that anaesthetic research has focused primarily on gastric emptying and that withholding of food does not necessarily ensure an empty stomach or reduce the acidity of stomach contents. They concluded that, although death due to aspiration pneumonitis is rare, there was little difference on labour and birth outcomes between women who fasted or who did not fast in labour and there was no evidence that fasting improved the outcome for woman and baby. Enkin et al (2000) suggest that there is no need to prevent women from eating and drinking sensible amounts in labour unless there is a reason why an epidural analgesia cannot be administered. Gyte & Richens' (2006) systematic review explored the use of the effects of antacids, H_2 receptor antagonists and dopamine antagonists given routinely to labouring women to prevent gastric aspiration syndrome. They advocate that there is no evidence to support the routine use of these drugs in normal labour to prevent gastric aspiration syndrome.

Policies for eating and drinking in labour may vary between maternity units. Some units continue to have restrictions on eating and drinking in labour, whereas women in other units may be allowed a low-residue, low-fat diet. On the subject of oral nutrition in labour, women who are considered high risk should have clear fluids only. Women considered low risk in the first stage of normal labour can eat and drink from a restricted range of food with characteristics such as low-fat, high-carbohydrate/high-energy, low-fibre and near-isosmolar (Micklewright & Champion 2002). Suggested food and drink includes toast with low-fat spread, jam or honey; cereals with skimmed milk; clear soup; tea with skimmed milk; squash drinks (dilute); and water.

A sensible protocol would be:

- Where there is no risk of general anaesthetic or instrumental delivery, women should be allowed to eat a light diet and isotonic drink as required.
- When narcotic analgesia has been given, oral food should be withheld and sips of water given (NICE 2007).

Hydration

In the early 1990s, work was undertaken to examine four of the situations which may lead to the administration of intravenous fluids in labour (Millns 1991). It was advocated that any administration of fluid in labour should be given intravenously. The following four situations remain relevant for current practice:

1. During the administration of epidural analgesia.

2. For the administration of oxytocic drugs.

3. To correct ketonuria which has occurred because of metabolism of fat stores.

4. To correct dehydration.

Nordstrom et al (1995) examined the effects of maternal glucose administration in labour by comparing continuous infusion of 5% dextrose with 0.9% saline solution. They found a significant rise in maternal and neonatal plasma glucose levels and maternal insulin levels during the administration of 5% dextrose but did not find evidence of fetal hyperinsulinism in healthy term fetuses. No differences were found in either maternal or fetal lactate levels and both regimens seemed to present no risk of increased fetal lactate levels or fetal hypoglycaemia. However, Stratton et al (1995) carried out similar research in women who required the administration of oxytocin. They found significantly lowered serum sodium levels in both women and babies where the oxytocin had been infused in 5% dextrose, suggesting that non-electrolyte solutions administered in labour may lead to hyponatraemia.

Monitoring the maternal condition

Local protocols may vary but observations for maternal monitoring should include the following:

- Maternal temperature should be recorded 4-hourly and the pulse hourly unless there is an indication for more frequent recording.
- In the early part of labour, blood pressure can be taken every 2 h and then hourly as labour progresses.
- Fluid intake should be encouraged and the woman should be encouraged to pass urine regularly to ensure the bladder is empty. Where a woman is compromised— for example, in the case of pre-eclampsia/eclampsia— input and output should be accurately measured and recorded hourly.
- The urine is tested for protein, glucose and ketones. Small amounts of protein in the absence of known hypertensive or renal disease may indicate contamination by show or amniotic fluid. A small amount of ketosis is expected in normal labour and can be

considered part of the physiological adaptation. Large amounts of ketones indicate exhaustion of the energy stores and may lead to uterine inertia if not corrected.

- The psychological response to labour and to pain should be assessed as any stress may interfere with the course of labour (NICE 2007).

Monitoring the fetal condition

The fetus in the first stage of labour

Blood vessels in the myometrium, which supply the fetus with oxygen and nutrients, are compressed during each uterine contraction. Delivery of nutrients and oxygen is impeded when the strength of a contraction exceeds 40 mmHg. Therefore, increased myometrial tone or rapidly occurring contractions may cause fetal hypoxia and distress. When the membranes remain intact, the pressure of each contraction is exerted on the fluid and, as fluid is not compressible, pressure is equalised throughout the uterus; this is known as **general fluid pressure** (see Fig. 37.3).

If the membranes are ruptured and the amniotic fluid is reduced, the pressure of contractions is applied directly to the fetus and the placenta is compressed between the uterine wall and the fetus, further reducing the oxygen supply to the fetus. Although there is a theoretical improvement in oxygenation by the avoidance of aortocaval compression, no research supports a clinical advantage to the fetus from any position taken in labour. The fetus is subjected to compression and hypoxic stress during uterine contractions and, if healthy, tolerates these conditions without a change in heart rate.

Distress in the fetus is indicated by alterations in heart rate, development of acidosis, passage of meconium, presence of excessive moulding and excessive movements. Information about fetal well-being is mainly obtained by recording fetal heart rate and rhythm, either intermittently or continuously. Amniotic fluid is inspected for the presence of meconium and, where the fetal heart rate is abnormal, a fetal blood sample is taken to check the pH of the fetal blood. A pH below 7.2 indicates fetal distress.

Heart rate

Intermittent monitoring

Intermittent monitoring of the fetal heart can be undertaken using Pinard's fetal stethoscope or a Doppler ultrasound apparatus such as Sonicaid. The **rate** is

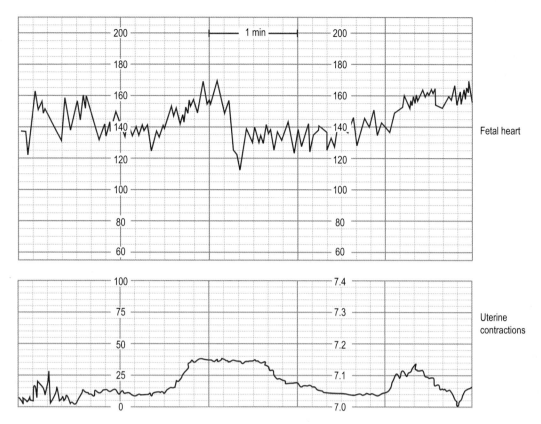

Figure 37.17 • Normal cardiotocograph. The fetal heart rate is normal and reactive. (Courtesy of J A Jordan, Birmingham Maternity Hospital.)

best counted over a full minute after each contraction (NICE 2007) to allow for variations, and should be between 110 and 160 beats/min (bpm). The maternal pulse should also be taken and documented to differentiate between the two heart rates. This is recommended practice (NICE 2007). If a Doppler apparatus is used, the heart rate can be monitored throughout a contraction and the rate should usually be within normal limits. If there is bradycardia, hypoxia may be a problem. The **rhythm** of the fetal heart, as for any heart, is coupled and should remain steady. Any irregularity needs prompt action to establish the cause.

Continuous fetal heart recording

Continuous recording of the fetal heart (**cardiography**) is usually combined with continuous monitoring of maternal uterine activity (**tocography**) by using a **cardiotocograph (CTG) apparatus**. This allows a graphic response of the fetal heart to uterine activity to be recorded (Fig. 37.17). Prior to any form of fetal monitoring being conducted the midwife must listen in with a fetal (pinard) stethoscope to clarify fetal pulse rate (Gauge & Henderson 2005) as sometimes the maternal pulse can be mistaken for the fetal pulse if solely electronic devices are used. A baseline CTG is done for about 20 min, followed by intermittent auscultation. If the fetus is thought to be compromised, continuous monitoring is performed. It is important that an explanation is given to the woman if there is a need for continuous fetal heart monitoring. The woman should discuss antenatally what her feelings are concerning an urgent need to monitor the fetus arising in the course of her labour. National guidelines such as NICE (2007) should be used as a basis for fetal heart monitoring.

External cardiotocography involves strapping on an ultrasound transducer to the abdominal wall over the point of maximum intensity of the fetal heart and the contraction transducer to the fundus of the uterus. The reading can be affected by maternal or fetal movement, the thickness of the abdominal wall and uterine contractions but is non-invasive. Internal cardiography (electrocardiogram) can be used by the application of a fetal scalp electrode to the fetal scalp. Membranes must be ruptured and the cervix should be at least 2–3 cm dilated. Wiring attaches the electrode to the CTG.

Telemetry

If available, internal cardiography can be recorded by a portable battery-operated transmitter used to pick up

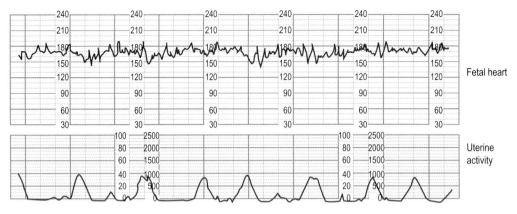

Figure 37.18 • Uncomplicated baseline tachycardia. (Courtesy of Sonicaid, Abingdon, Oxon.)

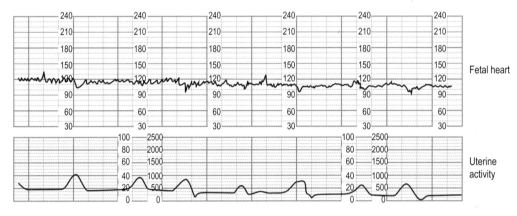

Figure 37.19 • Normal baseline bradycardia. (Courtesy of Sonicaid, Abingdon, Oxon.)

the signal from the fetal heart and the woman can be ambulant (telemetry). However, no recording of uterine activity can be made and the woman is requested to press a button at the onset of each contraction, which will mark the strip chart accordingly.

Findings

The cardiotocograph provides information about:

- Baseline fetal heart rate (FHR).
- Baseline variability.
- Fetal heart response to uterine contractions, i.e. accelerations or decelerations.

Each of the above measurements is now discussed and graphs are used to demonstrate the points and to begin to develop the skills of reading and interpreting recordings.

Baseline fetal heart rate

The definition of the normal range of FHR is 120–160 bpm, but in labour this is often accepted as being 110–160 bpm (NICE 2007). The baseline FHR is the mean level of the FHR between contractions. If the heart rate is more than 160 bpm, it is termed **baseline** tachycardia (Fig. 37.18), while a baseline of less than 110 bpm is called **baseline bradycardia** (Fig. 37.19). These two features, with no other alteration, may indicate hypoxia, but tachycardia may be a response to maternal ketosis, infection or pyrexia. Some fetuses have a normal baseline of between 110 and 120 bpm. However, continuous compression of the cord will cause a prolonged severe bradycardia.

Baseline variability

It is a normal function of the heart to have minute variations in the length of each beat. This is caused by electrical activity varying as a response to the environment and will produce a jagged rather than a smooth line on the graph called **baseline variability** (Fig. 37.20). The baseline rate should vary by at least 5 beats over a period of 1 min. Loss of this (Fig. 37.21) may indicate fetal hypoxia but has also been noted for a short period following the administration of an opioid to the woman, which depresses the cardiac centre in the fetal brain. Gibb (1988) found that periods of 'fetal sleep' will cause a loss of baseline variability lasting for about 20–30 min; sometimes this period can be longer than

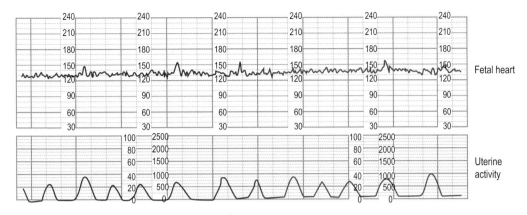

Figure 37.20 • ECG trace showing variability in fetal heart rate. (Courtesy of Sonicaid, Abingdon, Oxon.)

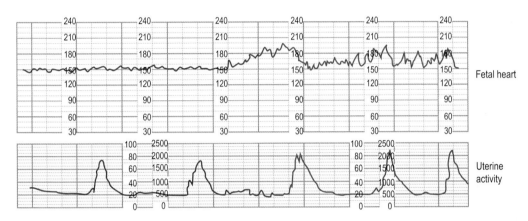

Figure 37.21 • Physiological reduction of baseline variability in fetal heart rate (left). Normal baseline variability (right). (Courtesy of Sonicaid, Abingdon, Oxon.)

30 min. Where there is very poor baseline variability in the absence of accelerations, the obstetrician will perform a fetal blood sampling procedure to ascertain the fetal blood pH. An acceleration is an increase in the fetal heart rate of 15 bpm or more, lasting for at least 15 s and related to fetal movement. Fetal hypoxia may also be indicated in cases of severe accelerations greater than 15 bpm (Gauge & Henderson 2005).

Response of the fetal heart to uterine contractions

It is normal for the fetal heart rate to remain steady or to accelerate during contractions (Fig. 37.22). The relationship of decelerations to the occurrence of uterine contractions must be considered closely to assess their significance. **Early decelerations** (Fig. 37.23) begin at or after the onset of a contraction, reach their lowest point at the peak of the contraction and return to the baseline rate by the time the contraction has finished. They are commonly associated with compression of the fetal head but may be an early sign of hypoxia.

Variable decelerations are inconsistent in shape and in their relationship to uterine contractions. They tend to have an amplitude of 40 bpm or more and accelerations often precede and follow the deceleration (termed shouldering). Variable decelerations are often mistakenly identified as early. These decelerations are related to cord compression (Gauge & Henderson 2005). Management would be to change maternal position and refer as appropriately. If variable decelerations continue they can lead to fetal hypoxia and late decelerations.

A **late deceleration** (Fig. 37.24) begins during or after a contraction, reaches its lowest point after the peak of the contraction and has not recovered by the time the contraction ends. These decelerations are related to uteroplacental insufficiency (Gauge & Henderson 2005). In severe deceleration the heart rate may not have returned to normal by the onset of the next contraction. The **time lag** between the peak of the contraction and the low point of the deceleration is more significant than the actual fall in rate. This always indicates fetal hypoxia and should be treated as an emergency. It is sensible to perform a vaginal examination to

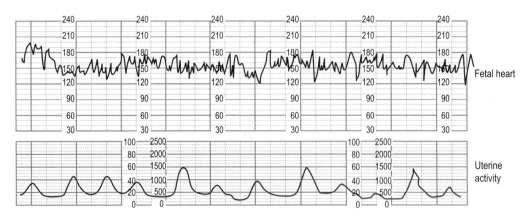

Figure 37.22 • Fetal heart rate accelerations. (Courtesy of Sonicaid, Abingdon, Oxon.)

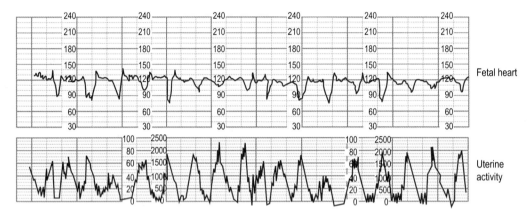

Figure 37.23 • Early fetal heart rate decelerations. (Courtesy of Sonicaid, Abingdon, Oxon.)

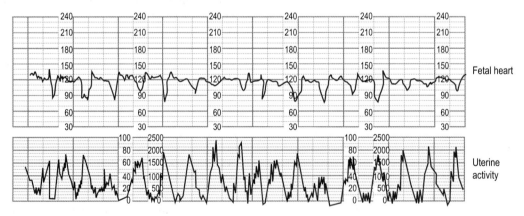

Figure 37.24 • Late fetal heart rate decelerations. (Courtesy of Sonicaid, Abingdon, Oxon.)

assess dilatation of the cervix and exclude cord prolapse prior to informing the obstetrician. The obstetrician will always do a fetal blood sampling procedure in all cases where there are late decelerations.

Fetal blood sampling

Hypoxia will lead to respiratory acidosis and a lowering of blood pH. The normal pH of fetal blood should be 7.35 or above. In the first stage of labour a pH of 7.25 calls for urgent action; in the second stage of labour a level of 7.2 can be accepted if delivery is imminent. Blood is taken by passing an amnioscope through the cervix and using a small blade to puncture the scalp skin (Fig. 37.25). A heparinised capillary tube is used to collect a blood sample for immediate analysis. The blood must not be allowed to clot or come into contact with atmospheric oxygen.

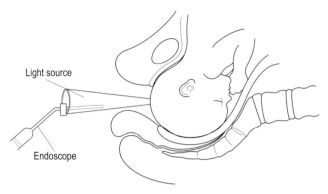

Figure 37.25 • Fetal blood sampling.

Amniotic fluid

If the membranes have ruptured there is a continuous escape of amniotic fluids available for inspection. The fluid should normally remain clear but the fetus may pass meconium; this is common at term but may also be due to fetal hypoxia. Fresh meconium stains the amniotic fluid green and it is likely that the fetus is hypoxic at that time; a muddy yellow colour indicates old meconium. A full discussion on fetal distress and neonatal asphyxia is presented in Chapter 46.

Main points

- In early labour, contractions may be 15–20 min apart and are fairly weak, each lasting about 30 s. In established labour, the uterus contracts every 2.5–3 min, and in advanced labour each contraction may last 50–60 s, with contractions being powerful. Contractions can be measured in mmHg by the pressure they exert on the amniotic fluid.

- Fundal dominance allows progressive dilatation of the cervix and, as the upper segment thickens and shortens, the fetus is propelled down the birth canal. Polarity during contractions allows the upper and lower poles of the uterus to act in harmony with contraction and retraction of the upper pole and dilation of the lower pole. Contraction and retraction of the uterine muscle leads to the progressive shortening and thickening of the UUS and diminishing of the uterine cavity. A retraction ring forms between the UUS and the LUS. The external os dilates until it is large enough for the widest diameter of the presenting part to pass through.

- When the membranes remain intact there is general fluid pressure. If the membranes are ruptured the placenta is compressed between the uterine wall and the fetus, reducing fetal oxygen supply.

- During each contraction, fetal axis pressure causes increasing flexion of the head. This is more significant during the second stage of labour. Upright postures facilitate engagement of the presenting part. Gravity may lead to better application of the presenting part to the cervix, promoting the Ferguson reflex and a rapid cervical dilatation.

- The process of labour uses energy. If insufficient carbohydrate is available, body fat will be utilised, with the release of ketones and the development of ketoacidosis. The main problem with food intake in labour is the possible need for a general anaesthetic and the subsequent risk of inhalation of acid gastric reflux, resulting in Mendelson's syndrome. The practice for eating and drinking in labour varies between maternity units.

- Blood vessels in the myometrium are compressed during each uterine contraction with impeded delivery of nutrients and oxygen when the strength of a contraction exceeds 40 mmHg. Fetal hypoxia and distress may occur, especially if the membranes are ruptured.

- Cardiotocography (CTG) allows recording of the response of the fetal heart rhythm and rate to uterine activity. No research findings support the value of CTG in normal labour. In the first stage of labour, fetal blood with a pH of 7.25 calls for urgent action; in the second stage of labour a pH of 7.2 may be accepted if delivery is imminent.

- If the membranes have ruptured, there is a continuous escape of amniotic fluid, which should normally remain clear. During episodes of fetal distress in labour, hypoxia results and the fetus passes meconium, which stains the fluid green. Presence of meconium requires closer vigilance on the condition of the fetus and the paediatrician should always be present at hospital delivery.

References

Bowen, R., Taylor, W., 2005. Skills for Midwifery Practice, second edn. Elsevier, London.

Byrne, D.L., Edmonds, D.K., 1990. Clinical method for evaluating the first stage of labour. Lancet 335 (8681), 122.

Cluett, E.R., Nikodem, V.C., McCandlish, R.E., Burns, E.E., 2002. Immersion in water in pregnancy, labour and birth. Cochrane Database Syst. Rev. (2) Update Software 2008, Oxford.

Downe, S., 2003. Transition and second stage of labour. In: Fraser, D.M., Cooper, M.A. (Eds.), Myles Textbook for Midwives, fourteenth edn. Churchill Livingstone, Edinburgh.

de Graaf, J.H., Haringa, M.P., Zweens, M.J., 1999. Rupture of umbilical cord in water. Br. Med. J. 319, 483–487.

Enkin, M., Keirse, J., Neilson, J., et al., 2000. A Guide to Effective Care in Pregnancy and Childbirth, third edn. Oxford University Press, Oxford.

Gauge, S., Henderson, C., 2005. CTG Made Easy, third edn. Elsevier, Edinburgh.

Gibb, D., 1988. A Practical Guide to Labour Management. Blackwell Science, Oxford.

Gilbert, R., Tookey, P., 1999. Perinatal mortality and morbidity among babies delivered in water. Br. Med. J. 319, 483–487.

Gould, D., 2000. Normal labour: a concept analysis. J. Adv. Nurs. 31 (2), 418–427.

Gyte, G.M.L., Richens, Y., 2006. Routine prophylactic drugs in normal labour for reducing gastric aspiration and its effects. Cochrane Database Syst. Rev. (3) Update Software 2008, Oxford.

Hall, S., Holloway, M., 1998. Staying in control: women's experiences of labour in water. Midwifery 14 (1), 30–36.

Henderson, C., Macdonald, S. (Eds.), 2004. Mayes' Midwifery: A Textbook for Midwives, Thirteenth edn. Baillière Tindall, London.

Hobbs, L., 2003. Assessing cervical dilatation without VEs. In: Wickam, S. (Ed.), Midwives Best Practice. Elsevier, Edinburgh.

Hughes, D., 2003. Midwives and women: coping with pain together. In: Wickham, S. (Ed.), Midwifery: Best Practice. Elsevier, London.

Lai, C.Y., Levy, V., 2005. Hong Kong chinese women's experiences of vaginal examinations in labour. In: Wickam, S. (Ed.), Midwifery Best Practice, Vol. 3. Elsevier Butterworth-Heineman, Edinburgh.

McCormick, C., Champion, P., 2002. Cultural and historic perspectives on eating and drinking in labour. In: Champion, P., McCormick, C. (Eds.), Eating and Drinking in Labour. Books for Midwives Press, Cheshire.

Micklewright, A., Champion, P., 2002. Labouring over food: the dietician's view. In: Champion, P., McCormick, C. (Eds.), Eating and Drinking in Labour. Books for Midwives Press, Cheshire.

Millns, J.P., 1991. Fluid balance in labour. Curr. Obstet. Gynaecol. 1 (1), 35–40.

NICE, 2007. Intrapartum Care: Care of Healthy Women and their Babies During Childbirth Nice Guideline 55. NICE, London. <http://www.nice.org.uk/>.

Nikodem, V., 2002. Immersion in water during pregnancy, labour and birth. Cochrane Database Syst. Rev. (1) Update Software 2003, Oxford.

Nordstrom, L., Arulkumaran, S., Chua, S., et al., 1995. Continuous maternal glucose infusion during labour: effects on maternal and fetal glucose and lactate levels. Am. J. Perinatol. 12 (5), 357–362.

Odent, M., 1998. Labouring women are not marathon runners. Pract. Midwife 1 (9), 16–18.

Otigbah, C., Dhanjal, M., Harmsworth, G., 2000. A retrospective comparison of water births and conventional vaginal deliveries. Eur. J. Obstet. Gynecol. Reprod. Biol. 9 (1), 15–20.

Schorn, M.N., McCallister, J.L., Blanco, J.D., 1993. Water immersion and the effect on labour. J. Nurse Midwifery 38 (6), 338–342.

Simkin, P., Ancheta, R., 2005. The Labor Progress Handbook, second edn. Blackwell, Oxford.

Sleutal, M., Golden, S., 1998. Fasting in labour: relic or requirement. J. Obstet. Gynecol. Neonat. Nurs. 28 (5), 507–512.

Smyth, R.M.D., Alldred, S.K., Markham, C., 2007. Amniotomy for shortening spontaneous labour. Cochrane Database Syst. Rev. (4) Update Software 2008, Oxford.

Stratton, J.F., Stronge, J., Boylan, P.C., 1995. Hyponatraemia and non-electrolyte solutions in labouring primigravidae. Eur. J. Obstet. Gynecol. Reprod. Biol. 59 (2), 149–151.

Stuart, C.C., 2003. Invasive actions in labour: where have all the 'old tricks' gone? In: Wickham, S. (Ed.), Midwifery: Best Practice. Elsevier, London.

Viccars, A., 2003. Antenatal care. In: Fraser, D.M., Cooper, M.A. (Eds.), Myles Textbook for Midwives, fourteenth edn. Churchill Livingstone, Edinburgh.

Walsh, D., 2000. Evidence based care series 5: Why should we reject the bed myth? Br. J. Midwifery 8 (9), 554–559.

Annotated recommended reading

Byrne, D.L., Edmonds, D.K., 1990. Clinical method for evaluating the first stage of labour. Lancet 335 (8681), 122.
This reference provides further information about the 'purple line' as a non-intervention method for assessing cervical dilatation in labour.

Hobbs, L., 2003. Assessing cervical dilatation without VEs. In: Wickam, S. (Ed.), Midwives Best Practice. Elsevier, Edinburgh.
This chapter provides further information for midwives about the 'purple line' as a non-intervention method for assessing cervical dilatation in labour.

Liu, D.T.Y., 2003. Labour Ward Manual, third edn. Churchill Livingstone, Edinburgh.
This book is a useful reference book for all those working on, or managing, the labour ward.

NICE, 2007. Intrapartum care: Care of healthy women and their babies during childbirth. NICE Clinical Guideline 55. <http://www.nice.org.uk/>.

The guidelines agree with the midwifery concept that childbirth is a normal physiological experience. It informs on caring for low-risk intrapartum women but also highlights high-risk care. The responsibility of maternal and fetal surveillance still remains with health care professionals responsible for the care of labouring woman. These guidelines published by RCOG were reprinted in 2008. There is affiliation with the International Confederation of Midwives (ICM).

Chapter Thirty-Eight

38

Pain relief in labour

Introduction

The experience of pain can be discussed on three levels: pain transmission and perception; pain reception; and pain modulation. Pain is a complex process and is experienced differently depending on the following factors: the physiological process, the context and the previous experience of an individual. Pain can be modulated at different points in the physiological pathway and by education aimed at achieving an understanding of the accompanying events and the meanings attached to them by individuals and by their culture. Walsh (2007) highlights two models of dealing with labour pain (Table 38.1) and informs us that the 'working with the pain relief approach' rather than the 'pain relief approach' would be an important model for midwives to adopt when caring for labouring women. The terminology and philosophy underpinning the approach takes into consideration that pain is a normal physiological process when it comes to childbirth. However, this does not always alter people's perception of pain related to birth.

Pain perception

The nature of pain depends not just on physiological parameters such as the part of the body affected and the extent of the injury but also on the psychological reaction to the pain (Allan et al 1996). McCaffery (1983) reminded us of the cognitive and emotional inputs into pain perception, stating that pain is what the patient says it is and exists when he says it does. Bryant & Yerby (2004) wrote that pain 'is a complex, personal, subjective, multifactorial phenomenon which is influenced by psychological, physiological and sociocultural factors'. In similar fashion, Carlson (2004) reminds us that pain is not purely physical. Pain can be modified by placebo drugs, emotions and other stimuli such as acupuncture. The translation of pain messages into unpleasant feelings ensures that an individual avoids repeating the experience if possible. These are important factors in the management of pain.

Whereas the physiological threshold for pain sensation appears to be similar in all people, the cognitive

Table 38.1 Models of labour pain

Pain relief approach	Working with pain approach
Language suggestive of pain as a problem	Language suggestive of pain as normative
Paternalistic 'we can protect you from uneccessary stress'	Egalitarian empowerment 'we are alongside you'
Techno/rationalism age, pain is preventable/treatable	Labour pain timeless component of 'rite-of-passage' transitions
Neutral impact of environment	Seminal impact of environment
Clinical expertise of professional companions	Supportive role of birth carers
Special session/focus in antenatal education	Woven throughout labour preparation sessions
'Menu approach' to options for coping with pain	Supportive strategies for journey of labour
Pain as a management issue for assembly-line birth	Pain as one dimension of labour care in one-to-one, small-scale birth setting
Contributes to trend of rising birth rates	Contributes to trend of less pharmacological analgesia
Risks of pharmacological agents outweighed by benefits	'Cascade of intervention' dynamic
First birth special case for 'menu approach'	First birth optimal opportunity for 'working with pain'
Informed choice means all options must be presented	Informed choice within context of birthing plan and philosophy

and emotive factors alter the individual's reaction to pain and the meaning attached to the experience. The anticipation of pain increases anxiety levels and the perceived intensity of pain. Hayward (1975) demonstrated that knowledge of events reduces anxiety and pain and this applies to pain in labour. Interesting work has been done by Walding (1991) on the 'locus of control' theory which suggests that pain is perceived as less threatening and with less intensity if women believe they are in control of events. Placing the woman at the centre of her care should therefore make labour less painful and less traumatic, even if problems such as occipitoposterior position occur.

Pain may also increase the level of catecholamines released into the blood. This in turn has the usual result of increased heart and respiration rate with decreased blood flow to the internal organs such as the uterus. The uterus in labour needs a good delivery of oxygen and nutrients to enable efficient contractions, and thus anxiety and fear increase pain, reduce uterine blood supply and may prolong labour.

Pain reception

The principle of pain reception is that several million bare sensory nerve endings weave their way through all the tissues and organs of the body (except the brain) and respond to noxious stimuli.

Marieb & Hoehn 2008

A chemical released from damaged tissue seems to act as a universal pain stimulus. This is **bradykinin**, which in turn releases inflammatory chemicals such as **histamine** and **prostaglandin**. Bradykinin is thought to bind to receptor endings, resulting in an action potential. However, pain perception is much more than the simple sensation relayed by neurons.

Classification of pain

Pain can be classified as somatic or visceral. Somatic pain arising from skin, muscles or joints can be deep or superficial. **Superficial pain** tends to be brief, highly localisable and sharp or pricking in character. This pain is transmitted along large myelinated fibres—the Aδ fibres. **Deep somatic pain** is more likely to be described as burning or aching; it is more diffuse and longer lasting and always indicates tissue destruction. Impulses travel along small unmyelinated fibres called C fibres. A third type of fibre, the myelinated Aβ fibre, relays light touch.

Pain pathways

Visceral pain results from the body's viscera or organs; it is described as burning, gnawing or aching. **Visceral sensory neurons** (afferents) accompany autonomic sympathetic and parasympathetic fibres and send information about chemical changes, distension or irritation of the viscera. Both somatic and visceral pain stimuli pass along the **dendrites** of the **first-order neurons** to their cell bodies in the **dorsal root ganglia**. Their **axons** leave the dorsal root ganglia to enter the spinal cord and synapse with **second-order neurons** in the dorsal horns of the spinal cord. The pain impulse causes the release of the pain neurotransmitter, **substance P**, from the presynaptic membrane into the synaptic cleft.

The anatomy of the dorsal horn

The cells in the spinal cord are arranged in **laminae** (layers) in a dorsal–ventral direction and running the full

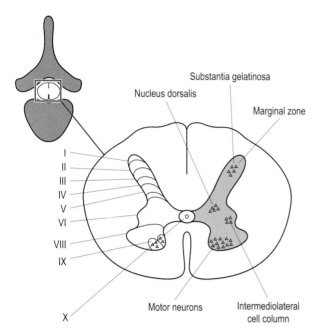

Figure 38.1 • Laminae (I–X) and named cell groups at midthoracic level. (From Montague S E, Watson R, Herbert R A 2005, with kind permission of Elsevier.)

length of the spinal cord (Fig. 38.1). The **dorsal horn** contains six laminae numbered from the tip of the horn inwards. The **ventral horn** contains three other laminae and another column of cells, lamina X, is clustered around the central canal. Laminae I and II are visible to the naked eye as a clear zone and are together called the **substantia gelatinosa**.

Ascending pathways

Sensory fibres returning to the dorsal horns do so in an orderly fashion (Fig. 38.2). The rule is that the thicker the fibre, the deeper it penetrates. The unmyelinated C fibres do not penetrate past lamina II; the small myelinated Aδ fibres mainly terminate in laminae I and II although a few make it to lamina V. The large myelinated fibres from the skin end mainly in laminae IV, V and VI. The specialised large muscle stretch afferents reach level VI (Melzack & Wall 1988).

The axons of most of the second-order neurons cross the cord and enter the **anterolateral spinothalamic tracts** to ascend to the thalamus (Fitzgerald & Folan-Curran 2002). There they synapse with **third-order neurons** to pass the pain message to the **sensory cortex** for interpretation. The second-order fibres may make abundant synapses in the brainstem, hypothalamus and limbic system before reaching the thalamus. This will add a state of arousal and emotion to the perception of pain. The limbic system is the affective (emotional) part of the brain, where emotions and thoughts are closely linked (Marieb & Hoehn 2008). This would explain

why Walsh (2007) argues that 'working with the pain relief approach' model is more advantageous as it deals with these aspects.

Pain modulation

Control systems descending from the brain

Nerve fibres descending in the white matter penetrate into the grey matter and innervate the nearest cells. The dorsolateral column is therefore able to send axons to the most dorsal laminae. In particular, fibres from the **raphe**, the **locus caeruleus** in the reticular formation and from the **hypothalamus** as well as the **pyramidal tract** from the cortex innervate the dorsal laminae III–VI. Descending fibres synapse in the dorsal horns and further modify the final ascending message by releasing endogenous opiates such as endorphins and encephalins into the synaptic cleft (Hughes et al 1975). Endogenous opiates have been shown to inhibit prostaglandin production. Prostaglandin is thought to be a key chemical necessary for pain perception.

The gate control theory of pain

In order to understand the theory of Melzack & Wall (1988), it is necessary to keep the following in mind:

- The ascending and descending tracts in the spinal cord.
- The relative conduction speeds of sensory nerve fibres returning to the spinal cord.
- The anatomy of the dorsal horns of the spinal cord.

Any theory of pain must explain several facts about pain perception (Melzack & Wall 1988):

- The high variability between injury and pain.
- The production of pain by innocuous stimuli.
- The perception of pain in areas seemingly removed from the area of damage.
- The persistence of pain in the absence of injury or after healing.
- The change in the location and nature of pain over time.
- The multidimensional nature of pain.
- The lack of treatment for some types of pain such as arthritic pain and migraines.

Melzack & Wall (1988) described their updated **gate control theory of pain** which they first proposed in 1965 (Fig. 38.3). Although they would emphasise that there is still work to be done to complete their understanding, most people would agree that the gate control theory offers satisfactory explanations for some of the above unusual phenomena.

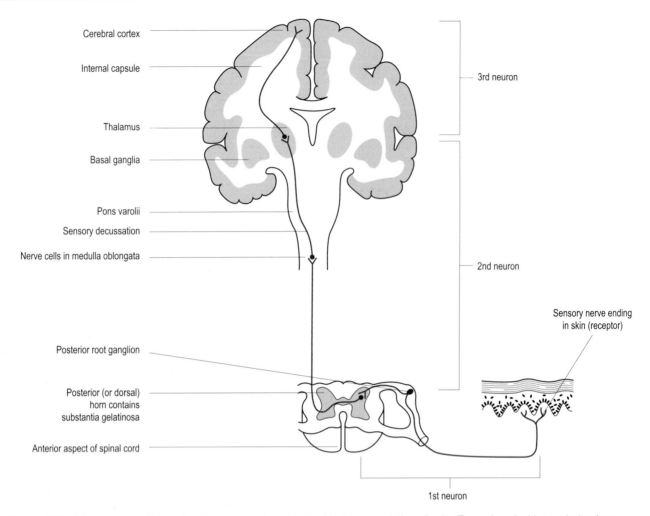

Figure 38.2 • The sensory pathway showing the structures involved in the appreciation of pain. (Reproduced with permission from Bevis 1984.)

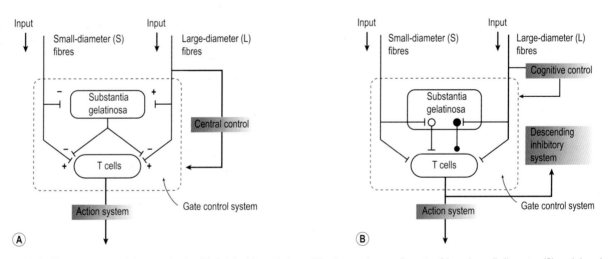

Figure 38.3 • The gate control theory of pain. (A) Original formulation of the theory. Large diameter (L) and small diameter (S) peripheral nerve fibres input to the substantia gelatinosa (SG) and to the first central transmission (T) cells of the spinal cord. The inhibitory effect exerted by the SG on the T cells is increased by activity of the S fibres (pain fibres). The central control mechanisms are represented as running from the L fibre system and feeding back to the gate control. (B) Updated model. On the basis of subsequent evidence, Melzack & Wall formulated the gate control theory to include excitatory (white circle) links from the SG to the T cells, as well as descending inhibitory control from the brainstem. All synaptic connections are excitatory except the inhibitory link from SG to T. The round knob at this inhibitory synapse implies that its action may be presynaptic, postsynaptic or both. (Reproduced with permission from Melzack & Wall 1988.)

The essence of the gate control theory

Gating of the spinothalamic tract response to C fibre activity can be achieved by stimulating large myelinated mechanoreceptor afferents by rub or tickle. These impulses inhibit the ascending pain impulse. Inputs from the large myelinated fibres conveying touch and smaller Aδ and C fibres conveying pain interact at the level of the spinal cord. The large-diameter sensory nerve impulses come into the spinal cord more rapidly. This normally inhibits the slower smaller fibre pain impulses presynaptically. This inhibition constitutes the gate that is normally closed against small-diameter fibre impulses unless the stimulation is so great that it overcomes the gate (Fig. 38.3).

Other modifications of the ascending pain impulse take place in the substantia gelatinosa:

- Interneurons in the substantia gelatinosa can regulate and amplify the impulse conducted to the brain via the ascending pathways.
- Descending fibres synapse in the same area of the spinal cord and further modify the final ascending message by releasing endogenous opiates such as endorphins and encephalins into the synaptic cleft (see above text).
- Virtually all of the brain plays a part in pain perception; the thalamus, reticular system, limbic system and cortex add their effects to the physical, emotional and cognitive experience of pain.

Knowledge of the multidimensional nature of pain perception allows the management of pain to be approached in an equally multidimensional manner. Techniques to inhibit the gate include stimulation of the large nerve fibres so that the pain impulses from the smaller fibres are blocked. Methods include heat, massage and pressure. Transcutaneous electrical nerve stimulation (TENS) works by applying a stimulating electrode to the skin at the level of the noxious C fibre activity and delivering an electrical current sufficient to cause a buzzing sensation (Fitzgerald & Folan-Curran 2002). **Descending fibre impulses** can also inhibit transmission of pain by release of natural opiates and concentration techniques may work in this way (Blackburn 2007).

Visceral sensory neurons

Although the autonomic nervous system (ANS) is considered to be a motor system, there are sensory neurons, mainly visceral pain afferents, in autonomic nerves. These visceral pain afferents travel along the same pathways as somatic pain fibres. Pain perception is referred to the somatic area of the specific dermatome of the surface of the body: for example, the pain of a heart attack is felt in the chest and along the medial aspect of the left arm.

Pain pathways in labour

Both visceral and somatic pain are perceived in labour. Visceral pain is caused by the uterine contractions, the dilatation of the cervix and, later, by the stretching of the vagina and pelvic floor. The body of the uterus is served by autonomic nerves originating in thoracic 11 and 12 and lumbar 1 vertebrae (Fig. 38.4). Sensation from the body of the uterus is perceived as pain in response to stretch, infection and contraction and possibly ischaemia.

The cervix is innervated by the sacral plexus from sacral 2, 3 and 4 vertebrae nerves (Fig. 38.4), which then pass through the transcervical nerve plexi. Pain sensation from the cervix is in response to rapid dilatation. Somatic pain is caused by the pressure of the fetus as it distends the birth canal, vulva and perineum. Sensations from the pelvic floor are relayed from the pudendal nerve to the sacral plexus. Pain during the first stage of labour may be referred as nerve impulses from the uterus and cervix stimulate spinal cord neurons that innervate the abdominal wall. Pain may be felt between the umbilicus and the symphysis pubis, and around the iliac crests to the buttocks. It may radiate down the thighs and into the lumbar and sacral regions of the back.

The effect of pain

Besides the physical, emotional and cognitive factors affecting pain perception, abnormalities of labour may cause an increase in the pain perceived. Pain may be increased in labour complicated by prolongation, occipitoposterior position and borderline cephalopelvic disproportion.

Pain is a form of stress and may cause increased levels of catecholamine secretion; these substances will cause the following signs (Hamilton 2003):

- Increased cardiac output.
- Increased heart rate.
- A rise in blood pressure.
- Hyperventilation.
- Maternal alkalosis.
- Decreased cerebral and uterine blood flow due to vasoconstriction.
- Decreased uterine contractions.
- Delayed stomach emptying, leading to nausea and vomiting.
- Delayed bladder emptying.

Management of pain

Understanding of pain pathways and perception leads to the offering of a reasonable range of interventions. Care

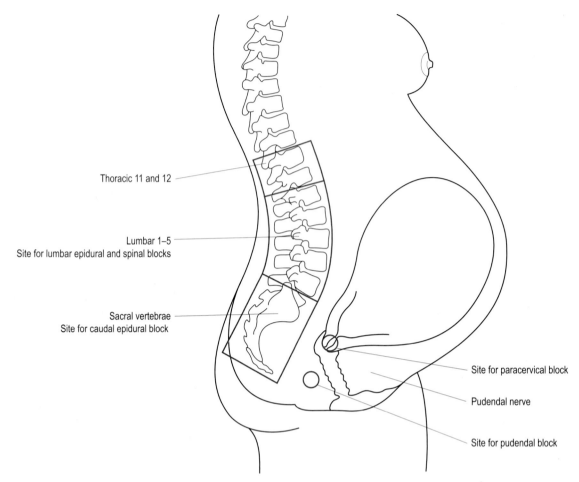

Thoracic 11 and 12

Lumbar 1–5
Site for lumbar epidural and spinal blocks

Sacral vertebrae
Site for caudal epidural block

Site for paracervical block

Pudendal nerve

Site for pudendal block

Figure 38.4 • Pain pathways in labour, showing the sites at which pain may be intercepted by local anaesthetic technique. (Reproduced with permission from Bevis 1984.)

may include pharmacological and non-pharmacological methods of pain relief. Carers can offer:

- Non-pharmacological support.
- Transcutaneous electrical nerve stimulation (TENS).
- Systemic analgesia.
- Tranquillisers.
- Inhalational analgesia.
- Regional and local analgesia.
- Alternative methods.

Non-pharmacological support

Antenatal preparation

Pain management ideally begins during the antenatal period. Women should be given the opportunity to discuss their anxieties and fears and be given information about pain relief at a level they are able to understand. Every person's needs are different but all women should participate in the planning of care in labour, including the choice of pain relief. There should be no feeling of

finality in the choice made: women need to understand and feel reassured that they can change their minds during the course of labour, depending on their actual experience of pain. Some women may wish to attend preparation classes.

During labour

Environment

The environment is important. When women and their partners enter the labour environment it is essential that they find the atmosphere and attitude of staff to be relaxed, friendly and welcoming. This is often more powerful at putting them at ease than the physical surroundings themselves, which also have a role to play (Simkin & Ancheta 2005). The room should be furnished comfortably but in such a way that any emergency treatment needed can be carried out swiftly and efficiently (Hamilton 2003). Wallpaper, curtains and screens can be useful in creating a restful atmosphere. There is a move towards informal furnishings such as beanbags, reclining chairs and rocking chairs in many units. Music and television can provide pleasure and distraction for some women in early labour (Simkin & Ancheta 2005).

Companionship

A companion of the woman's choice should be able to stay with her throughout labour. This may or may not be her partner as some men find the situation uncomfortable. Women may choose to give birth supported by a female relative or friend. If possible, a midwife known to the woman prior to labour should be available and should form a supportive relationship with the woman and her chosen companion.

Freedom of movement

Freedom to move about as and when she wants can give the woman control of her situation and shorten the process of birth (Simkin & Ancheta 2005). The perception of active participation in the birth is very important. The woman should be helped to find the position in which she is most comfortable, making full use of the range of furniture and equipment provided. Thus, she may walk about, lie down, sit astride a chair or kneel as she wishes. Massage has been demonstrated to be a useful technique for women in labour and it also includes the birth partner (Walsh 2005).

Relaxation techniques

Breathing and relaxation techniques are useful strategies to adopt in labour (Bryant & Yerby 2004). Relaxation techniques should be encouraged if the woman has learned them antenatally. It is also possible to teach women simple breathing techniques during the course of labour. Hypnobirthing is another concept, which some women practise and utilise.

Communication of information

Communication of information about progress and encouragement to keep going will also reduce anxiety and add to the feeling of being in control. The woman and her companion should participate in any decision making, such as the need for pain relief. Communication also includes physical contact, but care should be taken to ascertain what the woman is comfortable with. Some women may appreciate hand-holding, back-rubbing, massage and cuddling while others prefer to be left alone.

Birthing in water or bathing

Birthing in water or bathing may be soothing for some women both as a direct reliever of pain and indirectly through making her feel fresher. The systematic review of Cluett & Burns (2008) of eight trials (2939 women) found evidence that women who laboured in water for the first stage of labour reported less pain and used less analgesia (epidural and spinal anaesthesia/paracervical

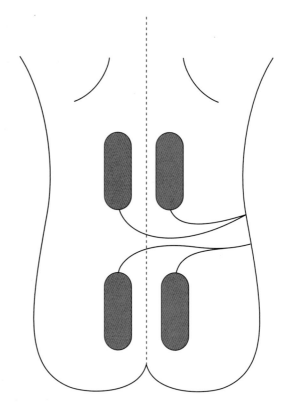

Figure 38.5 • Positions of TENS electrodes for pain relief in labour. (From Henderson C, Macdonald S 2004, with kind permission of Elsevier.)

analgesia). The reviewers also reported that there was no difference in vaginal operative deliveries, duration of labour or neonatal outcomes. This has demonstrated that labouring immersed in water alters the women's perception of pain and reduces intervention.

Transcutaneous electrical nerve stimulation

This non-pharmacological method of pain relief is based upon two hypotheses of pain physiology. First, is the gate control theory, according to which cells in the posterior horn of the spinal grey matter have a gate function. Electrical stimulation by TENS is thought to increase Aβ fibre input to the central pain pathways, thus producing inhibitory neurotransmitters which cause presynaptic inhibition—the closing of the 'gate' (Melzack & Wall 1965). Secondly, TENS is also thought to cause the production of endogenous opiates, which act as neuromoderators. A TENS unit is an electronic stimulus generator which transmits pulses of various configurations to electrodes which are attached to the skin. Electrodes are placed over the areas of the skin on the woman's back which overlie the thoracic (T10) and lumbar (L1) nerve endings and over the sacral nerves (S2–S4) (Fig. 38.5).

Accurate placing of electrodes is important for maximising the pain relief. The woman operates the equipment herself and she should have been able to practise with it in the antenatal period. Pressing a button causes a small electrical current to pass through the electrodes. The current may be pulsed—i.e. intermittent and low frequency—or it may be continuous and high frequency. Low-frequency TENS is thought to stimulate the release of endogenous opiates, while high-frequency TENS closes the pain gate (Hamilton 2003). TENS is most effective when commenced early in labour but may not provide adequate analgesia for some women if used on its own. It is probably most useful in the shorter multigravid labours although many primigravidae find it useful. The TENS equipment may interfere with the electrical mechanism within the heart if a woman has a cardiac pacemaker; this is really the only situation in which it cannot be utilised (other than immersion in water).

The use of TENS is within the midwives' sphere of practice and practitioners should be responsible for keeping themselves updated in the use of TENS, the contraindications for its use, and that equipment conforms to current safety standards. This is reiterated by the Code, which stipulates that midwives must deliver up-to-date evidence-based practice to a high standard (NMC 2008).

Systemic analgesia

An analgesic is a substance that reduces sensibility to pain without loss of consciousness and sense of touch. In labour the substance should not compromise the safety of mother or fetus and it is advisable that there should be a specific antagonist (Bryant & Yerby 2004). A strong analgesic drug is called a narcotic and these include opioid drugs. The two most commonly used drugs within the UK are **pethidine** and **diamorphine**, although **meptazinol** is also used (Tuckey et al 2008).

Pethidine is a synthetic drug which has powerful analgesic, sedative and antispasmodic effects. The effect of intramuscular injection of pethidine is rapid and lasts up to 4 h. The dose is from 50 to 200 mg, depending on the route of administration, the mother's weight, the progress of labour and the degree of pain. Pethidine may be given by intramuscular injection, by intravenous injection or by self-administered infusion. In the case of self-administered infusion, there is a built-in time limit so that the woman does not take an overdose.

Side-effects of pethidine include nausea, loss of self-control, a fall in blood pressure and perspiration. Pethidine crosses the placental membrane to affect the fetus, and changes in fetal heart rate pattern, with a loss of baseline variability, may be seen within 40 min of administration. As it also depresses the fetal respiratory centre, it is preferably not given if delivery is expected within 2–3 h. Given within 1 h of delivery, or more than 6 h before delivery, its effect on the neonate's respiration is minimal.

Diamorphine is an opioid analgesic used for acute pain and is administered by subcutaneous or intramuscular injection. The dose is 5 mg 4-hourly, up to 10 mg for heavier well-muscled patients (BNF 2008).

Morphine is an opioid analgesic used to relieve moderate to severe pain particularly of visceral origin. Morphine along with the analgesic effect produces an effect of euphoria and mental detachment. It is not suitable for long-term use as repeated doses cause dependence and tolerance (BNF 2008). It would therefore seem an appropriate drug of choice for short-term use such as an obstetric labour. Morphine is administered by intramuscular injection; the dose is 5–10 mg depending on hospital protocol.

The side effects of diamorphine and morphine are similar. These are nausea and vomiting, constipation and drowsiness, and can cause respiratory depression and hypotension if used in large doses. Morphine crosses the placental barrier and will affect the fetal heart rate pattern, with a loss of baseline variability. It will also depress the respiratory centre and, depending on the timing of administration, will interfere with initiation of respirations of the baby at birth. Appropriate resuscitation methods must be in place and used should this occur.

However, Barrett (1983) found that changes in sleep and arousal patterns, attention, motor competence and sucking and feeding patterns followed the administration of analgesics, especially of pethidine. Babies were less alert, more likely to cry when disturbed and more difficult to settle. They were more difficult to attach to the nipple and sucked less efficiently. The antidote for pethidine, diamorphine and morphine is naloxone hydrochloride (Narcan); the neonatal dose is 200 μg, although this is no longer commonly used within neonatal resuscitation practices.

Meptazinol is an analgesic that has little effect on cardiovascular and respiratory function. The dose is 100–150 mg and it is administered intramuscularly. There is little difference in the analgesic properties of pethidine and meptazinol and both may cause vomiting in the woman.

If an opioid analgesic is being administered, anti-emetic drugs are used to decrease the side effects of nausea and vomiting. The main drug used is prochlorperazine (Stemetil) 12.5 mg, administered by intramuscular injection 6-hourly if required, or metoclopramide hydrochloride (Maxalon) 10 mg administered intramuscularly or intravenously 8-hourly. Side effects of both of these drugs can be extrapyramidal effects, especially in young adults (BNF 2008).

Inhalational analgesia

The inhalation of a low dose of an anaesthetic agent will provide analgesia. **Entonox gas** contains a mixture of equal parts of oxygen and nitrous oxide (laughing gas) and is approved for use by midwives. Entonox may be available by cylinder or by piped supply (Fig. 38.6).

Entonox is colourless and odourless and the nitrous oxide is a heavier gas than oxygen. If stored at a temperature below $-7°C$, the gases may separate. Therefore, cylinders should always be stored above $10°C$ and on their side until needed, when the cylinder should be inverted several times to mix the contents. Entonox does not flow from the cylinder and must be obtained via the mouthpiece or face-mask by inspiratory efforts. The analgesic begins to take effect after about 20 s, with maximum effect after 50 s. The mother is instructed to begin to breathe the gas as soon as the uterus begins to contract and before the sensation of pain is felt. Entonox can be used in conjunction with narcotic drugs. It is excreted rapidly via the lungs as the mother exhales and therefore toxic levels do not build up to affect the fetus. Entonox does cross the placental barrier in both directions following a concentration gradient.

Anaesthetics are used to make a patient unaware of and unresponsive to painful stimulation (Rang et al 2007). They are given systemically and exert their effect on the central nervous system. In order to be a useful anaesthetic a drug must induce anaesthesia rapidly, be easily adjustable and reversible. The use of the inhaled gaseous agent nitrous oxide (laughing gas) was suggested by Humphrey Davy in 1800. Like ether, it was first used in dental extractions.

James Simpson used the agent chloroform to relieve the pain of childbirth, which was opposed at first by the clergy. The administration of chloroform to Queen Victoria during the birth of her seventh child silenced the opposition. Inhalation anaesthetics include a wide variety of substances with no common chemical structure such as halothane, nitrous oxide and xenon, and the mechanism for their action is not clear despite much research.

Stages of anaesthesia

When inhalational anaesthetics are given on their own, four well-defined stages are passed through as the blood concentration increases:

- **Stage 1: analgesia.** The person is conscious but drowsy and response to painful stimuli is reduced.
- **Stage II: excitement.** The subject loses consciousness and does not respond to non-painful stimuli but will respond in a reflex manner to painful stimuli. Cough and gag reflexes are also present. Irregular breathing may occur and this is a dangerous state that modern procedures are designed to eliminate.
- **Stage III: surgical anaesthesia.** Spontaneous movement ceases and respiration becomes regular. If the anaesthesia is light, some reflexes are still present and muscle tone is still good. As the anaesthesia deepens, muscles become flaccid and reflexes disappear. Respirations become progressively shallower.
- **Stage IV: medullary paralysis.** Respiration and vasomotor control disappear and death would occur in a few minutes.

Obstetric use of inhalational anaesthetics

An important characteristic of an inhalational anaesthetic is the rapidity with which the arterial blood concentration changes as the amount of drug inhaled changes. These drugs are generally used as anaesthetics in obstetrics in two ways: either as pain relief or as part of a combination of drugs to induce general anaesthesia during a caesarean section. Commonly, anaesthesia would be induced by an intravenous drug and then, to maintain the state, with an inhalational agent such as nitrous oxide or halothane. Muscle paralysis is obtained by the administration of a drug such as tubocurarine. Inhalation agents are time- and dose-dependent and may affect the fetus directly by being transported across the placenta or indirectly by altering uteroplacental blood flow.

Various factors, including the higher metabolic requirements and the presence of the fetus, make the pregnant woman more vulnerable to hypoxia should it occur during intubation. There is a rapid fall in Po_2, and hypoxia and respiratory acidosis may rapidly follow. Supine hypotensive syndrome may exaggerate the effect by reducing venous return and cardiac output so that the uteroplacental blood flow is poor; a left lateral tilt of the woman on the operating table will reduce the incidence of this problem. However, with safe techniques, light-to-moderate anaesthesia and adequate oxygen

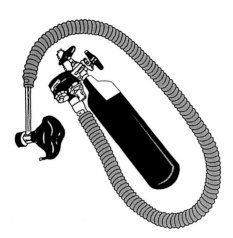

Figure 38.6 • The Entonox inhaler. (From Henderson C, Macdonald S 2004, with kind permission of Elsevier.)

administration, women with normal health should not have problems.

Epidural analgesia

Epidural analgesia involves the introduction of a local anaesthetic into the epidural space surrounding the spinal cord. A catheter is inserted so that further doses of local anaesthetic can be administered if needed. Epidural analgesia provides adequate pain relief in about 90% of women who are given the technique although the success rate may also depend on the experience of the anaesthetist. Anim-Somuah et al (2005) reviewed epidural anaesthesia compared to opioid analgesia. The evidence suggests that women received greater pain relief with an epidural compared to opioid analgesia. However, there were higher incidences of instrumental deliveries with the epidural group. The authors inform us that epidural analgesia had no statistically significant impact on the risk of caesarean section, maternal satisfaction with pain relief and long-term backache. Neonatal outcomes were also not affected from the use of Apgar scores. They conclude with recommendations for further research to explore rare but potentially severe adverse effects of epidural analgesia on women in labour and long-term neonatal outcomes.

Most women now choose epidural analgesia, especially primigravid women. Epidural and spinal analgesia are becoming more common as a method of pain relief for caesarean section.

Anatomy of the epidural space

The epidural space is a small space about 4 mm wide situated around the dura mater and contains blood vessels and fatty tissue (Figs 38.7, 38.8). The spinal nerves pass through it. Engorgement of the veins reduces the size of the space during pregnancy, and uterine contractions, which cause even more engorgement of the veins, reduce the epidural space even more. The aim is to surround specific fibres of the spinal nerves in order to remove the sensation of pain. The procedure is similar to a lumbar puncture but the meninges are not penetrated. Most commonly, the lumbar route is used and the alternative of caudal anaesthesia is not popular in Britain. The anaesthetic is introduced between lumbar vertebrae 3 and 4 or 2 and 3 (Fig. 38.9).

Preparation of the woman

The procedure and its risks are explained to the woman, who must give consent. Baseline readings of temperature, pulse, blood pressure and fetal heart are recorded. The woman is encouraged to empty her bladder. An intravenous infusion of a crystalloid solution such as

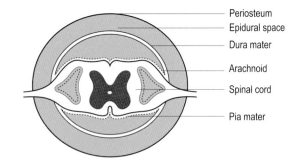

Figure 38.7 • The epidural space.

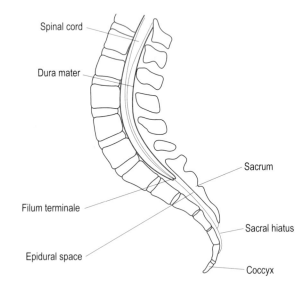

Figure 38.8 • The epidural space and sacral hiatus. (From Henderson C, Macdonald S 2004, with kind permission of Elsevier.)

Hartmann's is prepared and made ready for use. The epidural can cause sudden hypotension. If this occurs, the Hartmann's infusion is speeded up to restore normotension. Resuscitation equipment and drugs should always be available. Some maternity units administer preloading of fluids prior to administration of regional anaesthesia. Hofmeyr et al (2004) conducted a systematic review of six studies (473 women) to explore prophylactic preloading of intravenous fluids in labour prior to regional anaesthesia. They concluded that in healthy women preloading prior to a high-dose regional anaesthesia might have some benefits to prevent maternal hypotension and fetal heart rate abnormalities. Due to the small sample size for some of the studies more evidence is required to confirm whether or not preloading is beneficial for combined spinal epidural and low-dose epidural. During the siting of the epidural, the woman may be positioned on her left side or sitting up and asked to flex her back by drawing up her knees. This helps to separate the vertebrae and gives better access to the epidural space.

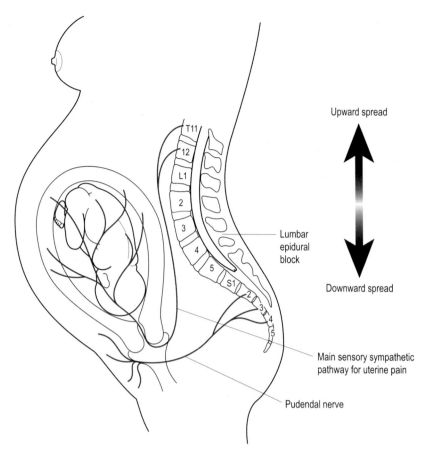

Figure 38.9 • Nerve supply in relation to epidural anaesthesia during labour. (From Henderson C, Macdonald S 2004, with kind permission of Elsevier.)

Procedure

Using an aseptic technique, the skin is cleaned and sterile towels are placed around the area of skin to be breached. A small amount of local anaesthetic is injected and a special epidural needle (**Tuohy needle**), which is a blunt needle with stilette, is inserted. The needle is advanced carefully until the resistance of the ligamentum flavum is reached, just before the epidural space. The stilette is removed and a syringe containing air or normal saline is attached to the needle. Further advancement of the needle brings it into the epidural space, which is recognised by a sudden loss of resistance when the plunger of the syringe is depressed. Any leakage of cerebrospinal fluid (CSF) would indicate that a dural tap has occurred.

If no blood or CSF is seen, the catheter is introduced through the epidural needle until its tip is in the epidural space. A test dose of 3–5 ml of local anaesthetic, usually bupivacaine (Marcain) 0.25%, is given. A bacterial filter is attached to the end of the catheter, which is taped securely in place. Observations of maternal blood pressure and pulse and fetal heart are recorded every 5 min for 20 min and then every 30 min. This is repeated with every top-up of the epidural.

Indications for epidural analgesia

- The woman's choice of pain relief.
- Effective analgesia.
- Hypertensive conditions, to prevent the rise of blood pressure (it may even cause a small fall in blood pressure).
- Preterm labour, to avoid the use of narcotic drugs.
- Prolonged labour, to allow rest and prevent exhaustion.
- Malpresentations such as breech, to prevent premature pushing and in case manipulations are needed in the second stage of labour.
- Malposition of occipitoposterior, to reduce pain and early pushing. However, there may be delay or no rotation of the head due to the reduced tone of the pelvic floor.
- Multiple pregnancy, to prevent the administration of narcotic drugs and in case manipulations are needed in the second stage of labour.
- Cardiac and respiratory disease.
- Operative deliveries such as caesarean section.
- Possible difficulties with intubation during administration of a general anaesthetic.

Contraindications

- Maternal reluctance for this form of pain relief.
- Sepsis near the site of the injection or systemic sepsis.
- Haemorrhagic disease or clotting disorder.
- Neurological disease.
- Hypovolaemia or hypotension.
- Spinal deformity.
- Chronic back problems.

Complications (Hamilton 2003)

Hypotension

Hypotension may occur because the local anaesthetic blocks the transmission of both motor and sensory nerves and affects the sympathetic nervous system. This causes vasodilation and a fall in blood pressure may occur unless blood volume is increased by infusion (a preload) prior to the epidural block, which is effective in high-dose regional anaesthesia (Hofmeyer et al 2004).

Dural tap

Dural tap may occur if the dura mater is punctured. It should be recognised by a few drops of CSF leaking through the Tuohy needle. If more CSF leaks, the woman may develop a severe headache, which often lasts a week. Lying flat will relieve the headache but also remove her ability to care for her baby. A blood patch of 10–20 ml of blood introduced into the epidural space usually cures the headache.

Total spinal block

Total spinal block is a rare complication and occurs if the anaesthetist fails to recognise a dural puncture and proceeds to inject the local anaesthetic. There is a profound motor and sensory block and a dramatic fall in blood pressure. The woman collapses and may have a cardiac arrest. Resuscitation and ventilatory support are needed immediately. Prevention of maternal hypoxia and restoration of normal blood pressure may allow the baby to be delivered safely as soon as feasible.

Bloody tap

A bloody tap occurs if the anaesthetist punctures an epidural vein. Blood will be seen in the epidural cannula. Resiting is necessary to avoid an intravenous injection of local anaesthetic. A patchy block with a better effect on one side of the body may occur, usually the right side. A top-up by the anaesthetist with the woman lying on the affected side may work but for a few women it may be impossible to provide total analgesia.

If utilising regional anaesthesia woman often have difficulty in bearing down due to the lack of sensation and have a higher incidence of assisted deliveries. A systematic review by Torvaldsen et al (2004) explored discontinuation of epidural anaesthesia to prevent incidence of instrumental delivery. There was insufficient evidence to support their hypothesis that 'discontinuing epidural analgesia late in labour reduced the rate of instrumental delivery'. The evidence highlights that if this practice is used women experience inadequate pain relief. The authors recommend that larger studies are required to review this factor.

Other drugs

Opiates have been injected into the epidural space, including diamorphine, morphine, pethidine and fentanyl. They do not produce a block so that there is little risk of hypotension but they may reduce the amount of pain perceived, especially postoperative pain. The use of a dilute combination of opiate with local anaesthetic may give a longer more effective analgesia with less motor blockade. The local anaesthetic blocks the Aδ fibres while the opiates remove pain transmitted by the smaller C fibres. This allows careful mobilisation of the woman and she can be more active in the second stage of labour. The drugs commonly used are **bupivacaine** and **fentanyl** and they may be given by epidural infusion as well as by bolus injection. Wild & Coyne (1992) report side-effects, including pruritus, urinary retention, postural hypotension, nausea, vomiting and respiratory depression.

Spinal anaesthesia

Spinal anaesthesia is different from epidural anaesthesia in that the local anaesthetic solution is injected into the subarachnoid space directly into the CSF rather than into the epidural space. It is quick, easy to perform and usually effective. It induces a total motor and sensory block below the anaesthetised area. There is more risk of profound hypotension occurring. It is useful for performing short procedures such as forceps delivery or manual removal of placenta. It can be used for performing a caesarean section but care must be taken that its effects do not wear off before the end of the surgery. Spinal anaesthesia may be combined with epidural anaesthesia to prevent the above risk (Hamilton 2003). The systematic review of Simmons et al (2007) focused on combined spinal–epidural (CSE) versus traditional epidural and CSE versus low-dose epidural in labour. From the evidence (19 trials, 2658 women) the reviewers concluded that both CSE and epidurals provide effective pain relief in labour. There was no difference in maternal satisfaction, maternal mobility or obstetric and fetal outcomes. One advantage highlighted was that CSE had a faster onset, although less pruritus was noted with epidurals. However, low-dose epidurals would be more appropriate as there was more urinary retention and rescue interventions with traditional techniques.

Pudendal block

This is the infiltration by the obstetrician of a local anaesthetic agent via a transvaginal route into an area around the pudendal nerve (Fig. 38.10). The pudendal nerve originates from S2–S4 and passes across the ischial spine. A special needle called a pudendal block needle, which has a guide, is used. Ten millilitres of lidocaine (lignocaine) 1% is introduced just below each ischial spine. Analgesia of the lower vagina and perineum results and is suitable for use in forceps or breech deliveries. Perineal repair may be carried out using the same analgesia although perineal infiltration would be more usual.

Perineal infiltration

This is the use of a local anaesthetic to infiltrate the perineum for either performance of an episiotomy or suturing: 10 ml of lidocaine (lignocaine) 1% solution is distributed by fan-like injections. Precautions are taken to avoid the inadvertent intravascular injection of the drug.

Complementary pain relief methods

Some women wish to avoid using pharmacological methods of pain relief or the invasive technique of epidural analgesia. Some midwives are keen to learn the techniques for complementary therapy so that they can offer a wider range of help to the women they care for, but they should ensure that they are trained and that the therapy has no hidden dangers for the mother (RCM 2007a,b). Some women choose to be accompanied in labour by their complementary therapist. Health professionals now accept many of the complementary therapies (Tiran & Mack 2000).

Some methods that are used and have been found to benefit women in labour are massage (Kimber 2003), acupuncture (Budd 1992), hypnosis (Jenkins & Pritchard 1993, Martin et al 2001), aromatherapy with oils placed in a warm bath (Burns & Blamey 1994),

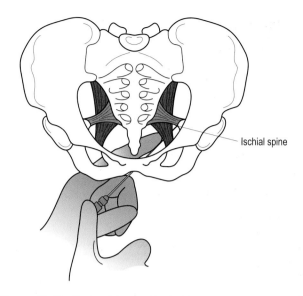

Figure 38.10 • Pudendal nerve block. (From Henderson C, Macdonald S 2004, with kind permission of Elsevier.)

Ischial spine

reflexology (Feder et al 1993) and biofeedback. Other allied therapies involve immersion in warm water, nipple stimulation to increase oxytocin production and listening to soothing music. The systematic review by Smith et al (2006) explored whether complementary and alternative therapies for managing pain in labour were effective. The authors conclude that acupuncture and hypnosis may be beneficial for the management of pain during labour. Hypnosis also demonstrated other benefits such as an increased rate of vaginal births, with a decreased use of oxytocin and greater maternal satisfaction. However, there were no differences in the groups of women who received aromatherapy or audio analgesia. The authors advocate for larger powered trials to ascertain the benefits of complementary therapies for women in labour.

It is important that all practitioners of complementary therapies have received training in their use. The Code (NMC 2008) provides guidance for practice (RCM 2007a,b, Yerby 2000).

Main points

- The chemicals bradykinin, prostaglandin and histamine are involved in the local production of inflammation and pain. The physiological threshold for pain sensation may be similar in all people but cognitive and emotive factors alter the individual's reaction to and experience of pain. The anticipation of pain increases anxiety levels and the perceived intensity of pain.

- Somatic pain may be deep or superficial. Superficial pain tends to be brief, highly localisable and sharp or pricking in character. Deep somatic pain is described as burning or aching, is more diffuse and longer lasting. Visceral pain results from the organs of the body cavities and is often described as burning, gnawing or aching. The brain plays a large part in the modulation of pain.

- Melzack & Wall (1988) updated their gate control theory of pain. Inputs from large myelinated fibres conveying touch and fibres conveying pain interact at the level of the spinal cord. The large-diameter sensory nerve impulses come into the spinal cord more rapidly, which inhibits the slower pain impulses presynaptically. This constitutes the gate against small-diameter fibre impulses.

- Besides the physical, emotional and cognitive factors affecting pain perception, abnormalities of labour may cause an increase in the pain perceived. Pain may be increased in labours complicated by prolongation, occipitoposterior position and borderline cephalopelvic disproportion.

- Pain may cause increased levels of catecholamine secretion, leading to increased cardiac output and heart rate, a rise in blood pressure, hyperventilation with maternal alkalosis, decreased cerebral and uterine blood flow due to vasoconstriction, decreased uterine contractions and delayed stomach and bladder emptying.

- Understanding of pain pathways and perception leads to both pharmacological and non-pharmacological methods of pain relief. The environment of the woman in labour is important and a companion of the woman's choice should stay with her throughout labour. The perception of active participation in the birth is very important. Communication of information about progress and encouragement will reduce anxiety and add to the feeling of being in control.

- Transcutaneous electrical nerve stimulation (TENS) depends on the physiology of the gate in the spinal cord. It works by interrupting the transmission of pain and is also thought to stimulate the release of endogenous opiates.

- In labour the most commonly used analgesics are morphine and pethidine. Entonox gas contains a mixture of equal parts of oxygen and nitrous oxide. It has no side-effects for the fetus and is commonly used in labour; it can be used in conjunction with other forms of analgesia.

- Epidural analgesia provides adequate pain relief in about 90% of women given the technique. There are numerous indications for epidural analgesia, including maternal choice, prolonged labour, malpresentations and malpositions, multiple pregnancy and hypertensive conditions.

- Some of the contraindications for epidural analgesia are maternal reluctance, sepsis, haemorrhagic disease or clotting disorder, and spinal deformity.

- The use of a dilute combination of opiate with local anaesthetic may give a longer, more effective analgesia with less motor blockade. This allows careful mobilisation of the woman and enables her to be more active in the second stage of labour.

- Pudendal block results in analgesia of the lower vagina and perineum and is suitable for use in forceps or breech deliveries. Perineal infiltration is used prior to performing an episiotomy or prior to suturing.

- Some women wish to use non-pharmacological methods of pain relief. Complementary therapies are now more accepted in labour. Midwives and others using these alternative therapies should be appropriately trained in their use.

References

Allan, D., Nie, V., Hunter, M., 1996. Control and co-ordination. In: Hinchliff, A.S.M., Montague, S.E., Watson, R. (Eds.), Physiology for Nursing Practice, third edn. Baillière Tindall, London.

Anim-Somuah, M., Smyth, R., Howell, C., 2005. Epidural versus non-epidural or no analgesia in labour. Cochrane Database Syst. Rev. (4) Update Software 2008, Oxford.

Barrett, J.W.H., 1983. Prenatal influences on adaptation in the newborn. In: Stratton, P. (Ed.), Psychobiology of the Human Newborn. Wiley, New York.

Blackburn, S.T., 2007. Maternal, Fetal and Neonatal Physiology: A Clinical Perspective, fourth edn. Elsevier Saunders, Missouri.

BNF (British National Formulary), 2008. No. 56. British Medical Association and British Pharmaceutical Society of Great Britain, London.

Bryant, H., Yerby, M., 2004. Relief of pain during labour. In: Henderson, C., Macdonald, S. (Eds.), Mayes' Midwifery: A Textbook for Midwifery, thirteenth edn. Baillière Tindall, London.

Budd, I.S., 1992. Traditional Chinese Medicine in Obstetrics. Midwives' Chron. 105, 140–143.

Burns, E., Blamey, C., 1994. Using aromatherapy in childbirth. Nurs. Times 9 (9), 54–60.

Carlson, N.R., 2004. Physiology of Behaviour, ninth edn. Pearson, Boston.

Cluett, E.R., Burns, E., 2008. Immersion in water in labour and birth. Cochrane Database Sys. Rev. (4) Art. No.: CD000111. DOI: 10.1002/14651858. CD000111.pub3.

Feder, E., Lisberg, G.B., Lenstrup, C., et al., 1993. Zone therapy in relation to birth. In: Midwives: Hear the Beat of the Future. Proceedings of the International Confederation of Midwives, 23rd International Congress. ICM, London.

Fitzgerald, M.J.T., Folan-Curran, J., 2002. Clinical Neuroanatomy and Neurosciences, fourth edn. Elsevier Saunders, Edinburgh.

Hamilton, A., 2003. Pain relief and comfort in labour. In: Fraser, D.M., Cooper, M.A. (Eds.), Myles Textbook for Midwives, fourteenth edn. Churchill Livingstone, Edinburgh.

Hayward, J., 1975. Information: A Prescription against Pain. Royal College of Nursing, London.

Henderson, C., Macdonald, S. (Eds.), 2004. Mayes' Midwifery: A textbook for Midwives, thirteenth edn. Baillière Tindall, London.

Hofmeyr, G.J., Cyna, A.M., Middleton, P., 2004. Prophylactic intravenous preloading for regional analgesia in labour. Cochrane Database Sys. Rev. (4) Update Software 2008, Oxford.

Hughes, J., Smith, T.W., Kosterlitz, H.W., et al., 1975. Identification of two related pentapeptides from the brain with opiate agonist activity. Nature 258, 577.

Jenkins, M.W., Pritchard, M., 1993. Practical appellations and theoretical considerations of hypnosis in normal labour. Br. J. Obstet. Gynaecol. 100, 221–226.

Kimber, L., 2003. How did it feel to you? An informal survey of massage techniques in labour. In: Wickham, S. (Ed.), Midwifery: Best Practice. Elsevier, London.

McCaffery, M., 1983. Understanding pain. In: Sofaer, B. (Ed.), The Patient in Pain. Lippincott, Philadelphia.

Marieb, E.N., Hoehn, K., 2008. Anatomy & Physiology, third edn. Pearson Benjamin Cummings, San Francisco.

Martin, A.A., Schauble, P.G., Surekha, H.R., Curry, R.W., 2001. The effects of hypnosis on the birth process and birth outcomes of pregnant adolescents. J. Fam. Pract. 50 (5), 441–443.

Melzack, R., Wall, P., 1965. Pain mechanisms: a new theory. Science 150 (3699), 971–979.

Melzack, R., Wall, P., 1988. The Challenge of Pain. Penguin, Harmondsworth.

NMC (Nursing and Midwifery Council), 2008. The Code: Standards of conduct, performance and ethics for nurses and midwives. <http://www.nmc-uk.org>.

Simkin, P., Ancheta, R., 2005. The Labor Progress Handbook, second edn. Blackwell, Oxford.

Simmons, S.W., Cyna, A.M., Dennis, A.T., Hughes, D., 2007. Combined spinal–epidural versus epidural analgesia in labour. Cochrane Database Syst. Rev. (3) Update Software 2008, Oxford.

Smith, C.A., Collins, C.T., Cyna, A.M., Crowther, C.A., 2006. Complementary and alternative therapies for pain management in labour. Cochrane Database Syst. Rev. (4) Update Software 2008, Oxford.

Rang, H.P., Dale, M.M., Ritter, J.M. (Eds.), et al., 2007. Pharmacology, sixth edn. Churchill Livingstone, Edinburgh.

RCM (Royal College of Midwives), 2007a. Complementary and Alternative Therapies. Guidance Paper No. 6. RCM, London.

RCM (Royal College of Midwives), 2007b. Complementary and Alternative Therapies. Position Statement No. 13. RCM, London.

Torvaldsen, S., Roberts, C.L., Bell, J.C., Raynes-Greenow, C.H., 2004. Discontinuation of epidural analgesia late in labour for reducing the adverse delivery outcomes associated with epidural analgesia. Cochrane Database Syst. Rev. (4) Update Software 2008, Oxford.

Tiran, D., Mack, S., 2000. Complementary Therapies and Childbearing, second edn. W B Saunders, Philadelphia.

Tuckey, J.P., Prout, R.E., Wee, M.Y.K., 2008. Prescribing intramuscular opioids for labour analgesia in consultant-led maternity units: a survey of UK practice. Int. J. Obstet. Anaesth. 17, 3–8.

Walding, M.F., 1991. Pain, anxiety and powerlessness. J. Adv. Nurs. 16, 338–397.

Walsh, D., 2005. NCT evidence based briefing: maternity care in birth centres Part 1. News Dig. 29, 18–23.

Walsh, D., 2007. Evidence-Based Care for Normal Labour and Birth: A Guide for Midwives. Routledge, London.

Wild, L., Coyne, C., 1992. The basics and beyond, epidural analgesia. Am. J. Nurs. April, 26–30.

Yerby, M., 2000. Pain in Childbearing: Key Issues in Management. Baillière Tindall, London.

Annotated recommended reading

Melzack, R., Wall, P., 1965. Pain mechanisms: A new theory. Science 150 (3699), 971–979.

This publication sites the original scientific paper on the 'Gate Control Theory' which is essential reading to those interested in understanding pain or studying pain management.

Melzack, R., Wall, P., 1988. The Challenge of Pain. Penguin Books, Harmondsworth (reprinted 1991).

A book that is easy to read and encompasses all the theories and principles of pain management. This is a reference book for those who require a deeper understanding of pain and its management.

Rang, H.P., Dale, M.M., Ritter, J.M. (Eds.), et al., 2007. Pharmacology, sixth edn. Churchill Livingstone, Edinburgh.

A very comprehensive textbook for science, medical, nursing and midwifery students. Its approach emphasises the mechanisms by which drugs act and relates these to the overall pharmacological effects and clinical issues.

Yerby, M., 2001. Pain in Childbearing: Key Issues in Management. Baillière Tindall, London.

A well-written book that covers key issues in pain in childbearing, facts and concepts that enable a deeper understanding of pain issues. This is an excellent reference book for pain management students.

Chapter Thirty-Nine

The second stage of labour

39

Introduction

NICE (2007) advocates that the duration of the second stage (2nd stage) should be 2 h in primigravidae and 1 h in multiparous women. However, women can be unpredictable and may have a second stage that lasts only a few minutes (Downe 2004). Irrespective of how we analyse, divide and measure the 2nd stage of labour, much physical effort is usually provided by the mother over a comparatively short period. The physiological changes that occur in the 2nd stage are a continuation of the forces that have been occurring in the first stage of labour but there is now no impediment to descent of the fetus through the birth canal and to its birth.

The 2nd stage of labour begins when the cervix is fully dilated (Fig. 39.1) and ends when the fetus is fully expelled from the birth canal. Both midwives and their medical colleagues have used this to base the management of the delivery of the baby according to a time regime. There have been challenges to the concept that the exact timing of the 2nd stage of labour is possible and progress rather than an estimated time limit is probably a more useful indicator of normality.

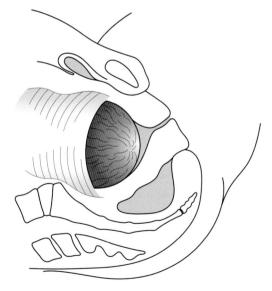

Figure 39.1 • The os uteri is fully dilated and the head enters the vagina.

Physiology of the second stage of labour

Contractions

There is often a brief lull in uterine activity at the end of the first stage (the **latent phase**) before the contractions take on their expulsive nature. The character of the contractions changes from that of the first stage. They become longer and stronger but may be less frequent so that the woman and her baby can recover between each expulsive effort. There is continued contraction and retraction of the upper uterine segment (UUS). The fetus descends the birth canal and fetal axis pressure increases flexion and reduces the size of the presenting part.

The secondary powers

As pressure is exerted on the rectum and pelvic floor, a reflex occurs which the woman feels as a compelling urge to push (the **active phase**). The 'Ferguson reflex' has been further explored in Chapter 36. Normal bearing-down efforts made by a woman if left to her own devices occur for about 5–6 s several times during the contraction. Compaction of the fetus occurs during the contraction, and pressure on the fetal head may evoke vagal stimuli, causing a transient fall in fetal heart rate with a rapid recovery. Reduction in oxygen supply due to compression of the placenta will add to this effect. Recent studies suggest that spontaneous pushing will prolong the 2nd stage of labour but cause fewer fetal heart rate changes, higher arterial pH and less damage to the birth canal.

Descent of the fetus

As the fetus descends the birth canal it displaces the soft tissues contained in the pelvis. Anteriorly, the bladder is pushed up into the abdominal cavity, which results in stretching and thinning of the urethra. Posteriorly, the rectum becomes flattened in the sacral curve and any faecal matter will be expelled. The levator ani muscles of the pelvic floor thin out and are displaced laterally. The perineal body is stretched and thinned.

The fetal head now becomes visible at the vulva and advances with each contraction to recede slightly between contractions until crowning of the head occurs (the **perineal phase**). The head is born and the shoulders and body of the baby are born with the next contraction, accompanied by a gush of amniotic fluid. The 2nd stage culminates as soon as the baby is completely born.

Onset of the second stage

There is often no clear demarcation between the end of the first stage and the beginning of the 2nd stage.

Several signs can be taken as indicative that the 2nd stage has begun but the midwife ought to have no difficulty in making the diagnosis. Downe (2003) outlines the **presumptive signs** of the onset of the 2nd stage of labour and differential diagnoses (Table 39.1). The appearance of several of the signs together may indicate that the 2nd stage of labour has begun but the midwife must use her skills to confirm this. It is sometimes necessary to confirm the absence of cervix by vaginal examination.

Duration of the second stage

The duration of the 2nd stage is difficult to predict and in multigravidae may last for as little as a few minutes whereas in primigravidae the process may take up to 2 h (Downe 2004, NICE 2007). There is no good evidence available to impose a time limit for this stage of labour and it is more relevant to base decisions on progress with evidence of adequate uterine contractions, descent and continuing good maternal and fetal well-being. However, NICE (2007) advocate referral of a primigravidae if she has not delivered within 2 h or 1 h for a multigravidae.

Two phases of the 2nd stage of labour can be described as in the first stage of labour: the **latent** and **active phases**. The latent phase begins at full dilatation of the cervix but the presenting part may not yet be visible at the pelvic outlet and the woman may not have an urge to bear down. As the fetal head descends due to the force of uterine contractions and stretches the tissues of the vagina and pelvic floor, it will become visible at the vaginal orifice. Once the fetal head is visible, pressure on the rectum will normally provide the reflex stimulus for maternal expulsive pushing and the active phase begins. Pressure of the fetus on the sacral nerves will result in the women experiencing pain from trauma to the tissue and sometimes leg cramp (Coad & Dunstall 2005).

Mechanisms of labour

The fetus is in effect a cylinder which has to negotiate the curved birth canal formed of the bony pelvis and soft tissues of the perineal body. There are two problems with being human and giving birth. One is the curve of the birth canal generated by the upright posture and walking on two legs (bipedalism) and the other is the large size of the baby's head due to the size of the human brain. Even so, the brain is only one-quarter of the size it will grow to in the adult. Moulding of the skull in order to reduce the presenting diameters is described elsewhere and this section will concern

Table 39.1 The presumptive signs of the 2nd stage of labour

Presumptive sign	Differential diagnosis
Expulsive uterine contractions	There may be an urge to push before full cervical dilatation if the rectum is full; this might be more a physiological response in some woman than a pathological response
Rupture of the forewaters	This may occur at any time in labour
Dilatation and gaping of the anus	Deep engagement of the presenting part and premature maternal pushing may be the cause
Anal cleft line	This is the purple-red line which is observed at the cleft of the buttock and climbs up the anal cleft as labour progresses; this requires further evidence
Rhomboid of Michaelis	A 'dome-shaped curve' is seen in the woman's lower back. This is displacement of the sacrum and coccyx as the occiput progresses into the sacral curve. The woman throws her buttocks forward, arches her back and throws her arms back to grasp onto something. This is thought to be a physiological response to optimise the process of the fetus through the birth canal by lengthening and straightening the curve of Carus
Upper abdominal pressure and epidural analgesia	Women have reported to have upper abdominal pressure when the 2nd stage occurs. More evidence is required to substantiate this finding
Appearance of the presenting part	Usually conclusive. However, excessive moulding and caput succedaneum formation may protrude through the cervix prior to full dilatation as may a breech presentation
Show	This must be distinguished from bleeding due to premature separation of the placenta

itself with the passive movements that the fetus makes in response to the forces exerted on it by the birth canal.

Collectively, these movements are called the **mechanisms of labour** and the fetus is turned slightly to take advantage of the widest part of each plane of the pelvis. The reader will remember that the plane of the inlet is widest in the transverse while the outlet is widest in the anteroposterior diameter. Knowledge of mechanisms enables the midwife to use skills in order to facilitate birth with least trauma to mother and fetus. Therefore it is important to take a fetal doll and pelvis and practise these mechanisms until they can be visualised in relation to the unseen movements during the birth of the baby. It is helpful to silently run through these when observing deliveries. It may be life-saving to understand what is occurring inside the woman's body so that external manoeuvres can be used to complete delivery.

Different mechanisms occur depending on the presentation and position of the fetus and there are principles common to all:

- Descent of the fetus takes place.
- The part of the fetus that leads and meets the resistance of the pelvic floor will rotate forwards to come to lie anteriorly under the symphysis pubis.
- Whatever part of the fetus emerges will pivot around the pubic bone.

The mechanism of a normal labour

There is a classical way of recalling the situation of a fetus at the commencement of the 2nd stage of labour. The terms are described in Chapter 37. The following is for a normal labour:

- **The lie** is longitudinal.
- **The attitude** is one of good flexion.

- The presentation is cephalic.
- **The position** is right or left occipitoanterior.
- **The denominator** is the occiput.
- **The presenting part** is the posterior part of the anterior parietal bone.

The movements

The movements involved in the normal mechanisms of labour are:

- Descent.
- Flexion.
- Internal rotation of the head.
- Crowning and extension of the head.
- Restitution.
- Internal rotation of the shoulders and external rotation of the head.
- Lateral flexion.

For illustrations of the movements see Figures 39.2–39.8.

Descent (Fig. 39.2)

Descent of the fetal head into the pelvis may have occurred in the antenatal period so that the woman, especially a primigravida, begins labour with the head engaged. This usually indicates that vaginal delivery is likely. The sagittal suture is in the transverse diameter of the pelvis. There is continued descent during the first stage of labour and this is speeded up by maternal effort during the 2nd stage of labour.

Flexion (Fig. 39.2)

The attitude determines which diameter will present in labour. The fetal head is in an attitude of natural flexion. Flexion of the fetal head on the trunk is increased during labour because the skull is attached to the fetal spine nearer the occiput than the sinciput. Pressure transmitted from the fundus of the uterus down the fetal spine will force the occiput lower than the sinciput, increasing flexion and resulting in the conversion of the suboccipitofrontal diameter of 10 cm to the favourable suboccipitobregmatic diameter of 9.5 cm.

Internal rotation of the head (Fig. 39.3)

As the leading part is driven onto the pelvic floor, the resistance of the muscular diaphragm and its gutter shape, sloping downwards anteriorly, cause the occiput to rotate forwards in the pelvis $\frac{1}{8}$th of a circle (45°) to lie under the symphysis pubis; the anteroposterior diameter of the head now lies in the anteroposterior diameter of the pelvis, which is the largest diameter. This causes a slight twist on the neck of the fetus so that the head is no longer aligned with the shoulders.

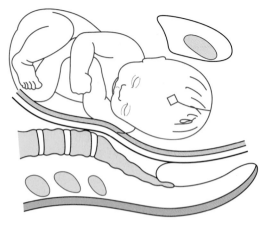

Figure 39.2 • Descent of a well-flexed head into the pelvis. The sagittal suture is in the transverse diameter of the pelvis.

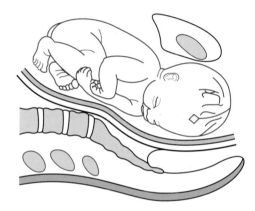

Figure 39.3 • Internal rotation. The sagittal suture is normally in the oblique diameter of the pelvis and as further descent occurs rotates into the anteroposterior diameter of the pelvis.

Crowning and extension of the head (Fig. 39.4)

The occiput escapes from beneath the subpubic arch and the smallest possible diameters, which are the suboccipitobregmatic diameter of 9.5 cm and the biparietal diameter of 9.5 cm, distend the vaginal orifice. This is termed 'crowning' and the head no longer retracts in between contractions. The head is now born by extension as it pivots on the suboccipital region around the pubic bone. The sinciput, face and chin sweep the perineum. The widest diameter to distend the vagina is the suboccipitofrontal 10 cm as the sinciput is born.

Restitution (Fig. 39.5)

Restitution is a movement made by the head following delivery which brings it into correct alignment with the shoulders. This will be $\frac{1}{8}$th of a circle towards the side from which it started.

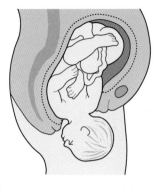
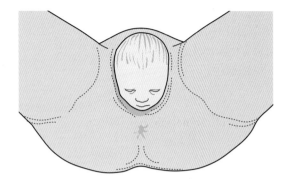

Figure 39.4 • Crowning and extension of the head.

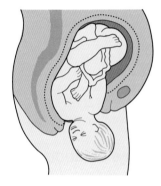
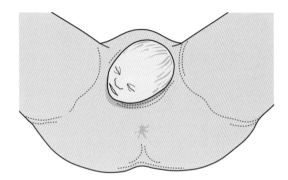

Figure 39.5 • Restitution of the head.

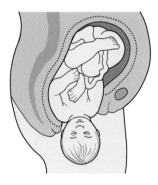
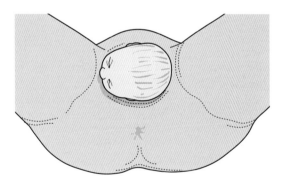

Figure 39.6 • Internal rotation of the shoulders and external rotation of the head.

Internal rotation of the shoulders and external rotation of the head (Fig. 39.6)

The anterior shoulder is the first to reach the pelvic floor and this now rotates forward to lie under the symphysis pubis. This movement is accompanied by external rotation of the head $\frac{1}{8}$th of a circle (45°) more in the direction of restitution. The occiput now lies laterally, turned towards the woman's thigh.

Lateral flexion (Figs 39.7, 39.8)

Shoulders are born sequentially, where the anterior shoulder is usually born first and slips under the pubic arch and then the posterior shoulder passes over the perineum. The remainder of the body is born by lateral flexion as the spine bends laterally on its way through the curved birth canal.

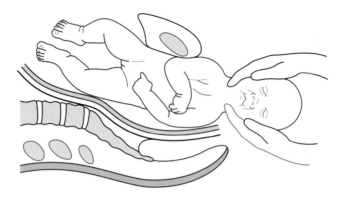

Figure 39.7 • Gentle downward traction is applied to deliver the anterior shoulder.

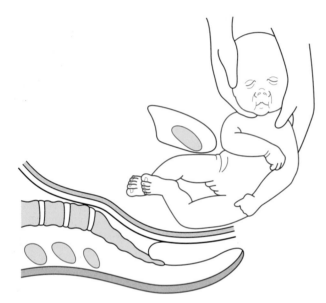

Figure 39.8 • The posterior shoulder is delivered and then the trunk by lateral flexion.

Physiological changes

Edwards (1995) outlines the physiological principles which should underlie the management of the 2nd stage of labour. These include:

- Fetal hormone secretion aimed at adaptation to independent life.
- The condition of mother and baby.
- The bearing-down reflex.
- Thinning of the perineum.
- Position of the mother.

Management

The 2nd stage of labour begins when the cervix is fully dilated and ends when the fetus is fully expelled from the birth canal. Midwives and medical colleagues have used this definition to base the management of the delivery of the baby according to a time regime. This suggests that the exact timing of the 2nd stage of labour is possible. This concept has been challenged and it is probable that progress rather than an estimated time limit is more useful as an indicator of normality (Enkin et al 2000). At the end of the day the question must be asked about stages and phases of labour as to whether they are physiological entities or human imagination. Before describing the physiology and management of the 2nd stage, the concepts need to be examined.

The second stage of labour: two or three phases?

Crawford (1983) believed that the division of labour into three stages and subdividing the stages into phases was contrary to the actual events of labour and that basing the management of labour on these concepts could lead to distress and hazard for mother and fetus. While he discussed the division of the first stage of labour into the latent and active phase, he stated that the 'distinction between the first and second stages leads to the greatest trouble in clinical practice'. He believed that the difficulty occurs because there is a lack of clear definition as to when the 2nd stage begins. If it begins with expulsive efforts by the woman, then some women wish to bear down before the cervix is fully dilated and sometimes a woman will not bear down until the presenting part is distending the perineum. Sometimes, if the woman has had epidural analgesia, she may not have an urge to bear down at all.

Aderhold & Roberts (1991) examined the concept of phases in the 2nd stage of labour with an in-depth study of four nulliparous women. They describe the above concepts of two phases to the 2nd stage as follows:

The early phase from complete dilation until the presenting part becomes visible which lasts 10 to 30 min and generally occurs with mild or no urge to bear down. Then the period of active bearing down…follows as the fetal scalp becomes visible, and proceeds until the birth of the baby. Pushing becomes more pronounced and there is a sudden change in the woman's demeanour.

They remind readers that some authorities have gone further and described **three phases** of the 2nd stage of labour: the latent phase or lull; the descent or active phase; and the perineal phase. In their small study of four nulliparous women, they found evidence to support the three phases.

The researchers suggest that, if further research verifies the phases of the 2nd stage, midwives and other obstetric care providers will be able to use this deeper understanding of spontaneous 2nd stage to inform their management. In particular, they agree with Crawford (1983) that forced expulsive efforts before the woman is ready could impose hypoxic stress on the fetus and maternal exhaustion could occur.

The length of the second stage of labour

Normal bearing-down efforts made by women if left to their own devices occur for about 5–6 s several times during the contraction (Caldeyro-Barcia 1979). Saunders et al (1992) investigated both neonatal and maternal morbidity in relation to the length of the 2nd stage of labour. They found no relation between the length of the 2nd stage of labour and the frequency of low Apgar scores or of admissions to the Special Care Baby Unit. They concluded that current management allowing spontaneous pushing, even in 2nd stages lasting up to 3 h, did not carry any undue risk to the fetus. Recent studies suggest that spontaneous pushing will prolong the 2nd stage of labour but will cause fewer fetal heart rate changes, higher arterial pH and less damage to the birth canal.

If the three factors discussed above are considered together and applied to clinical practice, it appears that the best way to manage the 2nd stage of labour is to allow the woman to push as and when she wishes as long as maternal and fetal condition remain good and progress is occurring (Enkin et al 2000). There is a need to take to heart the modifying statement by Chamberlain & Drife (1995) that, while there may be indications to change practice, further research must continue to be carried out, especially following up the infants into childhood.

Chamberlain & Drife (1995) summarised the previous decade of thinking:

…ideas about the length of the second stage of labour have swung from a regimented timetable to a go-as-you-please regime according to the attitudes of the mother, the midwife and possibly the fetus.

They add that the division between the first and 2nd stages cannot be timed, and go on to outline a possible history of why clinicians have been so keen to establish full dilatation of the cervix, concluding it is because that is the point at which vaginal delivery can be accomplished by the use of obstetrical forceps. They finally state that no rules can be laid down about the length of the 2nd stage of labour but that research should be continued into the effects on the fetus and long-term effects on the child. However, NICE (2007) state that the third stage of labour should be completed by 3 h in primigravidae and 2 h for multigravidae and advocate referral to an appropriate health care professional of a primigravida if she has not delivered within 2 h or 1 h for a multigravida.

The definition at the beginning of this chapter states that the 2nd stage begins with full cervical dilatation. At the time the woman is found to be 'fully dilated' it may be 3 or 4 h from the previous vaginal examination and it is not possible to know exactly when full dilatation occurred. This would therefore allow elements of bias in determining the actual overall length of the 2nd stage of labour.

Medical control

Crawford (1983) stated that clinicians believe they know when the 2nd stage of labour begins and that they have an 'entrenched opinion' about how long it should last. The problem is that the woman may be asked to bear down once full cervical dilatation is established, regardless of whether she feels she wants to. This creates a situation with developing maternal exhaustion, metabolic acidosis and ending in an instrumental delivery, resulting in possible birth trauma to the woman or her baby. Crawford believed that the woman should not be urged to bear down until she wished to or until the presenting part was distending the perineum and that if there was no maternal or fetal distress there was no need for instrumental delivery. These views were supported by Westcott (1984), who summarised them in an article looking at the wider issue of medical control of labour intended to be read by pregnant women.

In an attempt to clarify definitions, Westcott (1984) suggested that the first part of the 2nd stage begins at full cervical dilatation and ends when the mother voluntarily bears down. She found that there were two distinguishable parts and that the second part was more likely to lead to fetal acidosis and birth asphyxia than the first part. In her last paragraph she suggests that the first part of the 2nd stage should 'really be considered as the end of the first stage of labour'. Once again, the distinction between the end of the first stage and beginning of the 2nd stage is ill-defined.

Midwifery thinking

An important milestone for midwifery practice was a review of the management of women in the normal 2nd stage of labour undertaken by Thomson (1988). She described with feeling and accuracy the control exerted over the labouring woman, including position, forced expulsive efforts and the concentration on the vulva. She concluded that the available literature on managing the 2nd stage suggested an inter-relationship between three factors:

1. The position of the woman.

2. The means by which the woman exerts pressure to assist the uterus to expel the baby.

3. The length of the 2nd stage of labour.

These three factors still remain valid today and will be used as a plan for discussing the physiological management of labour.

Position of the woman

In most other cultures in the world and in Europe until the 18th century, women used a variety of positions during the 2nd stage of labour. Irrespective of the position used for delivery, women have tended to deliver with abducted thighs in an upright position. In most cases women adopt upright positions so that the third lumbar vertebra is above the fifth (Thomson 1988). Upright positions include standing, kneeling, sitting on birthing chairs and squatting. The lying down dorsal position may have originated in France because of the wish of Louis XIV to witness the delivery of the baby of his mistress but has been perpetuated for the ease of the medical profession. In Britain the left lateral position may have originated as the 'London position' advocated by Smellie in 1752 (Thomson 1988). The position a woman will adopt in labour is related to the context in which the birth is taking place (Walsh 2007). The majority of standard labour ward rooms have a bed as the central feature. Walsh (2007) advocates that measures could be taken to position the bed against a wall or remove it altogether from the room to decrease the bed's status in childbirth!

Although the recumbent position has been until the last few decades the most common position for delivery, it is known that it leads to supine hypotension, which may adversely affect fetal oxygenation (Enkin et al 2000). If the mother lies on her back there will be a significant reduction in maternal cardiac output and circulation of oxygenated blood through the placental tissue due to compression of the inferior vena cava and descending aorta although this does not happen if the woman lies on her side or if the uterus is tilted to the left. Rosser (2003) highlights that the upright posture has many beneficial physiological effects on the progress of the 2nd stage:

1. It allows gravity to play its part in the descent of the fetus.

2. It increases the diameters of the pelvic outlet by up to 1 cm in the transverse diameter and 2 cm in the anteroposterior diameter in the squatting position. This produces a 28% increase in the area of outlet compared with women delivered in the supine position.

3. There is better alignment of the fetus through the birth canal.

4. It increases the efficiency and strength of uterine contractions.

5. It reduces the incidence of aortocaval compression, which ultimately improves the acid–base balance of the baby.

Squatting

Squatting is probably the most common position for childbirth in the developing world. The mother may need the support of two people or she may support herself with her back to a wall or firm surface. The flexion and abduction of the thighs brought about by squatting has a number of advantages (Simkin & Ancheta 2005).

- It provides the advantage of gravity.
- It enlarges the pelvic outlet by increasing the intertuberous diameter.
- It allows freedom to shift weight comfortably.
- It provides mechanical advantage: upper trunk presses on fundus more than any other position.
- It may enhance the urge to push.
- It may hasten descent of the fetal head if it is engaged and well-aligned in an occipitoanterior position.
- It may relieve backache.

However, if the fetal head is at a relatively high station and asynclitic, squatting may impede correction of the angle of the head by reducing the space available for the fetus to move into synclitism. If squatting is continued for a prolonged period, the woman should lean back or rise after every contraction to prevent compression of the blood vessels and nerves located behind the knee joints.

Hands and knees/all-fours positions

Women may often adopt a kneeling position themselves. This position also has the following advantages:

- It aids fetal rotation from the occipitoposterior position.
- It may aid in reducing an anterior lip in the late first stage.

- It allows the woman freedom to sway, crawl or rock the pelvis, which can promote rotation and increase comfort.
- It reduces back pain and relieves haemorrhoids.
- It may resolve fetal heart problems that are mainly due to cord compression.

The position allows access for vaginal examination and provides an excellent view of the fetus and perineum and causes less perineal trauma. There may be an increase in vulval trauma.

Upright positions adopted by women for labour and birth have been noted to restore normality to prolonged labour (Simkin & Ancheta 2005).

Birthing chairs

Electronically controlled birthing chairs appeared to be an alternative for supporting women in the squatting position, giving the midwife good vision and access to the fetus. However, there have been problems associated with their use. There appears to be a higher mean blood loss and an increase in postpartum haemorrhage in multigravidae. This finding may be due to the increased accuracy in measuring blood loss or there may be more actual blood loss from perineal trauma caused by obstructed venous return because of pressure on the buttocks and perineum. This pressure may also be responsible for the increase in perineal oedema and haemorrhoids in women delivered in the upright position in birthing chairs.

Review of upright positions

For centuries there has been controversy about whether being upright or lying down has advantages for women delivering their babies. In a systematic review of research studies, Gupta et al (2004) considered the benefits and risks associated with the upright or lateral positions compared with supine or lithotomy positions. They concluded that the upright or lateral positions were associated with a reduced duration of 2nd stage, a reduction in both assisted deliveries and episiotomies, a smaller increase in 2nd degree tears and an increased risk of blood loss >500 ml. Women were also noted to perceive less severe pain and found bearing down to be easier. These are tentative findings and further well-controlled studies are required. In the meantime women should be encouraged to give birth in the position they find most comfortable.

Maternal effort in the second stage of labour

We may then accept that the 2nd stage of labour begins with full dilatation of the cervix but the presenting part may not yet be visible at the pelvic outlet and the woman may not have an urge to bear down. As the fetal head descends due to the force of uterine contractions and stretches the tissues of the vagina and pelvic floor, it will become visible at the vaginal orifice. Once the fetal head is visible, pressure on the rectum will normally provide the reflex stimulus for maternal expulsive pushing and the active phase begins.

Prior to the 1990s it was customary practice for birth attendants to give women formal instructions during the 2nd stage of labour (Watson 1994). The rationale for this was to reduce the length of the 2nd stage of labour and prevent too much stress for the fetus. Women were often encouraged to take a big breath at the start of each contraction and bear down as long and as hard as they could. This is known as the Valsalva manoeuvre and uses forced expiration against a closed glottis to increase intra-abdominal pressure to aid the uterus to expel the fetus. This manoeuvre causes the blood pressure to drop and rise again and women using the technique have shown alterations in heart rate and brain wave patterns. Forced pushing has been implicated as the cause of burst capillaries in the face and eyes and rarely cerebrovascular accidents (strokes) may occur.

There is no evidence to suggest that any benefits are gained from routine directed pushing and pushing from sustained bearing down, breath-holding or early bearing down (Enkin et al 2000). Current practice now recommends that directed pushing should be abandoned and women should be encouraged to follow their instincts. The midwife's role should be to affirm physiology, not control it or deny it, and to encourage women-centred approaches, which promote normality.

Effect on pelvic soft tissues

There are two ways of interpreting early pushing in the 2nd stage of labour: pushing in the early part of each contraction, as discussed above; and pushing in the latent phase. A classical paper by Beynon (1957) explains the effect that forceful pushing from the commencement of each contraction has on the soft tissues of the pelvic floor. He theorised that in the early part of a contraction the vaginal muscles are drawn taut to prevent the bladder supports and transverse cervical ligaments being pushed down in front of the baby's head. Early expulsive effort may lead to incontinence and prolapsed uterus later in life. Active pushing during the latent phase of the 2nd stage of labour may strain the uterine supports and the vaginal and perineal muscle before these tissues have a chance to stretch gradually.

Perineal lacerations

During the 2nd stage of labour, **perineal lacerations** may occur. Previously an episiotomy was conducted in order to control the extent of these lacerations; however, evidence does not support this practice (Carroli & Belizan 1999, Low et al 2000). Depending on the depth of tissue involved in the tear, perineal lacerations can be classified as follows:

- **First-degree tear**: a tear that only involves the skin of the fourchette.
- **Second-degree tear**: a tear that involves the skin of the fourchette, perineum and perineal body (superficial bulbocavernosus and transversus perinei muscles, deep pelvic floor pubococcygeus muscle).
- **Third-degree tear**: a tear that involves the skin of the fourchette, perineum, perineal body (superficial bulbocavernosus and transversus perinei muscles, deep pelvic floor pubococcygeus muscle) and the anal sphincter. Depending on the degree of anal sphincter involvement this category is further divided:
  - **3a**: less than 50% of external anal sphincter torn.
  - **3b**: more than 50% of external anal sphincter torn.
  - **3c**: internal anal sphincter torn.
- **Fourth-degree tear**: a tear that involves the skin of the fourchette, perineum and perineal body (superficial bulbocavernosus and transversus perinei muscles, deep pelvic floor ileococcygeus muscle) as well as the external anal sphincter, internal anal sphincter and anal epithelium (Downe 2003, Kettle 2004, RCOG 2004).

An **episiotomy** is a surgical incision of the perineum made to increase the diameter of the vulval outlet. The tissues that are involved are the same as a second-degree tear, namely the skin of the fourchette, perineum and perineal body (superficial bulbocavernosus and transversus perinei muscles, deep pelvic floor pubococcygeus muscle) (Downe 2003, Kettle 2004, RCOG 2004).

Other tissues may be lacerated during delivery. **Labial lacerations** are not usually severe enough to require suturing but can be very painful, especially during micturition. However, if they are bilateral labial laceration suturing might be required to prevent abnormal fusion of these tissues. **Vaginal** and **cervical lacerations** may bleed severely and need immediate pressure to control bleeding followed by suturing.

The episiotomy

An episiotomy, in a strict sense, is an incision of the pudendum. It is a deliberate incision of the perineum, through the structures involved in a second-degree tear. In common parlance, however, episiotomy is often used synonymously with perineotomy (Cunningham et al 2001). In the UK, it is an integral part of the midwife's role to perform an episiotomy and infiltrate the perineum with local anaesthetic when this procedure is required. The midwife must assess the need for this procedure and deliver evidence-based care to a high standard of practice (NMC 2008). The rationale for the incision is to enlarge the vulval outlet to facilitate delivery (Downe 2003, Kettle 2004). Early studies by Sleep (1984a,b) demonstrated that the performance of an episiotomy was not a valid reason to prevent perineal trauma. Findings indicated that there was no reduction in trauma to the pelvic floor nor did women suffer less pain or swelling; indeed, many women felt more pain. The perineal wound, whether tear or episiotomy, healed in a similar manner. Findings from recent studies and reviews support these findings and suggest that there is no evidence to suggest that episiotomies add any protection against perineal-related problems such as sphincter tears (Carroli & Belizan 1999, Low et al 2000).

More recently, the results of a study by Goldberg et al (2002) showed a trend in the reduction of episiotomies performed over almost two decades. The overall episiotomy rates in 34 048 vaginal births showed a significant reduction from 69.6% in 1983 to 19.4% in 2000.

Recommendations for performing an episiotomy

During the antenatal period women should be given a chance to discuss the possible need for the midwife to make an episiotomy to avoid confrontation situations in an emergency (Walsh 2000). It is unlikely that a woman will refuse if she is able to make an informed choice based on knowledge acquired calmly. Her wishes should be recorded on her birth plan.

Enkin et al (2000) state that there is no evidence from available studies to support the suggestion that the use of episiotomy minimises trauma to the fetal head. Recommendations for current practice should include the following:

- A reduction in the episiotomy rate for normal births to 10% or less (WHO 1996).
- Fetal indications are the only justification for performing an episiotomy (Walsh 2007): to expedite delivery if the fetal head is on the perineum and there is evidence of fetal distress or if the fetus is preterm or is presenting by the breech to reduce the risk of intracranial trauma.
- Elective episiotomies for previous third-degree tears should be discontinued and should not be mandatory for forceps or ventouse births.
- Documented consent should be obtained from the woman.

The incision

There are two types of incision: the mediolateral and the midline (Fig. 39.9). The mediolateral is most commonly used because it avoids damage to Bartholin's gland and is unlikely to extend in the midline to involve the anal sphincter.

The perineum is infiltrated along the line of the intended episiotomy using 5–10 ml of lidocaine (lignocaine) 1% (Fig. 39.10A). The practitioner should check carefully to avoid giving the injection intravenously to avoid the risk of causing bradycardia or collapse. The anaesthetic takes effect very quickly and the incision can then be made using episiotomy scissors. The incision is best made during a contraction when the perineum is thinned out and should be 3–4 cm long. The practitioner should protect the fetal head during the administration of the local anaesthetic and performing the episiotomy by inserting two fingers between the head and the perineum (Fig. 39.10B).

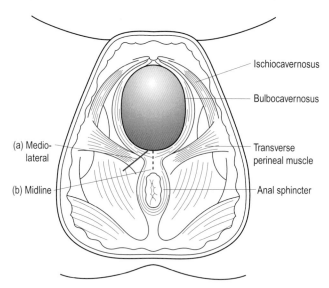

Figure 39.9 • Types of episiotomy incisions. (a) Mediolateral, (b) Midline.

Labels on figure:
(a) Mediolateral
(b) Midline
Ischiocavernosus
Bulbocavernosus
Transverse perineal muscle
Anal sphincter

Suturing the perineum

Approximately 85% of women in the UK who have a vaginal birth will have some degree of perineal trauma. Of these women 60–70% will require suturing (RCOG 2004). Repair of the perineum is now an integral part of the role of the midwife in intrapartum care. This includes being able to recognise situations where it is not appropriate for the midwife to suture: for instance, if a third-degree tear has unfortunately been sustained. The advantage to the woman is that the suturing is carried out immediately and she does not have to wait until a doctor is available. The midwife should comply with the local policies for the use of suture materials, which should be based on up-to-date research. Aseptic technique is universal. The most important point is to explore the depth of the wound and ensure that the first suture is placed above its apex to prevent the development of a vaginal haematoma.

Infiltration of the perineum

Using an aseptic technique infiltrate the perineum using 15–20 ml of lidocaine (lignocaine) 1% (the woman should be offered the use of Entonox inhalation analgesia if she has not got an effective epidural). Infiltration of the local anaesthetic can be inserted into the perineum using the following technique (Bowen & Taylor 2005) with reference to Figure 39.11:

1. The tissue at point A is held with a pair of tissue forceps. The needle of the local anaesthetic syringe is injected into point A of the laceration with the tip of the needle going through the tissues and ending at point B.

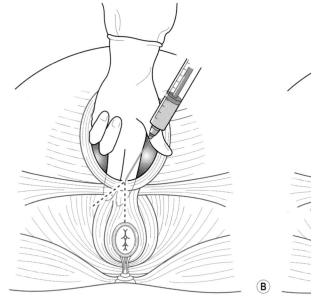
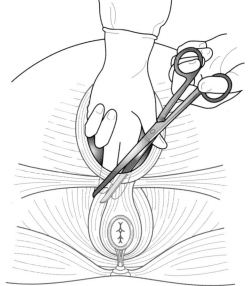

Figure 39.10 • (A) Infiltration of the perineum. (B) Making a mediolateral incision.

2. The plunger of the syringe is then withdrawn, making sure that the needle is not in a blood vessel (the same method that is used prior to administering an intramuscular injection).

3. The local anaesthetic is then infiltrated into the perineal tissue using the withdrawal technique (i.e. infiltrating the local anaesthetic while withdrawing the needle backwards through the tissue from point B to point A).

4. Without removing the needle from point A redirect the needle through the tissues so that the tip of

the needle is at point C and continue to infiltrate the perineal tissue using the previously explained infiltration withdrawal technique.

5. Repeat these steps for the other side of the laceration by removing the needle completely and reinserting it into point D of the laceration.

6. Infiltrate this side of the tear by following the same principles so that you infiltrate from B to D and from C to D using the previously explained withdrawal technique. Once adequate analgesia is effective suturing may commence. If at any point the woman still feels discomfort stop and reassess for more analgesia.

The perineum is then sutured in layers from the inside tissues outwards (Fig. 39.12). A loose continuous non-locking subcuticular method of suturing is recommended using polyglycolic sutures such as Vicryl (polyglactin 910) or Dexon (polyglycolic acid), as this can result in less suturing being required and less pain (Kettle & Johanson 1999, Kettle et al 2007); also, sutures dissolve in 42 days compared to previous suture material, which took up to 60–90 days (RCOG 2004). Following a systematic review of seven studies involving 3822 women, Kettle et al (2007) stated that the continuous suturing techniques for perineal closure, compared to interrupted methods, are associated with less short-term pain. They go on to further explain that if the continuous technique is used for all layers (vagina, perineal muscles and skin) compared to perineal skin only, the reduction in pain is even greater (Kettle et al 2007).

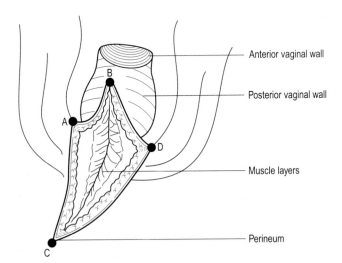

Figure 39.11 • Infiltration of perineum prior to suturing. (Adapted from Nisbet & Rouse 1992.)

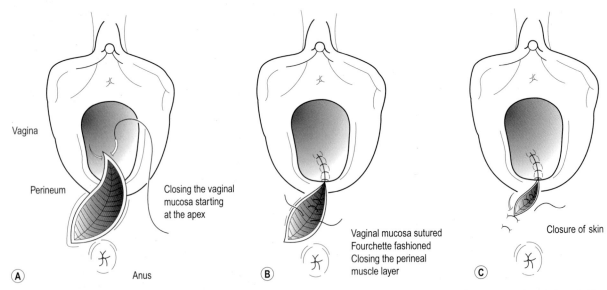

Figure 39.12 • Suturing the perineum. (A) Closing the vaginal mucosa, starting at the apex. (B) Vaginal mucosa sutured, fourchette fashioned, closing the perineal muscle layer. (C) Closure of the skin by continuous suture.

The fetus in the second stage of labour

It is traditional to view the 2nd stage of labour as the most dangerous stage for the fetus as there is an increased risk for the occurrence of asphyxia and trauma. This has led to attempts to deliver the baby as quickly as possible. Although the Valsalva manoeuvre will significantly shorten the 2nd stage of labour, studies have indicated that sustained breath-holding leads to abnormalities in the fetal heart (Caldeyro-Barcia 1979) and adversely affects fetal condition and neonatal outcome (Bassell et al 1980, Paine & Tinker 1992). Compaction of the fetus occurs during the contraction, and pressure on the fetal head may evoke vagal stimuli, causing a transient fall in fetal heart rate with a rapid recovery.

Reduction in oxygen supply due to compression of the placenta will add to this effect. This may cause prolongation of the normal fall in fetal heart rate seen after contractions in the 2nd stage of labour. Also, if the mother lies on her back there will be a significant reduction in cardiac output and circulation of oxygenated blood through the placental tissue due to compression of the inferior vena cava and descending aorta, although this does not happen if the woman lies on her side or if the uterus is tilted to the left.

Piquard et al (1988) examined the validity of fetal heart rate monitoring in the 2nd stage of labour and whether a time limit should be placed on the 2nd stage to safeguard the fetus. They cited evidence that umbilical artery pH decreased significantly if the 2nd stage exceeded 45 min. This aspect of care in the 2nd stage will be discussed more fully in Chapter 46. Piquard et al (1989) analysed fetal distress in relation to the concept of two biological parts to the 2nd stage of labour. They agreed with clinicians that the 2nd stage of labour is a time of risk for the fetus with distress related not only to hypoxia but also to mechanical stress.

Main points

- At the end of the first stage of labour there is often a brief lull in uterine activity before the contractions take on their expulsive nature, becoming longer and stronger but less frequent. The fetus descends the birth canal and increasing flexion reduces the size of the presenting part.

- The 2nd stage of labour begins with full dilatation of the cervix and ends when the fetus is fully expelled from the birth canal. Progress made during this stage rather than an estimated time limit is more useful as an indicator of normality.

- The duration of the 2nd stage in multigravidae may last for as little as 5 min, whereas in primigravidae the process may take up to 2 h. Two phases of the 2nd stage of labour can be described: the latent and active phases. The latent phase begins at full dilatation of the cervix but the woman may not have an urge to bear down. Pressure on the rectum normally provides the stimulus for maternal expulsive pushing and the active phase begins.

- The upright posture allows gravity to aid descent of the fetus, increases uterine contraction efficiency and reduces the incidence of fetal distress and neonatal asphyxia. The squatting position for labour and delivery has a number of additional advantages: it enlarges the pelvic outlet, allows freedom to shift weight comfortably, may enhance the urge to push and hasten descent of the head and may relieve backache. The hands and knees position appears to relieve backache, aids rotation and descent and causes less perineal trauma.

- Current practice recommends that directed pushing should be abandoned and women should be encouraged to follow their instincts. The midwife's role should be to affirm physiology, not control it or deny it, and to encourage women-centred approaches which promote normality.

- Perineal lacerations may occur during the 2nd stage of labour. Labial lacerations are not usually severe enough to require suturing but can be painful during micturition. Vaginal and cervical lacerations may bleed severely and may need to be sutured immediately to control bleeding.

- The rationale for the incision of an episiotomy is to enlarge the vulval outlet immediately before delivery. Fetal reasons are the only justification for performing an episiotomy. During the antenatal period, women should be given a chance to discuss the possible need for an episiotomy.

- Perineal repair is an integral part of the midwife's role. It is most important to explore the depth of the wound and ensure that the first suture is placed above its apex to prevent the development of a vaginal haematoma. The perineum is then sutured in layers from the inside tissues outwards with a continuous subcuticular method of suturing using polyglycolic sutures such as Vicryl or Dexon.

References

Aderhold, K.J., Roberts, J.E., 1991. Phases of second stage labor: four descriptive case studies. J. Nurse-Midwifery 36 (5), 267–275.

Bassell, G.M., Humayun, S.G., Marx, G.F., 1980. Maternal bearing-down efforts: another fetal risk? Obstet. Gynecol. 5 (1), 39–47.

Beynon, C., 1957. The normal second stage of labour. J. Obstet. Gynaecol. Br. Commonw. 64 (6), 815–820.

Bowen, R., Taylor, W., 2005. Skills for Midwifery Practice, second edn. Elsevier Churchill Livingstone, London.

Caldeyro-Barcia, R., 1979. The influence of maternal bearing-down efforts during second stage on fetal well-being. Birth Fam. J. 6 (1), 17–21.

Carroli, J., Belizan, J., 1999. Episiotomy for vaginal birth. Cochrane database Syst. Rev. (3) Update Software 2008, Oxford.

Chamberlain, G., Drife, J., 1995. What is a prolonged second stage of labour? Contemp. Rev. Obstet. Gynaecol. 7, 69–70.

Coad, J., Dunstall, M.J., 2005. Anatomy and Physiology for Midwives, second edn. Elsevier Churchill Livingstone, London.

Crawford, J.S., 1983. The stages and phases of labour: an outworn nomenclature that invites hazard. Lancet 321, 271–272.

Cunningham, F.G., MacDonald, P.C., Leveno, K.J., et al., 2001. Williams Obstetrics, twenty-first edn. Prentice-Hall International, New Jersey.

Downe, S., 2003. Transition and the second stage of labour. In: Fraser, D.M., Cooper, M.A. (Eds.), Myles Textbook for Midwives, 14th edn. Churchill Livingstone, Edinburgh.

Downe, S., 2004. Care in the second stage of labour. In: Henderson, C., Macdonald, S. (Eds.), Mayes' Midwifery: A Textbook for Midwifery, thirteenth edn. Ballière Tindall, London.

Edwards, N. P., 1995. Birthing your baby: The Second Stage. Association for Improvements in the Maternity Services, AIMS.

Enkin, M., Keirse, J., Neilson, J., et al., 2000. A Guide to Effective Care in Pregnancy and Childbirth, third edn. Oxford University Press, Oxford.

Goldberg, J., Holtz, D., Hyslop, J., 2002. Episiotomy rates. Obstet. Gynecol. 99 (3), 395–400.

Gupta, J.K., Hofmeyr, G.J., Smyth, R., 2004. Position in the second stage of labour for women without epidural anaesthesia. Cochrane database Syst. Rev. (1) Update Software 2008, Oxford.

Kettle, C., 2004. The pelvic floor. In: Henderson, C., Macdonald, S. (Eds.), Mayes' Midwifery: A Textbook for Midwifery, thirteenth edn. Ballière Tindall, London.

Kettle, C., Johanson, R.B., 1999. Absorbable synthetic versus catgut suture material for perineal repair. Cochrane Database Syst. Rev. (4) Update Software 2008, Oxford.

Kettle, C., Hills, R.K., Ismail, K.M.K., 2007. Continuous versus interrupted sutures for repair of episiotomy or second degree tears. Cochrane Database Syst. Rev. (4) Update Software 2008, Oxford.

Low, L., Seng, J., Murtland, T., et al., 2000. Clinical-specific episiotomy rates: impact on perineal outcomes. J. Midwifery Woman's Health 45 (2), 87–93.

NICE (National Institute for Health and Clinical Excellence), 2007. Intrapartum Care: Care of healthy women and their babies during childbirth. NICE Clin. Guidel. 55 http://www.nice.org.uk.

NMC (Nursing and Midwifery Council). (2008). The Code: Standards of conduct, performance and ethics for nurses and midwives. http://www.nmc-uk.org.

Paine, L.L., Tinker, D.D., 1992. The effect of maternal bearing-down efforts on arterial umbilical cord pH and length of the second stage of labor. J. Nurse-Midwifery 37 (1), 61–63.

Piquard, F., Hsiung, R., Schaefer, A., et al., 1988. The validity of fetal heart rate monitoring during the second stage of labor. Obstet. Gynecol. 72 (5), 746–751.

Piquard, F., Schaefer, A., Hsiung, R., et al., 1989. Are there two biological parts in the second stage of labor? Acta Obstetrica and Gynecologica Scandinavica 68, 713–718.

RCOG (Royal College of Obstetricians and Gynaecologists). (2004). Methods and Materials Used in Perineal Repair. Guideline No. 23. RCOG, London.

Rosser, J., 2003. Women's position in second stage. In: Wickam, S. (Ed.), Midwives Best Practice. Elsevier, Edinburgh.

Saunders, N.St.G., Paterson, C.M., Wadsworth, J., 1992. Neonatal and maternal morbidity in relation to the length of the second stage of labour. Br. J. Obstet. Gynaecol. 99, 381–385.

Simkin, P., Ancheta, R., 2005. The Labor Progress Handbook, second edn. Blackwell Publishing, Oxford.

Sleep, J., 1984a. Episiotomy in normal delivery 1. Nurs. Times 80 (47), 29–30.

Sleep, J., 1984b. Episiotomy in normal delivery 2: the management of the perineum. Nurs. Times 80 (48), 51–54.

Thomson, A.M., 1988. Management of the woman in normal second stage of labour: a review. Midwifery 4, 77–85.

Walsh, D., 2000. Evidence Based Care Series 8: Perineal care should be a feminist issue. Br. J. Midwifery 8 (12), 731–737.

Walsh, D., 2007. Evidence-Based Care for Normal Labour and Birth: A Guide for Midwives. Routledge, London.

Watson, V., 1994. Maternal position in the second stage of labour. Mod. Midwife 4 (7), 21–24.

Westcott, V.P., 1984. The revolution starts here. Mother and Baby April, 19–23.

WHO (World Health Organization) (1996). Care in Normal Birth: A practical guide. Report of a Technical Working Group, Maternal and Newborn Health/Safe Motherhood Unit, 1996, World Health Organization, Geneva.

Annotated recommended reading

Edwards, N. P., (1995). Birthing Your Baby: The Second Stage. Association for the Improvement in the Maternity Services (AIMS).

In this article Edwards outlines the physiological principles which should underlie the management of the second stage of labour.

Enkin, M., Keirse, J., Neilson, J., et al., 2000. A Guide to Effective Care in Pregnancy and Childbirth, third edn. Oxford University Press, Oxford.

This is a well-written book that covers 'effective care in pregnancy and childbirth'. It provides a research-based resource.

Chapter Forty

40

The third stage of labour

Introduction

The third stage (3rd stage) of labour is the period from the birth of the baby through to delivery of the placenta and membranes and ends with the control of bleeding. During this period vigilance is required as there are emergency situations that occur and can lead to maternal morbidity and mortality. An understanding of the normal physiology allows choice between the physiological management and active management of the 3rd stage. This will ultimately minimise the risk of complications by preventative management and rapid emergency treatment if necessary.

Physiology of the third stage of labour

During the 3rd stage, separation and expulsion of the placenta and membranes occur and bleeding from the placental site is minimised through normal haematological and physiological processes. This stage is most hazardous for the mother because of the risk of haemorrhage and other complications (discussed in Chapter 45). The physiological 3rd stage normally lasts from 5 to 30 min but may take up to an hour (NICE 2007). During the second stage of labour, the uterus is steadily emptied, accompanied by accelerated myometrial contraction and retraction.

Separation of the placenta

Separation of the placenta usually begins with the contraction that delivers the baby's body (Fig. 40.1). The sudden emptying of the uterus with the delivery of the baby rapidly reduces the surface area of the placental site to an area approximately 10 cm in diameter (Blackburn 2007). This reduction in the support base for the placenta leads to compression and shearing of the placenta from the uterine wall. The placenta is compressed so that blood in the intervillous spaces is forced back into the spongy layer of the decidua. Retraction of the oblique muscle fibres constricts the blood vessels supplying the placenta so that the blood cannot drain into the maternal vascular tree. This causes the congested veins to rupture, the villi to shear off the spongy decidua basalis, and the inelastic placenta to become wrinkled and peel away from the uterine wall. The weight of the placenta also increases due to congestion of blood and this helps to strip the membranes off the uterine wall. It is useful to note that the formation of the retroplacental clot is no longer believed to be a (natural) physiological event occurring in the separation process (Blackburn 2007, Wattis 2004).

The placenta may separate from the central area to the borders with inversion so that the fetal surface presents first. This is known as the **Schultze** mechanism of placental delivery (named after the German anatomist who first described this method). Generations of

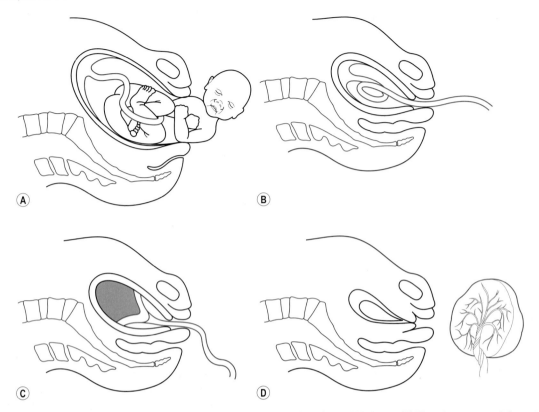

Figure 40.1 • The mechanism of placental separation. (A) The placenta before the child is born. (B) The placenta partially separated immediately after the birth of the child. (C) The placenta completely separated. (D) The placenta expelled and the uterus strongly contracted and retracted. (From Henderson C, Macdonald S 2004, with kind permission of Elsevier.)

midwives have termed this process as 'shiny Schultze', referring to the glistening appearance of the fetal surface of the placenta at the vulva.

Alternatively, the placenta may separate unevenly from the borders towards the centre with the maternal surface of the placenta appearing at the vulva. This process usually takes longer and there is more risk of incomplete expulsion of the membranes, often referred to as ragged membranes. This mechanism was first described by **Matthew Duncan** an eminent Scottish gynaecologist (1826–1890) and has been called 'dirty Duncan' as an aide-mémoire for students due to the bulky blood ingested at the maternal surface appearing first.

Placentas implanted in the fundus of the uterus are more likely to separate via Schultze mechanism; those implanted lower in the uterine wall usually separate by Duncan mechanism, although these placentas may invert before expulsion (Blackburn 2007).

Control of bleeding

Once separation is complete, the uterus contracts strongly (Fig. 40.2) and the placenta and membranes fall into the lower uterine segment and then into the vagina. It is important to remember that between 450 and 700 ml/min of blood flows to the uterus where

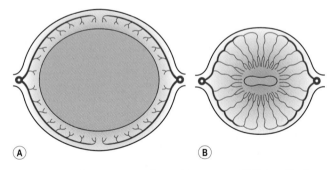

Figure 40.2 • Transverse sections of the uterus. (A) Relaxed before the 3rd stage. (B) Contracted and retracted after the 3rd stage; blood vessels are compressed and bleeding arrested. (From Henderson C, Macdonald S 2004, with kind permission of Elsevier.)

80% is perfusion for the placenta and 20% is perfusion for the myometrium (Murray 2003). This flow must be stopped in seconds to prevent serious haemorrhage. Three factors are involved in the process:

1. **Living ligatures**: The tortuous uterine blood vessels are surrounded by the oblique muscle fibres, which retract and act as 'living ligatures' (Fig. 40.3) and constrict the blood vessels.

2. **Pressure**: Once the placenta has left the upper segment, a vigorous contraction brings the walls of

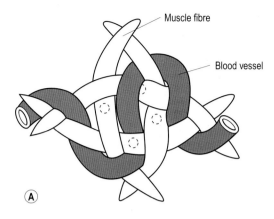

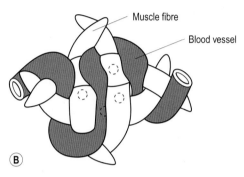

Figure 40.3 • How the blood vessels run between the interlacing muscle fibres of the uterus. (A) Muscle fibres relaxed and blood vessels not compressed. (B) Muscle fibres contracted, blood vessels compressed and bleeding arrested. (From Henderson C, Macdonald S 2004, with kind permission of Elsevier.)

the uterus in opposition, applying pressure to the placental site.

3. **Blood clotting**: There is a transitory increase in the activity of the coagulation system during and immediately after placental separation so that clot formation in the torn blood vessels is maximised. The placental site is rapidly covered by a fibrin mesh.

Attaching the baby on the breast will help achieve placental separation and assist with the control of bleeding by causing a release of oxytocin from the maternal posterior pituitary gland resulting in contraction of the uterus, whilst assisting with the above factors.

Management of the third stage of labour

The management of the 3rd stage of labour should be based on an understanding of the physiological process. For at least the last decade there has been as much discussion on the method of management of the 3rd stage of labour. The argument centres on the benefits of **active management** versus **physiological management** (also

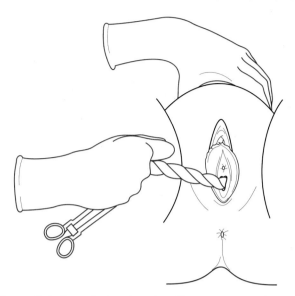

Figure 40.4 • Controlled cord traction. (From Henderson C, Macdonald S 2004, with kind permission of Elsevier.)

known as expectant or conservative management) of the 3rd stage. **Active management** involves using a prophylactic oxytocic drug followed by controlled cord traction (Fig. 40.4) to control the length of the 3rd stage and lessen the amount of bleeding. **Physiological management** involves letting nature take its course; it involves a 'hands-off approach', waiting for signs of placental separation and allowing the placenta to deliver spontaneously (possibly aided by gravity and nipple stimulation). The placenta and membranes are expelled by maternal effort but carefully retrieved by the midwife to avoid retention of placental tissue or membranes.

The development and use of oxytocic drugs to manage the third stage of labour

There has been a great deal of debate over the last decade about the optimum method for the safe expulsion of the placenta after childbirth (Anderson 2003). Active versus physiological management remains a controversial issue. Begley (1990) reminded us that in the first half of the last century postpartum haemorrhage (PPH) was a major cause of maternal death, with figures between 8% and 22%, depending on when and where the statistics were gathered. Increased availability of blood transfusions, the role of better antenatal care and nutrition in the prevention of anaemia and improved general health of women in westernised countries reduced this to between 4% and 7% by 1978. However, PPH still remains the most common cause of maternal mortality in the world with haemorrhage contributing to 11% of all global maternal deaths (Anderson 2003, Lewis 2007).

Van Dongen & de Groot (1995) wrote an informative historical paper on the use of ergot alkaloids. The alkaloid used in the management of the 3rd stage, ergometrine, was first isolated in 1932 and was synthesised in 1938. The World Health Organization (WHO) (1998) estimated that of over 500 000 (half a million) women who die during childbirth, PPH is one of the most common causes, accounting for 13% of maternal deaths in developed countries but 33% of deaths in developing countries. Latest WHO statistics (WHO 2007) estimate that 536 000 women die every year from complications of pregnancy and childbirth; 99% of these deaths occur in developing countries.

The first routine use of intramuscular ergometrine 0.5 mg was in 1951 and it was given as the head crowned. This shortened the 3rd stage of labour and reduced blood loss in all deliveries but, more significantly, it reduced the incidence of PPH. However, van Dongen & de Groot (1995) also mention that oxytocin is as efficient as ergometrine without its dangers. The risks associated with the administration of ergometrine are severe hypertension, nausea and vomiting, and side-effects due to vasoconstriction. Maternal deaths have occurred following its administration and for these reasons the writers considered that the administration of oxytocin may be safer.

Begley (1990) cited Embrey et al (1963), who compared the use of intramuscular ergometrine with intramuscular Syntometrine, a product combining ergometrine (500 μg) and synthetic oxytocin (5 IU), and this rapidly became the drug of choice in Britain. Figure 40.5 presents the speed of action of the drugs Syntocinon and ergometrine. During the 1980s women were better nourished, younger, of less parity and less anaemic than their mothers had been. They were also better informed and aware of the trend towards natural childbirth. It became part of the birth plan of many women to request that these oxytocic drugs should be omitted in the 3rd stage of labour unless thought necessary in an emergency. This led to a series of trials over recent years to ascertain the safety of this practice, which was named physiological management of the 3rd stage of labour.

In 1987 Gilbert et al studied the incidence and effect of PPH. They compared 86 women who had a PPH with 351 women whose blood loss at delivery was less than 350 ml and found risk factors of primiparity, induction of labour, forceps delivery, prolonged first and second stages of labour and the administration of oxytocin rather than Syntometrine. Epidural analgesia was an associated factor. They concluded that 'Changes in labour ward practices over the last 20 years have resulted in the re-emergence of PPH as a significant problem'. In particular they mentioned induction of labour, epidural analgesia and acceptance of a prolonged second stage as factors increasing the risk of PPH.

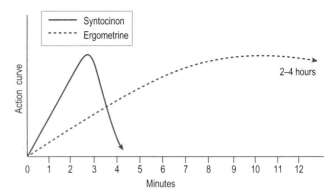

Figure 40.5 • Graph representing the relative speeds of action of the drugs Syntocinon and ergometrine.

Active versus physiological management

Prendiville et al (1988) reported on a major trial, called the Bristol Third Stage Trial. The rationale was the challenge of routine obstetric procedures and their effects on the natural process of labour. Inch (1985) had suggested that routine management of the 3rd stage of labour led to a 'cascade of intervention', leading to controlled cord traction, because:

- Women are delivered of their placentas without the aid of gravity.
- The umbilical cord is clamped early and routinely.
- A prophylactic oxytocic drug is administered.

In particular, the use of oxytocics, usually intramuscular Syntometrine, was challenged. The objective of the trial was to compare the effects on fetal and maternal morbidity of routine active management of the 3rd stage of labour and expectant (physiological) management, in particular to determine whether active management reduced the incidence of PPH. There were 1695 women of 4709 delivered between 1 January 1986 and 31 January 1987 included in the trial. They were allocated randomly to physiological management (849) and active (846) management.

After 5 months, a high level of PPH in the physiological group (16.5% versus 3.8%) made the researchers modify the protocol to exclude more women and allow those in the physiological group who needed some active management to be switched to fully active management. The physiological group continued to show a high rate of PPH and after the first 1500 deliveries the study was stopped.

Following criticism of their protocol, Prendiville et al (1988) reanalysed their results to exclude the risk categories mentioned in the Gilbert et al (1987) paper. They found that active management of the 3rd stage was preferable regardless of these first and second stage criteria. However, they also considered the effect of familiarity with the techniques of physiological management and also that midwives may find physiological management less acceptable because of their knowledge of the risks. They also considered the fact that women would have had no antenatal preparation for the maternal effort required. The main conclusion of the trial was still that active management of the 3rd stage of labour was justified.

Harding et al (1989) commented on the views of midwives and mothers participating in the trial and found that both mothers and midwives commented unfavourably about the length of the 3rd stage when it was managed physiologically. They were in favour of continuing the current practice of active management.

Following the Bristol Trial, a further study was set up, named the Dublin Trial. Begley (1990) gave the opposite point of view in a report of the findings of this randomised controlled trial of 1429 women, which compared active management of the 3rd stage of labour using intravenous ergometrine 0.5 mg with physiological management of women who had a low risk of PPH. The trial found that the use of ergometrine was associated with complications such as a greater need for manual removal of placenta, nausea, vomiting and severe after-pains, hypertension and secondary PPH. Although the incidence of PPH and postnatal haemoglobin <10 g/dl was higher in the physiologically managed group, there was no difference in the need for blood transfusion. The discussion stated that there was no need to use intravenous ergometrine in women at low risk for PPH and, in fact, more complications occurred because of its administration.

Thilaganathan et al (1993) reported on a further randomised controlled trial of active versus physiological management of the 3rd stage, called the Brighton Trial. Randomisation was achieved by consecutively numbered sealed envelopes and, like the other two trials, there were some post-randomisation withdrawals due to circumstances such as retained placenta. The high-risk categories were grand multiparity, previous PPH, previous caesarean section, pregnancy-induced hypertension, antepartum haemorrhage and premature rupture of the membranes. Women who had previously consented and who presented in spontaneous labour between 37 and 42 weeks of gestation were admitted to the trial. Women who then required augmentation of labour, operative delivery, cervical laceration or third-degree tear during delivery were withdrawn from the trial. It was found that active management of the 3rd stage of labour reduces the length of the 3rd stage of labour but may not reduce blood loss when compared to physiological management in women at low risk of PPH.

Rogers et al (1998) reported on the findings from the Hinchingbrooke Randomised Controlled Trial comparing active management with physiological management of the 3rd stage of labour. This trial was conducted to address those issues related to outcomes about the 3rd stage that had not been answered by either the Bristol Trial or the Dublin Trial. Active management included intramuscular Syntometrine (or Syntocinon for women with hypertension) within 2 min of birth, immediate cord clamping and cutting of the cord and delivery of the placenta by maternal effort or controlled cord traction. Physiological management involved no administration of a prophylactic drug, the cord was left intact until pulsation ceased and the placenta was delivered by maternal effort. Women (1512) were recruited to the trial if deemed to be low risk for PPH. Information was collected immediately after birth and up to 6 weeks postpartum and included subjective information from mothers. Midwives in this trial were already experienced in the practice of both active and physiological management. Results indicated that women who received physiological management had a PPH rate 2.5 times greater than women who were actively managed. There was more chance of these women requiring blood transfusion and the average length of the 3rd stage was 15 min compared with 8 min in the actively managed group who were also noted to have a raised number of side-effects. Women in the physiological group were three times more likely to make positive comments. Positive comments related to feelings of achievement; negative comments were related to the extra length of time.

Prendiville et al (2000) compared active versus expectant management of the 3rd stage of labour in a systematic review of the four main trials above. They concluded that routine active management of the 3rd stage is superior to expectant (physiological) management in terms of blood loss, PPH and other serious complications of the 3rd stage, which was reiterated by Cotter et al (2001). However, Prendiville et al (2000) found that active management was associated with unpleasant side-effects such as nausea and vomiting. They suggest that active management should be the routine management of choice for women expecting to deliver a baby by vaginal delivery in a maternity unit. The implications were found to be less clear for other birth settings, including domiciliary deliveries, developing countries and units where expectant management is the usual practice.

Soltani & Dickinson (2006) conducted a systematic review to explore placental cord drainage after spontaneous vaginal delivery as part of the management of the 3rd stage of labour. This review stated that it was not possible to draw any major conclusions from the research studies, due to the small numbers, poor quality and varied format of reporting, although they do argue that a statistically significant reduction in the length of the 3rd stage of labour was observed when performing cord drainage. They do, however, go on to emphasise that larger randomised controlled trials have to be conducted to explore cord drainage and the management of the 3rd stage specifically in relation to maternal removal of the placenta.

Syntometrine versus oxytocin

McDonald et al (2004) carried out a systematic review of six randomised controlled trials (9332 women) to compare the use of oxytocin and Syntometrine as prophylactic oxytocic drugs used in the active management of 3rd stage of labour. They concluded that the use of the combination preparation Syntometrine (oxytocin and ergometrine) was associated with a statistically significant reduction in the risk of PPH compared with oxytocin (5 units), but was found to be less so when 10 units were administered. No difference was found in relation to blood loss of greater than 1000 ml. Syntometrine was associated with adverse side-effects, including nausea, vomiting and raised blood pressure. However, there was no statistical difference between groups relating to retained placenta. Practice may vary across maternity units in relation to the administration of oxytocin and syntometrine.

Examination of the placenta

- The placenta and membranes must be examined carefully following the birth (Fig. 40.6):
  - To see whether or not the placenta and membranes have been completely expelled.
  - To detect abnormalities which might provide information about any intrauterine problems. This may be of help in planning neonatal care.
- Standard precautions should be taken (gloves, apron, goggles) to prevent the transmission of blood-borne diseases such as hepatitis or HIV.
- The number of cord vessels should be ascertained. The absence of one of the umbilical arteries is sometimes associated with renal agenesis.
- The placenta (fetal surface) should be held up by the cord top to inspect the membranes for completeness. There should be a single hole through which the fetus was delivered.
- The amnion is stripped back from the chorion to the cord insertion to ensure that both membranes are present.
- The maternal surface of the placenta should be examined to make sure all the cotyledons are present. Any abnormalities such as infarctions should be noted.

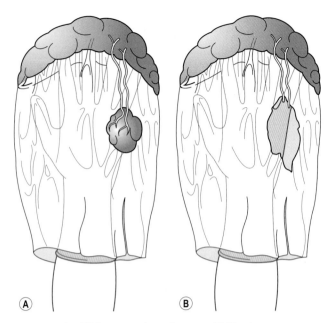

Figure 40.6 • (A) Succenturiate placenta. (B) The torn membrane; the missing lobe is in the uterus. (From Henderson C, Macdonald S 2004, with kind permission of Elsevier.)

- Blood loss is measured and added to the estimated loss present in the bed linen and pads. A blood loss of more than 500 ml is considered to be a PPH and should be reported to the obstetric team.
- Cord blood should be taken when the mother's blood group is rhesus negative, where antibodies have been found in maternal blood and for haemoglobinopathy investigations.

It is the midwife's responsibility to thoroughly examine the placenta and membranes and ensure that accurate contemporaneous documentation of the findings is executed.

The midwife should remain with the mother for at least 1 h following completion of the delivery, whether this is in the maternity unit or the home. The uterus should now be palpated gently to ensure that it remains well contracted and the lochia assessed. Maternal temperature, pulse and blood pressure should be recorded and the mother is encouraged to pass urine, attend to personal hygiene and have a light refreshment.

Main points

- In the 3rd stage of labour separation and expulsion of the placenta and membranes occur and bleeding from the placental site is minimal. This begins immediately following the birth of the baby and normally lasts from 5 to 30 min but may take up to an hour.

- The placental site rapidly diminishes in size and the placenta is compressed so that blood in the intervillous spaces is forced back into the spongy layer of the decidua. Retraction of the oblique muscle fibres constricts the blood vessels supplying the placenta, preventing blood from draining into the maternal vascular tree.

- The Shultze mechanism describes separation occurring from the centre of the placenta and results in the fetal surface of the placenta first appearing at the vulva. The Duncan mechanism describes separation occurring from the borders and results in the maternal surface of the placenta first appearing at the vulva.
- Three factors are involved in haemostasis: the action of the living ligatures; the walls of the uterus applying pressure to the placental site; and a transitory increase in the activity of the coagulation system.
- Active management involves using a prophylactic oxytocic drug followed by controlled cord traction to control the length of the 3rd stage and lessen the amount of bleeding. Physiological management involves a 'hands-off' approach, waiting for signs of placental separation and allowing the placenta to deliver spontaneously (possibly aided by gravity and nipple stimulation).

- Routine active management is superior to expectant (physiological) management in terms of blood loss, postpartum haemorrhage and other serious complications of the 3rd stage. However, active management (syntometrine) is associated with side-effects such as nausea and vomiting.
- The placenta and membranes should be examined following delivery. This is required to identify complete or incomplete delivery of the placenta and membranes and to detect abnormalities.
- The midwife should check that the uterus is well contracted and that lochia is minimal. Blood pressure, pulse and temperature are checked and recorded.

References

Anderson, T., 2003. Active versus expectant management of the third stage of labour. A Cochrane database review. In: Wickham, S. (Ed.), Midwifery: Best Practice. Elsevier, London.

Begley, C.M., 1990. A comparison of active and physiological management of the third stage of labour. Midwifery 6, 3–17.

Blackburn, S.T., 2007. Maternal, Fetal and Neonatal Physiology: A Clinical Perspective, fourth edn. Elsevier Saunders, Missouri.

Cotter, A., Ness, A., Tolosa, J., 2001. Prophylactic oxytocin for the third stage of labour. Cochrane Review. Cochrane Library Issue 4. Update Software 2008, Oxford.

Gilbert, L., Porter, W., Brown, V.A., 1987. Postpartum haemorrhage—a continuing problem. Br. J. Obstet. Gynaecol. 94, 67–71.

Harding, J.E., Elbourne, D.R., Prendiville, W.J., 1989. Views of mothers and midwives participating in the Bristol Randomised Controlled Trial of Active Management of the Third Stage of Labor. Birth 16 (1), 1–6.

Henderson, C., Macdonald, S. (Eds.), 2004. Mayes' Midwifery: A Textbook for Midwives, thirteenth edn. Baillière Tindall, London.

Inch, S., 1985. Management of the third stage of labour—another cascade of intervention? Midwifery 1, 114–122.

Lewis, G. (Ed.), 2007. Saving Mothers' Lives: The Seventh Report of the Confidential Enquiries into Maternal and Child Health. RCOG, London.

McDonald, S.J., Abbott, J.M., Higgins, S.P., 2004. Prophylactic ergometrine–oxytocin versus oxytocin for the third stage of labour. Cochrane Review. The Cochrane Library Issue 1. Update Software 2008, Oxford.

Murray, I., 2003. Changes and adaptation in pregnancy. In: Fraser, D.M., Cooper, M. A. (Eds.), Myles Textbook for Midwives, fourteenth edn. Churchill Livingstone, Edinburgh.

NICE (National Institute for Health and Clinical Excellence), 2007. Intrapartum Care: Care of healthy women and their babies during childbirth, NICE Clinical Guideline No. 55. RCOG Press, London.

Prendiville, W.J., Harding, J.E., Elbourne, D.R., et al., 1988. The Bristol Third Stage Trial: active versus physiological management of the third stage of labour. Br. Med. J. 297, 1295–1300.

Prendiville, W.J., Elbourne, D.R., McDonald, S., 2000. Active versus expectant management of the third stage of labour. Cochrane Review. Cochrane Library, Issue 4. Update Software 2002, Oxford.

Rogers, J., Wood, J., McCandlish, R., et al., 1998. Active versus expectant management of the third stage of labour: the Hinchingbrooke Randomised Controlled Trial. Lancet 351, 693–699.

Soltani, H., Dickinson, F., 2006. Timing of prophylactic oxytocics for the third stage of labour after vaginal birth (protocol). Cochrane Database of Syst. Rev. (4) Art. No.: CD006173. DOI: 10.1002/14651858. CD006173.

Thilaganathan, B., Cutner, A., Latimer, J., et al., 1993. Management of the third stage of labour in women at low risk of postpartum haemorrhage. Eur. J. Obstet. Gynecol. Reprod. Biol. 48, 19–22.

Van Dongen, P.W.J., de Groot, A.N.J.A., 1995. History of ergot alkaloids from ergotism to ergometrine. Eur. J. Obstet. Gynecol. Reprod. Biol. 60, 109–116.

Wattis, L., 2004. The third stage maze: which practice pathway for optimum outcomes? In: Wickes, S. (Ed.), Midwifery Best Practice 2. Elsevier, London.

World Health Organization (WHO), 1998. World Health Day highlights scandal of 600 000 maternal deaths each year. Press Release WHO/33.

World Health Organization (WHO), 2007. Maternal Mortality in 2005. WHO Press, Geneva.

Annotated recommended reading

Prendiville, W.J., Elbourne, D.R., McDonald, S., 2000. Active versus expectant management of the third stage of labour. Cochrane Review. Cochrane Library, Issue 4. Update Software 2009, Oxford.

This is the latest updated review of active versus physiological management of the 3rd stage of labour, and is essential reading for evidence-based intrapartum care.

Wattis, L., 2004. The third stage maze: which practice pathway for optimum outcomes? In: Wickes, S. (Ed.), Midwifery Best Practice 2. Elsevier, London.

This chapter provides a detailed overview of current issues related to 3rd stage, including choice of oxytocic drugs and cord clamping.

Yuen, P.M., Chan, N.S.T., Yim, S.F., et al., 1995. A randomised double blind comparison of Syntometrine and Syntocinon in the management of the third stage of labour. Br. J. Obstet. Gynaecol. 102, 277–380.

In this article Yuen et al compared the effectiveness of Syntometrine and Syntocinon and concluded that Syntometrine was the drug of choice as it was more effective than Syntocinon.

Section **3B**

Labour—Problems

SECTION CONTENTS

Although the majority of labours progress normally, problems may present at the onset or develop rapidly within labour that are life-threatening to both mother and fetus. The knowledge and experience required to recognise these problems and to summon help from the obstetric team is vital to the midwife. This section is concerned with abnormal labour. Traditionally, these problems can be grouped as the effects of the 'powers, passenger and passages' on the progress of labour. Chapter 41 examines the 'powers' and presents the problems of abnormal uterine action in detail. The following two chapters discuss problems with the 'passenger', i.e. the fetus. Chapter 42 is concerned with breech presentation, while Chapter 43 discusses all other abnormal positions and presentations. Except in extreme cases, it is artificial to discuss problems with the 'passages' as these almost always relate to the size, position and presentation of that particular fetus. However, Chapter 44 is concerned with cephalopelvic disproportion. The placenta and membranes are part of the passenger and problems with their delivery are considered in Chapter 45. Chapter 46 is about perinatal fetal asphyxia and sits at the junction between labour and neonatal care. Finally, Chapter 47 looks at operative procedures such as delivery by forceps, vacuum extraction and caesarean section.

Chapter Forty-One

Abnormalities of uterine action and onset of labour

Introduction

The length of labour is variable and is affected by different factors such as the type of uterine contractions, parity, birth interval, psychological state, presentation, position, pelvic shape and size of the fetus. This chapter discusses abnormalities of uterine action. Each of these factors must be considered in turn over the next few chapters, although in practice there may be interaction between them. This chapter on abnormal uterine action will include active management of labour. The association between the pattern of contractions and the progress of labour is highly variable and the outcome difficult to predict. Abnormal uterine action may be inefficient, resulting in prolongation of labour, or over-efficient, resulting in precipitate labour.

Normal labour begins spontaneously at term, i.e. after 37 completed weeks and before 42 completed weeks of pregnancy (McCormick 2003). The contractions increase in length, strength and frequency, resulting in progressive descent of the fetus and dilatation of the cervical os until the fetus, placenta and membranes are expelled from the uterus and bleeding is controlled. Normal labour is also characterised by harmonious interaction between the two poles of the uterus: the upper uterine segment contracts and retracts and the lower uterine segment thins out and the cervix dilates.

Abnormalities of uterine action

Prolonged labour

The first stage of labour can be described as having **latent**, **active** and **deceleration phases**. During the latent phase, the uterus contracts regularly and the cervix effaces and dilates and this will determine the progress (Simkin & Ancheta 2005). The latent phase lasts until cervical dilatation is about 3–4 cm; this can take 6–8 h in a primigravida. The active phase with rapid dilatation of the cervix is about 1 cm/h in a primigravida and 1.5 cm/h in a multigravida. Defining the term 'prolonged labour' is problematic and related to a chosen length, mainly because of a belief that, the longer labour lasts, the more danger there is for mother and fetus. It is important to remember that although prolonged labour is common in primigravidae it occurs less often in multigravidae and may be due to obstruction of labour, where rupture of the uterus may follow careless use of oxytocic drugs in a multigravid labour.

There has been a trend to reduce the accepted length of labour in a primigravida over the last 40 years from 24 to 12 h. If the length of the latent phase of the first stage of labour in a primigravida is accepted as 6 h, resulting in a dilatation of 4 cm, and average progress of dilatation up to 10 cm in the active and deceleration phases is 1 cm/h, it is easy to see how 12 h has become the accepted norm. Labour may be prolonged in the latent, active or deceleration phases. However, NICE (2007) advocate that the length of labour for a primigravida should be on average 8 h and not last more than 18 h, whereas a multigravida labour is shorter with an average of 5 h and not lasting more than 12 h. They stipulate that all aspects of labour progress should be assessed prior to diagnosing a delay in the first stage of labour such as: cervical dilatation of less than 2 cm in 4 h for both primigravida and multigravida or slowing down of labour in multigravida; a change in the frequency, duration and strength of uterine contractions; descent and rotation of the fetal head. This is echoed by Simkin & Ancheta (2005) who state that it is important that correct diagnosis is made. They highlight that, for labour to progress, six events must occur:

1. Posterior cervix changes to the anterior position.
2. Ripening and softening of the cervix.
3. Effacement of the cervix.
4. Dilatation of the cervix.
5. Flexion, rotation and moulding of fetal head.
6. Descent and further rotation of fetus and birth.

Timing of the onset of labour

A further difficulty is how to define the onset of labour. As discussed in Chapter 36, the timing is important as it allows decisions to be made about the progress and ongoing management of labour yet it is difficult to establish with accuracy. Gibb (1988) discusses the concept of **pre-labour**, meaning the changes that occur in the last few weeks of pregnancy. It is often difficult to decide when the transition from the painless uterine contractions of pre-labour develops into true labour. This is reiterated by Simkin & Ancheta (2005), who argue that most slow labours do progress into normal labour patterns so it is difficult to accurately state that a labour is dysfunctional until the active phase. A slow labour before women become established is sometimes referred to as a 'hesitant labour'.

Latent or active phase?

There is lack of agreement about whether to count the onset of labour from the onset of the latent phase or the active phase of the first stage of labour (Church & Hodgson 2004). The most frequently used marker for the commencement of labour is the onset of regular rhythmic painful uterine contractions. This is an arbitrary point in time rather than a biologically correct starting point (Enkin et al 2000). Vaginal examination of women at the time of admission demonstrates that

the decision to present for admission in labour varies, depending on the advice the woman has been given on recognising the onset of labour and her anxieties and expectations.

Dangers of prolonged labour to the mother and fetus

Maternal risks

The physical effort, pain and anxiety of a prolonged labour result in dehydration, ketosis and tiredness. If this were to be allowed to continue:

- Maternal distress could occur: the temperature, pulse and blood pressure rise; dehydration, oliguria and ketosis develop; and the woman may vomit.
- If undetected cephalopelvic disproportion is present, the uterus may rupture.
- Other risks include trauma to the bladder, operative interventions and postpartum haemorrhage.
- If the membranes are ruptured, intrauterine infection is a risk (Smyth et al 2007).
- Haemorrhage is also associated with prolonged labour (Smyth et al 2007).

Fetal risks

- Intrapartum hypoxia may cause acidosis, fetal distress, neonatal asphyxia and meconium aspiration, possibly leading to perinatal death.
- Cerebral trauma may occur due to excessive pounding of the fetal head against the bony pelvis or excessive moulding.
- Prolonged rupture of the membranes may result in neonatal infection, e.g. pneumonia.

The Stillbirth, Neonatal and Post-Neonatal Mortality Report still suggests that of the intrapartum causes of fetal mortality 1.1% are due to mechanical complications (CEMACH 2007).

Inefficient uterine action

Uterine contractions are inefficient if they do not result in dilatation of the cervix. Inefficient uterine action is the most common cause of abnormal labour in primigravidae. O'Driscoll et al (1993) showed that inefficient uterine action caused delay in 65% of 9018 nulliparous women with prolonged labour. The remaining cases were caused by persistent occipitoposterior position (24%) and cephalopelvic disproportion (CPD) (11%) (Malone et al 1996). There is slow progress and the length of labour is prolonged. Inefficiency may be because the contractions are too weak (**hypotonic uterine action**) or because there is loss of coordination between the upper and lower uterine segments (**incoordinate uterine action**).

Hypotonic uterine action

The uterine contractions are weak and short and there is slow dilatation or no dilatation of the cervix. The woman does not find the contractions too painful or distressing. The fetus remains in good condition. If hypotonic contractions occur from the commencement of labour, they are said to be **primary**. The cause of primary hypotonic uterine action is unknown but is more commonly seen in primigravidae. If they begin after a period of normal uterine action, they are said to be **secondary** and there may be abnormalities of labour such as CPD, malposition of the occiput, a malpresentation, maternal dehydration or ketosis. The commencement of epidural analgesia sometimes causes hypotonic uterine action (Church & Hodgson 2004) due to the relaxation of the pelvic floor, which interferes with the mechanisms of labour.

Incoordinate uterine action

There is loss of polarity and an increase in resting tone of the uterus. The contractions are frequent and painful and the woman feels pain between contractions. The woman feels the contraction before and after it is palpable abdominally. The cervix dilates slowly or not at all. Placental blood flow is decreased, which might lead to fetal distress. This type of uterine action is associated with malpositions of the occiput. If there is not maternal problems or fetal distress it is important to alleviate the woman's anxiety and try mobilisation first, which might aid progress in labour prior to active management and introduction of interventions (Church & Hodgson 2004).

Active management of labour

In the 1960s, O'Driscoll introduced active management of labour for the management of labour in primigravidae (O'Driscoll et al 1986). There must be accurate diagnosis of the onset of labour with painful uterine contractions and either complete effacement of the cervix, a show or spontaneous rupture of the membranes (Henderson 1996). Amniotomy is carried out shortly after admission with augmentation of labour with Syntocinon (oxytocin) if there is inadequate progress after 1 h. Some maternity units have a policy of putting up a Syntocinon infusion immediately after amniotomy. All women are given adequate emotional support and ongoing peer review to assess the efficiency and effectiveness of the protocol (Church & Hodgson 2004, Gerhardstein et al 1995).

Augmentation of labour

A Syntocinon infusion is used to manage prolonged labour when progress is slow but otherwise normal. This is acceleration or augmentation of labour. Once delay has been diagnosed and abnormalities of presentation or CPD ruled out, the membranes are ruptured and an intravenous infusion of Syntocinon is commenced to stimulate labour contractions. Any abnormality of fluid and electrolyte balance is corrected and both mother and fetus are monitored carefully. Adequate pain relief should be provided. Findings regarding the progress of labour should be recorded graphically on a partogram (Fig. 41.1) so that deviations from normal can be immediately

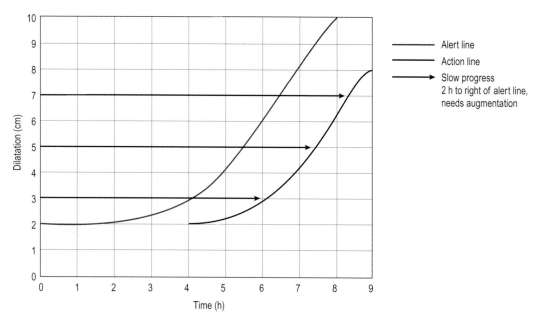

Figure 41.1 • Normogram/partogram of cervimetric progress commencing at 2 cm dilatation. 'Alert' line outlines normal progress. 'Action' line indicates when augmentation should be instituted. (After Studd 1973.)

recognised. There should be good psychological support of the woman. This should include explanation of what is happening and reassurance that everything is going as planned.

Amniotomy

The benefits of intact membranes throughout labour include reduced risk of intrauterine infection (Smyth et al 2007) and of fetal hypoxia because of less placental compression and less reduction of size of the placental site. Amniotomy is the artificial rupture of the fetal membranes that results in drainage of liquor (Shiers 2003). This procedure has been practiced for several decades and is usually performed to accelerate labour. Amniotomy may also be done to examine the amniotic fluid for the presence of meconium.

In a systematic review, Smyth et al (2007) studied the effects of amniotomy on the rate of caesarean sections and other indicators of maternal and neonatal morbidity. They concluded that amniotomy in spontaneous labour should not be routine practice. There was no difference in length of first stage of labour, maternal satisfaction or Apgar scores less than 7 at 5 min. The review showed an upward trend in the number of caesarean sections performed. The reviewers suggest that the findings from the paper should be discussed with women prior to amniotomy in labour being conducted. In similar fashion, Church & Hodgson (2004) believe there should be a clear indication of the need for amniotomy before it is carried out.

Oxytocic infusion

Church & Hodgson (2004) report that the use of oxytocin for labour varies, whereas O'Driscoll et al (1993) state the rates are as high as 45%. As described above, the benefits are correction of inefficient uterine action, a shorter labour, a reduced rate of caesarean section with a corresponding increase in vaginal delivery. Byrne et al (1993) found no evidence that an oxytocic infusion generated excessive intrauterine pressures. However, women experience more painful contractions and are restricted in their ability to move about.

The division of the first stage of labour into latent, active and deceleration phases must be considered as being important to the use and efficacy of oxytocin. Olah et al (1993) found that cervical muscle fibres constrict in response to oxytocin in the latent phase, leading to a poor response; they also described high intrauterine pressures and the possibility of fetal distress, although O'Driscoll et al (1993) found no evidence of this.

Expectations of childbirth have developed and the medicalisation of a normal physiological process was criticised in the 1980s (Walkinshaw 1994). There is now much variation in practice between units and, until recently, maternal satisfaction with delivery has not been considered in research protocols. Enkin et al (2000) summarised the evidence and did not think there was any benefit to women and their babies of liberal use of oxytocic infusions. They concluded that, although the use of an oxytocic infusion had its place in the management of women enduring a prolonged labour, other measures such as ambulation and allowing intake of appropriate nutrition should be considered before labelling a labour as abnormal and using medical intervention (Church & Hodgson 2004).

Prolonged second stage of labour

A discussion on the acceptable length of the second stage of labour is presented in Chapter 39. Delayed progress may be due to:

- Inefficient uterine action (primary powers).
- Inefficient maternal effort (secondary powers).
- A full bladder or rectum, a rigid perineum.
- A contracted pelvic outlet.
- A large baby.
- A fetal abnormality such as hydrocephaly or abdominal enlargement.
- Persistent occipitoposterior position.
- Deep transverse arrest of the head.
- Malpresentation.

Management

The condition of mother and fetus should be carefully assessed and as long as progress is being made, although slowly, more time may be given. Adopting an upright position, kneeling, standing or squatting may enlarge the pelvic outlet (Simkin & Ancheta 2005) and direct the presenting part against the posterior vaginal wall, utilising Ferguson's reflex with the release of oxytocin. If the maternal or fetal condition becomes worrying or there is no obvious progress, an assisted vaginal delivery or, more rarely, a caesarean section may be needed.

Over-efficient uterine action

Precipitate labour

A precipitate labour occurs when the uterine contractions occur frequently and are intense. There is rapid completion of the first and second stages of labour and delivery normally occurs within an hour. This condition is much more common in the multigravid woman and is usually caused by lack of resistance of the maternal soft tissues. There may have been minimal pain in the first stage of labour and the woman becomes aware of imminent delivery when the head is about to be born.

Dangers of precipitate labour

The woman may have lacerations to the cervix and perineum. Postpartum haemorrhage may follow. The baby may be hypoxic and may sustain intracranial injuries because of rapid descent through the birth canal. If the birth takes place in an inappropriate place, the baby may be injured. Any labouring woman with a history of a previous precipitate delivery should not be left alone and watched very closely when in labour.

Tonic contraction of the uterus

This rare event, where the tone of the uterus is continuously high and there is no relaxation of the uterine muscle, is accompanied by intense pain. The fetus becomes distressed as the placental circulation is grossly restricted. Intrauterine death may occur. Causes may be obstructed labour or misuse of oxytocic drugs such as Syntocinon and prostaglandins. This is an emergency and immediate treatment may save the baby's life and prevent uterine rupture:

- If an oxytocic infusion is in progress, discontinue (NICE 2008).
- Turn the mother onto her left side to enhance uteroplacental blood flow.
- Inform the obstetrician, who will review the woman with regards to caesarean section.

Administration of facial oxygen was common practice; however, there is no evidence to support either prophylaxis or short-term use of oxygen for fetal compromise (Fawole & Hofmeyr 2003, NICE 2008).

Cervical dystocia

Cervical dystocia, where the cervix dilates slowly if at all, may be congenital or acquired. Congenital problems may be fibrosis, stenosis or poor cervical development. Acquired cervical dystocia may be due to fibrosis and scarring of the cervix following surgery, cautery or irradiation. In the past when there was failure to recognise the condition, prolonged pressure would result in ischaemia and there would be annular detachment of the cervix.

If the anterior part of the cervix is trapped between the pelvic brim and the fetal head, venous return is restricted and the anterior lip may become swollen and oedematous and feel as thick as a finger during vaginal examination. The first stage of labour will be prolonged and occasionally the cervix may be seen blue and glistening between the fetal head and the symphysis pubis. This is caused by the woman bearing down before full cervical dilatation and it is commonly the result of a persistent occipitoposterior position (Simkin & Ancheta 2005). If the woman lies on her side and is encouraged to use inhalational analgesia, she will be helped to avoid pushing. Elevating the foot of her bed may also help. Epidural analgesia may occasionally be needed. It is sometimes possible to push an anterior lip of cervix up behind the fetal head but care must be taken not to tear the cervix.

Problems: timing of the onset of labour

Preterm onset of labour

Preterm labour is one that begins before the end of the 37th week of pregnancy. A baby born from such a labour is a preterm baby irrespective of birth weight. Not all preterm babies are of low birth weight (LBW), weighing less than 2000 g, but many babies are both preterm and of low birth weight. Babies weighing less than 1500 g are very low birth weight (VLBW), while those weighing less than 1000 g are named extremely low birth weight (ELBW). Preterm babies have different problems and needs to those babies who are of low weight because of growth retardation; the care of such babies will be discussed in the relevant chapter.

Kramer et al (1998) showed that between 1978 and 1996 the incidence of preterm delivery increased from 6.6% to 9.8% for births at less than 37 weeks' gestation, from 1.7% to 2.3% at less than 34 weeks and from 1.0% to 1.2% at less than 32 weeks. The incidence of preterm delivery as a proportion of all births ranges from 6% to 10% in developed countries and has changed little over the past few decades (Dodd et al 2006, Lindsay 2004). However, noticeably fetal morbidity remains high. Findings from the Confidential Enquiry into Maternal and Child Health (CEMACH 2005), which used the extended Wigglesworth Classification, showed that immaturity was found to be the main contributing factor in 49.7% of all neonatal deaths in 2003. Maternal mortality and morbidity is rarely affected by preterm onset of labour although women may suffer feelings of inadequacy as a result of perceiving themselves to have failed (Edmonds 2007).

Aetiology

Preterm births may follow a spontaneous onset of labour or be elective because of a problem for the woman or the fetus. The following conditions may lead to preterm delivery:

- Severe pre-eclampsia.
- Maternal disease such as renal disease, diabetes mellitus and maternal infection.
- Severe intrauterine growth retardation.
- Rhesus isoimmunisation.
- Premature rupture of the membranes.
- Prolapsed cord.
- Placental abruption.

In about 40% of cases onset of labour occurs spontaneously with no known cause. Lindsay (2004) summarises the **risk factors** associated with preterm labour (Table 41.1). While not directly causative, they may indicate which women have an increased risk of preterm delivery. Although the above list is comprehensive, it is difficult to predict which woman will begin labour before term. A further problem is that, even if the onset of preterm labour could be predicted, it is difficult to prevent the progress to delivery.

As the risk factors are so wide, attempts at reducing some of the physical or social factors have had limited success. Risk-scoring systems have been developed using the above factors but have been found to be poor predictors, especially in primigravid women. Home monitoring of uterine activity has had no effect on the rate of preterm birth. Cervical effacement can be assessed but it is not a good predictor of preterm birth and may also introduce infection.

Fetal fibrinectin

High levels of fetal fibrinectin, a component of the extracellular matrix secreted by the anchoring trophoblastic villi, have been found in cervical and vaginal secretions prior to the onset of preterm labour (Lockwood et al 1991). Separation of maternal and fetal tissue at the choriodecidual junction leads to a leakage of fibronectin and a test has been developed. The test is accurate in up to 80% of cases and can be carried out every 2 weeks after the 24th week of pregnancy. Both blood and amniotic fluid contain fibronectin and this limits the use of the test (Lindsay 2004).

Preterm rupture of the membranes

Spontaneous preterm pre-labour rupture of the membranes is associated with genital tract infection (Flenady & King 2002) and cervical incompetence. Labour may begin soon after the event, but, if delayed, bacteria may ascend the genital tract to colonise the uterus and fetus. The woman must be admitted to a hospital with a neonatal intensive care unit. No vaginal examination is performed in the absence of signs of labour and a speculum examination is carried out to visualise the cervix. A high vaginal swab is taken for culture and sensitivity testing (RCOG 2006a).

Table 41.1 A summary of the risk factors associated with preterm labour (Lindsay 2004)

Biological/medical factors	Reproductive history	Current pregnancy	Socioeconomic and psychological (Peacock et al 1995)	Cultural/behavioural
Age less than 16 or more than 35	History of previous preterm birth (two previous preterm births increases risk by 70%)	Poor nutrition and BMI less than 19.8	Poverty and social deprivation	Cigarette, alcohol or drug use
Low weight for height (low BMI)	Bleeding in previous pregnancy	Bleeding in this pregnancy	Psychological distress	Short interpregnancy interval
History of hypertension, renal disease or diabetes mellitus	Uterine abnormality (increases risk by 19%)	Retained intrauterine contraceptive device		Late antenatal booking and poor attendance for care
Generalised infections, especially viral		Abdominal surgery Infections, e.g. pyelonephritis Genital tract infection, e.g. bacterial vaginosis (Hillier et al 1995), Chlamydia, group B haemolytic streptococcus Fetal problems: multiple pregnancy, fetal malformation, rhesus disease, fetal death, polyhydramnios		

The use of drugs in preterm onset of labour and preterm rupture of the membranes

Corticosteroids

The risk of hyaline membrane disease for the neonate is high and the steroid dexamethasone is given to the mother to accelerate surfactant production in the lungs. Roberts & Dalziel (2006) have provided an extremely detailed review of the use of corticosteroids prior to preterm delivery, analysing 21 studies and 4269 babies. Their findings were that antenatal administration of corticosteroids to women expected to deliver preterm reduces mortality, respiratory distress syndrome and intraventricular haemorrhage in preterm infants. They concluded that it should be routine practice to administer a single dose of corticosteroids prior to preterm delivery, with few exceptions. A typical regimen is two doses of 12 mg given orally or by intramuscular injection 12 h apart. The effects of the drug take 24 h and it is effective for up to 7 days.

Antibiotics

Chorioamnionitis is the cause of preterm labour in up to 30% of cases. Intra-amniotic infection may exist without a rise in temperature, rise in white cell count, uterine tenderness or fetal tachycardia and the cause is poorly understood. Preterm labour possibly follows infection because of an increased production of prostaglandin by the decidua and the amnion. Prophylactic use of antibiotics has resulted in the reduction of the risk of preterm delivery occurring within 1 week and the prevention of infection in the mother or baby (Enkin et al 2000).

King & Flenady (2002) completed a systematic review to assess the effects of prophylactic antibiotics administered to women in preterm labour with intact membranes. This involved 7428 women over 11 trials, including the recent large Oracle II 2001 Trial. The review failed to demonstrate a clear overall benefit from the use of prophylactic antibiotic treatment for preterm labour with intact membranes on neonatal outcomes. In fact, the review raised concerns about the increased neonatal mortality in those who had received antibiotics. The findings could not currently recommend prophylactic antibiotics for routine practice.

In preterm prelabour rupture of the membranes with clear evidence of infection or vaginal colonisation with pathogenic bacteria, antibiotic therapy is commenced. There is evidence to suggest that routine use of antibiotics in preterm rupture of membranes is associated with a delay in delivery and a reduction in the factors contributing to neonatal morbidity (Kenyon et al 2003).

Tocolytic drugs

If preterm labour is diagnosed and the membranes are intact, β-adrenergic drugs such as ritodrine hydrochloride, salbutamol and terbutaline, which relax smooth muscle, may be administered by intravenous infusion. No effect on perinatal mortality has been found but the delay of onset of labour by 48 h gives time for the corticosteroids to be effective (BNF 2008).

These drugs affect all smooth muscle and the woman may suffer side-effects of tachycardia, cardiac dysrhythmias, palpitations and peripheral vasodilation, resulting in hypotension and flushing (Rang et al 2007). Nausea and muscle tremors can be a problem. Pulmonary oedema may occur because of increased permeability of the alveolar–capillary barrier (Watson & Morgan 1989). There may be stimulation of the renin–aldosterone system, with increased secretion of antidiuretic hormone, leading to fluid retention. No attempt should be made to stop labour if the fetus is more than 34 weeks' gestation or is estimated to be more than 2500 g (Pearce 1985).

Prostaglandin synthesis inhibitors such as indometacin may also be used; they block the production of the enzyme endoperoxide synthase, which is responsible for the conversion of arachidonic acid to prostaglandin. Maternal side-effects are nausea, vomiting, diarrhoea, dizziness and headaches. Fetal effects may be premature closing of the ductus arteriosus, right-side heart failure (RCOG 2002) and death in utero. Major et al (1994) found an increased incidence of necrotising enterocolitis in neonates following exposure to indometacin in utero. Indometacin may be the best current tocolytic agent but is not the first choice because of the side-effects on the fetus (Rang et al 2007).

Calcium channel blockers such as nifepidine inhibit muscle contraction (Marieb & Hoehn 2008). There must be careful observation of mother and fetus, including blood glucose monitoring, because of the side-effects of the drugs. Delivery is probably inevitable if cervical dilatation progresses to 4 cm or if the membranes rupture.

Labour and delivery

All tocolytic drugs are stopped and careful monitoring of the condition of the woman and her fetus carried out. Analgesic drugs such as pethidine and morphine should be avoided if possible and the preferred methods of pain relief are epidural anaesthesia or Entonox, neither of which affects the fetus adversely. An obstetrician and paediatrician should be present at the delivery and an elective episiotomy performed to reduce pressure on the fetal head and minimise cerebral trauma. Forceps may offer better protection. Some obstetricians prefer to deliver VLBW babies, especially if presenting by the breech, by caesarean section, but there is insufficient evidence to support this practice (RCOG 2002). The cord should be clamped at least 10 cm away from its insertion into the abdominal wall to facilitate care in the neonatal unit. Vitamin K 0.5–1.0 mg is usually given, intramuscularly, with informed parental consent to minimise the risk of haemorrhagic disease of the newborn.

Prolonged pregnancy

A pregnancy is considered to be post-term if the gestational age is accurate and it is prolonged beyond 42 completed weeks (294 days) (Gülmezoglu et al 2006). The risk of prolonged pregnancy is higher in primigravidae, being about 20% higher than in women who have given birth previously. Fetal maturity can be estimated by calculation if the first day of the last menstrual period is known and the woman has a regular cycle. Gülmezoglu et al (2006) inform us that 'There are currently no tests that can tell if a baby would be better to be left in the womb or be induced and born, so arbitrary time limits have been suggested'.

Abdominal examination is not an accurate way of measuring gestational age. An early ultrasound scan will provide good assessment of fetal age and serial scans later in pregnancy can monitor continuing fetal growth. Static maternal weight, abnormal fetal heart rate patterns and reduced fetal movements may indicate deterioration in fetal condition.

Risk factors

A post-term pregnancy has associated problems for both the woman and the fetus. For the woman, this involves interventions such as induction of labour with an unfavourable cervix and caesarean section, prolonged labour, postpartum haemorrhage and traumatic birth (Gülmezoglu et al 2006). Gülmezoglu et al (2006) suggest that some of these outcomes result from intervening when the uterus and cervix are not ready for labour. Post-term pregnancy also has a higher incidence of perinatal death and congenital malformation. After term, there may be progressive placental insufficiency and perinatal asphyxia is more common. The volume of amniotic fluid may diminish so that oxygen supply may be interrupted during contractions due to compression of the placenta. Meconium staining of the liquor is common, with the risk of meconium aspiration syndrome. Babies born after 42 weeks are more likely to weigh more than 4000 g and the increased size of the fetus may result in shoulder dystocia, accompanied by the typical trauma of brachial and facial palsy and fractured clavicle.

Management of post-term pregnancy

Conservative management of pregnancy is becoming more common if there are no complications. It is possible to monitor the well-being of the fetus by cardiotocography, ultrasound measurement of amniotic fluid volume (RCOG 2002, NICE 2008) and biophysical profile, but there is no evidence that their use improves the outcome for the fetus. Unrestricted breast stimulation and coitus after 39 weeks may decrease the incidence of post-term pregnancy although more robust evidence-based studies are required to support these factors (Kavanagh et al 2001, 2005). Digital separation of the membranes from the lower pole of the uterus (sweeping the membranes) may also help and should be discussed with and offered to women (RCOG 2002, NICE 2008). Induction of labour after 41 weeks has been shown to lessen the incidence of perinatal death but there is no support for the use of induction of labour in post-term pregnancies before 41 weeks (Enkin et al 2000).

Induction of labour

Induction of labour is defined as 'an intervention designed to artificially initiate uterine contraction, leading to progressive dilatation and effacement of the cervix and the birth of the baby' (NICE 2008). Induction is carried out for medical or obstetric reasons when it is thought that the health of the mother or fetus would be compromised by the continuation of pregnancy (Table 41.2).

Contraindications

Contraindications include placenta praevia, CPD, oblique or transverse lie, severe fetal compromise and lack of maternal consent.

Method

Induction should be timed when the presence of favourable factors indicates readiness. The success of induction depends on the state of the cervix (Enkin et al

Table 41.2 Some indications for induction of labour

Maternal indications	Fetal indications	Joint indications
Prolonged pregnancy	Placental insufficiency	Pre-eclampsia
Following spontaneous rupture of membranes	Rhesus isoimmunisation with haemolysis	Placental abruption
Medical conditions such as diabetes mellitus	Intrauterine death	Previous precipitate labour
Poor obstetric history such as a previous stillbirth	Severe congenital abnormalities	An unstable lie
Maternal request for social/psychological reasons		

2000), which can be assessed by the Bishop scoring system (NICE 2008) (Table 41.3). The prognosis for induction is good with a score of 6 or more.

Cervical ripening

Prostaglandins

There are few oxytocin receptors in the cervix, making oxytocin inefficient at ripening the cervix. There is a high failure of induction, leading to long labours and an increase in the need for caesarean section if the cervix is unfavourable at the commencement of induction. The introduction of vaginal administration of **prostaglandins** (PGE_2) or a smaller dose by the endocervical route for cervical ripening has increased the likelihood of a successful induction of labour, leading to spontaneous vaginal delivery within 12–24 h (Enkin et al 2000). However, uterine hypertonus occurs more often among women in whom prostaglandin ripening of the cervix has been used than in those women who received placebo or no prostaglandins. Abnormalities of fetal heart rate are also more likely to occur but neither trend appears to result in an increase in operative delivery (Enkin et al 2000). The systematic review of Kelly & Tan (2001) compared oxytocin alone with either intravaginal or intracervical PGE_2 and discovered that the prostaglandin agents with oxytocin were more beneficial, although it was noted in one subgroup that there was an increased rate of caesarean section. However, the authors do state that from the evidence the combined method is the recommended choice. In another systematic review (Luckas & Bricker 2000) of 13 trials (1165 women), which explored the use of intravenous prostaglandin compared to intravenous oxytocin, it was discovered that there was no difference in the rates of vaginal delivery but there were greater maternal side-effects such as pyrexia, thrombophlebitis and gastrointestinal disturbances and more uterine hyperstimulation from the use of prostaglandins compared to

the controls. French (2001) reiterates the side-effects from prostaglandin when he explored oral prostaglandins compared to oxytocin and argues that there is no clear advantage of oral prostaglandins over other methods of induction of labour.

Sweeping the membranes

Sweeping or stripping of the membranes is a relatively simple technique to perform during vaginal examination. The practitioner's finger is introduced into the cervical os and the inferior pole of the membranes is detached from the lower uterine segment by a circular movement of the finger. This procedure has the potential to initiate labour by increasing local production of prostaglandins. In a randomised controlled trial of 142 nulliparous and multiparous women, membrane stripping was found to be a safe and possibly effective way of avoiding induction by promoting spontaneous onset of labour at term (Berghella et al 1996). In a systematic review of 22 trials (2797 women), Boulvain et al (2005) conclude that, although routine sweeping of the membranes from 38 weeks was associated with reduced duration of pregnancy and reduced frequency of pregnancy continuing beyond 41 weeks, it does not seem to produce clinically proven benefits. There is agreement in the literature that a larger trial is necessary to judge the effectiveness of this procedure (Enkin et al 2000).

Amniotomy with or without oxytocin

Rupturing the membranes is a point of no return in obstetric management of labour. Once performed, the risk of intrauterine infection increases with the time interval before delivery. Amniotomy may be used on its own, accompanied by commencement of an oxytocic infusion if contractions do not commence after a few hours, or with the simultaneous commencement of an oxytocic infusion. Syntocinon infusion must be carefully

Table 41.3 Modified Bishop scoring system (RCOG 2001)

Assessment features	0	1	2	3
Dilatation of the cervix (cm)	0	1–2	3–4	5–6
Consistency of the cervix	Firm	Medium	Soft	–
Length of cervical canal (cm)	>2	1–2	0.5–1	<0.5
Position of cervix	Posterior	Mid	Anterior	–
Station of presenting part related to ischial spines	−3	−2	−1	+1, +2

regulated to avoid the complications of hyperstimulation of uterine action and water retention. Amniotic fluid embolism is a rare complication which follows hyperstimulation of uterine action.

Moldin & Sundell (1996) carried out a randomised controlled trial of amniotomy versus amniotomy with oxytocin infusion with 196 participants. All the women had a favourable Bishop score and were at term with an indication for induction. Group A had the combined induction regimen, whereas group B had amniotomy alone. The addition of an oxytocic drug led to a shorter induction–delivery interval due to a shorter latent phase of labour but no difference in the active phase of labour or the second stage of labour. Of the group B women who had amniotomy alone, 32% eventually received oxytocin although the length of time of oxytocin administration was nearly 5 times less than in group A where oxytocin had been commenced soon after the amniotomy. The authors concluded that the minor differences between the groups justified an individual management policy with attention paid to both the indication for induction of labour and the woman's choice. The evidence on this issue is sparse, which is highlighted by the systematic review of Bricker & Luckas (2000). They argue that there are insufficient data to concur that although there may be situations where amniotomy alone would be desirable this topic is worthy of more research. Howarth & Botha (2001) reiterate this finding and argue that data on the effectiveness and safety of amniotomy and intravenous oxytocin are lacking. They specify that if the combined method of amniotomy plus intravenous oxytocin is to be continued in practice it is important to compare the effectiveness and safety of these methods, and to define under which clinical circumstances one may be preferable to another.

Main points

- The type of uterine contractions, parity, birth interval, psychological state, presentation and position, pelvic shape and size all affect the length of labour. Each factor must be considered, although there may be interaction between them.

- The first stage of labour can be described as having latent, active and deceleration phases. The term 'prolonged labour' is used because of the belief that, the longer labour lasts, the more danger there is for mother and fetus.

- The dangers of prolonged labour to the mother are the physical effort, pain and anxiety, dehydration, ketosis and tiredness. Maternal distress could lead to maternal morbidity and mortality. Risks to the baby include intrapartum acidosis, fetal distress, neonatal asphyxia and meconium aspiration, perinatal death, cerebral trauma and ascending neonatal infections.

- Uterine contractions are inefficient if they do not result in dilatation of the cervix. The most common cause of abnormal labour in primigravidae is inefficient uterine action due to hypotonic uterine action or incoordinate uterine action. Progress is slow and labour is prolonged. The administration of oxytocin corrects inefficient uterine action and shortens labour. However, women experience more painful contractions and are restricted in their ability to move about.

- Delayed progress in the second stage of labour may be due to inefficient uterine action or inefficient maternal effort, a full bladder or rectum, cephalopelvic disproportion or obstructed labour. Adopting an upright position may enlarge the pelvic outlet and directs the presenting part against the posterior vaginal wall, bringing about increased uterine action.

- In precipitate labour, uterine contractions occur frequently and are intense, delivery occurring within an hour. It is most common in multigravid women and is usually caused by lack of resistance of the maternal soft tissues. The woman may have lacerations to the cervix or perineum and postpartum haemorrhage may follow. The baby may sustain intracranial injuries.

- Tonic uterine action is usually accompanied by intense pain. The fetus becomes distressed as the placental circulation is grossly restricted and intrauterine death may occur. Causes may be obstructed labour or misuse of oxytocic drugs such as Syntocinon or prostaglandins. Immediate treatment will prevent uterine rupture and save the baby's life.

- If preterm labour is diagnosed and the membranes are intact, tocolytic drugs may be administered. The delay of onset of labour by 48 h gives time for the corticosteroids to be effective in maturation of the fetal lungs. If delivery is inevitable, tocolytic drugs are discontinued. Analgesic drugs such as pethidine and morphine should be avoided if possible. Prophylactic antibiotic therapy is recommended for use in preterm rupture of membranes, as it is associated with a delay in delivery and benefits for neonatal morbidity.

- The introduction of vaginal or endocervical administration of prostaglandins (PGE_2) for cervical ripening has increased the likelihood of a successful induction of labour. Stripping the membranes from the lower uterine segment possibly produces increased amounts of prostaglandin and may be a safe way of avoiding induction by promoting spontaneous onset of labour at term.

References

Berghella, V., Rogers, R.A., Lescale, K., 1996. Stripping of membranes as a safe method to reduce prolonged pregnancies. Obstet. Gynecol. 87 (6), 927–931.

BNF (British National Formulary), 2008. No. 56. British Medical Association and the Royal Pharmaceutical Society of Great Britain, London.

Boulvain, M., Stan, C., Irion, O., 2005. Membrane sweeping for induction of labour. Cochrane Review. Cochrane Library, Issue (1) Update Software 2008, Oxford.

Bricker, L., Luckas, M., 2000. Amniotomy alone for induction of labour. Cochrane Review. Cochrane Library, Issue (4) Update Software 2008, Oxford.

Byrne, B.M., Keane, D., Boylan, P., et al., 1993. Intra-uterine pressure and the active management of labour. J. Obstet. Gynaecol. 13, 433–436.

CEMACH (Confidential Enquiry into Maternal and Child Health), 2005. Stillbirth, Neonatal and Post-Neonatal Mortality 2000–2003 Report. RCOG Press, London.

CEMACH (Confidential Enquiry into Maternal and Child Health), 2007. Stillbirth, Neonatal and Post-Neonatal Mortality 2003–2005 Report. RCOG Press, London.

Church, S., Hodgson, T., 2004. Prolonged labour and disordered uterine action, Ch. 49. In: Mayes' Textbook for Midwives, fourteenth edn. Elsevier, Edinburgh.

Dodd, J.M., Flenady, V., Cincotta, R., Crowther, C.A., 2006. Prenatal administration of progesterone for preventing preterm birth. Cochrane Review. Cochrane Library, Issue (1) Update Software 2008, Oxford.

Edmonds, D.K., 2007. Puerperium and lactation. In: Edmonds, D.K. (Ed.), Dewhurst's Textbook of Obstetrics, seventh edn. Blackwell Science, Oxford.

Enkin, M., Keirse, J., Neilson, J., et al., 2000. A Guide to Effective Care in Pregnancy and Childbirth, third edn. Oxford University Press, Oxford.

Fawole, B., Hofmeyr, G.J., 2003. Maternal oxygen administration for fetal distress. Cochrane Review. Cochrane Library, Issue (4) Update Software 2008, Oxford.

French, L., 2001. Oral prostaglandin E_2 for induction of labour. Cochrane Review. Cochrane Library, Issue (2) Update Software 2008, Oxford.

Gerhardstein, L.P., Allswede, M.T., Sloan, C.T., et al., 1995. Reduction in caesarean birth with active management of labor

and intermediate-dose oxytocin. J. Reprod. Med. 40 (1), 4–8.

Gibb, D., 1988. A Practical Guide to Labour Management. Blackwell Science, Oxford.

Gülmezoglu, A.M., Crowther, C.A., Middleton, P., 2006. Induction of labour for improving birth outcomes for women at or beyond term. Cochrane Review. Cochrane Library, Issue (4) Update Software 2008, Oxford.

Henderson, J., 1996. Active management of labour and caesarean section rates. Br. J. Midwifery, 4 (3), 132–149.

Hillier, S.L., Nugent, R.P., Eschenbach, D.A., 1995. Association between a bacterial vaginosis and preterm delivery of a low birth-weight infant. N. Engl. J. Med. 333 (26), 1736–1742.

Howarth, G.R., Botha, D.J., 2001. Amniotomy plus intravenous oxytocin for induction of labour. Cochrane Review. Cochrane Library, Issue (3) Update Software 2008, Oxford.

Flenady, V., King, J., 2002. Antibiotics for prelabour rupture of membranes at or near term. Cochrane Review. Chochrane Library, Issue (3) Update Software 2008, Oxford.

Kavanagh, J., Kelly, A.J., Thomas, J., 2001. Sexual intercourse for cervical ripening and induction of labour. Cochrane Review. Cochrane Library, Issue (2) Update Software 2008, Oxford.

Kavanagh, J., Kelly, A.J., Thomas, J., 2005. Breast stimulation for cervical ripening and induction of labour. Cochrane Review. Cochrane Library, Issue (3) Update Software 2008, Oxford.

Kelly, A.J., Tan, B., 2001. Intravenous oxytocin alone for cervical ripening and induction of labour. Cochrane Review. Cochrane Library, Issue (3) Update Software 2008, Oxford.

Kenyon, S., Boulvain, M., Neilson, J., 2003. Antibiotics for preterm rupture of membranes. Cochrane Review. Cochrane Library, Issue (2) Update Software 2008, Oxford.

King, J., Flenady, V., 2002. Prophylactic antibiotics for inhibiting preterm labour with intact membranes. Cochrane Review. Cochrane Library, Issue (2) Update Software 2008, Oxford.

Kramer, M.S., Platt, R., Yang, H., et al., 1998. Secular trends in preterm birth: a hospital-based cohort study. J. Am. Med. Assoc. 280, 1849–1854.

Lindsay, P., 2004. Preterm labour. In: Henderson, C., Macdonald, S. (Eds.) Mayes' Midwifery: A Textbook for

Midwifery, thirteenth edn. Baillière Tindall, London.

Lockwood, C., Senyei, A., Dishe, M., et al., 1991. Fetal fibronectin in cervical and vaginal secretions as a predictor of preterm delivery. N. Engl. Med. J. 325 (10), 669–674.

Luckas, M., Bricker, L., 2000. Intravenous prostaglandin for induction of labour. Cochrane Review. Cochrane Library, Issue (4) Update Software 2008, Oxford.

McCormick, C., 2003. The first stage of labour: physiology and early care. In: Fraser, D.M., Cooper, M.A. (Eds.) Myles Textbook for Midwives, fourteenth edn. Churchill Livingstone, Edinburgh.

Major, C., Lewis, D., Harding, J., et al., 1994. Tocolysis with indomethacin increases the incidence of necrotising enterocolitis in the low weight neonate. Am. J. Obstet. Gynecol. 170 (1), 102–106.

Malone, F.D., Geary, M., Chelmow, D., et al., 1996. Prolonged labor in nulliparas: lessons from the active management of labor. Obstet. Gynecol. 88 (2), 211–215.

Marieb, E.N., Hoehn, K., 2008. Anatomy & Physiology, third edn. Pearson/Benjamin Cummings, New York.

Moldin, P.G., Sundell, G., 1996. Induction of labour: a randomised clinical trial of amniotomy versus amniotomy with oxytocin infusion. Br. J. Obstet. Gynaecol. 103 (4), 306–312.

NICE (National Institute for Health and Clinical Excellence), 2007. Intrapartum Care: Care of healthy women and their babies during labour and childbirth. Clinical Guideline 55. RCOG, London. <http://www.nice.org.uk/>.

NICE (National Institute for Health and Clinical Excellence), 2008. Induction of Labour. Clinical Guideline 70. RCOG, London. <http://www.nice.org.uk/>.

O'Driscoll, K., Meagher, D., Boylan, P., 1986. Active Management of Labour, second edn. Mosby, London.

O'Driscoll, K., Meagher, D., Boylan, P., 1993. Active Management of Labour, third edn. Mosby, London.

Olah, K.S.J., Gee, A., Brown, J.S., 1993. Cervical contractions: the response of the cervix to oxytocic stimulation in the latent phase of labour. Br. J. Obstet. Gynaecol. 100, 535–640.

Peacock, J.L., Bland, J.M., Anderson, H.R., 1995. Preterm delivery: effects of socio-economic factors, psychological stress, smoking, alcohol and caffeine. Br. Med. J. 311 (7004), 532–536.

Pearce, M.J., 1985. The management of preterm labour. In: Studd, T. (Ed.), The Management of Labour. Blackwell Science, Oxford.

Rang, H.P., Dale, M.M., Ritter, J.M. (Eds.), et al., 2007. Pharmacology, sixth edn. Churchill Livingstone, Edinburgh.

RCOG (Royal College of Obstetricians and Gynaecologists), 2001. Induction of Labour. Guideline No. 9. RCOG, London.

RCOG (Royal College of Obstetricians and Gynaecologists), 2002. Tocolytic Drugs for Women in Preterm Labour. Guideline No. 1B. RCOG, London.

RCOG (Royal College of Obstetricians and Gynaecologists), 2006a. Preterm Prelabour Rupture of Membranes. Guideline No. 44. RCOG, London.

RCOG (Royal College of Obstetricians and Gynaecologists), 2006b. The Management of Breech Presentation. Guideline No. 20B. RCOG, London.

Roberts, D., Dalziel, S., 2006. Antenatal corticosteroids for accelerating fetal lung maturation for women at risk of preterm birth. Cochrane Review. Cochrane Library, Issue (3) Update Software 2008, Oxford.

Shiers, C.V., 2003. Prolonged pregnancy and disorders of uterine action. In: Fraser, D.M., Cooper, M.A. (Eds.), Myles Textbook for Midwives, fourteenth edn. Churchill Livingstone, Edinburgh.

Simkin, P., Ancheta, R., 2005. The Labour Progress Handbook, second edn. Blackwell Publishing, Oxford.

Smyth, R.M.D., Alldred, S.K., Markham, C., 2007. Amniotomy for shortening spontaneous labour. Cochrane Review. Cochrane Library, Issue (4) Update Software 2008, Oxford.

Walkinshaw, S.A., 1994. Is routine active intervention in spontaneous labour beneficial? Contem. Rev. Obstet. Gynaecol. 6 (January), 13–17.

Watson, N., Morgan, B., 1989. Pulmonary oedema and salbutamol in preterm labour. Br. J. Obstet. Gynaecol. 96 (12), 1445–1448.

Annotated recommended reading

National Institute for Health and Clinical Excellence (NICE), 2007. Intrapartum care: Care of healthy women and their babies during childbirth. NICE Clinical Guideline 55. <http://www.nice.org.uk/>.

This document sets out research-based guidelines for care in labour. It is essential reading for midwives and obstetricians. The overall responsibility for care remains with the lead professional caring for the woman.

National Institute for Health and Clinical Excellence (NICE), 2008. Induction of labour. Clinical Guideline 70. RCOG, London.

This document sets out research-based guidelines for induction of labour. These provide an excellent resource for midwives and obstetricians.

Shiers, C.V., 2003. Prolonged pregnancy and disorders of uterine action. In: Fraser, D.M., Cooper, M.A. (Eds.), Myles Textbook for Midwives, fourteenth ed. Churchill Livingstone, Edinburgh.

In this chapter Shiers has written comprehensively about prolonged pregnancy, disorders of uterine action and subsequent management.

Chapter Forty-Two

Breech presentation

Introduction

Any presentation of the fetus other than a vertex is called a **malpresentation**, which includes breech, face, brow and shoulder. These presentations have in common an ill-fitting presenting part which may be associated with early rupture of the membranes. There is also the likelihood of poor uterine action, leading to prolongation of labour. Each malpresentation leads to a different mechanism for descent and there may be difficulties in delivery; an understanding of the movements made by the fetus in response to the maternal pelvis will help to prevent injury to the woman or her baby. The risk of morbidity and mortality for the fetus is increased and malpresentations may result in operative delivery. Breech presentation is discussed in this chapter and the other malpresentations in Chapter 43.

Breech presentation

Breech presentation is where the lie is longitudinal but the fetal buttocks lie in the lower segment of the uterus. This presentation is found in 3–4% of all deliveries at term (RCOG 2006a,b). One in four fetuses will present by the breech at some stage in pregnancy but as pregnancy progresses spontaneous version to a vertex presentation is likely to occur, especially in multigravidae. In many cases there is no known cause; however, certain factors contribute to breech presentation such as extended legs, multiple pregnancy, preterm labour, polyhydramnios, hydrocephaly, uterine abnormality and placenta praevia (Coates 2003).

Types of breech presentation

Depending on the relationship of the lower limb(s) to the fetal trunk, four types of breech presentation can be described (Fig. 42.1). This can influence the diagnosis of breech presentation antenatally and the complications likely to occur at delivery:

1. **Complete or flexed breech (Fig. 42.1A):** the thighs and knees are flexed and the feet are close to the buttocks (tailor sitting or squatting), which occurs in 10–15% and is most common in multigravidae.

2. **Extended or frank breech (Fig. 42.1B):** the fetal thighs are flexed and the legs extended at the knees. The legs lie alongside the trunk with the feet near the head. This is the most common of the four types of breech presentation, occurring in 45–50%, and is seen most commonly in primigravidae near to term. The firm uterine and abdominal muscles prevent fetal movement so that the fetus is unable to flex

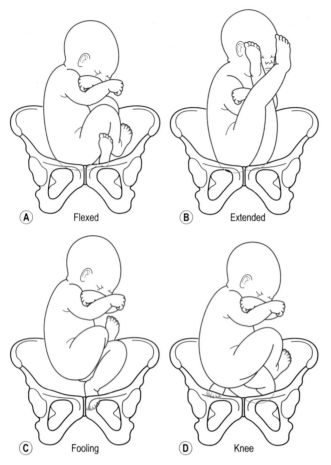

Figure 42.1 • Types of breech presentations. (From Henderson C, Macdonald S 2004, with kind permission of Elsevier.)

The figure shows four types labelled: (A) Flexed, (B) Extended, (C) Fooling, (D) Knee.

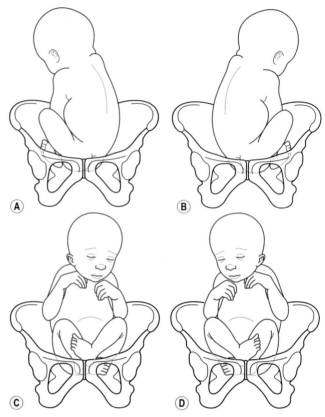

Figure 42.2 • Breech positions. (A) Left sacroanterior. (B) Right sacroanterior. (C) Right sacroposterior. (D) Left sacroposterior. (From Henderson C, Macdonald S 2004, with kind permission of Elsevier.)

its knees and there is limited likelihood of a turn to cephalic presentation.

3. **Footling presentation (Fig. 42.1C):** one or both hips and knees are extended and the feet present below the buttocks. This rare complication is more common in preterm labour.

4. **Knee presentation (Fig. 42.1D):** one or both hips are extended and the knees flexed. The knee(s) present below the buttocks. This is the rarest of the four presentations.

As in vertex presentations, the baby presenting by the breech can take up different positions (Fig. 42.2).

Aetiology

Many of the causes of persistent breech presentation are associated with conditions which either restrict the movement of the fetus or allow excessive movement of the fetus. Others involve the health of the fetus (see Table 42.1).

Table 42.1 Possible causes of breech presentation

Restricted space	Excessive intrauterine space	Fetal causes
Primigravidae with firm uterine and abdominal muscles	Grande multiparity because of lax uterine and abdominal muscles	Fetal abnormalities
Uterine malformations such as bicornuate uterus	Polyhydramnios	Fetal death in utero
Uterine fibroids		Decreased fetal activity
Contracted pelvis preventing engagement of the presenting part		Impaired fetal growth
Multiple pregnancy		Short umbilical cord
Placenta praevia		
Oligohydramnios		

BOX 42.1 ABDOMINAL PALPATION OF BREECH

Although abdominal examination is the main diagnostic tool it may be difficult to recognise in the primigravid woman with an extended breech. The breech may be deep in the pelvis and simulate an engaged head. The feet lie alongside the head and both prevent identification by palpation and prevent movement of the head on the neck elicited by ballottement. Finally, if the breech is engaged, the fetal heart may be heard in the expected position for a vertex presentation.

Diagnosis of breech presentation

On discussion

A past history of a previous breech presentation could suggest a uterine anomaly and an increased risk of repeated breech. If the woman complains of discomfort under the ribs it may be due to the presence in the fundus of the hard fetal head. The woman may also be aware of fetal kicking movements below the umbilicus.

On abdominal examination

Findings are:

- **Inspection:** usually reveals nothing unusual.
- **Palpation:** the presenting part feels firm but not hard or smooth. The head may be felt in the fundus, hard, round and ballottable. Box 42.1 presents possible findings on abdominal palpation of breech presentation.
- **Auscultation:** fetal heart sounds may be heard above the umbilicus.

On vaginal examination

On vaginal examination, either small parts or the breech itself may be detected. It is essential to distinguish between a hand and a foot if small parts are felt (a hand might grasp the examiner's finger, whereas a foot will not!). The breech itself is smooth and rounded and may feel like a vertex. A vaginal examination will also exclude a deeply engaged head either in pregnancy or labour. It is sometimes difficult to differentiate the shoulders, which lie at the level of the pelvic brim, from the breech.

Ultrasound scan

Diagnosis in a suspected breech presentation can be made by ultrasound. The fetus should be examined for anomalies at the same time.

Associated risk factors

The increased risk of morbidity and mortality in breech deliveries may be four times that of cephalic presentation but is partly dependent on associated factors. These factors include prematurity, congenital abnormalities, placenta praevia and placental abruption (Enkin et al 2000). Prolapse of the umbilical cord may lead to anoxia and fetal death, as may entrapment of the fetal head behind an incompletely dilated cervix. The woman is also placed at risk because of the possible delivery by caesarean section (CS).

Congenital abnormality

The presence of a congenital abnormality occurs more frequently with a breech presentation than with a vertex. The risk of congenital abnormality may be as high as 15% in babies of less than 1500 g (Arias 1993). The most common major abnormality is a defect of the neural tube such as meningomyelocele, hydrocephaly or anencephaly. Anomalies of the internal systems such as the gastrointestinal, respiratory, cardiovascular and urinary systems are also found. Congenital dislocation of the hip is the most common problem, occurring in three times as many girls as boys.

Risks at delivery

The fetus is at risk from the following:

- **Intrauterine and extrauterine asphyxia**, because of the delay in delivery of the head after the birth of the thorax and arms. Placental separation may occur before the birth is complete and cord compression is inevitable. Hypoxia may stimulate breathing with the inhalation of blood, liquor and mucus.
- **Intracranial haemorrhage**, which used to be thought to be due to rapid compression and decompression of the brain as the head descended through the pelvis, resulting in a torn tentorium cerebelli. However, it is now thought that the main cause of cerebral haemorrhage is anoxia and congestion of the cerebral vessels.
- **Skeletal fractures and dislocations**, damage to muscles and nerves and rupture of abdominal organs due to difficulties arising during delivery or to faulty delivery technique.
- **Genital oedema and bruising**, because of the formation of a caput succedaneum.

Management of pregnancy

Any woman found to have a breech presentation after 32 weeks should be seen by an obstetrician. With her full involvement, a decision needs to be made about the safest option for delivery. NICE (2004) state that in an uncomplicated singleton breech pregnancy at 36 weeks' gestation, women should be offered external cephalic version (ECV). However, women excluded would be labouring women, women with ruptured membranes, vaginal bleeding, uterine scar or abnormality, medical conditions and fetal compromise. If ECV is contraindicated or has been unsuccessful to reduce perinatal mortality and morbidity then women with a singleton breech presentation at term should be offered CS (NICE 2004).

Cephalic version

Promotion of spontaneous cephalic version

Various exercises and positions have been tried in an attempt to turn a breech. Hofmeyr & Kulier (2000) systematically reviewed the postural techniques 'used by doctors, midwives and birth attendants to promote cephalic version'. The review cited the following five studies involving 392 women:

- **Chenia & Crowther (1987)**, who modified Elkin's procedure asking women to adopt the posture three times a day for 7 days with a full bladder.
- **Bung et al (1987)**, who used a different technique—the 'Indian' version—where women are encouraged to lie down once or twice a day in a supine head-down position with the pelvis supported on a wedge-shaped cushion.
- **Hartadottir & Thornton (1992)**, who carried out a randomised controlled trial with women with a diagnosed breech presentation after 34 weeks. One group were taught how to take up the knee–chest position for 15 min twice a day. The results were compared to a control group of normally managed women.
- **Obwegeser et al (1999)**, who asked women to adopt the supine position with the pelvis elevated by a 30–35 cm high cushion for periods of 10 min twice a day.
- **Smith et al (1999)**, who asked women to assume the knee–chest position for 15 min, three times a day for 1 week.

There is insufficient evidence from well-controlled trials to support the use of postural management for breech presentation and larger trials are needed to assess the clinical value of these techniques. However, these exercises do not do any harm and there are no contraindications.

Moxibustion

Moxibustion (burning herbs to stimulate acupuncture points) is a traditional Chinese method used to help version of a fetus in breech presentation (Coyle et al 2005, Lewis 2004). In this technique a practitioner inserts heated acupuncture needles, then places small cones of moxa on the needle heads and ignites them. The acupuncture point Bladder 67 (BL67) is located at the tip of the fifth toe; its Chinese name is Zhiyin (Coyle et al 2005). It is a way of applying heat locally to regulate, tone and supplement the body's flow of Qi (vital energy). This method is popular in China and Japan.

The systematic review of Coyle et al (2005) evaluated the evidence from three trials; their aim was 'to examine the effectiveness and safety of moxibustion on changing the presentation of an unborn baby in the breech position, the need for ECV, mode of birth, and perinatal morbidity and mortality for breech presentation'. Meta-analysis was unable to be conducted due to the difference in interventions and overall small sample size (579 women in total). Only one trial reported on other outcome measures relevant to the review and stated that moxibustion reduced the need for ECV and resulted in decreased use of oxytocin before or during labour for women who had vaginal deliveries. However, there is insufficient evidence to support the use of moxibustion to correct a breech presentation. Moxibustion may be beneficial in reducing the need for ECV and decreasing the use of oxytocin; however, further well-designed randomised controlled trials to evaluate moxibustion for breech presentation which report on clinically relevant outcomes as well as the safety of the intervention are required.

External cephalic version

During ECV the fetus is manipulated through the abdominal wall to turn it from a breech to a cephalic presentation (RCOG 2006a) (Fig. 42.3). This manual manoeuvre has always been controversial, especially if carried out before 36 weeks. There are risks attached to the procedure: bleeding from the placental site, cord entanglement, causing fetal distress, converting the lie and presentation to an undeliverable one and initiating preterm labour. To reduce these risks to a minimum, the following contraindications are described:

- History of infertility.
- Elderly primigravida.
- Hypertension.
- Rhesus-negative mother.
- Cephalopelvic disproportion.
- Uterine scar.
- Placenta praevia or placental abruption.
- Multiple pregnancy.
- Congenital malformations.
- Intrauterine fetal death.

The role of ECV in three different situations has been systematically reviewed:

1. External cephalic version before term (Hutton & Hofmeyr 2006).

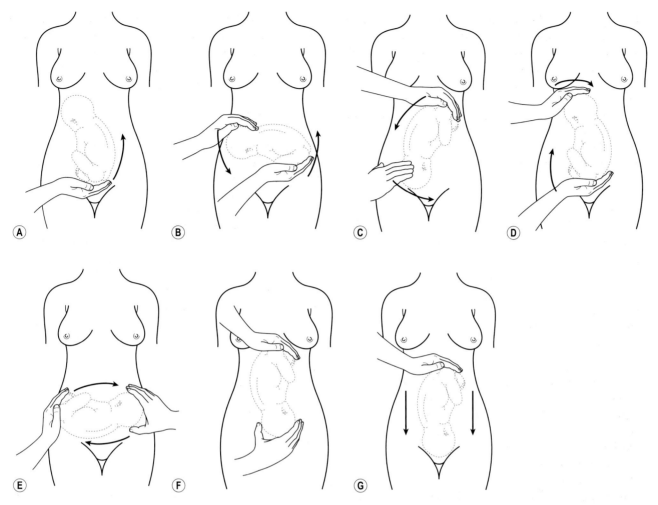

Figure 42.3 • External cephalic version. (A) Palpation and mobilisation of the breech. (B) Manual forward rotation using both hands, one to push the breech and the other to guide the vertex. (C) Completion of forward roll. (D) Backward flip using both hands. (E) Quarter turn accomplished. Continue to push breech upwards and vertex downwards. (F) Completion of external version. (G) Gently push the breech downwards to direct vertex into pelvis. (Reproduced with permission from Clay et al 1993.)

2. External cephalic version at term (Hofmeyr & Kulier 1996).

3. Interventions to help external cephalic version at term (Hofmeyr & Gyte 2004).

ECV before term appears to improve pregnancy outcomes in relation to the incidence of breech presentation and rates of CS. However, Hutton & Hofmeyr (2006) concluded that although ECV at 34–35 weeks did have these benefits, they would recommend that practice is not changed. They inform us that ECV should continue to be conducted at 37 weeks' gestation until further studies have explored the incidence of associated preterm labour and fetal outcome. This reiterates the systematic review of Hofmeyer & Kulier (1996), which found evidence to support the use of attempting ECV at term. This procedure was found to reduce the chance of non-cephalic births and CSs. In individual cases the risk of ECV needs to be weighed against the current and future risks of continued breech presentation to mother and fetus.

The interventions reviewed by Hofmeyr & Gyte (2004) for ECV included routine tocolysis, fetal acoustic stimulation, epidural or spinal analgesia and transabdominal amnioinfusion. Tocolysis involves the use of drugs that act as relaxants to the uterine musculature, such as salbutamol and ritodrine, prior to carrying out ECV. Hofmeyr & Gyte (2004) found that routine tocolysis appears to reduce the failure rate of ECV at term. However, there was not enough evidence to evaluate the other types of intervention although some of the findings appeared promising. No randomised trials were found for transabdominal amnioinfusion for ECV at term.

The advantages of delaying ECV until term include:

• The delay will give more time for spontaneous version to occur.

• Less reversions to breech presentation.

- A reduction in fetal mortality.
- Other pregnancy complications, excluding ECV, may become apparent.
- If complications occur, the fetus is mature enough to be delivered.
- Reducing the incidence of breech deliveries.
- Reducing the incidence of CS.

Disadvantages are that the membranes may rupture and labour commences before version is attempted.

The procedure for ECV

A skilled and experienced practitioner should carry out the procedure, where facilities for monitoring and immediate delivery are available (RCOG 2006a). A successful procedure not only depends on the practitioner but also on the position and engagement of the fetus, volume of liquor and maternal parity. The position of the breech should be confirmed by ultrasound scan and the woman should give prior consent for the procedure. The woman should be 'nil by mouth' in preparation for a potential CS if complications arise. A cardiotocographic recording of the fetal heart should always be obtained prior to the procedure. The woman should be asked to empty her bladder and she then lies flat on a couch or bed. A tocolytic drug may be used although there is no firm evidence to support the use of these drugs. The obstetrician disimpacts the breech from the pelvis and then, applying pressure to both poles of the fetus, the fetus is rotated into a cephalic presentation (Fig. 42.3). It is safer to achieve this by making the fetus turn a forward somersault or to 'follow its nose'! A backward somersault may sometimes achieve the version more easily but there is a risk of extension of the neck, resulting in a brow presentation. On completion of the manoeuvre, the fetal heart should be recorded for 30 min to ensure there is no fetal distress. Uterine contractions, signs of rupture of the membranes and any vaginal bleeding are watched for and reported to the obstetrician immediately. If the woman's blood group is rhesus negative, 500 IU of anti-D immunoglobulin is administered following ECV.

The role of planned caesarean section at term

Over the last 25 years it has been accepted that CS should be the mode of delivery for fetuses presenting by the breech, but few studies have been carried out to evaluate this use of planned CS. In a systematic review, Hofmeyr & Hannah (2003) suggest that there is sufficient evidence to evaluate the use of a policy of planned CS for breech presentation and argue that 'planned caesarean section compared with planned vaginal birth reduced perinatal or neonatal death or serious neonatal morbidity, at the expense of somewhat increased maternal morbidity'. However, it was also noteworthy that planned CS will decrease the number of skilled operators of breech delivery and place women electing for a vaginal breech delivery at increased risk (Hofmeyr & Hannah 2003).

Conversely, a multicentre international, randomised controlled trial compared elective CS to vaginal delivery for selected breech presentations, including frank or complete breech, greater than 37 weeks' gestation and less than 4000 g estimated fetal weight (Hannah 2000, SOGC 2000). The trial was stopped earlier than planned due to preliminary data showing a significant reduction in perinatal mortality and morbidity and no increase in serious maternal complications in the elective CS group (Hannah 2000).

In a study of long-term outcomes of children with breech presentation at term, Danelian et al (1996) reviewed data on preschool children and found that planned delivery by CS was not associated with better long-term outcomes. A handicap rate of 19.4% in 1387 children whose records were available was present in both CS and vaginal delivery groups, suggesting that planned vaginal delivery is as safe as elective CS when long-term outcome is considered. A further problem with more breech babies delivered by CS is that practitioners lose their skills, thus endangering the fetus. What appears to be more certain is the role of elective CS in the delivery of the preterm breech. A trend towards increased risk of neonatal death has been found when the baby weighs less than 1750 g (Kiely 1991) and 1600 g (Gilady & Cols 1996). Babies with birth weights over 3000 g are also at risk.

Vaginal delivery

In the event of a persistent breech presentation, the following factors are considered prior to vaginal delivery:

- **Maternal age and parity**: there is an increased risk of failure with young women with low vaginal parity.
- **Period of gestation**: any gestation taking into account the risk factors for the mother.
- **History of the present pregnancy**: this should be a healthy pregnancy with no obstetric or medical problems.
- **Past obstetric history**.
- **Size and shape of the pelvis**: should be large enough for the particular fetus.
- **Condition of the fetus**.

There are fundamental differences in delivery between cephalic and breech presentations. With cephalic or vertex presentation, the largest part of the fetus, the head, delivers first. Moulding of the cranium can occur over several hours. In a breech delivery, the breech is first delivered followed by the shoulders and then the head. Each part of the fetus is larger and less compressible than the previous part. The after-coming head has not had time to mould because it enters the pelvis with the base of the skull leading and this cannot mould (ALSO 2005). In a vaginal breech delivery the biggest challenge is that the head might not fit through the pelvis as it is the last and largest part to deliver. However, RCOG (2006b) argue that if the fetal trunk and thighs pass through the pelvis simultaneously with ease then cephalopelvic disproportion is improbable.

If women are selected carefully so that the pelvis is of adequate dimensions in relation to the fetus and there are no other adverse factors, they should be able to deliver safely per vaginam. It is essential to understand the mechanism of a breech delivery so that management of the delivery can be completed without trauma. In ideal conditions vaginal breech delivery should be performed by an experienced midwife or under the supervision of a senior obstetrician. A paediatrician should be present at delivery. The practice in normal spontaneous breech birth is to keep hands off and allow the breech to delivery spontaneously. However, the practitioner must be able to intervene if necessary and it is important to know the normal mechanisms of breech delivery.

Management

The mechanism of a breech delivery

There are six possible positions for a breech delivery. These are right or left sacroanterior, right or left sacroposterior, right or left sacrolateral. The mechanism of the **left sacroanterior position** will be described in full:

- The **lie** is longitudinal.
- The **presentation** is breech.
- The **denominator** is the sacrum.
- The **attitude** is one of complete flexion.
- The **presenting part** is the anterior (left) buttock.
- The **bitrochanteric diameter**, 10 cm, enters the pelvis in the left oblique diameter of the pelvic brim.

The movements

It is necessary to consider the birth of the fetus in three main stages: the buttocks, the shoulders and the head.

Compaction and flexion
Descent takes place with increasing compaction due to increased flexion of the limbs on the trunk.

Internal rotation of the buttocks
The anterior buttock reaches the pelvic floor and rotates forwards in the pelvis $\frac{1}{8}$th of a circle to lie under the symphysis pubis. The bitrochanteric diameter now lies in the anteroposterior diameter of the pelvis.

Lateral flexion of the trunk
The anterior buttock escapes under the symphysis pubis, the posterior buttock sweeps the perineum and the buttocks are born by a movement of lateral flexion (Fig. 42.4).

Restitution
The anterior buttock turns slightly to the mother's right side.

Internal rotation of the shoulders
With the birth of the buttocks, the bisacromial diameter (11 cm) of the shoulders enters the pelvis in the same diameter of the pelvis as the buttocks, the left oblique. The anterior (left) shoulder reaches the pelvic floor and rotates forwards $\frac{1}{8}$th of a circle to lie behind the symphysis pubis.

Birth of the shoulders
The anterior shoulder and arm escape under the symphysis pubis and the posterior shoulder and arm pass over the perineum.

Internal rotation and delivery of the head
The flexed head engages with the suboccipitobregmatic diameter of 9.5 cm or the suboccipitofrontal diameter of 10 cm lying in the right oblique or transverse diameter of the pelvic brim. Internal rotation of the head carries the occiput behind the symphysis pubis. The face lies in the hollow of the sacrum. Internal rotation of the

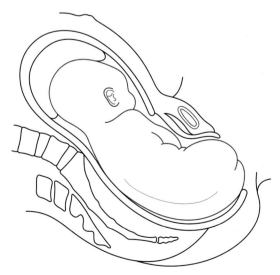

Figure 42.4 • Lateral flexion and birth of the buttocks. (From Henderson C, Macdonald S 2004, with kind permission of Elsevier.)

head is accompanied by external rotation of the trunk. The chin, face, vertex and occiput are born over the perineum by a movement of flexion.

The first stage of labour

The first stage does not differ from normal labour and may be allowed to continue spontaneously if there is progressive dilatation and descent with no fetal or maternal complications. However, the risks of the delivery mean that the birth should take place in a consultant unit with an anaesthetist and paediatrician being available. Labour is normally induced at term and some obstetricians prefer to induce labour at 38 weeks when the fetus will be smaller. If the breech is flexed and not engaged, there may be early rupture of the membranes with the risk of prolapse of the umbilical cord. If the legs are extended, the breech is likely to be engaged and the risk of cord prolapse is minimal.

Epidural analgesia is the analgesia of choice from the obstetric point of view, because it prevents the desire to push too early when the buttocks slip through the incompletely dilated cervical os with a risk of entrapment of the head (Al-Azzawi 1998). There is also the possibility of delivery of the head by forceps. However, Chadha et al (1992) found that the contractions in both first and second stages of labour decrease in intensity following the commencement of epidural analgesia. This appeared to increase the frequency of breech extraction (see below) or CS and its use is not advocated by all. 'Low-dose' epidurals give effective pain relief and the woman is able to push effectively when the cervix is fully dilated. If the woman has minimal analgesics then she can labour standing up or on all fours which facilitates the delivery of the breech. Careful monitoring of the fetal heart would be important as part of the continual assessment of the woman's progress in labour (Coates 2003, Lewis 2004) and to prevent morbidity and mortality (RCOG 2006b). Continuous electronic fetal monitoring by cardiotocography should be offered to women throughout labour (RCOG 2006b).

The second stage of labour

The woman must be encouraged not to push until the cervix is confirmed as fully dilated by vaginal examination. An experienced midwife or obstetrician will normally conduct the delivery. In hospital, the woman's legs are usually placed in lithotomy position for the actual delivery. All midwives should be familiar with the manoeuvres necessary to deliver the baby in case of an emergency. Simulated practice is essential. An anaesthetist and paediatrician should be present at the delivery in case of a sudden need for intervention.

Breech delivery may be spontaneous with little help needed, usually in a multigravida or with a preterm baby, where the woman adopts a standing or all-fours position and assisted delivery where the manoeuvres are performed to help the birth of the baby. Breech extraction may be occasionally necessary where the fetus is extracted from the birth canal by manipulation rather than by assisting the normal mechanism. This is dangerous and is not often used in developed countries. The breech is engaged when the bitrochanteric diameter (10 cm) is at the pelvic brim, which is the diameter between the greater trochanters of the femora of the fetus.

Assisted breech delivery

The woman's bladder is emptied prior to commencement. Although episiotomy is routinely conducted to allow the practitioner to perform various manipulations as required, there is no evidence to support this (RCOG 2006b).

The buttocks

No handling is necessary and delivery should proceed spontaneously until the fetal umbilicus appears at the introitus. When the umbilicus delivers, a loop of several inches of cord should be gently pulled down to prevent tension on the cord as the body delivers. This will also allow easy monitoring of the fetal pulse by palpation (ALSO 2005). The legs should normally deliver themselves.

The body

After the umbilicus is born, gentle downward traction may be used to deliver the body. The practitioner's fingers should be used to carefully grasp the fetal pelvis, with the thumbs placed on the sacroiliac regions to avoid injuring the abdominal organs. Traction should be in a 45° downwards direction. The body may deliver quickly with little effort.

The head

There are two alternative methods for delivering the head: the Burns–Marshall manoeuvre (Fig. 42.5) and the modified Mauriceau–Smellie–Veit manoeuvre (Fig. 42.6).

Burns–Marshall manoeuvre

The baby is allowed to hang by his own weight to encourage descent and flexion of the head, taking care not to let sudden delivery of the head. Once the nape of the neck and hairline can be seen, the baby's ankles are grasped and with slight traction the trunk is carried in a wide arc up over the mother's abdomen. The other hand should support the perineum to prevent sudden delivery of the head. Once the mouth is clear, the baby can breathe and time should be taken to complete the delivery of the cranium.

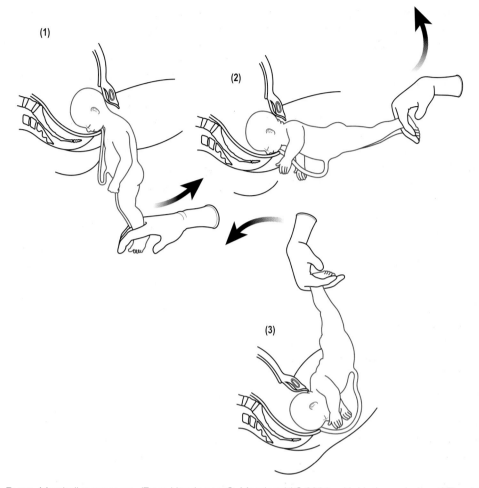

Figure 42.5 • The Burns–Marshall manoeuvre. (From Henderson C, Macdonald S 2004, with kind permission of Elsevier.)

Mauriceau–Smellie–Veit (modified) manoeuvre

This method is recommended for delivery of the head and all the movements promote head flexion. One of the practitioner's hands should be placed above the fetus, with one finger inserted into the vagina and placed on the occiput and one finger on each of the fetal shoulders. The other hand is placed beneath the fetus. The classical Mauriceau–Smellie–Veit manoeuvre describes placing a finger in the mouth as seen in Fig. 42.6. However, traction on the lower jaw has been found to cause dislocation. As an alternative the modified manoeuvre involves placing two fingers on the maxilla instead. An assistant should follow the head abdominally and be prepared to apply suprapubic pressure to flex the head through the pelvis. The fetus may be draped on the practitioner's lower arm.

Delivery of the head commences and is flexed through the pelvis by four separate mechanisms:

1. The occipital finger applies flexing pressure on the occiput.

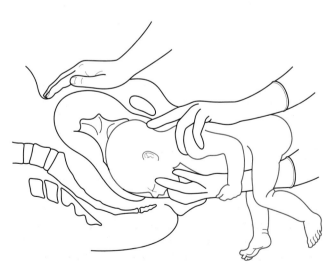

Figure 42.6 • The Mauriceau–Smellie–Veit manoeuvre. (From Henderson C, Macdonald S 2004, with kind permission of Elsevier.)

2. The assistant applies suprapubic pressure on the occiput as required.

3. The fingers on the maxillae apply pressure on the lower face, which tends to promote flexion.

4. Some traction is also required for the delivery by downward pressure of the fingers on the shoulders.

Oropharyngeal suction is not required as the mouth and nose appear over the perineum. The baby's head is carefully delivered following the curve of the birth canal.

Extended legs

If the legs are extended, they may splint the body and prevent lateral flexion of the trunk. The legs of a frank breech may be delivered by inserting a finger behind the knee to flex the knee and abduct the thigh. Active efforts to deliver the legs are not mandatory, as the legs will deliver spontaneously and the feet will become free eventually (ALSO 2005).

Extended arms

If the baby's arms cannot be found crossed over the chest, they may be extended alongside the head, making the total diameter of the presenting part too large to descend into the pelvis. This often happens when the breech is pulled on to deliver the legs and trunk. The arms must be brought down before the head can be delivered and this is done by the Lövset's manoeuvre (Fig. 42.7). The success of the manoeuvre arises from the relative positions of the two shoulders. The posterior shoulder is below the sacral promontory while the anterior shoulder is above the symphysis pubis.

The baby's thighs are grasped with thumbs placed over the sacrum. The baby is gently pulled downwards and it is critical to keep the back uppermost to allow the fetal head to enter the pelvis with the occiput anterior. The baby is rotated through 180° to bring the posterior shoulder to the anterior position but beneath the symphysis pubis. Friction of the arm against the pelvic walls will bring the arm down and it can be released. The manoeuvre is repeated in the opposite direction to release the second arm.

Extended head

If the hairline does not become visible after a few seconds of allowing the baby to hang by its weight, the

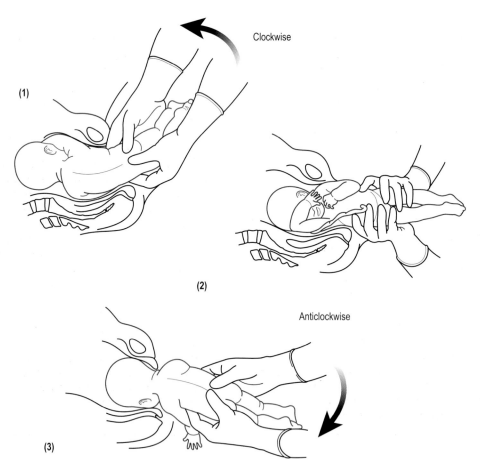

Figure 42.7 • Birth of the arms using Lövset's manoeuvre. (From Henderson C, Macdonald S 2004, with kind permission of Elsevier.)

head is probably extended. Forceps are usually used to deliver the head but the modified Mauriceau–Smellie–Veit manoeuvre may be used if the midwife has to conduct the delivery.

Entrapment of the fetal head

This dangerous situation arises when the fetal body slips through an incompletely dilated cervix and the head is partially trapped behind the cervix. In the immediate absence of medical aid it may be possible to make an airway for the baby by placing fingers or a Simm's speculum in the vagina, thus holding maternal tissues away from the baby's mouth and nose.

The obstetrician will try to release the baby's head from the cervix and one method that may help is the McRobert's manoeuvre, which is also useful in the delivery of a fetus with shoulder dystocia. The woman lies on her back, lifts her knees up to her chest and raises her buttocks off the bed. Arias (1993) stated that 'There is no adequate description in the literature of the incidence, methods of management and outcome of infants when the fetal head is entrapped during a breech delivery'. He

suggested incisions into the cervix as the quickest way of freeing the head, although these are known to extend into the lower segment and cause cervical incompetence. He also suggests trying an injection of diazoxide or other drugs to relax the cervix. However, mortality and morbidity rates for the neonate are high.

Undiagnosed cephalopelvic disproportion

In an unbooked woman or where there has been failure to diagnose a degree of hydrocephaly, this dire emergency may arise as the delivery proceeds. If the breech is delivered up to the head, there is usually difficulty in performing a CS. Symphysiotomy may save the baby's life.

Posterior rotation of the occiput

This is a rare complication. In this situation the back of the baby is turned towards the mother's buttocks. To deliver the head the chin and face are allowed to escape under the symphysis pubis as far as the root of the nose, and then the baby is lifted towards the mother's abdomen to allow the occiput to sweep the perineum.

Main points

- One in four fetuses will present by the breech at some stage in pregnancy but spontaneous version to a vertex presentation is likely to occur, especially in multigravidae. Depending on the relationship of the lower limb(s) to the trunk of the fetus, breech presentation may be complete or flexed, extended or frank, footling or knee presentation.

- There is an increased risk of morbidity and mortality in breech deliveries. Associated factors include prematurity, congenital abnormalities, placenta praevia and placental abruption, prolapse of the umbilical cord and entrapment of the fetal head behind an incompletely dilated cervix.

- At delivery, the fetus is at risk from asphyxia, intracranial haemorrhage, skeletal fractures and dislocations, damage to muscles and nerves and rupture of abdominal organs, genital oedema and bruising. Long-term problems are thought to include growth hormone deficiency.

- An obstetrician should see any woman with a breech presentation after 32 weeks. A decision needs to be made with her about the safest option for delivery. NICE (2004) recommend that ECV should

be offered at 36 weeks' gestation to women with an uncomplicated singleton breech pregnancy.

- The risks of a vaginal breech delivery mean that the birth should take place in a consultant unit. Labour is normally induced at term and some obstetricians prefer to induce labour at 38 weeks when the fetus will be smaller. If the breech is flexed and not engaged there may be early rupture of the membranes with the risk of prolapse of the umbilical cord.

- An experienced midwife or obstetrician will conduct the delivery. All midwives should be familiar with the manoeuvres necessary to deliver the baby presenting by the breech, in case of an emergency. The modified Mauriceau–Smellie–Veit manoeuvre is recommended for delivery of the head as the movements all promote flexion.

- An anaesthetist and paediatrician should be present at the delivery in case of a sudden need for intervention. Dangerous but rare complications such as entrapment of the fetal head, late diagnosis of cephalopelvic disproportion and posterior rotation of the occiput may lead to fetal death.

References

Al-Azzawi, F., 1998. Childbirth and Obstetric Techniques, second edn. Mosby, St Louis.

ALSO, 2005. Malpresentations, Malpositions, and Multiple Gestation Advanced Life Support in Obstetrics, Registered Charity No. 1024554, fifth edn. UK Office, Newcastle-upon-Tyne.

Arias, F., 1993. Practical Guide to High Risk Pregnancy and Delivery, second edn. Mosby Year Book, Chicago.

Bung, P., Huch, R., Huch, A., 1987. Is Indian version a successful method of lowering the incidence of breech presentation? Gerbultshilfe und Frauenheilkunde 47, 202–205.

Chadha, Y.C., Mahmood, T.A., Dick, M.J., et al., 1992. Breech delivery and epidural analgesia. Br. J. Obstet. Gynaecol. 99, 96–100.

Chenia, F., Crowther, C.A., 1987. Does advice to assume the knee-chest position reduce the incidence of breech presentation at delivery? A randomized controlled trial. Birth 14, 75–78.

Coates, T., 2003. Malpositions of the occiput and malpresentations. In: Fraser, D.M., Cooper, M.A. (Eds.) Myles Textbook for Midwives, fourteenth edn. Churchill Livingstone, Edinburgh.

Coyle, M.E., Smith, C.A., Peat, B., 2005. Cephalic version by moxibustion for breech presentation. Cochrane Review. Cochrane Library, Issue 2. Update Software 2008, Oxford.

Danelian, P.J., Wang, J., Hall, M.H., 1996. Long-term outcome of term breech presentation by method of delivery. Br. J. Med. 312 (7044), 1451–1453.

Enkin, M., Keirse, J., Neilson, J., et al., 2000. A Guide to Effective Care in Pregnancy and Childbirth, third edn. Oxford University Press, Oxford.

Gilady, Y., Cols, E., 1996. The delivery of very low birthweight breech. What is the best way for the baby? Isr. J. Med. Sci. 32 (2), 116–120.

Hannah, M., 2000. The Term Breech Collaborative Group. What is the best way to deliver a breech baby? Lancet 356, 1375–1383.

Hartadottir, T., Thornton, J. G. (1992). A randomized trial of the knee-chest position to encourage spontaneous version of breech pregnancies. Proceeding of the 26th British Congress of Obstetricians and Gynaecologists, Manchester, 1992, 356.

Henderson, C., Macdonald, S. (Eds.), 2004. Mayes' Midwifery: A Textbook for Midwives, thirteenth edn. Baillière Tindall, London.

Hofmeyr G J, Gyte G 2004 Interventions to help external cephalic version for breech presentation at term. Cochrane Review. Cochrane Library, Issue 1. Update Software 2008, Oxford.

Hofmeyr G J, Hannah M E 2003 Planned caesarean section for term breech delivery. Cochrane Review. Cochrane Library, Issue 2. Update Software 2008, Oxford.

Hofmeyr G J, Kulier R 1996 External cephalic version for breech presentation at term. Cochrane Review. Cochrane Library, Issue 1. Update Software 2008, Oxford.

Hofmeyr G J, Kulier R 2000 Cephalic version by postural management for breech presentation. Cochrane Review. Cochrane Library, Issue 2. Update Software 2008, Oxford.

Hutton E K, Hofmeyr G J 2006 External cephalic version for breech presentation before term. Cochrane Review. Cochrane Library, Issue 1. Update Software 2008, Oxford.

Kiely, J.L., 1991. Mode of delivery and neonatal death in 17587 infants presenting by the breech. Br. J. Obstet. Gynaecol. 98 (9), 898–904.

Lewis, P., 2004. Malpositions and malpresentations. In: Henderson, C., Macdonald, S. (Eds.) Mayes' Midwifery: A Textbook for Midwifery, thirteenth edn. Baillière Tindall, London.

NICE (National Institute for Clinical Excellence), 2004. Caesarean Section. Clinical Guideline. RCOG Press, London.

Obwegeser, R., Hohlagschwandtner, M., Aurbach, L., et al., 1999. Management of breech presentation by Indian version: a prospective randomized trial. Zeitschrift für Gerbultschilfe und Neonatologie 203, 161–165.

RCOG (Royal College of Obstetricians and Gynaecologists), 2006a. External Cephalic Version and Reducing the Incidence of Breech Presentation Guideline No. 20A. RCOG, London.

RCOG (Royal College of Obstetricians and Gynaecologists), 2006b. The Management of Breech Presentation. Guideline No. 20B. RCOG, London.

Smith, C., Crowther, C., Wilkinson, C., et al., 1999. Knee-chest postural management for breech delivery at term: a randomized controlled trial. Birth 26, 71–75.

SOGC (Society of Obstetricians and Gynaecologists of Canada), Interim Position on Management of Term Breech, 2000 September. SOGC 27.

Annotated recommended reading

Al-Azzawi, F., 1998. Childbirth and Obstetric Techniques, second edn. Mosby, St Louis.

This atlas contains a superb collection of colour photographs, a pictorial demonstration of normal childbirth and its variations and a breech delivery.

Enkin, M., Keirse, J., Neilson, J., et al., 2000. A Guide to Effective Care in Pregnancy and Childbirth, third edn. Oxford University Press, Oxford.

This book is based on systematic reviews of research literature on pregnancy and childbirth and includes sections on breech delivery and external cephalic version.

Gilady, Y., Cols, E., 1996. The delivery of very low birth weight breech. What is the best way for the baby? Isr. J. Med. Sci. 32 (2), 116–120.

In this article, Gilady & Cols review the literature on the delivery of the preterm breech. They found that babies weighing less than 1700 g were at risk of neonatal death if delivered by the breech.

RCOG (Royal College of Obstetricians and Gynaecologists), 2006. External Cephalic Version and Reducing the Incidence of Breech Presentation Guideline No. 20A. RCOG, London.

RCOG (Royal College of Obstetricians and Gynaecologists), 2006. The Management of Breech Presentation. Guideline No. 20B. RCOG, London.

These two guidelines are recommended reading for practitioners working within obstetrics. They provide important information and guidance.

Chapter Forty-Three

Malposition and cephalic malpresentations

Introduction

If the vertex is the denominator in a cephalic presentation, the term malpresentation is not used. The correct word to use for occipitoposterior position of the vertex is **malposition**. True cephalic malpresentations are face and brow. Also included is a shoulder presentation resulting from oblique or transverse lie; this is a rare but dangerous event. Each of these situations may affect the length and outcome of the labour and require vigilance to prevent maternal and fetal morbidity and, rarely, mortality. The more common occipitoposterior position will be discussed first as it may lead to secondary brow or face presentation.

Occipitoposterior position of the vertex

In occipitoposterior position of the vertex, the occiput occupies one of the two posterior quadrants of the mother's pelvis and the sinciput points towards the opposite anterior quadrant (Fig. 43.1). Malposition is common and affects about 10% of all labours. The outcome of such labours is generally normal with rotation of the occiput to the anterior and normal vertex delivery. However, there may be prolonged labour and mechanical difficulties associated with the delivery.

Causes

There is no single satisfactory cause for occipitoposterior position. However, if the forepelvis is small, as found in android and anthropoid pelves, the head may take up a posterior position. Other possible causes include a pendulous abdomen, a flat sacrum or an anterior placenta (Lewis 2004).

Attitude

Instead of the normal well-flexed attitude with the limbs and head flexed on the trunk and the rounded back pointing towards the mother's soft abdominal wall, the fetal spine faces the forward curve of the maternal lumbar spine and good flexion is not possible. The fetal spine is straightened, the head is held in a deflexed position known as the 'military position' and the anterior fontanelle is found directly over the internal os. The term 'bregmatic presentation' is sometimes used (Lewis 2004). This position of the head brings larger diameters into relationship with the pelvic brim and engagement of the head may not occur.

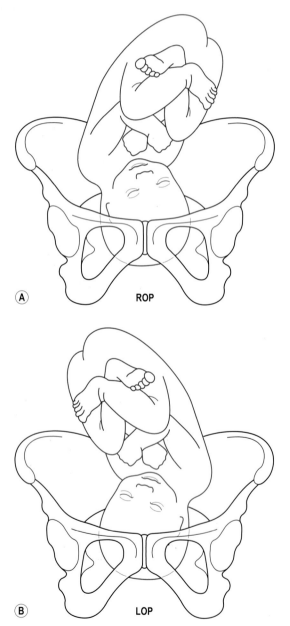

Figure 43.1 • Right and left occipitoposterior positions. (From Henderson C, Macdonald S 2004, with kind permission of Elsevier.)

Risks

- Obstructed labour if either deep transverse arrest or brow presentation result.
- Maternal perineal trauma such as a third-degree tear and bruising.
- Cord prolapse if there is early spontaneous rupture of the membranes and ill-fitting presenting part.
- Neonatal cerebral haemorrhage due to upward moulding of the fetal skull. The falx cerebri may be pulled away from the tentorium cerebelli, resulting in a tear of the great vein of Galen.
- Chronic fetal hypoxia, if present, results in venous distension, which increases the likelihood of haemorrhage.

Diagnosis in pregnancy

Occipitoposterior position is the most common cause of a non-engaged head in late pregnancy in primigravidae. The woman may complain that the baby has too many hands and feet and that she has to pass urine more frequently in the absence of infection (El Halta 1996). Abdominal examination will confirm the diagnosis:

- On **inspection**: the abdomen appears flattened. There may be a saucer-shaped depression below the umbilicus between the fetal head and limbs (Fig. 43.2A).

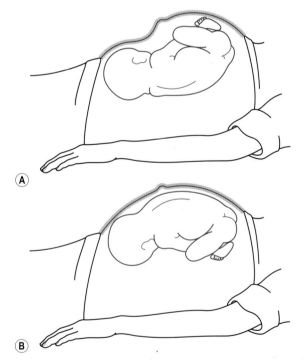

Figure 43.2 • (A) Abdominal contour with occipitoposterior position, showing depression at umbilicus. (B) Rounded abdominal contour with occipitoanterior position. (From Henderson C, Macdonald S 2004, with kind permission of Elsevier.)

- On **palpation**: the fetal head is high and deflexed. It may feel large if the occiput is more lateral but small if the occiput is quite posterior and the bitemporal diameter is palpated. Fetal limbs may be felt on both sides of the midline of the uterus and the fetal back may be felt out in the flank (Fig. 43.3).
- On **auscultation**: the fetal heart may be heard at or just above the umbilicus or out in one flank.

Diagnosis in labour

Abdominal examination, as described above, will indicate the presence of an occipitoposterior position although the head may be flexed and become engaged.

On vaginal examination, palpation of the anterior fontanelle is a diagnostic aid in determining occipitoposterior position (ALSO 2005). If the head is reasonably well flexed, the anterior fontanelle will be felt anteriorly and it may be possible to feel the posterior fontanelle. When the head is deflexed, the anterior fontanelle is almost central and easy to feel by its shape and size (Fig. 43.4B).

The first stage of labour

Fetal malposition of occipitoposterior is associated with more painful, prolonged and obstructed labour and a difficult delivery (Hunter et al 2007). The course of labour partly depends on the degree of descent and flexion that takes place (Fig. 43.5). This in turn is influenced by the strength of uterine contractions. If the head flexes, it is likely that labour will proceed normally. The engaging diameter is the suboccipitofrontal (10 cm). When the occiput reaches the pelvic floor and rotates $\frac{3}{8}$ths of a circle, the baby is born with the occiput anterior.

If the head remains deflexed, problems may arise. The engaging diameter is the occipitofrontal (11.5 cm). The head may be non-engaged at the commencement of labour and early rupture of the membranes may occur. If the presenting part is high and not well applied to the cervix, there is a risk of cord prolapse.

Labour is prolonged because of poor stimulation of the cervix and dilation is slow and uneven. Contractions

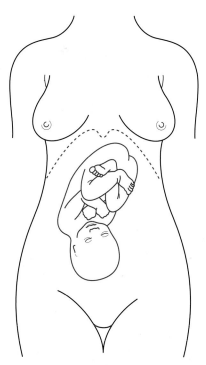

Figure 43.3 • In occipitoposterior positions the anterior shoulder is well out from the midline and fetal limbs are readily palpable. This may cause a mistaken diagnosis of multiple pregnancy. (From Beischer N A, Mackay E V 1986 Obstetrics and the Newborn. Baillière Tindall, London, with kind permission of Elsevier.)

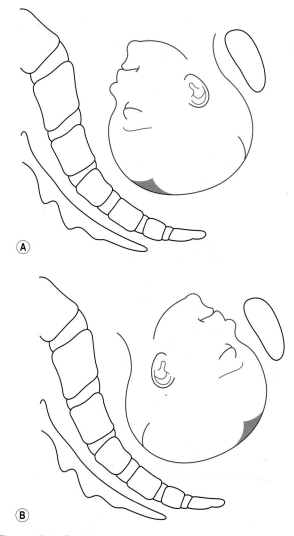

Figure 43.4 • Position of the anterior and posterior fontanelles. (A) Occipitoanterior. (B) Occipitoposterior. (From Henderson C, Macdonald S 2004, with kind permission of Elsevier.)

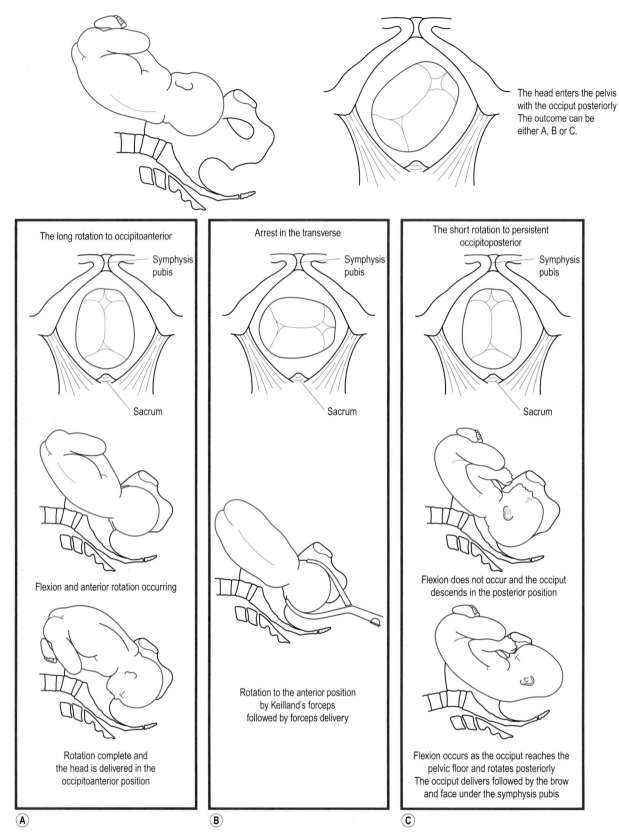

Figure 43.5 • Outcome of an occipitoposterior position. The head enters the pelvis with the occiput posteriorly. The outcome can be A, B or C. (From Henderson C, Macdonald S 2004, with kind permission of Elsevier.)

may be excessive but uncoordinated and painful and the woman experiences severe backache. Encouraging the mother to take up a knee–chest position for 45 min may help rotation of the vertex to an anterior position (El Halta 1996). Augmentation of labour may be necessary (see Chapter 41). Care must be taken to prevent maternal loss of confidence, ketosis and dehydration and fetal distress. There may be difficulty in micturition with retention of urine and the woman needs encouragement to empty her bladder frequently. Catheterisation may be necessary if the woman is unable to pass urine.

The role of maternal position

Hunter et al (2007) discuss the benefits of upright and leaning-forward postures in order to encourage the fetal head to engage in the optimal occipitoanterior position. Avoidance of a reclining position with the knees higher than the hips will reduce the incidence of occipitoposterior position of the fetal head at the commencement of labour (Sutton 2001). Taking up an all-fours posture may reduce the pressure of the fetus on the maternal spine and help to reduce backache. It may also aid rotation of the fetus to an occipitoanterior position (Simkin & Ancheta 2005).

It has been suggested that in the antenatal period if a woman adopts a hands-and-knees posture leaning forward then this might promote a favourable position of the baby (Hunter et al 2007). Three trials (2794 women) were included in a systematic review (Hunter et al 2007) to explore this issue. Two trials were focused on the antenatal period. In one trial (100 women), four different postures (four groups of 20 women) were combined for comparison with the control group of 20 women. Findings were that in the lateral or posterior position the presenting part of the fetus was less likely to persist following 10 min in the hands-and-knees position compared to a sitting position. In a second trial (2547 women), advice to assume the hands-and-knees posture for 10 min twice daily in the last weeks of pregnancy had no effect on the baby's position at delivery or on any of the other pregnancy outcomes.

Simkin & Ancheta (2005) detail the advantages of ambulation and forward-leaning positions in labour. Freedom to move around in the first stage of labour and the maintenance of an upright position such as can be achieved by sitting astride a chair and leaning on its back have been shown to be beneficial to women with an occipitoposterior presentation. Descent of the fetal head is encouraged and good uterine contractions should follow. Progress is more likely to be normal, culminating in long internal rotation of the occiput (see below). In the second stage of labour, the squatting position increases the anteroposterior diameter of the outlet and may aid rotation, descent and delivery.

The third trial in the systematic review of Hunter et al studied the use of hands-and-knees position in labour. The sample comprised 147 labouring women at 37 or more weeks' gestation, where the fetal occipitoposterior position was confirmed by ultrasound. Randomisation occurred: 70 women (intervention group) assumed hands-and-knees positioning for a period of at least 30 min compared to 77 women (control group) who did not assume hands-and-knees positioning in labour. There was no statistical significance in the reduction of occipitoposterior or transverse positions at delivery and operative deliveries. However, there was a significant reduction in back pain. The authors conclude from the evidence in the systematic review (Hunter et al 2007) that adopting these positions as a recommended intervention could not be endorsed. However, they stated that if the women find these positions comfortable then they should adopt them and especially in labour where maternal backache is reduced.

Relieving backache

To relieve the backache, many women find the kneeling position beneficial. This position may also aid rotation of the head to an occipitoanterior position. Massaging the woman's back in the lumbosacral region may also help to relieve the backache and a warm bath has been found to be helpful. Epidural analgesia is the most effective method of relieving the pain. In the second stage of labour, perineal trauma is minimised by an upright position (Aasheim et al 2007).

A difficult problem for the woman in the late first stage of labour is feeling a strong urge to push before full cervical dilatation. Pushing presses the fetal head against the cervix and oedema may occur, thus lengthening the transitional stage of labour. Simkin & Ancheta (2005) suggest that the adoption of the kneeling position with the head resting on the forearms may lessen the pressure on the cervix.

The second stage of labour

The five main possible outcomes of an occipitoposterior position are:

1. Long internal rotation of the occiput and delivery as an occipitoanterior.
2. Deep transverse arrest of the head.
3. Short internal rotation of the sinciput and delivery as 'face to pubes'.
4. Partial extension of the head to a brow presentation.
5. Full extension of the head to a mentoposterior face presentation.

Mechanism of long internal rotation of a right occipitoposterior position

- The lie is longitudinal.
- The attitude of the head is deflexed.
- The presentation is vertex.
- The position is right occipitoposterior.
- The denominator is the occiput.
- The presenting part is the middle to anterior area of the left parietal bone.

The movements

Descent and flexion

There is continued descent with flexion during the first stage of labour and the presenting diameter of occipitofrontal (11.5 cm) is converted to suboccipitofrontal (10 cm).

Internal rotation of the head

The occiput reaches the pelvic floor first and rotates forwards along the right side of the pelvis $\frac{3}{8}$ths of a circle to lie under the symphysis pubis. The anteroposterior diameter of the head now lies in the anteroposterior diameter of the pelvis. The shoulders follow and rotate $\frac{2}{8}$ths of a circle. The occiput escapes from beneath the subpubic arch.

Extension of the head

The head is now born by extension as it pivots on the suboccipital region around the pubic bone. The sinciput, face and chin sweep the perineum.

Restitution

Restitution is a movement made by the head following delivery which brings it into correct alignment with the shoulders. This will be $\frac{1}{8}$th of a circle towards the side of the occiput.

Internal rotation of the shoulders

The anterior shoulder is the first to reach the pelvic floor and rotates forwards to lie under the symphysis pubis. This movement is accompanied by **external rotation of the head** $\frac{1}{8}$th of a circle more in the direction of restitution. The occiput now lies laterally turned towards the woman's thigh.

Lateral flexion

The anterior shoulder is usually born first and slips under the pubic arch and the posterior shoulder passes over the perineum. The remainder of the body is born by lateral flexion. This outcome is the most common, occurring in about 65% of births.

Deep transverse arrest of the head

If the head remains deflexed, deep transverse arrest may occur. The fetal head has begun long internal rotation but there is insufficient flexion to complete the process. The occipitofrontal diameter is caught above the ischial spines in the bispinous diameter. Labour becomes obstructed. Weak contractions, or a straight sacrum with narrow outlet (as found in the android pelvis), may lead to this.

Diagnosis and management

Diagnosis is made by finding the sagittal suture in the transverse diameter of the pelvis with a fontanelle at each end of the suture. Caput succedaneum may obscure the landmarks. It will be necessary to rotate the head to an occipitoanterior position either manually or with Kielland's forceps prior to delivery by forceps. An alternative way of rotating and delivering the fetal head is by vacuum extraction. Some obstetricians would be unwilling to do an instrumental delivery when the head has not descended below the ischial spines.

The use of the vacuum extractor is preferable to the forceps as it reduces the incidence of maternal injuries (Enkin et al 2000). Johanson & Menon (1999) found that, although vacuum extraction was related to increased incidence of neonatal cephalhaematoma and retinal haemorrhage, there was less incidence of maternal trauma and caesarean section (CS). In the light of their review, they recommended the use of vacuum extraction.

Short internal rotation of the sinciput and delivery as 'face to pubes'

In about 5% of labours the occiput fails to rotate spontaneously to an anterior position (Arias 1993). This is known as persistent occipitoposterior position or POP. The head remains deflexed and the sinciput reaches the pelvic floor first and rotates forwards. The occiput comes to lie in the hollow of the sacrum and the head of the baby is born facing the pubic bone. Incidentally, this is the normal birth position of the great apes such as chimpanzees.

Diagnosis

- There may be delay in the second stage of labour.
- There is gaping of the vagina and dilatation of the anus due to the presence of the large occiput.
- Confirmation is by finding the anterior fontanelle directly behind the symphysis pubis. This may be masked by caput succedaneum and feeling for the pinna of the ear will aid confirmation. In a POP, the pinna will point towards the maternal sacrum.

Management of the spontaneous delivery

The second stage is likely to be prolonged and, even when the woman wishes to push, there may be incomplete cervical dilatation (Kuo et al 1996). The squatting position may assist descent of the presenting part (Simkin & Ancheta 2005). Once the perineal phase of delivery is reached, to maintain the smallest possible diameters distending the perineum, the sinciput is allowed to emerge under the symphysis pubis as far as the root of the nose. Flexion is maintained and the occiput is allowed to sweep the perineum. The rest of the face is brought down from under the symphysis pubis. There is a high risk of perineal trauma, especially a 'buttonhole' tear in the centre of the perineum. An episiotomy may be required.

Face presentation

The incidence of face presentation at term is about 1 in 500. In this presentation, the head and spine are fully extended and the limbs fully flexed. The fetal occiput lies against its shoulder blades and the face is directly above the internal os (Fig. 43.6). Face presentation can lead to prolonged labours (Lanni & Seeds 2007).

Causes

Face presentation may be described as primary when it is present before the onset of labour (Lanni & Seeds 2007). The fetus is often abnormal and anencephaly is common, while a rarer cause is due to fetal goitre which prevents the head from flexing. A secondary face presentation is one that develops as labour proceeds (Lanni & Seeds 2007). In a deflexed occipitoposterior position, the biparietal diameter of the fetal head may be unable to pass through the sacrocotyloid diameter (9.5 cm) of the pelvic brim (sacrocotyloid diameter is from the sacral promontory to the nearest point of the illeopectineal eminence). The bitemporal diameter descends more quickly and the

head extends first to a brow presentation and ultimately to a face presentation. Other causes of face presentation include a flat pelvis, poor uterine muscle tone, prematurity, polyhydramnios or multiple pregnancy.

Risks

- Obstructed labour if either deep transverse arrest or brow presentation result.
- Maternal perineal trauma such as a third- or fourth-degree tear and bruising.
- Cord prolapse if there is early spontaneous rupture of the membranes.
- Facial bruising as the caput forms over the face.
- Cerebral haemorrhage due to excessive moulding of the cranium.

Diagnosis

Per abdomen

In pregnancy, face presentation is rarely found as the majority of cases develop in labour (Coates 2003). It may be difficult to diagnose face presentation. A deep groove may be palpated between the fetal head and back. The chest wall may be pressed up against the anterior wall of the uterus and heart sounds are heard clearly on the side where limbs are palpated. However, in mentoposterior positions where the chest faces posteriorly, heart sounds may be difficult to hear. In women who have a late ultrasound, a face presentation is sometimes found.

Per vaginam

In labour, the possibility of a face presentation should be suspected if the head remains high. On vaginal

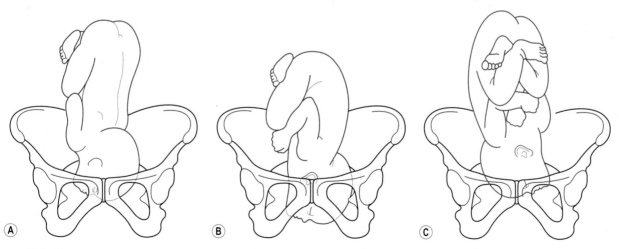

Figure 43.6 • Face presentations. (A) Right mentoposterior. (B) Right mentolateral. (C) Left mentoanterior. (From Henderson C, Macdonald S 2004, with kind permission of Elsevier.)

examination, feeling orbital ridges and a mouth with gum margins will confirm the diagnosis. The fetus may suck the examining finger. The mouth feels very different from the soft and clinging anal orifice, which would be found if the presentation was breech. Also, the examining finger may have meconium coating it if the breech was presenting. It is important to determine whether the fetus is presenting in a mentoposterior or mentoanterior position. Unless a posterior face rotates to anterior, there will be an obstructed labour. The position of the chin is the important diagnostic tool.

Progress and outcomes of labour

As in many labours where there is an irregular high presenting part, there may be early spontaneous rupture of the membranes with the risk of cord prolapse and contractions may be inefficient, leading to a prolonged labour. The face bones cannot mould and large diameters must enter the pelvis.

Mentoanterior position

In mentoanterior position if contractions are good, descent and rotation of the head occur and labour progresses to a spontaneous delivery (Barger 2002).

Mechanism of a left mentoanterior position

There are six possible positions: right mentoanterior, mentolateral and mentoposterior; and left mentoanterior, mentolateral and mentoposterior. The mechanisms are:

- The **lie** is longitudinal.
- The **attitude** of the head and back is one of extension.
- The **presentation** is face.
- The **position** is left mentoanterior.
- The **denominator** is the mentum.
- The **presenting part** is the left malar bone.

The movements

Descent
There is continued descent with increasing extension; the mentum is the leading part.

Internal rotation of the head
The mentum reaches the pelvic floor first and rotates forwards $\frac{1}{8}$th of a circle to lie under the symphysis pubis. The chin escapes from beneath the subpubic arch (Fig. 43.7).

Flexion of the head
The head is now born by flexion. The sinciput, vertex and occiput sweep the perineum.

Restitution
Restitution occurs as the chin turns $\frac{1}{8}$th of a circle towards the left side of the woman.

Internal rotation of the shoulders
The anterior shoulder is the first to reach the pelvic floor and rotates forwards to lie under the symphysis pubis. This movement is accompanied by **external rotation of the head** $\frac{1}{8}$th of a circle more in the direction of restitution.

Lateral flexion
The anterior shoulder is usually born first and slips under the pubic arch and the posterior shoulder passes over the perineum. The remainder of the body is born by lateral flexion.

Mentoposterior position

If the head is completely extended and the mentum reaches the pelvic floor first, the mentum rotates forwards into a mentoanterior position and delivery is possible. If the head is incompletely extended, there is a persistent mentoposterior position and the sinciput reaches the pelvic floor first. The chin comes to lie in the hollow of the pelvis and there can be no further progress. For further progress, the head and shoulders of the fetus would have to be in the pelvic cavity together. In order to be born, the presenting fetal part must pivot round the subpubic arch either by flexion or extension. If the chin is posterior, this cannot happen as the fully extended head cannot extend further and labour is obstructed.

Management of labour

The **first stage** of labour is managed according to the risks. During vaginal examination, note should be taken of the descent of the mentum. If the head remains high

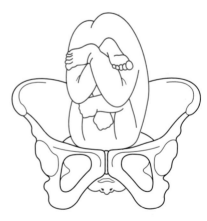

Figure 43.7 • The face at the outlet, the chin passing under the pubic arch. (From Henderson C, Macdonald S 2004, with kind permission of Elsevier.)

or there is a suspicion of cephalopelvic disproportion, the fetus should normally be delivered by CS.

In the **second stage**, when the face appears at the vulva, the sinciput must be held back to permit extension. This allows the mentum to escape under the pubic arch before the occiput sweeps the perineum. This ensures that the smallest possible diameter, which is the submentovertical (11.5 cm), distends the vaginal orifice rather than the large mentovertical diameter (13.5 cm). An elective episiotomy must be made because of the large diameters distending the vaginal orifice. The chin escapes under the pubic arch and the head is born by flexion. If there is delay in descent or if the fetus remains in a persistent mentoposterior position, a forceps delivery, with rotation if necessary, may be successful. Otherwise, a CS will be needed to reduce maternal and fetal morbidity and mortality.

Brow presentation

Brow presentation occurs in about 1 in 2000 deliveries. Except for anencephaly, the causes are the same as for face presentation. The head is an attitude midway between full flexion and full extension (or face). The largest diameter of the head, the mentovertical (13.5 cm), cannot enter the widest possible diameter of the pelvic brim, which is the transverse (13 cm) (Fig. 43.8). Unless the brow presentation extends fully to a face presentation and the mentum comes anterior, labour is obstructed.

Diagnosis

Per abdomen

The head is very high and the presenting diameter is very wide. A groove may be felt between the occiput and the back.

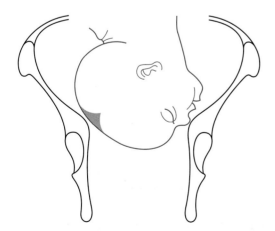

Figure 43.8 • Brow presentation. (From Henderson C, Macdonald S 2004, with kind permission of Elsevier.)

Per vaginam

The presenting part may be so high it cannot be reached. If the brow is within reach, the orbital ridges are felt at one side and the anterior fontanelle on the other with the frontal suture running between them. Frequently, the examination is confusing because of the oedema and unfamiliarity of the presenting features (ALSO 2005). Diagnosis can be confirmed by ultrasound.

Management

If the brow presentation is diagnosed early in labour and both maternal and fetal conditions are satisfactory, time may be allowed to see if the head will flex to a vertex or extend to a face presentation. If the brow presentation persists, a CS will be necessary.

Shoulder presentation

Shoulder presentation in labour is the result of an uncorrected abnormal lie in pregnancy. Instead of the normal longitudinal lie, the fetus lies across the uterus in either an oblique or a transverse lie. The lie may be unstable. In a shoulder presentation where the fetus is in the transverse lie the risk of cord prolapse is 20 times higher than in a vertex presentation (Lewis 2004). A shoulder presentation leads to obstructed labour and delivery should normally be by CS.

Causes

The most common cause is grande multiparity. Grande multiparous women often have lax uterine and abdominal muscles; in this case, the fetus takes the transverse lie. More than 80% of cases occur in women with three or more previous pregnancies (Lanni & Seeds 2007). Other causes include anything that prevents the fetus from adopting a longitudinal lie or the fetal head from engaging. These include placenta praevia, multiple pregnancy, polyhydramnios, uterine abnormality, large uterine fibroid or contracted pelvis. When the fetus dies in utero it may slump into an abnormal lie.

Diagnosis

Per abdomen

A transverse lie is easy to diagnose in pregnancy because of the abnormal shape of the uterus. The uterus is broader and the fundal height lower than normal and there may be a discernible bulge at either side of the uterus. On palpation, the fetal head will be felt on one side of the uterus and the breech on the other. The fetal back may be anterior (dorsoanterior) or posterior (dorso-posterior). There is no presenting part entering the pelvis (Fig. 43.9). In an oblique lie the shape of the uterus may be indicative and one or other pole of the fetus is found in one or other iliac fossa. Ultrasound is useful both to confirm the diagnosis and detect the cause.

Per vaginam

A vaginal examination should not be done if a transverse lie is suspected on abdominal examination in case there is a placenta praevia. Rarely, a woman will be admitted already in labour with the shoulder impacted at the brim of the pelvis. It may be mistaken for a breech presentation. The fetal cord and arm may prolapse (Fig. 43.9) into the vagina. On vaginal examination the shoulder is recognised by feeling the fetal ribs and the hand, which must be differentiated from a foot by the length of the digits and the presence of a heel. The safest method of delivery is by CS, even if the fetus is dead.

Management

A full examination is made during pregnancy to exclude causes such as placenta praevia. If no major pregnancy abnormality is found, the obstetrician may attempt to correct the lie to a longitudinal lie and cephalic presentation. However, reversion to the original lie is common and some doctors do not perform repeated external cephalic version (ECV) before the onset of labour, planned or otherwise. As pregnancy progresses, some lies will stabilise as longitudinal. However, 0.4% of all births will be a shoulder presentation (Lewis 2004).

The woman should be admitted to hospital at 37–38 weeks, when the fetus is mature for ECV and induction of labour. There is a risk of labour commencing spontaneously with early rupture of the membranes and cord prolapse. When the contractions are established and the fetal head enters the pelvis, the membranes can be ruptured.

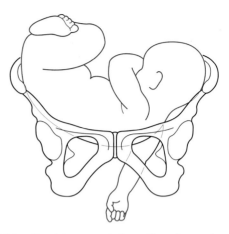

Figure 43.9 • Shoulder presentation with prolapse of one arm. (From Henderson C, Macdonald S 2004, with kind permission of Elsevier.)

If complications arise or if the woman has a poor obstetric history, a CS is performed.

In the case of twins, if after the birth of the first twin, the second twin takes up a transverse or oblique lie, the fetus must be turned by ECV, the second set of membranes ruptured and the delivery completed.

Compound presentation

This is a presentation where a hand or foot lies alongside the head. It is a rare complication and the incidence is about 0.1% of all deliveries (Lanni & Seeds 2007). Cord prolapse may occur in up to 20% of cases. It is more likely to happen if the fetus is small and the pelvis large or there is any condition that prevents the descent of the head such as contracted pelvis, prematurity or multiple pregnancy. The limb may recede as the head advances and the delivery proceeds normally. If the limb does not recede, it will be impossible for the head and hand to be delivered simultaneously; in this case, a CS is performed.

Main points

- There is no single cause for occipitoposterior position of the vertex but if the forepelvis is small, as found in android and anthropoid pelves, the head may take up a posterior position. Other causes include a pendulous abdomen, a flat sacrum or an anterior placenta. Risks include obstructed labour, maternal perineal trauma, cord prolapse and neonatal cerebral haemorrhage.

- Antenatally, occipitoposterior position is the most common cause of a non-engaged head in late pregnancy in primigravidae. It may be detected by a combination of maternal complaints and abdominal examination. In labour, during a vaginal examination, palpation of the anterior fontanelle confirms the diagnosis.

- The possible outcomes of an occipitoposterior position are long internal rotation of the occiput and delivery as an occipitoanterior, deep transverse arrest of the head, short internal rotation of the sinciput and delivery as 'face to pubes', partial extension of the head to a brow presentation or full extension of the head to a mentoposterior face presentation.

- If there is deep transverse arrest, the head must be rotated to an occipitoanterior position either manually or with Kielland's forceps prior to delivery by forceps.
- Face presentation may be primary when it is present before the onset of labour or secondary when it develops as labour proceeds. Risks include obstructed labour, maternal perineal trauma, cord prolapse, facial bruising and cerebral haemorrhage.
- In labour it is important to determine whether the fetus is presenting in a mentoposterior or mentoanterior position. The position of the chin is the important diagnostic tool. In a mentoanterior position with good contractions, descent and rotation of the head occurs and labour progresses to a spontaneous delivery. In a mentoposterior position, the usual outcome is that the fully extended head cannot extend further and labour is obstructed.
- In brow presentation, the mentovertical diameter is too large to enter the transverse widest possible diameter of the pelvic brim. Unless the head extends fully to a face presentation and the mentum becomes anterior, labour is obstructed. If brow presentation is diagnosed early in labour and maternal and fetal conditions are satisfactory, time may be allowed to see if the head will flex to a vertex or extend to a face presentation. If brow presentation persists, CS is necessary.
- Shoulder presentation in labour is the result of an uncorrected abnormal lie in pregnancy. The fetus lies across the uterus either in an oblique or a transverse lie. Shoulder presentation leads to obstructed labour and must be prevented. The most common cause is laxity of the uterine and abdominal muscles most often in multiparous women.
- In compound presentation, a hand or foot lies alongside the head. It is more likely to occur if the fetus is small and the pelvis large or there is any condition that prevents the descent of the head. The limb may recede as the head advances and the delivery proceeds normally. If the limb does not recede, it will be impossible to deliver the head and hand simultaneously; in this case, a CS is performed.

References

Aasheim, V., Nilsen, A.B.V., Lukasse, M., Reinar, L.M., 2007. Perineal Techniques During the Second Stage of Labour for Reducing Perineal Trauma (Protocol). Cochrane Review. Cochrane Library, Issue (3). Update Software 2008, Oxford.

ALSO 2005. Malpresentations, Malpositions, and Multiple Gestation, 6th edn. Advanced Life Support in Obstetrics, Registered Charity No. 1024554, UK Office, Newcastle-upon-Tyne.

Arias, F., 1993. Practical Guide to High Risk Pregnancy and Delivery, second edn. Mosby Year Book, Chicago.

Barger, M.K., 2002. What do you do when the baby is winking at you? Case report of a face presentation. J. Midwifery Women's Health 47 (6), 487–489.

Coates, T., 2003. Malpositions of the occiput and malpresentations. In: Fraser, D.M., Cooper, M.A. (Eds.), Myles Textbook for Midwives, fourteenth edn. Churchill Livingstone, Edinburgh.

El Halta, V., 1996. Posterior labor: a pain in the back! Its prevention and cure. Clarion 11 (1), 12–13.

Enkin, M., Keirse, J., Neilson, J., et al., 2000. A Guide to Effective Care in Pregnancy and Childbirth, third edn. Oxford University Press, Oxford.

Hunter, S., Hofmeyr, G.J., Kulier, R., 2007. Hands and knees posture in late pregnancy or labour for fetal malposition (lateral or posterior). Cochrane Review. Cochrane Library, (4). Update Software 2008, Oxford.

Johanson, R.B., Menon, V., 1999. Vacuum extraction versus forceps for assisted vaginal delivery. Cochrane Review. Cochrane Library, (2). Update Software 2008, Oxford.

Kuo, Y.-C., Chen, C.-P., Wong, K.-G., 1996. Factors influencing the prolonged second stage and the effects on perinatal and maternal outcomes. J. Obstet. Gynaecol. Res. 22 (3), 253–257.

Lanni, S.M., Seeds, J.W., et al., 2007. Malpresentations. In: Gabbe, S.G., Simpson, J.L., Niebyl, J.R. (Eds.) Obstetrics: Normal and Problem Pregnancies, fifth edn. Churchill Livingstone.

Lewis, P., 2004. Malpositions and malpresentation. In: Henderson, C., Macdonald, S. (Eds.), Mayes' Midwifery: A Textbook for Midwifery, thirteenth edn. Baillière Tindall, London.

Simkin, P., Ancheta, R., 2005. The Labor Progress Handbook, second edn. Blackwell Publishing, Oxford.

Sutton, J., 1996. A midwife's observations of how the birth process is influenced by the relationship of the maternal pelvis and the foetal head. J. Assoc. Chart. Phys. Women's Health 79, 31–33.

Annotated recommended reading

Coates, T., 2003. Malpositions of the occiput and malpresentations. In: Fraser, D.M., Cooper, M.A. (Eds.), Myles Textbook for Midwives, fourteenth edn. Churchill Livingstone, Edinburgh.

A chapter in an edited book in which Coates describes abnormal presentations and their management. It is an invaluable reference for those who provide intrapartum care.

Enkin, M., Keirse, J., Neilson, J., et al., 2000. A Guide to Effective Care in Pregnancy and Childbirth, third edn. Oxford University Press, Oxford.

A well-written book based on authoritative evidence available on all aspects of care during pregnancy and childbirth. An invaluable resource for intrapartum care.

Chapter Forty-Four

Cephalopelvic disproportion, obstructed labour and other obstetric emergencies

44

Introduction

Two evolutionary adaptations lead to problems between the female pelvis and the fetal head fitting.

First, the birth canal and the pathway taken by the fetus are complex as the human pelvis is adapted to a bipedal posture (Morgan 1994). Compared to other primates such as the chimpanzee:

- The anteroposterior diameter is reduced at the brim, cavity and outlet.
- There is widening of the transverse diameters.
- The sacral promontory protrudes into the pelvic inlet.
- The sacrum makes an angle with the lumbar spine—the **lumbosacral angle**.
- There is inward protrusion of the ischial spines in order to support the strong pelvic floor.
- The sacrum is curved.
- The superior ramus is thinned and elongated with widening of the subpubic angle.

Second, the fetal head is able to negotiate the pelvis successfully because of three features:

1. Spheroid shape of the vertex.
2. Mobility of the head on the neck, allowing flexion or extension.
3. Moulding of the bones of the vault (Abitol 1993).

Cephalopelvic disproportion

Any condition leading to a misfit between the fetal head and the maternal pelvis, with failure of descent of the head into the pelvis despite good contractions, results in **cephalopelvic disproportion** (CPD). Ultimately CPD interferes with the natural mechanisms of labour. The presenting diameters of the fetal head are larger than the diameters of the pelvis (Neilson et al 2003). The shape of the pelvis may be abnormal but, as long as the diameters allow passage of the fetal head, delivery should follow as there should be no problem with the rest of the fetus. CPD is an absolute cause of obstructed labour and there are tremendous dangers for mother and fetus (Neilson et al 2003).

Diagnosis

In a primigravida it is expected that the fetal head should engage in the last 2–3 weeks of pregnancy. If the head does not engage, an attempt to make it engage is tried and, if unsuccessful, CPD should be suspected. The most common cause for non-engagement of the head is **occipitoposterior position**, with deflexed head and a presenting occipitofrontal diameter (11.5 cm). However, in most of these cases the head flexes and descent occurs in labour. Other causes of a non-engaged head include **pelvic tumours**, **placenta praevia** and **polyhydramnios**. A steep **angle of inclination** between the pelvic brim and the horizontal is found in some Afro-Caribbean women and may delay engagement until late in labour.

Maternal indications of possible CPD

These indications include:

- Bone conditions such as rickets or osteomalacia, which may have resulted in alterations in the size and shape of the pelvis (Neilson et al 2003).
- Spinal deformities such as scoliosis.
- Pelvic trauma and fractures which may have altered the size and shape of the pelvis.
- Previous obstetric conditions such as prolonged labour, difficult delivery or CS.
- Short stature of the woman. Mahmood et al (1988) found that the height of the woman was a better predictor of CPD than the shoe size, although 80% of women under 1.6 m still achieved vaginal delivery.

Fetal conditions leading to CPD

These conditions include:

- Fetal abnormalities such as hydrocephalus.
- Size of the fetus in relation to the maternal pelvis. In a multigravida with deliveries of normal-sized infants, CPD is less likely, but in the event of a larger fetus there may be a problem. Abdominal palpation is an inaccurate method of judging fetal size, although experienced practitioners may become quite adept. Estimation of fetal size is becoming easier as ultrasound technology advances, although Hofmeyr (2004) argues that neither clinical nor ultrasound examination is good at estimating fetal weight and ultimately diagnosing obstructed labour.

Assessing the pelvis

A combination of careful history taking and clinical expertise backed up by technology should enable selection of women at risk. **Head fitting** or **pelvic assessment** examinations may be carried out. However, Enkin et al (2000) write that there is:

reasonable correlation between clinical and radiological assessment of pelvic dimensions but neither is particularly accurate in predicting the outcome of labour and opinion varies about the value of pre-labour assessments.

Head fitting

In head fitting, the technique is to attempt to cause engagement of the non-engaged head. The woman is asked to empty her bladder and to lie flat on the examination couch. The symphysis pubis is located with the fingers of the right hand and the fetal head is held between the thumb and fingers of the left hand. The woman takes a deep breath and as she breathes out the head is pushed downwards and backwards into the brim of the pelvis. The fingers of the right hand palpate to assess whether the widest diameter of the head has entered the pelvic brim.

Pelvic assessment

Pelvic assessment of the shape and size of the pelvis is carried out by the obstetrician in the last few weeks of pregnancy if the head cannot be made to engage. The tissues will be softer, allowing ease of examination, and the fetus is large enough to relate to the size of the pelvis. The aim is to assess the brim, cavity and outlet of the pelvis. An attempt is made to measure the diagonal conjugate which runs from the lower border of the symphysis pubis to the sacral promontory and thus assess the anteroposterior diameter of the pelvic brim, also known as the **true** or **obstetric conjugate**, through which the fetus has to pass.

During a vaginal examination an attempt is made to reach the sacral promontory but in a good-sized pelvis it is unlikely to be reached as the diagonal conjugate measures 12–13 cm. If it is reached, 2 cm are subtracted to allow for the depth of the pubic bone and the obstetric conjugate is estimated. The size of the pelvic cavity is assessed by examination of the length and curve of the sacrum and by feeling the length of the sacrospinous ligament, which should accommodate two fingers.

Finally, the shape and size of the pelvic outlet can then be assessed. The ischial spines are located to see whether or not they are prominent, which may suggest a narrow transverse diameter of the outlet. The subpubic angle should be more than 90° and should accommodate the width of two fingers. One external measurement is made with the fist: the distance between the ischial tuberosities should accommodate a large fist.

X-ray pelvimetry

Erect lateral X-ray pelvimetry provides information about the size and shape of the pelvis and the relationship of the fetal head to the pelvic brim. However, there has been criticism of its use because of an association between prenatal irradiation and childhood leukaemia. It may also be a poor predictor of CPD and the results do not appear to affect the management; therefore, X-ray pelvimetry should seldom if ever be necessary in pregnancy (Enkin et al 2000). This is reiterated by Pattison & Farrell (1997) and Hofmeyr (2004), who inform us that in the four 'randomised trials' reviewed of 1000 women X-ray pelvimetry led to more caesarean sections (CSs) but no increase in perinatal outcomes and the evidence does not support the use of pelvimetry in women with cephalic presentations. Pattinson & Farrell (1997) further stress that there were insufficient sample sizes to truly assess perinatal outcomes and more studies to evaluate this are required.

If X-ray pelvimetry is conducted, the following details can be noted:

- The shape of the pelvis.
- The shape of the sacrum.
- The inclination between the sacrum and pelvic brim.
- The anteroposterior diameters of the brim, cavity and outlet.
- The width of the sacrosciatic notch.
- The depth of the pelvic cavity.

Request for pelvimetry

Pelvimetry may be requested for the following:

- Any primigravida with the fetal head not engaged at term in whom clinical assessment suggests pelvic contraction.
- A primigravida with a breech presentation if external cephalic version has failed or is contraindicated and vaginal delivery is being considered.
- Any multipara with a history of difficult labour such as failure to progress in labour, prolonged labour and operative delivery, although these women should be offered pelvimetry in the postnatal period to avoid the risks of radiation to the fetus. A previous CS for any reason other than CPD is not a contraindication for trial of labour (Flamm et al 1994).
- Women with a history of injury or disease of the pelvis and spine or any limp or deformity.

A very small study (n = 48) by Sporri et al (2002) examined the benefits of magnetic resonance imaging (MRI). More accurate measurements of the pelvic outlet without the danger of radiation may be achievable but due to the insufficient sample size no conclusion can be drawn from this evidence on labour outcome. More research is needed to explore the issue. Retrospective data analysis of MRI pelvimetric data in 781 women by Keller et al (2003) highlighted that women who had undergone a CS or assisted delivery had smaller pelvimetric dimensions compared to women who had a vaginal delivery. Depending on the antenatal findings discussed above, there are three possibilities: disproportion is not present and vaginal delivery will be possible; there is CPD of such a degree that vaginal delivery will not be possible; and there is a degree of CPD which may be overcome in labour.

Trial of vaginal delivery

If there are no obstetric or medical complications, the woman can be admitted to hospital for a trial of labour. The aim is to allow time for the contractions of labour, aided by the abdominal and pelvic floor muscles, to cause sufficient flexion and moulding of the fetal head so that descent occurs (Abitol 1993). Engagement of the head is likely to be followed by vaginal delivery. All primigravidae with a non-engaged head are considered to be undergoing a trial of labour (Brock 2004). An old but probably useful saying is that the fetal head is the best pelvimeter!

Selection of women for trial of vaginal delivery

- The presentation must be cephalic.
- There should be no major degree of CPD.
- The woman should be healthy with a good obstetric and medical history.
- There should be no pregnancy complications such as hypertension.

Management

There must be careful monitoring of mother and fetus and facilities for the immediate carrying out of a CS if needed. All observations are plotted on a partogram and any changes in the conditions of mother, fetus or progress noted by the midwife must be reported to the obstetrician, who is the decision maker (Shiers 2003). The obstetrician may wish to conduct all vaginal examinations. Ambulation and adoption of an upright position encourages flexion and descent of the head, maintenance of good uterine action and cervical dilatation (Simkin & Ancheta 2005).

Assessment of progress

Successful progression to a vaginal delivery should occur if the contractions are good, the fetal head flexes and the skull bones mould, the pelvic joints relax and maternal and fetal heart remain satisfactory. Progress is assessed by observation of descent of the fetal head by abdominal palpation. The dilatation of the cervix is assessed by vaginal examination. Progress in dilatation should follow that of 1 cm/h.

If progress is slow due to inefficient uterine action and thought to be unrelated to CPD, active management of labour can be undertaken and oxytocic drugs can be used. However, it is important to remember that the injudicious use of oxytocic drugs in the presence of more than a minor degree of CPD may lead to rupture of the uterus. If hyperstimulation occurs, the Syntocinon (oxytocin) infusion should be stopped immediately and the obstetrician informed. A CS may be necessary if:

- The progress of labour remains slow following the commencement of the oxytocin infusion.
- The head fails to descend in the presence of efficient contractions.
- Fetal distress arises.

Obstructed labour

Obstructed labour occurs when there is no advance of the presenting part despite strong uterine contractions (Shiers 2003). There is a large increase in maternal and fetal morbidity and mortality if labour is allowed to proceed in the presence of unrecognised obstructed labour. The situation is more common in remote areas of the world such as villages in Africa or India where women do not have access to trained personnel, but it can also occur in a developed country such as in the UK if a woman fails to disclose her pregnancy or to present herself for care in labour.

Causes

- Cephalopelvic disproportion is a cause of obstructed labour that is unresolvable except by CS (in remote areas of the world, division of the symphysis pubis— symphysiotomy—or a fetal destructive operation may save the life of the mother).
- Malpositions and malpresentations of the head, such as brow, posterior face or deep transverse arrest of the head.
- Fetal abnormalities such as hydrocephalus.
- Maternal tumours.
- Fibroids.

Signs and symptoms

Early signs

- There is little progress in labour, with no descent of the head despite efficient uterine action.
- On vaginal examination, the presenting part is high.
- The cervix dilates slowly and is not well applied to the presenting part (Brock 2004).

- The membranes have usually ruptured early and there is an ever-present risk of cord prolapse.
- In a primigravida there may be active phase arrest and the contractions stop for a while, finally restarting with increased strength. The woman may complain of severe and continuous pain.
- The multiparous woman may have tumultuous contractions that proceed rapidly to uterine rupture.

Late signs

- If nothing was done for the woman or, much more likely in the UK, if she presented herself for care late in labour, she may progress to having a raised temperature, rapid pulse and dehydration.
- On abdominal inspection, the uterus would appear to be moulded around the fetus because of tonic contraction and loss of liquor amnii.
- A Bandl's pathological retraction ring may be seen as a ridge of tissue running obliquely across the abdomen. This denotes an extremely thinned lower uterine segment and imminent rupture of the uterus.
- There will be a cutting off of the fetoplacental blood supply and fetal oxygen supply and the fetus will die.
- On examination the vagina feels hot and dry and the presenting part is high. There may be excessive moulding and a large caput succedaneum obscuring the presenting part in a cephalic presentation.
- Urinary output is reduced and a vesicovaginal fistula may occur due to sloughing off tissue due to prolonged pressure.

Management

Prevention, by achieving a high standard of antenatal care and observations in early labour, would be the best management to allow early detection of likely difficulties and treatment before obstructed labour occurs. Removal of an ovarian cyst, correction of an abnormal lie or performing a planned CS are examples of actions that minimise the chances of obstructed labour occurring. There should also be caution in the use of amniotomy in obstructed labours. The systematic review of Smyth et al (2007) of 14 studies ($n = 4893$) explored amniotomy for shortening spontaneous labour. They advocate that routine amniotomy is not recommended for normal labours nor is it recommended in prolonged labours as it increases the risk of CS. If labour is advanced when the woman is first seen, an emergency CS is carried out regardless of whether the fetus is dead or alive. Rarely, especially in developing countries, if the fetus is dead and the cervix is fully dilated destructive operations such as cleidotomy (division of the clavicles) or craniotomy (perforation of the skull) may allow vaginal delivery but there is risk of perforation of the thin lower uterine segment (Gupta & Chitra 1994).

Uterine rupture

Rupture of the uterus is an obstetric emergency and the fetus and mother may die. Rupture of the uterus may involve a previous scar, spontaneous rupture of an intact uterus or traumatic rupture. Deaths from uterine trauma have reduced to two between 1997 and 1999 compared with five deaths in the previous triennial report of the Confidential Enquiry into Maternal Deaths in the UK (Lewis 2007). However, the latest CEMACH report still highlights that there were three cases of uterine rupture (Lewis 2007). The incidence of uterine rupture appears to be consistent in developed countries but may be rising in the developing countries due to vaginal delivery following a previous CS and due to inappropriate use of oxytocic infusions (Grace et al 1993).

Types of uterine rupture

Scar rupture is usually due to a previous CS. A longitudinal scar in the uterus (classical incision) is more likely to rupture than a transverse scar in the lower segment. Rupture of the classical scar occurs in about 2% of cases and is more likely to occur in late pregnancy when the upper segment is stretched to its limit. Performing a CS at 38 weeks may reduce this rate. Rupture of a transverse lower segment scar is more likely to happen in labour as the lower segment is thinned and extended. Uterine rupture following a lower segment CS is less than 1%.

Traumatic rupture of the uterus may be caused by the use of obstetric instruments such as forceps. These can cause tearing of the cervix which extends into the lower segment. Intrauterine manipulations such as internal podalic version, where the foot of the fetus is grasped at delivery to convert a transverse lie—usually of the second twin—to breech or correction of a shoulder presentation in labour, may lead to uterine rupture as may the misuse of oxytocic drugs.

Spontaneous rupture of the uterus may follow strong spontaneous uterine action such as that occurring in obstructed labour. The rupture is found most often in the lower segment. Abruptio placentae where there is extravasation of blood into the uterine muscle (Couvelaire uterus) facilitates such a rupture.

Signs and symptoms

Complete rupture

Rupture of the uterus may be complete or true, involving the full thickness of the uterine wall and the pelvic peritoneum. This is usually an acute event associated with sudden intense pain, blood loss and collapse followed by maternal and fetal death. The uterine contractions cease and there is vaginal bleeding. The fetus may pass into the abdominal cavity and be palpable outside the uterus directly under the abdominal wall.

Incomplete rupture

Incomplete or silent rupture involves the myometrium but the peritoneum remains intact. It is more frequently associated with a previous lower segment CS. Because scar tissue tends to be avascular, there are less dramatic signs. The mother's condition deteriorates slowly. Abdominal pain or scar tenderness may be present and a rise in maternal heart rate may be an indicator of impending rupture.

Management

If a ruptured uterus is diagnosed, obstetric, anaesthetic and theatre emergency teams must be alerted and the mother immediately transferred to theatre. The anaesthetist will establish venous access and start resuscitative measures while the surgeons and the theatre teams scrub up for emergency CS. A blood transfusion will be necessary. The baby is delivered and the uterus repaired if possible. A hysterectomy may be necessary if the rupture is severe and bleeding difficult to control. Postoperative treatment should include observation of severe side-effects of haemorrhage such as renal failure or, later, onset of Sheehan's syndrome. The psychological effect of the experience on the woman and her family should be anticipated and explanations and counselling made available.

Shoulder dystocia

This term is used to describe a range of difficulties encountered with delivering the shoulders after delivering the head. Shoulder dystocia occurs when either the anterior or, less commonly, the posterior fetal shoulder impacts on the maternal symphysis or sacral promontory (RCOG 2005) (Fig. 44.1).

Definition

Shoulder dystocia is a condition requiring special manoeuvres to deliver shoulders following an unsuccessful attempt to apply downward traction.

Shoulder dystocia is another obstetric emergency which may end in fetal and maternal morbidity and mortality. There is difficulty in delivering the anterior shoulder and urgent manoeuvres are necessary. It is important to remember that this is a bony obstruction problem and NOT a soft tissue obstruction! There are two causes:

1. A large baby;

2. Failure of the shoulders to rotate into the anteroposterior diameter following delivery of the head.

The incidence of shoulder dystocia is about 0.6% (RCOG 2005) and the risk rises as pregnancy becomes prolonged with increasing birth weight.

Discrepancies in the definition, the degree of difficulty and the manoeuvres used have resulted in variations between 0.15% and 2% of all vaginal deliveries in the reported incidence of this obstetric emergency.

Recognition

The head fails to advance and the fetus looks to be burying its chin in the perineum. This happens because the anterior shoulder is wedged firmly behind the symphysis pubis. Difficulty in delivering the face and the chin are warning signs (Shiers & Coates 2003). The baby's head may fail to rotate or allow restitution to occur. This is sometimes referred to as a 'turtle' sign! (Medford et al 2006).

Risk factors

It is important to remember that shoulder dystocia can be an unpredictable event. However, the following factors, most of them associated with a large fetus, should be taken into consideration so that the woman can be delivered in an appropriate setting:

- If the mother is over 35 years there may be an associated increase in birth weight.

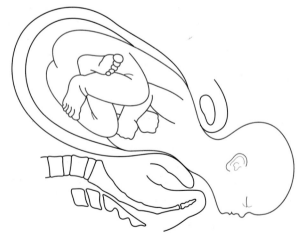

Figure 44.1 • Shoulder dystocia. (From Henderson C, Macdonald S 2004, with kind permission of Elsevier.)

- A maternal BMI of >30 is the most frequently associated factor.
- Maternal diabetes mellitus, whether insulin-dependent or gestational, is associated with fetal macrosomia and difficulty in delivering the shoulders.
- Infants of increased birth weight in non-diabetic mothers have less incidence of shoulder dystocia, with a 10% risk rather than the 31% risk of the diabetic woman (Spellacy et al 1985).
- Maternal high birth weight is associated with high birth weight of her own fetus.
- In women with a platypelloid pelvis, where the anteroposterior diameter is reduced, shoulder dystocia may develop with a normal-sized infant.

Management

Excessive force must not be applied to the fetal head or neck and fundal pressure must be avoided (ALSO 2005). These activities are unlikely to free the impaction and may cause maternal and fetal injury and may lead to uterine rupture (RCOG 2005). Routine traction should be applied to the neck rather than a downwards traction so as to decrease the risk of fetal nerve injury (RCOG 2005). If possible, the midwife should summon an obstetrician, paediatrician and anaesthetist. However, there is little time to save the life of the baby and the woman may be in her own home so the midwife must attempt to complete the delivery. Woodward et al (2005) advocate that the help must be appropriate for the setting, and could take the form of a second midwife, general practitioner or paramedic. It may be necessary to try more than one manoeuvre so it is necessary to keep calm and think clearly about what is happening inside the mother's pelvis. Shoulder dystocia should be treated as an obstetric emergency to prevent fetal morbidity as 47% of babies die within 5 min of the head being delivered (RCOG 2005).

Manoeuvres

The HELPERR(S) mnemonic is a clinical tool that can provide practitioners with a structured framework to deal with this extremely difficult situation:

H   Call for help

E   Evaluate for episiotomy

L   Legs (the McRoberts' position)

P   Pressure (suprapubic)

E   Enter (internal manoeuvres)

R   Remove the posterior arm

R   Roll the woman (onto 'all fours' position)

S   Start all over again!

The manoeuvres (ALSO 2005) will be dealt with individually but this does not imply that any one technique is superior to any other; together they are a valuable tool to help practitioners take effective steps to overcome this situation. The steps should be carried out efficiently and appropriately as the time element is vital. An assistant should maintain relevant recordings of the events.

The three main aims of the manoeuvres are to:

1. Increase the functional size of the bony pelvis.
2. Decrease the bisacromial diameter (12 cm).
3. Change the relationship of the bisacromial diameter within the bony pelvis.

It is recommended that an episiotomy be performed, if possible. However, it is important to be aware that although an episiotomy will make room for the internal manoeuvres and prevent maternal trauma the obstruction is bony. Delivery of the baby should be attempted following each manoeuvre.

The McRoberts' position

This is a simple manoeuvre and its effectiveness makes it appropriate for the first step in the management. The woman is helped to lie on her back with her knees drawn up to her chest (Fig. 44.2), which simulates the squatting position. This manoeuvre can help to deliver the shoulders by:

- Opening the pelvic inlet to its maximum possible diameter.
- Flexing the fetal spine and pushing the posterior shoulder over the sacral promontory and into the hollow of the sacrum.
- Rotating the symphysis pubis superiorly over the impacted shoulder.
- Elevating the anterior shoulder.
- Straightening any maternal lumbosacral lordosis and flattening the sacral promontory to reduce this obstruction.

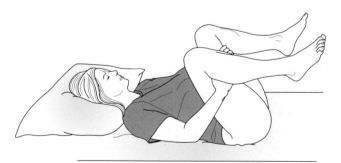

Figure 44.2 • McRoberts' position. (From Henderson C, Macdonald S 2004, with kind permission of Elsevier.)

- Bringing the inlet perpendicular to the maximum expulsive force.
- Removing the weight-bearing forces from the sacrum.
- Allowing the direction of the maternal force to be perpendicular to the plane of the inlet.

This manoeuvre is attempted for 30 s, while the delivering practitioner continues gentle traction on the baby.

Suprapubic pressure

This is the **P** or **Pressure** component as described in the mnemonic. An assistant should attempt external manual suprapubic pressure for 30–60 s while the delivering practitioner continues gentle traction. The suprapubic hand should be placed over the posterior aspect of the fetus's anterior shoulder and pressure should be applied in a 'CPR' style in such a way as to adduct or collapse the shoulder anteriorly and pass under the pubic symphysis. Initially, the pressure should be continuous but, if not accomplished, a rocking motion is recommended to dislodge the shoulder from behind the pubic symphysis. McRoberts' manoeuvre can also be maintained simultaneously.

Internal manoeuvres

The following two manoeuvres attempt to manipulate the fetus to rotate the anterior shoulder into an oblique plane and under the maternal symphysis pubis. If at any time the manoeuvres are successful delivery of the baby is attempted by gentle traction. Each of the manoeuvres is conducted for up to 30 s; if unsuccessful the practitioner will move on to the next manoeuvre.

Rubin's manoeuvre

Rubin's manoeuvre is carried out to reduce the diameter of the shoulder girdle and is the basis of the first part of the **E** or **Enter** component. The fingers of one hand are inserted into the vagina at either 5 or 7 o'clock on the side of the fetal back and manoeuvred behind the anterior shoulder (11 or 1 o'clock position). The shoulder is pushed towards the fetus's chest to reduce the diameter. If both shoulders are adducted, the circumference of the baby's body is greatly reduced (we use this position to squeeze through narrow spaces by bringing our shoulders forward to make ourselves smaller). This may free the shoulders from the symphysis pubis to allow delivery. The McRoberts' manoeuvre can still be applied to facilitate delivery. If unsuccessful, the practitioner should proceed to the next movement.

Wood's screw manoeuvre

This next manoeuvre can be combined with the Rubin's manoeuvre. The practitioner keeps the first hand behind the anterior shoulder at either the 11 or 1 o'clock position and inserts two fingers of the other hand into the vagina to the front of the posterior shoulder at the 5 or 7 o'clock position. The practitioner rotates the shoulder towards the symphysis in the same direction as with the Rubin's manoeuvre. The practitioner now has two fingers behind the anterior shoulder and two fingers of the other hand in front of the posterior shoulder. The Rubin manoeuvre adducts or flexes the anterior shoulder while the Wood's screw manoeuvre abducts or extends the posterior shoulder. This is why the combination of the two manoeuvres may be more successful.

If these manoeuvres fail, then the **reverse Wood's screw** manoeuvre may be tried. The fingers of the entering hand are placed on the posterior shoulder from behind and the attempt is to rotate the fetus in the opposite direction as the Wood's screw manoeuvre. This rotates the shoulders out of the impacted position to allow delivery. This manoeuvre is identical to the Rubin's when performed on the posterior shoulder.

There remains a lot of confusion in obstetrics about performing these manoeuvres. They can occasionally be difficult to perform particularly when the anterior shoulder is partially wedged underneath the symphysis. At times it may be necessary to push the posterior shoulder, or sometimes the anterior shoulder, back up into the pelvis slightly in order to accomplish the manoeuvre (ALSO 2005). Since this is an obstetric emergency it is important that practitioners are prepared to perform all the practical skills of the different manoeuvres. These should be practised in work-group situations using dolls and pelvis or other similar models for simulation purposes.

Remove the posterior arm

This is the **R** or **Remove the posterior arm** component. A hand is inserted into the vagina along the sacral curve to locate the posterior arm or hand (Fig. 44.3A). Once located, the elbow should be flexed (Fig. 44.3B) so that the forearm can be delivered in a sweeping motion over the anterior chest wall of the fetus, thus shortening the bisacromial diameter (12 cm) (Fig. 44.3C). This allows the anterior shoulder to collapse as the fetus drops into the pelvic hollow, freeing the impaction anteriorly.

Roll the woman

This is the **R** or **Roll the woman**. The woman should be rolled onto the 'all-fours' position. This is a safe, rapid and effective technique for the reduction of shoulder dystocia. By rotating to this position, the true obstetrical conjugate increases by as much as 10 mm and the sagittal measurement of the pelvic outlet increases up to 20 mm. The fetal shoulders often dislodge during the act

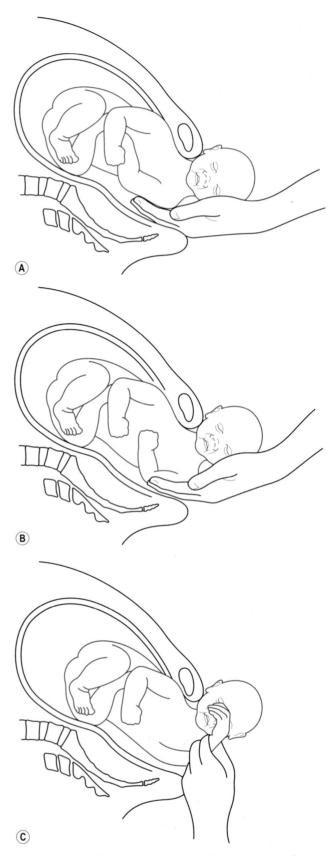

Figure 44.3 • Delivery of posterior arm. (From Henderson C, Macdonald S 2004, with kind permission of Elsevier.)

of turning from supine to this position. This would not be an appropriate manoeuvre to consider if the woman was anaesthetised with an epidural.

Other manoeuvres

Cleidotomy

This is a deliberate fracture of the clavicle but is difficult and rarely done. Spontaneous fracture may occur and facilitate delivery.

Symphysiotomy

This is a minimally invasive surgical procedure where a scalpel is inserted through the skin overlying the symphysis pubis and the joint and supporting ligaments are incised using a pivoting movement (Björklund 2002). Björklund (2002) states that for a minimally invasive procedure it can relieve a moderately obstructed labour and questions whether or not this would be an appropriate method to relieve an obstruction where CS is not available.

Zavanelli manoeuvre

This manoeuvre of cephalic replacement followed by CS involves returning the head to its pre-restitution position, flexing the head and pushing it back into the birth canal. Continuous upward pressure is maintained until the CS can be performed. This manoeuvre has a high mortality rate and should only be used as a last resort when all other methods have failed (Vollebergh & van Dongen 2000).

Outcome for mother and fetus

Maternal death is rare but can happen. Maternal morbidity is more common, with perineal, vaginal and cervical lacerations, uterine rupture, vaginal haematoma and haemorrhage possibly occurring. Postpartum haemorrhage should be anticipated and the genitalia carefully examined for lacerations.

For the baby, birth asphyxia is a complication of shoulder dystocia. Meconium aspiration may occur due to the asphyxia. Birth injury is also commonly reported with brachial plexus injury.

Cord presentation and prolapse

Campbell & Lees (2000) state that 1 in 300 births are complicated by presentation of the umbilical cord when the cord lies in front of the presenting part with the fetal membranes still intact. If a loop of cord lies alongside the fetal presenting part, it is an **occult cord presentation**. If the membranes rupture, the cord is prolapsed. Murphy & MacKenzie (1995) found an incidence of cord prolapse in 132 babies born in the John Radcliffe Hospital, Oxford, between 1984 and 1992. This gave a rate of 1 in 426 total births. There were 6 stillbirths and 6 neonatal deaths, giving an uncorrected perinatal mortality rate of 91 per 1000. Of 120 survivors, only one baby was known to have developed a major neurological handicap.

Causes of cord presentation and prolapse

The characteristics of pregnancy that increase the risk of cord presentation and cord prolapse are not generally avoidable. Fetomaternal factors that lead to the maternal pelvis not being completely filled by the fetus and obstetric intervention are the two key risk factors. Common risk factors include:

- A high presenting part, multiparous women, malposition of the occiput and malpresentations such as brow, face, shoulder presentation and breech presentation.
- Transverse and oblique lie of the fetus.
- The high assimilation pelvis found in Afro-Caribbean women.
- Preterm labour because of the increased ratio of liquor amnii to fetus and the prevalence of malpresentations.
- Multiple births, especially following the birth of the first baby.
- Polyhydramnios.
- An unusually long cord.
- Following obstetric manipulations such as external cephalic version.

Diagnosis and management

Cord presentation may be diagnosed in pregnancy by ultrasound scanning, especially in women with any of the risk factors mentioned above (Lange et al 1985). However, the RCOG (2008) do not recommend that routine ultrasound scans to diagnose cord presentation can predict a cord prolapse as there is insufficient evidence to support it. In early labour vaginal examination may occasionally find the rope-like cord between the presenting part and the membranes. It will be pulsating in time with the fetal heart rate. If cord presentation is suspected, it is essential to ensure that the membranes do not rupture. If there has been altered heart rate patterns following amniotomy or spontaneous rupture of membranes then cord prolapse should be suspected and a vaginal examination conducted in term pregnancies or speculum examination in preterm pregnancies (RCOG 2008). Routine vaginal examination is not required if there are no risk factors or signs of fetal distress following spontaneous rupture of membranes with clear amniotic fluid (RCOG 2008).

If cord prolapse is suspected or diagnosed then the mother is best placed in an exaggerated Simm's position with her pelvis, hips and buttocks elevated to take pressure off the cord and membranes (Fig. 44.4) or in the Trendelenberg position (elevate the bottom of the bed). This is an obstetric emergency and medical assistance should be obtained immediately. If cord presentation persists, an emergency CS will be needed. If the membranes have ruptured, the cord may have prolapsed through the cervix, into the vagina or even outside of the vulva.

If the cord is prolapsed it may be felt in the vagina or seen at the vulva. The cord may be compressed, especially if the presentation is cephalic because of the hardness of the fetal head, and the fetal oxygen supply cut off. If the cord is external to the vagina, cooling, drying and handling may precipitate spasm in the umbilical vessels. If the woman is in hospital the prognosis can be good. However, if the woman is at home fetal loss may be high.

Factors to take into consideration are the stage in labour and whether or not the fetus is dead. If fetal death is confirmed, labour can be allowed to continue unless other conditions such as obstructed labour contraindicate vaginal delivery. If the fetus is thought to be alive, the treatment is immediate delivery. In the first stage of labour an emergency CS is arranged. In the meantime, pressure must be kept off the cord by positioning the woman in a knee–chest all-fours posture with buttocks raised (Fig. 44.5) or exaggerated Simm's position (Fig. 44.4). The cord can be replaced gently back in the vagina although minimal handling of the cord is advocated to

prevent vasoconstriction from spasm (RCOG 2008). Oxygen therapy may be of use but there is limited evidence to support its administration for use in fetal distress (Fawole & Hofmeyr 2003).

In the early part of the second stage of labour with no cephalopelvic disproportion or malpresentation, a forceps delivery is performed. If the woman is multiparous and in late second stage an episiotomy may allow early delivery.

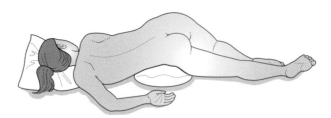

Figure 44.4 • Exaggerated Sim's position. Pillows or wedges are used to elevate the woman's buttocks to relieve pressure on the umbilical cord. (From Fraser & Cooper 2009, with kind permission of Elsevier.)

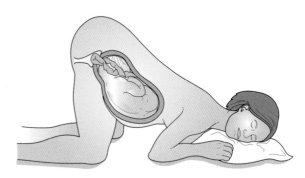

Figure 44.5 • Knee–chest position. Pressure on the umbilical cord is relieved as the fetus gravitates towards the fundus. (From Fraser & Cooper 2009, with kind permission of Elsevier.)

Main points

- Any condition leading to a misfit between the fetal head and the maternal pelvis with failure of descent of the head into the pelvis despite good contractions results in cephalopelvic disproportion (CPD). CPD is an absolute cause of obstructed labour and there are dangers for mother and fetus.

- Maternal indications of possible CPD include bone conditions which may have resulted in alterations in the size and shape of the pelvis, spinal deformities, pelvic trauma and fractures, previous difficulties with delivery and short stature. Fetal conditions leading to CPD include size of the fetus in relation to the maternal pelvis.

- A combination of careful history taking and clinical expertise backed up by technology should enable selection of women at risk. Head fitting and clinical

or radiological pelvic assessment examinations may be carried out. Erect lateral X-ray pelvimetry provides information about the size and shape of the pelvis and the relationship of the fetal head to the pelvic brim. Magnetic resonance imaging (MRI) may allow more accurate measurements of the pelvis.

- Obstructed labour occurs whenever there is an impassable barrier to the descent of the fetus through the birth canal in spite of efficient uterine action. There is a large increase in maternal and fetal morbidity and mortality if labour is allowed to proceed. Causes of obstructed labour are CPD, malpositions and malpresentations of the head, such as brow, posterior face or deep transverse arrest of the head, fetal abnormalities such as hydrocephalus and maternal tumours.

- Rupture of the uterus may involve a previous scar, spontaneous rupture of an intact uterus or traumatic rupture. Rupture of the uterus may be complete. This is usually an acute event associated with sudden intense pain, blood loss and collapse followed by maternal and fetal death. Incomplete or silent rupture is more frequently associated with a previous lower segment CS.
- Shoulder dystocia is an obstetric emergency which may end in fetal and maternal morbidity and mortality. It may be due to a large baby or failure of the shoulders to rotate into the anteroposterior diameter following delivery of the head.

- Causes of cord presentation and prolapse include high presenting part, breech presentation, cephalopelvic disproportion, placenta praevia, fibroids, preterm labour, multiple births, polyhydramnios, a long cord and external cephalic version. If the membranes rupture, the cord may prolapse and may become compressed, cutting off the fetal oxygen supply. If the cord is outside the vagina, cooling, drying and handling may precipitate umbilical vessel spasm which should be avoided.

References

Abitol, M.M., 1993. Adjustment of the fetal head and adult pelvis in modern humans. J. Hum. Evol. 8 (3), 167–185.

ALSO, 2005. Shoulder Dystocia, fifth edn. Advanced Life Support in Obstetrics, Newcastle-upon-Tyne, Registered Charity No. 1024554, UK Office.

Björklund, K., 2002. Minimally invasive surgery for obstructed labour: a review of symphysiotomy during the twentieth century (including 5000 cases). BJOG 109, 236–248.

Brock, M., 2004. Disproportion, obstructed labour and uterine rupture. In: Henderson, C., Macdonald, S. (Eds.). Mayes' Midwifery: A Textbook for Midwifery, thirteenth edn. Baillière Tindall, London.

Campbell, S., Lees, C., 2000. Obstetrics by Ten Teachers, seventeenth edn. Hodder, London.

Enkin, M., Keirse, J., Neilson, J., et al., 2000. A Guide to Effective Care in Pregnancy and Childbirth, third edn. Oxford University Press, Oxford.

Fawole, B., Hofmeyr, G.J., 2003. Maternal oxygen administration for fetal distress. Cochrane Review. Cochrane Library 4. Update Software 2008, Oxford.

Flamm, B.L., Goings, J.R., Liu, Y., et al., 1994. Elective repeat caesarean delivery versus trial of labour: a prospective multi-centre study. Obstet. Gynecol. 83 (6), 927–932.

Grace, D., Lavery, G., Loughran, P.G., 1993. Acute uterine rupture and its sequelae. Int. J. Obstet. Anaesth. 2, 41–44.

Gupta, U., Chitra, R., 1994. Destructive operations still have a place in developing countries. Int. J. Gynaecol. Obstet. 44 (1), 15–19.

Hofmeyr, G.J., 2004. Obstructed labour: using better technologies to reduce mortality. Int. J. Gynaecol. Obstet. 85 (1), S63–S72.

Keller, T.M., Rake, A., Michel, S.C.A., et al., 2003. Obstetric MR pelvimetry: reference values and evaluation of inter- and intraobserver error and intraindividual variability. Radiology 227 (1), 37–43.

Lange, I.R., Manning, F.A., Morrison, I., et al., 1985. Cord prolapse: is antenatal diagnosis possible? Am. J. Obstet. Gynecol. 1512, 1083–1085.

Lewis, G. (Ed.), 2007. Saving Mothers' Lives: The Seventh Report of the Confidential Enquiries into the Maternal and Child Health Report. RCOG, London.

Mahmood, T.A., Campbell, D.M., Wilson, A.W., 1988. Maternal height, shoe size, and outcome of labour in white primigravidas: a prospective study. Br. Med. J. 297, 515–517.

Medford, J., Battersby, S., Evans, M., 2006. Oxford Handbook of Midwifery. Oxford University Press, Oxford.

Morgan, E., 1994. The Descent of the Child. Souvenir Press, London.

Murphy, D.J., MacKenzie, I.Z., 1995. The mortality and morbidity associated with umbilical cord prolapse. Br. J. Obstet. Gynaecol. 102 (10), 826–830.

Neilson, J.P., Lavender, T., Quenby, S., et al., 2003. Obstructed labour. Br. Med. Bull. 67, 91–204.

Pattinson, R.C., Farrell, E-M.E., 1997. Pelvimetry for fetal cephalic presentations at or near term. Cochrane Database Syst. Rev. 2007 (2) Art. No.: CD000161. DOI: 10.1002/14651858. CD000161.

RCOG (Royal College of Obstetricians and Gynaecologists), 2005. Shoulder Dystocia Guideline No. 42. RCOG, London.

RCOG (Royal College of Obstetricians and Gynaecologists), 2008. Umbilical Cord Prolapse Guideline No. 50. RCOG, London.

Shiers, C., 2003. Prolonged pregnancy and disorders of uterine action. In: Fraser, D.M., Cooper, M.A. (Eds.). Myles Textbook for Midwives, fourteenth edn. Churchill Livingstone, Edinburgh.

Shiers, C., Coates, T., 2003. Midwifery and obstetric emergencies. In: Fraser, D.M., Cooper, M.A. (Eds.). Myles Textbook for Midwives, fourteenth edn. Churchill Livingstone, Edinburgh.

Simkin, P., Ancheta, R., 2005. The Labor Progress Handbook, second edn. Blackwell Publishing, Oxford.

Smyth, R.M.D., Alldred, S.K., Markham, C. 2007. Amniotomy for shortening spontaneous labour. Cochrane Review. Cochrane Library Issue 4. Update Software 2008, Oxford.

Spellacy, W.N., Miller, S., Winegar, A., et al., 1985. Macrosomia, maternal characteristics and infant complications. Obstet. Gynaecol. 66 (2), 158–161.

Sporri, S., Thoeny, H.C., Raio, L., et al., 2002. MR imaging pelvimetry: A useful adjunct in the treatment of women at risk of dystocia? Am. J. Roentgenol. 179 (1), 137–144.

Vollebergh, J.H.A., van Dongen, P.W.J., 2000. The Zavanelli manoeuvre in shoulder dystocia: a case report and review of published cases. Eur. J. Obstet. Gynecol. Reprod. Biol. 89, 81–84.

Woodward, V., Bates, K., Young, N., 2005. Managing Childbirth Emergencies in Community Settings. Palgrave Macmillan, Hampshire.

Annotated recommended reading

Lewis, G. (Ed.), 2007. Saving Mothers Lives: The Seventh Report of the Confidential Enquiries into the Maternal and Child Health Report. RCOG, London.

This triennial report was produced for the Confidential Enquiries into Maternal Deaths in the UK. All health professionals providing care for women during pregnancy and childbirth are encouraged to read the full report.

Royal College of Obstetricians and Gynaecologists (RCOG), 2005. Shoulder Dystocia Guideline No. 42. RCOG, London.

Royal College of Obstetricians and Gynaecologists (RCOG), 2008. Umbilical Cord Prolapse Guideline No. 50. London, RCOG.

These two RCOG guidelines are recommended reading for practitioners working within obstetrics.

Postpartum haemorrhage and other third-stage problems

Introduction

Once the baby has been born, delivery of the placenta and membranes may seem an anticlimax. However, the third (3rd) stage of labour is hazardous for the mother because of the risk of haemorrhage and other complications. The management of the 3rd stage should be aimed at minimising these possible serious complications but interfering as little as possible with the physiological process (discussed in Chapter 40) and the mother's enjoyment of her baby (Enkin et al 2000). A major role of the midwife is to explain the need for active interventions, such as the giving of an oxytocic drug or commencing an intravenous infusion, to the mothers, prior to labour so that women are enabled to make informed choices should the need suddenly arise.

Postpartum haemorrhage

Definition

Postpartum haemorrhage (PPH) is defined as excessive bleeding from the genital tract following the birth of the child. PPH occurs in the period extending from the time of birth to the end of the puerperium. If bleeding occurs in the first 24 h, it is called **primary PPH** (Mousa & Alfirevic 2007) and complicates about 6% of labours. If the bleeding occurs after the first 24 h and before the end of the 6th week, it is called **secondary PPH** (Alexander et al 2008), a much less common occurrence that complicates less than 1% of deliveries.

Postpartum haemorrhage is also classified according to the site of bleeding. Most commonly, the bleeding is from the placental site and there is poor tone of the uterine muscle. This is **atonic haemorrhage**. Bleeding may also be traumatic due to a laceration of the genital tract. In primary PPH, bleeding is said to be excessive if the amount exceeds 500 ml or is sufficient to cause deterioration in the woman's condition. Because of the diuresis and haemoconcentration that follow delivery, smaller amounts of blood loss are detrimental in secondary PPH.

Primary PPH is one of the most serious complications of labour that a midwife has to deal with until medical aid arrives. At term, maternal circulating blood flow to the uterus is 450–700 ml/min, where 80% is perfusion for the placenta and 20% is perfusion for the myometrium (Murray 2003). The blood loss may be rapid and devastating if the bleeding is not controlled. PPH is still a significant cause of maternal mortality, especially following a caesarean section (CS) (Lewis 2007). The most recent CEMACH Report stipulates that there were 14 maternal deaths related to obstetric haemorrhage and 9 of these were due to PPH (Lewis 2007). Measuring blood loss at delivery can be difficult. It is important to remember that blood soaks into sheets and towels and that it separates into clot and serum. Any clot placed in a jug and measured will only be 40% of the total loss so that it is easy to underestimate the total loss by up to 50%.

Primary postpartum haemorrhage from the placental site

Causes

Uterine atony, which is failure of the uterine muscle fibres to contract and retract to compress the blood vessels is the most common cause (Mousa & Alfirevic 2007). Risk factors are:

- A history of previous postpartum haemorrhage.
- High parity: para 3 or more.
- Overdistension of the uterus in multiple pregnancy, polyhydramnios and a large fetus.
- Fibroids may interfere with efficient contraction and retraction.
- Antepartum haemorrhage: the bleeding that occurs into the muscle during placental abruption will reduce the fibres' ability to contract and retract and in placenta praevia there is little contractile ability in the lower uterine segment.
- Prolonged labour with weak or uncoordinated contractions.
- Atony caused by drugs such as antihypertensives, general anaesthesia and tocolytics.
- Retained placenta.
- Anaemia because even a small amount of blood loss may precipitate shock.
- Inversion of the uterus.
- Mismanagement of the 3rd stage of labour by fiddling with the uterus.
- Coagulation defects: disseminated intravascular coagulation may complicate concealed placental abruption, amniotic fluid embolus, severe pre-eclampsia and eclampsia and intrauterine death.
- Medical disorders of clotting may also lead to primary PPH.

Despite the long list of risk factors outlined above, many cases of primary PPH occur in normal labours with no explanation.

Management of primary postpartum haemorrhage

In the antenatal period prevention is the best form of management and this begins with the booking interview. The following reports highlight the importance of good history taking and a crucial part of risk assessment: Maternal History Taking (NHS Quality Improvement Scotland 2004) and CEMACH 'Saving Mothers' Lives' (Lewis 2007). If any of the risk factors described above are present, the woman should be delivered in hospital so that if bleeding does occur then treatment is immediately available. As pregnancy progresses detection and treatment of anaemia is important (RCOG 2009) and it would be advantageous to raise the haemoglobin (Hb) level to at least 11 g/dl before delivery (Lindsay 2004).

In labour

Women at risk of PPH must be managed carefully to minimise the likelihood of bleeding. When labour commences an intravenous cannula (size 14 or 16 gauge) is inserted and blood is taken for a full blood count (FBC) and confirmation of blood group. Serum is saved for 'cross-matching' blood should it become necessary to give the woman a blood transfusion. Prolonged labour, with its problems of dehydration and exhaustion, should be avoided. A Syntocinon (oxytocin) infusion should be started if labour progress is slow. The woman's bladder should be kept empty by encouraging micturition or by catheterisation, as a full bladder may inhibit uterine muscle activity and add to the risk of atony.

Management of the 3rd stage should be discussed with the woman antenatally so that previous verbal consent can be given for any intervention, should it arise. She should be advised that the potential for PPH is greater with physiological management of the 3rd stage than it is with 'active management'. It should be explained to her that the medical view is that it is safer to manage the 3rd stage of labour actively. In active management, an intramuscular injection of Syntocinon 10 IU or Syntometrine 1 ml, which contains Syntocinon 5 units and ergometrine 500 μg, is given with the birth of the anterior shoulder. The placenta is then delivered by controlled cord traction. An intravenous or intramuscular injection of Syntometrine 1 ml or ergometrine 500 μg would be prescribed if the woman starts to bleed, depending on what had been administered previously.

One intervention advocated by the RCOG (2007) is prophylactic radiology. This process involves inserting an arterial balloon into the blood vessels causing occlusion and embolisation to prevent major blood loss. This intervention should be used in the event of a PPH if the cause is secondary to:

- Atonic uterus following normal or prolonged labour, with or without caesarean section.
- Surgical complications or uterine tears at the time of caesarean section.
- Bleeding continues on the postnatal ward or in the postoperative recovery area following a normal delivery or a caesarean section.
- Bleeding following a hysterectomy.

This process involves inserting a balloon into the vessels and occlusion or embolisation occurs to prevent blood loss.

Signs of postpartum haemorrhage

It would be difficult to miss the visible bleeding and maternal collapse that can occur. Other signs that may be present if blood loss is not visible (e.g. if clots are retained in an atonic uterus) are:

- Pallor.
- A rising pulse rate and falling blood pressure.
- Altered levels of consciousness.
- Air hunger.
- An enlarged 'boggy'-feeling uterus.

Management of primary postpartum haemorrhage: treatment

It is important that a midwife is familiar with the sequence of actions needed to deal with a PPH and to minimise the effects of blood loss.

If bleeding begins **before the placenta is delivered**, the following actions should be taken:

1. Ensure that medical aid is available.
2. Massage the fundus of the uterus firmly by a smooth circular motion to stimulate a uterine contraction, i.e. to 'rub up' a contraction. Bleeding indicates that the placenta has begun to separate and it is no longer necessary to await events.
3. Give an oxytocic drug. Intramuscular Syntometrine 1 ml will act to contract the uterus in 2.5 min and an intravenous injection of either Syntometrine 1 ml or ergometrine 500 μg will act in 45 s. Note that the midwife should not give more than two injections of ergometrine 500 μg as the drug may cause severe peripheral vasoconstriction and a sudden rise in blood pressure.
4. Pass a catheter into the bladder and ensure that it is completely empty.
5. Palpate to ensure the uterus is contracted, and then attempt to deliver the placenta by controlled cord traction.
6. If all else fails, the obstetrician should be asked to review. The obstetrician will try to deliver the placenta by cord traction. If this fails, the woman will need a manual removal of the placenta under spinal or epidural anaesthesia.

If the uterus is well contracted, the bleeding is likely to be from traumatic injury to the soft tissues. Locate the bleeding site and try to stem the bleeding using pressure.

If bleeding begins **after delivery of the placenta**, massage the uterus to obtain a contraction and expel any blood clots remaining in the uterus. An injection of an oxytocic drug, either intramuscular Syntometrine 1 ml or ergometrine 500 μg, should then stop bleeding by achieving a sustained contraction. Ensure that the urinary bladder is empty. If bleeding continues, it is necessary to carry out bimanual compression of the uterus. Following delivery of the placenta and membranes, they should be examined for completeness. If the placenta appears incomplete, the doctor will carry out an exploration and evacuation of the uterus under spinal or epidural anaesthesia.

Bimanual compression of the uterus

Bimanual compression may be performed externally or internally. In **external bimanual compression**, one hand is dipped down as far as possible behind the uterus while the other is placed flat on the abdomen. The uterus is compressed between the two hands and pulled upwards in the abdomen. This ensures that the bleeding area of the placental site is compressed while the uterine veins are straightened out to allow free drainage, relieve congestion and decrease the bleeding (Lindsay 2004).

Internal bimanual compression is carried out if the mother is anaesthetised and still bleeding after manual removal of placenta. One hand is closed to form a fist, inserted into the anterior vaginal fornix and pushed up towards the body of the uterus. The other hand is placed on the abdominal wall behind the uterus and compresses the uterus downwards against the hand in the vagina. This applies compression to the placental site until the uterus is felt to contract (Fig. 45.1).

Once bleeding is controlled, an intravenous infusion containing Syntocinon (oxytocin) is started to maintain uterine contraction. If blood loss is excessive or if the woman had a low haemoglobin level before delivery, a blood transfusion may be necessary. There are approximately 4000 cases of obstetric haemorrhage a year. The majority will require a blood transfusion (RCOG 2009). Therefore it is important not to underestimate the amount of blood lost. Brant (1967) found

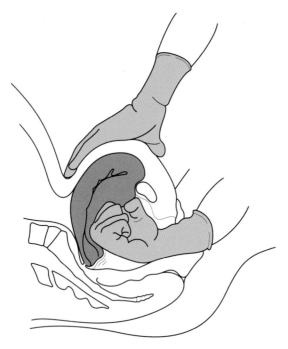

Figure 45.1 • Internal bimanual compression of the uterus. (From Henderson C, Macdonald S 2004, with kind permission of Elsevier.)

that estimates of blood loss became more inaccurate as the amount lost increased. In the case of serious PPH, the obstetrician and anaesthetist will agree on the management of fluid replacement. It is recommended that each obstetric unit should have a protocol on managing PPH, which should be followed and 'fire-drill' scenarios conducted to train and update practitioners on the protocol (RCOG 2009). Group O rhesus-negative blood should be available on the labour ward for use in emergencies. Where large volumes of blood are to be transfused, blood-warming coils should be used. Appropriate personnel must be included and there should be early involvement of consultant obstetrician, anaesthetist, haematologist and blood bank (RCOG 2005).

If the uterus fails to contract even though oxytocic drugs have been used, a deep intramuscular injection of the prostanoid carboprost, which is 15-methyl-PGF$_{2\alpha}$ (Rang et al 2007), can be given in a dose of 250 µg and repeated at intervals of 1.5 h. Carboprost is contraindicated in women with cardiac, renal, pulmonary and hepatic disease as well as in acute pelvic inflammation. It should be used with care in women who have asthma, hypertension, diabetes, epilepsy, hypotension or hypertension (BNF 2008). Different maternity units, according to their guidelines, may use different methods for controlling bleeding. In continuing haemorrhage, internal iliac artery ligation and uterine packing may be needed and, if all fails, a hysterectomy may be performed to save the woman's life. A systematic review by Mousa & Alfirevic (2007) argues that there is not enough robust evidence

in which to alter the present treatment of primary PPH, which is the combined use of oxytocin and ergometrine with misoprostol. Further controlled trials are required to assess the effectiveness and safety of pharmacological, interventional radiology and surgical interventions used for the treatment of PPH (Mousa & Alfirevic 2007).

Observations

Once blood loss is controlled, the total loss is estimated remembering how difficult this can be and that estimates become less accurate as blood loss increases. Fluid intake is recorded, as is the hourly urine output. Central venous pressure measurement may be required, depending on the blood loss and the severity of the woman's condition, which may require correct fluid replacement. Maternal pulse and blood pressure are recorded every 15 min to ensure her condition remains satisfactory. The uterine fundus is palpated frequently to ensure it remains contracted and the lochia are observed. All findings can be recorded using a modified early warning system (e.g. MEWS).

If the problem involves failure of blood coagulation, a haematologist should be involved. Fresh blood is usually the best treatment as it contains both platelets and coagulation factors but fresh frozen plasma, containing factors V and VIII and fibrinogen, can be used. This is guided by the results from the blood coagulation screen (RCOG 2007).

Traumatic postpartum haemorrhage

If the blood loss is from a laceration of the genital tract, bleeding should be stopped by direct pressure if possible and then sutured. Bleeding from a cervical or lower uterine tear should be suspected if the uterus is well contracted, no superficial bleeding can be seen and the blood loss is slow and steady. Tears of the upper part of the vagina, the cervix and lower uterine segment should be sutured under spinal or epidural anaesthesia. If severe bleeding is from the uterus and cannot be stopped, a hysterectomy may be necessary to save the woman's life.

Secondary postpartum haemorrhage

Secondary PPH is any abnormal bleeding or excessive bleeding from the birth canal occurring 24 h and 12 weeks postnatally (Alexander et al 2002). This is a complication of the puerperium and is most often seen between days 4 and 14. It is usually due to a retained piece of placenta but other causes include the presence of blood clot or a fibroid in the uterine wall. Secondary PPH is also commonly associated with infection. There may have been warning signs of heavy, red, offensive lochia and subinvolution. If infection is present, pyrexia and tachycardia may be present.

Management

If the uterus is palpable it is massaged to make it contract. Any clots are expelled and the bladder must be emptied. If bleeding is slight it may be managed at home with antibiotics and oral ergometrine tablets.

If bleeding is severe, an intravenous injection of ergometrine 500 μg or intramuscular Syntometrine 1 ml is given. If the woman is at home she should be transferred to hospital once her condition is under control. A blood transfusion may be given, depending on the blood loss and the antenatal Hb. The uterus is evacuated under spinal or epidural anaesthesia. However, currently there is no robust evidence from randomised controlled trials to inform practice (Alexander et al 2002). Alexander et al (2002) recommend that further robust randomised controlled trials are conducted to explore the different therapies for secondary PPH.

Complications of postpartum haemorrhage

Unless adequately treated, the woman is likely to develop **chronic iron-deficiency anaemia**. Infection is more common and lactation may be poor. If shock develops, acute renal tubular necrosis may present with anuria. Anterior pituitary necrosis leading to Sheehan's syndrome may occur if the haemorrhage was severe. All women who have suffered a postpartum haemorrhage should be advised to book into hospital for any subsequent deliveries.

Haematoma formation

Postpartum haemorrhage may be concealed if progressive haematoma formation occurs in the perineum or lower vagina. A site of haematoma formation more difficult to diagnose is bleeding into the broad ligament. Up to 1 litre of blood may collect in the tissues, leading to increasing maternal pain due to pressure. The mother may collapse with signs of shock.

Management

The woman will have to be taken to theatre so that the haematoma can be drained and haemostasis achieved under spinal or general anaesthetic. Replacement of the lost blood may be necessary. Infection is a risk and antibiotics are usually prescribed.

Prolonged third stage

Failure of the placenta to deliver spontaneously remains an important cause of postpartum haemorrhage (Lewis 2007). If labour is managed actively, the placenta and membranes should be delivered within 10 min.

If the placenta is not delivered within 30 min, the 3rd stage is considered to be prolonged. With physiological management of the 3rd stage, up to 1 h may be allowed before considering the procedure to be prolonged. The placenta may be separated but retained, trapped behind the reforming cervix, and bleeding is likely. Alternatively, the placenta may be morbidly adherent to the uterine wall and, if there is no separation, bleeding will not occur.

Causes

- Uterine inertia.
- Full bladder.
- Mismanagement of the 3rd stage where 'fiddling' with the fundus causes irregular contractions and partial separation of the placenta.
- The formation of a constriction ring or spasm between the upper and lower uterine segments.
- A uterine abnormality such as bicornuate uterus.
- Morbid adherence of the placenta, more likely to occur in women who have had a previous CS or placenta praevia.

Types of adherent placenta

1. **Placenta accreta**, where the decidua basalis is deficient and the chorionic villi have attached to the myometrium.

2. **Placenta increta**, where the villi penetrate deeply into the myometrium.

3. **Placenta percreta**, where the villi have penetrated to the serous external coat of the uterus.

Management

As long as the placenta remains in the uterus, haemorrhage is a threat. If there is no success in delivering the placenta after emptying the bladder, manual removal of the placenta by the obstetrician will be necessary (Fig. 45.2). The procedure may cause shock if conducted without adequate anaesthesia.

The obstetrician has two choices in deeply adherent placentae. A CS can be performed or the placenta can be left in situ to be reabsorbed. The drug methotrexate has been used to hasten the absorption of the placental tissue but is not always successful (Lindsay 2004). An intravenous oxytocic injection is given following successful manual removal followed by an intravenous infusion of Syntocinon (oxytocin). Different hospitals have different protocols for the amount of Syntocinon to be used after manual removal of placenta. Prophylactic antibiotic therapy is commenced, as manual removal of placenta may have introduced organisms into the uterus.

Acute inversion of the uterus

In this rare condition, which occurs in about 1 in 100 000 deliveries, the uterus is partly or completely turned inside out (Fig. 45.3). In **partial inversion**, the inner surface of the fundus is drawn down into the uterine cavity; in **severe inversion**, the inside of the fundus protrudes through the cervix into the vagina. If the uterus is fully turned inside out, it may appear outside the vulva. Profound neurogenic shock due to traction

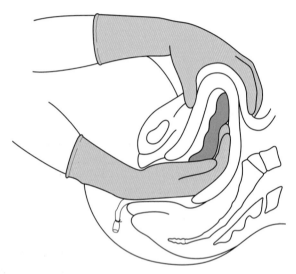

Figure 45.2 ● Manual removal of the placenta. (From Henderson C, Macdonald S 2004, with kind permission of Elsevier.)

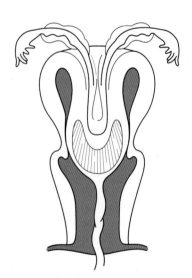

Figure 45.3 ● Inversion of the uterus. (From Henderson C, Macdonald S 2004, with kind permission of Elsevier.)

on the uterine supportive ligaments is likely to occur. There will be pain and possibly haemorrhage if there is partial placental separation.

Causes

*   Mismanagement of the 3rd stage by applying fundal pressure or cord traction with the uterus relaxed.
*   A short cord, where the fundus descends with the fetus.
*   Manual removal of placenta if the operator withdraws the hand in the uterus while still applying fundal pressure.
*   Spontaneous inversion, possibly due to straining, which raises intra-abdominal pressure, such as a sudden cough or sneeze.

Diagnosis and management

The woman will complain of pain and may collapse suddenly. Cardiac arrest may occur. On palpation of the uterus, it will be difficult to find the fundus of the uterus. A distinct hollow in the fundus may be felt. The woman may complain of a feeling that something is in her vagina.

The rapid replacement of the uterus will prevent the development of shock. Replacement is easier if it is carried out immediately, before uterine congestion and oedema develop. Pressure is applied first to the part of the lower segment nearest the cervix, gently proceeding upwards towards the fundus. If replacement is not possible, the uterus should be replaced in the vagina and the foot of the bed elevated to reduce traction on the uterine ligaments, fallopian tubes and ovaries. An injection of morphine 15 mg will reduce pain. If the placenta is still attached to the uterine wall, it should not be removed.

Methods of replacement

If there has been delay, the woman is anaesthetised and the uterus replaced manually, as described above, by pressure in the fornices to replace the lower segment, which was last to invert, and the fundus last. If a retraction ring has developed between the upper and lower uterine segments, the replacement may be difficult. Inhalation of amyl nitrite vapour or a deep general anaesthetic may be needed to relax the uterine muscle.

O'Sullivan's hydrostatic method is preferred by some obstetricians. Two to three litres of warm normal saline are infused via a douche nozzle into the vagina while the introitus is sealed around the forearm by the other hand (Lindsay 2004). The fluid container is held about 1 m above the level of the uterus with the woman in the lithotomy position. The pressure of the liquid distends the vagina and the uterus replaces itself quite quickly. Following replacement, an intravenous injection of ergometrine 500μg will ensure it remains in its correct position. The placenta may now be removed if necessary.

Amniotic fluid embolism

This obstetric emergency occurs when amniotic fluid is forced from the uterine venous sinuses of the placental bed into the maternal circulation. It usually follows uterine hyperactivity but may also occur near to term, before labour begins or in the 3rd stage as a result of a tear in the lower uterine segment. The embolus travels around the systemic circulation, through the heart and into the pulmonary circulation to obstruct pulmonary arterioles or alveolar capillaries. This causes sudden maternal collapse and respiratory and cardiac arrest.

Risk factors

Amniotic embolism is more likely to occur in women where intra-amniotic pressures are raised:

- Hypertonic uterine action, spontaneous or induced by oxytocic drugs.
- Older multiparous women with rapid labours.
- Multiple pregnancy.
- Polyhydramnios.
- Uterine trauma such as CS, ruptured uterus, internal podalic version or manual removal of placenta.

Clinical signs and symptoms

The diagnosis can only be made with certainty if amniotic fluid is detected in the maternal circulation and often this is post mortem when fetal desquamated skin and lanugo are also found in the lungs. There is usually sudden onset of **maternal respiratory distress** with cyanosis, chest pain, dyspnoea, blood-stained frothy sputum and collapse. **Cardiovascular collapse** soon follows with tachycardia and hypotension. Amniotic fluid is rich in thromboplastins and its release into the blood may cause **disseminated intravascular coagulation** (DIC) and coagulation failure (Davies & Harrison 1992). DIC is most likely to occur within 30 min of the initial collapse (Shiers & Coates 2003).

Management

This is an obstetric emergency. The uterus must be emptied as quickly as possible and a CS performed if necessary. Unfortunately, this rare complication often results in the death of the woman and her baby despite active treatment. Oxygen is given by face mask and cardiopulmonary resuscitation commenced if the woman collapses. Intravenous aminophylline may help relieve bronchospasm and hydrocortisone will relieve the inflammatory effect of amniotic fluid on lung tissue. An attempt is made to reverse the DIC and control haemorrhage should they occur. If the woman survives there may be **renal failure** and dialysis may be necessary if the kidneys do not respond to diuretic drugs such as mannitol.

Shock in obstetrics

McCance & Huether (2001) define shock as being a condition in which the cardiovascular system fails to perfuse the tissues adequately, resulting in widespread impairment of cellular metabolism. Three functions of the cardiovascular system may be altered and result in shock. If the heart is thought of as a pump, these can be summarised as:

1. **Heart function**: loss of the pump.
2. **Blood volume**: nothing to pump.
3. **Blood pressure**: no force in the pump.

   Shock from any condition will inevitably cause progress to organ failure and death unless some compensatory mechanisms occur to reverse the situation or clinical treatments are successful.

If shock remains untreated, the body's compensatory mechanisms are overwhelmed and a downward spiral towards death will occur. The compensatory mechanisms function to maintain blood pressure and blood flow to vital organs such as the brain and the heart (Marieb & Hoehn 2008).

Recognition of shock

Because the body has many systems, all involving cells at the microscopic level, shock presents with many signs and symptoms. Tissue damage is diverse and subjective symptoms can be vague. A person may report nausea, weakness, feeling cold or hot, dizziness, confusion, fear and anxiety, thirst and shortage of breath with air hunger. Clinical measurements will find pulse and respiration rate increased, blood pressure and cardiac output decreased, diminished urinary output, cold, clammy skin, pallor and reduced core temperature.

Classification of shock

There are various ways of classifying shock: for example, by pathophysiological processes, by clinical manifestations or by cause. Classification by cause is the

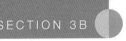

most useful as it will also indicate the likely patho-physiology underlying the shock and highlight the disorder that will need treating to reverse the shock (Tables 45.1, 45.2). The three main cardiovascular functions that are impaired are obvious. All of the following types of shock may occur in childbearing women and will first be described in detail. Possible causes of obstetric shock will then be discussed. The danger is that the compensatory mechanisms may mask the signs of shock until maternal and fetal lives are at risk.

Cardiogenic shock

Heart failure is the cause of cardiogenic shock and most cases are due to myocardial infarction. Shock may also occur in congestive cardiac failure, myocardial ischaemia and drug toxicity. It is not very responsive to treatment and often leads to death.

Table 45.1 Types of shock and their immediate cause

Type	Cause
Cardiogenic	Heart failure
Hypovolaemic	Reduced blood volume
Neurogenic	Neural alterations of smooth muscle tone resulting in vasodilation
Anaphylactic	Immune system pathology resulting in vasodilation
Septic	Resulting in cardiac depression and dilatation with vasodilation

Compensatory sequence of events

- As cardiac output begins to decrease, renin produced by the kidneys stimulates aldosterone release so that sodium and water are retained.
- Hypothalamic responses cause catecholamine release from the adrenal glands, resulting in vasoconstriction to maintain blood pressure.
- Cardiac performance is enhanced but there is increased demand for oxygen and nutrients.
- Tissue perfusion begins to fall and nutrient and oxygen delivery to the cells decreases.
- Cellular metabolism is impaired and signs of shock appear.

Hypovolaemic shock

Hypovolaemic shock with inadequate blood volume is the most common form. Shock begins to develop when intravascular volume is decreased by 15%. The first sign is a thready pulse as intense vasoconstriction attempts to move blood from the periphery to supply the vital organs. A sharp decline in blood pressure is a late and serious sign (Marieb & Hoehn 2008). It may occur because of:

- Loss of whole blood in haemorrhage.
- Loss of plasma as in burns.
- Loss of interstitial fluid.
- Diabetes mellitus.
- Excessive vomiting or diarrhoea.

Compensatory sequence of events

- Adrenals release catecholamines, which increase heart rate and systemic vascular resistance (SVR).
- Interstitial fluid moves into the vascular compartment.

Table 45.2 Pathophysiological causes of shock in childbearing

Cardiogenic shock	Hypovolaemic shock	Neurogenic shock	Anaphylactic shock	Septic shock
Pulmonary embolism	Haemorrhage associated with childbearing	Acute inversion of the uterus	Adverse drug reactions	Infection in septic abortion and puerperal infection
Severe anaemia	Ruptured ectopic pregnancy	Aspiration of acid gastric contents (Mendelson's syndrome)		
Cardiac disorders such as valvular or congenital problems	Ruptured uterus	Intrauterine manipulations without adequate anaesthesia		
Severe hypertension	Coagulopathy hypertension following amniotic fluid embolism Diabetic crisis			

- The liver and spleen disgorge stored red blood cells and plasma into the circulation.
- Renin produced by the kidneys stimulates aldosterone release and sodium and water are retained.
- Tissue perfusion begins to fall and nutrient and oxygen delivery to the cells decreases.
- Cellular metabolism is impaired and signs of shock appear.

Management of hypovolaemic shock

The crucial factor is to restore circulating blood volume. It is an obstetric emergency and requires immediate resuscitative measures (Dougherty & Lister 2004, Lindsay 2004, Shiers & Coates 2003):

1. Summon help as time is of the essence. If hypovalaemic shock is not acted on promptly it can lead to maternal death. Appropriate staff would be senior midwifery staff, obstetrician and anaesthetist.

2. Reassure the woman and her partner/birthing partner of what is happening.

3. Remember the important concepts of ABC—airway, breathing and circulation.

4. Maintain or secure an airway. Intubation may be necessary if the woman is collapsed.
   - Oxygen via a Hudson mask (15 L/min).
   - Cannulate with two large-bore venflons (gauge 14 or 16) and commence an intravenous infusion using crystalloid or normal saline solution.
   - Laboratory blood tests:
     - Blood type (group and cross-match).
     - Full blood count.
     - Coagulation screen.
   - Prepare for blood transfusion (uncross-matched O negative or ABO cross-matched).

5. Assess maternal condition (when woman is stable move to a high-dependency environment).
   - Observations: blood pressure, pulse, SaO_2 and temperature.
   - BP, pulse and SaO_2 recorded every 5 min.
   - Document findings on acute care or MEWS chart.

6. Assess and stop cause of haemorrhage.

Neurogenic shock

Another name for neurogenic shock is **vasogenic shock**, referring to the massive vasodilation that results because of a loss of balance between the sympathetic and parasympathetic stimulation of vascular smooth muscle.

Although blood volume does not change, the vascular compartment is increased drastically, resulting in relative hypovolaemia with a decrease in SVR. Vascular resistance is normally maintained by the sympathetic stimulus and if this is interrupted or inhibited for any length of time, neurogenic shock will follow. It may occur because of:

- Trauma to the spinal cord.
- Cerebral hypoxia.
- Medullary hypoglycaemia.
- Anaesthetics and other depressive drugs.
- Pain and severe emotional distress.

Compensatory sequence of events

- An increase in sympathetic activity will correct the bradycardia and very low SVR.
- Fainting ensures that the person is prevented from maintaining an upright posture so that blood pressure is equalised from head to toe and cerebral blood supply is maximised.

Anaphylactic shock

Anaphylactic shock results from a widespread hypersensitivity reaction. The pathophysiology is similar to that of neurogenic shock, with widespread vasodilation and pooling of blood in the periphery. This type of shock is very serious because it involves multiple body systems. It begins as an allergic reaction with an immune and inflammatory response to a proteinaceous substance such as insect venom, pollen, shellfish, penicillin or foreign serum. The vascular component of this response includes vasodilation and increased vascular permeability so that the relative hypovolaemia brought about by peripheral pooling is exacerbated by tissue oedema. There is bronchoconstriction so that the ability to provide oxygen to the tissues is severely compromised.

The onset of anaphylactic shock is rapid and can progress to death in minutes unless emergency treatment is available. The effects to a few people of ingesting peanuts have been widely reported in the press and illustrate the condition well. The signs are anxiety, difficulty in breathing, gastrointestinal cramps, oedema and urticaria with severe itching and burning sensations in the skin (McCance & Huether 2001). A steep fall in blood pressure follows with confusion and coma.

Emergency management

There is little time for spontaneous compensatory mechanisms and the person may die unless medical intervention is possible:

- Adrenaline (epinephrine) injection will reverse airway constriction and cause vasoconstriction.

- Volume expanders intravenously will reverse the relative hypovolaemia.
- Steroids will end the inflammatory process.

Septic shock

Septic shock is a very complex process and the explanations for its progress are still being investigated. Gram-negative bacteria cause more than half the cases and in the non-pregnant population the most common sources of infection are the respiratory tract and the gastrointestinal tract. Infections of the genital tract are of prime importance in the childbearing woman.

Septic shock is triggered by bacteraemia and bacteria may be present in the blood for quite a long time before shock develops. It is most likely to be the elderly, critically ill or immunocompromised who develop bacteraemic shock. An example could be related to a women becoming severely ill following insertion of an intrauterine contraceptive device. Uterine infection was followed by generalised infection and bacteraemia.

Four major body chemicals have been implicated in the development of bacteraemic shock (McCance & Huether 2001):

1. **Interleukins (ILs)** are cytokines produced by the white blood cells and cause vasodilation and increase vascular permeability. They also influence the hypothalamus to cause fever, initiate the complement cascade and stimulate the release of TNF.

2. **Tumour necrosis factor (TNF)** is a cytokine produced by macrophages, natural killer cells and mast cells. It activates both clotting and complement cascades. In addition, TNF causes vasodilation and increases vascular permeability.

3. **Platelet-activating factor (PAF)** is released from mononuclear phagocytes, platelets and some endothelial cells in response to the presence of an endotoxin. It is directly toxic to multiple organs and causes vasodilation and increased vascular permeability. PAF also mobilises white cells, activates platelets and stimulates the release of TNF.

4. **Myocardial depressant substance (MDS)** is secreted by white blood cells in response to an endotoxin. The heart responds to MDS by becoming depressed and dilated, which results in pump failure and hypotension.

As shock increases, carbohydrate metabolism is altered, with a serum increase in both insulin and glucagon. Serum glucose levels fluctuate and glucose usage by the tissues is enhanced. Glucose and glycogen stores become depleted. Depletion of glucose leads to heart failure and oxygen shortage and **multiple organ dysfunction syndrome (MODS)** may develop.

Multiple organ dysfunction syndrome

MODS is present if there is failure of two or more organ systems after severe illness or injury (Fig. 45.4). Sepsis and septic shock are the most common precipitating causes. Mortality is high and it is the most common cause of death following sepsis, trauma and burns. The following processes occur:

- Release of the stress hormones cortisol, adrenaline (epinephrine), noradrenaline (norepinephrine) and endorphins.
- Stimulation of the sympathetic nervous system.
- Vascular endothelial damage by endotoxins or inflammatory substances.
- Interstitial oedema.
- Disseminated intravascular coagulation with microvascular thrombi and capillary obstruction.
- Hyperdynamic circulation with increased venous return.

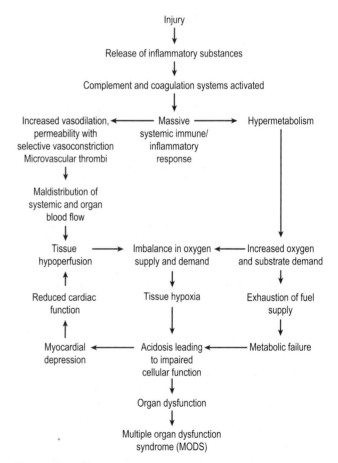

Figure 45.4 • The pathogenesis of multiple organ dysfunction. (Reproduced with permission from McCance & Huether 1994.)

- Hypermetabolism with elevated carbohydrate, lipid and protein breakdown to provide energy, leading to weight loss.

Failure of the lungs develops first with adult respiratory distress syndrome (ARDS). If this occurs, there is a mortality of over 80% (Pearlman & Tintinalli 1998). Renal and liver failure follow and there is gastrointestinal and immune system failure. Cardiovascular collapse with myocardial depression of function causes the death of the patient after about 3 weeks if treatment is unsuccessful. The normal supply of oxygen to the tissues is based on need and is met by alterations in blood flow distribution. This system fails and oxygen supply depends only on how much the circulation is able to deliver. This is known as **supply-dependent oxygen consumption**.

Outline of the management of MODS

The reader is referred to McCance & Huether (2001) for a fuller description of the management of MODS. Briefly, early recognition is extremely important followed by treatment of the precipitating cause: for example, removing the source of infection. Restoration of tissue oxygenation and nutrition is very important. Individual organs such as the kidney may need supporting through the crisis.

Shock in childbearing

The above causes of shock can all be related to specific emergencies arising in childbearing; a summary is presented in Tables 45.1 and 45.2.

Main points

- In primary postpartum haemorrhage (PPH), the bleeding may be from the placental site but may occasionally be due to a laceration of the genital tract. Risk factors include previous PPH, high parity, overdistension of the uterus, fibroids, retained products of conception, inverted uterus, 3rd stage mismanagement and coagulation defects. If any of the risk factors are present, the woman should be delivered in hospital. Physiological management of the 3rd stage is considered unsafe.

- If bleeding commences before the placenta is delivered, the uterus is massaged to encourage contractions, an oxytocic drug is given and an attempt to deliver the placenta is made. A manual removal of placenta under anaesthesia will be necessary if the placenta cannot be delivered by controlled cord traction. If bleeding begins after delivery of the placenta, the uterus is massaged to obtain a contraction and expel any blood clots remaining in the uterus. An injection of an oxytocic drug should sustain contractions and stop bleeding.

- If the placenta is incomplete, evacuation of the uterus under spinal or general anaesthesia will be carried out. Once bleeding is controlled, an intravenous infusion containing oxytocin is commenced to maintain uterine contraction. Blood transfusion and fluid replacement may be required if bleeding is excessive. Prophylactic antibiotics will be prescribed following any operative intervention. If severe bleeding is from a tear in the uterus and bleeding cannot be controlled, a hysterectomy will save the woman's life.

- Secondary PPH is usually due to a retained piece of placenta or membrane. Other causes include the presence of blood clots, a fibroid or infection. If the uterus is palpable it is massaged until it contracts, clots are expelled and the bladder emptied. An intravenous

- injection of an oxytocic drug is given if bleeding is severe followed by evacuation of the uterus.

- Bleeding in the puerperium should always be reported to the obstetrician. Inadequate treatment may lead to iron-deficiency anaemia, acute renal tubular necrosis or anterior pituitary necrosis and Sheehan's syndrome.

- Failure of the placenta to deliver spontaneously is one of the main causes of PPH. The placenta may be separated but retained, when bleeding is likely, or morbidly adherent to the uterine wall and bleeding will not occur. Manual removal may be necessary. In deeply adherent placentae, a CS can be performed.

- Causes of acute inversion of the uterus include mismanagement of the 3rd stage but spontaneous inversion does occur. Rapid replacement of the uterus will prevent shock.

- An amniotic fluid embolus travels into the pulmonary circulation to obstruct pulmonary arterioles or capillaries. It is more likely to occur where intra-amniotic pressures are raised and in uterine trauma. Sudden onset of maternal respiratory distress is followed by cardiovascular collapse and possibly disseminated intravascular coagulation (DIC). Oxygen is given and cardiopulmonary resuscitation commenced if needed. Intravenous fluids are administered. Mortality is high and renal failure may be a complication.

- Three functions of the cardiovascular system may be altered and result in shock: heart function, blood volume and blood pressure. Shock progresses to organ failure and death unless compensatory mechanisms or clinical treatments can reverse the pathology.

- Classification of shock by cause is the most useful as it will also indicate the likely pathophysiology and highlight the underlying disorder that will need treating. Types of shock are cardiogenic, hypovolaemic, neurogenic, anaphylactic and septic.

References

Alexander, J., Thomas, P.W., Sanghera, J., 2008. Treatments for secondary postpartum haemorrhage. Cochrane Database Syst. Rev. (1) 2008, Art. No.: CD002867. DOI: 10.1002/14651858. CD002867.

BNF (British National Formulary), September 2008. Number 56, British Medical Association and Royal Pharmaceutical Society of Great Britain, London.

Brant, H., 1967. Precise estimation of postpartum haemorrhage: difficulties and importance. Br. Med. J. 1, 389–400.

Davies, M., Harrison, J., 1992. Amniotic fluid embolism: maternal mortality revisited. Br. J. Hosp. Med. 14 (10), 775–776.

Dougherty, L., Lister, S. (Eds.), 2004. The Royal Marsden Hospital Manual of Clinical Nursing Procedures, sixth edn. Blackwell Publishing, Oxford.

Enkin, M., Keirse, J., Neilson, J., et al., 2000. A Guide to Effective Care in Pregnancy and Childbirth, third edn. Oxford University Press, Oxford.

Lewis, G. (Ed.), 2007. Saving Mothers' Lives: The Seventh Report of the Confidential Enquiries into Maternal and Child Health Report. RCOG, London.

Lindsay, P., 2004. Complications of the third stage of labour. In: Henderson, C., Macdonald, S. (Eds.), Mayes' Midwifery: A Textbook for Midwifery, thirteenth edn. Baillière Tindall, London.

McCance, K.L., Huether, S.E. (Eds.), 2001. Pathophysiology: The Biologic Basis for Disease in Adults and Children, fourth edn. Mosby, St Louis.

Marieb, E.N., Hoehn, K., 2008. Anatomy & Physiology, third edn. Pearson/Benjamin Cummings, New York.

Mousa, H.A., Alfirevic, Z., 2007. Treatment for primary postpartum haemorrhage. Cochrane Database Syst. Rev. (1) Update Software 2008, Oxford.

NHS Quality Improvement Scotland (NHS QIS), 2004. Maternal History Taking. Best Practice Statement. NHS QIS, Edinburgh.

Pearlman, M.D., Tintinalli, J.E. (Eds.), 1998. Emergency Care of the Woman. McGraw-Hill, New York.

Rang, H.P., Dale, M.M., Ritter, J.M. (Eds.), et al., 2007. Pharmacology, sixth edn. Churchill Livingstone, Edinburgh.

RCOG (Royal College of Obstetricians and Gynaecologists), 2005. Blood Transfusion in Obstetrics. Guideline No. 47. RCOG, London.

RCOG (Royal College of Obstetricians and Gynaecologists), 2007. The Role of Emergency and Elective Interventional Radiology in Postpartum Haemorrhage, Good Practice No. 6. RCOG, London.

RCOG (Royal College of Obstetricians and Gynaecologists), 2009. Prevention and Management of Postpartum haemorrhage. Green Top Guideline No. 52. RCOG, London.

Shiers, C., Coates, T., 2003. Midwifery and obstetric emergencies. In: Fraser, D.M., Cooper, M.A. (Eds.) Myles Textbook for Midwives, fourteenth edn. Churchill Livingstone, Edinburgh.

Annotated recommended reading

Lewis, G. (Ed.), 2007. Saving Mothers' Lives: The Seventh Report of the Confidential Enquiries into Maternal and Child Health Report. RCOG, London.

This report is produced from the confidential enquiries into maternal deaths taking place between 2003 and 2005. The report discusses individual cases in detail and provides a section for midwives to facilitate the safe outcome of pregnancy for all women. All midwives are encouraged to read either the midwives summary or the full report.

Royal College of Obstetricians and Gynaecologists (RCOG) (2005). Blood Transfusion in Obstetrics. Guideline No. 47. RCOG, London.

This guideline is recommended reading for practitioners working within obstetrics. It provides valuable information about using blood transfusions in obstetrics.

Chapter Forty-Six

46

Perinatal fetal asphyxia

Introduction

It has been known for centuries that labour can be dangerous for the fetus. Uterine contractions interfere with umbilical and uteroplacental blood flow and affect fetal gas exchange. The result is a normal tendency to mild metabolic acidosis in the active phase of the first stage and in the early second stage of labour. At the end of the second stage of labour there may be transient respiratory acidosis (Agrawal et al 2004).

Definitions

- **Fetal distress** is a general purpose term to indicate the fetus is in jeopardy, sometimes but not always because of hypoxia.
- **Acidosis** is an increased concentration of hydrogen ions (H^+) in blood and at the cellular level, resulting from an accumulation of acid or loss of base with a blood pH of less than 7.2.
- **Hypoxia** is a decreased concentration of oxygen in blood (hypoxaemia) and at the cellular level.
- **Hypercapnia (hypercarbia)** is an increased concentration of carbon dioxide in blood and at the cellular level.
- **Asphyxia**, from the Greek word 'pulseless', is a severe abnormality of gas exchange which results in hypoxia, hypercapnia and acidosis. Asphyxia is characterised by profound acidaemia that is both metabolic and respiratory in nature (Blackburn 2007). The term **fetal asphyxia** is preferred to that of **fetal distress**, which refers to a state of fetal danger that may or may not be caused by asphyxia.

Fetal gas exchange and pH regulation

The bicarbonate buffer system which regulates fetal acid–base balance is not as efficient as in the neonate because of a decreased ability to eliminate carbon dioxide (CO_2). As carbon dioxide cannot be expelled by the fetus into the air, it must be eliminated as molecular CO_2 via the placenta to be removed by the maternal respiratory system.

Respiratory acidosis

In the placenta there is a gradient between maternal and fetal circulations down which fetal CO_2 can diffuse. Fetal scalp blood Pco_2 is about 38–44 mmHg and maternal blood Pco_2 is 18–24 mmHg. In most cases interference with fetal gas exchange involves a problem of elimination of CO_2, resulting in respiratory acidosis. An excessive rise in fetal Pco_2 causes fetal H^+ ions to be released from the unstable carbonic acid (H_2CO_3), which lowers fetal blood pH (acidosis). The buffering bicarbonate ions, which are also released, are insufficient to correct the acidosis. The full equation is:

$$CO_2 + H_2O \rightleftharpoons H_2CO_3 \rightleftharpoons H^+ + HCO_3^- \quad (46.1)$$

Metabolic acidosis

Decreased oxygen transfer to the fetus will also cause acidosis. Oxygen deficiency causes cells to switch to anaerobic respiration, with the release of lactic acid and H^+ ions into the blood. If hypoxia persists, the excess H^+ ions cause CO_2 and water (H_2O) to be released from the buffer bicarbonate to add respiratory acidosis to the metabolic acidosis. Water is transferred across the placenta to the maternal circulation but there is a delay in removing the CO_2. Anaerobic respiration is inefficient and utilises more energy, resulting in a decrease in glucose.

Intrauterine hypoxia

Oxygenation of the fetus depends on maternal oxygenation, perfusion of the placental site, the fetoplacental circulation and adequate fetal haemoglobin (Blackburn 2007). Disruption or impairment to the flow of oxygen from the air to the fetus will result in fetal hypoxia.

Possible causes of intrauterine hypoxia

- Oxygenation of the mother may be impaired by respiratory or cardiovascular disease.
- Perfusion of the placental site may be reduced in:
  - Hypertension because of vasoconstriction.
  - Hypotension due to blood loss.
  - Aortocaval occlusion.
  - Shock.
  - Excessive uterine contractions.
- Prolapse, compression or a true knot in the umbilical cord may cause fetal hypoxia.
- Placental disease.

- There may be a reduction in fetal red cells caused by haemolysis.

Fetal response to hypoxia

The fetal response to hypoxia is an acceleration of heart rate to maintain oxygen supply to the brain and delivery of excess CO_2 to the placenta. As glycogen reserves become depleted, the increased supply of glucose demanded by the heart muscle because of the **tachycardia** cannot be met and the heart slows (**bradycardia**). The anal sphincter relaxes and fresh meconium is passed into the amniotic fluid. Hypoxia may stimulate the fetus to make gasping movements and meconium may be inhaled.

Physiological control of the fetal heart

The cardiac regulatory centre is situated in the medulla oblongata. Baroreceptors found in the arch of the aorta and carotid sinus are responsive to changes in blood pressure, and chemoreceptors in the same blood vessels respond to changes in blood gas tensions (Blackburn 2007). These receptors send messages to the cardiac regulatory centre, which in turn sends messages via the sympathetic and parasympathetic nervous systems to the heart. Sympathetic stimulation via the sinoatrial node will increase the heart rate whereas parasympathetic stimulation via the vagus nerve will decrease the heart rate. The continuous interaction between these two branches of the autonomic system causes small fluctuations in heart rate which lead to variability on heart rate tracings.

Monitoring the fetus in labour

The fetal response to labour may be monitored clinically by observing the amniotic fluid and the rate and rhythm of the fetal heart, either intermittently using a Pinard fetal stethoscope or Doppler ultrasound fetal heart rate detector or by continuous cardiotocographic monitoring (see Chapter 37). Where it is difficult to monitor the fetal heart from the maternal abdomen, for example in obese women, the fetal heart can be monitored electronically using a fetal scalp electrode, which is attached to the fetal skull and it produces a direct **fetal electrocardiogram**. Contraction length, strength and frequency can also be monitored externally by a transducer or internally by an intrauterine catheter pressure device.

Meconium

The presence of meconium in amniotic fluid is only suggestive of intrapartum asphyxia in the fetus. Between 15% and 20% of term pregnancies are associated with meconium-stained liquor which in the majority of cases is not a concern (NICE 2007). Meconium is a non-specific finding that may be associated with fetal problems other than asphyxia (Clark & Clark 2002). Meconium-stained amniotic fluid is associated with cardiovascular malformations, rhesus isoimmunisation, chorioamnionitis and pre-eclampsia. However, if the pregnancy is known to be high risk and the meconium is freshly passed, as indicated by it being dark green or black, thick and tenacious, its predictive value of asphyxia is high. Old or stale meconium giving rise to lightly stained yellowish or greenish amniotic fluid does not correlate well with fetal asphyxia.

Meconium-stained liquor

Meiss et al (1978) **classified** meconium into early light, early heavy and late meconium staining. Early staining was present from during the active phase of labour and late meconium was newly passed in the second stage of labour. Early heavy staining and late staining were associated with a significant increase in meconium aspiration. Similarly, thick fresh meconium at the onset of labour is associated with increased morbidity from meconium aspiration (Blackburn 2007). Thick undiluted meconium reflects reduced amniotic fluid volume, which is itself a risk factor (Enkin et al 2000).

The routine use of amniotomy to visualise the amniotic fluid for meconium staining remains a controversial issue. The outcome of a well-recognised randomised controlled trial (RCT) which included nulliparous women found that routine amniotomy had little effect on the important outcomes of labour and was not to be recommended (UK Amniotomy Group 1994). The study of prophylactic amnioinfusion has been found to dilute meconium but did not improve perinatal outcome and increased the risk of chorioamnionitis and endometritis (Spong et al 1994). They suggested that the benefit of amnioinfusion resulted from the alleviation of variable fetal heart rate decelerations rather than meconium dilution. Studies and systematic reviews of the use of amnioinfusion for meconium-stained liquor in labour suggested that any associated benefits were more likely to be due to an improvement in oligohydramnios than in dilution of meconium (Fraser et al 2005, Hofmeyr 2002). Guidelines recommend that amnioinfusion should not be used for the treatment of women with meconium-stained liquor (NICE 2007).

Fetal heart monitoring

Intermittent auscultation

The frequency of monitoring of the fetal heart by the midwife is decided by the frequency and strength of the uterine contractions and the effects on the fetus. Other risk factors likely to affect fetal oxygenation were also taken into account. Intermittent auscultation is usually carried out hourly in early labour, every 15 min as contractions increase and between each contraction in the late first stage and second stage of labour. The heart rate and rhythm should be listened to, commencing immediately after a contraction and counted over a full minute, to assess whether decelerations are present. The normal fetal heart rate range (reassuring) recommended is between 110 and 150 beats per minute (bpm) (NICE 2007). The faster rate is found in preterm babies and the lower in term and post-term babies. The rhythm is regular with a coupled beat.

Electronic fetal monitoring

Continuous electronic fetal heart rate monitoring was introduced in the 1970s and adopted enthusiastically by obstetricians as 'a significant improvement in intrapartum fetal assessment'. The technique was introduced before evidence of its efficacy or safety had been sought. Electronic fetal monitoring (EFM) (see Chapter 37) is used in the monitoring of labour in 3 out of 4 pregnancies in the USA. EFM can be used continuously or intermittently: for instance, for 15–30 min periodically.

Implications for practice

Concerns have been raised about the safety and efficiency of continuous EFM. Alfirevic et al (2006) compared EFM with intermittent auscultation during labour using the results of 12 randomised and quasi-RCTs involving a comparison of continuous cardiotocography (with and without fetal blood sampling) with no fetal monitoring, intermittent auscultation, intermittent cardiotocography. The studies included over 37 000 women of which only two studies were of a high quality. The review found no measurable impact on morbidity or mortality, with the exception of reduced incidence of neonatal seizures. However, continuous cardiotocography was found to be associated with an increase in caesarean sections and instrumental vaginal births. Overall the real challenge for practice is how best to convey this uncertainty to women to enable them to make an informed choice without compromising the normality of labour and unduly worrying the woman of the increased risk of operative delivery. NICE (2007) guidelines and expert panels in the USA and Canada have advised against routine EFM in low-risk pregnancies and have found weak evidence for its inclusion in high-risk pregnancies. Some believe the technology was introduced before it was well developed and that more research is needed.

Waveform analysis

Hypoxaemia during labour can alter the shape of the fetal electrocardiogram (ECG) waveform, notably the relaxation of the PR to RR intervals, and elevation or depression of the ST segment. Technical systems have been developed to monitor the fetal ECG during labour as an adjunct to continuous electronic fetal heart rate monitoring with a view to improving fetal outcome and minimising obstetric intervention. Neilson (2006) conducted a systematic review of five RCTs (10628 women) comparing fetal ECG waveform analysis with alternative methods of fetal monitoring during labour. The reviewer concluded that there was some report for the use of fetal ST waveform analysis when undertaking continuous electronic fetal heart rate monitoring during labour. However, the advantages need to be considered along with the disadvantages of the need to use an internal scalp electrode for ECG waveform recordings after membrane rupture.

Fetal heart patterns on electronic monitoring

The following terms are used to interpret conventional cardiotocographic readings.

Baseline fetal heart rate

There is a baseline rate of beats per minute (bpm) of 110–160 (NICE 2007), which is the rate present between periods of acceleration and deceleration. A rate over 160 bpm is called **baseline tachycardia** and below 110 bpm is **baseline bradycardia**. Both tachycardia and bradycardia may be associated with fetal hypoxia. Tachycardia may be seen if the woman is ketotic or pyrexial. Some fetuses normally have a heart rate of 110–120 bpm. A prolonged bradycardia occurs when there is continuous compression of the umbilical cord.

Baseline variability

Continuous adjustments in the autonomic nervous stimulation of the heart due to fetal response to the environment lead to minute variations in the length of each heart beat. This leads to the tracing having a jagged appearance, as the baseline rate is continuously adjusting, rather than being a straight line because each beat is the same length. There should be variance in the baseline rate of at least 5 bpm. Loss of variance may be due to hypoxia. It is also seen after the administration of some opiate analgesics because of depression of the cardiac regulatory centre in the fetal brain. Fetal sleep lasting 20–30 min may also cause a reduction in variability.

Response to uterine contractions

The fetal heart normally remains steady or **accelerates** during a contraction. Accelerations of 15 bpm above the baseline are associated with fetal activity and stimulation. The presence of two accelerations within a 20-min period is a sign of fetal health and the tracing is said to

be reactive. **Decelerations**, dips of more than 15 bpm below baseline, are more worrying.

- An **early deceleration** mirrors the pattern of the contraction. It commences at or after the onset of a contraction, reaches its lowest point at the peak of the contraction and then returns to normal by the end of the contraction. It is associated with compression of the fetal head and vagal response but may also indicate early fetal hypoxia.
- A **late deceleration** begins during or just after a contraction, reaches its lowest point after the peak of the contraction and may not recover until the onset of the next contraction. This time lag between the peak of the contraction and the low point of the deceleration is more significant than the drop in heart rate. It indicates fetal hypoxia and inadequate fetal brain oxygenation (Aldrich et al 1995) and is suggestive of cord compression. Prolapse of the cord should be excluded by vaginal examination and the obstetrician should be informed.
- **Variable decelerations**, where the heart rate varies in timing, frequency and amplitude, are associated with cord compression where there is obstruction to venous flow and a corresponding rise in fetal blood pressure. Both early and late decelerations are present. This pattern can be considered benign but if the decelerations are below 60 bpm, 60 bpm below the baseline or last for longer than 1 min the fetus may be in danger.

Two other unusual and rare patterns are observed: first, a sinusoidal pattern where there is a regular trace with a wave pattern of 3–6 per min with amplitude of 5–30 bpm—this is associated with rhesus isoimmunisation, fetal anaemia and asphyxia; secondly, a saltatory pattern with excessive variability of more than 25 bpm—this may be associated with fetal acidosis but the cause is unclear.

Fetal blood sampling

Cardiotocography can suggest the presence of fetal hypoxia but acidosis can only be confirmed by fetal blood sampling (Nickelsen 2002). The normal pH of fetal blood is 7.25–7.45 in labour. If this falls below 7.25 in the first stage of labour or below 7.2 in the second stage of labour, the fetus may be in danger and must be delivered immediately (NICE 2007). In order to carry out a fetal blood sampling procedure, the membranes need to be ruptured and the cervix needs to be at least 3 cm dilated. An amnioscope is passed through the cervix to access the fetal scalp. The scalp is sprayed with ethyl chloride to produce a reactive hyperaemia and a thin layer of silicone gel applied to ensure blood collects in a droplet. The skin is punctured and blood is collected in a heparinised capillary tube for immediate analysis of blood pH (see Fig. 37.25).

Management of confirmed fetal asphyxia

Severe hypoxia may result in the baby being stillborn, asphyxiated at birth or suffering brain damage. If the condition of the fetus monitored by the above findings suggests a major problem, the obstetrician must be called to see the woman and her fetus. If labour is being augmented by administration of Syntocinon (oxytocin), it is sensible to reduce the force of the uterine contractions by discontinuing the infusion. Administration of oxygen to the mother may be useful if the underlying cause of the fetal hypoxia is maternal disease. Delivery will probably be either by caesarean section in the first stage of labour or by instrumental delivery in the second stage. If delivery is imminent, an episiotomy may be all that is required. A resuscitaire should be present and a paediatrician should be called to the delivery room in all cases of fetal distress in preparation for resuscitation, if required.

Neonatal asphyxia and resuscitation

Initiation of respirations at birth

From about 22 weeks surfactant is produced in the fetal lung. The amount present increases until birth and there is a surge of production at about 34 weeks gestation. Surfactant has two main functions: to reduce surface tension in the alveoli so that they can expand more easily and to help prevent the alveoli collapsing at the end of each expiration. Fetal breathing movements have been identified as early as 11 weeks gestation and these increase in strength and frequency until they are present over 50% of the time. The rate varies between 30 and 70 breaths/min.

Establishing respiration at birth

This topic is summarised below and fully explored in Chapter 48.
- As the fetal chest is compressed by the birth canal, it is squeezed and lung and amniotic fluid are forced out of the alveoli into the upper respiratory tract. Passive recoil of the chest after delivery helps to draw air into the lungs and push the remaining fluid into the lymphatic system.
- Hypoxia during the late stage of delivery occurs with the birth of the head and the beginning of placental separation. The oxygen content of the blood falls and the carbon dioxide content rises, stimulating chemoreceptors to send a message to the respiratory centre and causing onset of breathing.
- The respiratory centre is also bombarded with stimuli from handling of the baby and the temperature changes found in the nasopharynx and on the skin.
- Circulatory changes direct the blood away from the placental circulation to the pulmonary circulation and lungs for oxygenation.
- Effective oxygenation is achieved by respiratory exchange in the alveoli and by adequate circulation. Most neonates establish respirations within 1 min of birth.

Birth asphyxia

Failure to initiate or sustain respirations at birth is called **birth asphyxia** or **asphyxia neonatorum**.

Causes

- Obstruction of the airway by mucus, blood, meconium or amniotic fluid may occur, especially if intrauterine anoxia has been present. Because of stimulation of the respiratory centre the fetus may have gasped in utero, drawing the above substances into the trachea and bronchi.
- The airways may not be patent due to congenital anomalies such as choanal atresia, hypoplastic lungs or diaphragmatic hernia.
- Lung function may be compromised by abnormalities in the cardiovascular system or central nervous system.
- Pain-relieving drugs such as pethidine and morphine and narcotic drugs such as diazepam, as well as general anaesthetics, if given in large doses, may depress the fetal respiratory centre.
- Intracranial haemorrhage may cause pressure on the cerebellum and medulla, affecting the cardiovascular and respiratory centres.
- Severe intrauterine infections following prolonged rupture of the membranes, leading to pneumonia, meningitis and septicaemia, may inhibit the efficient establishment of respiration.
- Immaturity of the neonate may lead to mechanical dysfunction because of poor lung development, lack of surfactant and a soft rib cage.

Recognition

Birth asphyxia may be classified as mild, moderate or severe, depending on scoring systems such as that devised by Virginia Apgar in 1953. **Apgar scores** are

Sign	Score		
	0	1	2
Heart rate	Absent	Slow – below 100	Fast – above 100
Respiratory effort	Absent	Slow, irregular	Good, crying
Muscle tone	Limp	Some flexion of the extremities	Active
Reflex irritability	No response	Grimace	Crying, cough
Colour	Blue, pale	Body pink, extremities blue	Completely pink

Figure 46.1 • The Apgar scoring system based on points being awarded for five physiological signs.

well known to be poor predictors of hypoxia and acidosis; however, they continue to be widely used in delivery suites. The principle of scoring systems such as Apgar score (Fig. 46.1) is to assess the condition of the baby at birth and may be affected by all the above causes of neonatal asphyxia. It follows that babies may not always have shown pre-delivery signs of impending asphyxia, many of the causes arising suddenly after delivery. Respiratory depression by fetal hypoxia is only one factor that may cause a baby to fail to breathe at birth (Richmond 2006).

For each of the vital signs in Fig. 46.1 the neonate may be given a score of 0, 1 or 2 depending on the descriptors. The Apgar score at 1 min is recorded; the suggested parameters for asphyxia are:

- 7–10: no asphyxia (healthy baby).
- 4–6: mild to moderate asphyxia, response to treatment usually good (a less healthy baby).
- 3 or less: severe asphyxia, requires urgent resuscitation (an ill baby).

Management of birth asphyxia

Newborn life support (NLS) provides detailed step-by-step guidelines which all practitioners should be familiar with (Resuscitation Council, www.resus.org.uk/pages/guide.htm). These guidelines are intended to provide help to establish normal breathing and comprise the following elements (see Fig. 46.2):

- Drying and covering the newborn baby to conserve heat.
- Assessing the need for any intervention.
- Opening the airway.
- Lung aeration (i.e. inflation breaths).
- Rescue breathing (i.e. ventilation breaths).
- Chest compression.
- Administration of drugs (rarely).

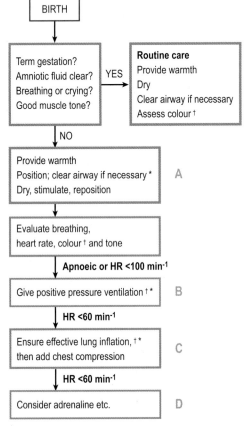

Figure 46.2 • Newborn life support algorithm. (Reproduced from Resuscitation Guidelines 2005, with kind permission of the Resuscitation Council (UK).)

A simple way to remember an overview of the steps in resuscitation is the **ABC method** (with **D** added):

A Airway: ensure patency.

B Breathing: ensure that oxygen enters the lungs.

C Cardiac function: ensure there is an adequate heart beat and circulation.

D Drugs: ensure that the resuscitation trolley with all its required components is available.

Summary of the sequence of actions

1. Keep the baby warm and assess, making sure the cord is securely clamped:

   - Drying the baby will provide significant stimulation and will allow time to assess colour, tone, breathing and heart rate. Reassess these observations every 30 s (particularly heart rate which will be the first sign of improvement).

   Consider asking for help immediately:

   - A healthy baby will be born blue with good tone, will cry within a few seconds and have a good heart rate (120–150 bpm) and will rapidly become pink during the first 90 s.

   - A less healthy baby will be blue at birth, will have less good tone, may have a slow heart rate (less than 100 bpm) and may not establish adequate breathing by 90–120 s.

   - An ill baby will be born pale and floppy, not breathing and with a slow heart rate.

   The heart rate of a baby is more accurately recorded and judged by using a stethoscope.

2. Airway. Before the baby can breathe effectively the airway must be open:

   - The best way to achieve this is to place the baby on its back with the head in the neutral position, i.e. with the head neither flexed nor extended.

   - If the baby is very floppy it may be necessary to apply chin lift or jaw thrust.

3. Breathing:

   - If the baby is not breathing adequately by about 90 s give 5 inflation breaths. Until now the baby's lungs will have been filled with fluid. Aeration of the lungs in these circumstances is likely to require sustained application of pressures of about 30 cmH$_2$O for 2–3 s: these are 'inflation breaths'.

   - If the heart rate was below 100 bpm initially then it should rapidly increase as oxygenated blood reaches the heart. If the heart rate does increase then it has to be assumed that the lungs have been successfully aerated. If the heart rate increases but the baby does not start breathing for itself, then continue to provide regular (ventilation) breaths at a rate of about 30–40 per min until the baby starts to breathe on its own.

   - If the heart rate does not increase following inflation breaths, then either the lungs are not aerated or the baby needs more than lung aeration alone. The most likely reason is that the lungs have failed to be effectively aerated. If the heart rate does not increase, and the chest does not passively move with each inflation breath, then the lungs are not aerated.

   - Do not progress to chest compression if you have not had good chest wall movement from the inflation breaths.

     - Check that the baby's head is in the neutral position;

     - Consider additional airway manoeuvre such as jaw thrust or insertion of an airway;

     - Consider obstruction in the oropharynx;

     - Ask for assistance.

4. Chest compression:

   - Almost all babies needing help at birth will respond to successful lung inflation with an increase in heart rate followed quickly by normal breathing. However, in some cases chest compression is necessary.

   - Chest compression should be started only when the lungs have been aerated successfully. In babies, the most efficient method of delivering chest compression is to grip the chest in both hands in such a way that the two thumbs can press on the lower third of the sternum, just below an imaginary line joining the nipples, with the fingers over the spine at the back. Compress the chest quickly and firmly, reducing the anteroposterior diameter of the chest by about one-third.

   The ratio of compressions to inflations in newborn resuscitation is 3:1.

   Chest compressions move oxygenated blood from the lungs back to the heart. Allow enough time during the relaxation phase of each compression cycle for the heart to refill with blood. Ensure the chest has inflated with each breath. Drugs may be required for a very few babies where inflation of the lungs and chest compression has not been sufficient to produce effective circulation.

5. Drugs:

   - Drugs are needed only if there is no significant cardiac output despite effective lung inflation and chest compression.

   - The drugs used are adrenaline (epinephrine) (1:10 000), sodium bicarbonate (ideally 4.2%) and dextrose (10%). They are best delivered close to the heart, usually via an umbilical venous catheter. The recommended doses are detailed in the guidelines (Resuscitation Council, www.resus.org/uk).

Meconium

The practice of attempting to aspirate meconium from the nose and mouth of the unborn baby while the head is still on the perineum is no longer recommended. This recommendation is based on the findings from a multicentred RCT study that concluded that this practice did not prevent meconium aspiration syndrome (Vain et al 2004). An RCT study has shown that attempts to remove meconium from the airways of vigorous babies after birth also fail to prevent this syndrome (Wiswell et al 2000).

If babies are born through thick meconium and are unresponsive (or not vigorous) at birth, the oropharynx should be inspected and cleared of meconium. If the practitioner has intubation skills then the larynx and trachea should be inspected and cleared of meconium.

All midwives and paediatric practitioners should be up to date with NLS but only trained practitioners should attempt intubation and drug administration. The midwife should ensure that the baby has a clear airway and start IPPV (intermittent positive pressure ventilation) with bag and mask until a trained practitioner arrives. More harm can be done to the baby if an inexperienced practitioner attempts to perform intubation. For midwives practising in the community it is reassuring to remember that severe neonatal asphyxia rarely occurs unannounced and warning signs identified during fetal monitoring in labour should result in the woman being transferred to a maternity unit to safeguard the fetus.

Transfer to the neonatal unit

A baby who has suffered severe asphyxia should be transferred to the neonatal unit for further observation.

Complications such as cerebral oedema, hypoglycaemia, hypothermia and electrolyte disturbance should be anticipated and prevented if possible and treated if they occur. Paediatric follow-up is important to detect long-term problems such as developmental delay or cerebral palsy.

Correction of acidosis

If only one of the two types of acidosis is present, the other system can be used to compensate. The lungs are central to the control of carbon dioxide level in respiratory acidosis while the kidneys control bicarbonate level in metabolic acidosis. Acidosis in neonates tends to be mixed and the buffering systems may fail. As stated above, the administration of sodium bicarbonate is controversial and should always follow blood gas analysis. The bicarbonate combines with hydrogen ions to form carbonic acid. This then dissociates into water and carbon dioxide:

$$H^+ + HCO_3^- \rightleftharpoons H_2CO_3 \rightleftharpoons CO_2 + H_2O \quad (46.2)$$

If the carbon dioxide can leave the body by the lungs, there is no problem but in respiratory difficulties it may accumulate in the body. It crosses cell membranes and the blood–brain barrier to cause intracellular acidosis, even if there seems to be a blood picture improvement in acidosis. This is because the bicarbonate buffer cannot cross cell membranes as readily as the carbon dioxide. The sodium content in sodium bicarbonate may result in an overloading of the baby's vascular system, resulting in cellular overhydration and damage.

Main points

- Impairment of the distribution of oxygen to the fetus will result in fetal hypoxia with acceleration of heart rate to maintain oxygen supply to the brain and deliver excess CO_2 to the placenta.
- Both tachycardia and bradycardia may be associated with fetal hypoxia. A prolonged bradycardia suggests continuous compression of the umbilical cord.
- Fetal acidosis can be confirmed by fetal blood sampling. Severe hypoxia may result in the baby being stillborn, asphyxiated at birth and suffering brain damage.
- A healthy baby will have good tone, a good heart rate (120–150 bpm) and will rapidly become pink. A less healthy baby will have less good tone, may have a slow heart rate of <100 bpm and may not establish adequate breathing by 90–120 s. An ill baby will be born pale and floppy, not breathing and with a slow heart rate.

- The sequence of actions in neonatal resuscitation include: keep the baby warm and assess; make sure the airway is open; place the baby's head in the neutral position; deal with breathing;—5 inflation breaths to aerate the lungs, ventilation breaths 30–40 per min (if required); ratio of chest compression (if required) to inflations is 3:1; drugs may be required.
- Assess the baby at each stage in line with Newborn Life Support (NLS) guideline—www.resusc-org.uk/.
- A baby who has suffered severe asphyxia should be transferred to the neonatal unit for further observation. Complications such as cerebral oedema, hypoglycaemia, hypothermia and electrolyte disturbance should be anticipated, prevented if possible and treated if they occur.

References

Agrawal, S.K., Doucette, F., Gratton, R., et al., 2004. Intrapartum computerized fetal heart rate parameters and metabolic acidosis at birth. Obstet. Gynecol. 103 (5), 1002–1003.

Aldrich, C.J., D'Antona, D., Spencer, J.A., 1995. Late fetal heart decelerations and changes in cerebral oxygenation during the first stage of labour. Br. J. Obstet. Gynaecol. 102 (1), 9–13.

Alfirevic, Z., Devane, D., Gyte, G.M.L., 2006. Continuous cardiotocography (CTG) as a form of electronic fetal monitoring (EFM) for fetal assessment during labour. Cochrane Database Syst. Rev. (3) Art. No. CD006066. DOI: 10.1002/14651858.CD006066.

Blackburn, S.T., 2007. Maternal, Fetal and Neonatal Physiology: A Clinical Perspective, fourth edn. Elsevier Saunders, Missouri.

Clark, D.A., Clark, M.B., 2002. Meconium aspiration syndrome. e-Med. J. 3 (1).

Enkin, M., Keirse, M.J.N.C., Renfrew, M., et al., 2000. A Guide to Effective Care in Pregnancy and Childbirth, third edn. Oxford University Press, Oxford.

Fraser, W.D., Hofmeyr, J., Lede, R., et al., 2005. Amnioinfusion for the prevention of the meconium aspiration syndrome. N Engl. J. Med. 353 (9), 909–917.

Hofmeyr, G.J., 2002. Amnioinfusion for meconium-stained liquor in labour. Cochrane Review. Cochrane Library, Issue 2. Update Software 2003, Oxford.

Meiss, P.J., Hall, M., Marshall, J.R., et al., 1978. Meconium passage: a new classification for risk assessment during labor. Am. J. Obstet. Gynecol. 131, 509.

Neilson, J.P., 2006. Fetal electrocardiogram (ECG) for fetal monitoring during labour. Cochrane Database Syst. Rev. (3) Art. No. CD000116. DOI:10.1002/14651858.

NICE (National Institute for Health and Clinical Excellence), 2007. Intrapartum Care: Care of Healthy Women and their Babies during Labour and Childbirth. RCOG, London.

Nickelsen, C.N., 2002. Fetal capillary blood pH. Blood Gas News 11 (1), 44–46.

Richmond, S. (Ed.), 2006. Newborn Life Support: Resuscitation at birth, second edn. Resuscitation Council (UK), London.

Spong, C.Y., Ogundipe, O.A., Ross, M.G., 1994. Prophylactic amnioinfusion for meconium-stained amniotic fluid. Am. J. Obstet. Gynecol. 171, 931–935.

UK Amniotomy Group. 1994. Comparing routine versus delayed amniotomy in spontaneous first labour at term. A multicentre randomised trial. Online Journal of Current Clinical Trials. Document No. 122, 1 April.

Vain, N.E., Szyld, E.G., Prudent, L.M., et al., 2004. Oropharyngeal and nasopharyngeal suctioning of meconium-stained neonates before delivery of their shoulders: multicentre, randomized controlled trial. Lancet 364, 597–602.

Wiswell, T.E., Gannon, C.M., Jacob, J., et al., 2000. Delivery room management of the apparently vigorous meconium-stained neonate: results of the multicenter international collaborative trial. Pediatrics 105, 1–7.

Annotated recommended reading

National Institute for Health and Clinical Excellence, 2007. Intrapartum Care: Care of Healthy Women and Their Babies during Labour and Childbirth. RCOG, London.

This publication sets out evidence-based guidelines and recommendations for intrapartum care.

Resuscitation Council. www.resus.org.uk

This site provides clear guidelines for resuscitation of the newborn.

Vain, N.E., Szyld, E.G., Prudent, L.M., et al., 2004. Oropharyngeal and nasopharyngeal suctioning of meconium-stained neonates before delivery of their shoulders: multicentre, randomized controlled trial. Lancet 364, 597–602.

This is an interesting RCT study which is pertinent to everyday intrapartum care.

Chapter Forty-Seven

Operative delivery

Introduction

An operative delivery is performed if a spontaneous birth is judged to pose a greater risk to mother and baby. Operations are divided into vaginal assisted methods (forceps and vacuum extraction deliveries) and abdominal methods (caesarean section).

Achievement of a safe vaginal delivery depends, in many cases, on the ability of the obstetrician to effect an operative delivery with forceps or vacuum.

Arias 1993

The RCOG (2005) further reiterate that the operator must have the appropriate skill and knowledge not only to be able to conduct the instrumental delivery but also to be able to manage any complications, should they occur. They advocate that obstetricians should also have previous experience of vaginal deliveries prior to training in operative procedures. Vaginal assisted deliveries should be undertaken for four basic reasons (Chamberlain & Steer 1999):

1. Fetal or maternal distress in second stage of labour.

2. Lack of advancement in second stage of labour.

3. Control of the after-coming head in a breech delivery.

4. Prophylactic shortening of second stage in, for example, heart disease.

The only absolute indications for caesarean section (CS) are cephalopelvic disproportion and major degrees of placenta praevia. Other indications demand a judgement by the obstetrician that the risk of vaginal delivery exceeds the risk of the operation or that the mother's perception is that it does (Chamberlain & Steer 1999).

Forceps delivery

Obstetric forceps have been known and utilised in difficult deliveries since their invention by the Chamberlen family in the 17th century (Dunn 1999). Since then, there have been attempts to modify and improve their effectiveness and safety, leading to a variety of instruments available for use in different obstetric situations (Fig. 47.1). Obstetric forceps consist of two blades, each with a handle and a shank. The blades are marked 'L' left or 'R' right, according to the side of the mother's

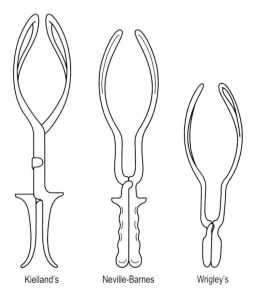

Kielland's   Neville-Barnes   Wrigley's

Figure 47.1 • Obstetric forceps. (From Henderson C, Macdonald S 2004, with kind permission of Elsevier.)

pelvis in which they lie when applied. There may be a locking or traction device incorporated into the mechanism (Hamilton 2003a). Whatever the variation in shape, two considerations are important leading to the addition of **pelvic** and **cephalic curves**:

*   The shape and size of the fetal head.
*   The curve, shape and size of the bony pelvis.

The use of forceps

The shape and size of forceps depend on its use. Forceps may be applied in mid-cavity or at the pelvic outlet. They may be used to **rotate** the fetal head followed by **traction** in the direction of the curve of Carus to complete the delivery or to apply traction only.

*   For traction without rotation, non-rotational forceps such as those designed by **Wrigley** or **Simpson** are used for low-cavity delivery, mainly now for delivery of the aftercoming head of the breech. **Neville-Barnes** or **Haig-Ferguson** forceps for mid-cavity delivery have a pelvic and cephalic curve although these are now used exclusively for low-cavity non-rotational delivery and the axis traction attachments are rarely used.
*   It is important to understand that mid- and high-cavity forceps deliveries (when the fetal head is higher than station +2 cm) are no longer undertaken because of the possibility of trauma. CS is more likely to be the method of choice in those cases.
*   To correct malposition from occipitolateral or occipitoposterior to occipitoanterior prior to traction, rotational forceps such as **Kielland's forceps** are the design commonly used (RCOG 2005). These forceps

have no pelvic curve (straight) so that they can be rotated in the confines of the birth canal. In malpositions there is often **asynclitism** (tilting of the fetal head). Kielland's forceps have a sliding lock so that asynclitism can be corrected prior to rotation and traction. There is a gap between the handles when the blades are applied and there is a danger that too much pressure may be applied to the fetal head with the risk of cerebral trauma.

Applying the forceps

Positioning the forceps

The blades are inserted separately on either side of the fetal head so that they are located alongside the head and over the ears (Fig. 47.2). They should be situated symmetrically between the eye orbits and the ears, reaching from the parietal eminences to the malar area and cheeks (Vacca 1999). They should come together and lock easily without the use of strength if they are applied correctly. Baskett et al (2007) described the line of application extending from the point of the chin to a point on the sagittal suture near the posterior fontanelle.

The skill of the operator

The operator is a major determinant of the success or failure of instrumental delivery and should have appropriate training prior to conducting operative procedures (RCOG 2005). Unfavourable results are almost always caused by the user's unfamiliarity with either the instrument or the rules governing its use (Enkin et al 2000). It is important that the skills of using any instrument are acquired under supervision because of the devastating consequences that could arise if mother or baby is damaged during the operation.

Prerequisites for forceps delivery (Chamberlain & Steer 1999)

No obstruction to the descent of the fetus

*   The cervix must be fully dilated; attempts to apply forceps blades with an undilated cervix will lead to trauma without successful delivery.
*   The membranes should be ruptured.
*   The bladder must be empty to prevent trauma.
*   No obvious bar should exist such as cephalopelvic disproportion.
*   Engagement of the head.

Safeguarding the mother

*   Adequate anaesthesia must be available by epidural or pudendal block.
*   A full explanation of the procedure should be given to the woman and her partner and consent obtained.

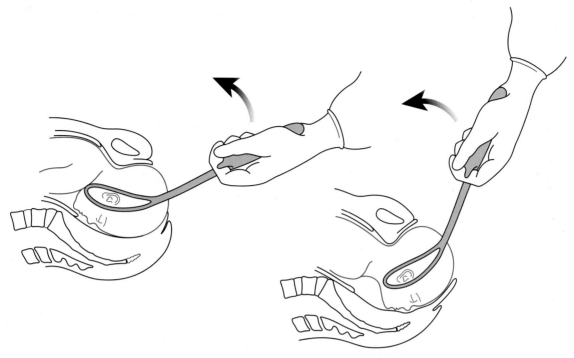

Figure 47.2 • Forceps delivery. (From Henderson C, Macdonald S 2004, with kind permission of Elsevier.)

- An episiotomy is usually performed, to allow space for the posterior pull.

The RCOG (2005) evaluated a study in the USA, which linked more perineal trauma with vacuum extraction and use of episiotomy compared to forceps delivery. However, they go on to argue that it is not possible to relate these results to UK practice, as within the UK a mediolateral episiotomy is used compared with the midline episiotomy in the USA. The RCOG (2005) acknowledges that the use of episiotomy 'has crept into clinical practice without formal evaluation' and advocate for further research to be conducted to explore this issue.

There should be as much safety, comfort and dignity for the woman as possible although the lithotomy position is essential. The procedure is carried out aseptically using sterile instruments.

Safeguarding the baby

- There should be careful and accurate identification of the presentation and position of the fetal head.
- The forceps blades should be applied correctly and their position checked before rotation and/or traction is commenced.
- A paediatrician should be present at the delivery.
- Neonatal resuscitation equipment should be available.
- Some obstetricians prefer manual rotation of the head as it is thought to be less traumatic than instrumental

rotation (Hamilton 2003a). Rotational forceps delivery may cause a significant deterioration in fetal acid–base balance (Baker & Johnson 1994).

Complications of forceps delivery

Maternal

- There may be soft tissue damage to the lower uterine segment, cervix, vagina and perineum.
- Bleeding from tissue trauma may lead to postpartum haemorrhage and shock.
- Retention of urine may occur if there is bruising and oedema of the urethra and neck of the bladder.
- Perineal pain may be present once the anaesthesia has worn off.
- Dyspareunia may occur in the long term.
- Psychological effects may lead to avoidance of future pregnancy.

Neonatal

- A cephalhaematoma may form due to friction between the fetal head and the blades or pelvic walls.
- Facial or scalp abrasions are common.
- Bruising of the scalp may lead to neonatal jaundice.
- Intracranial haemorrhage is a rare but serious problem, which may lead to convulsions.

- These problems are more often seen in rotational forceps as is failed forceps delivery resulting in emergency CS (Johanson et al 1992).

Vacuum extraction (ventouse delivery)

Use of the vacuum extractor

Delivery by the use of **vacuum extraction** has a history as long as that of forceps delivery and is not new. The modern version was developed by **Malmström** in the 1950s and has been modified by others (Vacca 1999). Originally, the vacuum extractor consisted of a rounded metal cup in three sizes—40, 50 and 60 mm in diameter (Bird 1969)—and this type of cup is still in use. The cup was attached to a **chain** and handle and a suction pump to extract air and create a vacuum. The largest cup size that can be passed through the cervix was chosen.

Cups now available are made of silastic, silicone rubber and plastic. Johanson & Menon (2000) compared soft versus rigid vacuum extractor cups. They found that soft cups were significantly more likely to fail to achieve a vaginal delivery than metal cups, although soft cups had better outcomes in a well-flexed vertex. They also found that soft cups were associated with less scalp injury. Metal cups appeared to be more suitable for occipitoposterior, transverse or difficult occipitoanterior position deliveries whereas soft cups seemed to be appropriate for uncomplicated deliveries needing assistance in the second stage. Soft cups deform to follow the contours of the baby's head during application but the application is poor if there is moderate to severe caput succedaneum. However, Johanson & Menon (2000) advocate more evidence on the use of both soft and metal cups on fetal outcomes. Another form of cup for ventouse delivery is the Kiwi Omnicup. The Omnicup is made of rigid plastic and can be used for malpresentations such as occipitoposterior as well as occipitoanterior positions (Vacca 1999). The Omnicup

forms a chignon similar to that formed by metal cups but without the associated scalp injury.

Applying the vacuum extractor

Positioning

The cup is attached by suction to the fetal scalp as near to the occiput as possible and taking care to avoid the anterior fontanelle (Fig. 47.3). A **vacuum** is created with a negative pressure of 0.2 kg/cm, drawing an artificial caput (chignon) into the cup (Meakin 2004). The cup is checked for position and to ensure that no maternal soft tissue such as the cervix has been included within the rim. The vacuum pressure is increased to 0.8 kg/cm. This can either be done in stages or in one step. One to two minutes should be allowed for the **chignon** to develop. There is limited evidence on this issue and currently there is a protocol for a future systematic review on rapid versus stepwise negative pressure application for vacuum extraction assisted vaginal delivery (Suwannachat et al 2007). Traction is then applied following the curve of Carus to enhance the natural forces of uterine contractions and maternal expulsive effort (Figs 47.4A,B).

The skill of the operator

Used skilfully, the advantages of the **ventouse** are that there is no increase to the presenting diameters

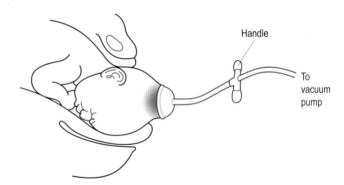

Figure 47.3 • Vacuum extraction. (From Henderson C, Macdonald S 2004, with kind permission of Elsevier.)

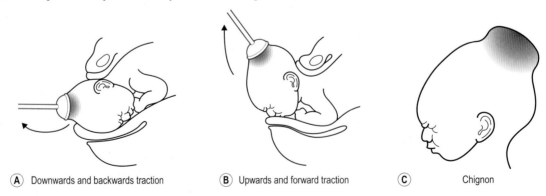

(A) Downwards and backwards traction   (B) Upwards and forward traction   (C) Chignon

Figure 47.4 • Formation of chignon and direction of traction in vacuum extraction. (A) Downwards and backwards traction, (B) Upwards and forward traction, (C) Chignon.

and the instrument can be used to flex and rotate the head and to assist the mother to deliver her infant. However, some operators may be too hasty or unskilled and apply traction before suction has been achieved, resulting in the cup coming away from the scalp. Some maternity units have trained midwives to perform ventouse deliveries. The technique is also useful where midwives work alone, without obstetric colleagues, in remote areas of the world. It is important that a midwife is properly trained and is confident in the use of this device and that their employing authority approves the use of ventouse equipment by midwives.

Prerequisites

- These are as for forceps delivery.
- The vacuum extractor is not suitable for application in babies with suspected coagulability.
- It should not be used where contractions are weak or maternal effort is poor.

Complications

Maternal

There is less trauma to maternal tissues than that caused by forceps if the cup has been applied correctly to the fetal head (Johanson & Menon 1999).

There is a tendency for more bleeding due to the abrupt distension of the lower birth canal caused by traction and friction of the fetal head.

Neonatal

- Trauma to the fetal scalp is the most common complication although this is reduced if soft cups compared to rigid vacuum cups are used for assisted vaginal delivery (Johanson & Menon 2000).
- All babies will have a chignon, which is a combination of oedema and bruising (Fig. 47.4C).
- Abrasions of the scalp may be caused by the cup being pulled off during inexpert traction.
- Jaundice, usually mild and responding to phototherapy, may be due to the reabsorption of the red cells which have escaped the circulatory system during bruise formation.
- Neonatal retinal haemorrhages are more common following vacuum extraction than forceps delivery but there are no long-term problems.
- Vacuum extraction has been found to be associated with umbilical cord blood acid–base changes but these changes in pH and Pco_2 were not associated with increased perinatal morbidity or mortality or acidaemia at birth. These findings suggest that

vacuum extraction can be used to deliver babies with fetal distress in the second stage of labour.

Comparison of forceps and vacuum extraction

Although **assisted vaginal delivery** is performed worldwide, there is a large variation in its application, ranging from 1.5% of all deliveries in the Czech Republic to 15% in Australia and Canada (Stephenson 1992). In the UK the rates for operative vaginal delivery have remained stable at between 10% and 15% (RCOG 2005). In a systematic review of 10 studies, Johanson & Menon (1999) compared assisted vaginal delivery by obstetric forceps versus ventouse extraction. The reviewers concluded that the use of vacuum extractor appears to reduce maternal morbidity. However, there was a reduction in cephalhaematoma and retinal haemorrhage for the fetus with forceps delivery and this was seen to be a compensatory benefit.

This area remains controversial, although the benefits to the mother of vacuum extraction have been established. Further research using larger studies is required to provide further information about major adverse neonatal effects of both methods and improving operator skill.

Caesarean section

Overview

Caesarean section (CS) is a surgical procedure in which the abdomen and uterus are incised to facilitate the birth of the baby. There are records of this procedure being performed prior to the discovery of anaesthetic drugs, and usually for delivery of the fetus when the mother has died. Caesarean section may be carried out as an emergency in response to adverse conditions developing in late pregnancy or in labour. Elective CS is a planned event where the timing is chosen to maximise safety for mother and fetus.

Current rates

Rates of CS worldwide have increased steadily over the last few decades (Savage 1996). In the UK rates have doubled and in the USA and Canada they have tripled. The World Health Organization (WHO 1985) said that CS rates should not need to be more than 10–15%, while Savage believes that this rate should not need to be more than 6–8%. The rate in England and Wales has been observed to increase: 11.3% in 1989–90 to 22.7% in 2003–2004 (DoH 2001, 2005). Within

Scotland the rate has also markedly risen from 8.6% in 1976 to 23.9% in 2005 (Information Statistics Division Scotland (ISD) 2008). Figures for Ireland are consistent with the rates throughout the UK, with rates being quoted between 20% and 25% (VHI Healthcare 2008). Within the UK the figures for caesarean rates in relation to maternal mortalities is startling. Of the 230 maternal deaths reported, 141 (61%) woman were delivered by caesarean section (Lewis 2007) of which the majority of the sections were conducted for maternal medical conditions (73 women) (Lewis 2007).

Indications

Countries in the UK compile and review statistics and offer some explanations as to why caesarean rates continue to rise, such as: changes in demographics, changes in clinical practice, availability of resources, one-to-one support in labour (ISD 2008). Black et al (2005) also highlight that women's choices in childbirth are contributing to the increasing caesarean rates in the UK. Findings suggest that the reasons for conducting caesarean sections are: breech presentation, repeat caesarean section (Black et al 2005), delivery of twins and preterm babies (ISD 2008). Increased maternal age and weight is also thought to correlate to a rise in caesarean section (ISD 2008). The setting up of post-traumatic stress clinics for women who have had previous traumatic 'normal deliveries' may also have contributed to the rising numbers of CSs, as the women involved may opt for a CS for subsequent deliveries. Table 47.1 summarises the indications for CS.

Method

The operation of CS is a technique whereby the course of childbirth is interrupted, and delivery via the natural passage is skirted in favour of the abdominal route (Al-Azzawi 1998).

Any person called on to assist at a CS must be aware of the surgical techniques involved. Technically, there are two types of CS according to the incision in the uterus: the **lower segment** and the **classical**. There is no association with the type of abdominal wall incision, although a lower segment CS is most often performed through a transverse incision, also called the **Pfannenstiel** or **bikini-line incision** (Hamilton 2003a). The lower segment forms from about 32 weeks of pregnancy and is less muscular than the upper segment. A transverse incision into the lower uterine segment heals more rapidly than a vertical incision into the upper uterine segment and there is less risk of rupture of the uterus in a subsequent pregnancy. For this reason, classical CS is rarely performed unless the fetus is to be delivered prior to the 32nd week of pregnancy or there is an anterior placenta praevia.

Anatomical layers incised and sutured in a caesarean section

- Skin.
- Fat.
- Rectus sheath.
- Muscle (rectus abdominis).
- Abdominal peritoneum.

Table 47.1 Maternal and fetal indications for caesarean section

Maternal	Fetal	Maternal and fetal
Severe pregnancy-induced hypertension	Severe rhesus isoimmunisation	Cephalopelvic disproportion
Previous vaginal reconstructive surgery	Cord prolapse	Pelvic tumours
Previous third-degree tears	Multiple fetuses (3 or more)	High-risk obstetric history
A large-for-dates fetus (with previous shoulder dystocia)	Breech presentation	Antepartum haemorrhage
Eclampsia	Brow or shoulder presentation	Uterine rupture
Terminal illness of the mother	Severe intrauterine growth retardation (which may be complicated by maternal disease)	Failure to progress in labour
	Fetal distress in labour	Placenta praevia
	Fetal abnormality where damage may be increased by vaginal delivery	Fetal macrosomia
	Active genital herpes	Tumours

- Pelvic (visceral peritoneum or perimetrium).
- Uterine muscle (sutured in two layers).

As the uterus is incised, the membranes are ruptured with the escape of amniotic fluid. There is likely to be substantial bleeding because of the increased blood supply to the uterus. Immediate postoperative care is as for any surgery but the woman will wish to see and have contact with her baby as soon as possible and to breastfeed if that is her intended method of feeding. Even though the woman has had a CS the baby can still be placed skin-to-skin to initiate that first breastfeed if both the mother and baby's condition allow. Due to the proximity of the bladder to the lower uterine segment, urine output must be observed closely. A urinary catheter is inserted in the bladder for at least 24h after the CS as there may be difficulty in micturition at first. Any presence of haematuria must be reported to the obstetrician.

Types of anaesthesia used for caesarean section

Types of anaesthesia used for CS will depend on the reason why the CS is being performed. In the case of fetal distress, where a woman already has a working epidural, the epidural will be topped-up with a stronger anaesthetic with or without an opiate drug such as morphine or fentanyl. Spinal anaesthesia is used for an elective CS or when an epidural is ineffective. In the case of severe fetal bradycardia, where the fetus has to be delivered quickly, a general anaesthetic is usually given. A general anaesthetic is also given when a patient who has had a spinal or epidural complains of pain during the operation. Women with clotting disorders will always have a general anaesthetic as there is a high risk of bleeding.

Postoperative analgesia

The anaesthetist should prescribe adequate and effective analgesia which should include:

- Intramuscular or subcuticular analgesia, e.g. morphine sulphate injections.
- If the woman's condition allows, non-steroidal anti-inflammatory drugs, e.g. diclofenac (Voltarol) 100mg per rectum or oral tablets (Brufen 600mg), are prescribed as recommended in the British National Formulary (BNF 2008).
- Oral tablets, e.g. paracetamol 1g, four times a day, or co-codamol, two tablets taken 6-hourly.
- Patient-controlled analgesia may be prescribed, if a woman has coagulation problems, to avoid frequent intramuscular injections, and may also be necessary for women who have had a general anaesthetic for an emergency CS.

If the woman is having opioid analgesia an antiemetic is usually given simultaneously. Antiemetics of choice would be Stemitil 12.5mg (prochloperazine) or Maxalon (metochlopramide).

Safety

Lilford (1990) warned that any increase in the proportions of elective CS would lead to an increase in the CS rate and probably in maternal mortality. CS carried out for the safety of the fetus puts the mother's life at risk (Hillan 1991). Even with the benefit of modern surgical techniques, CS is still less safe for the woman than a vaginal delivery. The major hazard is **pulmonary embolism**, which is difficult to prevent (Savage 1996). **Haemorrhage** and **infection** as well as thromboembolic disorders may occur (Francome et al 1993). Long-term morbidity with **infertility**, voluntary or involuntary, may be a problem. The Confidential Enquiry into Maternal Deaths (CEMD) for the years 1994–96 reported that 48.8% of all direct deaths were following CS. The subsequent CEMD report noted that from 1997 to 1999 there was a dramatic fall in the number of direct deaths following CS (Lewis 2001). However, the most recent CEMACH 'Saving Mothers Lives' Report (CEMACH 2007, formerly the CEMD) highlighted that from 2003 to 2005 the majority of maternal deaths were delivered by caesarean section (61%) (Lewis 2007). This is a noticeable rise from previous years.

Neonatal behaviour

There is a profound effect on neonatal behaviour attributable to at least the following four factors (Trevathen 1987):

1. Caesarean section is often carried out before term.

2. Maternal medication is greater than in vaginal births.

3. In elective CS the baby is not subjected to the stress of labour.

4. Hormonal influences vary depending on the time and mode of delivery.

Babies are less active if delivered by CS; they sleep more and cry less. The influence of drugs in labour on neonatal behaviour will be examined in more detail in Chapter 57.

Liston et al (2008) conducted a population-based cohort study ($n = 142929$) from 1988 to 2002, which included low- and high-risk women. Regression analysis was used. There were 142929 deliveries and 27263 were caesarean sections of which 61% were conducted in labour. There was an increased risk of the baby having respiratory conditions if there had been a caesarean section following labour compared to babies who were delivered by caesarean section with no labour. Liston et al advocate that the findings can be generalised to a wider population because the sample comprised both low- and high-risk women.

General anaesthesia in pregnancy and childbirth

Reversible anaesthesia, which is a state of unconsciousness and muscle relaxation, is brought about by pharmacological preparations. There is a great difference in obstetric anaesthesia from general surgery as two lives have to be cared for—the mother and the fetus. The recent CEMACH report recommends the need for vigilance in the care of the pregnant woman undergoing general anaesthesia (Lewis 2007).

The altered physiology of the woman increases the danger and includes raised maternal intragastric pressure, acidity of gastric contents and delayed gastric emptying, leading to the risk of acid aspiration syndrome. Aortocaval compression, the effect of drugs on the fetus, maternal hypoxia or hypotension, placental insufficiency and intrapartum fetal hypoxia also increase the risk of neonatal respiratory depression (Meakin 2004).

General anaesthetic agents

For a drug to be used as an **anaesthetic agent**, it must affect the central nervous system appropriately and be rapidly controllable so that anaesthesia can be induced rapidly, be adjusted during the operation to provide the correct level of consciousness and the effects quickly reversible after the operation (Rang et al 2007). Humphrey Davy suggested the use of the gas **nitrous oxide** for relieving the pain of surgery in 1800. He tested its effects on himself and a few others including the then prime minister. It was found to cause euphoria, analgesia and loss of consciousness but became famous as 'laughing gas' until an American dentist, Horace Wells, had a tooth extracted under its influence.

Inhalational anaesthetics were used in surgery in 1846 when William Morton used ether to extract a tooth. He persuaded the chief surgeon at Massachusetts General Hospital to use it during a surgical procedure on the 16th October 1846 and it was successful; subsequently, planned protracted surgical procedures could be carried out. The famous American Oliver Wendell Holmes invented the word 'anaesthesia'. In 1847 James Simpson, professor of obstetrics in Glasgow, used the agent **chloroform** to relieve pain in childbirth, but it only became popular after Queen Victoria gave birth to her seventh child under the influence of chloroform in 1853.

The modern drugs

Although many CSs are now performed under epidural anaesthesia (see Ch. 38), general anaesthesia is still used. It is now common practice to preoxygenate pregnant women prior to induction of a general anaesthetic although this may lead to stress for the woman (Hamilton 2003b). The choice made by the woman is important. Holdcroft et al (1995) found that one-third of the women in their small study opted to be unconscious during CS. Induction agents used to initiate anaesthesia include barbiturates such as **thiopental**, which causes loss of consciousness in 20s if given intravenously (Rang et al 2001), or **propofol**, which appears to be a good alternative to thiopental. Maternal unconsciousness follows rapidly with minimal side-effects and fetal respiratory depression can be avoided.

Anaesthesia is then maintained by inhalational anaesthetic agents such as nitrous oxide combined with a volatile agent such as **halothane** (Fluothane) or **enflurane** (Ethrane). Halothane has limited usefulness as an obstetric anaesthetic agent as it causes relaxation of the uterine muscle (Rang et al 2007). These agents deepen the anaesthesia, improve uterine blood flow by reducing circulating catecholamines and improve fetal acid–base status (Capogna & Celluno 1993).

Problems

Failed intubation

Failed intubation is an obstetric emergency requiring prompt and calm action. Most maternal deaths attributed directly to anaesthesia have been reported to be due to a misplaced endotracheal tube. It is usual to have a failed intubation drill (Hamilton 2003). The anaesthetist may choose to maintain an airway with a Guedel airway and face mask, with an assistant maintaining cricoid pressure throughout the anaesthetic, or **spinal anaesthesia** may be chosen. The Royal College of Anaesthetists (RCA 2004) inform us that maternity units that have general anaesthetic facilities should have the necessary protocols to implement when failed intubation occurs. It is also pertinent that there are appropriately trained and skilled anaesthetists and anaesthetic assistants working within these facilities to deal with situations should they occur.

Effect of anaesthetics on the nervous system

The mode of action of drugs that create a state of anaesthesia is as yet unexplained. The brain has a large blood flow and the blood–brain barrier is freely permeable to anaesthetic agents (Rang et al 2007). Theories involve interaction with the lipid bilayer of the cell membrane or with hydrophobic binding sites on protein molecules.

Anaesthetics inhibit the conduction of cellular action potentials and synaptic transmission.

It is probable that **anaesthetics act** on two main parts of the brain: the **reticular formation** and the **hippocampus**. Loss of consciousness is probably due to the effect of the drug on the reticular formation of the brain. Anaesthetics also cause short-term amnesia and the hippocampus is likely to be the site for this action. Many other brain functions are affected such as motor control and reflex action. It is not helpful to look for one site of action as all neurons are affected.

Muscle relaxation is achieved by drugs which **depolarise** neuromuscular messages postsynaptically such as suxamethonium (Scoline) or **non-polarising agents** which act postsynaptically such as pancuronium (Pavulon) (Rang et al 2007).

Acid aspiration syndrome (Mendelson's syndrome)

This life-threatening syndrome arises from the inhalation of acid gastric contents and was first described by Mendelson in 1946. The result of such aspiration is a chemical pneumonitis leading to **adult respiratory distress syndrome (ARDS)** with acute bronchospasm, dyspnoea, cyanosis, wheezing and tachycardia (Meakin 2004). The factors predisposing to this arise from the physiological effect of progesterone on the smooth muscle of the stomach which causes delayed emptying, decreased lower oesophageal tone, which leads to reflux, and the altered position of the stomach due to the enlarged uterus. There is also gastric hypersecretion in labour and there is still no consensus on nil-by-mouth policies. There is no firm evidence to support the policy of restricting food intake for all women in labour. Most maternity units now only restrict food intake in those women who have a higher risk of having an emergency CS.

Prevention of acid aspiration syndrome

Prevention of this syndrome is essential. The administration of **antacid preparations** such as sodium citrate 30 ml prior to anaesthetic induction and **histamine-2 (H$_2$) antagonists** such as ranitidine 150 mg are recommended. Other drugs such as **metoclopramide** act centrally in the nervous system and also locally in the gastrointestinal tract. These are antiemetic drugs, and they act as stimulants to gastric motility, accelerating emptying without stimulating gastric juice production. They increase tone in the lower oesophagus and prevent gastro-oesophageal reflux (Rang et al 2007).

During induction of the general anaesthetic and intubation, **cricoid pressure (Sellick's manoeuvre)**, part of which is referred to as 'crash induction', along with the immediate passing of a cuffed endotracheal tube, is essential to prevent aspiration of acid stomach contents. The cricoid cartilage is compressed between the thumb and finger towards the cervical spine in order to occlude the oesophagus. Deaths have occurred due to inexperience of the practitioner and it is recommended that only an experienced anaesthetist should be involved in obstetric anaesthesia (Lewis 2007). The RCA (2004) and RCOG Press (2007) also stipulate that not only is it important to have the experienced obstetric anaesthetists, but there must also be the appropriate facilities for high-dependency monitoring and regular training updates for multidisciplinary staff on emergency drills.

Aortocaval compression

The alternative name for **aortocaval compression** is supine hypotensive syndrome, which Hamilton (2003a) believes to be misleading as the fall in blood pressure is a late sign and placental perfusion will have occurred before the drop in maternal blood pressure. A reduction in venous return and a fall in cardiac output are produced by the weight of the gravid uterus pressing on and partly occluding the inferior vena cava. It will occur whenever the woman lies supine in late pregnancy. If fetal distress is present, the interference with placental circulation will increase the severity of hypoxia.

Prevention of aortocaval compression

If the woman has to lie supine, the sequence of events can be avoided by placing a folded blanket or a small rubber wedge under the mattress to tilt the woman's body about 15° to the left. Modern operating tables and delivery beds have this function built into their design. Wilkinson & Enkin (1997) reviewed the use of **lateral tilt** during CS but found the data to be poor. However, they stated that low Apgar scores were fewer and neonatal pH measurements and oxygen tensions appeared to be better if lateral tilt was used.

Main points

- Forceps may be used to rotate the fetal head before traction is applied to complete the delivery or to apply traction only to complete delivery. It is necessary to confirm that there is no obstruction to the descent of the fetus before performing a forceps delivery.

- Maternal complications following forceps delivery include: soft tissue damage to the lower uterine segment, cervix, vagina and perineum; bleeding from tissue trauma; retention of urine; post-delivery perineal pain; and dyspareunia in the long term. Neonatal complications are more often seen in rotational forceps and include cephalhaematoma, abrasions, neonatal jaundice and intracranial haemorrhage.

- Equipment for vacuum extraction delivery has been modified. Cups are now available made of silastic, silicone rubber and plastic as well as the original metal. Soft cups deform to follow the contours of the baby's head during application and are less likely to be associated with scalp trauma.

- Midwives can be specially trained to perform this technique and can use the ventouse equipment for delivery if it is approved by their employing authority.

- Worldwide CS rates have risen over the last 25 years. In the UK the majority of operations are performed for hypertensive disorders of pregnancy, antepartum haemorrhage or fetal distress. Even with modern surgical techniques it is still less safe for the woman than a vaginal delivery. During CS, the altered physiology of the woman increases the danger of acid aspiration syndrome but the major hazard is pulmonary embolism.

- Although many CSs are now performed under spinal or epidural anaesthesia, general anaesthesia is still used. Acid aspiration syndrome arises from the inhalation of acid gastric contents, resulting in chemical pneumonitis and adult respiratory distress syndrome. Prevention is essential and antacid preparations and histamine-2 (H_2) antagonists are recommended. Most maternal deaths attributed directly to anaesthesia are due to a misplaced endotracheal tube. During induction of the general anaesthetic and intubation, cricoid pressure is essential to prevent aspiration of acid stomach contents.

References

Al-Azzawi, F., 1998. Childbirth & Obstetric Techniques, second edn. Mosby, St Louis.

Arias, F., 1993. Practical Guide to High Risk Pregnancy and Delivery, second edn. Mosby Year Book, Chicago.

Baker, N., Johnson, I.R., 1994. A study of rotational forceps delivery on fetal acid–base balance. Acta Obstet. Gynecol. Scand. 73, 787–789.

Baskett, T.F., Cader, A.A., Sabaratnam, A., 2007. Munro Kerr's Operative Obstetrics, eleventh edn. Baillière Tindall.

Black, C., Kaye, J.A., Hershel, J., 2005. Cesarean delivery in the United Kingdom: time trends in the General Practice Research Database. Obstet. Gynecol. 106 (1), 151–155.

Bird, G.C., 1969. Modification of Malmström's vacuum extractor. Br. Med. J. 3, 526.

BNF (British National Formulary), 2008. Number 56 (September). British Medical Association and Royal Pharmaceutical Society of Great Britain, London.

Capogna, G., Celluno, D., 1993. The effects of anaesthetic agents on the newborn. In: Reynolds, F. (Ed.), Effects on the Baby of Maternal Analgesia and Anaesthesia. W B Saunders, London.

CEMACH (Confidential Enquiry into Maternal and Child Health), 2007. Saving Mothers' Lives 2003–2005. RCOG Press, London.

Chamberlain, G., Steer, P., 1999. ABC of labour care: operative delivery. Br. Med. J. 318, 1260–1264.

DoH (Department of Health), 2001. NHS Maternity Statistics, England 1995–1996 to 1997–1998. Department of Health, London.

DoH (Department of Health), 2005. NHS Maternity Statistics, England 2003–2004. Department of Health, London.

Dunn, P.M., 1999. The Chamberlen family (1560–1728) and obstetric forceps. Arch. Dis. Child. Fetal Neonat. Ed. 81, F232–F235.

Enkin, M., Keirse, J., Neilson, J., et al., 2000. A Guide to Effective Care in Pregnancy and Childbirth, third edn. Oxford University Press, Oxford.

Francome, C., Savage, W., Churchill, H., et al., 1993. Caesarean Birth in Britain. Middlesex University Press, National Childbirth Trust, London.

Hamilton, A., 2003a. Operative deliveries. In: Fraser, D.M., Cooper, M.A. (Eds.), Myles Textbook for Midwives, fourteenth edn. Churchill Livingstone, Edinburgh.

Hamilton, A., 2003b. Pain relief and comfort in labour. In: Fraser, D.M., Cooper, M.A. (Eds.), Myles Textbook for Midwives, fourteenth edn. Churchill Livingstone, Edinburgh.

Holdcroft, A., Parshall, A.M., Knowles, M.G., et al., 1995. Factors associated with mothers selecting general anaesthesia for lower segment caesarean section. J. Psychosom. Obstet. Gynaecol. 16 (3), 167–170.

Information Statistics Division Scotland (ISD Scotland), 2008. Scottish Health Statistics Births & Babies—Mode of Delivery. Online. <http://www.extras. isd.scotland.org/>. accessed 25/6/08.

Johanson, R.B., Menon, V., 1999. Vacuum extraction versus forceps for assisted vaginal delivery. Cochrane Review. Cochrane Library, Issue (2) Update Software 2008, Oxford.

Johanson, R.B., Menon, V., 2000. Soft versus rigid vacuum extractor cups for assisted vaginal delivery. Cochrane Review. Cochrane Library, Issue (2) Update Software 2008, Oxford.

Johanson, R.B., Rice, C., Doyle, M., et al., 1992. A randomised prospective study comparing the new vacuum extractor policy with forceps delivery. Br. J. Obstet. Gynaecol. 100, 524–530.

Lewis, G. (Ed.), 2001. The Confidential Enquiries into Maternal Deaths in the United Kingdom: Why Mothers Die 1997–1999. RCOG, London.

Lewis, G. (Ed.), 2007. Saving Mothers, Lives: The Seventh Report of the Confidential Enquiries into Maternal and Child Health Report 2003–2005. RCOG, London.

Lilford, R., 1990. Maternal mortality and caesarean section. Br. J. Obstet. Gynaecol. 97, 883–892.

Liston, F.A., Allen, V.M., O'Connell, C.M., Jangaard, K.A., 2008. Neonatal outcomes with caesarean delivery at term. Arch. Dis. Child. Fetal Neonat. Ed. 93 (3), F176–F182.

Meakin, S., 2004. Procedures in obstetrics. In: Henderson, C., Macdonald, S. (Eds.) Mayes' Midwifery: A Textbook for Midwifery, thirteenth edn. Baillière Tindall, London.

Rang, H.P., Dale, M.M., Ritter, J.M. (Eds.), et al., 2007. Pharmacology, sixth edn. Churchill Livingstone, Edinburgh.

RCA (Royal College of Anaesthetists), 2004. Guidelines for the Provision of Anaesthetic Services. Royal College of Anaesthetists, London.

RCOG (Royal College of Obstetricians and Gynaecologists), 2005. Operative Vaginal Delivery. Guideline No. 26. RCOG, London.

RCOG Press (Royal College of Anaesthetists, Royal College of Midwives, Royal College of Obstetricians and Gynaecologists, Royal College of Paediatrics and Child Health), 2007. Safer Childbirth: Delivery of Care in Labour. RCOG Press, London.

Suwannachat, B., Lumbiganon, P., Laopaiboon, M., 2007. Rapid versus stepwise negative pressure application for vacuum extraction assisted vaginal delivery (Protocol). Cochrane Review. Cochrane Library, Issue (3) Update Software 2008, Oxford.

Savage, W., 1996. The caesarean section epidemic: a psychological problem?

J. Assoc. Chart. Physiotherapists Women's Health 79, 13–16.

Stephenson, P.A., 1992. International Differences in the Use of Obstetrical Interventions. World Health Organization, Copenhagen WHO (EUR/ICP/MCH):112.

Trevathen, W., 1987. Human Birth: An Evolutionary Perspective. Aldine de Gruyter, New York.

Vacca, A., 1999. Handbook of Vacuum Extraction in Obstetric Practice. Vacca Research, Brisbane.

VHI Healthcare, 2008. Caesarean deliveries more dangerous—study. <http://www.vhi.ie/>, accessed 25/6/08.

WHO (World Health Organization) Appropriate technology for birth, 1985. Lancet ii, 436–437.

Wilkinson, C., Enkin, M.W., 1997. Lateral tilt during caesarean section. Cochrane Database Syst. Rev. (2) Update Software 2008, Oxford.

Annotated recommended reading

Chalmers, B., 1992. WHO, Appropriate technology for birth revisited. Br. J. Obstet. Gynaecol. 99, 709–710.

In this article, Chalmers questions the basis of the WHO's 1985 recommendations (appropriate technology for birth). Do they match up to today's research findings? The documents require critical analysis by both practitioners and decision makers.

Johanson, R.B., Menon, V., 1999. Vacuum extraction versus forceps for assisted vaginal delivery. Cochrane Database Syst. Rev. (2) Update Software 2008, Oxford.

This systematic review on the use of ventouse versus forceps provides useful information for those who perform instrumental deliveries and those responsible for giving advice to women and their partners.

World Health Organization (WHO) Appropriate technology for birth,1985. Lancet ii, 436–437.

As a result of debates at the United Nations of increasing caesarean sections in 1979, the WHO undertook research into perinatal services and developed recommendations for appropriate technology for birth. This document includes the recommendations.

Section **4A**

Puerperium—The Baby as a Neonate

SECTION CONTENTS

Section 4 considers the mother and her baby during the puerperium. Midwives care for mothers and their babies for up to 28 days and it is imperative that they are able to distinguish between normal appearances and behaviours of the mother and her baby and deal responsibly with any deviations present. Section 4A is about the baby. Chapters 48 and 49 provide a detailed account of the adaptation of the fetus to independent extrauterine life. The remaining chapters provide an introduction to some commonly encountered serious disorders that neonates can present with. Chapter 50 is about the care of the low-birth-weight baby, Chapter 51 examines cardiac and respiratory problems, Chapter 52 is concerned with neonatal jaundice and some common metabolic disorders, while Chapter 53 discusses problems arising from infection or trauma. These chapters cannot take the place of a specifically written textbook on neonatal care and the reader is referred to one of the many excellent books available and the papers given within the chapter reference lists.

Adaptation to extrauterine life 1: haematological, cardiovascular, respiratory and genitourinary considerations

Introduction

Chapters 48–53 explore some of the physiological mechanisms fundamental to the adaptation to extrauterine life and highlight common pathophysiological changes that augment adaptation to extrauterine life. Understanding these complex anatomical features and physiological processes provides a foundation for competent assessment of neonates and enables practitioners to draw conclusions about neonatal health. To ensure clarity in the ensuing discussion the masculine pronoun is used to distinguish the neonate from his mother.

This chapter considers many anatomical, physiological and biochemical adaptations that characterise the transition of a term fetus to an independent neonate (birth to 28 days). Throughout intrauterine life, fetal survival is dependent on the mother; however, at birth anatomical, physiological and biochemical changes contribute to independent extrauterine life. Every system contributes to the ever-changing homeostatic conditions crucial to independence. The respiratory and cardiovascular systems are amongst the first to respond and initiate changes leading to a considerable rise in the neonate's blood partial pressure of carbon dioxide (Pco_2). This initiates the respiratory drive that enables the neonate to take the first breath and maintain effective respiration. Blood oxygen content increases and favourable haemodynamic changes support and adjust cardiovascular and respiratory functions, impacting on oxygen perfusion of every organ and system. Oxygen supports cell metabolism and the production of energy whilst metabolic waste, including water, urea, salts and acids, is efficiently eliminated. It is important that health care practitioners caring for mothers and their neonates understand the complex changes that occur at this stage of life.

The appearance of the normal neonate

General appearance and the skin and hair at birth

At 40 weeks gestation the **neonate** (Fig. 48.1) weighs about 3500–4000 g and averages 50–55 cm in length. His occipitofrontal head circumference averages 35 cm making his head almost 25% of total body mass; the

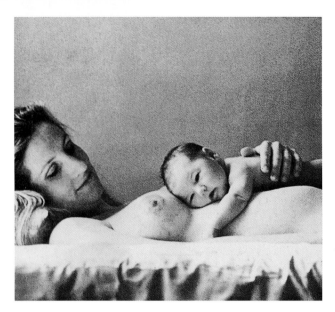

Figure 48.1 • Skin-to-skin contact in a warm labour ward. (Courtesy of Professor J Hedgecoe.)

brain weighs between 300 and 400 g (Collins 2004). A healthy neonate appears plump with a rounded abdomen, largely due to deposition of subcutaneous fat and water. At birth the upper and lower limbs are of a similar length although primary ossification is present only in the upper limbs. Term neonates cannot achieve full elbow extension but flexion up to 145° is possible. They have a strong palmar grasp within a few days of birth. All four limbs should have five separated digits with well-formed nails and well-defined palmar and sole features.

Fine but dishevelled, silky hair covers the scalp. Some neonates appear fairly bald but others have luxuriant straight or curly hair. Abnormally unruly hair on the forehead or the back of the head and neck, especially when accompanied by unusual facies, may imply underlying genetic or chromosomal problems (Avery et al 1999). Remnants of **lanugo**, the fine hair that covers the entire body during the second and third trimesters of pregnancy, may be present on the shoulders, the forehead, in the axilla, the groins and other parts of the body, especially if the neonate is premature. The degree of skin pigmentation is determined by the neonate's gestation as well as the race of his natural parents.

In healthy neonates the skin, mucous membranes and nails should be a good colour, indicating favourable tissue perfusion and oxygenation. Generally, pigmentation of the nipples and genitalia is deeper in neonates with darker skin complexions. A **linea nigra** may be present in the lower abdominal midline and, depending on racial origin, diffuse bluish-black skin colouration known as the **Mongolian blue spot** may be present, usually over the sacrum.

Humans are unique amongst primates in having large **sebaceous glands** which produce **sebum** over the scalp, face and upper back. These glands are very active in utero, producing waxy substances that mix with dead skin cells and form **vernix caseosa**, which initially covers the entire fetal skin. Term neonates only show residual vernix caseosa being present in the groins, the axillae and sometimes the scalp. A few distended sebaceous glands called **milia** may present over the nose, forehead and chin.

Eccrine glands (sweat glands) first appear in fetuses at 5 months of gestation on the palms and the soles of its feet. At the same time, **apocrine glands** (scent glands), used by many mammals for cooling, develop throughout the body. By 7 months the apocrine glands disappear except for in the armpits, pubic area, around the nipples and lips while the eccrine glands continue to spread all over the body. In humans, but no other primates, these glands are used for **sweat cooling** when the body temperature rises above a critical physiological point (Carlton 2003). Although the eccrine glands are inactive for the first few days of life most neonates experience a regional eccrine gland maturation in the craniocaudal direction, with the earliest perspiration occurring on the forehead followed by the chest, upper arms and then the rest of the body (Collins 2004).

Posture and crying

After birth most neonates lie in a flexed position emulating the fetal position and resisting limb extension. Once their arms are extended, neonates show a tendency, possibly by reflex, to move both arms outwards. When placed on their back, there is a distinctive tendency to turn their heads spontaneously to one side, usually the right side, elevating the left shoulder. Conversely, when placed in the prone position neonates tend to draw their knees under their abdomen, elevating their buttocks and turning their head to one side. At term, healthy neonates are active and should move all four limbs spontaneously. These postural phenomena may not be evident in premature neonates due to the structural immaturity of the neural and locomotor systems. Neonates that hold their arm(s) alongside the body in internal rotation may be manifesting Erb–Duchenne paralysis which is caused by damage to the upper root of the brachial plexus involving the 5th and 6th cranial roots.

Crying is a physiological response to hunger, discomfort and distress and serves to alert the mother. The duration and type of crying vary with the severity of the distress (see Ch. 57) and attentive mothers quickly learn to discern between the different types of crying. Overby (2003) suggests that a 2-week-old neonate may cry intermittently on average 2 h per day, increasing these episodes to a total of 3 h per day by 6 weeks of age. From then on most healthy babies are physically more comfortable, more secure, and crying reduces to about 1 h per day.

Eyes

Competent examination of a neonate's eyes requires knowledge, skills and patience. The external appearance of the eyes can reflect racial origins as seen in Oriental neonates. Neonates born with Down syndrome also have **epicanthic folds** (vertical pleats of skin that overlap the medial angles of the eyes), although epicanthic folds are common in other neonates, especially those of Asian origin. It is important to establish the structural features of the eyes and gentle attempts should be made to establish their presence, position, relative size and shape. Gross structural anomalies should be ruled out, and if present must be proactively treated. The colour of the neonate's eyes may be attributed to the poorly defined iris generally appearing dark blue-grey, although some dark-skinned neonates tend to have brown eyes at birth. Permanent colouring of the iris may take several years to develop.

Assessing a neonate's vision by an observed reaction to light is adequate unless significant structural anomalies warrant a fuller assessment. This requires a relatively dark room and a moderately bright beam of light in order to avoid stimulating reflex eye closure. The pupil size of term neonates should be equal, average in diameter within a range of 1.8 mm (when constricted) and 5.4 mm (when dilated). Measurements that fall outside these parameters should be further investigated, especially if a space-occupying lesion is suspected. Assessment of vision is best achieved when the neonate is content but alert, although neonates startle in response to a bright light even if their eyelids are closed, indicating that the optic pathways are functioning (Avery et al 1999).

Neonates cannot generally produce tears, which provide a natural lubricant and antiseptic for the eyes. This contributes to a higher incidence of eye infections such as conjunctivitis, often further complicated by temporary blockage of the lacrimal ducts, which under normal conditions help to keep the conjunctiva moist and clean. Avery et al (1999) advocate that any symptoms of tearing or persistent discharge from the eyes appearing after the 2nd day after birth should be investigated to exclude unsuspected lesions, abrasions, glaucoma and congenital or acquired infection.

Ears

A considerable range of factors, including the amounts of cartilage and activity of the auricular muscles, determine the shape, position and resistance to deformation of the external ears. Both ears should be placed symmetrically on either side of head. The position of the ear lobes generally approximates with the vertical distance from the arch of the brow to the lower parts of the nose (Avery et al 1999). Preauricular pits and skin appendages are fairly common (Carlton 2003) but more significant malformations, low-set ears and other dysmorphic features tend to be associated with urogenital malformations, deafness and autosomal dominant problems. Alert neonates with normal auditory capability generally react to a ringing bell, are startled or cry in response to sudden, unaccustomed loud noise and turn spontaneously towards human speech. The absence of such behaviours requires more systematic audiometry assessments.

Nose

Most neonates are obligate nose-breathers and their respiratory function depends on the patency of both nares. Nasal deformities and nasolacrimal duct obstructions should be ruled out. Although unilateral or bilateral anatomical obstructions caused by choanal atresia are rare these must be ruled out, especially in neonates who develop respiratory difficulties and cyanosis soon after birth.

Mouth and throat

The shape of the mouth and oral cavity is partly determined by neuromotor activity that occurs during fetal life. The tongue, buccal surfaces, palate, uvula and posterior aspects of the oral cavity should be inspected visually but the gum and hard palate are best examined by gentle finger palpation. Healthy neonates should have a gag reflex and usually suckle vigorously on a finger. In some neonates the tongue may be attached to a short central frenulum but this anomaly rarely interferes with feeding or later speech development. The presence of facial asymmetries on feeding or crying may suggest facial nerve paresis.

Neck and chest

Mature neonates have a full range of spontaneous neck movements although the neck is short and the muscles are incapable of supporting the weight of the head. The absence of, or abnormalities in, spontaneous movements may indicate cervical spine abnormalities or the presence of space-occupying lesions such as goitre or cystic hygromas which may compress and distort the central position of the trachea causing inspiratory obstruction. Neck trauma occurring at birth where the cervical nerves are damaged may lead to the neonate developing Horner's syndrome. In instances where the phrenic nerve(s) is damaged the neonate will develop corresponding paralysis of the diaphragm with respiratory difficulties. The chest at term should be symmetrical, barrel-shaped with a prominent xiphoid sternum and compliant ribs. The chest circumference is generally 1–2 cm less than the head circumference. The neonate's lung sounds are more tubular than vesicular due to better sound transmission from the large airways across the small chest.

Major systemic characteristics of the neonate

The haematological system

Circulatory volume

The separation of the fetus from the placental circulation following birth is a major physiological event. The **umbilical arteries** taking deoxygenated blood from fetus to placenta for oxygenation constrict whilst the umbilical vein remains dilated limiting fetal blood loss. Fetal–placental blood volume varies from 110 to 120 ml/kg (Padbury 2003) throughout the latter parts of pregnancy, although approximately 80 ml/kg of this blood is probably in the neonate. At delivery, if the umbilical cord is cut immediately or there is low intrauterine pressure or the neonate is held above the uterus, placental transfusion does not occur. However, Padbury (2003) suggests that within 5–15 s of delivery 5–15 ml/kg of placental blood may be transfused with the uterine contraction that initiates the 3rd stage of labour. If umbilical cord clamping is delayed for 60–90 s or the neonate is held below the uterus, more than 25–30 ml/kg of placental blood is transfused to the neonate. Conversely, neonates held more than 50 cm above the introitus may receive negligible amounts of placental blood and it is conceivable that small amounts of neonatal blood could transfuse into the placenta. Clamping of the umbilical cord, which stops all blood flow (Fig. 48.2) is an important haemodynamic step for the neonate.

Early versus late clamping of the umbilical cord

There are associated advantages and disadvantages. In general the umbilical cord is clamped early to avert systemic difficulties especially seen in premature neonates whose cardiovascular and respiratory systems are less well equipped to deal with additional volumes, high erythrocyte values and subsequent **hyperbilirubinaemia.** As any increase in plasma volume expands the vascular compartment, especially in the immature lungs, transfusion of 80 ml of placental blood may pose a significant risk to the neonate.

Controversially, some evidence suggests that late clamping of the umbilical cord (30 s following birth) may be beneficial in some premature neonates. The ensuing increase in circulating blood volume may improve cardiac output, enhance oxygen transportation, support renal perfusion and maintain acid–base balance. However, such practices should generally be avoided in neonates who are born with a history of **hydrops fetalis** or **rhesus isoimmunisation** (see Ch. 52) and those at risk of developing polycythaemia because of **cyanotic heart disease** (see Ch. 51). Caution should also be exercised in neonates born with **severe systemic immaturity** caused by maternal diabetes mellitus (see Ch. 50). Finally, in multiple births, the cord of the first-born neonate should be clamped **early** to prevent blood loss from the unborn fetus to the newborn sibling through any communicating placental circulation.

Adaptations in the neonate's haematological parameters

Circulating blood volume at term averages 85–90 ml/kg of body weight (Padbury 2003). Haemopoiesis proceeds at a relatively steady pace ensuring that all cell types remain in circulation within narrow limits. Haemopoiesis is highly responsive, with a unique capacity to up-regulate or down-regulate the production of any cell type on demand. This responsiveness is also crucial in ensuring that the transition in the composition of the neonate's blood is successful. Changes continue to occur during the transitional period of the 1st week of life

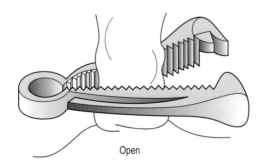
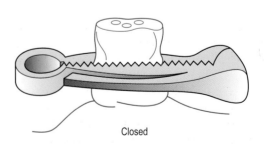

Open   Closed

Figure 48.2 • A cord clamp. (From Henderson C, Macdonald S 2004, with kind permission of Elsevier.)

when the type and quantities of haemoglobin change, with fetal haemoglobin being gradually replaced by adult haemoglobin more suited to extrauterine life.

The complex microanatomical and physiological processes that regulate haemopoiesis lead to equilibrium between cell production, maturation, function and biodegradation. The neonate's blood cells gradually change from their fetal state to that of the child in whom mature **erythrocytes** function for 120 days, **platelets** for 10 days and **neutrophils** for 6–8 h. Genetic, epigenetic and a range of physiological variables influence the differentiation of the red bone marrow's pleuripotent stem cells into mature blood (Pocock & Richards 2006). These include haemopoietic growth factors, such as granulocyte colony-stimulating factor (**G-CSF**), granulocyte–macrophage colony-stimulating factor (**GM-CSF**), **interleukin 6** (IL-6) and **interleukin 8** (IL-8). For example, **GM-CSF** stimulates myeloid progenitor cell cycling, clonal development of neutrophils and enhances neutrophil function as phagocytic cells (see Ch. 29).

The erythrocyte count at birth averages 5.3×10^{-6}, generating a mean packed cell volume of 56% and a haemoglobin of 18.5 g/dl (Avery et al 1999). As many of these erythrocytes are nucleate or contain fetal haemoglobin they are fairly rapidly biodegraded by the reticuloendothelial system and it is unusual to find nucleated erythrocytes in circulation after the first week of extrauterine life. The earliest erythrocytes are **normoblasts**, which differentiate into **reticulocytes** and subsequently mature into erythrocytes containing predominantly adult haemoglobin (HbA).

The maturation of precursor cells into competent erythrocytes is controlled by a vast range of factors including **erythropoietin**, which is produced in the liver during fetal life and the kidneys after birth. Erythropoietin binds to specific receptor sites found in the membrane of myelocytic cells and erythroblasts, accelerating their differentiation and maturation respectively, by mechanisms that are not fully understood (Pocock & Richards 2006). Normal erythropoiesis also depends on the presence of iron, vitamin C and the vitamin B group.

The relative increase in erythrocytes due to **plasma reduction** and **haemoconcentration** which occurs in the first few hours/days of life is a transitional phenomenon, corrected by the rapid destruction of excess erythrocytes which occurs following birth. A more physiological erythrocyte count is achieved by 6 months (Pearson 2003). Nucleated, immature erythrocytes are seen in large numbers during the first 24 h following birth, possibly due to stressors associated with birth, but these usually disappear within 4 days. Significantly, the fetal blood erythropoietin values observed during intrauterine life fall within the first 24 h, but gradually return to physiological values during the first 2–3 months

after birth. This coincides with the steady resumption of erythropoiesis. Erythrocytes are more specialised in composition than most other cells because of the presence of haemoglobin, which accounts for 95% of total cellular protein content.

Cord blood haemoglobin content varies with gestational age but broad parameters are suggested by Avery et al (1999). In healthy mature neonates haemoglobin averages 16.5–18.5 g/dl. This may increase by a further 6 g/dl over the first 24 h due to a shift in fluid distribution, associated diuresis, reduction in circulating blood volume and haemoconcentration. There is a gradual reduction in haemoglobin (HbF) concentration back to umbilical cord blood values by the end of the 1st week of life. By 3 months, the haemoglobin level in healthy infants tends to fall to 12 g/dl (Pearson 2003) which contrasts sharply with the varied cord blood haemoglobin content shown in the following résumé:

- Fetal haemoglobin (HbF): 50–85%.
- Adult haemoglobin (HbA): 15–40%.
- Haemoglobin A_2 (HbA$_2$): <2%.

As new erythrocytes are produced the rate of HbF production is reduced and the rate of HbA production increases so that at 4 months of age the average healthy child has less than 20% of HbF.

A primary function of haemoglobin is to combine reversibly with oxygen and carbon dioxide, thereby allowing the delivery of oxygen from the lungs to the tissues to support cellular metabolism. This function is best demonstrated by the oxygen dissociation curve, whereby the oxygen saturation of the blood is plotted against oxygen tension or partial pressure of the whole blood (Pocock & Richards 2006). Due to the high concentration of HbF in healthy neonates, the oxygen dissociation curve is placed firmly to the left, denoting high affinity of HbF for oxygen. This phenomenon is necessary for efficient extraction of oxygen from the maternal circulation during fetal life; however, after birth, HbF whilst capable of extracting large quantities of oxygen in the lungs releases oxygen to the tissues only as needed.

Affinity of HbF and HbA to oxygen is influenced by pH, P_{CO_2}, 2,3-diphosphoglycerate (2,3-DPG) and blood temperature. After birth the shift in the **oxygen dissociation curve** to the right is partly attributable to organic phosphates which decrease the affinity of HbA to oxygen by competing for the same binding sites.

2,3-DPG is formed during anaerobic glycolysis (mature erythrocytes lack mitochondria and their glucose metabolism is anaerobic) and enhances the release of oxygen from haemoglobin. HbF has a lower affinity for 2,3-DPG than HbA and is able to bind oxygen more tenaciously. This accounts for the shift of the oxygen dissociation curve to the left in the fetus and neonate. Finally, the postnatal shift of the oxygen dissociation curve to the right is directly attributable to the gradual replacement of HbF by HbA which has a lower affinity for oxygen and greater capacity for oxygen to dissociate, thus enhancing oxygen release to the tissues (Marieb 2008).

White blood cells (WBCs) defend the body against genetically different antigens (see Ch. 29). At birth most neonates show an initial increase in the number of circulating white blood cells, possibly due to their displacement from other sites provoked by the stress of birth. However, gradual reduction in these cells brings about normal WBC values by the 5th day after birth. The two main functions of WBCs are **phagocytosis** and **competent immune response** (see Ch 29). In neonates neutrophils make up approximately 50% and lymphocytes about 30% of the total WBCs. However, the proportion of lymphocytes increases rapidly within the first few months to an average of 60%, and this value persists for the first 2 years of life. Monocytes are the most abundant cells in the first few weeks of extrauterine life but gradually decline to the much lower adult value.

Theorists who attempt to explain neonates' susceptibility to topical and systemic infections consider the variations in WBC differentials relative to the immaturity of the immune system. A range of structural, and biochemical, differences exist in the immature neutrophils and lymphocytes which may contribute to their less effective response to infection. For instance, cell immaturity may interfere with intracellular signal transduction, or hinder cell mobility as a consequence of cytoskeletal rigidity and poor microfilament contraction. These factors could also affect neutrophil migration from capillary blood into the surrounding tissue which may compromise tissue healing following injury.

Haemostasis (see Ch. 16) depends on the interaction between injured vessels, **platelets** and a group of **clot-promoting factors (coagulation system)**. However, neonates are most likely considered to be at risk of spontaneous bleeding between the 3rd and 6th days of life due to the relative deficiency of **vitamin K** (Box 48.1), which amongst other functions plays important roles in the synthesis of important clotting factors within the

BOX 48.1 VITAMIN K AND HAEMORRHAGIC DISEASE OF THE NEWBORN

The reduction of vitamin K and clotting factors results from poor placental transfer of vitamin K to the fetus and the absence of appropriate fetal intestinal flora. There is a further decline in these factors over the first few days following birth, particularly in breastfed babies, as breast milk contains very low levels of vitamin K. However, colostrum and hind milk contain high concentrations of vitamin K and mothers should feed this kind of milk to their neonate. The content of vitamin K in cow's milk and formula milk is greater than in human breast milk (Enkin et al 2000). Breastfed babies may eventually develop prolonged prothrombin deficiency which could contribute to haemorrhagic disease of the newborn which occurs in 0.4–1.7% of all babies in the 1st week of life (Merenstein et al 1993). However, many early studies were carried out when breastfeeding practices were restricted and neonates did not always receive as much colostrum and hind milk due to supplementary milk feeding, thus the above evidence may not be fully dependable without further systematic reviews.

The awareness of some of the benefits of vitamin K has resulted in its prophylactic administration (since the 1950s) to neonates at risk of spontaneous haemorrhage, especially within the gastrointestinal tract, resulting in **haematemesis** and the passage of **melaena stools**. Bleed from the umbilical cord and the more serious risk of **intracranial**

haemorrhage in susceptible premature and hypoxic neonates must also be guarded against.

The British Paediatric Association recommended that oral vitamin K 0.5 mg was given with a repeat dose at 8 days. However, by 1993 there was evidence that late **haemorrhagic disease** was occurring in neonates who had been given oral vitamin K. Giving premature babies and others at risk of haemorrhage, intramuscular or intravenous vitamin K 0.5–1 mg was considered and those with haemorrhagic disease could be given Konakion (vitamin K_1 or phytomenadione) 1 mg intravenously. Most paediatricians recommended giving 0.5–1 mg vitamin K to all neonates at birth, as it is difficult to predict which are likely to be at risk of developing systemic or multisystemic haemorrhage. Enkin et al (2000) recommend giving vitamin K to all babies that are breastfed until further research is carried out. If bleeding is severe, **fresh** blood transfusion may be necessary, but normal coagulation mechanisms must be established to limit the severity of bleeding and other pathophysiological events.

Golding et al (1992) suggested a link between the intramuscular administration of vitamin K and childhood cancer although this was not substantiated by Hull (1992) nor did the American Academy of Pediatrics find a correlation between the administration

BOX 48.1 (CONTINUED)

of prophylactic vitamin K and any increase in the incidence of childhood leukaemia (Ekelund et al 1993, Merenstein et al 1993, Rudolph et al 2003).

Administration of vitamin K to mothers

Nishiguchi et al (1996) examined three strategies for prevention of vitamin K deficiency in neonates:

1. Routine oral prophylaxis at birth.
2. Additional vitamin K for breastfeeding mothers as well as routine oral prophylaxis.
3. Screening and treatment of babies at greatest risk.

They found that giving babies two doses of oral vitamin K did not totally abolish the risk of haemorrhagic disease. In the group where the mothers took a 15 mg capsule of vitamin K daily for 2 weeks starting 2 weeks following delivery, no babies were found to be vitamin K-deficient. However, Crowther & Henderson-Smart (2000) reviewed five trials and found no evidence that vitamin K administered to expectant mothers prior to preterm birth prevented neonatal periventricular

haemorrhage. Because there was no link found between vitamin K and childhood leukaemia and the inadequacy of oral administration, Puckett & Offringa (2000) reinforced the earlier recommendation of the use of intramuscular vitamin K.

Arguments against the policy

The need for the prophylactic administration of vitamin K for all neonates has been questioned. Some studies suggest that the neonate is not vitamin K-deficient and that concentrations of vitamin K-dependent factors do not always increase after the administration of vitamin K. In particular, the route of administration has come under scrutiny. To assess the vitamin status in neonates against that observed in the adult norm may be inappropriate. Furthermore, in evolutionary terms, to suggest that an entire group of a given population is disadvantaged could be misleading and yet this is what the policy for the prophylactic use of vitamin K does. Clearly, there is a need for a long-term clinical trial and review of the empirical evidence about the prophylactic administration of vitamin K to all neonates.

---

liver. Vitamin K is often administered to neonates at birth. However, as a constant supply of vitamin K is required, milk feeding is the best means of colonising the neonate's sterile gastrointestinal tract by bacteria capable of synthesising it. It is worth noting that, when the neonate requires treatment with broad-spectrum antimicrobials, the vitamin K-producing bacteria may be destroyed, leaving the neonate with low vitamin K and increased risk of bleeding.

Mature **platelets** (see Ch. 16) are complex fragments of megakaryocytes released into circulation when required to support normal coagulation. Platelets enjoy a life span of 10 days when structurally intact. The platelet surface properties as well as their internal constituents play crucial roles in haemostasis. Platelet counts in adults range between 150 and 400×10^9/L and, although term neonates show similar values, premature neonates frequently have lower values (Avery et al 1999). Furthermore, the release of stored substances enhancing the clotting cascade may be reduced, further compromising the neonate's ability to form indissolvable clots in injured blood vessels. For instance, the lack of vitamin K reduces **prothrombin** values, and clotting factors such as **factors VII, IX and X**. Neonatal fibrinogen levels are similar to those of adults so it is important that an effective fibrinolytic system exists to limit blood clot formation either at any vessel injury or within intact blood vessels. To achieve a balance between clot formation and fibrinolysis the fibrinolytic

system is activated simultaneously with the coagulation system (Manco-Johnson 2003).

The cardiovascular system

The fundamentals of fetal circulation

Successful transition from fetal to extrauterine life is dependent on gradual adaptation of the **fetal circulation** (Fig. 48.3) to the anatomical configuration that characterises the adult cardiovascular system (Fig. 48.4). Under normal conditions, immediate changes take place within the first 60 s although full cardiovascular transformation can take up to several weeks or months. The neonate's first breath followed by sustained spontaneous respiration contributes to the successful transition by ensuring that the lungs hold sufficient oxygenated air required to support pulmonary gas exchange. However, as fetal circulation differs significantly from that of the older child or adult, several anatomical modifications need to be made closing specific cardiovascular structures and establishing a dual circulatory network capable of supporting the uniqueness of the pulmonary and systemic circulation.

The blood vessels that transport blood between the fetus and placenta are:

1. The ductus venosus.
2. Two hypogastric arteries.

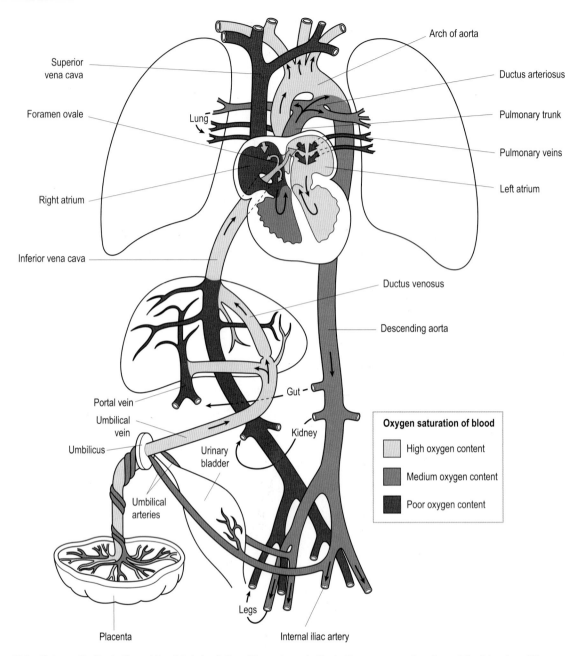

Figure 48.3 • Schematic illustration of the fetal circulation. The colours indicate the oxygen saturation of the blood and the arrows show the course of the blood from the placenta to the heart. The organs are not drawn to scale. Observe that three shunts permit most of the blood to bypass the liver and lungs: ductus venosus, foramen ovale, and ductus arteriosus. The poorly oxygenated blood returns to the placenta for oxygen and nutrients through the umbilical arteries. (Reproduced with permission from Moore 1989.)

Right-to-left shunts that allow 90% of blood flow to bypass the lungs are created by:

3. The **ductus arteriosus**, which is located between the pulmonary artery and aorta.

4. The **foramen ovale**, which is located in the membranous septum that divides the right and left atria.

The ductus venosus lies between the layers of the lesser omentum in a groove between the left and caudate lobes of the liver (Collins 2004). It connects the umbilical vein to the left hepatic vein or the inferior vena cava. Obliteration of this vessel is gradual, initiated in the 2nd week following birth at the portal vein end and moves gradually towards the vena cava. Its lumen tends to be completely closed by the 2nd or 3rd month. The hypogastric arteries branch off from the internal iliac arteries, enter the umbilical cord and become the umbilical arteries. The ductus arteriosus leads from the bifurcation of the pulmonary arteries to the aortic arch, entering it just after the exit of the subclavian

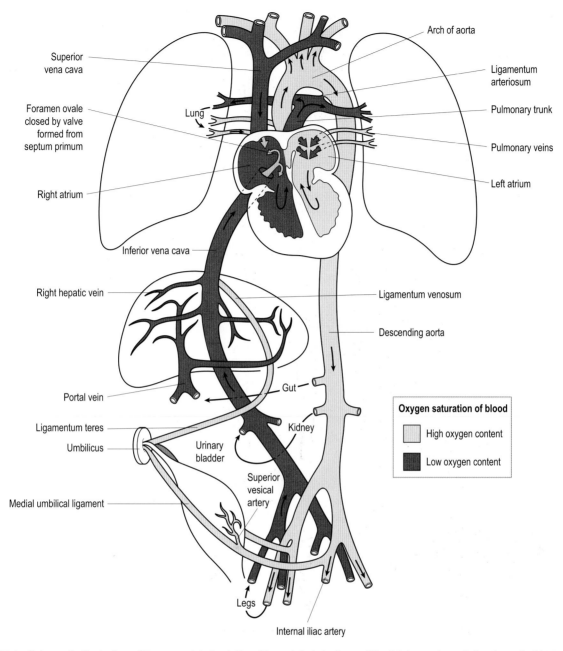

Figure 48.4 • Schematic illustration of the neonatal circulation. The adult derivatives of the fetal vessels and structures that become non-functional at birth are also shown. The arrows indicate the course of the blood in the infant. The organs are not drawn to scale. After birth, the three shunts that short-circuited the blood during fetal life cease to function and the pulmonary and systemic circulations become separated. (Reproduced with permission from Moore 1989.)

and carotid arteries. The membranous foramen ovale is about 4–6 mm in length and 3–4 mm in width (Collins 2004), located within the atrial septum and diverts blood away from the lungs during intrauterine life.

The path taken by the fetal blood flow, referred to as the fetal circulation, begins at the placenta. The sequence of events are best understood by reading the following résumé and referring to Fig. 48.3:

- Oxygenated blood flows from the placenta to the fetus via a single umbilical vein.

- Some of this blood enters the liver directly reaching the inferior vena cava via the hepatic veins. A considerable amount of blood circulates through the liver with the portal venous blood before also entering the hepatic veins.

- Blood from the ductus venosus and hepatic veins mixes in the inferior vena cava with the deoxygenated blood returning from the lower limbs and abdominal wall. This reduces the oxygen content of the blood contained in the upper parts of the inferior vena cava.

- As the inferior vena cava enters the heart, its position is aligned with the foramen ovale. The free edge of the atrial septum (the crista dividens) separates the blood flow into two streams. Most of this blood passes from the right atrium through the foramen ovale to the left atrium, creating a right-to-left shunt. From the left atrium the blood flows to the left ventricle and then to the aorta which distributes the oxygenated blood to the head, trunk and limbs.

- Significant amounts of the right atrial blood pass through the tricuspid valve into the right ventricle. This engagement of the right ventricle contributes to the morphological development of the ventricle, the pulmonary artery and their respective valves, and ensures that the pulmonary artery directs a small quantity (10%) of oxygenated blood to the lung tissue. The remaining 90% of this blood is directed into the aorta via the second right-to-left shunt, the ductus arteriosus found between the pulmonary artery and aorta. As oxygenated and deoxygenated blood mix along the different sections of the fetal circulation, the upper part of the descending aorta carries mixed oxygenated blood which is distributed via the iliac arteries to the lower limbs and some abdominal and pelvic organs.

- Deoxygenated blood from the head and neck returns to the right atrium via the superior vena cava. Here this stream of blood crosses the stream of blood coming from the inferior vena cava en route to the right ventricle, thus reducing the oxygen content of that blood even further. The two streams in the right atrium remain separate due to the atrial shape although there is some mixing of about 25% of the blood allowing oxygen and nutrients to be taken to the lungs.

- By the time the circulating blood enters the internal iliac arteries its oxygen content is significantly reduced as it returns to the placenta via the two umbilical arteries for reoxygenation, uptake of nutrients and elimination of metabolic waste products. Fetal metabolic waste such as potassium, urea, uric acid and water are removed via the placental circulation into the maternal circulation and then eliminated via the mother's kidneys.

Résumé of cardiovascular and haemodynamic changes at birth

Some of the unique features of the fetal circulation must adapt at birth, or shortly thereafter if the neonate is to survive independently. This adaptation to extrauterine life depends largely on the interplay between the cardiovascular and respiratory systems:

- The separation of the neonate from the placental circulation results in the cessation of blood flow which contributes to the collapse of the umbilical vein and arteries. The ductus venosus and the hypogastric arteries gradually fibrose giving rise to supporting ligaments.

- The resulting reduction in blood flow to the right atrium causes a fall in the right atrial pressure. As blood flow through the hypogastric arteries ceases, a significant volume of blood is contained in smaller systemic compartments which increases systemic vascular resistance (SVR) and improves venous and arterial returns to the heart and lungs. As larger quantities of blood are returned from the lungs to the left atrium via the pulmonary veins, the left atrial pressure rises closing the foramen ovale.

- The initial equalising of pressures in the two atria holds the flap of the foramen ovale in position stopping the shunting of blood from the right-to-left atrium. However, the foramen ovale can reopen and remain patent for a few days or weeks, especially if left atrial pressure falls.

- As the baby takes his first breath, the lungs expand and oxygenated air is inspired. This displaces the pulmonary fluid further and triggers mechanisms essential to effective respiration and pulmonary gas exchange. Oxygen content of the blood increases, causing vasodilation in the pulmonary vascular bed. As a consequence the pulmonary vascular resistance (PVR) falls by 80%, dramatically increasing pulmonary blood flow.

- At the same time the amount of blood being shunted via the ductus arteriosus decreases and, as oxygen tension in the blood rises, the oxygen-sensitive fibromuscular tissue in this ductus constricts, eventually closing this short vessel. In some neonates the patency of the ductus arteriosus may persist for a few days or weeks, especially in premature infants and those born with cardiovascular and respiratory anomalies.

The obsolete structures reform and serve as ligaments in the following manner:

- The umbilical vein becomes the ligamentum teres.
- The ductus venosus becomes the ligamentum venosum.
- The ductus arteriosus becomes the ligamentum arteriosum.
- The foramen ovale becomes the fossa ovalis.
- The hypogastric arteries are known as the obliterated hypogastric arteries.

A small number of infants with unresolved respiratory or cardiac disorders (Box 48.2) will experience various degrees of persistent fetal circulation that will require careful diagnostic and therapeutic interventions.

It is now appreciated that neonates should undergo thorough cardiovascular assessment in conjunction with the Apgar score. At birth most neonates will manifest heart murmurs although these may disappear within 12 h.

BOX 48.2 PERSISTENT FETAL CIRCULATION

When the neonate presents with respiratory or cardiac disorders, frequently accompanied by hypoxia and acidosis, a modified form of fetal circulation may persist. The ductus arteriosus remains patent, and in some circumstances the neonate may experience a reversal of the earlier cardiovascular and pulmonary changes (Rudolph et al 2003). This exacerbates the problem of hypoxia as deoxygenated blood from the right side of the heart is able to mix with the oxygenated blood returning from the lungs to the left side of the heart. The resulting reduction in oxygen tension relaxes the fibromuscular tissue of the ductus arteriosus and interferes with its normal closure.

Throughout fetal life the patency of the ductus arteriosus is maintained by high circulating levels of prostaglandins such as PGE_2 and local release of prostacyclins such as PGI_2. Therefore, when the closure of the ductus arteriosus is compromised, prostaglandin synthetase inhibitors such as indometacin may be used to facilitate its closure pharmacologically. Indometacin may reduce urinary output and it may be necessary to administer furosemide (frusemide) to ensure renal tissue perfusion and urine formation (Avery et al 1999). If the pharmacological method fails, mechanical or surgical intervention may eventually be necessary.

The heart rate varies between 110 and 160 beats/min and blood pressure may average at 80/40 mmHg (Padbury 2003). Most neonates experience a gradual reduction in heart rate and increase in blood pressure within the first few days following birth.

The respiratory system

At term, the acinar portion of the fetal lung is well developed and more than 25% of **true alveoli** are present (Fig. 48.5). However, as the pulmonary blood vessels are quite narrow, only a small amount of blood perfuses the lungs. This is adequate for meeting the metabolic needs of pulmonary tissue because the fetus obtains oxygen and excretes carbon dioxide via the placenta and maternal circulation; the fetal lungs are not required for gas exchange. At term, the lungs hold about 25 ml/kg of **pulmonary fluid**, which is partially expelled when the chest is compressed during vaginal delivery. The remaining fluid is absorbed by the lymphatic and pulmonary vessels and returned into the cardiovascular system. The fetus exercises its muscles of respiration, particularly the diaphragm, by making irregular fetal breathing movements. This activity may encourage muscle development to prepare for independent respiration.

Surfactant

From about 32 weeks gestation, increasing amounts of **surfactant,** produced by alveolar type II pneumocytes, prepare the lungs for effective gas exchange after birth. Surfactant is composed of a number of **phospholipids** and specialised **protein molecules** (Fig. 48.6). After the successful first breath, these jointly reduce the **surface tension** of the alveolar fluid, thin out the alveolar membrane and increase the surface area for gas exchange.

Glucocorticoids and thyroid hormones regulate the synthesis of surfactant in late fetal life (Smith & Sabry 1983). A **platelet-activating factor** (PAF) stimulates the production of the phospholipids by triggering enzyme activities within the type II pneumocytes (Andreeva et al 2007). At term, surfactant forms a monolayer lining within the alveoli which acts as an air–liquid interface, reducing the surface tension within the terminal alveolar sacs (imagine blowing a soap bubble). This facilitates inspiration and prevents the alveoli from collapsing with each expiration.

Onset of respirations

Most neonates gasp within the first few seconds of birth and establish regular respiration within minutes. It is important that this adaptation happens without delay to support the body's cellular metabolic needs by providing oxygen and removing carbon dioxide. The **respiratory centre** in the medulla oblongata matches respiratory effort to metabolic needs. **Chemoreceptors** and **stretch reflexes** influence the medulla oblongata's contribution to respiration although the neonate's response to chemoreceptor stimulus is generally weak.

During birth a reduction in blood oxygen values **(physiological hypoxia)** accompanied by a simultaneous accumulation of carbon dioxide **(physiological hypercarbia)** establishes a new respiratory drive within the medulla oblongata capable of sustaining successful pulmonary ventilation. Furthermore, the gradual elimination of the pulmonary fluid combined with the expansion of the pulmonary vascular bed and the elastic recoil of the respiratory muscles and the rib cage generates a negative pressure of up to 9.8 kPa, which assists in the taking of the first breath and subsequent sustained respiratory function (Michie 1999). At the first inspiration

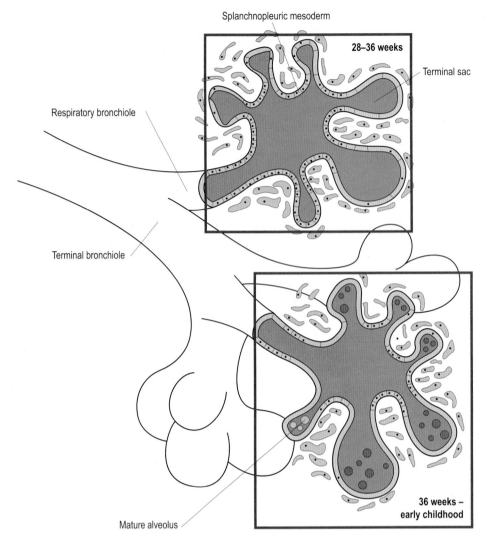

Figure 48.5 • Maturation of the lung tissue. Terminal sacs (primitive alveoli) begin to form between weeks 28 and 36 and begin to mature between 36 weeks and birth. Only 5–20% of all terminal sacs produced by the age of 8 years, however, are formed prior to birth. (Reproduced with permission from Larsen 1993.)

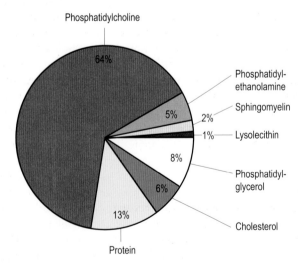

Figure 48.6 • Composition of pulmonary surfactant. (Reproduced with permission from Blackburn & Loper 1992.)

the diaphragm contracts strongly and the compliant ribs and sternum are pulled into a concave shape, but subsequent breaths require much less active work. The factors that initiate the first breath and lung expansion are:

- Compression of the chest wall during vaginal delivery and the recoil of the chest wall immediately after birth.
- Chemoreceptor stimulation by the reduction in oxygen and increase in carbon dioxide in the blood.
- Sensory stimuli on the skin, such as touch, pressure and low environmental temperature.
- Stimulation of the senses by light, noise and touch.

Neonatal respiratory rate averages 50 breaths/min although in healthy neonates this falls to 40 breaths/min. The initial high respiratory rate may result from increased activities within the excitatory respiratory neural synapses which increase respiratory motor activity (Avery et al 1999).

However, neonatal respiration is characteristically **irregular** with short periods of **apnoea**, and involves the abdominal muscles. Although initially inspiration and expiration are energy-dependent once established, the control of respiratory effort is thought to be similar to that in older children. However, the inspiratory and expiratory time ratios in neonates and infants average 1:1; i.e. the inspiration phase equals the expiratory phase.

Inflation of a normal lung in a term neonate is completed within the first few breaths and most alveoli are expanded within the first few hours, establishing a lung volume of approximately 25 ml/kg body weight. The rhythmic inflation of the lungs encourages the **intra-alveolar fluid** to move into the peribronchial and perivascular spaces from which the pulmonary fluid is absorbed into the local blood and lymph vessels and sent to the heart. Delays in the removal of this fluid interfere with the efficiency of respiratory gas transfer, compromise lung compliance and functional residual capacity and eventually cause significant cardiorespiratory distress, especially in immature neonates.

The urinary system

Neonatal kidneys differ from that of the older child in both **glomerular** and **tubular function** and its lobular appearance is different to the mature kidney. By 35 weeks gestation the fetal kidney has a full complement of **nephrons**, although these may be shorter and not as functionally mature. The **cortex** is morphologically more mature than the **medulla** by the end of the 36th week of gestation and at this time **nephrogenesis** is believed to cease, with each kidney having a complement of between 850 000 and 1 000 000 nephrons (Rudolph et al 2003). In premature babies nephrogenesis appears to continue for a variable period of time.

Postnatal development of the kidneys

At birth the kidneys are lobulated, rounded in shape, but capable of responding rapidly to haemodynamic changes and to endogenous and exogenous stressors. The clamping of the umbilical cord is one signal that increases renal function and the kidneys take over the control of fluid, electrolyte, acid–base balance and the excretion of metabolic wastes. From a value of 10 ml/min/m^2 in term neonates, **glomerular filtration rate** (GFR) doubles during the neonate's first 2 weeks. The GFR is lower in very premature neonates, but is gradually corrected as the glomeruli mature.

Although clamping of the umbilical cord is fundamental, the most likely factors enhancing renal maturation and function are the haemodynamic changes occurring at birth (Collins 2004). These culminate in a decrease in **renal vascular resistance** and a corresponding increase in **systemic blood pressure**, so improving filtration pressure. **Vasoactive substances** such as prostaglandins and prostacyclins also help to mediate the renal haemodynamic changes and facilitate renal blood flow to enhance GFR.

Renal growth in early infancy depends on hypertrophy of existing microstructures within the pyramids. Kidney size correlates well with age and somatic growth but the rate of glomerular growth varies and immature glomeruli may be present for months after birth, especially in premature neonates (Collins 2004). Development of the lobulated kidneys proceeds from the corticomedullary junction out towards the periphery in a **centrifugal pattern** (Brenner & Rector 1991). This contributes to a process of budding from the ends of the collecting ducts to ensure that new nephrons are added to the outermost parts of the kidney. Recently formed nephrons are fitted into the developing cortical matrix which eventually reshapes the external surface of the kidneys.

Neonatal renal physiology

Neonatal tubular functions are either effective at birth or mature rapidly to lower urinary osmolality and regulation of acid–base balance within acceptable values. Mechanisms involved in blood pressure control such as the **renin–angiotensin system** are very active at birth, possibly due to stimulation by excessive fetal **catecholamines** produced in response to the stress of birth. As catecholamines enhance cardiac output and renal blood flow it is likely that these enhance renal function. Another variable that may enhance renal function is the kidneys' capability to consume 7% of the total body oxygen.

Rapid renal growth ensures a functional relationship between the glomeruli and the nephrons. The average glomerular size of 100 μm, present at birth, increases to 300 μm. This is important for the transport and processing of vast amounts of solutes and water. In most neonates tubular thresholds for the absorption of some solutes are lower, which can result in unwanted loss of sodium, glucose and other solutes in the urine. Although both full-term and premature neonates can excrete normal quantities of acid and bases via their kidneys their reserve to cope with acidosis is limited. A lower corticomedullary gradient may contribute to limited excretion of urea and haphazard sodium chloride transport mechanisms in the **loop of Henle**. However, neonates maintain a reasonable plasma sodium balance by the 3rd day. The blunted response to sodium loading may be attributed to a high concentration of circulating aldosterone, which falls only gradually, in conjunction with similar decreases in renin and angiotensin, after the 1st week of life. Whilst the tubules are sensitive to

antidiuretic hormone, which facilitates absorption of water thereby preventing life-threatening diuresis, the neonate's ability to dilute or concentrate urine is limited compared to that of older children, possibly due to the lower corticomedullary gradient and immature long loops of Henle. This may adversely affect the neonate's ability to excrete drugs such as gentamicin efficiently.

The urinary bladder and micturition

The bladder in neonates is fusiform (cigar-shaped) or egg-shaped (Collins 2004) rather than pyramidal as in older children. It is situated almost entirely in the abdominal cavity and when full its apex extends to the umbilicus. The bladder descends gradually, locating in the pelvic cavity when the child is about 6 years old. This is accompanied by lengthening of the ureters, extending the distance to the kidneys. In neonates the bladder empties by reflex action and any distension will increase the intra-abdominal pressure and may exacerbate respiratory difficulties.

Most term neonates pass urine at or shortly after birth although this may pass unobserved and unrecorded. The use of magnesium sulphate to control eclampsia or lidocaine (lignocaine) to induce epidural analgesia may delay the neonate's ability to void. Some delays may occur in premature neonates and those who experience perinatal asphyxia or severe stress. The neonate's overall haemodynamics, state of hydration/nutrition, cardiac output and renal perfusion must always be considered in evaluating urinary output. Term neonates excrete between 15 and 60 ml/kg of urine daily, increasing this four-fold by the end of the 1st week as fluid intake increases and the redundant pulmonary fluid is excreted. The urine is dilute, straw-coloured and odourless. It is important to observe the force and direction of the stream of urine and in boys whether the stream leaves the tip of the penis. In boys

effective voiding can be compromised by the presence of posterior urethral valves or a tight prepuce. The smallest quantity of urine that neonates should pass averages 0.5–1.0 ml/kg of body weight per hour.

Body composition

For clinical convenience, **total body water** is divided into discrete compartments which provides a basis for interpreting changes that occur in the distribution and composition of body fluids and electrolytes. **Intracellular fluid** is separated by cell membranes from **extracellular fluid**, which is divided into **intravascular** and **extravascular** components (see Ch. 2). Transcellular fluids formed by secretory activities of organs such as the biliary system are called **specialised (third space) fluids**.

The proportion and distribution of the body water varies with age, maturity, gender and white adipose tissue. The total water content of the normal neonate averages 77%, falling to approximately 65% by 6 months (Rudolph et al 2003). The distributions of body fluids in infants and adults are compared in Tables 48.1 and 48.2. In comparison to adults, neonates have considerably more interstitial fluid. The gradual translocation of intracellular fluid into the interstitial compartment after birth may be attributed to withdrawal of maternal hormones. In any event, neonates are slightly oedematous although a significant **diuresis** adjusts the distribution of water across the fluid compartments. In term neonates a loss of 5–10% of body weight in the 1st week is attributed to this diuresis. Sedin & Bland (2003) believe that extracellular fluid loss during the first week of life is an adaptation fundamental to vital organ function.

Maintenance of normal body water equilibrium also depends on a balanced fluid intake and output. During the first few days of extrauterine life, when neonates consume small volumes of liquid, a significant transfer of water from the intracellular fluid to the extracellular

Table 48.1 Total body water content of infants (3.0 kg in body weight, body surface area 0.2 m^2)

Body fluid compartment	Total body water content		
	Percent of body weight	**Litres**	**Litres/m^2**
Intracellular	38	1.14	5.7
Extracellular:			
—Interstitial	40	0.99	4.95
—Plasma	5	0.15	0.75
Total	83	2.28	11.4

Table 48.2 Total body water content of adults (70.0 kg in body weight, body surface area 1.85 m^2)

Body fluid compartment	Total body water content		
	Percent of body weight	**Litres**	**Litres/m^2**
Intracellular	40	28	15.2
Extracellular:			
—Interstitial	16	11.2	6
—Plasma	4	2.8	1.5
Total	60	42	22.7

fluid compartment expands the already large extracellular fluid volume. This potentially protects neonates against dehydration during the episodes of physiologically induced diuresis. Whilst healthy neonates seldom perspire they are vulnerable to water loss because of their large body surface area which enhances water evaporation.

Healthy neonates can exchange 50% of the total extracellular fluid volume over 24h in comparison to the 14–15% seen in adults. Midwives must remember that significant differences exist between the size of fluid compartments in neonates, pregnant mothers and newly delivered mothers and use this knowledge in caring for them. Fluid therapies and nutritional support must take into account individual physiological differences to avoid iatrogenic problems that compromise cardiovascular and respiratory functions.

Sexual characteristics

Both sexes have a small nodule of breast tissue averaging 1 cm in diameter surrounding the nipples. Initially, the breast tissue may be enlarged due to high plasma maternal oestrogens, and briefly a milky fluid, traditionally referred to as **witches' milk,** may be discharged. No attempt should be made to remove this milk as squeezing the nipple or breast tissue may lead to bruising and abscess formation.

In boys born at term the testes are descended into the scrotum but remain undescended in premature neonates. Though the foreskin adheres to the glans penis this will not obstruct the voiding of urine unless there is obstruction caused by such anatomical problems as posterior urethral valves (usually diagnosed in pregnancy). In girls, fat deposition in the genital area ensures that the labia majora covers and conceals the labia minora, a feature not present in premature neonates. As a consequence, the urethral and vaginal orifices can be seen when the labia minora are parted. Some female neonates also manifest a thick white vaginal discharge which is probably a response to maternal oestrogens. As the linings of the uterus and vagina consist of fairly mature epithelium some girls may have a small **pseudomenstrual bleed**, although, as the maternal oestrogen levels in the neonate's blood fall, the genital tract returns to an infantile state.

Main points

- A fetus depends on his mother for survival using the placenta as a life-supporting unit. At birth he must adapt to an independent life and this involves every body system establishing and maintaining new homeostatic values. The respiratory and cardiovascular systems ensure oxygen uptake from the surrounding air whilst carbon dioxide and other metabolites are eliminated.

- Term neonates have a barrel chest and rounded abdomen. Varying amounts of fine silky hair cover the scalp, lanugo is sometimes found on the face, arms and shoulders and vernix caseosa in the groins and axillae. The ear cartilage is well formed and the palm and sole creases are well defined. Both boys and girls have a small nodule of breast tissue. In boys the testes are descended into the scrotum and the foreskin still adheres to the glans penis. In girls the labia majora covers the labia minora.

- Neonatal circulating blood volume varies from 75 to 125 ml/kg depending on the direction and amount of blood flow between fetus and placenta at birth, the gestation of the infant and the time of clamping of the umbilical cord. Erythrocyte count at birth averages about 5 million/ml. The average haemoglobin is 16.5–17.5 g/dl.

- A lack of vitamin K predisposes neonates to spontaneous bleeding between the 3rd and 6th days of life and breastfed babies may develop significant prothrombin deficiency. Prophylactic administration of vitamin K to prevent the risk of spontaneous haemorrhage is common.

- Fetal circulation differs from that of an adult as cardiovascular modifications bypass the lungs transferring blood to and from the placenta for exchange of gases. Adaptations in the cardiovascular and respiratory system at birth culminate in the establishment of cardiovascular and respiratory functions comparable to those in adults. Respiratory or cardiac disorders accompanied by hypoxia and acidosis may lead to persistent fetal circulation with a patent ductus arteriosus.

- By 38–40 weeks gestation, surfactant forms a monolayer lining for the alveoli, creating an air–liquid interface and reducing surface tension in the terminal sacs. This prevents the alveoli from collapsing at the end of expiration.

- Nephrogenesis is complete by 35 weeks of gestation but in premature babies continues for a variable period of time. Renal growth depends on hypertrophy of existing units. Clamping the umbilical cord may increase renal function but the most likely contributing factors are haemodynamic such as good cardiac output mediated by vasoactive substances such as prostaglandins.

- Neonates have larger total body water content with greater proportions forming extracellular fluid. They become slightly oedematous because of a shift of intracellular fluid into the extracellular fluid compartment after birth. Diuresis results in a loss of 5–10% of body weight in the 1st week. Renal perfusion, glomerular filtration rate and tubular filtration adjust to neonatal metabolic demands by the end of the 2nd week.

- Tubular thresholds for solute reabsorption are lower in neonates, resulting in loss of sodium, glucose and other solutes in the urine. Infants are able to excrete normal quantities of acid via the kidneys but have little reserve to cope with

increased levels that may occur in cardiorespiratory disturbances.

- The neonate's ability to dilute or concentrate urine is also limited. Most babies pass urine within 12 h of birth. It is important to observe the force and direction of the stream of urine and, in boys, whether the stream leaves the tip of the penis.

References

Avery, G., Fletcher, M., MacDonald, M., 1999. Neonatology: Pathophysiology and Management of the Newborn. Lippincott Williams and Wilkinson, Philadelphia.

Andreeva, A., Kutuzov, M., Voyno-Yasenetskaya, T., 2007. Regulation of Surfactant Secretion in Alveolar Type II Cells. Am. J. Physiol. Lung Cell Mol. Physiol. 293, 259–271.

Brenner, B., Rector, F., 1991. The Kidney. W B Saunders, Philadelphia.

Carlton, D., et al., 2003. Transitional changes in the newborn infant around the time of birth. In: Rudolph, A., Hoffman, J., Rudolph, C. (Eds.), Rudolph's Pediatrics. Prentice-Hall, New Jersey.

Collins, P., 2009. Neonatal anatomy and growth. In: Gray's Anatomy. Churchill Livingstone, New York.

Crowther C. A, Henderson-Smart D. J. 2000. Vitamin K prior to preterm birth for preventing neonatal periventricular haemorrhage. Cochrane Review. Cochrane Library, Issue 2. Update Software 2003, Oxford.

Ekelund, H., Finnstrom, O., Gunnarskog, I., Kallen, B., Larsson, Y., 1993. Administration of vitamin K to newborn infants and childhood cancer. Br. Med. J. 301, 89–91.

Enkin, M., Keirse, M.J.N.C., Renfrew, M., et al., 2000. A Guide to Effective Care in Pregnancy and Childbirth, second edn. Oxford University Press, Oxford.

Golding, J., Greenwood, R., Birmingham, K., Mott, M., 1992. Childhood cancer, intramuscular vitamin K, and pethidine given in labour. Br. Med. J. 305, 341–346.

Hull, D., 1992. Vitamin K and childhood cancer: the risk of haemorrhagic disease is certain; that of cancer is not. Br. Med. J. 305, 326–327.

Manco-Johnson, M., et al., 2003. Hemostasis. In: Rudolph, J., Hoffman, J., Rudolph, C. (Eds.), Rudolph's Pediatrics. Prentice-Hall, New Jersey.

Marieb, E.N., 2008. Human Anatomy and Physiology, fifth edn. Benjamin/Cummings, New York.

Merenstein, K., Hathaway, W.E., Miller, R.W., et al., 1993. Controversies concerning vitamin K and the newborn. Pediatrics 91, 1001–1002.

Michie, M.M., 1999. The baby at birth. In: Bennett, V.R., Brown, L.K. (Eds.), Myles Textbook for Midwives. Churchill Livingstone, Edinburgh.

Nishiguchi, T., Saga, K., Sumimito, K., et al., 1996. Vitamin K prophylaxis to prevent neonatal vitamin K deficient intracranial haemorrhage in Shizuoka prefecture. Br. J. Obstet. Gynaecol. 8 (11), 1078–1084.

Overby, K., et al., 2003. Pediatric health supervision. In: Rudolph, A., Hoffman, J., Rudolph, C. (Eds.), Rudolph's Pediatrics. Prentice-Hall, New Jersey.

Padbury, J., et al., 2003. Hemodynamic adaptation at birth. In: Rudolph, A., Hoffman, J., Rudolph, C. (Eds.), Rudolph's Pediatrics. Prentice-Hall, New Jersey.

Pearson, H., Dallman, P., et al., 2003. Anaemia: Diagnosis and Classification. In: Rudolph, A., Hoffman, J., Rudolph, C. (Eds.), Rudolph's Pediatrics. Prentice-Hall, New Jersey.

Pocock, G., Richards, R., 2006. Human Physiology: The Basis of Medicine. Oxford University Press, Oxford.

Puckett R M, Offringa M., 2000. Prophylactic vitamin K for vitamin K deficiency bleeding in neonates. Cochrane Review. Cochrane Library, Issue 2. Update Software 2003, Oxford.

Rudolph, A., Hoffman, J., Rudolph, C. (Eds.), et al., 2003. Rudolph's Pediatrics. Prentice-Hall, New Jersey.

Sedin, G., Bland, R., et al., 2003. Supportive care of the preterm infant. In: Rudolph, A., Hoffman, J., Rudolph, C. (Eds.), Rudolph's Pediatrics. Prentice-Hall, New Jersey.

Smith, B., Sabry, K., 1983. Glucocorticoid–thyroid synergism in lung maturation: A mechanism involving epithelial–mesenchymal interaction. Dev. Biol. 80, 1951–1954.

Annotated recommended reading

Boxwell, G., 2000. Neonatal Intensive Care Nursing. Routledge, London.

This textbook outlines a range of common and challenging neonatal problems and provides helpful and directive suggestions for neonatal intensive care nursing. Critical analysis and reflection on the identified neonatal nursing concepts would reinforce best practice.

Hull, D., 1992. Vitamin K and childhood cancer: the risk of haemorrhagic disease is certain; that of cancer is not. Br. Med. J. 305, 326–327.

This article provides a balanced consideration of the benefits of neonatal vitamin K administration, particularly in circumstances where there is a risk of haemorrhagic disease and intracranial bleeding.

Polin, R., Fox, W., 2006. Fetal and Neonatal Physiology. W B Saunders, Philadelphia.

This textbook offers detailed accounts of important bioscientific concepts in fetal and neonatal care. A résumé of genetics underpins a more detailed exploration of normal embryonic development. The exploration of biochemical,

physiological, nutritional and pathophysiological principles contributes to clinical practice and research.

Wong, D., 2007. Nursing Care of Infants and Children. Mosby, St Louis.

This textbook offers detailed accounts of the biophysical, psychosocial and nursing issues relevant in managing the care of infants and children. It has a range of helpful appendices, including excellent developmental screening tools and biophysical nomograms and parameters invaluable in child care.

Chapter Forty-Nine

49

Adaptation to extrauterine life 2: gastrointestinal, metabolic, neural and immunological considerations

CHAPTER CONTENTS

Introduction

The human placenta is a discoid haemochorial organ that usually connects to a small part of the internal aspects of the uterus (see Ch. 12). It has many functions including serving as a metabolic unit capable of exchanging nutrients and metabolic waste products between mother and embryo/fetus. At term, in a single pregnancy, a normal placenta and its membranes weigh 450–500 g averaging 12% of the neonate's body weight. After birth, these physiological processes are supported by the neonate's own systems.

The gastrointestinal tract

Neonatal characteristics

The embryological development of the gut is described in Chapter 11 and it may be necessary to revise this before reading on. Significant anatomical and physiological limitations exist in the neonatal gastrointestinal (GI) tract, many of which may be partly attributed to the requirement of the fetus to swallow amniotic fluid (Polin & Fox 2004). The swallowing of small boluses of amniotic fluid may be fundamental to the patency of the GI tract. Although the fetal GI tract seems not to serve any nutritional purposes, it must process nutrients after birth.

The oral cavity
The walls of the oral cavity should be well formed with a central, short, broad but freely moveable tongue accommodated comfortably within it. The hard palate is slightly arched and gently corrugated by 5 or 6 irregular transverse folds which assist with suckling. Neonates have a high epiglottis that makes direct contact with the soft palate. As milk passes from the mouth to the pharynx, the larynx is elevated so that its opening is above the level of the oral cavity. The high position of the larynx, further elevated during suckling, directs its opening into the nasopharynx enabling neonates to breath when they suckle. Although neonates are thought to be obligate nose breathers, oral breathing occurs in the presence of nasal occlusion (Rodenstein 1985).

The stomach at birth

The neonate's stomach has a small capacity, holding only 15–30 ml at birth, but increasing rapidly within the first few weeks. Neonatal swallowing may distend/enlarge the stomach capacity by 4 or 5 times and shift its position relative to other viscera. **Gastric emptying time** is initially slow, averaging 2–3 h. This is influenced by nutrient digestibility: for example, carbohydrates increase emptying time while fats decrease it. The presence of mucus in the stomach during the first 24–48 h can delay gastric emptying, whereas weakness of the **cardiac sphincter** contributes to milk regurgitation.

Gastric acidity at birth equals that of an adult, but the pH rises gradually to alkaline values because of a fall in hydrochloric acid production. This rise in pH allows commensals essential to the production of vitamin K and vitamin B complex to colonise the large bowel but also allows pathogens to survive, making the baby vulnerable to infection (Michie 1999). Furthermore during the first 6 months the intestinal mucosal barrier remains immature, allowing the transport of **antigens** and other **macromolecules** across the epithelium into the systemic circulation. However, maternal **colostrum** is rich in antibodies and helps the passage of **meconium** so that the risk of systemic infection is reduced. Postnatal maturation of the gut is stimulated by increases in peptide hormones such as **gastrin** and **motilin** (see Ch. 21), which are secreted following the commencement of feeding.

At term the neonate's small intestine averages 300 cm in length and the large intestine averages 66 cm in length (Collins 2004); both intestines share a diameter of about 1 cm. Both forms of intestine have many secretory glands and villi but the muscular structures are weak and poorly developed. The villi increase the intestine's absorptive surface area. As the haustra are not present for 6 months, the external surface of the large intestine appears smooth. Term neonates have a relatively long rectum that should connect to a patent anus. Digestive enzymes are synthesised and released as required. However, the relative deficiency of **amylase** and **lipase** causes difficulties in digesting carbohydrates and fats. The entry of food into the stomach induces a **gastrocolic reflex**, resulting in **ileocaecal valve** opening. As the ileal contents enter the colon they stimulate forceful **peristalsis** accompanied by a reflex emptying of the **rectum** (Michie 1999).

Meconium

Meconium is a dark, rather sticky substance that collects in the intestines of the fetus from the 16th week and forms the first stools of the neonate. Its presence may ensure the patency of the intestine. Its characteristic viscid consistency and greenish-black colour is attributed to the accumulation of digestive enzymes, intestinal gland secretions, bile salts and components of amniotic fluid such as vernix, lanugo, fatty acids, epithelial cells, mucus and blood cells (Blackburn 2003). Initially, meconium is sterile but within 24 h of birth it begins to be colonised with bacteria, largely in response to enteral feeding. Most neonates pass meconium within 24 h of birth and failure to do so could be an early indication of intestinal malformation, malfunction, obstruction such as imperforate anus or cystic fibrosis.

Milk feeding induces a change in the neonate's stools. As digested milk enters the colon, a gradual **transition** results in stools that are fairly liquid and yellow-brownish in appearance. Following this, the consistency and frequency of the stools depends on the type of feeding. Breastfed babies pass loose, bright yellow, inoffensive stools on average 6–10 times in 24 h in the earlier days to once a day when feeding is established. By contrast, bottle-fed babies pass paler, more formed stools with a recognisable smell and generally less frequently with a tendency towards constipation.

The liver

The fetal liver is a proportionally large organ and the liver in mature neonates accounts for 4–5% of total body weight. Although immature, it is considered to be the central organ of homeostasis. The neonatal liver has less than 20% of the **hepatocytes** found in an adult liver and ongoing mitosis is critical to the development of a functionally mature organ.

At birth, although physiologically immature, the liver produces small quantities of enzymes which metabolise substances by utilising **oxidative** and **conjugation processes**. One of the major functions that the liver must be capable of is the synthesis of glucuronyl transferase, which is essential for bilirubin conjugation. Shortfalls in this enzyme lead to a rise in plasma values of **unconjugated bilirubin**. This situation is often exacerbated by the breakdown of superfluous erythrocytes during the first 6 weeks of postnatal life. Binding of unconjugated bilirubin to fatty tissue contributes to a transient neonatal jaundice on the 3rd–5th days. Feeding stimulates liver function and bacterial colonisation of the gut which in turn stimulates vitamin K production crucial to normal coagulation.

Metabolism

Fetal metabolic processes are mainly **anabolic**, required to support rapid growth. After birth neonates must support their own metabolic needs by utilising essential nutrients and gases as fuels. These adaptive changes are energy demanding. The fetus prepares for independence by laying down a store of glycogen and lipids during the last few weeks of gestation; fetal blood glucose during the last trimester averages 80% of maternal blood glucose concentration (Carlton 2003). However, nutrient reserves are fairly limited and most neonates require an intake of glucose, protein, fat and water within the first few hours of birth. The risk of a neonate developing **hypoglycaemia** is considerable. The relative excess water in neonates confers no protection against dehydration since the daily turnover of water equals 15–20%. Evaporative water loss is also costly in energy terms as the loss of 1 g of water causes the loss of 0.6 kcal of heat.

After birth, body heat production is attributed to **brown adipose tissue** and hepatic **tri-iodothyronine** synthesis which facilitates the transition from a net anabolic state to a **catabolic** state as glycogen and lipid reserves are mobilised to meet the metabolic increase (Blackburn 2003). These adaptations are influenced by factors such as maternal nutrition in late pregnancy, neonatal maturity, respiratory function and the ambient humidity and temperature.

Glucose metabolism

Glucose is the major **substrate** for carbohydrate metabolism in newborn babies (Garrow & James 2006). At birth, neonatal plasma glucose concentration depends upon such factors as the timing of the last maternal meal, the duration and nature of labour and delivery and the type and quantity of intravenous fluid administered to the labouring mother. After birth, as the neonate loses the maternal glucose source, falling **plasma insulin levels** and slow production of insulin prevent cellular uptake of glucose. This is coupled with an increase in **serum glucagon levels** which mobilise glucose from the intracellular **glycogen stores**.

Hepatic glycogen stores decrease rapidly as 90% is utilised by the neonate within the first 24 h after birth. Muscle glycogen is also reduced by 50–80%. After birth, **gluconeogenesis** is regulated by changes in the serum insulin:glucose ratio, catecholamine release, fatty acid oxidation and activation of liver gluconeogenic enzymes. The concentration of hepatic enzymes increases for the next 1–4 days. Lactose is the principal carbohydrate in human milk and many milk formulae, and term neonates consume 10–12 g/100 kcal/day.

Neonatal blood glucose falls to the lowest values between 2 and 6 h after birth, stabilises, then rises and equilibrates at about 3.6 mmol/L as he adapts to the extrauterine environment (Dodds 1996). Most paediatricians believe that the lowest safe level for neonatal blood glucose is not less than 2 mmol/L (Koh & Vong 1996). The method of feeding can influence neonatal blood glucose levels. The average neonatal blood glucose level in 132 breastfed term babies was found to be 3.6 mmol/L with a range of 1.5–5.3 mmol/L (Hawdon et al 1992). These values are significantly lower than blood glucose values found in bottle-fed neonates.

Fat metabolism

Lipolysis increases rapidly after birth, reaching a maximum within a few hours of birth and adult levels by 24 h, resulting in a rise in plasma **free fatty acids**. During this time about two-thirds of neonatal energy is produced from fat oxidation, the major form of neonatal stored calories.

The major differences between human milk and formula milk are the absence of **long-chain unsaturated fatty acids** in formulae compared with high concentrations of long-chain unsaturated fatty acids and cholesterol in mature human milk (see Ch. 56). The fat content in colostrum averages 2%, but phospholipids and **cholesterol** are found in higher concentrations. Mature human milk has a fat content of 3.5–4.5% contained within membrane-enclosed fat globules, whose core consists of **triglycerides** which permits dispersion of the lipids in the milk and protects them from hydrolysis by milk lipase.

Alternative fat stores and **ketone body** release are stimulated by the release of catecholamines associated with the body cooling following birth. Ketone bodies are produced during fatty acid metabolism and these form important metabolites. Similarly, acetate is metabolised by the mitochondria and contributes to further energy release. Ketone bodies may be a major energy source for the developing brain and the myocardium (Polin & Fox 2004).

Protein metabolism

Whereas the basic fetal cellular building blocks are supplied by the placenta, the neonate has to digest milk proteins into **amino acids** and **oligopeptides** which requires **proteolytic enzymes**. The relatively high concentration of free amino acids and peptides in human milk probably enhances the release of **gastrin** and **cholecystokinin**, which promotes the release of the proteolytic enzymes. The neonate's ability to synthesise protein is limited, due to hepatic immaturity. As a consequence, serum amino acid levels are higher in the first few weeks and there is significant urinary amino acid excretion. Protein synthesis in mature fetuses and neonates is greater than later in life and this excessive protein turnover could be attributed to the significant remodelling during a period of rapid cell differentiation and tissue growth (Philipps & Sherman 2003).

Calcium, phosphorus and magnesium balance

Compared with maternal blood values, most neonates manifest **hypercalcaemia** and **hyperphosphataemia**.

Calcium

Calcium is the most abundant mineral in the body and at term most newborn babies have accumulated between 20 and 30 g of it, 80% of which is accrued in the last trimester of pregnancy (Polin & Fox 2004). Of this, 99% is located in the neonate's developing skeleton. Serum calcium exists in three separate fractions:

1. Protein-bound calcium represents approximately 40% of the total serum concentration, with albumin serving as the primary binding protein.

2. Calcium is also bound to other anions such as citrate, phosphate, bicarbonate and sulphate.

3. Free, ionised calcium, which is the physiologically active form of calcium.

The ultimate balance in plasma calcium is partly determined by an ongoing exchange between the skeletal system, muscles, the intestine and the kidneys (Garrow & James 2006). This movement of calcium is controlled by **parathyroid hormone**, **1,25-dihydroxycholecalciferol** and **calcitonin**. Calcium metabolism is also influenced by growth hormones, corticosteroids and some locally acting hormones and co-factors including **cytokines**.

The normal range for blood calcium in a neonate is 1.8–2.2 mmol/L. During the first 2 days of life serum calcium levels fall and there is a physiological hypocalcaemia, increasing back to normal between 5 and 10 mmol/L once intestinal absorption of calcium matures. Renal excretion of calcium is efficient and continues to increase in conjunction with glomerular filtration rate.

Neonatal aspects of calcium metabolism

- As serum calcium levels decrease parathyroid hormone (PTH) levels increase. By 3–4 days the parathyroid glands are responding adequately to calcium levels.
- Calcitonin levels are normal at birth but this is followed by a surge in the next 24 h returning back to normal values within the following 36 h. This may protect the neonate from the effects of increased PTH and reabsorption of calcium from bone. Neither oral nor intravenous calcium administration affects calcitonin levels.
- Term neonates metabolise vitamin D in the liver and the kidneys, although absorption of exogenous vitamin D may be limited due to reduced fat absorption. Human breast milk has very limited stores of vitamins K and D; availability seems a problem rather than absorption.

Phosphorus

Approximately 80% of the phosphorus in term neonates is accumulated by the fetus during the last trimester of pregnancy. The total amounts of phosphorus are divided into three component parts:

1. At least 85% of the infant's total phosphorus is contained in the skeletal system.

2. Phosphorus in body fluids is divided between an organic fraction composed of phospholipids and phosphoesters.

3. Inorganic phosphate.

Although phosphorus levels decrease in the first 2 days after birth, they still remain higher than in the adult. This may be partly attributed to delayed renal excretion of phosphorus caused by an initial decrease in glomerular filtration rate (GFR) and increase in tubular reabsorption rate. Furthermore, increased cellular energy manufacture with conversion of adenosine triphosphate (ATP) to adenosine diphosphate (ADP) releases additional phosphate. If feeding is delayed, this catabolic process is increased even further.

Magnesium

Magnesium is the second most common **intracellular cation** in the body. Mature neonates contain about 20 mg of magnesium/100 g of fat-free weight (Polin & Fox 2004). As usual, the total body magnesium is divided between three compartments:

1. The skeletal system, which contains about 60%.

2. Muscle tissue, which holds about 29%.

3. The remainder is distributed through other forms of soft and connective tissue.

Only 1% of total body magnesium is located in the extracellular space. The normal range for plasma magnesium is 0.7–1.0 mmol/L. About 60% of this exists as **free ion** while 20% is bound to various **anions** such as phosphate and oxalate. The remainder is bound to serum proteins and not easily measured. However, plasma protein-binding capacity maintains the free magnesium within quite tight limits. As no specific hormones have yet been identified as responsible for fine-tuning plasma magnesium, the kidneys are considered the primary regulators for reabsorption and loss of this ion.

The neonatal nervous system

The mature central nervous system consists of approximately 100 billion **neurons** which interact to make consciousness, thought, learning, memory, vision and other nervous system properties possible. Although neural development is nutrient-dependent, the adult neural pattern is partly dependent on early environmental stimulation (Shatz 1992). The nervous system and special sense organs originate from neural ectoderm which forms the notochord and then the neural tube. This creates a range of specialised cells that form the nervous system. The term neonate is capable of processing incoming information from the environment and producing age-appropriate behaviours. The functions of the nervous system can be divided into three parts: the autonomic, sensory and motor state.

Autonomic functions

At birth the neonate's nervous system takes over control of functions such as hunger, thirst and satiety, which are balanced by hypothalamic centres which are also thought to influence nutritive sucking and swallowing. Homeostasis is achieved by the regulation of respiration, heart beat, body temperature and metabolic activity and is adjusted to ensure the body generates sufficient heat to support important enzyme activity and off-loads redundant heat (see thermoregulation).

Sensory functions

The neonate can detect odour, differentiate between tastes, see and observe preferential stimuli and hear and discriminate sounds, all sensory modalities that are useful in the interaction with his carers (see Ch. 57). Many of these functions would have already been exercised in utero.

Motor functions

Movements in neonates, as in adults, may be reflexive or volitional. Volitional movement is under the control of the motor cortex. At first, the neonate appears to make few volitional movements but gradual motor control becomes evident as myelination of the major central and peripheral nerve tracts progresses. It is likely that environmental stimulation encourages skeletal muscle movements and these contribute to the generation of new dendrites (Fig. 49.1), motor neurons and interneuron connections. These ultimately contribute to the complexity of the many integrated functions of the central nervous system.

Ongoing neural development

The neonate's nervous system has a considerable complement of neurons but many of these will be lost by **apoptosis** and a new complement of neurons will be generated over the next 2 years (Shaffer 2002). The significant increase in the size of the brain in the 1st year is attributed to the development of **neuroglia** and **myelin**. During infancy the brain and spinal cord have

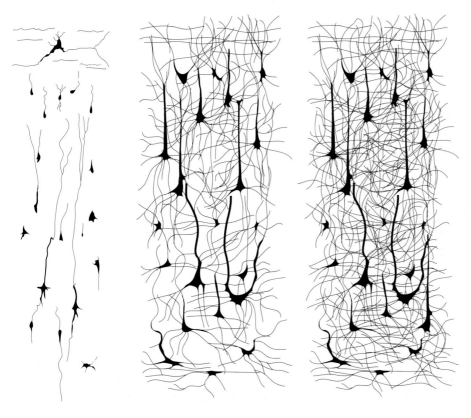

Figure 49.1 • Dendritic growth. (Reproduced with permission from Blackburn & Loper 1992.)

a considerable degree of **plasticity**, so that the developing nervous system can respond to environmental stimuli and balanced nutrition with ongoing modifications. Neonates learn by receiving, processing and responding to a vast range of sensory stimuli.

The characteristic neural development contributes significantly to the neonate's typical pattern of muscle tone which causes ongoing neuromuscular growth and development. At first there is active **flexion** and **extension** but these are replaced by purposeful movement allowing greater control and accuracy. Neuromuscular control proceeds in a **cephalocaudal** direction and amongst the first to develop are head and neck control, turning over, reaching, grasping and then crawling and walking.

Reflexes

Reflexes are autonomic, 'built-in' motor behaviours which generally occur in the spinal cord and are critical to safety and survival. These provide opportunities for assessing neonatal motor capabilities, responsiveness and needs. The absence, exaggerated state or persistence of many reflexes may signify brain damage:

- The **Moro (startle) reflex** involves adduction and extension of the arms with the fingers fanned out followed by abduction of the arms with flexed elbows in an 'embrace' position. The neonate's legs initiate a similar response. This response may be accompanied by crying. Generally, this primitive reflex disappears by the 8th week of life.
- The nasal reflexes produce apnoea by utilising the primitive diving reflexes. Reflex responses to changes in temperature of the face and nasopharynx may be a prerequisite to the onset of respiration and pulmonary gas exchange (Collins 2004).
- The **palmar grasp reflex** involves a neonate closing his fingers tightly around any object placed in his palm. Trevathan (1987) suggests that the Moro, grasp reflex, walking and crawling movements evolved to help the infant readjust to different carrying positions.
- **Rooting reflex** is seen when the side of the mouth or cheek is gently stroked. The neonate will turn his head towards the source of the stimulus and open his mouth ready to suckle.
- **Sucking and swallowing reflexes** are well developed in the term neonate. Sucking and swallowing are coordinated with respiration, including gag, cough and sneeze reflexes.
- The **tonic neck (fencing) reflex** is apparent when the neonate's head is turned to one side. He will extend the arm and leg on the side of body the head is turned to, and flex the arm and leg on the other side. This helps to stabilise the neonate and prevent him from rolling over.

- **Traction response** is observed when the neonate is held by the wrists and pulled into a sitting position. The head lags at first, then rights itself, deploying neck muscles, before falling forward.
- The **stepping reflex** is seen when the neonate is held upright with his feet touching a solid surface, in response to which alternating stepping movements are made.
- Healthy term neonates should show considerable symmetry in **tendon reflexes** and any asymmetry or absent reflexes could be indicative of serious central or peripheral nervous system anomalies.

Behavioural state regulation

An excellent description of **behavioural states** is given by Prechtl & O'Brien (1982); this term refers to the recognisable combination of behaviours repeated by the neonate over time. Such behavioural states have been investigated by observational studies, electroencephalography and polygraphy where physiological signals are studied. Prechtl defined five states using the four parameters of eyes open, respiration regular, gross movements and vocalisation. Brazelton (1984) uses similar criteria, as outlined in Michie (1999).

Sleep states

Deep sleep

The eyes are closed, respirations are regular, no eye movements are present and response to stimuli is delayed. Jerky movements may be present.

Light sleep

Rapid eye movements (REM) occur, respiration is irregular, non-nutritive sucking movements may occur, response to stimuli is rapid and may result in an alteration of sleep state, and random movements are noticed.

Awake states

Drowsy state

The eyes may be open or closed with some eyelid flutter, smiling may occur, smooth limb movements interspersed with startle responses may be present and alteration of state occurs readily following stimulation.

Quiet but alert state

Motor activity is minimal but the baby is alert to visual and auditory stimuli.

Active alert state

The baby is active and reactive to the environment. It is in this state he will mimic facial expressions.

Active crying state

The baby cries vigorously and may be difficult to console. There is considerable muscular activity. Neonates cry for different reasons such as hunger, thirst, pain, a need to change position or unsatisfactory room temperature. This is their only means of attracting attention to their needs. Although crying causes anxiety, mothers usually learn to recognise and respond to the different cries. Understanding these different behavioural states may lessen anxiety and allow greater parental enjoyment.

The essence of immunocompetence

Perhaps the most important components of the evolving **immune system** are the red bone marrow, the thymus gland and peripheral lymph nodes. The thymus gland weighs approximately 10 g and then grows steadily until puberty when it weights approximately 30 g. **Lymphopoiesis** (see Ch. 29) produces **immunocytes** capable of distinguishing between foreign and self-antigens, facilitating the elimination of foreign antigens and maintaining a memory of previous exposure to them. The development of lymphoid tissue proceeds along two classical pathways culminating in the formation of:

1. Naïve B lymphocytes which on exposure to antigens become plasma cells capable of mounting **antibody-mediated immunity**.

2. **T lymphocytes**, which are predominantly responsible for coordinating **cell-mediated immunity**.

Both fetus and neonate are compromised by their immature immune systems. Also, lack of exposure to common pathogens and antigens contributes to significant delay in mounting an immune response. Since both pathways are functionally immature, the inflammatory response and complement cascade are limited. Immune system immaturity may also predispose to allergy formation and susceptibility to gastrointestinal infections.

At birth the fetus enters an environment containing potentially harmful pathogens. The skin, respiratory system and gastrointestinal tract must acquire normal microbe commensal populations and respond appropriately to pathogens and allergens. The initial colonisation is via the mother's genital tract during birth, then her skin organisms, especially during breastfeeding, and finally environmental organisms.

Organisms such as *Lactobacillus* sp., *Escherichia coli* and protective anaerobes are derived from the mother's genital tract along with pathogens such as group B streptococcus and *Chlamydia trachomatis*. As neonatal skin and mucous membranes are fragile and easily breached, the colonisation that initially occurs on the skin, umbilical stump and genitalia followed by mucous membranes

of the eyes, nose and throat can result in potentially dangerous systemic infections.

Gastrointestinal perspectives

The initial mild acidity of the stomach secretions may afford some protection against ingested pathogens and the colonisation of meconium, which occurs within a few hours of birth and increases rapidly over the next few days, rarely leads to infection. Breastfed babies develop a different pattern of bacterial colonisation to that of neonates fed with formula milk. The acid environment in the gut in which protective organisms such as *Lactobacillus* can grow appears to prevent colonisation by more harmful pathogenic organisms. Eventually, the development of gut defence mechanisms such as 'gut closure', accompanied by the development of the mucosal barrier and other defences, renders the epithelium impermeable to pathogens. As further immune defence, the tonsils and peritoneal Peyer's patches develop.

Specific immune responses

Two specific immune responses concern immunoglobulin IgA (humoral-mediated immunity) and maturation of T cells (cell-mediated immunity).

Humoral-mediated immunity

During fetal life there is transfer of IgG via the placenta from mother to fetus, affording the fetus passive immunity. However, IgA does not cross the placenta and neonatal levels are low. Colonising IgA is transferred in the colostrum and milk, which protect it from the acidic contents and proteolytic enzymes present in the baby's gastrointestinal tract. IgM is too large a molecule to cross the placental barrier. However, the neonate is capable of producing sufficient amounts of IgM in response to a challenge by micro-organisms such as the TORCH organisms (Toxoplasmosis, Other viruses, Rubella, Cytomegalovirus, Herpes simplex).

Cell-mediated immunity

At birth, T cell numbers are similar to those found in the adult but their function is decreased. Cytotoxic activity of T cells is only 30–60% of that found in the adult. These T cells are naïve and require significant maturation before they can mount minimal protection.

Thermoregulation

Thermoregulation is the balance between the body's ability to produce heat and lose heat under physiologically appropriate conditions.

Adult mechanisms

Humans are **homeotherms,** maintaining a constant body temperature independent of their environment. Skin receptors send signals to the **hypothalamus,** triggering autonomic nervous system responses. The transfer of these signals to the cerebral cortex triggers learned behavioural responses. Consequently, a rise in normal body temperature in humans is accompanied by an autonomically triggered **peripheral vasodilation,** sweating and a behavioural response of searching for a cooler environment and wearing appropriate clothing. If the body temperature falls there is usually a reflex **peripheral vasoconstriction** and shivering and the person seeks a warmer environment and more suitable clothing (Guyton & Hall 2006).

Neonatal mechanisms

At birth the neonate passes from a thermoconstant intrauterine temperature of 37.7°C to an environment where the room temperature averages between 21°C and 25°C. This contributes to rapid heat loss due to the wet, warm skin. Heat may be transferred down the internal gradient from the body core to the skin surface and to the environment at a speed dependent on capillary blood flow and the amount of subcutaneous fat present. In contrast, the loss of heat down the external gradient depends on the difference between the skin temperature and the external environment which involves mechanisms of evaporation, convection, radiation and conduction. The balance between heat gain and heat loss in the neonate is shown in Table 49.1.

Table 49.1 Sources of heat gain and heat loss in the neonate

Heat gain	Heat loss
Metabolic processes such as oxidative metabolism of glucose, fats and proteins	Evaporation: water loss from the skin and respiratory tract, most common at birth Heat is also lost in urine and faeces
Physical activity such as crying, restlessness and hyperactivity	Convection: heat lost into the air around the baby
Non-shivering thermogenesis generated through metabolism in brown adipose tissue	Radiation: heat radiated to nearby cold solid surfaces, most common after the first week of life
	Conduction: heat lost by direct contact with cold surfaces touching the baby

Thermoregulation is a common physiological problem amongst neonates largely due to immaturity and inefficiency of the control mechanisms observed in adults. In the first few days, neonates lose sweat only from their head region. The neonate has a much larger head surface area than an adult as the head makes up 25% of the **body mass**. Normally a neonate's rectal temperature may average 36.0–37.2°C, and skin temperature (peripheral temperature) may average 35.5–37.4°C (Wilkinson et al 2003).

Neonates are generally unable to shiver and are limited in their ability to generate heat from muscle action, so they are at a disadvantage. They can decrease their surface area exposed to the environment by flexing their limbs and taking up the fetal position. During the first 24 h after birth healthy term neonates will increase their heat production by 2.5 times as a physiological response to cold. This process appears to be activated by catecholamine release which induces **lipolysis** in the brown adipose tissue (BAT), small amounts of which are also found in most human adults, other animal neonates and hibernating animals.

Heat production and BAT

About 2–7% of the weight of a newborn infant probably consists of BAT which is mainly situated around the kidneys, in the mediastinum, around the nape of the neck and scapulae, along the spinal column and around the large blood vessels in the neck (Fig. 49.2). **Brown adipocytes** (fat cells) begin to proliferate at 26–30 weeks gestation and continue to increase in number for some months after birth. A small amount of BAT persists throughout life, with greater quantities being present in slender individuals.

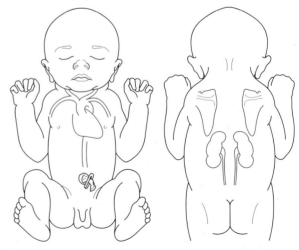

Figure 49.2 • The areas where brown fat is found. (Reproduced with permission from Wallis & Harvey 1979.)

BAT adipocytes differ from those in white adipose tissue by their scope for enhanced metabolic activity and heat production. The cells contain many small fat vacuoles, numerous mitochondria and other active organelles. BAT has extensive capillary perfusion, giving it a brownish colour. Activity of the sympathetic nerve fibres during cold stress causes the adrenal glands to release catecholamines, such as **noradrenaline** (norepinephrine), which stimulate the anterior pituitary gland to release **thyroid-stimulating hormone** (TSH). This causes the thyroid gland to increases production of **thyroxine** (T_4). **Adrenaline** (epinephrine) and thyroxine increase metabolic activity within BAT and heat is produced, providing adequate oxygen and glucose are available.

Care of the neonate

It is important that parents as well as professionals caring for neonates are aware of the need to keep the head and nape of the neck warm and to adjust both the environmental temperature and the amount of clothing worn by neonates in order to maximise heat regulation. At the time of birth the baby should be dried, covered and given to the mother to hold if possible. Initially, the best source of heat is from the mother's body. Implications for the care of small and sick neonates are discussed in a later chapter.

Main points

- The nutritional, excretory and metabolic needs of the fetus and its protection against pathogenic organisms and toxins are met by the placenta. After birth these processes must function independently.

- At birth, the gastrointestinal system of the neonate manifests some anatomical and physiological limitations, partly influenced by fetal swallowing of amniotic fluid. The swallowing actions of the small bolus of amniotic fluid may be important in the development and maintenance of gastrointestinal patency.

- In term neonates sucking and swallowing reflexes are present at birth. The small stomach capacity increases rapidly within the first few weeks of life, allowing the infant to take larger feeds. The cardiac sphincter remains weak and milk regurgitation is common.

- The intestinal mucosal barrier remains immature so that antigens and other macromolecules can be transported across the epithelium into the systemic circulation. Colostrum is rich in antibodies and helps the elimination of meconium. The relative deficiency of the enzymes amylase and lipase can result in neonates having difficulties digesting carbohydrates and fats.

- A gastrocolic reflex ensures that feeding is often accompanied by reflex emptying of the bowel. Most neonates pass meconium within 24 h of birth. Failure to do so could be a sign of intestinal obstruction, anal atresia or early signs of meconium ileus.

- The immature liver has low production of enzymes such as glucuronyl transferase. Enteral feeding stimulates liver function and bacterial colonisation of the gut, allowing vitamin K to be produced.

- The fetus lays down a fuel store of glycogen and lipids during the last few weeks of pregnancy. After birth these glycogen and fat stores are used as metabolic fuel. Catecholamines released in response to body cooling stimulate the release of alternative fat stores and ketone bodies.

- Neonatal blood glucose levels fall to a lowest level between 2 and 6 h after birth, become stable and then rise as the baby adapts to his extrauterine environment. The feeding method can influence neonatal blood glucose levels.

- Lipolysis increases rapidly after birth, reaching a maximum within a few hours. In the first 24 h two-thirds of the baby's energy is derived from fat oxidation. The neonate's ability to synthesise protein is limited due to immaturity of liver enzyme systems resulting in higher serum amino acid levels and urinary amino acid excretion.

- During the first 2 days of life serum calcium levels fall leading to physiological hypocalcaemia. This rises to normal values between 5 and 10 days as intestinal absorption of calcium increases. Renal excretion of calcium is efficient. Neonates metabolise vitamin D in the liver and kidneys. Absorption of exogenous vitamin D is limited because of immature fat absorption mechanisms.

- The decreased glomerular filtration rate and increased tubular reabsorption rate delay renal excretion of phosphorus. Increased energy needs with conversion of ATP to ADP may contribute to greater phosphate release.

- Only 1% of total body magnesium is located in the extracellular space. In plasma about 60% of the magnesium exists as free ion while 20% is bound to various anions. The remaining plasma magnesium is bound to serum proteins. The kidneys are the primary organs for serum magnesium regulation.

- Nervous system activity increases steadily throughout gestation. At term the neonate processes incoming information from the environment and produces behaviour appropriate for its status. Plasticity of the brain ensures that new neural connections can be established and modified by environmental stimuli.

- The term neonate demonstrates a typical muscle tone which changes, giving rise to strong passive flexion and eventually to purposive movement. Reflexes are critical for the baby's safety and survival. The absence of such reflexes or unusual persistence may indicate brain damage.

- Neonatal behaviours include two sleep states (deep and light) and four awake states (drowsy, quiet alert, active alert and active crying). Helping parents to recognise these different behavioural states may contribute to better parenting skills.
- Naïve B and T lymphocytes mature on exposure to antigens. Neonates are susceptible to infections. At birth the neonate's skin, respiratory system and gastrointestinal tract must acquire normal microbe commensal populations and respond appropriately to pathogens and allergens. Colonisation is via the mother's genital tract during birth, then her skin micro-organisms and finally environmental organisms.
- Breastfed babies develop a different pattern of bacterial colonisation than artificially fed babies. The acid environment in the gut facilitates the growth of *Lactobacillus*, preventing colonisation by pathogenic micro-organisms. Neonates eventually develop gut closure to render the epithelium impermeable to such micro-organisms.
- Neonatal thermoregulation can be a problem as the large body surface area contributes to greater heat loss. Neonates can increase their heat production by 2.5 times in response to cold by BAT lipolysis.

References

Blackburn, S.T., 2003. Maternal, Fetal and Neonatal Physiology: A clinical perspective, second edn. W B Saunders, Philadelphia.

Brazelton, T.B., 1984. Neonatal Behaviour Assessment Scale, second edn. Spastics International Medical Publications, Blackwell Scientific, Oxford.

Carlton, D., et al., 2003. Transitional changes in the newborn infant around the time of birth. In: Rudolph, C., Rudolph, A., Hostetter, M. (Eds.), Rudolph's Pediatrics. McGraw-Hill, New York.

Collins, P., et al., 2004. Neonatal anatomy and growth. In: Bannister, L., Berry, M., Collins, P. (Eds.), Gray's Anatomy. Churchill Livingstone, New York.

Dodds, R., 1996. When policies collide: breastfeeding and hypoglycaemia. MIDIRS Midwifery Dig. 6 (4), 382–386.

Garrow, J., James, W., 2006. Human Nutrition and Dietetics. Churchill Livingstone, Edinburgh.

Guyton, A., Hall, J., 2006. Medical Physiology. Elsevier Saunders, London.

Hawdon, J.M., Platt, M.P.W., Aynsley-Green, A., 1992. Patterns of metabolic adaptation for preterm and term infants in the first neonatal week. Arch. Child. Fetal Neonatal 67 (4), 357–365.

Koh, T., Vong, S.K., 1996. Definition of neonatal hypoglycaemia: is there a change? J. Paediatr. Child Health 344 (4), 302–305.

Michie, M.M., 1999. The baby at birth. In: Bennett, V.R., Brown, S. (Eds.), Myles Textbook for Midwives, thirteenth edn. Churchill Livingstone, Edinburgh.

Philipps, A., Sherman, M., et al., 2003. Neonatal nutrition and Gastrointestinal function. In: Rudolph, C., Rudolph, A., Hostetter, M. (Eds.), Rudolph's Pediatrics. McGraw-Hill, New York.

Polin, R., Fox, W., 2004. Fetal and Neonatal Physiology. W B Saunders, Philadelphia.

Prechtl, H.F.R., O'Brien, M.J., 1982. Behavioural states of the full-term newborn. The emergence of concept. In: Stratton, P. (Ed.), Psychobiology of the Human Newborn. Wiley, Chichester.

Rodenstein, D., 1985. Infants are not obligatory nasal breathers. Am. Rev. Respir. Dis. 131, 343–347.

Shaffer, D., 2002. Developmental Psychology: Childhood and adolescence. Wadsworth, Belmont, California.

Shatz, C., 1992. The developing brain. Sci. Am. 9, 35–41.

Trevathan, W.R., 1987. Human Birth: An Evolutionary Perspective. Aldine de Gruyter, New York.

Wilkinson, A., Charlton, V., Phibbs, R., Amiel-Tison, C.M., et al., 2003. Examination of the newborn infant. In: Rudolph, C., Rudolph, A., Hostetter, M. (Eds.), Rudolph's Pediatrics. McGraw-Hill, New York.

Annotated recommended reading

Boxwell, G., 2000. Neonatal Intensive Care Nursing. Routledge, London.

This textbook outlines a range of common and challenging neonatal problems and provides helpful and directive suggestions for neonatal intensive care nursing. Critical analysis and reflection on the identified neonatal concepts reinforce best practice.

Dodds, R., 1996. When policies collide: breastfeeding and hypoglycaemia. MIDIRS Midwifery Dig. 6 (4), 382–386.

This paper discusses why giving babies who are to be breastfed unnecessary artificial feeds is based on non-scientific physiological interpretations of blood glucose levels.

Hockenberry, M., Wilson, D., 2007. Wong's Nursing Care of Infants and Children. Mosby Elsevier, St Louis.

This textbook offers detailed accounts of the relevant biophysical, psychosocial and nursing issues in managing the care of infants and children. It contains helpful appendices, including excellent developmental screening tools and biophysical nomograms and parameters.

Polin, R., Fox, W., 2004. Fetal and Neonatal Physiology. W B Saunders, Philadelphia.

This two-volume textbook offers detailed accounts of bioscientific concepts important in fetal and neonatal care. A résumé of genetics acts as a basis for a detailed exploration of normal embryonic development. The systematic exploration of biochemical, physiological, nutritional and pathophysiological principles makes a significant contribution to clinical practice and research.

Chapter Fifty

50

Health challenges and problems in neonates of low birth weight

CONTENT CHAPTERS

Introduction

This chapter aims to define low birth weight, consider some of the common causes and address some of the most prevalent health challenges and problems that may occur in such neonates. The complexity and diversity of health problems require all those caring for these neonates to have specialist knowledge and expertise and this chapter aims to offer a résumé of relevant biological principles that may guide practice. The chapter will also build on some of the diagnostic accounts of congenital abnormalities in Chapter 15, giving due consideration to relevant aspects of physiology, pathophysiology and, where appropriate, therapeutic caring interventions.

Defining low birth weight

The term **low birth weight** applies to all neonates, regardless of gestational age, whose body weight at birth is less than 2500g. The improved survival of neonates weighing less than 1000g required the introduction of the term **extremely low birth weight** in order to contextualise the challenges and outcomes related to these very small neonates. Given that about 70% of **perinatal mortality** (total of stillbirths and neonatal deaths) occurs in the 7% of babies whose birth weight is low or very low, this group of neonates clearly encounters complex problems. Regardless of the cause, these neonates are often grouped according to their birth weight in the following manner (England 2003):

- Low birth weight (LBW) includes neonates weighing 2500g or less at birth.
- Very low birth weight (VLBW) includes neonates weighing 1500g or less at birth.
- Extremely low birth weight (ELBW) includes neonates weighing under 1000g at birth.

Causes of low birth weight

The two most dominate reasons for a neonate's low birth weight are **prematurity** and **intrauterine growth retardation** (IUGR) (Fig. 50.1). Premature neonates are born before 37 completed weeks of pregnancy and the term prematurity is used regardless of birth weight. Neonates who are **small for gestational age** (SFGA) weigh less at birth than would be predicted for their gestational age. This group usually includes neonates born below the **10th centile**. As these two groups of neonates are likely to present with a range of problems requiring specialist intervention, practitioners must be capable of assessing them at birth and identifying and

Preterm baby   Small-for-gestational-age baby

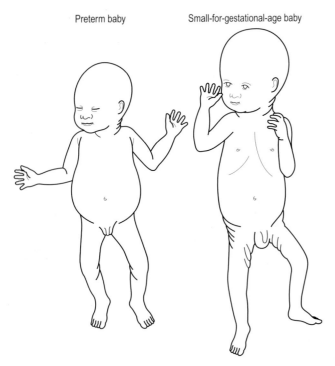

Figure 50.1 • Low-birth-weight babies. (From Henderson C, Macdonald S 2004, with kind permission of Elsevier.)

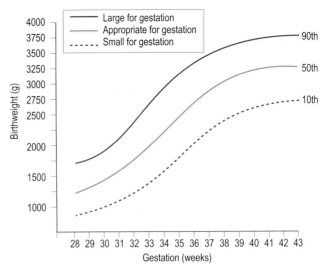

Figure 50.2 • A centile chart, showing weight and gestation. (From Henderson C, Macdonald S 2004, with kind permission of Elsevier.)

managing problems which are present. Ongoing vigilance is needed in recognising new problems which evolve in the first few days or even weeks of life. Specialist knowledge, clinical expertise and vigilance are crucial in providing optimal care.

Assessment of gestational age

One of the tools commonly used in assessing such neonates is **centile** charts (Fig. 50.2) which help to define the small-for-gestational-age neonates by using their birth weight which is invariably more than two **standard deviations** below the mean or less than the 10th percentile of a population-specific birth weight for gestational age. Whilst variations in fetal growth exist, birth weight is frequently used to distinguish between neonates who are small for gestational age from those who are small but normal for gestational age. Assessments of fetal growth, development and maturation must take into consideration variations in **genetic** and **environmental factors** which are known to impact on the expectant mother's health as well as the growth of her fetus(es).

In most instances, assessment of fetal growth would be based on the length of gestation by taking into account the onset of the last menstrual period, the size and shape of the growing uterus and maternofetal hormone profile. **Ultrasonic studies**, and in some instances, **amniocentesis**, provide additional information when required. Most fetuses fall into a **symmetric** or **asymmetric growth**

pattern. Symmetric growth implies that both brain and body growths are limited, whereas asymmetric growth implies that body growth is restricted to a greater extent than head and brain growth. The mechanisms for such asynchronous growth are not understood although Anderson & Hay (1999) suggest that increased cerebral blood flow relative to the remainder of the systemic circulation may contribute. The birth of low-birth-weight neonates generally warrants the presence of experienced paediatricians at the delivery.

In addition to establishing the birth weight, length, head circumference and gestational age, all small neonates must undergo a thorough physical assessment that may include **scoring** of neurological and neuromuscular capabilities initially devised by Dubowitz et al (1970) but used widely in the United Kingdom (Fig. 50.3). However, as this scale awards points for neurological states as well as external criteria, it is not always suitable for assessing the gestational age of sick neonates. The Parkin score (Parkin et al 1976), which uses exclusively external criteria, is quicker to use, though less accurate (Fig. 50.4). However, assessments may have adverse effects on the stability of the neonate's condition. They are less useful with the more sophisticated fetal assessments using ultrasound, unless the mother is seen for the first time in labour (England 2003).

The preterm neonate

Health challenges experienced by premature neonates can, to a large extent, be attributed to immaturity of body systems (Fig. 50.5), which means that some organs and systems have not reached the fully functional state required for adaptation to extrauterine life.

External (superficial) criteria					
EXTERNAL SIGN	**SCORE 0**	**1**	**2**	**3**	**4**
OEDEMA	Obvious oedema hands and feet; pitting over tibia	No obvious oedema hands and feet; pitting over tibia	No oedema		
SKIN TEXTURE	Very thin, gelatinous	Thin and smooth	Smooth: medium thickness. Rash or superficial peeling	Slight thickening. Superficial cracking and peeling esp. hand and feet	Thick and parchment-like: superficial or deep cracking
SKIN COLOUR (Infant not crying)	Dark red	Uniformly pink	Pale pink: variable over body	Pale. Only pink over ears, lips, palms or soles	
SKIN OPACITY (trunk)	Numerous veins and venules clearly seen, especially over abdomen	Veins and tributaries seen	A few large vessels clearly seen over abdomen	A few large vessels seen indistinctly over abdomen	No blood vessels seen
LANUGO (over back)	No lanugo	Abundant; long and thick over whole back	Hair thinning especially over lower back	Small amount of lanugo and bald areas	At least half of back devoid of lanugo
PLANTAR CREASES	No skin creases	Faint red marks over anterior half of sole	Definite red marks over more than anterior half; indentations over less than anterior third	Indentations over more than anterior third	Definite deep indentations over more than anterior third
NIPPLE FORMATION	Nipple barely visible; no areola	Nipple well defined; areola smooth and flat diameter <0.75 cm	Areola stippled, edge not raised; diameter <0.75 cm	Areola stippled, edge raised diameter >0.75 cm	
BREAST SIZE	No breast tissue palpable	Breast tissue on one or both sides <0.5 cm diameter	Breast tissue both sides; one or both 0.5–1.0 cm	Breast tissue both sides; one or both >1 cm	
EAR FORM	Pinna flat and shapeless, little or no incurving edge	Incurving of part of edge of pinna	Partial incurving whole of upper pinna	Well-defined incurving whole of upper pinna	
EAR FIRMNESS	Pinna soft, easily folded, no recoil	Pinna soft, easily folded, slow recoil	Cartilage to edge of pinna, but soft in places, ready recoil	Pinna firm, cartilage to edge, instant recoil	
GENITALIA MALE	Neither testis in scrotum	At least one testis high in scrotum	At least one testis right down		
FEMALE (With hips half abducted)	Labia majora widely separated, labia minora protruding	Labia majora almost cover labia minora	Labia majora completely cover labia minora		

(A)

Figure 50.3 • (A)–(C) Dubowitz scoring system. (Adapted from Dubowitz L M S, Dubowitz V, Goldberg C 1970.)

Characteristics of the premature neonate

- A large head and small face in proportion to the body.
- Brain and spinal cord tissue is fragile and much more susceptible to injury.
- Soft skull bones with widely spaced sutures and large fontanelles.
- Neonates born before 24 weeks may present with fused eyelids.
- The skin is red and thin, subcutaneous fat is almost absent and surface veins are prominent.
- Lanugo is present, depending on the gestational age.
- A small narrow chest with little breast tissue.
- A large prominent abdomen with a low-set umbilicus.
- Thin limbs with soft nails not reaching the ends of the digits.
- Small genitalia: in girls, the labia majora do not cover the labia minora; in boys, the testes have not descended into the scrotum.
- Muscle tone is poor and all four limbs may be held in the extended position.
- Normal reflexes, including sucking, gagging and coughing may be absent or feeble.

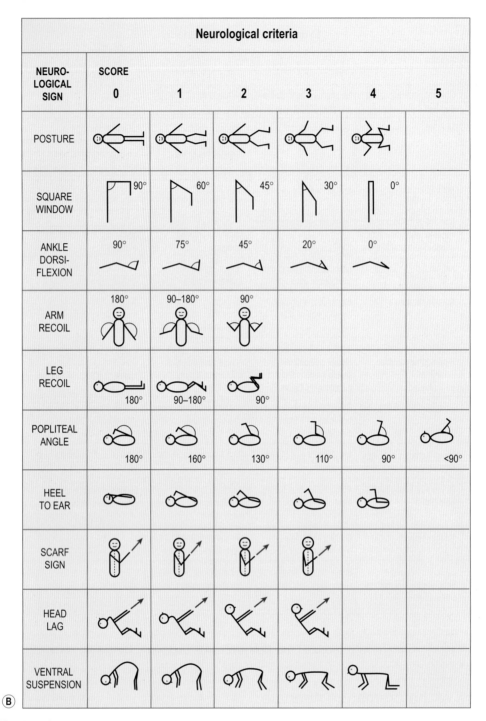

Figure 50.3 • (Continued)

Causes of preterm birth

Although preterm births occur spontaneously, in many circumstances the sequence of events may be medically controlled for maternal or fetal safety. Whilst 40% of such births have no established causes, a range of contributing factors such as physical disorders in the fetus or the mother, or the mother's social class, may play a key role (Table 50.1). This is not surprising as

many suboptimal health problems appear to be the consequence of interplays between genetic and environmental factors (see Chs 8 and 15).

Immediate management

Proactive care of the premature neonate aims at supporting the physiological shortfalls which are apparent at birth. Usually this care is initiated before or during labour

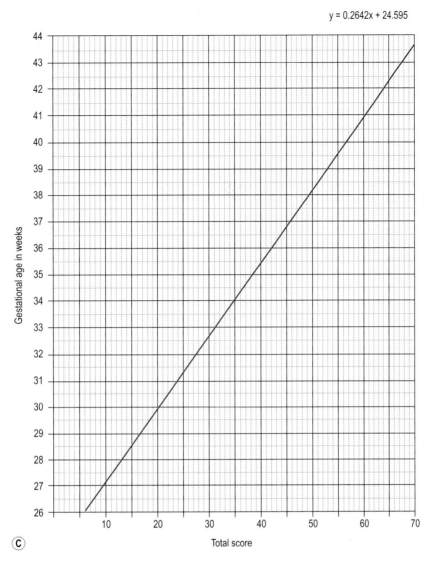

$y = 0.2642x + 24.595$

Figure 50.3 • (Continued)

to ensure the neonate's survival. Ideally all premature neonates should be delivered in maternity departments with specialist neonatal care facilities as the transfer of such small neonates is fraught with problems and increased risks.

In labour

Ideally, **prophylactic corticosteroids** should be administered to a mother who is in early labour and likely to give birth. Such practice is reviewed by Roberts & Dalziel (2006) who recommend that the administration of 24 mg betamethasone or dexamethasone or 2 g hydrocortisone administered as a single course in divided dosages will **reduce the severity of respiratory distress syndrome** and **intraventricular haemorrhage** with no apparent adverse effects to the fetus/neonate. The **pharmacodynamic effects** of such corticosteroid administration are not fully understood although Hansen & Hawgood (2003) suggest that such therapeutic interventions vastly outweigh any potential risks to the neonate possibly by stimulating lung maturation and facilitating gas exchange which reduces the hypoxia thought to contribute to intraventricular bleeding. The positive clinical outcomes in preterm neonates support this practice.

The delivery of the fetus must be given careful consideration. Some have advocated delivery of the fetus by elective caesarean section because this mode of delivery may improve the outcome for VLBW neonates, particularly where the fetus is a breech presentation (Gilady et al 1996). However, Grant & Glazener (2003) conclude that there is 'not enough evidence to evaluate a policy for elective caesarean delivery for small neonates'.

In cases where vaginal delivery is the elected choice, an episiotomy is generally advocated and forceps may

Parkin, Hey and Clowes score

This is quicker to perform but may not be quite so accurate as the Dubowitz scoring system.

Skin texture.   Tested by picking up a fold of abdominal skin between finger and thumb, and by inspection.
0 Very thin with a gelatinous feel.
1 Thin and smooth.
2 Smooth and of medium thickness, irritation and rash and superficial peeling may be present.
3 Slight thickening and stiff feeling with superficial cracking and peeling especially evident on the hands and feet.
4 Thick and parchment-like with superficial or deep cracking.

Skin colour.   Estimated by inspection when the baby is quiet.
0 Dark red.
1 Uniformly pink.
2 Pale pink, though the colour may vary over different parts of the body, some parts may be very pale.
3 Pale, nowhere really pink except on the ears, lips, palms and soles.

Breast size.   Measured by picking up the breast tissue between finger and thumb.
0 No breast tissue palpable.
1 Breast tissue palpable on one or both sides, neither being more than 0.5 cm in diameter.
2 Breast tissue palpable on both sides, one or both being 0.5–1 cm in diameter.
3 Breast tissue palpable on both sides, one or both being more than 1 cm in diameter.

Ear firmness.   Tested by palpation and folding of the upper pinna.
0 Pinna feels soft and is easily folded into bizarre positions without springing back into position spontaneously.
1 Pinna feels soft along the edge and is easily folded but returns slowly to the correct position spontaneously.
2 Cartilage can be felt to the edge of the pinna though it is thin in places and the pinna springs back readily after being folded.
3 Pinna firm with definite cartilage extending to the periphery and springs back immediately into position after being folded.

Score each external sign in turn. Add them up. Read off the baby's gestational age on the following chart.

	Gestational age	
Score	Days	Weeks
1	190	27
2	210	30
3	230	33
4	240	34.5
5	250	36
6	260	37
7	270	38.5
8	276	39.5
9	281	40
10	285	41
11	290	41.5
12	295	42

Figure 50.4 • Parkin, Hey and Clowes scoring system. (Reproduced from Parkin et al 1976.)

be used to facilitate the birth and so lessen the risk of intracranial haemorrhage. In these circumstances care must be taken to ensure that the maternal medication such as analgesia does not compromise the fetus's scope for initiation of spontaneous respiration at birth.

At birth

The delivery suite must be equipped for resuscitation of the neonate if this is needed. Ideally, an experienced paediatric team should be present during the delivery. Some neonates have weak respiratory muscles and immature respiratory centres both of which may cause difficulties in establishing effective respiration. In such circumstances, elective **endotracheal intubation** may improve the neonate's chances of survival and well-being. Many of these neonates, although well at birth, go on develop respiratory, cardiovascular and gastrointestinal problems and a timely elective intervention may be advantageous.

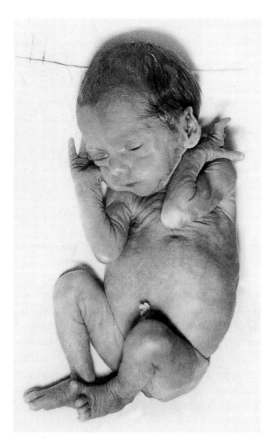

Figure 50.5 • A preterm baby born in 1954 at 28 weeks gestation and weighing 1.1 kg. He was discharged in good health after 11 weeks in hospital. (From Kelnar C, Harvey D, Simpson C 1995, with permission.)

Table 50.1 Causes of preterm birth

Fetal causes	Maternal causes
Multiple pregnancy	Pre-eclampsia
Polyhydramnios	Antepartum haemorrhage
Congenital abnormalities	Rhesus incompatibility
	Systemic maternal disease such as diabetes mellitus
	Pyrexia associated with viral infections
	Smoking, alcohol and drug abuse
	Maternal short stature
	Cervical incompetence
	Maternal age and parity
	Inappropriate maternal nutrition

The ambient temperature of the delivery suite and the neonatal unit should be no less than 24°C. As most of these neonates have limited or no subcutaneous adipose tissue, thermoregulation will be a problem and effective drying and warm swaddling are advocated. If the neonate's respiratory and cardiovascular functions are satisfactory, the parents should be allowed to hold their baby. However, if the mother wishes to have a more direct skin-to-skin contact with her baby, then warm protective blankets may be required. If the neonate needs **cardiopulmonary resuscitation**, an overhead radiant heater should be used to ensure that the immediate vicinity is warm to prevent heat loss.

Ongoing care of premature neonates

Potential problems

Premature neonates may present with a potential for a range of problems which may include:

- Respiratory problems such as apnoea, respiratory distress syndrome and later bronchopulmonary dysplasia.
- Metabolic problems such as hypoglycaemia and hypocalcaemia.
- Structural organic problems such as necrotising enterocolitis and periventricular and intraventricular haemorrhage.
- Haematological problems such as jaundice and anaemia.
- Haemodynamic problems such as persistent fetal circulation.

Any clinical evidence that some of the above problems exist or could develop will require the premature neonate to receive specialist supportive care which should include:

- Maintenance of ambient and body temperature.
- Proactive support for respiratory and cardiovascular and potential neurological dysfunction.
- Proactive support for gastrointestinal function, supportive nutrition and supportive intervention.
- Proactive management of metabolic problems.
- Proactive support to maintain effective renal perfusion and glomerular filtration.
- Prevention of infection.
- Monitoring of excretion: urine, meconium, changing stool patterns.
- Supportive intervention that fosters bonding between the parents and their baby.

Maintenance of temperature

Compared with term infants, premature infants have a narrower thermoneutral range where heat production cannot always match the rate of heat loss. This is further compromised by considerable heat loss due to a larger head-to-body ratio and the exaggerated body surface area that is characteristic of all premature and small-for-gestational-age neonates. The greater heat loss makes additional metabolic demands on the neonate whose ability to assimilate nutrients and exchange gases can be compromised by multi-organ immaturity. Therefore, although neonates are dependent on oxygen and glucose as energy, delivery of these substrates must not exceed the physiological norm.

To ensure that the neonate's body temperature is kept within the very narrow physiological range, ambient temperatures are held between 26°C and 28°C and the incubator temperature at about 36°C to maintain the neonate's body temperature at about 37°C. A temperature-monitoring skin probe (skin servocontrol) can be used to control the incubator temperature, allowing it to adjust automatically in response to changes in the neonate's temperature. Neonates born before 30 weeks of gestation have porous skin, allowing water to evaporate and increase heat loss. Such neonates should be nursed in a humid atmosphere for the 1st week of their life.

Respiration

Premature neonates generally have a respiratory rate that averages between 60 and 80 breaths/min (Hansen & Hawgood 2003) with equal time for inspiration and expiration (ratio of 1:1). To ensure energy-efficient gas exchange, premature neonates use the apnoeic form of respiration: for instance, 5 short breaths are followed by a rest period. This physiological apnoea permits gas diffusion across the inflated alveolae and the pulmonary capillary interface. Ongoing observation and hourly monitoring should ensure that neonate's respiratory functions are assessed and distress is noted, including:

- The shape of the chest, its symmetry, inflation and contour; asymmetrical chest expansion.
- The colour of the skin; evidence of central and peripheral cyanosis.
- The rate and rhythm and effort on respiration; evidence of sternal and subcostal recession.

- Breath sounds on chest auscultation; evidence of expiratory or inspiratory wheeze.

Oxygen therapy

Oxygen therapy may be required in circumstances where respiratory distress and cyanosis develop (see Ch. 51). In such instances the temperature, humidity, flow rate and concentration of inspired oxygen must be monitored (Anderson et al 2006) to minimize the risks of oxygen toxicity. Oxygen-enriched air may be delivered into the neonate's head box (Fig. 50.6) or in more severe circumstances by assisted mechanical ventilation. The amount of oxygen given must be adjusted to maintain arterial oxygen tension within a normal physiological range.

Too high concentrations of oxygen can have adverse effects, especially in premature neonates, contributing to the development of **retinopathy of prematurity** (Quinn 2003) and **bronchopulmonary damage**. Inadequate oxygenation or hypoxia can also be detrimental, particularly by contributing to episodes of profound bradycardia and cerebral hypoxia. Monitoring of oxygen administration by means of **transcutaneous oxygen monitoring** and **arterial blood sampling** is therefore crucial, especially in very ill neonates. As continuous transcutaneous monitoring has many advantages over the intermittent sampling, it is the method of choice in most neonatal (intensive) care units. **Assisted mechanical ventilation** is an effective means of life support where reliable spontaneous ventilation and effective gas exchange cannot be sustained, although this should be curtailed when the neonate's clinical condition allows.

Nutrition

The neonate's specific nutritional requirements depend partly on his total body stores of fat, protein, glycogen, water and micronutrients. **Hypoglycaemia** is one of the most common problems of premature and LBW neonates, especially in the first 3 days of life (Hansen &

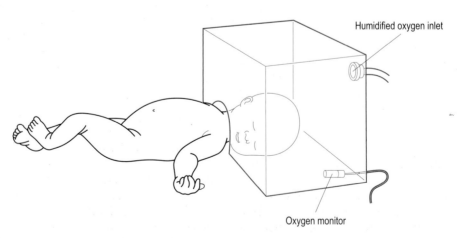

Humidified oxygen inlet

Oxygen monitor

Figure 50.6 • Baby being nursed in a headbox (incubator not shown). (From Henderson C, Macdonald S 2004, with kind permission of Elsevier.)

Hawgood 2003). When planning a nutritional programme, intestinal uptake, assimilation of nutrients, energy expenditure and elimination must be taken into consideration in conjunction with the neonate's physical maturity and health.

For practical reasons, the neonate's energy requirements may be divided into two major roles: to support **physical growth** and **development** and to support metabolic activities and energy expenditure associated with **ill-health**. In general, the energy requirements for metabolic activities take precedence over that required for growth. This becomes evident in circumstances where compromised nutrition and energy supply fail to meet the metabolic demands resulting in poor growth.

Term neonates should be breastfed where circumstances allow. However, the energy reserves and nutritional needs of premature and LBW neonates are more challenging. Milk expressed from the mothers of preterm infants has the correct whey:casein ratio and is preferable (Anderson et al 2006). Ideally, appropriate nutritional support should commence within minutes of birth. However, since the initial period tends to be complicated by a range of acute medical problems that require intervention, nutritional support is sometimes viewed as less important. Premature and small-for-gestational-age neonates should receive intravenous hydration and glucose within 30 min of their birth if homeostatic problems are to be avoided (Anderson & Hay 1999). There is a need to be careful to prevent fluid overload, especially in infants whose mothers were given corticosteroids in labour (Kerr et al 2006).

Fats

Fats are the main dietary source of energy in neonates, providing up to 50% of the total caloric needs. Yet all premature and LBW neonates have poor fat stores for energy production and for thermogenesis and lower plasma free fatty acid levels in comparison to term neonates (Anderson et al 2006). Anderson & Hay (1999) reported that these neonates appear to have deficient oxidation of free fatty acids and utilisation of triglycerides, which could partly contribute to hypoglycaemia. Since fats are essential to the formation of cell membranes and contribute to the development of the nervous system, it seems logical that nutrition must contain the right kinds and quantities of fats to support the neonate's multifactorial needs.

Proteins

Although dietary proteins supply less than 10–14% of the daily caloric needs, a daily intake of proteins is critical for growth, particularly in premature and LBW neonates whose muscle mass is deficient. Metabolic studies have shown that there is a need for higher protein intakes in the preterm neonate than in the term infant and protein supplementation is generally necessary. Protein loss may average 11–14% of the total body protein per day. Although neonates can synthesise some amino acids, some **essential amino acids** such as histidine, isoleucine, leucine, lysine, methionine, phenylalanine, threonine, tryptophan, taurine and valine must be given (Anderson et al 2006).

Carbohydrates

Enterally fed neonates use carbohydrates, and glucose in particular, as a major source of energy. The minimal 24-h glucose utilisation rate by the resting term neonate is estimated to be 4 mg/kg/min. An intake of glucose less than that rate may result in **gluconeogenesis** from non-carbohydrate sources such as amino acids. Conversely, excess glucose can be stored in the liver as glycogen and converted into glucose when required to support metabolic demands. However, in LBW neonates, glycogen stores are usually low in the early neonatal period and this is a major contributing factor to the hypoglycaemia observed in these neonates. Other contributing factors may include deficient catecholamine release and decreased hepatic and muscle glycogen stores.

Method of feeding

The best method of feeding neonates depends on size, maturity and physical condition. Whenever possible, his inclination to suck should be used as an indication that breast or bottle feeding could be offered carefully. However, premature neonates may have poor sucking and swallowing abilities so that **enteral tube feeding**, either **nasojejunal** (Fig. 50.7) or **nasogastric**, may be necessary. Such feeding may be continuous or intermittent in circumstances where abdominal distension or severe regurgitation become apparent.

Neonates who require assisted mechanical ventilation may have the additional risk of milk aspiration or the presence of milk in the stomach may embarrass respiratory function. In such instances **total parenteral nutrition** may be more suitable for providing nutritional support. It is usual to commence with intravenous water and dextrose with the addition of salts such as sodium, phosphate and calcium. If parenteral feeding is to be continued, amino acids, lipids and vitamins and trace elements must be added. As the neonate's clinical condition improves, enteral feeding is introduced and gradually increased as the intravenous feeding regimen is reduced and discontinued.

Small and sick neonates will have additional nutritional requirements. Irrespective of whether enteral or parenteral feeding is chosen, the amount of fluid in which the nutrients are given must not exceed the kidney's ability to excrete metabolic waste products. Premature neonates grow more rapidly than

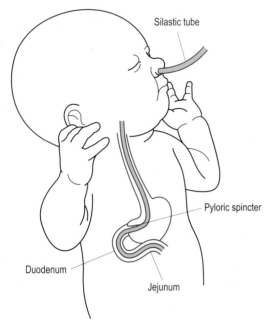

Figure 50.7 • Baby with nasojejunal tube in situ. (From Henderson C, Macdonald S 2004, with kind permission of Elsevier.)

term neonates and need on average 600 kJ/kg/day. To achieve this, 180–200 ml/kg/day of breast milk or standard formula milk is necessary. Since this volume is excessive, the neonate's energy needs may be met by giving smaller amounts of low-birth-weight formula milk or adding calorific supplements to standard formula milk.

Supplements

Growing neonates require **nutritional supplements**. These include vitamins A and D from the age of 1 month to 2 years because premature babies have limited fat stores which may have an impact on the neonate's ability to store and utilise fat-soluble vitamins. Vitamin C, a water-soluble vitamin, is also needed to support growth and healing and to aid iron absorption. As there is a delay in the production of erythrocytes by the bone marrow, premature neonates can become very anaemic, sometimes requiring blood transfusion. In most instances, iron supplements are recommended from about the 4th week after birth until weaning.

The treatments themselves may contribute to problems. For instance, blood transfusion may suppress erythrocyte production and iron supplementation can increase the risk of infection by inhibiting the anti-infective properties of lactoferrin, allowing *Escherichia coli* to multiply. Very small babies may also require folic acid supplements. Calcium and phosphate supplementation may be required in order to increase the rate of bone mineralisation.

Excretion

As with all neonates, premature neonates should pass urine within 24 h of birth and the amount should increase as fluid intake increases. All neonates cared for in a neonatal unit should have their urine output measured and the urine tested for glucose and **osmolality**. Glycosuria may indicate a lower renal threshold for glucose. This will require a review of the amount of glucose administered in order to avoid dehydration. The osmolality of the urine will indicate whether there is fluid retention or normal excretion, giving an indication of the amounts of fluids needing to be administered. Failure to produce urine as well as failure to micturate may be indicative of some haemodynamic problems such as hypotension, acute renal failure or urinary obstruction. Each of these problems is potentially life-threatening and care must be taken to intervene in the earliest stages.

The passage of meconium may be delayed in small premature neonates, especially in those with moderately severe respiratory distress syndrome or suspected cystic fibrosis. Testing of the first meconium stool for the presence of abnormal constituents is important. The presence of blood and mucus in the stools may be indicative of a serious disorder such as necrotising enterocolitis (Kitterman 2003) and must therefore be attended to immediately.

Pain

For many years clinicians took little account of the pain suffered by neonates and small babies. Many believed neonates felt little pain (Gardner et al 2006). This view has now been largely dismissed by multiple studies showing that fetuses, neonates and small infants feel and respond to painful stimuli. From an evolutionary point of view this would seem to be an essential adaptation to extrauterine life!

McClain & Kain (2005), as Gardner et al (2006), draw attention to the need for using adequate pain assessment tools and being proactive in the management of pain in neonates. Response to pain stimuli may be: behavioural, such as crying, grimacing and startle or withdrawing limbs; physiological, such as tachycardia, bradycardia, hypertension and increased oxygen requirements; or metabolic, manifesting as increased metabolic rate in response to decreased insulin secretion and increased corticosteroid release, leading to hyperglycaemia and in some instances glycosuria, proteinuria, ketonuria and a raised urine pH.

The relief of pain includes caring for the environment. Staff should develop expertise in techniques such as heel prick and intravenous line siting, procedures known to induce pain. Comfort interventions such as stroking, non-nutritive sucking, positioning and cuddling can reduce pain. Analgesia where required must be used with caution and anaesthesia should be used when invasive techniques and surgery are being carried out. Most neonates require postoperative analgesia, although care must be taken not to suppress the neonate's respiratory drive and compromise respiratory function. Neonates whose respiratory function is supported by assisted mechanical ventilation may, if required, receive sedatives and, as an adjunct to analgesia, muscle-paralysing agents.

Environmental neonatology

The premature neonate is adapted to the intrauterine environment, and the effects of **noise**, **light**, **handling** and **positioning** may influence its well-being in the neonatal unit and beyond. Such neonates require a vast amount of sleep yet neonatal units are not necessarily the most restful places for this. Noise and light levels can be high and care often necessitates frequent handling disturbance. These factors are thought to contribute to apnoea and bradycardia and, in some instances, poor growth.

Noise

Noise levels are measured in logarithmic units called **decibels** (dB). The human ear is very sensitive and can hear sound over a wide range from a pin dropping to a shrieking steam whistle—a range from 0.1 dB to 120 dB. In adults, noise of 130 dB is invariably associated with inducing pain and therefore this level acts as a threshold. It must, however, be recognised that severe hearing dysfunction and loss can occur with continuous exposure to sound over 90 dB. Common sound levels include the background noise in a home (50 dB), a noisy restaurant (80 dB) and amplified rock music (over 90 dB) (Marieb 2008).

Ongoing research into the effects of noise on these babies, such as the continuous noise levels inside an incubator, suggests that care should be taken to minimise all sounds. The mean recommended noise should not exceed 50 dB and yet many incubator alarms can exceed 60 dB (Gardner & Goldson 2006). Sudden loud noise can cause sleep disturbance, crying, tachycardia, hypoxaemia and raised intracranial pressure (Long et al 1980). This suggests that extra care must be taken when closing portholes, cupboard doors and moving incubators.

In order to observe neonates adequately, the level of light in neonatal intensive care units has increased 5- or 10-fold in the last two decades. The use of phototherapy lamps increases the risk for premature neonates of developing **retinopathy** (Glass et al 1985) whilst rising free and unbound bilirubin may cause **changes in brain stem responses** and **auditory neuropathy** (Stevenson &

Madan 2003). Establishing a day/night pattern of lighting and dimming lights when not in use can reduce some of these harmful effects. Mann et al (1986) found that when noise and light stimuli were reduced at night neonates slept on average 2 h/day longer and increased their weight gain more rapidly than neonates without conventional day/night cycling. It is important to cover the neonate's eyes when undergoing **phototherapy** and bright sunlight should be avoided. Phototherapy must be used vigilantly if the risks of encephalopathy caused by free or bound bilirubin is to be avoided.

Positioning

One significant problem in most neonatal units is the need to carry out invasive investigations whilst providing comforting care. Thoughtful planning to ensure that interventions are carried out systematically and in a coordinated manner should ensure longer rest periods. Soothing and comforting interventions include massage and 'kangaroo care' evaluated by Lacy & Ohlsson (1993). **Facilitated tucking** (containment of the infant's arms and legs in a flexed position close to his trunk) is often used to comfort neonates with mild pain (Corff et al 1995, McClain & Kain 2005).

Kelnar & Harvey (1995) cited various studies on the effects of faulty positioning in premature neonates (Fig. 50.8). Prolonged nursing in the **prone position** can result in externally rotated hips and everted feet, both of which may delay standing and walking (Bottos & Stefani 1982). A lack of careful positioning that mimics the flexed position and extension normally adopted by fetuses during the last few weeks in utero may result in developmental delay (Fetters 1986). Premature neonates often develop flattened, elongated and asymmetrically shaped heads. This can be minimised by altering the resting position of the head and taking care that the neonate's prone position is interspersed with lying in a lateral position with the hips and knees in optimal positions.

Infection

Exposure to pathogens is a major problem for premature neonates whose immune system cannot mount a full defence. Therefore, it is important to prevent infection by careful hand/forearm washing both before and after attending to each neonate, in conjunction with upholding the highest standards of hygiene. Appropriate liquid cleansing agents must be used, jewellery should be removed and strict hand-washing procedures should be followed. Gloves, and in some instances protective gowns, may need to be worn if body secretions are thought to be infectious.

Overcrowding must be avoided and each neonate must have a personal set of caring equipment stored in the vicinity of the incubator or cot. Care must be

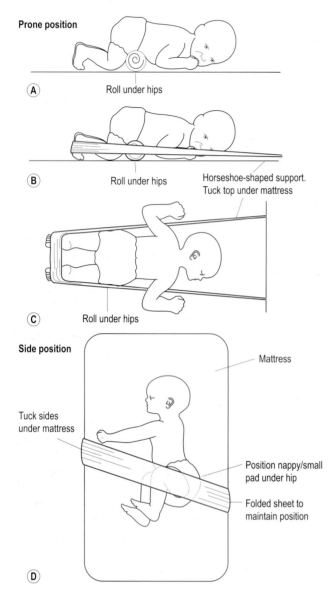

Prone position

(A) Roll under hips

(B) Roll under hips   Horseshoe-shaped support. Tuck top under mattress

(C) Roll under hips

Side position

Tuck sides under mattress

Mattress

Position nappy/small pad under hip

Folded sheet to maintain position

(D)

Figure 50.8 • Prone positioning and side lying. (From Kelnar C, Harvey D, Simpson C 1995, with permission.)

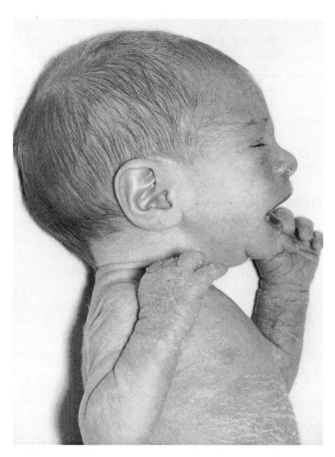

Figure 50.9 • The small-for-gestational-age (SFGA or dysmature) baby. (From Kelnar C, Harvey D, Simpson C 1995, with permission.)

taken to allow sufficient space between cots or incubators to prevent cross-infection. Disposable items should be used where these are available and continuous vigilance with cleaning of equipment is essential. Staff or visitors, including parents and siblings, with infections such as herpes simplex, upper respiratory tract infections, gastroenteritis or septic wounds should not enter a neonatal unit until their treatment is concluded and the infectious source eliminated.

The small-for-gestational-age baby

Neonates who are SFGA are sometimes referred to as '**light for dates**' who manifest symptoms of asymmetrical growth retardation or symmetrical growth retardation (see Ch. 13). Most of them are born after the 37th week of gestation and are frequently neurologically mature though lacking subcutaneous fat (Fig. 50.9). Their birth weight falls below the 10th percentile for gestational age (Hay 2003). As the fetal brain generally undergoes a growth spurt in the last trimester of pregnancy, there is sometimes a risk that this might have been compromised because of nutrient and oxygen deficiencies. Lack of energy stores can also compromise fetal ability to cope with the process of labour and birth. The risk of **hypoxia** during labour and **hypoglycaemia** after birth is high. Other health problems which may later be attributed to the condition of these fetuses in utero are **hypertension** and **cardiovascular disease** and **mature-onset diabetes mellitus** (Barker 1992).

Asymmetrical growth retardation

Asymmetrical growth retardation indicates that body growth is restricted to a much greater extent than growth of the head and the brain. In such cases brain growth is considered '**spared**'. Maternal conditions such as preeclampsia may be a contributing factor as it frequently affects placental function to the detriment of the fetus. Fetal malnutrition may in such instances present as:

- The birth weight is low but the head circumference and length of the baby are normal for gestational age.
- There is a lack of subcutaneous fat and the body and limbs appear wasted.
- The ribs are visible and the abdomen is flat or hollow due to the small size of the liver.
- The skin is dry, loose and peeling and may be stained with meconium.
- The umbilical cord is thin and may also be stained with meconium.
- The face often looks old and wizened with large eyes and an anxious and hungry expression.
- Muscle tone is generally good and the neonate is active.
- The neonate is very hungry and sucks his fist.

Symmetrical growth retardation

Symmetrical growth retardation implies that the fetal brain and body growth are limited, a phenomenon which may be apparent throughout the pregnancy (Anderson & Hay 1999). In this instance, the most common contributing factors could include intrauterine infections, maternal illness, fetal genetic or chromosomal abnormalities and maternal substance abuse. Characteristically, the neonate's head circumference is in proportion to body size and weight. These neonates may experience greater morbidity and mortality in comparison to neonates who present with asymmetrical growth retardation.

Immediate management

Small-for-gestational-age fetuses should be delivered in a maternity hospital with a suitably equipped neonatal unit capable of providing appropriate immediate care. Complications may include perinatal asphyxia (see Ch. 46), meconium aspiration syndrome, hypothermia, hypoglycaemia, **polycythaemia** and **pulmonary haemorrhage**. Most of these neonates also present with **immunological deficiencies** such as reduction in lymphocyte number and function. As can be anticipated, some of these physical problems may extend beyond the neonatal period and therefore early specialist intervention is invaluable in limiting undesirable outcomes. Some of these problems are discussed in Chapter 51.

Labour and delivery

Recognition of fetal growth retardation in utero allows anticipation of poor energy reserves, including limited fat, muscle and glycogen stores. It is essential, therefore, particularly during labour, to monitor fetal fitness by continuously observing fetal heart rate patterns and noting the presence of fresh meconium in the liquor. A paediatrician or midwife skilled in resuscitation should be present at the delivery and initiate appropriate therapeutic and supportive intervention when required. Since these neonates lack subcutaneous fat, loss of body heat can be rapid and the risks of hypothermia can be high. These neonates must therefore always be dried quickly and wrapped warmly as soon as practicable.

Ongoing care of small-for-gestational-age babies

Many SFGA neonates have different health-related problems from the premature neonate. However, certain aspects of care such as the maintenance of body temperature, respiration, cardiac and renal function, nutrition and excretion require individual attention. Prevention of infection is a priority for both groups of babies. As these babies are usually active, vigorous and alert and feed well, they may not require specialist care in a neonatal unit.

Transitional care

Transitional care wards have been developed in many maternity units, ideally situated near to the neonatal unit, to allow mothers to care for neonates with minor problems, such as heat loss, who benefit from being cared for by their mothers supervised by experienced staff. Mothers and babies are not separated and the mother is able to develop caring skills. Most of these neonates, regardless of their weight, are likely to be transferred home once they are well, providing that the home environment is suitable to their needs.

Early care (during the first 48 h) for such neonates is aimed at preventing complications such as hypoglycaemia, which is more likely to present following asphyxia or hypothermia. Frequent (3–4 hourly) recordings of blood glucose level are therefore important during the first 48 h or until plasma glucose values are stable. Since these neonates may develop transient neonatal diabetes mellitus, presenting with hyperglycaemia and glycosuria but no ketones in the urine, care must be taken to guard against **dehydration** and **failure to thrive**. Although breastfeeding reduces the risk of infection, there is some advantage in offering such neonates LBW formula milk, which is energy dense.

All neonates require follow-up care to ensure that their growth and **developmental milestones** are monitored, especially when growth has been symmetrically retarded. Since intrauterine growth retardation may be associated with ongoing and later health problems and complications, careful monitoring of these babies may be a considerable advantage.

Main points

- About 70% of perinatal mortality occurs in the 7% of babies of low birth weight. Such neonates may be small because of prematurity or as a consequence of being small for gestational age (SFGA) due to other factors such as infection. Assessment of gestational age by using the Dubowitz scale or Parkin score is sometimes fundamental to clinical management.

- Expectant mothers in preterm labour must not be given drugs that could depress the fetal respiratory centre and experienced paediatricians should be present at the time of delivery. The neonate's weak respiratory muscles and immature lungs and respiratory centres may compromise spontaneous respiration and gas exchange.

- Respiratory rate and effort should be adequate to keep the neonate well oxygenated. Carefully controlled oxygen therapy may be necessary to relieve cyanosis when respiratory or cardiovascular problems develop.

- Care must be taken to minimise the neonate's excessive heat loss and body temperature should be maintained by creating a thermoneutral environment.

- Nutritional requirements will depend on total body stores of fat, protein, glycogen and ongoing energy expenditure. Intestinal uptake and assimilation of nutrients and elimination of the by-products of digestion must be carefully considered when planning any nutritional programme.

- Premature neonates are poorly equipped in terms of maintenance of metabolic and nutritional homeostasis. Fats are the main dietary source of energy and provide up to 50% of the total caloric needs. Proteins supply less than 14% of daily caloric needs but are essential to ensure a steady supply of amino acids to replace nitrogen lost in protein turnover.

- Enterally fed neonates use carbohydrates as a major source of energy. A deficient glucose intake may result in gluconeogenesis from non-carbohydrate sources. In low-birth-weight (LBW) infants glycogen stores are usually lower in the early neonatal period and this may contribute to hypoglycaemia.

- The method of feeding of neonates is determined by their maturity, size and state of health. If possible, breast or bottle feeds should be offered but premature neonates have poor sucking and swallowing ability and nasogastric or nasojejunal tube feeding may be necessary. Ill neonates may require total parenteral nutrition. Hydration is a critical component of the overall nutritional management. Some neonates also require nutritional supplements.

- All premature neonates should pass urine within 24 h of delivery and the amount should increase as fluid intake increases. Urinary output should be measured and the urine tested for glucose and osmolality. The presence of glycosuria suggests reducing the amount of glucose that is being administered. Urine osmolality gives an indication of the volume of fluid required.

- The passage of meconium may be delayed by a number of days in small premature neonates, especially if they experience respiratory difficulties. However, the presence of abdominal pain, blood and mucus in the stools may be indicative of the presence of necrotising enterocolitis.

- The nervous system is sufficiently developed to allow neonates to feel and react to painful stimuli. Painful responses must be monitored and analgesia given if necessary. Comforting interventions such as stroking can sometimes reduce pain.

- The premature neonate gradually adapts to the extrauterine environment and the effect of noise, light, handling and positioning may influence this experience. Noise and light levels should be minimised to avoid noise-induced sleep problems and light-induced retinopathy problems.

- Prolonged nursing in the prone position may contribute to external rotation of hips and everted feet, which may delay standing and walking. Gentle changes in the position of the neonate's head will minimise the development of an elongated and asymmetrical head shape.

- The immune system in all premature neonates is immature which contributes to the ongoing risk of infection. High standards of hygiene and careful handwashing and drying as well as incubator care are essential.

- Small-for-gestational-age neonates may present with asymmetrical or symmetrical growth retardation.

- Most neonates are born after the 37th week of gestation and are neurologically mature. Complications such as asphyxia, hypoglycaemia, meconium aspiration syndrome, hypothermia, polycythaemia and pulmonary haemorrhage may present after birth. They lack subcutaneous fat and lose heat rapidly but their active, alert behaviour usually poses no feeding problems.

- Small-for-gestational-age neonates may develop long-term problems (as adults) such as hypertension, cardiovascular disease and mature-onset diabetes mellitus.

- Small neonates may be cared for in transitional care wards by their mothers. It is essential to offer follow-up care to ensure that these neonates meet their growth and developmental milestones.

References

Anderson, M., Hay, W., 1999. Intrauterine growth restriction and the small for gestational age infant. In: Avery, G., Fletcher, M., MacDonald, M. (Eds.), Neonatology: Pathophysiology and Management of the Newborn. Lippincott Williams and Wilkins, Philadelphia.

Anderson, M.S., et al., 2006. Enteral nutrition. In: Merenstein, G.B., Gardner, S.L. (Eds.), Handbook of Neonatal Intensive Care. Elsevier Mosby, St Louis, Missouri.

Barker, D.J.P., 1992. Fetal and Infant Origins of Adult Disease. BMJ Books, London.

Bottos, M., Stefani, D., 1982. Postural and motor care of the premature baby. Dev. Med. Child Neurol. 24, 706–707.

Corff, K.E., Seideman, R., Venkataraman, P. S., et al., 1995. Facilitated tucking: a non-pharmacological comfort measure for pain in preterm infants. J. Obstet. Gynecol. Neonatal Nurs. 24 (2), 143–147.

Dubowitz, L.M.S., Dubowitz, V., Goldberg., 1970. Clinical assessment of gestational age in the newborn infant. J. Paediatr. 77, 1–10.

Fetters, L., 1986. Sensory-motor management of the high risk neonate. Phys. Occup. Ther. Pediatr. 6, 217–229.

Fraser, D.M., Cooper, M.A. (Eds.), 2003. Myles Textbook for Midwives, fourteenth edn. Churchill Livingstone, Edinburgh.

Gardner, S.L., Goldson, E., 2006. The neonate and the environment: impact on development. In: Merenstein, G.B., Gardner, S.L. (Eds.), Handbook of Neonatal Intensive Care. Elsevier Mosby, St Louis, Missouri.

Gardner, S.L., Hagedorn, M.I., Dickey, L.A., 2006. Pain and pain relief. In: Merenstein, G.B., Gardner, S.L. (Eds.), Handbook of Neonatal Intensive Care. Elsevier Mosby, St Louis, Missouri.

Gilady, Y., Battino, S., Reich, D., et al., 1996. Delivery of the very low birth weight breech: what is the best way for the baby? Isr. J. Med. Sci. 32 (2), 116–120.

Glass, P., Avery, G.B., Subramanian, K.N., et al., 1985. Effect of bright light in the hospital nursery on the incidence of retinopathy of prematurity. N Engl. J. Med. 313, 7.

Grant, A., Glazener, C.M.A., 2003. Elective caesarean section versus expectant management for delivery of the small baby. Cochrane Database Syst. Rev. (4) Update Software 2003, Oxford.

Hansen, T., Hawgood, S., et al., 2003. Disorders specifically related to premature birth. In: Rudolph, C., Rudolph, A., Hostetter, M. (Eds.), Rudolph's Pediatrics. McGraw-Hill, London.

Hay, W., et al., 2003. The small for gestational age infant. In: Rudolph, C., Rudolph, A., Hostetter, M. (Eds.), Rudolph's Pediatrics. McGraw-Hill, London.

Kerr, B.A., Starbuck, A.L., Block, S.M., 2006. Fluid and electrolyte measurement. In: Merenstein, G.B., Gardner, S.L. (Eds.), Handbook of Neonatal Intensive Care. Mosby Elsevier, St Louis, Missouri.

Kitterman, J., et al., 2003. Necrotizing enterocolitis. In: Rudolph, C., Rudolph, A.,

Hostetter, M. (Eds.), Rudolph's Pediatrics. McGraw-Hill, London.

Lacy, J.B., Ohlsson, A., 1993. Behavioural outcomes of environmental or care-giving hospital-based interventions for preterm infants: a critical overview. Acta Paediatr. 82, 408–415.

Long, G.J., Lucey, J.F., Philip, A.G.S., 1980. Noise and hypoxaemia in the intensive care unit. Pediatrics 65, 143–145.

Mann, N.P., Haddow, R., Stokes, L., et al., 1986. Effect of night and day on preterm infants in a newborn nursery: randomised trial. Br. Med. J. 293, 1265–1267.

Marieb, E.N., 2008. Human Anatomy and Physiology, fifth edn. Benjamin/ Cummings, New York.

McClain, B., Kain, Z., 2005. Procedural pain in neonates: the new millennium. Paediatrics 115, 1073–1075.

Parkin, J.M., Hey, E.N., Clowes, J.S., 1976. Rapid assessment of gestational age at birth. Arch. Dis. Child. 51, 259.

Quinn, G., et al., 2003. Retinopathy of prematurity. In: Rudolph, C., Rudolph, A., Hostetter, M. (Eds.), Rudolph's Pediatrics. McGraw-Hill, London.

Roberts, D., Dalziel, S.R., 2006. Antenatal corticosteroids for accelerating fetal lung maturation for women at risk of preterm birth. Cochrane Database Syst. Rev. (3).

Stevenson, D., Madan, A., et al., 2003. Jaundice in the newborn. In: Rudolph, C., Rudolph, A., Hostetter, M. (Eds.), Rudolph's Pediatrics. McGraw-Hill, London.

Annotated recommended reading

Barker, D.J.P., 1992. Fetal and Infant Origins of Adult Disease. BMJ Books, London.

This textbook provides an invaluable account of the possible links between genetic inheritance, fetal growth and development, and the origins of disease in adults. The empirical evidence and the analytical style make a significant contribution to the practice of midwifery.

Grant, A., Glazener, C.M.A., 2000. Elective caesarean section versus expectant management for delivery of the small baby. Cochrane Database Syst. Rev. (2) Update Software 2003, Oxford.

The Cochrane Database offers a useful source for care in pregnancy, labour and the puerperium. Each research review is updated as necessary and the data are easily accessible in most colleges

of nursing and midwifery. This update concludes that there is insufficient evidence to support elective caesarean section for small babies.

Merenstein, G.B., Gardner, S.L., 2006. Handbook of Neonatal Intensive Care. Elsevier Mosby, St. Louis, Missouri.

This textbook offers informative, highly readable systems-based accounts of common problems encountered by neonates and suggests a range of management and therapeutic interventions. The text is suitable for all students of nursing, midwifery and medicine when considering neonatal care.

Polin, R., Fox, W., Abman, S., 2004. Fetal and Neonatal Physiology. W B Saunders, Philadelphia.

These textbooks discuss bioscientific concepts important in fetal and neonatal care. The résumé of genetics leads to a more detailed exploration of normal and abnormal embryonic and fetal development. Overall, these books make a significant contribution to clinical practice and research.

Wong, D., 2004. Nursing Care of Infants and Children. Mosby, St Louis.

This textbook offers detailed accounts of the biophysical, psychosocial and nursing issues relevant in managing the care of infants and children. It concludes with a range of helpful appendices, which include excellent developmental screening tools and biophysical nomograms and parameters.

Developmental anatomy: related cardiovascular and respiratory disorders

CHAPTER CONTENTS

Introduction

This chapter considers common neonatal **cardiovascular** and **respiratory problems**. Specialist textbooks such as those by Taeusch et al (2005) and McCance & Huether (2007) and current research give fuller accounts of a wider range of pathophysiological developments and relevant clinical management. Neonates become ill very quickly and all neonates that cause concern should be referred to skilled paediatricians or a neonatal specialist so that any evolving problems are managed in a proactive manner thus minimising short- and long-term problems.

Aspects of cardiovascular development

The embryology of the anatomical structures of the heart is explained in Chapter 11 and the student should refer to the appropriate section. Of importance also is the conducting system of the heart. Prior to the septation of the atria and the ventricles, specialised conducting cells form the sinoatrial ventriculobulbar and bulbotruncal junctions. This specialised conduction tissue is thought to originate from the cardiac myocytes, possibly in response to specialised, although not as yet understood, signals (Bristow 2003). The looping of the primitive heart allows the atrioventricular ring to invaginate so that it lies at the base of the atrial septum; this allows some of the specialised conduction cells to establish continuity between the atrioventricular node and the bundle of His. Failure in the various segments of these specialised conducting cells to make contact with each other causes congenital heart block.

Cardiovascular problems

Cardiovascular abnormalities

Cardiovascular malformations make up the largest group (approx. 30%) of congenital anomalies. This averages about 8% per 1000 live births (Flanagan et al 1999). Neonates may be born with **acyanotic** or **cyanotic cardiovascular anomalies** which will require expert intervention. Although the specific cause of cardiac anomalies is unknown, the occurrence of many of them is linked with chromosomal and genetic aberrations and poorly understood syndromes.

For example, **atrioventricular** and **endocardial cushion defects** are associated with trisomy 21—Down syndrome. The affected chromosomes/genes in some syndromes have been identified as in trisomy 21, genetic mutations encoding for **extracellular matrix proteins**, **fibrillin-1** being responsible for Marfan syndrome and **elastin** being responsible for Williams syndrome. Genetic mutations on chromosome 22q11 may contribute to **aortic arch anomalies**, including **Fallot's tetralogy**. As many of these anomalies are potentially life threatening, parents will seek an explanation for these problems and any risks for re-occurrence in future pregnancies.

In general, cardiovascular anomalies are grouped according to the direction of blood flow; thus defects that cause '**right-to-left shunts**' in the **heart** or **great vessels** almost always cause **central cyanosis**. In contrast, defects that cause '**left-to-right shunts**' in the **heart** or **great vessels** initially allow the neonate to be **acyanotic** (Table 51.1). Some cardiovascular anomalies cause obstruction, inhibiting either the right or the left ventricular outflow tract as seen in neonates with pulmonary and aortic valve hypoplasias. Those neonates that develop **heart failure** eventually present with considerable peripheral and central cyanosis.

Risk factors

Contributory factors thought to play a role in the development of some of the cardiovascular anomalies are:

- Maternal diabetes mellitus: ventricular septal defect (VSD), coarctation of the aorta and transposition of the great vessels.
- Chromosomal abnormalities such as Down syndrome (40%): atrioventricular defect (AVD), Fallot's tetralogy, VSDs and patent ductus arteriosus (PDA).
- Genetic problems such as Williams syndrome.
- Family history, where siblings or a parent have a cardiac defect.
- Infectious agents such as those causing rubella or toxoplasmosis infection in pregnancy.
- Nutritional/vitamin deficiencies such as folic acid deficiency (Chien 2000).
- Environmental factors and maternal drug abuse.

Presenting features in a neonate

Some of the following features may be present in neonates with cardiovascular anomalies although some of these features may also be suggestive of respiratory problems:

- Tachypnoea/dyspnoea.
- Grunting.
- Pulmonary plethora.
- Peripheral/central cyanosis.
- Tachycardia.
- Heart murmurs.
- Poor feeding ability.
- Poor weight gain and growth retardation.
- Hepatomegaly.
- Cachexia.

A paediatrician must examine all neonates presenting with any of the above symptoms; however, as some cardiovascular symptoms can be vague the actual anomaly may not be diagnosed for several days or weeks and usually following extensive investigations in a specialist centre.

Investigations

Persistent tachypnoea may be the first indication of a cardiovascular or pulmonary anomaly. Generally, cardiovascular anomalies that cause excessive pulmonary arterial blood flow and **pulmonary venous hypertension** enlarge the pulmonary vessels causing **pulmonary oedema**, decreasing the neonate's lung compliance. The cumulative effects of all these events manifest in significant respiratory difficulties and cyanosis. In contrast, cardiovascular anomalies resulting in a decrease in pulmonary blood flow tend to contribute to intense cyanosis that elicits tachypnoea without significant respiratory distress. A persistent respiratory rate of 60 breaths/min or greater accompanied by increased respiratory depth commonly precedes clinical deterioration.

Chest radiograph

A chest X-ray will establish the size and position of the heart in relation to the lungs and mediastinum as some

Table 51.1 Cardiac defects and their relative percentage occurrence

Right-to-left shunt	%	Left-to-right shunt	%	Obstructive disease	%
Transposition of the great vessels	4	Ventricular septal defect	33	Aortic stenosis	6
Tricuspid atresia	1–2	Patent ductus arteriosus	10	Pulmonary stenosis	8
Total anomalous pulmonary venous drainage	1–2	Atrial septal defect	8	Coarctation of the aorta	6

cardiovascular defects and anomalies alter the normal size, shape and position of the heart. Any deviations from the normal appearance of the mediastinum, the heart, greater blood vessels and lungs contribute to the diagnosis.

Electrocardiography

Electrocardiography is extremely valuable when neonates present with cardiac arrhythmia of any origin. ECG recordings often reflect the degree of neonatal adaptation to extrauterine life. Specialist practitioners should interpret the recorded evidence, distinguishing between the gradual transition in right ventricular dominance noticeable in the first 72 h and electrophysiological anomalies that may help towards the overall diagnostic assessment.

Echocardiography

Exploration of the cardiovascular system by two-dimensional **echocardiography** involves ultrasound scanning (Fig. 51.1) and contributes to the analysis of cardiovascular and intracardiac structures (Knight & Washington 2006). Neonates are good candidates for echocardiographic imaging because of their thin thoracic walls. Images of the heart chambers, and valves and dimensions of the large vessels can be easily identified. Although many abnormalities can be identified in the fetus from 16 weeks of gestation, new images are required after birth to confirm diagnosis.

Colour images help to visualise the presence and direction of blood flow in neonates with persistent patent ductus arteriosus, septal defects, systemic venous anomalies and arteriovenous malformations. Pulsed and continuous-wave **Doppler techniques** can estimate pressure gradients across stenotic valves, septal defects and abnormal vessel structures such as the dimensions

of patent ductus arteriosus and coarctation of the aorta. Palliative and corrective surgery is sometimes initiated solely on the basis of echocardiographic findings, without more invasive investigations such as cardiac catheterisation, but such decisions are dependent on the nature and severity of the cardiovascular anomaly.

Magnetic resonance imaging

MRI detects intrathoracic abnormalities of the aortic arch, the peripheral pulmonary arteries and the systematic collateral vessels, which are not adequately evaluated by echocardiography.

Cardiac catheterisation and angiocardiography

These are invasive procedures that are required in neonates with complex cardiovascular defects when explicit details are needed about the size of the defects and related haemodynamics. A fine catheter is inserted into the femoral vein, inferior vena cava, and the right side of the heart, the pulmonary artery and its branches. In general, such procedures have diagnostic purposes although occasionally cardiac catheterisation can be used to provide **palliative treatment** for neonates born with **transposition of the great arteries** or **tricuspid atresia**, whose life is dependent on interatrial blood flow. Then the catheterisation is carried out under general anaesthesia and the intracardiac catheter is used to carry out a **balloon atrial septostomy** which enhances systemic and pulmonary blood flow. If a septal defect is present, it may be possible to pass the catheter into the left side of the heart. Abnormal tracts can be identified and blood pressure and oxygen saturation within the heart and great vessels can be measured (Feinstein & Moore 2003).

Arterial blood gases

Measurement of arterial blood gases from a baby breathing air followed by 100% oxygen can provide evidence for a differential diagnosis of a right-to-left shunt in cyanotic heart disease. Po_2 seldom exceeds 25 kPa in a baby with cyanotic heart disease breathing 100% oxygen, whereas a baby with cyanosis caused by lung disorders will usually have a higher level of arterial oxygen. However, this test may provoke closure of the ductus arteriosus with disastrous consequences in neonates dependent on ductal blood flow.

Some common disorders: acyanotic lesions

Patent ductus arteriosus

The incidence of isolated persistent **patency of the ductus arteriosus** is about 10–12% of all congenital heart disease (Friedman & Silverman 2001), although Hoffman (2003)

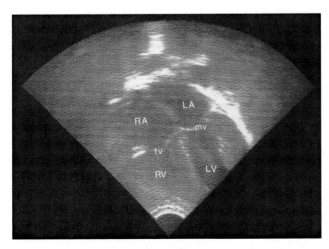

Figure 51.1 • A four chamber echo of the normal heart. LA, left atrium; LV, left ventricle; RA, right atrium; RV, right ventricle; tv, tricuspid valve; mv, mitral valve. (From Kelnar C, Harvey D, Simpson C 1995, with permission.)

suggests a lower percentage at 7.1%. It is twice as common in females as in males. In a term neonate the ductus arteriosus usually closes within the first few hours of birth in response to increased blood oxygen saturation. This functional closure is then followed by an anatomical occlusion several days later. Premature neonates may take up to 3 months to achieve such spontaneous closures which are attributed to the development of specialised contractile smooth muscle tissue and intimal thickening and fibrosis.

Where the patency of the ductus arteriosus persists, the fall in the neonate's pulmonary resistance reverses the direction of blood flow through the ductus from the aorta (left) shunting the oxygenated blood back into the pulmonary circulation (right). In some neonates the ductus arteriosus remains open when cardiac anomalies such as pulmonary stenosis are present (Fig. 51.2). In such instances the additional pulmonary blood flow is advantageous until the anomaly is surgically corrected. In the absence of the more complex cardiac anomalies, failure of spontaneous closure of the ductus arteriosus in premature neonates can contribute to persistence of respiratory distress syndrome (RDS). In term neonates it may lead to congestive cardiac failure, pulmonary hypertension and subacute bacterial endocarditis.

Symptoms of persistent ductus arteriosus develop between the 3rd and 7th days following birth. The neonate develops tachypnoea, dyspnoea and lethargy. Systolic and diastolic murmurs are almost always present. Therapeutic intervention includes restriction of fluids, adequate oxygenation and, where necessary, treatment for congestive cardiac failure (CCF) with **digitalis, furosemide (frusemide)** and **potassium supplementation.**

Indometacin may be used to induce ductus closure in premature neonates although term neonates are not as responsive to this drug, possibly due to its quicker clearance through the kidneys (Clyman 2005). As indometacin binds to plasma albumin, its presence may displace bilirubin and contribute to jaundice. Where appropriate expertise is available, transcatheter device occlusion may be the method of choice for ductal closure; however, more invasive methods of closure by means of a thoracotomy or thoracoscopy (Hoffman 2003) which facilitate ligation may be necessary if the earlier medical management fails.

Ventricular septal defects

Ventricular septal defects (VSDs) are common and account for 20% of congenital heart malformations (Friedman & Silverman 2001). A VSD can occur as an isolated intracardiac abnormality or it can be an adjunct to other cardiovascular lesions as is the case in about 50% of neonates born with congenital cardiovascular abnormalities. The defect usually occurs in the **membranous septum** but can present anywhere within the muscular part of the **interventricular septum** (Fig. 51.3).

The size and complexity of such defects varies from minute openings to almost complete absence of the interventricular septum. Knowledge of the precise size and position of the defect(s) is critical to successful therapeutic management. The incidence of spontaneous closure of the muscular defect is high, averaging 70%, although surgical repair is required where larger defects fail to close or membranous defects persist. Infants with small defects may be asymptomatic and eventually experience spontaneous closure, resulting in normal cardiac anatomy.

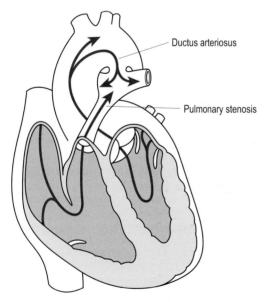

Figure 51.2 • Persistent ductus arteriosus in the presence of pulmonary stenosis. (From Fitzgerald M J T, Fitzgerald M 1994, with permission.)

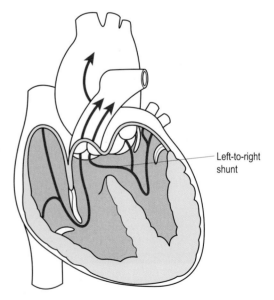

Figure 51.3 • Ventricular septal defect. (From Fitzgerald M J T, Fitzgerald M 1994, with permission.)

Larger defects are likely to lead to CCF, feeding problems and delays in growth. For this reason, VSDs are classified as acyanotic heart lesions with increased pulmonary blood flow caused by the increasing left ventricular pressure occurring after birth. The defect generates a left-to-right interventricular flow of blood. The presence of multiple VSDs or a large VSD allows the left-to-right shunt to equalise the pressure in both ventricles due to the shunting of oxygenated blood from the left ventricle into the right ventricle. This shunting will eventually lead to right ventricular volume overload, **pulmonary plethora** and CCF. Furthermore, the persistent increase in pulmonary blood volume increases pulmonary venous return to the left side of the heart. This eventually results in left ventricular volume overload, exacerbation of the left-to-right shunt and left ventricular hypertrophy.

For a time, the enlarged left ventricle pumps more efficiently, but eventually the heart fails and pulmonary hypertension develops. If untreated, the persistent problems contribute to the development of **Eisenmenger's syndrome** (McCance & Huether 2007). Pre-emptive therapeutic interventions are important if long-term problems are to be averted or minimised. Early diagnosis and proactive management of CCF as above should be considered until the defect is closed surgically. Where necessary, surgery is delayed until the infant is at least 12–18 months old but all defects must ideally be closed, surgically if necessary, by the time the child enters school.

Atrial septal defects

Atrial septal defects are relatively common congenital cardiac malformations occurring in 1:1000 of live births (Wernovsky & Gruber 2005). Interferences with the sequential atrial septal development may cause a variety of atrial septal defects (Srivastava & Olson 2000) some of which may be simple, involving only the **foramen ovale**, while others may be complex. Severe atrioventricular defects may extend to the ventricular septum, the **mitral** and **tricuspid** valves.

The most common of these defects are:

- **Septum primum** with endocardial cushion defects. This defect is generally associated with abnormalities of the mitral and tricuspid valves and atrioventricular canals (Fig. 51.4A). Although this defect may occur in isolation in otherwise normal neonates, 30% of cases occur in neonates with Down syndrome in whom the involvement of the endocardial cushions may also contribute to the defective formation of the upper portion of the intraventricular septum.
- **Ostium secundum.** This defect is found in the central portion of the atrial septum. Because of its close anatomical association with the fossa ovalis, it is often referred to as the fossa ovalis defect (Fig. 51.4B).
- **Sinus venosus** defect. This defect is characteristically found in the superior portion of the atrial septum and generally extends into the superior vena cava.

Simple defects cause few problems and, if spontaneous closure does not occur, surgical repairs are carried out by about 4–5 years of age. As these defects cause a left-to-right intracardiac shunt, no cyanosis occurs. However, for neonates born with atrioventricular defects (AVD), the prognosis is less favourable as they may experience conduction problems. Complex atrial septal defects are usually diagnosed in the first few days of life as these neonates develop tachypnoea, mild cyanosis, abnormal heart sounds and systolic murmurs, poor feeding and later fail to gain weight (Rudolph et al 2003).

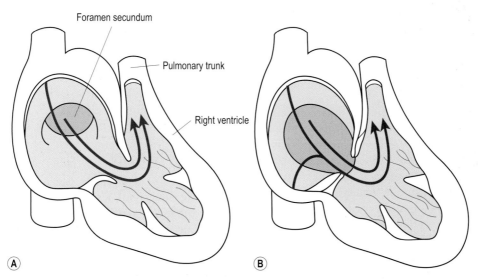

Figure 51.4 • (A) Septum primum lesion. (B) Ostium secundum lesion. (From Fitzgerald M J T, Fitzgerald M 1994, with permission.)

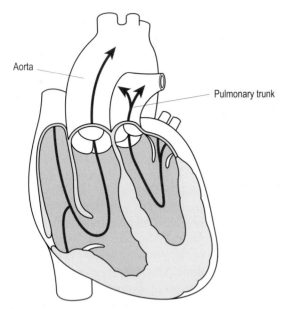

Figure 51.5 • Transposition of great arteries. (From Fitzgerald M J T, Fitzgerald M 1994, with permission.)

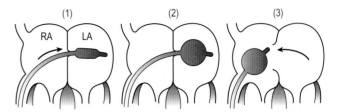

Figure 51.6 • Rashkind's atrial septostomy. (1) A catheter is passed into the right atrium (RA) and pushed through the foramen ovale into the left atrium (LA). (2) A balloon at the tip of the catheter is inflated. (3) The catheter is withdrawn sharply so that the inflated balloon tears the atrial septum, allowing oxygenated blood to reach the systemic circulation. (Reproduced with permission from Wallis & Harvey 1979.)

Some common disorders: cyanotic lesions

Transposition of the great arteries

Complete transposition of the great arteries (TGA) is the most common cardiovascular cause of peripheral and central cyanosis in neonates; the aorta arises from the right ventricle and the pulmonary artery from the left ventricle. This complete switch of the great vessels (Fig. 51.5) leads to the formation of **two separate closed circulatory systems**, whereby the blood from the pulmonary circulation cannot enter the systemic circulation and vice versa. Survival of these neonates depends on the patency of the right-to-left shunts in the ductus arteriosus and/or the foramen ovale. The presence of a concurrent VSD also permits mixing of the oxygenated and deoxygenated blood at the interventricular level. Boys appear to be affected twice as often as girls (Flanagan et al 1999).

A neonate with complete TGA and no accompanying ventricular defect will become increasingly cyanotic as the ductus arteriosus begins to close. This cyanosis is not relieved by administration of 100% oxygen and urgent life-saving intervention is needed. This is likely to consist of **prostaglandin infusion** to maintain the PDA open until palliative or corrective **surgery** can be carried out.

The palliative intervention may consist of a balloon septostomy (e.g. **Rashkind's**), generally carried out as an emergency to enlarge the foramen ovale and increase the interatrial mixing of blood. When possible, corrective surgery will be carried out some weeks/months later (Fig. 51.6). This consists of switching the pulmonary artery and the aorta to the correct ventricles and closing any remaining cardiovascular defects. Care is taken to ensure that the **coronary arteries** can sustain **normal myocardial perfusion**. Most surgical corrections are successful with a survival rate of up to 90% (McCance & Huether 2007).

Total anomalous pulmonary venous drainage

Total anomalous pulmonary venous connection occurs in 1:150 000 and is characterised by the absence of any direct connection of the **pulmonary veins** to the **left atrium**. Instead, the pulmonary veins connect either to the right atrium, various systemic veins or the liver. Depending on these unusual connections, oxygenated blood is returned into the right atrium, via the superior vena cava, the coronary sinus or the ductus venosus. About 30% of neonates born with total anomalous pulmonary venous drainage have other cardiac anomalies that must be considered in the overall management. Almost all surviving neonates present with a right-to-left shunt of blood at atrial or ventricular level, allowing mixed arterial and venous blood to circulate to the lungs and body. Central cyanosis, dyspnoea, tachypnoea and CCF occur and urgent, life-saving surgical correction is necessary. Mortality can be between 5% and 25% (Knight & Washington 2006).

Tetralogy of Fallot

The tetralogy of Fallot is the most common form of cyanotic congenital lesion in infants beyond the first year of life. Neonates can sometimes be asymptomatic. The four anatomic defects are (Fig. 51.7):

1. A high, large VSD.

2. An overriding aorta which straddles the VSD.

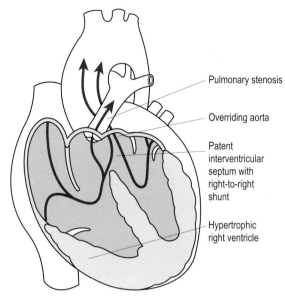

Figure 51.7 • Tetralogy of Fallot. (From Fitzgerald M J T, Fitzgerald M 1994, with permission.)

Labels on figure:
- Pulmonary stenosis
- Overriding aorta
- Patent interventricular septum with right-to-right shunt
- Hypertrophic right ventricle

3. Pulmonary stenosis: a funnel-shaped opening at the entrance to the pulmonary artery. The pulmonary artery and valve may rarely be completely obliterated.

4. Right ventricular hypertrophy, developing because of the obstruction to blood flow.

These defects can be associated with Down syndrome, first trimester rubella infection, Noonan's syndrome, Turner's syndrome and other undefined genetic mutations (Srivastava & Olson 2000). The clinical features of this defect relate to the neonate's pulmonary blood flow, which depends on:

1. The severity of the right ventricular outflow tract obstruction.

2. The relative resistance to ventricular outflow imposed by the systemic and pulmonary circulations.

3. The presence of systemic-to-pulmonary collateral blood flow through the bronchial arteries or, rarely, a PDA.

The symptoms vary depending on the degree of pulmonary stenosis, although the size of the VSD is important. Pulmonary stenosis decreases blood flow to the lungs as well as the return of oxygenated blood to the left atrium. With a large VSD, blood may shunt from the right ventricle to the left ventricle, causing further reduction in systemic oxygen content and an increase in central and peripheral cyanosis. However, giving oxygen in this instance may result in the closure of the PDA, further increasing cyanosis. Hypoxia stimulates the kidneys to produce erythropoietin so most children develop polycythaemia. Older children may have sudden spells of dyspnoea, cyanosis and restlessness and squat to alleviate these hypoxic spells.

Infants born with tetralogy of Fallot and pulmonary atresia usually require specialist surgical intervention of a corrective and/or palliative nature in the first few days or weeks of life. As most such infants will have a history of CCF which might impair their growth and development, management in a specialist cardiac centre is advocated.

Some common disorders: obstructive lesions

Coarctation of the aorta

Coarctation of the aorta occurs in 1:30 000 live births (Wernovsky & Gruber 2005) and is characterised by an abnormal segmental narrowing of the aorta anywhere from the aortic arch to the bifurcation of the abdominal aorta at its lower end. However, 98% occur at the junction with the ductus arteriosus. The narrowing may occur at (**preductal**) (Fig. 51.8) or after (**postductal**) the opening of the ductus arteriosus. Generally, coarctations of the aorta obstruct left ventricular outflow leading to left ventricular failure. Although **collateral arteries** may develop, bypassing the obstruction, many neonates present with life-threatening haemodynamic disturbances that lead to acute myocardial and renal failure.

In neonates presenting with postductal coarctation of the aorta, blood is delivered to the upper body from the ascending aorta via the subclavian arteries; this increases the blood pressure to the upper parts of the body. However, as the aortic narrowing reduces blood flow to the descending aorta, the lower parts of the body are not so well perfused so that the blood pressure in the lower limbs is low and **femoral pulses** are weak and sometimes absent.

Preductal coarctation is often associated with other anomalies. The ductus arteriosus may remain patent, creating a shunt allowing blood flow in either direction depending on the pressure differences between the aorta and the main pulmonary artery. If blood flows from the right to the left, the right ventricle acts as a systemic pump and the blood pressure and pulse differences between the upper and lower extremities disappear. If the blood flow is directed from the left to the right, more than the normal amount of blood will be sent to the lungs, causing CCF with left ventricular hypertrophy.

CCF may be one of the first features manifested by such neonates, and must be managed accordingly. However, **high oxygen levels must be avoided** and prostaglandin (PGE_1) may be given intravenously to maintain patency of the ductus arteriosus until the coarctation of the aorta is surgically corrected. Diuretics such as furosemide (frusemide) 1 mg/kg body weight may be

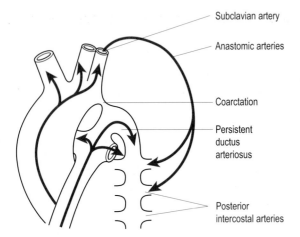

Figure 51.8 • Preductal coarctation of the aorta. (From Fitzgerald M J T, Fitzgerald M 1994, with permission.)

Labels on figure:
- Subclavian artery
- Anastomic arteries
- Coarctation
- Persistent ductus arteriosus
- Posterior intercostal arteries

given to decrease fluid overload and correct pulmonary and systemic oedema. Surgery with correction and reconstruction of the defective segment of the aorta will be carried out as the neonate's clinical condition is stabilised.

Pulmonary valve stenosis and aortic valve stenosis

Narrowing of the **pulmonary valve** occurs on its own in about 8% and **aortic stenosis** in about 6% of children born with congenital cardiac abnormalities. Mild valvular stenosis improves with age although more severe narrowing produces symptoms in neonates, most commonly pulmonary oedema and CCF. Surgical correction or, less commonly, valve replacement may be necessary in early infancy or childhood if cardiorespiratory function is compromising the child's growth and exercise tolerance.

Tricuspid atresia

Tricuspid atresia is uncommon and manifests in the first few hours or days of life. A distinctive clinical feature is extreme central cyanosis caused by the entire systemic venous return entering the right atrium and exiting through the foramen ovale into the left side of the heart. As the systemic and pulmonary venous blood mix in the left atrium, the left ventricle receives only mixed oxygenated and deoxygenated blood which is then pumped to the entire body, including the lungs. A variable but small amount of blood will enter the pulmonary artery through an existing VSD. The diminutive right ventricle and pulmonary valve and pulmonary artery tend to control the pulmonary blood flow. Although an existing PDA will support the pulmonary blood flow initially, long-term survival depends on the success of palliative and corrective surgery.

Hypoplastic left heart syndrome

This syndrome is the consequence of specific cardiovascular malformations such as severe obstruction or atresia of the mitral valve, diminutive left ventricle, aortic atresia and malalignments of the **atrioventricular canals**. These neonates become symptomatic within the first few hours or days of life, developing CCF (see below). Cardiac enlargement, pulmonary plethora, hypotension and bradycardia require supportive intervention. Surviving neonates will require palliative surgery. Despite advances in paediatric cardiothoracic surgery, the mortality rate is high as no successful corrective surgery is possible (Knight & Washington 2006). **Cardiac transplantation** might be considered.

Congestive cardiac failure

Congestive cardiac failure is a syndrome in which the failing heart cannot sustain a normal cardiac output or supply adequate oxygenated blood to the tissues. The major causes in neonates are **excessive volume overload, excessive pressure load** and **abnormal myocardial function**.

Excessive volume overload

Large valve incompetence or left-to-right shunts are the most common causes of volume overload and in the neonate the cause is likely to be attributed to a PDA, large VSDs or endocardial cushion defects with gross valve incompetence. Less commonly, volume overload may be initiated by excessive placental transfusion at birth.

Excessive pressure load

Severe forms of aortic stenosis and coarctation of the aorta, commonly referred to as **left ventricular outflow tract obstruction**, lead to CCF in the first weeks of life. Infants with either of these lesions may present with very poor pulses and a large left-to-right shunt at the atrial level. The moderately severe pulmonary hypertension can be attributed to early CCF. Once the intra-atrial left-to-right shunt reverses or a large right-to-left shunt develops through the ductus arteriosus, neonates present with moderately severe peripheral and central cyanosis.

Myocardial dysfunction

Bristow (1996) argues that the fetal and neonatal myocardium develops much less **active tension** during **isometric contraction** than that of an adult. In the adult 60% of the myocardium is a contractile mass, whereas in fetuses and neonates the myocardium holds more water, fewer contractile proteins and is less compliant, reducing myocardial contractile force. The sparse **myofibrils** are randomly organised and surrounded by considerable amounts of interstitial fluid (Larsen 2008). Therefore, the filling pressures in the neonatal heart may need to be higher than the values seen in adults to optimise myofilament alignment.

Normal myocardial function in neonates

At birth the structure of the two ventricles is similar. However, as the neonate's physiological pulmonary vascular resistance falls, the right ventricle gradually adapts, losing power as it pumps to a low-resistance system that doesn't require such muscular effort. This physiological adaptation culminates in the typically disproportional developments of the two ventricles.

Mature myocardium has a **sarcoplasmic reticulum** which stores and releases calcium to support contractility. Since the neonatal myocardium has less sarcoplasmic reticulum and reduced calcium storage facilities, it depends more on **trans-sarcolemmal calcium influx** than the adult myocardium. Gradual maturation of the myocardium increases the amounts of sarcoplasmic reticulum, although most neonates show a short-lived increase in ventricular performance when calcium is given to support myocardial contractility. The neonatal myocardium is much less susceptible to hypoxia than the adult myocardium (Hatch et al 1995). This reflects the greater neonatal capacity for **anaerobic metabolism**.

Causes of myocardial dysfunction in neonates

The most likely cause of neonatal myocardial dysfunction is **myocardial ischaemia** caused by severe perinatal asphyxia (Rychik & Cohen 2005) and the presence of an anomalous coronary artery (Friedman & Silverman 2001). However, in neonates the myocardium can also be severely depressed by **metabolic problems** such as severe postpartum asphyxia, hypoglycaemia, hypocalcaemia and hypomagnesaemia. **Arrhythmias** such as congenital heart block, paroxysmal tachycardia or bradycardia can cause cardiac failure in both fetus and neonate. However, neonatal tachycardias are often intermittent and difficulties may occur in diagnosing these conditions. The causes of CCF must be identified and used as indicators in the management of the haemodynamic disturbances so that permanent damage to the heart or the entire cardiorespiratory system is averted or minimised.

Common manifestations of CCF

These include tachypnoea, pulmonary oedema, cyanosis, diaphoresis, feeding difficulties and, occasionally, periorbital or peripheral oedema (Friedman & Silverman 2001), cold extremities, low blood pressure and recurrent chest infections (Sharma et al 2003). As the causes of CCF can be extensive and complex, it is essential to establish an early diagnosis and efficient treatment. The neonate's survival and quality of life will depend on this.

Lower respiratory tract problems in neonates

Breathing difficulties are the most common clinical problems encountered in neonates and it is often difficult to make a clear diagnosis, even after examining chest X-rays together with other diagnostic results. Lung infections are difficult to rule out and many neonates are given antibiotics until microbiology results are available. Birth records detailing neonatal respiratory effort and the time of onset of respiratory difficulties are important in formulating a diagnosis. A major difficulty is to establish whether the neonate's cyanosis is caused by respiratory disorders or congenital heart disease (Flanagan et al 1999), although a distinction must be made if treatment is to succeed. Neonates with significant respiratory dysfunction accompanied by cyanosis should be cared for in neonatal intensive care units (Fig. 51.9).

Respiratory distress syndrome

Most neonates initiate spontaneous respiration at birth. The inspired air gradually displaces the alveolar and interstitial fluid, increasing pulmonary compliance and a greater pulmonary blood flow as the vascular tree expands. The 10-fold increase in pulmonary capillary blood facilitates an acceptable gas exchange across alveolar walls, providing the lungs are sufficiently mature and capable of synthesising **surfactant**.

Surfactant, a lipoprotein complex secreted by type II pneumocytes, consists of 90% **lipids**, including **lecithin**, **sphingomyelin** and **cholesterol**. The remainder is made up of substances such as specific proteins and some carbohydrates. Surfactant is extruded into the alveolar spaces where it unravels, forming complex lipid structures called **tubular myelin**. These form the **surface monolayer** at the alveolar air–liquid interface.

The fetal lungs secrete surfactant from about the 22nd week, with considerable surges at 33 weeks of gestation and at birth. Surfactant coats the inner aspect of the alveoli and reduces surface tension created by the alveolar fluid, ensuring that the alveoli do not collapse at the end of expiration. The ratio of lecithin to sphingomyelin (**L:S ratio**) is 1:1 at about 34 weeks of gestation, but the amount of lecithin increases until the ratio is 2:1, comparable to a mature lung. Amniotic fluid can be tested for these two substances to establish fetal lung maturity.

RDS (or **hyaline membrane disease**) occurs predominantly in premature neonates due to immature lung anatomy and physiology (Enzman Hagedorn et al 2006). This severe lung disorder causes more neonatal deaths than any other condition. The incidence is inversely proportional to gestational age, occurring in about 70% of neonates born at 29 weeks of gestation and declining sharply to near 0%

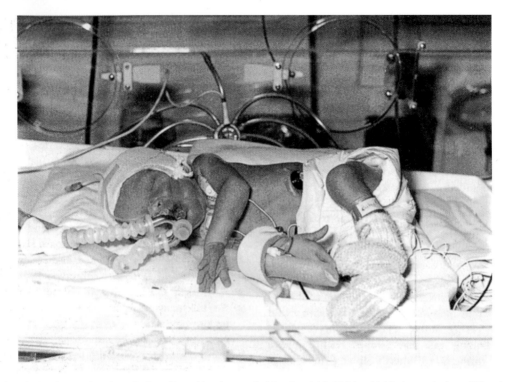

Figure 51.9 • A baby having assisted ventilation. (From Henderson C, Macdonald S 2004, with kind permission of Elsevier.)

at 39 weeks (Ariagno 1995) although it is fairly common in term neonates born to mothers suffering from diabetes mellitus. The cause is multifactorial, but insufficient active pulmonary surfactant is the major contributing factor. Predisposing factors include:

- Immature lungs, especially in male neonates.
- Surfactant inactivation caused by endothelial damage.
- Birth by caesarean section prior to the onset of labour.
- Asphyxia neonatorum, as respiratory and metabolic acidosis interferes with surfactant synthesis.
- Hypovolaemia or hypervolaemia.
- Mother has a history of diabetes mellitus (this seems to delay lung maturity).
- Premature/prolonged rupture of membranes.
- Maternal antepartum haemorrhage.
- Maternal haemodynamic instability.
- Maternal substance abuse.

Pathophysiology

RDS is due to the absence or immaturity of type II pneumocytes and their incapacity to produce sufficient amounts of functional surfactant. A greater inspiratory effort is needed to keep the alveoli open. Poor alveolar stability contributes to poor lung compliance, limited lung distensibility and reduced functional residual capacity. This impacts directly on **pulmonary perfusion** and most neonates develop a right-to-left shunt, which contributes to significant hypoxia with a depressing effect on myocardial function. A moderate PDA may also add to the existing respiratory problems due to the additional pulmonary blood flow which compromises pulmonary function. Some neonates will eventually develop myocardial failure, hypotension and poor renal and peripheral perfusion.

Other problems such as **respiratory acidosis** and **atelectasis** (inadequate alveolar expansion and collapse of lung tissue) further compromise respiratory gas exchange. The atelectasis is generally attributed to unequal pressures and filling capacity in some alveoli. The normal alveoli become overdistended and the smaller alveoli collapse, reducing the functional residual capacity and creating a significant **dead space** within the lungs (Blackburn 2007).

The resulting **hypoxia** and **hypercapnia** lead to pulmonary vasoconstriction and, sometimes, **persistent fetal circulation** with significant intracardiac right-to-left shunting of blood through the foramen ovale and ductus arteriosus. Lung ischaemia exacerbates the damage to the alveolar epithelial surfaces and capillaries. Metabolic and respiratory acidosis further suppresses the production of surfactant. Increased alveolar surface tension combined with the low plasma protein levels present in the premature neonates lead to a shift of interstitial fluid towards the alveolar space. As the exudate is rich in **fibrinogen**,

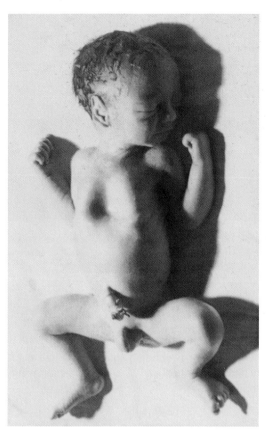

Figure 51.10 • A baby with respiratory distress syndrome. Note marked sternal recession. (From Kelnar C, Harvey D, Simpson C 1995, with permission.)

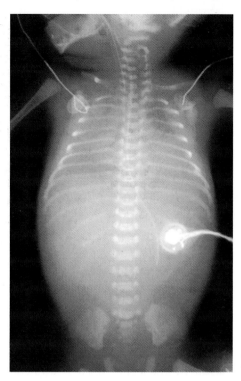

Figure 51.11 • Chest X-ray showing 'ground-glass' appearance of lungs in hyaline membrane disease. (From Kelnar C, Harvey D, Simpson C 1995, with permission.)

it is converted to **fibrin** as it lines the alveoli. Blood products and cellular debris present within the alveoli bind the fibrin forming the **hyaline membrane**, which further reduces lung surface area (Blackburn 2007) and makes the lungs less compliant.

Clinical symptoms

Affected neonates gradually develop symptoms of RDS typically about 4h after birth, with tachypnoea, increased respiratory effort and grunting on expiration. There is evidence of chest wall recession, peripheral and later central cyanosis (Fig. 51.10). A chest X-ray shows a 'ground-glass' appearance to the lungs (Fig. 51.11), whereas an air bronchogram shows air in the larger airways against the background opaqueness (Enzman Hagedorn et al 2006).

Management of respiratory distress syndrome

Prebirth maternal treatment with corticosteroids

Management of RDS includes prevention and treatment. The production of surfactant in the fetal lung can be increased by treating the mother with a **corticosteroid** such as betamethasone for at least 24h before birth. Indications for commencing corticosteroid administration may be a low L:S ratio or, if this invasive test is not possible, the anticipated premature birth. Roberts & Dalziel's (2006) review of the research concluded that this proactive management reduces the severity of RDS in susceptible premature neonates with significant reduction in morbidity and mortality.

Surfactant therapy

The use of natural and artificial surfactant postdelivery has been effective in the management of affected neonates. Soll & Blanco (2001) updated earlier research reviews concerning **surfactant therapy**, comparing the benefits and drawbacks of natural versus synthetic surfactant and multiple versus single dose of natural surfactant. Both natural and artificial surfactants were effective in the treatment of established RDS. There was earlier improvement in neonates who required assisted ventilatory support (Stevens et al 2002), with fewer instances of **pneumothorax** occurring in neonates treated with natural surfactant extract. Multiple doses of natural surfactant extract also resulted in greater improvements in respiratory function and oxygen levels, reducing the occurrence of pneumothorax. Multiple doses of natural surfactant extract appear to be the most effective treatment (Taeusch et al 2005).

Oxygen therapy

Oxygen therapy is necessary to avert hypoxia which can lead to brain damage. Some neonates only require a low concentration of humidified oxygen administered in a head box. Others may require **continuous positive airway pressure** (CPAP) to reduce the work of breathing by maintaining a constant alveolar end-expiratory pressure of 5–10 cmH$_2$O. However, very small neonates and those with severe RDS may require mechanical ventilation by **intermittent positive pressure ventilation** (IPPV) (Welty et al 2005) and this group of neonates may also benefit from the use of surfactant therapies.

Complications associated with excessive use of oxygen therapy and IPPV include:

- Pneumothorax, pulmonary interstitial fibrosis and later bronchopulmonary dysplasia.
- Periventricular haemorrhage when oxygen saturation is badly controlled or excessive.
- Infection and secondary pneumonia may follow endotracheal intubation and periodic lavage to keep the tube patent.
- Retinopathy (retrolental fibroplasia) most common in premature neonates exposed to high O$_2$ tension.
- Myopia and cataracts.
- Cellular damage due to the excessive production of oxygen-derived free radicals.
- Central nervous system toxicity and seizures.

Bronchopulmonary dysplasia

Bronchopulmonary dysplasia is a form of subacute or chronic **fibrosis of the lungs** associated with severe hyaline membrane disease, prolonged assisted mechanical ventilation and high oxygen requirement. This disorder affects infants weighing less than 1500 g at birth (Banks-Randall & Ballard 2005, Enzman Hagedorn et al 2006). Affected infants remain oxygen-dependent, have respiratory symptoms such as tachypnoea and intercostal recession and abnormal lung findings on radiography (Fig. 51.12) after 28 days (McCance & Huether 2007).

Scarring of the lung tissue, **emphysema**, failure of the alveoli to multiply and inflammatory destruction of the epithelial lining of the lungs and ciliated epithelial surfaces in the bronchi are characteristic features. In addition, mucous plugs and debris clog the small-diameter airways, contributing to recurrent pulmonary infection. Many of the affected neonates experience some of the events shown in Table 51.2 (deMello & Reid 1995). The clinical picture may persist for some months or years and, whilst some infants recover with minimal residual lung damage, others die.

Therapy involves maintenance of normal oxygen saturation, prevention of infection and adequate nutrition.

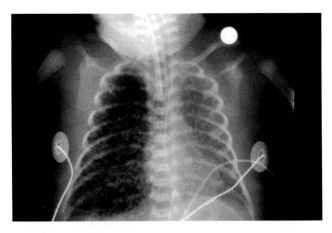

Figure 51.12 • Chest X-ray showing early stages of bronchopulmonary dysplasia. (From Kelnar C, Harvey D, Simpson C 1995, with permission.)

Table 51.2 Some events occurring in infants with bronchopulmonary dysplasia

Pulmonary injury and barotrauma	Resolution and healing	Catch-up growth in surviving lung tissue
Pulmonary oedema	Phagocytosis and absorption of inflammatory products	Alveolar multiplication
Cell necrosis	Scarring of lung tissue	Pulmonary vascular remodelling
Hyaline membrane formation	Overinflation of the intervening lung	
Atelectasis	Increased resting volume	

Dexamethasone may be used to reduce the inflammatory changes and improve oxygenation without increasing the risk of infection (Ng 1993). Antibiotics can be used to control infection. Once the infant's condition is stabilised and the parents can manage the oxygen therapy and other supportive interventions, home care is encouraged. Ideally, a community specialist paediatric nurse and health visitor should support the family. Administration of vitamin A to extremely LBW babies is associated with a reduction in death or oxygen requirement at 1 month of age (Enzman Hagedorn et al 2006).

Meconium aspiration syndrome

When a fetus suffers from intrapartum asphyxia, meconium is passed into the amniotic fluid and inhaled as gasping movements are made. At birth, prompt clearing of the mouth and upper airways must be carried out to avoid the consequences of such inhalation. If possible any meconium present must be removed.

Management

Meconium encourages growth of micro-organisms and any neonate suspected of having inhaled meconium must be observed for the next 24–48 h for signs of respiratory distress manifesting as tachypnoea and cyanosis. Oxygen therapy may be required and a prophylactic course of antibiotics may be given to avert the onset of **pneumonia**. More severely affected neonates may show signs of persistent fetal circulation, resulting in cardiopulmonary problems such as pulmonary hypertension, systemic hypotension and hypoxia. Pneumothoraxes are a relatively common complication (Ballard et al 2005).

Surfactant treatment

The presence of meconium in the lung may inactivate surfactant and short-term administration of surfactant (four doses every 6 h), commenced within 6 h of birth, improves oxygenation and reduced respiratory morbidity. However, where persistent fetal circulation and pulmonary hypertension are severe, more drastic measures involve assisted ventilatory support using high-frequency oscillatory ventilation and nitric oxide. The relative efficacy of surfactant therapy, either alone or in conjunction with **nitric oxide** or ventilation, needs more research (Soll & Dargaville 1999).

Pneumothorax

A pneumothorax occurs as a result of injury to the pleural membranes, allowing air to leak into the pleural space. In neonates the most likely cause is alveolar rupture and associated damage to the visceral layer of the **pleural membrane**. The affected lung collapses, causing a mediastinal shift and displacing the normal position of heart and greater vessels. This in turn compromises cardiac function, initiating low cardiac output, hypotension and bradycardia. Recently, the selective use of surfactant therapy has contributed to a significant reduction in the number of neonates developing a pneumothorax and requiring additional supportive interventions.

Management

A pneumothorax does not present with the classical symptoms seen in the adult and may be difficult to diagnose. The neonate suddenly collapses and becomes cyanotic with bradycardia. There may be cardiac displacement and **transillumination**; shining a cold light against the thorax may demonstrate air around the lung. Chest radiography will

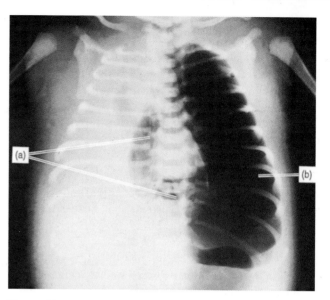

Figure 51.13 • Pneumopericardium (a) with a large left pneumothorax (b). (From Kelnar C, Harvey D, Simpson C 1995, with permission.)

confirm the diagnosis (Fig. 51.13). If the neonate is otherwise in good health, draining the air may not be necessary as it will be gradually reabsorbed. However, neonates who experience respiratory distress and haemodynamic changes will require the insertion of a pleural drain connected to underwater sealed drainage which allows the air to escape and the lung to re-expand.

Transient tachypnoea of the newborn

Transient tachypnoea of the newborn is relatively common in term neonates who present with tachypnoea, intercostal retraction, slight grunting and possibly cyanoses. A chest X-ray shows enlarged lymph vessels and signs of **pulmonary interstitial oedema** (Welty et al 2005). This may persist from 2 to 5 days. Although the precise cause remains unknown, the most obvious factor is a mild immaturity in the surfactant system which may be responsible for surfactant deficiency or failure to absorb lung fluid following delivery. Most neonates require less than 40% oxygen to maintain systemic oxygenation.

Sudden infant death syndrome

A **sudden infant death** is the unexpected death of an otherwise healthy infant. These deaths almost always occur during sleep, most commonly at night, during winter and are usually unexplained by postmortem examination (Hansen & Corbet 2005). The term sudden infant death syndrome (SIDS) should only be used when it is the sole cause of death stated on the death certificate. The peak incidence of such deaths is between 2 and 4 months of age. Less than 1% of such deaths occur under the age of 2 months. Boys are more likely to die than girls, and low-birth-weight babies are at higher risk. SIDS is 'the greatest single cause of death amongst infants between 1 week and 1 year of age' (McCance & Huether 2007).

The causes of sudden infant death syndrome

SIDS is a complex phenomenon and key contributory factors include the infant's sleeping position, overheating, sudden illness, cardiac arrhythmias such as prolonged Q-T syndrome (Hansen & Corbet 2005) and possible effects of smoking by the parents, but further research is required.

Position of the larynx

The position of the infant's larynx and its close contact with the soft palate, which normally facilitates the infant's ability to breathe and swallow simultaneously, may be a contributing factor (Morgan 1994). From the 3rd month the **larynx** moves to a position below the back of the tongue, an arrangement necessary for speech production. Crelin (1973) first postulated that this may influence the occurrence of SIDS. The risk is highest during the transitional period and once the larynx has reached its new position at 6 months the risk of death falls. This is unlikely to be the sole cause but should be considered by researchers. Morgan (1994) also postulates that, when neonates lie in the prone position, the **uvula** may enter the larynx and block the airway. If the infant is ill, weak and cannot change the position of his head and neck, he may suffocate. Hansen & Corbet (2005) draw attention to inappropriate 'laryngeal chemoreflex' activities, positioning and sleep patterns.

Sleeping position

The fashion for placing babies in the **prone position** for sleeping was introduced in the Netherlands in the 1970s. Babies lying in the prone position were thought to be less likely to inhale regurgitated feeds. However, this practice led to a 3-fold increase in SIDS and enhanced research interest in the effects of sleeping position on the occurrence of SIDS. The studies of the 1980s concluded that death rates were lowered if infants were placed on their backs when sleeping. Fleming et al (1990) found an 8-fold increase in risk if a baby was placed prone for sleeping rather than on its side or back. Placing an infant on his side doubles the risk, possibly because babies can easily roll onto their stomachs.

Overheating

Tuffnell et al (1996) found that deep body temperature in infants who co-sleep with their parents was higher than in infants who slept alone. Parents are advised to separate their bodies from the baby by making a separate 'nest' for the baby with pillows. Mothers tend to wrap up their babies in the winter months or during illness. The occurrence of SIDS tended to coincide with infants being heavily wrapped, lain prone and allowed to sleep in an overheated room (Fleming et al 1990).

Smoking

Studies have shown that active and passive smoking in pregnancy increases the risk of SIDS (Schoendorf & Kiely 1992). There may be an increased risk if both parents smoke. Because of a steady rise in SIDS in England and Wales, peaking at 2.3:1000 in 1988, campaigns to reduce the deaths were introduced in 1991 by the Foundation for the Study of Infant Deaths and the Department of Health. Between 1991 and 1995 the SIDS rate in England and Wales, which had already fallen from the high point of 1988, fell 50% from 1.4 to 0.6:1000 live births (Office for National Statistics 1996). The recommendations were:

1. Babies should not be placed upon their fronts to sleep.

2. Babies should not be overheated.

3. If babies are unwell, medical help should be sought without delay.

4. Babies should not be exposed to nicotine.

Main points

- Cardiovascular anomalies are the most common forms of congenital malformations. Neonates may present with tachypnoea, dyspnoea, cyanosis, tachycardia, bradycardia, hypo- and hypertension, heart murmurs, poor feeding, grunting and systemic oedema.
- Closure of the ductus arteriosus in the preterm infant may take up to 3 months. Therapeutic interventions may include restriction of fluids, oxygen therapy, a course of indometacin or invasive ligation if medical management fails.
- Ventricular septal defects may be asymptomatic and close spontaneously, although large defects can lead to haemodynamic problems and congestive cardiac failure which must be treated prior to surgical closure.
- Simple atrial septal defects cause few problems although surgical closure is advisable before the child

enters school. Neonates born with atrioventricular canal defects may experience conduction problems prior to and following surgical correction.

- Transposition of the great vessels leads to the formation of two separate circulatory systems preventing the transfer of oxygenated blood into the systemic circulation. Neonatal survival depends on the patency of the ductus arteriosus, the foramen ovale and the existence of a VSD which must be preserved until corrective surgery is possible.

- Total anomalous pulmonary venous connection interferes with normal pulmonary venous return to the left atrium. As oxygenated blood returns to the right side of the heart, the baby rapidly develops cyanosis, tachypnoea and other haemodynamic problems requiring urgent surgical correction.

- The classical features of tetralogy of Fallot are: a high, large ventricular septal defect; an overriding aorta, which straddles the VSD; pulmonary stenosis; and right ventricular hypertrophy. Surgical correction is always necessary.

- Coarctation of the aorta commonly occurs at the junction with the ductus arteriosus. Collateral arteries can develop to bypass the obstruction. Abnormal blood pressure and pulses can be the first sign. Prostaglandin administration may maintain patency of the ductus arteriosus to sustain the systemic circulation to the lower part of the body until a surgical correction is possible.

- The major causes of neonatal congestive cardiac failure are excessive volume overload, excessive pressure load and abnormal myocardial function. Early diagnosis of the primary cause and effective evidence-based management are crucial to the neonate's survival and quality of life.

- In respiratory distress syndrome, increasing inspiratory effort and expiratory difficulties may lead to respiratory failure and atelectasis. Hypoxia and hypercapnia lead to pulmonary vasoconstriction and persistent fetal circulation. Natural/synthetic surfactant administration to combat severe respiratory distress has significantly reduced neonatal morbidity and mortality.

- In bronchopulmonary dysplasia neonates/infants may remain oxygen-dependent. Dexamethasone may reduce pulmonary inflammation. Some infants show considerable recovery in pulmonary function whereas others experience permanent pulmonary scarring and ongoing respiratory problems.

- Inhalation of meconium may cause respiratory difficulties. Oxygen therapy and antibiotics may be needed to avoid pneumonia. Surfactant therapy commenced within 6 h of birth may improve prognosis.

- A pneumothorax occasionally occurs as a result of other primary respiratory problems. As this can influence haemodynamic stability, it will require invasive therapeutic intervention.

- Transient tachypnoea of the newborn may be caused by mild surfactant deficiency or failure to absorb lung fluid following birth. Oxygen therapy generally aids gradual recovery.

- Sudden infant death almost always occurs during sleep, with a peak incidence in the winter. Low-birth-weight babies are at higher risk. Causative factors include sleeping position, overheating, undetected illness and parental smoking. To date, no single common factor has been isolated. Successful campaigns aimed at reducing SIDS in England and Wales were introduced in 1991.

References

Ariagno, R., 1995. Respiratory problems in the preterm infant. In: Reed, G., Claireaux, A., Cockburn, F. (Eds.), Diseases of the Fetus and Newborn: Pathology, Imaging Genetics and Management, Vol. 2. Chapman and Hall Medical, London.

Banks-Randall, B., Ballard, R., 2005. Bronchopulmonary dysplasia. In: Taeusch, W., Ballard, R., Gleason, C. (Eds.), Avery's Diseases of the Newborn. Elsevier Saunders, London.

Blackburn, S.T., 2007. Maternal, Fetal and Neonatal Physiology: A Clinical Perspective, third edn. W B Saunders, Philadelphia.

Bristow, J., 1996. Cardiac and myocardial structure and myocardial cellular and molecular function. In: Gluckman, P., Heyman, M. (Eds.), Paediatric

Perinatology: The Scientific Basis. Arnold, London.

Bristow, J., et al., 2003. Overview of cardiac development. In: Rudolph, C., Rudolph, A., Hostetter, M. (Eds.), Rudolph's Pediatrics. McGraw-Hill, London.

Chien, K., 2000. Genomic circuits and the integrative biology of cardiac disease. Nature 407, 227–232.

Clyman, R., 2005. Patent ductus arteriosus in the premature infant. In: Tauesch, W., Ballard, R., Gleason, C. (Eds.), Avery's Diseases of the Newborn. Elsevier Saunders, London.

Crelin, E., 1973. Functional Anatomy of the Newborn. Yale University Press, New Haven, Connecticut.

DeMello, D., Reid, L., 1995. Respiratory tract and lungs. In: Reed, G., Claireaux, A.,

Cockburn, F. (Eds.), Diseases of the Fetus and Newborn: Pathology, Imaging, Genetics and Management, Vol. 2. Chapman and Hall Medical, London.

Enzman Hagedorn, M.I., Gardner, S.L., Dickey, L.A., Abman, S.H., 2006. Respiratory diseases, 2006. In: Merenstein, G.B., Gardner, S.L. (Eds.), Handbook of Neonatal Intensive Care, sixth edn. Mosby Elsevier, St Louis, Missouri.

Feinstein, J., Moore, P., et al., 2003. Cardiac catheterization. In: Rudolph, C., Rudolph, A., Hostetter, M. (Eds.), Rudolph's Pediatrics. McGraw-Hill, London.

Flanagan, M., Yeager, S., Weidling, S., 1999. Cardiac disease. In: Avery, G., Fletcher, M., MacDonald, M. (Eds.), Neonatal Pathophysiology and Management of the Newborn. Lippincott, Williams and Wilkins, Philadelphia.

Fleming, P.J., Gilbert, R., Azaz, Y., et al., 1990. Interaction between bedding and sleeping position in sudden infant death syndrome: a population based case-control study. Br. Med. J. 301, 85–89.

Friedman, W., Silverman, N., 2001. Diseases of the heart, pericardium and pulmonary vascular beds: congenital heart disease in infancy and childhood. In: Braunwald, E., Zipes, D., Libby, P. (Eds.), Heart Disease: A Textbook of Cardiovascular Medicine, Vol. 2. W B Saunders, Philadelphia.

Hansen, T., Corbet, A., 2005. Control of breathing. In: Taeusch, W., Ballard, R., Gleason, C. (Eds.), Avery's Diseases of the Newborn. Elsevier Saunders, London.

Hatch, D., Somner, E., Hellman, J., et al., 1995. The Surgical Neonate: Anaesthesia and Intensive Care. Edward Arnold, London.

Hoffman, J., 2003. Congenital heart disease incidence and recurrence. In: Rudolph, C., Rudolph, A., Hostetter, M. (Eds.), Rudolph's Pediatrics. McGraw-Hill, London.

Knight, S.E., Washington, R.L., 2006. Cardiovascular and surgical interventions 2006. In: Merenstein, G.B., Gardber, S.L. (Eds.), Handbook of Neonatal Care. Elsevier Mosby, St Louis Missouri.

Larsen, W., 2008. Human Embryology. Churchill Livingstone, New York.

McCance, K.L., Huether, S.E., 2007. Pathophysiology: The biologic basis for disease in adults and children, third edn. Mosby, St Louis.

Morgan, E., 1994. The Descent of the Child. Souvenir Press, London.

Ng, P.C., 1993. The effectiveness and side effects of dexamethasone in preterm infants with bronchopulmonary dysplasia. Arch. Dis. Child. 68, 330–336.

Roberts, D., Dalziel, S.R., 2006. Antenatal corticosteroids for accelerating fetal lung maturation for women at risk of preterm birth. Cochrane Database of Syst. Rev. (3) 2006.

Rudolph, C., Rudolph, A., Hostetter, M., et al., 2003. Rudolph's Pediatrics. McGraw-Hill, London.

Rychik, J., Cohen, M., 2005. Echocardiography in the neonatal intensive care unit. In: Taeusch, W., Ballard, R., Gleason, C. (Eds.), Avery's Diseases of the Newborn. Elsevier Saunders, London.

Schoendorf, K.C., Kiely, J.L., 1992. Relationship of sudden infant death syndrome to maternal smoking during and after pregnancy. Pediatrics 90, 905–908.

Sharma, M., Nair, M., Jatana, S., Shahi, B., 2003. Congestive heart failure in infants and children. MJAFI 59 (3), 228–233.

Soll, R.F., Blanco, F., 2001. Natural surfactant extract versus synthetic surfactant for neonatal respiratory distress syndrome. Cochrane Review. Cochrane Library, Issue (1) Update Software 2003, Oxford.

Soll, R.F., Dargaville, P., 1999. Surfactant for meconium aspiration syndrome in full term infants. Cochrane Review. Cochrane Library, Issue (1) Update Software 2003, Oxford.

Srivastava, D., Olson, E., 2000. A genetic blueprint for cardiac development. Nature 47, 221–226.

Stevens, T.P., Blennow, M., Soll, R.F., 2002. Early surfactant administration with brief ventilation vs. selective surfactant and continued mechanical ventilation for preterm infants with or at risk for RDS. Cochrane Review. Cochrane Library, Issue (1) Update Software 2003, Oxford.

Taeusch, W., Ramierez-Schrempp, D., Laing, I., 2005. Surfactant treatment of respiratory disorders. In: Taeusch, W., Ballard, R., Gleason, C. (Eds.), Avery's Diseases of the Newborn. Elsevier Saunders, London.

Tuffnell, C.S., Petersen, S.A., Wailoo, M.P., 1996. Higher rectal temperatures in co-sleeping infants. Arch. Dis. Child. 75 (3), 249–250.

Welty, S., Hansen, T., Corbet, A., 2005. Respiratory distress in preterm infants. In: Taeusch, W., Ballard, R., Gleason, C. (Eds.), Avery's Diseases of the Newborn. Elsevier Saunders, London.

Wernovsky, G., Gruber, P., 2005. Common congenital heart disease: presentation, management and outcomes. In: Taeusch, W., Ballard, R., Gleason, C. (Eds.), Avery's Diseases of the Newborn. Elsevier Saunders, London.

Annotated recommended reading

Boxwell, G., 2000. Neonatal Intensive Care Nursing. Routledge, London.

This textbook outlines a range of common and challenging neonatal problems and then provides helpful and directive suggestions for neonatal intensive care nursing which allows critical analysis and reflection on the identified neonatal nursing concepts and reinforces best practice.

Friedman, W., Silverman, N., 2001. Diseases of the heart, pericardium and pulmonary vascular bed: congenital heart disease in infancy and childhood. In: Braunwald, E., Zipes, D., Libby, P. (Eds.) Heart Disease: A Textbook of Cardiovascular Medicine, Vol. 2. W B Saunders, Philadelphia.

This chapter describes congenital cardiovascular disease in infants and children. The authors distinguish between acyanotic and cyanotic lesions and detail the specific presenting features of the most common lesions that occur in infancy and childhood. They also offer a credible rationale for diagnostic and therapeutic interventions.

Polin, R., Fox, W., Abman, S., 2004. Fetal and Neonatal Physiology. W B Saunders, Philadelphia.

These textbooks discuss bioscientific concepts important in fetal and neonatal care. The résumé of genetics leads to a more detailed exploration of normal and abnormal embryonic and fetal development. Overall, these books make a significant contribution to clinical practice and research.

Roberts, D., Dalziel, S.R., 2006. Antenatal corticosteroids for accelerating fetal lung maturation for women at risk of preterm birth. Cochrane Database of Syst. Rev. (3) 2006.

This article provides an invaluable review of empirical evidence concerning the use of corticosteroids as a preventative measure against respiratory distress syndrome. The overall conclusions are supportive of such prophylactic administrations of the chosen corticosteroids.

Wong, D., 2004. Nursing Care of Infants and Children. Mosby, St Louis.

This textbook offers detailed accounts of the relevant biophysical, psychosocial and nursing issues in managing the care of infants and children. It concludes with a range of helpful appendices, which include excellent developmental screening tools and biophysical nomograms and parameters invaluable in all aspects of child care.

Chapter Fifty-Two

52

Jaundice and common metabolic problems in neonates

Introduction

Transition to extrauterine life occurs normally when fetal organs are sufficiently mature to support neonatal survival. The liver plays vital roles in this transition. This chapter explores the developmental features of the liver, its contribution to the synthesis and excretion of bilirubin and draws attention to common metabolic problems that can occur in neonates.

Neonatal jaundice

Morphological factors

Details of the structure and function of the mature liver are given in Chapter 22. As hepatic immaturity, hepatic disease and jaundice are common in neonates it is important to understand the morphological features and functional scope of the liver and its biliary tract. The liver is one of the largest visceral organs in neonates and normally extends from the right hypochondrium, through the epigastrium into the left hypochondrium, descending 2.5–3 cm below the costal margin. As an outgrowth of the caudal part of the foregut, the liver retains its connection with the gastrointestinal system via the biliary tree. In mature livers the hepatocytes are arranged into plates which are usually one cell thick (until the age of 7 years these plates are two cells thick) and separated by venous sinusoids which anastomose with each other forming larger veins which join corresponding central veins. The hepatic parenchyma is supplied by nerves arising from the hepatic plexus and containing sympathetic and parasympathetic (vagal) fibres. Distension or disruption of the liver capsule may cause localised sharp pain (Borley et al 2008).

A complex network of systemic and portal vessels ensures that the liver benefits from good blood supply and venous and lymphatic drainage. The portal venous system ensures that most of the blood from the gastrointestinal system is returned to the liver. In contrast, the hepatic venous system returns blood from the liver into the inferior vena cava. The protein-rich lymph is drained from the liver into the thoracic duct.

Synthesis and metabolism of bilirubin

Small amounts of **bilirubin** are detected in the amniotic fluid between the 13th and 37th weeks of gestation, possibly as a consequence of the limitations of the immature fetal liver to remove and conjugate it. This implies that the major route for fetal bilirubin excretion is across the placenta. Because most of the fetal plasma bilirubin is unconjugated it is easily transferred across the placenta into the maternal circulation and to the maternal liver for conjugation and excretion. Therefore fetuses seldom manifest jaundice unless they suffer severe haemolytic disease.

In neonates, 75% of bilirubin is a by-product of haemoglobin of which 1 g yields 35 mg of bilirubin (Frank & Frank 2006) (Fig. 52.1). About 25% is generated from other non-erythropoietic haem protein sources, principally in the liver and the destruction of immature erythrocytes in the bone marrow. Senescent erythrocytes are removed and destroyed by the reticuloendothelial system where haemoglobin is catabolised and converted into bilirubin. The iron atoms at the centre of the haem skeleton are reused. On leaving the reticuloendothelial system unconjugated bilirubin is transported in the plasma tightly bound to albumin. Although hepatocytes easily take up the unbound lipid-soluble bilirubin a carrier molecule is needed to take up any bound complexes. Once in the hepatocytes, bilirubin binds to ligandin and possibly other cytoplasmic binding proteins. The unconjugated bilirubin is conjugated with a sugar/glucuronic acid by enzymes to form bilirubin monoglucuronide and diglucuronide pigments which are more water-soluble and can be excreted into the bile or through the kidneys into the urine (Fig. 52.2). Bilirubin conjugation requires oxygen and glucose, and hypoxia or hypoglycaemia may slow down the conjugation process.

Some of the conjugated bilirubin is carried in bile to the duodenum and metabolised in the terminal ileum and colon by bacterial enzymes to produce **urobilinogen** (**stercobilinogen** in the gut), which gives faeces the yellowish colour in infants and brown colour in adults. In its absence faeces are greyish white. Small quantities of urobilinogen re-enter the circulation and are excreted by the liver and the kidneys as hydrophilic urobilinogen.

Bilirubin in the neonate

After birth the neonate's liver must take over bilirubin metabolism and clearance. Most of this bilirubin is diverted into the meconium; 200 g of meconium contains about 175 g of bilirubin, 50% of which is conjugated. Delays in meconium excretion, which occur in premature neonates and neonates with **cystic fibrosis**, may contribute to the return of some unconjugated bilirubin into the systemic circulation.

Term neonates hold about 137–171 μmol of bilirubin per litre of plasma (Maisels 1999). These high values compared to bilirubin values in adults are attributed to higher circulating erythrocytes at birth which are gradually biodegraded. The shorter erythrocyte life span of 80 days, as opposed to 120 days in adults, and a corresponding increase in immature or fragile erythrocytes means that more erythrocytes must be degraded (Madan et al 2005). The less-effective bilirubin binding

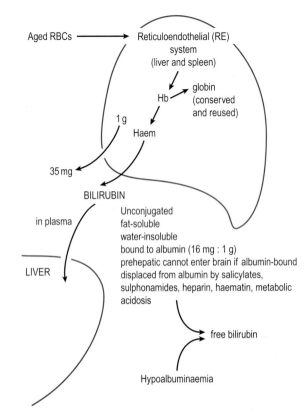

Figure 52.1 • The formation of bilirubin. (From Kelnar C, Harvey D, Simpson C 1995, with permission.)

to albumin, enhanced absorption of bilirubin through the enterohepatic circulation and the somewhat dormant hepatic conjugating system further complicate bilirubin conjugation and excretion. All neonates manifest a progressive rise in unconjugated bilirubin, which peaks at 180 μmol/L on the 3rd or 4th day of life, giving rise to **physiological jaundice**. The increase in unconjugated bilirubin, a relatively low liver uptake of bilirubin and the transient deficiency of the glucuronyl transferase enzyme culminate in reduced excretion of conjugated bilirubin. Although healthy neonates produce almost twice as much bilirubin as adults, their plasma bilirubin values fall to physiological norms within 6 weeks of birth.

Whilst the mechanisms involved in bilirubin conjugation are not fully understood, evidence shows that bilirubin is synthesised by, and released from, the **reticuloendothelial system** into the plasma and binds to plasma albumin. The higher levels of unconjugated bilirubin in neonates are attributed to lower plasma albumin values and lower albumin affinity for bilirubin. This is possibly due to the undeveloped molecular structure of the albumin (Blackburn 2007) and that some albumin-binding sites may be **occupied by other molecular substances** such as **drugs**, including heparin and chloramphenicol (Maisels 1999).

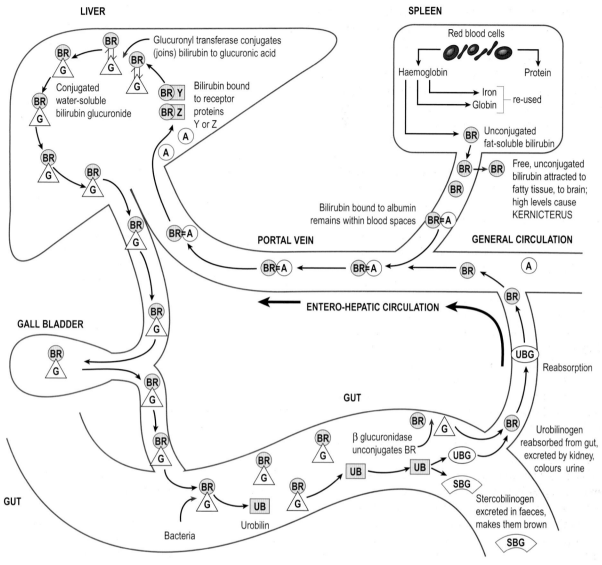

Figure 52.2 • Schematic diagram showing the conjugation of bilirubin. BR, bilirubin; =, bound to; A, albumin; G, glucuronic acid; UB, urobilin; UBG, urobilinogen; SBG, stercobilinogen. (From Bennett VR, Brown L 1993, with permission.)

Kernicterus

Although bilirubin plays important physiological roles as an **antioxidant** and a **free radical scavenger**, its tendency to aggregate increases the risks of neurotoxicity. Plasma pH affects significantly the solubility of bilirubin and its binding to tissue sites: solubility decreases as plasma pH falls. Bilirubin may bind to cell membranes, compromise Na^+–K^+ exchange, lower cell membrane potential, reduce mitochondrial viability, augment the basal ganglia and decrease activity in the auditory brain stem (Cashor 1990, cited by Maisels 1999). Bilirubin is preferentially deposited in the basal ganglia; Maisels (1999) suggests this may be because bilirubin attaches first to nerve terminals where it may lower membrane potentials. This may decrease nerve conduction and allow a retrograde uptake of bilirubin into cell bodies where it binds with various cellular components, staining these and augmenting their function.

Delays in bilirubin conjugation are of concern as unbound, unconjugated fat-soluble bilirubin deposits in neural tissue and visceral organs. Although under normal circumstances bilirubin flows constantly into and out of the brain, it is difficult under experimental conditions to keep bilirubin in the brain of 'healthy animals' or produce significant electrophysiological changes. However, asphyxiated animals and those who have a defective blood–brain barrier experienced 'gross staining of the brain and electrophysiological changes' (Maisels 1999). An intact blood–brain barrier probably excludes most water-soluble substances and protein but is permeable to lipid-soluble substances that are not protein-bound. Large proteins such as albumin are excluded from the brain but may cross the blood–brain barrier when its impermeability is compromised.

However, modest elevation of unconjugated serum bilirubin can produce reversible clinical and electrophysiological alterations in healthy full-term infants (Bratlid 1990). The second mechanism for bilirubin entry into the brain occurs when there is a marked increase in unbound bilirubin. Acidosis may facilitate the transfer of bilirubin across the blood–brain barrier and its subsequent deposition in the neural tissue of the brain (Maisels 1999). Although neural mitochondria contain the enzyme bilirubin oxidase, which converts bilirubin to biliverdin and other non-toxic products, the risk of irreversible brain damage caused by unconjugated bilirubin is high.

The risk of **bilirubin encephalopathy** (occuring in neonates with mild, reversible **hyperbilirubinaemia**) is increased in low-birth-weight neonates and those who experience hypoxic ischaemic insults. However, autopsy reports on jaundiced neonates also reveal bilirubin staining of the aorta, pleural fluid and visceral organs (Maisels 1999). In the brain unconjugated bilirubin leads to irreversible staining, especially in the basal ganglia and cerebellum, and causes **kernicterus** (yellow kernel). Deposition of larger quantities of unconjugated bilirubin may cause irreversible neural damage with long-term sequelae of **cerebral athetosis** and significant **mental retardation**. Such events are most likely to occur when the neonate's serum bilirubin level rises above 350 μmol/L although concerns are raised when the bilirubin level rises above 250 μmol/L. Kernicterus is preventable in all but very small, sick neonates where the blood–brain barrier may be ineffective and quite low levels of bilirubin may damage the fragile tissues.

A résumé of common causes of neonatal jaundice

Jaundice (yellow discoloration of the skin and sclera caused by deposits of conjugated and unconjugated bilirubin) becomes visible when the serum bilirubin rises above 85 μmol/L. Bilirubin is a yellowish-green bile pigment which, prior to conjugation, is a weak acid. It is very soluble in lipid but only slightly soluble in water, making its excretion difficult. About 75% of bilirubin is released along with biliverdin when red blood cells are broken down in the liver and spleen, releasing haem and globin to the body stores. The remainder is derived from other haem products. Excessive bilirubin may enter the bloodstream in three ways (McCance & Huether 2006), all of which may affect the neonate:

1. During excessive haemolysis of red blood cells (prehepatic).

2. Where liver disease affects the metabolism and excretion of bile (hepatic).

3. Congenital obstruction of a component of the biliary system, e.g. congenital biliary atresia (post-hepatic).

As each of the above problems requires different therapeutic interventions, an appropriate range of investigations is needed if the:

- Jaundice appears within the first 24 h after birth.
- Jaundice persists for longer than 2 weeks.
- Neonate's total bilirubin level is >250 μmol/L.
- Conjugated hyperbilirubinaemia is >300 μmol/L.
- Jaundice appears in an ill baby irrespective of its age and fails to respond to treatment.

It is important to distinguish between unconjugated and conjugated forms of bilirubin. The common causes of neonatal jaundice are shown in Table 52.1; Figure 52.3 illustrates the sites of events leading to jaundice.

Prehepatic: unconjugated bilirubin

Physiological jaundice usually appears in otherwise healthy infants around the 3rd day of life and fades gradually over the next 10 days. It is attributed to the increase in erythrocyte breakdown leading to greater bilirubin production and greater enteric reabsorption and enterohepatic circulation of bilirubin. The immature liver cannot synthesise sufficient glucuronyl transferase to metabolise fat-soluble unconjugated bilirubin into water-soluble conjugated bilirubin. As the unconjugated bilirubin cannot be excreted readily it diffuses into body tissues. The less-efficient binding of unconjugated bilirubin to plasma albumin increases diffusion and the presence of meconium increases enteric reabsorption of unconjugated bilirubin. Late umbilical cord clamping may increase the **circulating blood volume** and **haematocrit,** both of which can exacerbate the rise in bilirubin. Neonates who present with physiological jaundice may be helped with periodic phototherapy and increased hydration.

Jaundice of prematurity is a more serious form of physiological jaundice. Due to a greater immaturity of the liver, premature neonates may manifest a more exaggerated form of jaundice which begins earlier, lasts longer and is more severe. Therapeutic interventions should be directed at minimising the risks of bilirubin encephalopathy. If **phototherapy** only marginally improves bilirubin conjugation, **exchange fresh blood transfusion** may be required.

The two main causes of erythrocyte haemolysis are **rhesus isoimmunisation**, a clinically serious problem, and **ABO incompatibility**, which is rarely severe (see Ch. 12). Both clinical problems cause **haemolytic jaundice** generally in the first 24 h of life.

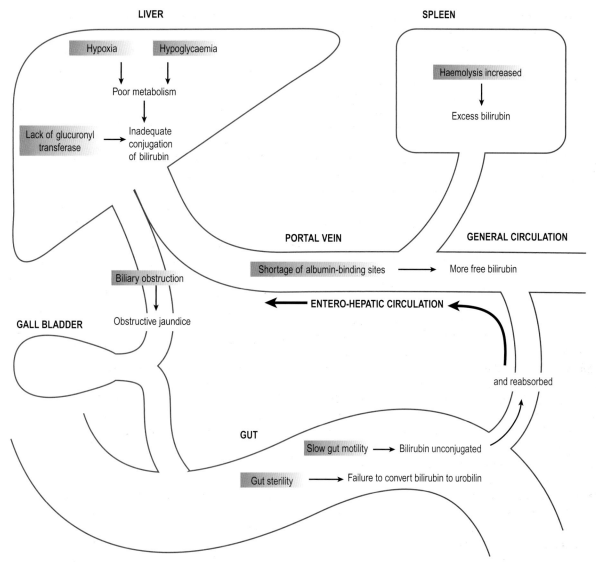

Figure 52.3 • Sites of events leading to jaundice. (From Bennett V R, Brown L 1993, with permission.)

Bruising and haematomas such as cephalhaematoma will lead to significant erythrocyte breakdown during the resolution of the bruise and cause jaundice which may last for several weeks.

Polycythaemia with excess erythrocytes that must be haemolysed will increase bilirubin synthesis. This may occur in **twin transfusion syndrome**, delayed cord clamping and neonates of diabetic mothers.

Infections such as septicaemia, urinary tract infections, meningitis and ventriculitis may also cause significant haemolysis of erythrocytes which leads to jaundice.

Congenital hypothyroidism may cause prolonged (unconjugated) hyperbilirubinaemia possibly as a consequence of the delay in the maturation of the bilirubin-conjugating enzymes.

Neonates with **glucose-6-phosphate dehydrogenase (G6PD) deficiency** may be particularly susceptible to the haemolytic action of vitamin K analogues. G6PD deficiency is a heterogeneous sex-linked recessive trait whose occurrence has its greatest prevalence in Africa and Mediterranean and Asian countries. Because of this enzyme deficiency, erythrocytes cannot activate the pentose phosphate metabolic pathway and therefore are unable to defend adequately against oxidative stress. Haemolytic reactions and hyperbilirubinaemia may occur in response to certain drugs and vitamin K analogues as well as other chemical and household products (Madan et al 2005).

Hepatic: unconjugated bilirubin

Breast milk jaundice occurs in 1–2% of breastfed babies who are significantly more likely to develop hyperbilirubinaemia than bottle-fed neonates. It may occur early

Table 52.1 Causes of neonatal jaundice

Prehepatic: unconjugated bilirubin	Hepatic: unconjugated bilirubin	Hepatic: mixed unconjugated and conjugated bilirubin	Posthepatic: unconjugated mixed and conjugated bilirubin	Posthepatic: unconjugated bilirubin
Physiological jaundice/ jaundice of prematurity Haemolytic jaundice Bruising and haematoma Polycythaemia Postnatal infections	Breast milk jaundice	Congenital hypothyroidism Inborn errors of metabolism: galactosaemia Hepatitis, due to transplacental infections (TORCH organisms)	Congenital biliary atresia Bile plug syndrome	Paralytic ileus High intestinal obstruction such as duodenal atresia

at 3–4 days and persist for up to 14 days after which there is a gradual decline in bilirubin levels. It causes no ill-effects and should not lead to discontinuation of breastfeeding. It sometimes creates anxiety for parents who see it as an illness. The cause of breast milk jaundice has not been established although it may involve:

- Inhibition of glucuronyl transferase by substances found in breast milk such as the maternal hormone pregnanediol and unsaturated fatty acids.
- The presence, in breast milk, of lipase, which releases free fatty acids into the neonate's intestines.
- The presence in breast milk of the enzyme β-glucuronidase, which splits conjugated bilirubin and increases shunting of unconjugated bilirubin from intestine back to liver.
- The delay in the passage of meconium seen in fully breastfed babies. Early breastfeeding with adequate colostrum intake will act as a laxative and, at least in part, reduce the severity of breast milk jaundice (Blackburn 2007).

Hepatic: mixed unconjugated and conjugated bilirubin

Congenital hypothyroidism contributes to jaundice and the primary disorder must be treated as well as the jaundice to avert neurological problems. Neonatal screening using the Guthrie blood test should alert clinicians early to this major endocrine problem. Sometimes neonates present early with other features of hypothyroidism as well as jaundice and these must be taken into consideration when using investigative procedures and planning treatment with levothyroxine (thyroxine) to avert developmental problems and mental retardation.

Some **inborn errors of metabolism** such as cystic fibrosis and galactosaemia may cause severe jaundice due to adversely affected metabolic pathways releasing metabolites that alter or compromise liver function.

Hepatitis is often part of a syndrome accompanying transplacental infection by pathogens such as toxoplasmosis, cytomegalovirus and herpes simplex. The source and extent of the primary infection must be identified and treated in conjunction with any therapeutic interventions that may be required to minimize the severity of the jaundice.

Posthepatic: mixed unconjugated and conjugated bilirubin

Congenital structural anomalies of the biliary ducts interfere with normal bile flow and often lead to significant cholestasis. Some biliary malformations are extrahepatic biliary atresias, intrahepatic biliary hypoplasia, cystic dilatation of the major intrahepatic bile ducts and duodenal atresia. It is important to distinguish between these disorders as surgical correction of biliary malformations may be life-saving. If cholestasis is caused by inflammatory response, infections or metabolic disorders surgery is not needed.

Extrahepatic biliary atresia is the most common form of biliary malformation, with an incidence of 5–10 babies per 100 000 live births. It is more common in females. Associated histological features are proliferation of the hepatic interlobular bile ducts and periportal fibrosis. Such neonates develop a deep bronze jaundice in the 2nd week of life, the stools are putty coloured and the urine contains bilirubin. The liver becomes firm and enlarged. Because the bilirubin is conjugated, the neonate is not at risk of developing kernicterus although if the intrahepatic accumulation of bile is untreated the liver will be damaged and such infants will go on to develop varying degrees of biliary cirrhosis, portal hypertension and liver failure.

Surgical intervention is usually required to reconstruct the defective biliary tree but the prognosis is poor because only a few such neonates are suitable for early surgery before the liver is irreparably damaged. **Liver transplantation** is a long-term solution for some but is generally only carried out in older infants. When liver transplantation is not a realistic option, 80% of affected children die before the age of 3 years (McCance & Huether 2006).

Management of jaundice

Investigations

Depending on the history, clinical evidence and gestational age, investigations may include serum conjugated and unconjugated bilirubin monitoring, blood group establishment, haemoglobin estimation, rhesus antibodies, screening for infection, monitoring of metabolic functions including thyroid function, digestive enzyme assays and enzyme deficiencies such as G6PD deficiency.

Phototherapy

If jaundice persists, the first line of treatment to prevent the development of kernicterus is phototherapy. When a light of wavelength 400–500 nm is shone on the skin, any unconjugated bilirubin is converted to a non-toxic water-soluble substance which is more easily excreted through the kidneys and gastrointestinal tract. Phototherapy may work by inducing **photo-oxidation**, **structural isomerisation** and **configurational isomerisation** (Dennery et al 2001).

- Photo-oxidation is the reaction of bilirubin with singlet oxygen, leading to readily excreted colourless non-reactive products.
- Structural isomerisation involves the molecule lumirubin, formed by intramolecular cyclisation of the bilirubin molecule at the third carbon, leading to a polar compound.
- Configuration isomerisation involves structural changes in the bilirubin molecules. The isomers are readily taken up by the liver and transported into the bile.

Phototherapy is not risk-free. Bilirubin is a **photosensitiser** and may sometimes induce skin blistering and bronze baby syndrome. The phototherapy light may initiate retinal damage if the neonate's eyes are not protected although the **photodecomposition products** have no known neurotoxic effects (Maisels 1999).

Clinical evidence and literature reviewed by Maisels (1999) suggest it is safe to withhold treatment in healthy term infants until the serum bilirubin reaches 320 μmol/L. However, premature neonates born around 28 weeks of gestation require phototherapy treatment when the unconjugated bilirubin level exceeds 150–180 μmol/L and for neonates born about 34 weeks of gestation at 200–240 μmol/L (Madan et al 2005). As phototherapy breaks down unconjugated bilirubin into the conjugated form, its excretion through the gastrointestinal tract is increased along with bile salts. This results in frequent loose stools, which increase the risk of dehydration which can be reduced by giving extra fluids.

Exchange blood transfusion

This procedure is mainly carried out in neonates with rhesus haemolytic disease where excess bilirubin and antibodies must be removed from the blood. Reducing the plasma bilirubin levels lowers the risk of kernicterus and a reduction in antibodies lessens the severity of erythrocyte haemolysis. This intervention carries a mortality risk of 0.5% due to complications such as vascular complications, electrolyte and glucose disturbances and bleeding but these can be minimised by careful procedure (Frank & Frank 2006).

Common metabolic disorders

The scope of this book does not allow exploration of the mainly recessively inherited **inborn errors of metabolism**. Detailed accounts of conditions such as **phenylketonuria, cystic fibrosis** and **galactosaemia** can be found in McCance & Huether (2006). Preconception, antenatal and neonatal screening tests should be carried out where metabolic problems are anticipated. Disturbances in common substances such as glucose, calcium and sodium can alter cerebral tissue function and cause permanent neurological damage that could be avoided by proactive screening and prompt treatment.

Hypoglycaemia

Glucose homeostasis relies on the net balance in intake, production, storage and utilisation of glucose. Since neonatal glucose homeostasis is less than optimal due to metabolic transitions around birth, problems occur when glucose utilisation exceeds its availability or synthesis by the body leading to a fall in plasma glucose concentration. Conversely, glucose production can exceed utilisation, resulting in an abnormal rise in plasma glucose. Regulation of hepatic glucose production is critical to homeostatic maintenance. Although the kidneys are capable of glycogen synthesis, **glycoge-nolysis** and **gluconeogenesis**, their glucose contribution is insufficient to maintain homeostatic balance except in prolonged starvation and metabolic acidosis. Most neonates who develop hypoglycaemia in the first 24 h have a history of:

- A mother who suffers from diabetes mellitus.
- A mother who developed pregnancy-induced hypertension.
- Stress related to neonatal asphyxia.
- Being large or small for gestational age.
- Hyperinsulinism.

Most hypoglycaemic infants make a gradual but spontaneous recovery. However, recurrent or persistent hypoglycaemia may be caused by hepatic enzyme defects, endocrine deficiencies or hyperinsulinism. A plasma glucose of 2.6 mmol/L in a symptomatic baby may lead to neurological dysfunction, manifesting as tremors and seizures (Ogata 1999). Although hypoglycaemia is more common in low-birth-weight babies and in babies of diabetic mothers, it also occurs in neonates with a history of birth asphyxia, respiratory distress syndrome, hypothermia, cerebral damage, severe haemolytic disease or an inborn error of metabolism.

The clinical evidence

Hypoglycaemia may be asymptomatic or may be associated with other clinical problems such as lethargy, hypotonia, shallow respirations with periods of apnoea, cyanosis, muscle twitching, convulsions and coma. Prolonged hypoglycaemia may be associated with brain damage, and associated seizures may worsen the neonate's overall prognosis (Ogata 1999, Rudolph et al 2003).

Management

Prevention is the best form of management, especially if the neonate is at risk of developing hypoglycaemia. Early feeding and repeated blood monitoring are essential. In neonates whose blood glucose level is 1.7 mmol/L or more, immediate milk feed should be given. However, where the plasma glucose level is below 1.7 mmol/L a feed consisting of 10% glucose should be offered. If this is impossible, an intravenous infusion of 10% glucose solution may be necessary. If symptoms reappear, the neonate must have regular neurological and metabolic checks to identify or exclude more sinister problems.

Hypocalcaemia and hypomagnesaemia

During the last trimester of pregnancy, free calcium diffuses from the mother to fetus, ensuring that by term his skeleton is mineralised. A manifestation of this positive calcium movement in favour of the fetus is reflected by calcium levels in the fetal blood, which are usually 10% higher than maternal values.

This **fetal hypercalcaemia** suppresses fetal **parathyroid secretion** and stimulates **calcitonin** release, favouring mineral deposition in the fetal skeletal system. This relative suppression of parathyroid function at birth contributes to the onset of a **transient hypoparathyroid state** with a fall in plasma calcium levels. The term neonate may show decreasing plasma calcium levels during the 24–72 h following birth, reaching levels of 1.75–2.0 mmol/L. This physiologically induced **hypocalcaemia** may result in stimulation of the parathyroid glands and suppression of calcitonin secretion.

Plasma calcium levels increase to acceptable levels within 5 days of birth. If the transition to normal calcium metabolism fails to happen, symptomatic hypocalcaemia develops. **Neonatal tetany** may occur when the plasma calcium level is less than 1.7 mmol/L. Hypocalcaemia may occur in the first 3 days of life in premature neonates with a history of birth asphyxia, hypothermia or respiratory distress syndrome.

Late hypocalcaemia, 5–6 days after birth, is usually associated with feeding the neonate unmodified cow's milk and is rare in developed countries. Cow's milk is high in **phosphorus** and the increase in serum phosphate causes the serum calcium to fall. Some immigrant mothers and mothers in lower socioeconomic groups may have **vitamin D** and **calcium deficiencies** due to inadequate nutrition, leading to hypocalcaemia in pregnancy. Their babies may experience lower plasma calcium levels and higher risks of developing tetany.

Signs of tetany

Neonatal tetany results in irritability followed by muscle twitching, apnoea and convulsions. The neonate is generally conscious and alert between convulsions.

Management

Prevention is by advising expectant mothers to increase their calcium intake. Breastfeeding is encouraged whenever possible and modified cow's milk is only given when breastfeeding is unachievable. If a neonate experiences muscle twitching and convulsions, an infusion of **10% calcium gluconate** diluted in a ratio of 1:4 with sterile water or **dextrose** 10% is considered. Oral calcium gluconate supplements may be continued when normal plasma calcium levels are restored. Intravenous administration of calcium gluconate must be given slowly, over 20 min (not into a peripheral vein). As calcium has a direct impact on heart rate, rhythm and contractility, arrhythmias such as bradycardia may develop. If the neonate is asymptomatic, oral calcium supplements will usually be adequate (Rubin 2005).

Associated hypomagnesaemia

Failure of plasma calcium concentration to respond to administration of intravenous calcium salts should raise the suspicion of coexisting **hypomagnesaemia**. In such circumstances an intramuscular injection of 0.2 mmol/kg of **50% magnesium sulphate** is required to correct both metabolic conditions. Hypomagnesaemia is often associated with hypocalcaemia when the serum magnesium levels may be below 0.6 mmol/L (normal 0.6–1.0 mmol/L). Its homeostasis is probably controlled by the kidneys and gastrointestinal tract. Long-term calcium and magnesium instabilities may contribute to hypoplasia of tooth enamel in the primary teeth.

Hypernatraemia

Neonatal hypernatraemia is almost always the consequence of **water depletion** and is defined by a plasma sodium level exceeding 143 mmol/L. It may be provoked by excessive fluid loss: e.g. during phototherapy or as a consequence of vomiting and diarrhoea. It may also follow excessive sodium intake, sometimes in intravenous solutions such as sodium bicarbonate. Any neonate receiving intensive care should have **plasma electrolytes** checked at least once a day.

Inappropriate infant feeding may lead to hypernatraemia. Where possible, breastfeeding should be encouraged. Mothers should be taught the principles of feed preparation and helped to understand the balanced hydration and nutrition that infants require. In hot weather, infants perspire, become thirsty and cry, but if mothers misinterpret the cry as hunger, more sodium is added to the existing high plasma levels. Adding extra scoops of powdered milk when mixing formula feeds will increase the sodium content. Babies cannot excrete a high solute load by concentrating their urine. More dilute urine is produced and water is lost as it passively follows the excess sodium along the kidney tubules.

Signs of hypernatraemia

The infant may appear fretful and thirsty at first, followed by dehydration, pyrexia, hypertension and a bulging pulsatile fontanelle. If the condition remains untreated, convulsions occur. Sometimes the infant may present with encephalopathy and other neurological problems which could be life-threatening. There may also be failure to gain weight, irritability, hypertonicity and convulsions, especially when plasma sodium levels exceed 150 mmol/L. As the osmotic gradient favours maintenance of extracellular fluid at the expense of intracellular fluid, it may be difficult to establish the true diagnosis.

Management of hypernatraemia

Management of persistent hypernatraemia may be difficult because of its association with **cerebral haemorrhage** and **renal vein thrombosis**. Overaggressive correction may cause cellular overhydration which can affect the structural integrity of the brain tissue. Generally, the baby is slowly rehydrated with an infusion of an isotonic solution such as 0.9% saline. Sedation may be necessary to control convulsions. Any other electrolyte imbalance or hypoglycaemia must be treated. Follow-up care should observe for signs of potential neurological damage.

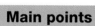

Main points

- Neonates produce twice as much bilirubin as adults due to the excessive haemolysis of erythrocytes containing fetal haemoglobin. Although bilirubin is thought to have antioxidant properties, excessive quantities of unconjugated bilirubin can be neurotoxic.

- As the unconjugated fat-soluble bilirubin binds to tissue with high fat content, particularly the central nervous system, if left untreated it may cause kernicterus and related long-term sequelae including cerebral athetosis and delays in cognitive development. Kernicterus is a preventable problem in all but very small, sick neonates.

- Prehepatic causes of neonatal jaundice with an excess of unconjugated bilirubin include physiological jaundice, jaundice of prematurity, haemolytic jaundice, bruising and haematoma, polycythaemia and some postnatal infections.

- Hepatic causes of jaundice include breast milk feeding and congenital hypothyroidism. High values of mixed unconjugated and conjugated bilirubin may be attributed to such problems as inborn errors of metabolism and hepatitis due to transplacental infections. Breast milk jaundice should not be a reason to discontinue breastfeeding.

- Posthepatic jaundice caused by high mixed unconjugated and conjugated bilirubin values is generally caused by congenital biliary atresia and high intestinal obstruction such as duodenal atresia.

- Phototherapy and additional hydration are occasionally necessary in physiological jaundice, especially in premature infants; phototherapy minimises the risks of hyperbilirubinaemia. Exchange blood transfusion may have to be considered for neonates at risk.

- Bruising and haematomas can delay the onset and resolution of jaundice because of erythrocyte breakdown during the resolution of the bruise. Polycythaemia caused by twin transfusion syndrome or delayed cord clamping will induce a more extensive form of physiological jaundice.

- Neonates with biliary atresia present with deep bronze jaundice in the 2nd week of life, often accompanied by light-coloured stools and dark urine containing bilirubin. The high concentrations of bile salts in the liver lead to progressive destruction of hepatocytes, biliary cirrhosis, portal hypertension and liver failure. Surgical intervention is necessary to minimise problems.

- Disturbances in glucose, calcium, magnesium and sodium homeostasis may lead to neurological changes and permanent neural tissue damage. Plasma glucose levels of 2.6 mmol/L in jaundiced neonates may lead to neurological changes.

- Hypoglycaemia is more common in low-birth-weight babies and in babies of diabetic mothers. Regular milk feeds normally restore normoglycaemia although neonates with plasma glucose values of 1.7 mmol/L may require intravenous infusion of 10% glucose in 0.9% saline to correct any deficits.

- Early symptoms of hypocalcaemia occur in premature neonates or those with a history of birth asphyxia, hypothermia or respiratory distress syndrome. Late hypocalcaemia is usually associated with feeding neonates with unmodified cow's milk.

- Pregnant mothers with deficient intake of vitamin D and calcium may develop hypocalcaemia which predisposes their neonates to tetany. Oral calcium supplements may be given to such neonates but in instances where the neonate convulses infusion of 10% calcium gluconate diluted in a ratio of 1:4 with sterile water or 10% dextrose must be considered.

- Hypernatraemia may be caused by excessive fluid loss or excessive sodium intake as neonates cannot excrete high solute loads by concentrating urine; their urine is almost always dilute.

References

Blackburn, S.T., 2007. Maternal, Fetal and Neonatal Physiology: A Clinical Perspective, third edn. W B Saunders, Philadelphia.

Borley, N., Collins, P., Healy, J., Wigley, C., et al., 2008. Abdominal viscera: liver. In: Borley, N. (Eds.), Gray's Anatomy: The Anatomical Basis of Clinical Practice. Elsevier Churchill Livingstone, London.

Bratlid, D., 1990. How bilirubin gets into the brain. Clin. Perinatol. 17, 459.

Dennery, P., Seidman, D., Stevenson, D., 2001. Neonatal hyperbilirubinemia. N. Engl. J. Med. 344, 581–590.

Frank, C.G., Frank, P.H., 2006. Jaundice. In: Merenstein, G.B., Gardner, S.L. (Eds.), Handbook of Neonatal Intensive Care. Mosby, St Louis, Missouri.

Madan, A., MacMahon, J., Stevenson, D., 2005. Neonatal hyperbilirubinaemia. In: Taeusch, H., Ballard, R., Gleason, C. (Eds.), Avery's Diseases of the Newborn. Elsevier Saunders, London.

Maisels, M., 1999. Jaundice. In: Avery, G., Fletcher, M., MacDonald, M. (Eds.), Neonatology: Pathophysiology and Management of the Newborn. Lippincott, Williams and Wilkins, Philadelphia.

McCance, K.L., Huether, S.E., 2006. Pathophysiology: The Biologic Basis for Disease in Adults and Children, second ed. Mosby, St Louis.

Ogata, E., 1999. Carbohydrate homeostasis. In: Avery, G., Fletcher, M., MacDonald, M. (Eds.), Neonatology: Pathophysiology and Management of the Newborn. Lippincott, Williams and Wilkins, Philadelphia.

Rubin, L., 2005. Disorders of calcium and phosphorus metabolism. In: Taeusch, H., Ballard, R., Gleason, C. (Eds.), Avery's Diseases of the Newborn. Elsevier Saunders, London.

Rudolph, C., Rudolph, A., Hostetter, M., et al., 2003. Rudolph's Paediatrics. McGraw-Hill, London.

Annotated recommended reading

Merenstein, G.B., Gardner, S.L., 2006. Handbook of Neonatal Intensive Care. Mosby, St Louis, Missouri.
This textbook offers a succinct update of a range of concepts, with emphasis on the biophysical and pathophysiological issues, central to competent neonatal care.

Polin, R., Fox, W., Abman, S., 2004. Fetal and Neonatal Physiology. W B Saunders, Philadelphia.

These textbooks discuss bioscientific concepts important in fetal and neonatal care. The résumé of genetics leads to a more detailed exploration of normal and abnormal embryonic and fetal development. Overall, these books make a significant contribution to clinical practice and research.

Wong, D., 2004. Nursing Care of Infants and Children. Mosby, St Louis.

This textbook offers detailed accounts of the relevant biophysical, psychosocial and nursing issues in managing the care of infants and children. It concludes with a range of helpful appendices, which include excellent developmental screening tools and biophysical nomograms and parameters invaluable in all aspects of child care.

Chapter Fifty-Three

53

Risks of infection and trauma in neonates

Infections

Fetal and neonatal immunocompetence

Although not fully developed, the **neonatal immune system** is capable of mounting considerable defence against pathogens, removing worn out and damaged host cells, monitoring and destroying mutant cells. The term immune system subsumes both innate and specific immunity. Innate immune mechanisms are generally well developed at birth, always vigilant, rapidly activated and encoded in the individual's genome. Components of innate immunity such as the neutrophils are responsible for immediate recognition, isolation and initiation of pathogen destruction. In contrast, the specific immune mechanisms are activated on exposure to specific pathogens (or vaccines), but these mechanisms require days or weeks for development and are invariably dependent on somatic gene rearrangements (Giroir 2003). The most important components of the specific immune system are the B and T lymphocytes. Both these naïve cell lineages must be exposed to and programmed by specific antigens. In response, the mature B lymphocytes are converted into antibody-producing plasma cells whereas the activated T cells synthesise and release cytokines such as interferons.

Bellanti et al (1999) define **immaturity** of the immune mechanisms as 'the inability of the immune system to mount a genetically programmed immune response to antigens such as bacteria, viruses and mutant cells'. In fetuses, as in neonates, the functional immaturity of the immune system is generally attributed to the limited exposure of the B and T lymphocytes to antigens and pathogens capable of activating appropriate immunological mechanisms critical to the generation of competent, specific immune responses. Those wishing to review the immune system should read Chapter 29. Although most neonates have some specific immunity obtained by passive means from colostrum and breast milk, the relative immaturity of the acquired immune mechanisms can predispose some neonates to infection (Table 53.1).

Sources of neonatal infection can be divided into three categories (Venkatesh 2006):

1. Transplacental acquisition.

2. Perinatal acquisition.

3. Postnatal infection.

Fetuses are vulnerable to pathogenic infections due to their relatively immature and inexperienced immune systems. Many of these conditions are covered in Chapter 14. Some of the prevalent fetal infections are:

- TORCH pathogens which cross the placenta relatively uninhibited (see Ch. 14).

- Any pathogens that may be introduced during invasive procedures such as amniocentesis.

Table 53.1 Factors predisposing to neonatal infection

Possible barriers	Deficiencies in host defence mechanisms
Anatomical barriers	Skin abrasions sustained during delivery
	Invasive procedures: airway lavage, endotracheal intubation, umbilical artery catheterisation
Phagocytic cells	Small numbers of polymorphonuclear leucocytes
	Decreased polymorphonuclear cell activity
	Slow up-regulation in neutrophil production
	Poor transmission of neutrophils into the tissue
Complement mechanisms	Decreased levels of complement proteins in the blood, possibly due to immaturity of the liver
Cellular immunity	Possible defects in T-cell immunoregulation
Humoral immunity	Low levels of immunoglobulins IgA and IgM
	Low levels of IgG in premature infants
	Impaired antibody function
	Low levels of cytokines, e.g. interferon and tumour necrosis factor

- Any pathogens ascending the maternal reproductive tract, especially if the fetal membranes rupture early during the perinatal period.
- Other infections acquired during pregnancy from organisms such as *Candida albicans*, *Neisseria gonorrhoeae*, *Chlamydia trachomatis*, *Listeria monocytogenes*, herpes simplex, HIV infection (see Ch. 14).

Perinatal and postnatal infections

Neonates are colonised by **commensals** and **pathogens** during labour as well as after birth when they are exposed to new environments. Some of these pathogens are most likely to cause neonatal systemic and topical infections. Neonatal infections are difficult to recognise as early signs may be non-specific. The neonate may be lethargic, reluctant to feed, fretful, develop jaundice and have unexplained vomiting and unusual stool pattern with significant weight loss. Poor temperature control, manifesting as either pyrexia or more commonly hypothermia, accompanied by tachypnoea, apnoea, cyanosis and bradycardia must be carefully monitored. A neonate's cold peripheries, mottled skin and grey or pale appearance are often late signs of systemic infection. Because in some instances such neonates collapse suddenly, **differential diagnoses** such as metabolic disturbances, respiratory or cardiovascular problems or intracranial bleeding cannot be ruled out.

Apparently healthy neonates who suddenly deteriorate must therefore be examined for evidence of infection. This should include **microbiology screening** and **haemodynamic monitoring** until a diagnosis is established. Early supportive and antimicrobial therapy may limit the severity of the infection, although delaying the diagnosis and deferring appropriate therapeutic interventions may contribute to the spread of pathogens and the development of **septicaemia**. In cases of doubt, neonates will undergo **systematic screening**, usually including obtaining nasal, throat, umbilical and skin swabs for microbiology cultures. A **full blood profile**, including white cell count, platelet count and blood cultures, is carried out. Cerebrospinal fluid obtained by lumbar puncture provides the means for screening neonates for evidence of **meningitis** and **ventriculitis**. Collection of **urine** and **stool samples** for microbial culture and pathogen sensitivity to antimicrobial drugs can provide an indication of the source of infection and influence the therapeutic management.

It is often expedient to administer **broad-spectrum antimicrobials**, frequently intravenously, until a diagnosis is confirmed and the pathogens and their sensitivity identified. Most neonatal units use specific combinations of antimicrobials such as **amoxicillin** and **gentamicin**, depending on which pathogens are present in that environment. Such neonates will also require supportive care to ensure that their body temperature is maintained, that they are well hydrated, adequately nourished and any risks of hypoglycaemia and acidosis are minimised (Giroir 2003). Fluid intake must be carefully managed as studies indicate that overhydration may lead to patent ductus arteriosus and **necrotising enterocolitis** (Bell & Acarregui 2001). Seriously ill neonates may require assisted mechanical ventilation.

Skin and surface infections

All neonatal skin lesions must be considered potentially abnormal, particularly if they are associated with **staphylococcal infections**, which may spread from the ear, nose, mouth and skin of a carer, another neonate or child. Due to the immaturity of the neonate's immune system, simple lesions can rapidly lead to serious systemic infections. For instance, **pyoderma**, the appearance of small spots or pustules on the skin, and **paronychia**, a localised staphylococcal nail-bed infection, may spread rapidly in premature and ill neonates causing systemic infections. Both infections may require early antimicrobial therapy to minimise the risk of systemic infection.

Staphylococcal scalded skin syndrome is a serious skin infection caused by staphylococci entering the superficial soft tissue through a broken skin surface such as a scratch. Such infections are highly contagious and may lead to epidemics that result in closure of maternity units; therefore any blisters appearing on the neonate's skin should be notified early to paediatricians as they may be due to **exfoliative toxins** produced by staphylococci (Hanakawa et al 2002). Generally these lesions appear on the head and the trunk and, if unattended, fill with pus, break and leave raw skin surfaces open to further infection. Extensive blisters may coalesce, giving a 'scalded skin' appearance. The neonate may become seriously ill with dehydration and may develop septicaemia. Affected neonates are cared for in an isolated environment. Supportive interventions include antibiotic therapy and rehydration. It is important to be aware of the prevalence of **meticillin-resistant** organisms that may not respond to the usual antibiotics.

Omphalitis or infection of the umbilicus can be serious because of a possible spread of common staphylococcal pathogens through the umbilical vein to the liver and kidneys (Fig. 53.1). Widespread erythema around the umbilicus or discharge of fluid or pus indicates local infection and must be treated with appropriate antibiotics and meticulous hygiene.

Ophthalmia neonatorum means the presence of a purulent discharge from the neonate's eye(s). Such infections may develop within 21 days of birth. Both eyes must be treated with appropriate antimicrobial therapy in order to minimise the risks of blindness. In severe cases, systemic antimicrobials are required. Although such severe eye infections are now rarely seen, pathogens such as the penicillin-resistant strains of *Neisseria gonorrhoeae*, staphylococci species, *Escherichia coli* and *Chlamydia trachomatis* can induce them. Care needs to be taken to ensure that neonates with such ocular infections are nursed with the affected eye in a downward position to ensure that the pathogens do not spread to the clean eye.

Serious infections

The most serious infections encountered in neonates are septicaemia, meningitis and pneumonia. In general, these infections present with non-specific signs such as

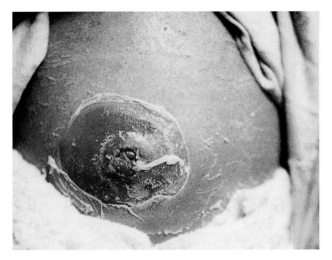

Figure 53.1 • Severe periumbilical infection. (From Kelnar C, Harvey D, Simpson C 1995, with permission.)

thermoregulation problems, lethargy, apnoea, poor feeding and vomiting. Group B β-haemolytic *Streptococcus aureus* is frequently implicated in such neonatal sepsis (Oddie & Embleton 2002).

Septicaemia is a serious end-result of topical infection which, in most instances, is confirmed by blood culture. Besides the non-specific signs, abdominal distension, increased white blood cell count, hypotonia, unexplained metabolic acidosis and hypoglycaemia and hyperglycaemia may occur in premature and low-birthweight neonates. Occasionally, the pathogens cause disseminated intravascular coagulopathy (DIC) in which case the septicaemia and coagulopathy require life-saving supportive and therapeutic interventions.

Meningitis is most likely to occur in premature neonates or those born after difficult pregnancies and deliveries. Group B β-haemolytic streptococcus and *Escherichia coli* are the most likely pathogens although *Listeria monocytogenes*, pneumococci, staphylococci and *Candida albicans* may be detected in cerebrospinal fluid cultures. The incidence of bacterial meningitis averages 0.4 per 1000 live births. Convulsions, bulging fontanelle, head retraction and hypothermia present in some neonates in the early stages of infection. Such symptoms must always be taken seriously and following investigative protocols managed proactively if mortality and the risks of long-term morbidity such as deafness, blindness and nerve palsies are to be minimised (Polin et al 2005).

Neonatal pneumonia may follow the inhalation of infected amniotic fluid or meconium causing respiratory distress within hours of birth. Conversely, **aspiration pneumonia** occurs in neonates who inhale milk or fluids given by nasogastric tube. This is most likely to occur in premature neonates whose swallowing and coughing reflexes are absent or weak. A range of pathogens can cause pneumonia with development of respiratory distress and cyanosis. All neonates require antimicrobial intervention and chest physiotherapy during the resolution phase of pneumonia. In milder forms of pneumonia, and where the neonate is relatively strong, being nursed in an incubator with humidified oxygen may be sufficient to ensure recovery. However, premature and very small neonates may require mechanical respiratory support. Nasogastric feeding is continued if possible, although neonates who manifest a degree of respiratory distress may benefit from intravenous hydration and nutrition.

Necrotising enterocolitis

Necrotising enterocolitis (NEC) is an acute inflammatory change affecting the small and large bowel in predominantly premature neonates (Anderson et al 2006, Berseth & Poenaru 2005). Although the aetiology remains unclear (Berseth & Poenaru 2005, Caplan & Jilling 2001), stress, infection, hypoxia, hypoglycaemia and inappropriate feeding may be contributing factors. Lucas & Cole (1990) showed that NEC is up to 10 times more common in exclusively formula-fed babies than those fed with breast milk alone, and three times more prevalent in those receiving both formula and breast milk feeds. The prevention of pathogenic presence by the early colonisation of the gut by **lactobacilli** may be crucial. If the neonate is not breastfed, factors such as **IgA** and **lymphocytes** from colostrum are absent, which allows invasion of the bowel wall, portal system and bowel lymphatic glands by bacteria such as *Klebsiella*, *Clostridium* and *E. coli*.

Partial- or full-thickness intestinal **ischaemia** usually involves the terminal ileum. The sloughing of the ischaemic mucosal layer (Berseth & Poenaru 2005) contributes to gas formation within the muscular layers and the formation of **pneumatosis cystoides intestinalis**, detectable on abdominal X-ray films. Full-thickness **necrosis** leads to gut perforation and **peritonitis** and the neonate becomes critically ill. **Disseminated intravascular coagulopathy**, septicaemia and peritonitis may develop. Hepatic portal venous gas collection usually implies that an extensive form of necrosis is present and that the neonate requires surgery.

Other clinical manifestations of NEC

- Abdominal distension.
- Acute severe abdominal pain.
- Retained gastric contents and vomiting.
- Fresh blood in stools.
- Thermal instability.
- Poor activity.
- Apnoea.
- Haemodynamic instability.

Therapeutic interventions

In mild forms of NEC early **conservative treatment** consists of analgesia, no gastric feeding, gastric decompression and intravenous antimicrobials. This may avert the severe form of gut necrosis and perforation. **Intravenous fluids** are used to maintain hydration, acceptable blood glucose and electrolyte values. Regular **analgesia** such as morphine or fentanyl is administered. It is often advantageous to establish **assisted mechanical ventilation**, particularly if respiratory distress and metabolic acidosis are evident. All affected neonates will require **antimicrobials** against Gram-negative and Gram-positive pathogens.

The presence of fresh blood in the stool usually confirms the diagnosis, although a stool specimen must be sent for culture and sensitivity screening. **Surgical interventions** are required if conservative medical interventions fail and the neonate shows signs of bowel perforation and peritonitis. Removal of the affected segments of the bowel with reanastomosis of the healthy segments of bowel later may have to be considered. If a functioning **ileostomy** is created, it is closed when the infant has recovered from the acute illness and surgery. Since the mortality rate averages 40% for neonates who require surgery, the onset of this acute stage of the illness must be prevented (Berseth & Poenaru 2005).

Gastroenteritis

Gastroenteritis is rare in breastfed babies and outbreaks are commonly caused by **rotavirus**, which spreads rapidly and has a high risk of mortality. Every effort must be taken to contain infection. *Salmonella* and certain strains of *E. coli* may also cause an outbreak. Most neonates deteriorate rapidly, as vomiting and frequent watery stools lead to severe dehydration. The gastrointestinal inflammatory changes may cause severe, spasmodic abdominal pain, requiring careful management. Segregation of the infected neonate is essential and, where more than one neonate is affected, the neonatal unit should be closed to new admissions. Affected neonates must be rehydrated and have their electrolyte imbalance and haemodynamic disturbances restored. Antimicrobial treatment is usually life-saving. An affected neonatal unit may only reopen following treatment and discharge of all neonates followed by disinfection of the clinical areas.

Birth trauma

Uncomplicated labour rarely results in maternal or **neonatal trauma** and severe birth traumas are therefore now rare and avoidable (Greig 2003, Rudolph et al 2003), but minor injuries may occur during difficult deliveries such as rotational forceps, ventouse extraction, shoulder dystocia or breech presentation. Neonates who are large in relation to the mother's pelvis, of low birth weight, multiple fetuses and those born by precipitate birth are also at risk. **Neural tissue injuries** (Madan et al 2005) and **fractures** of the long bones of the arm or leg may follow **shoulder dystocia** or **vaginal breech delivery**.

Head injuries

Premature neonates are at great risk of sustaining head injuries, leading to **intracranial haemorrhage** as a result of damage to protective layers around the brain (Fig. 53.2). The most severe forms of intracranial bleeding are a major cause of perinatal death. A **tentorial tear** involving the great vein of Galen, a **subaponeurotic haemorrhage** or **subdural haemorrhage** (see below) may be fatal (Madan et al 2005, Rudolph et al 2003).

Cephalhaematoma

A **cephalhaematoma** is a swelling on a baby's head caused by an effusion of blood under the periosteum of the affected skull bone (Fig. 53.3). Friction between the fetal head and the hard bone of the maternal pelvis or forceps may cause lacerations in the **periosteum**, leading to bleeding and haematoma formation. It may contribute to late onset of jaundice, as the excessive extravasated blood cells are reabsorbed. The cephalhaematoma is differentiated from the superficial oedema caused by **caput succedaneum** (see Ch. 24) by characteristic features (Table 53.2).

Subaponeurotic haemorrhage

Subaponeurotic haemorrhage is a serious birth injury commonly associated with births assisted by vacuum extraction (Greig 2003, Madan et al 2005). Bleeding occurs from beneath the **epicranial aponeurosis**, giving

rise to a swelling which can cross suture lines. This problem must be differentiated from caput succedaneum. A subaponeurotic haematoma is present at birth and continues to increase in size. Haemorrhage is extensive and may extend into the subcutaneous tissues of the neck or eyelids, giving rise to painful swellings. The blood loss may cause anaemia and a blood transfusion may be required. Clinical resolution is slow, extending over 2–3 weeks or longer, depending on extent and severity.

Intracranial haemorrhage

Bleeding into the **periventricular space** and other parts of brain tissue is relatively common in premature and low-birth-weight neonates. Ultrasound scanning, computed tomography (CT) scanning and lumbar puncture may help provide a differential diagnosis. The time of onset, duration and severity of bleeding are significant

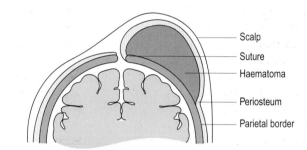

Figure 53.3 • Cross-section of a cephalhaematoma. (From Henderson C, Macdonald S 2004, with kind permission of Elsevier.)

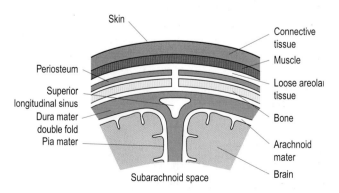

Figure 53.2 • A cross-section through the skull. (From Henderson C, Macdonald S 2004, with kind permission of Elsevier.)

Table 53.2 Differentiation between cephalhaematoma and caput succedaneum

Cephalhaematoma	Caput succedaneum
It appears in the first 12 h after birth	It is present at birth
It is clearly circumscribed and confined to one bone, never crossing a suture line	It may cross suture lines
It does not pit	As it is oedematous, pitting can occur
It tends to grow larger rather than disappear	It resolves within the first few days of life
No treatment is needed and the swelling usually disappears within 6–9 weeks, but may ossify	No treatment is necessary in normal circumstances

in planning a neonate's management. Intracranial haemorrhage is most likely to occur in premature neonates with a history of birth trauma, asphyxia or hypoxia. Poor autoregulation of cerebral blood flow may contribute. **Meningeal** and vessel tears occur in the **falx cerebri** or **tentorium cerebelli** (Fig. 53.4) although fragility of other cerebral blood vessels may be significant. The classical definitions of neonatal intracranial haemorrhage according to the site of bleeding are:

- Subdural haemorrhage.
- Subarachnoid haemorrhage.
- Intraparenchymal haemorrhage.
- Periventricular/intraventricular haemorrhage.

Subdural haemorrhage is almost exclusively associated with trauma. A tear in the tentorium cerebelli at its junction with the falx cerebri causes rupture of the venous sinuses and the great vein of Galen. Initially the neonate may appear sleepy, but becomes irritable with a high-pitched cry, vomiting and a bulging anterior fontanelle. Convulsions may occur, requiring the use of anticonvulsant drugs and dexamethasone. A subdural tap may be performed to alleviate rising intracranial pressure and prevent the development of meningeal adhesions, which could contribute to later development of hydrocephalus (Madan et al 2005, Rudolph et al 2003).

In **subarachnoid haemorrhage** there is bleeding from small vessels into the subarachnoid space following mild trauma or asphyxia. It may be asymptomatic and undetectable on ultrasound scan and is therefore more common than realised. There is often blood-stained cerebrospinal fluid (CSF). The presence of blood may initiate local inflammatory changes, which may ultimately lead to **hydrocephalus**.

Intraparenchymal haemorrhage is bleeding into the cerebral tissue associated with birth asphyxia or with disseminated intravascular coagulopathy. The presence of blood within the cerebral tissue will cause local irritation, possibly leading to generalised or localised convulsions. Distortion and destruction of affected cerebral tissue leads eventually to the formation of **porencephalic cysts** (Greig 2003, Madan et al 2005) although these are eventually reabsorbed. Many such neonates make a slow but full recovery.

Periventricular/intraventricular haemorrhage (PVH/IVH) is the most common and most serious type of intracranial haemorrhage (Fig. 53.5) in premature neonates with a history of birth asphyxia, respiratory distress syndrome and stress. It is associated with direct trauma to neurons caused by accumulating blood, rising intracranial pressure and inflammatory changes. The accumulation of blood and inflammatory cells also interferes with normal production and circulation of cerebrospinal fluid, which may lead to hydrocephalus. Long-term outcomes may include motor and sensory disabilities and cognitive developmental delay (Blackburn 2007, Madan et al 2005, Rudolph et al 2003). This form of haemorrhage is one of the most common causes of death in neonates born before 32 weeks.

The site of bleeding is generally related to the gestation and developmental stage of the brain. The **subependymal germinal matrix** in the premature neonate is located adjacent to the lateral ventricles and contains actively dividing cells. From 24 to 32 weeks of gestation a large capillary bed supplies these cells. The large cerebral blood flow contained in relatively fragile blood vessels is incapable of autoregulation and the fragile capillary and related arteriovenous network is easily disrupted by hypoxia and hypercapnia, both capable of inducing cerebrovasodilation. This matrix almost disappears

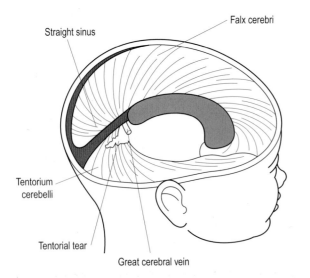

Figure 53.4 • A tentorial tear. (From Henderson C, Macdonald S 2004, with kind permission of Elsevier.)

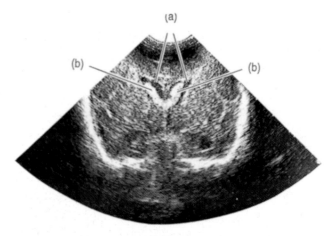

Figure 53.5 • Coronal cranial ultrasound scan showing intraventricular haemorrhages (b) in dilated lateral ventricles (a). (From Kelnar C, Harvey D, Simpson C 1995, with permission.)

in term neonates and the risk of periventricular and intraventricular bleeding is reduced as the brain matures. In full-term neonates intracranial haemorrhage is mainly from the **choroid plexus**, contrasting sharply with the predominantly **capillary bleeding** in the subependymal germinal matrix observed in premature neonates.

The neonate with a sudden, large periventricular or intraventricular haemorrhage presents with apnoea and circulatory collapse characterised by marked bradycardia. The **anterior fontanelle** may be enlarged and tense. Active resuscitation (Greig 2003) and respiratory support may be required. Balanced hydration and nutrition are administered intravenously, although fluids may have to be restricted if there is raised intracranial pressure. The prognosis for neonates with small haemorrhages is good but neonates with massive haemorrhages may suffer from convulsions, localised **cerebral atrophy** and hydrocephalus (Madan et al 2005, Rudolph et al 2003).

In **periventricular leucomalacia** (PVL), cerebral tissue ischaemia leads to necrotic changes in the white matter surrounding the ventricles where blood flow may be interrupted due to hypotension. This area of the brain is vulnerable because it forms a boundary zone requiring blood supply from different arterial trees (Blackburn 2007). PVL destroys neural tissue of the corticospinal motor pathways, resulting in **spastic cerebral palsy** (Fig. 53.6).

Nerve palsies

Facial palsy

Facial palsy is commonly attributed to damage of the **seventh cranial nerve** by pressure applied to the facial nerve as it emerges near the angle of the jaw. The affected side of the face shows no spontaneous movement, the eye remains open and the corner of the mouth droops (Fig. 53.7). The neonate almost always recovers complete facial muscle movement.

Erb's palsy

Erb's palsy results from damage to the **fifth** and **sixth cervical nerves** caused by **compression of the upper brachial plexus** by traction or rotation applied to the neck in a breech or difficult cephalic delivery. This results in paralysis of the arm, which is inwardly rotated and hangs limply at the side, and the half closed hand is turned outwards, the characteristic 'waiter's tip position' (Fig. 53.8). As these nerves control the arm and some neck and chest muscles, any superficial or deep nerve injury will manifest in neuromuscular changes, but full recovery is often possible.

Klumpke's palsy

Klumpke's palsy is an uncommon problem caused by traction on the arm with damage to the **eighth cervical** and **first thoracic nerve roots** of the lower brachial plexus. The neonate presents with paralysis of the hand and 'wrist drop', although the upper arm generally has a normal range of movement. Physical assessment and radiographic screening rule out fractures to the humerus and clavicle and identify dislocated joints. Where fractures or joint problems are present, the neonate generally cannot move his affected arm. Most neonates make a slow recovery, which may take up to 2 years. **Analgesia** will limit pain and induce local muscle relaxation to aid healing. **Physiotherapy** encourages normal muscle movement and prevents contractures. Where the neonate does not make a spontaneous recovery, **surgical**

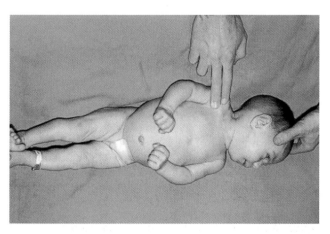

Figure 53.6 • Hypertonic baby with cerebral palsy. (From Kelnar C, Harvey D, Simpson C 1995, with permission.)

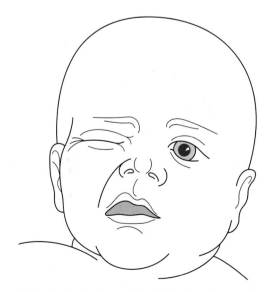

Figure 53.7 • Left-sided facial palsy. The right side is active when the baby cries but the left side is relaxed. (From Henderson C, Macdonald S 2004, with kind permission of Elsevier.)

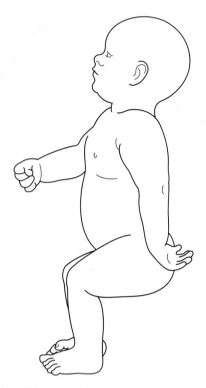

Figure 53.8 • Erb's palsy. (From Henderson C, Macdonald S 2004, with kind permission of Elsevier.)

intervention, including nerve graft or repair, may be considered.

Soft tissue injuries

The most common cause of soft tissue injuries is vaginal breech delivery. Injuries include:

- Superficial bruising.
- Injury to liver and spleen.
- Injury to the kidneys and adrenal glands.
- Injury to the intestines.

Although painful superficial bruising is obvious, other more life-threatening complications may develop. This is particularly so where injury to the liver, spleen or adrenal glands results in bleeding and hypovolaemic circulatory collapse. Ultrasound scanning should establish the diagnosis. Where the neonate develops haemodynamic instability that could compromise vital organs, supportive interventions are necessary.

Main points

- Fetal infection may be acquired transplacentally or during invasive procedures such as amniocentesis. Some infections are acquired perinatally due to pathogens ascending through the maternal reproductive tract, especially once the fetal membranes rupture early.

- Early signs of systemic infection in neonates are non-specific and include lethargy, poor feeding, jaundice, vomiting, diarrhoea and weight loss. Hypothermia, pyrexia, tachypnoea, apnoea, cyanosis, bradycardia and haemodynamic instability indicate severe infection.

- Delays in diagnosing and treating local infections may contribute to the spread of the pathogens causing severe systemic infection such as meningitis and septicaemia. All infections must be treated with broad-spectrum antimicrobials. Early diagnosis and treatment reduces mortality and severe complications.

- Group B β-haemolytic streptococci and staphylococci are the most common pathogens in septicaemia. Meningitis is frequently caused by the group B β-haemolytic *Staphylococcus aureus*. Most neonates who develop pneumonia are very ill and require assisted mechanical ventilation, broad-spectrum

antimicrobials and timely frequent but gentle physiotherapy.

- Gastroenteritis is rare in the breastfed baby. Outbreaks are commonly caused by rotavirus and are associated with a high mortality. *Salmonella* and some strains of *E. coli* may also cause an outbreak. Antibiotic therapy, rehydration and segregation of infectious neonates are necessary.

- Pemphigus neonatorum may lead to more serious systemic infection. Infectious neonates are isolated and treated with antimicrobials. Omphalitis and ophthalmia neonatorum are potentially serious infections requiring antibiotic treatment and high standards of hygiene.

- Early diagnosis and swift medical intervention of necrotising enterocolitis may reduce its severity. Neonates who develop bowel necrosis and perforation require specialist surgery.

- Normal labour rarely results in birth injuries but minor soft tissue injuries may occur during a difficult labour. Friction between the fetal head and the maternal pelvis or forceps may cause a cephalhaematoma. No treatment is needed and the cephalhaematoma usually subsides within 6 weeks.

- Subaponeurotic haemorrhage is a serious birth injury commonly associated with vacuum extraction. Bleeding may extend into the subcutaneous tissues of the neck or eyelids, and in some instances blood will cross the suture lines.
- Intracranial haemorrhages are a major cause of perinatal death when prematurity is associated with hypoxia, asphyxia or trauma to the falx cerebri or tentorium cerebelli, resulting in subdural bleeding and subarachnoid bleeding, respectively. The time of onset, the duration and extent of the bleeding into the brain tissue are important in the overall prognosis.
- Intraparenchymal haemorrhage is frequently associated with birth asphyxia. Destruction of the affected cerebral tissue with formation of parencephalic cysts can be observed in some neonates.
- Periventricular/intraventricular haemorrhage is the most common and serious form of intracranial haemorrhage occurring in premature neonates. Some develop hydrocephalus and motor, sensory and cognitive disabilities. These neonates may develop leucomalacia. The destructive changes may result in permanent damage to the corticospinal motor pathways and cause spastic cerebral palsy.
- Nerve palsies include facial palsy, Erb's palsy and Klumpke's palsy. The most common causes of soft tissue injuries in neonates occur as a result of the fetus being in a breech position. Care must therefore be taken during such deliveries in order to avoid superficial and central organ trauma.

References

Anderson Jr., M.S., Wood, L.L., Keller, J., Hay, W.W., 2006. Enteral nutrition. In: Merenstein, G.B., Gardner, S.L. (Eds.), Handbook of Neonatal Intensive Care. Mosby, St Louis, Missouri.

Bell, E.F., Acarregui, M.J., 2001. Restricted versus liberal water intake for preventing morbidity and mortality in preterm infants. Cochrane Review. Cochrane Library, Issue (1) Update Software 2003, Oxford.

Bellanti, J., Zeling, B., Pung, Y., 1999. Immunology of the fetus and the newborn. In: Avery, G., Fletcher, M., MacDonald, M. (Eds.), Neonatology: Pathophysiology and Management of the Newborn. Lippincott, Williams and Wilkins, Philadelphia, pp. 1063–1122.

Berseth, C., Poenaru, D., 2005. Necrotizing enterocolitis and short bowel syndrome. In: Taeusch, H., Ballard, R., Gleason, C. (Eds.) Avery's Diseases of the Newborn. Elsevier Saunders, London.

Blackburn, S.T., 2007. Maternal, Fetal and Neonatal Physiology: A Clinical Perspective, second edn. W B Saunders, Philadelphia.

Caplan, M.S., Jilling, T., 2001. New concepts in necrotising enterocolitis. Curr. Opin. Pediatr. 13 (2), 111–115.

Giroir, B., et al., 2003. Pathophysiology of systemic inflammation. In: Rudolph, C., Rudolph, A., Hostetter, M. (Eds.), Rudolph's Pediatrics. McGraw-Hill, London.

Greig, C., 2003. Trauma and haemorrhage. In: Fraser, D.M., Cooper, M.A. (Eds.), Myles Textbook for Midwives, fourteenth edn. Churchill Livingstone, Edinburgh.

Hanakawa, Y., Schecter, N.M., Lin, C., et al., 2002. Molecular mechanisms of blister formation in bullous impetigo and staphylococcal scalded skin syndrome. J. Clin. Invest. 110 (1), 55–60.

Lucas, A., Cole, T., 1990. Breast milk and necrotizing enterocolitis. Lancet 336, 1519–1523.

Madan, A., Hamrick, S., Ferriero, D., 2005. Central nervous system injuries and neuroprotection. In: Taeusch, H., Ballard, R., Gleason, C. (Eds.), Avery's Diseases of the Newborn. Elsevier Saunders, London.

Oddie, S., Embleton, N.D., 2002. Risk factors for early onset neonatal group B streptococcal sepsis: case control study. Br. J. Med. 325 (7359), 308–311.

Polin, R., Paravicinin, E., Regan, J., Taeusch, H., 2005. Bacterial sepsis and meningitis. In: Taeusch, H., Ballard, R., Gleason, C. (Eds.), Avery's Diseases of the Newborn. Elsevier Saunders, London.

Rudolph, C., Rudolph, A., Hostetter, M., et al., 2003. Rudolph's Pediatrics. McGraw-Hill, London.

Venkatesh, M., 2006. Infection in the neonate. In: Merenstein, G.B., Gardner, S.L. (Eds.), Handbook of Neonatal Intensive Care. Mosby, St Louis, Missouri.

Annotated recommended reading

Hill, A., Volpe, J., 1999. Neurological and neuromuscular disorders. In: Avery, G., Fletcher, M., MacDonald, M. (Eds.), Neonatology: Pathophysiology and Management of the Newborn. Lippincott, Williams and Wilkins, Philadelphia.
This chapter of the book offers a comprehensive account of the neurophysiology and neuropathophysiology of common neonatal problems. It enriches the existing understanding of the neuromuscular problems which may occur in neonates.

MacLean, A., Regan, L., Carrington, D., 2001. Infection and Pregnancy. RCOG Press, London.
This textbook offers excellent current reviews of microbiology. It identifies the most common pathogens that may cause maternal and fetal infection. A few chapters focus on the likelihood of transmission of infectious pathogens from the mother to the neonate.

Polin, R., Fox, W., Abman, S., 2004. Fetal and Neonatal Physiology. W B Saunders, Philadelphia.

This textbook offers detailed accounts of bioscientific concepts important in fetal and neonatal care. A résumé of genetics underpins a more detailed exploration of normal embryonic development. The systematic exploration of relevant biochemical, physiological, nutritional and pathophysiological principles makes a significant contribution to clinical practice and research.

Wong, D., 2004. Nursing Care of Infants and Children. Mosby, St Louis.

This textbook offers detailed accounts of the biophysical, psychosocial and nursing issues relevant in managing the care of infants and children. It concludes with a range of helpful appendices, which include excellent developmental screening tools and biophysical nomograms and parameters invaluable in all aspects of child care.

Section 4B

Puerperium—The Mother

SECTION CONTENTS

This section examines the return to normal physiology of the woman following childbirth, the onset of lactation and the parent–baby relationship. The importance of breastfeeding cannot be overstated; breast anatomy and lactation are discussed in Chapter 54 while breastfeeding practice and problems are considered in Chapter 55. Advances in technology provide further opportunity to revisit structures in the body using sophisticated investigations and tests such as ultrasound imaging, histology and tomography. The recent findings in the gross structure of the lactating breast are exciting and provide valuable information to facilitate the understanding of the mechanisms of breastfeeding and practical advice given to lactating women. Chapter 56 is about the other physiological changes occurring in the puerperium and the pathological conditions that may affect the woman. Some pathological conditions not previously mentioned in the book are discussed, including puerperal infection. The last chapter in the book considers the development of mother–baby relationships in terms of biological theories. However, the student should not lose sight of the integration of biology, psychology and sociology which underpins human behaviour.

Chapter Fifty-Four

54

The breasts and lactation

Introduction

Lactation is the production of milk by specialised organs called **mammary glands**, named from the Latin word *mamma* for breast. Humans are classified as mammals and distinguished from other vertebrates because of their ability to produce milk for their young. Lactation was probably a key physiological feature that enabled mammals to survive the climatic changes that led to the demise of the dinosaurs about 65 million years ago (Czerkas & Czerkas 1990).

The human mammary gland, an exocrine gland, is the only organ not fully developed at birth. Dramatic changes occur in size, shape and function in the mammary glands from birth through pregnancy, lactation and ultimately involution. It is essential that all practitioners involved with women during pregnancy and childbirth have sound knowledge and understanding of the anatomy of the human breast and the physiological mechanisms of milk production. This knowledge will help them to encourage and support women to breastfeed their babies.

The anatomy of the breast

Situation, shape and size

The adult breasts are always paired and develop bilaterally on the ventral surface of the body. They possibly originate from modified apocrine sweat glands and subsequently form part of the skin. The shape of the breast varies from woman to woman but it tends to be dome-shaped in adolescence, becoming more hemispheric and finally pendulous in parous females (Lawrence & Lawrence 2005). The two breasts are situated on the anterior chest wall on either side of the midline and will vary in size depending on the amount of adipose tissue present. The mature breast extends between the second rib and the sixth intercostal cartilage and lies over the pectoralis major muscle from sternum to axilla. Mammary glandular tissue projects somewhat into the axillary region blending with the anterior axillary fold and this is known as the tail of Spence. The **nipple** is surrounded by areola and protrudes from the centre of each breast at the level of the fourth intercostal space.

Structure

The mammary glands are modified exocrine glands comprising skin, subcutaneous tissue and the corpus mammae (body of the breast). The corpus mammae is the breast mass remaining after the breast is freed from the deep attachments and the skin, subcutaneous connective tissue and adipose tissue are removed.

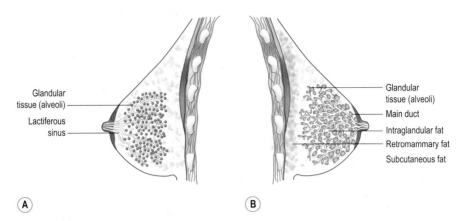

Glandular
tissue (alveoli)

Lactiferous
sinus

Glandular
tissue (alveoli)

Main duct

Intraglandular fat

Retromammary fat

Subcutaneous fat

(A)

(B)

Figure 54.1 • (A) Traditional schematic diagram of the anatomy of the breast. The main milk ducts below the nipple are depicted as dilated portions of lactiferous sinuses and the glandular tissue within the breast. (B) Schematic diagram of the ductal anatomy of the breast based on the findings of Ramsay et al (2005). Milk ducts are shown to be small and branch a short distance from the base of the nipple. The ductal system is erratic and glandular tissue is situated directly beneath the nipple. (Reproduced with permission from Geddes 2007.)

Table 54.1 Summary of the structure of the breast comparing traditional description with current description

Traditional descriptions	Current descriptions (based on recent research findings)
Approx. 22 ducts leading to the nipple	Approx. 9 ducts (range 4–18) in each lactating breast (Ramsay et al 2005)
15–20 lobes with each lobe being a separate entity and arranged in a structured way radiating out from the nipple	Lobes are merged and difficult to separate surgically (Ohtake et al 2001). Ducts are not always arranged systematically in a radial pattern and main ducts may lie under one another (Geddes 2007)
Alveoli connect to very small ducts that join to form larger ducts draining the lobules. Larger ducts finally merge into one milk duct for each lobe	Duct diameter emanates from the glandular tissue directly under the nipple. Duct enlargement occurs at points where multiple branches merge and ducts in the periphery of the breast are sometimes the same size as those near the nipple (Ramsay et al 2005)
Lactiferous ampulla (reservoir for milk). This milk is available to the infant before and during suckling	There is no evidence of an ampulla (reservoir for milk). Only small amounts of milk (1–10 ml) can be expressed prior to milk ejection (Kent et al 2002) and the infant consumes little milk prior to milk ejection (Ramsay et al 2004) The smaller number, size and shape of ducts observed suggest that the main function of the ducts is the transport rather than the storage of milk. Milk ducts at the base of the nipple are superficial and easily compressed (Ramsay et al 2004)
Predominantly glandular tissue and the proportion of glandular tissue increase relative to the adipose tissue. Calculated ratio of glandular tissue to adipose tissue is 2:1 for lactating women compared with 1:1 for non-lactating women (Heggie 1996, Jamal et al 2004)	Some women have an abundance of adipose tissue and it may consititute half the breast tissue There is a large amount of glandular tissue (2.5 times more) relative to adipose tissue close to the base of the nipple (approx. 2.5 times as much) (Ramsay et al 2005)

Corpus mammae (body of the breast)

The tissue of the mammary gland consists of two major divisions: the **parenchyma** and the **stroma**. The parenchyma or glandular (secretory) tissue is the functional component of the breast tissue. The stroma comprises adipose (fatty) tissue, blood and lymph vessels, nerve tissue and is supported by a loose framework of fibrous connective tissue called Cooper's ligaments.

The parenchyma consists of epithelial glandular tissue with an extensive system of branching ducts (Fig. 54.1B). The traditional description of breast anatomy has recently been replaced by findings emerging from recent research studies (Table 54.1).

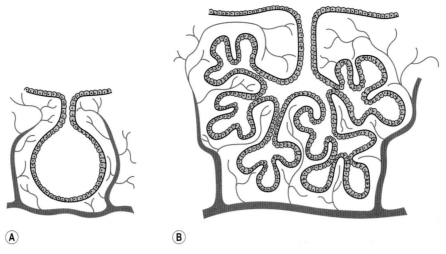

Figure 54.2 • The structure of the breast. (A) Single alveolus. (B) One lobule. (From Henderson C, Macdonald S 2004, with kind permission of Elsevier.)

The alveoli, ducts and lobes

As with all exocrine glands, the glandular tissue contains secretory and ductal tissue within a lobuloalveolar system (Fig. 54.2). Lobes are merged together and difficult to separate surgically (Ohtake et al 2001). The basic glandular unit, making up a lobe, consists of alveoli connected to ducts leading to the nipple. The alveolus is the site of milk synthesis and secretion and consists of clusters of epithelial secretory cells (lactocytes) surrounded by myoepithelial cells to form smooth muscle contractile units responsible for ejecting milk into the ducts from the lumen of the alveoli. Ductal epithelial cells line the interior of the branching ductal network in a single layer. Lactocytes secrete all the components of breast milk into the alveolar lumen. Ductal cells are of the same family as lactocytes and comprise many of the same structural and membrane-bound proteins. They are, however, less functionally complex than lactocytes in that these cells do not have the ability to synthesise milk. A recent study found that each breast contains about 9 milk ducts (range 4–18 ducts) arranged in a complex network and which converge at the nipple (Ramsay et al 2005).

The basal lamina

Each alveolus is surrounded by a **basement membrane** (basal lamina) made up of collagen, glycoprotein and glycosaminoglycans secreted by the epithelial cells where they are in contact with connective tissue. This provides a barrier between the epithelial and stromal components of breast tissue which cannot be crossed by cells other than leucocytes. Lymphocytes or monocytes are found wedged between the secretory cells of the alveoli and have migrated there. They play a role in local production of antibodies in the form of immunoglobulin A (IgA) for secretion into the breast milk.

The secretory cells

The secretory cells lining the alveoli are cuboidal and very polarised in structure (Fig. 54.3). The nucleus is situated at the base of the cell facing the circulation, and facing the lumen is a well-developed Golgi apparatus with layers of flattened vesicles. Most of the cell is occupied by rough endoplasmic reticulum and there are a large number of mitochondria. There are large fat droplets and vesicles containing granules of protein. The basal surface of the cell has numerous infoldings for the uptake of substrate for milk production while the surface facing the lumen is covered with microvilli for secretion of milk.

The stroma

Connective and adipose tissue, which form the largest part of the mammary glands in the non-pregnant state, separate and support the glandular tissue. The breasts are held in position by the suspensory ligaments of Astley Cooper which form from the interlobar connective tissue. These fibrous bands of tissue attach the breast to the underlying muscle fascia and to the overlying dermis.

The nipple and areola

The skin of the breast includes the nipple and surrounding areola which are all visible externally. The **nipple** or papilla mammae is a conic elevation located in the centre of the areola. The nipple contains about 4–18 milk ducts surrounded by a muscular fibroelastic tissue. The smooth muscle fibres in the nipple represent a closing mechanism for the milk ducts and the nipple is richly

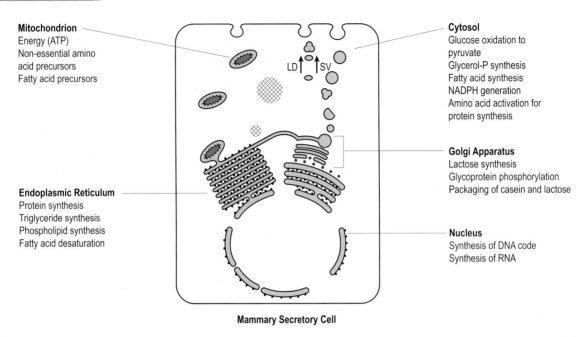

Mitochondrion
Energy (ATP)
Non-essential amino
acid precursors
Fatty acid precursors

Cytosol
Glucose oxidation to
pyruvate
Glycerol-P synthesis
Fatty acid synthesis
NADPH generation
Amino acid activation for
protein synthesis

Golgi Apparatus
Lactose synthesis
Glycoprotein phosphorylation
Packaging of casein and lactose

Endoplasmic Reticulum
Protein synthesis
Triglyceride synthesis
Phospholipid synthesis
Fatty acid desaturation

Nucleus
Synthesis of DNA code
Synthesis of RNA

Mammary Secretory Cell

Figure 54.3 • Schematic representation of cytological and biochemical interrelationships of secretory cell of mammary gland. LD, liquid droplet; SV, secretory vesicle. (Reproduced with permission from Lawrence & Lawrence 2005.)

innervated with sensory nerve endings. Nipple erection is induced by tactile, sensory or autonomic sympathetic stimuli. Local venostasis and hyperaemia occur to enhance the process of erection. The nipple and areola are extremely elastic due to the muscular fibroelastic system which functions to decrease the surface of the areola, produce nipple erection and empties the lactiferous sinuses during lactation. When the nipple erects, it becomes smaller, firmer and more prominent.

The **areola**, or areola mammae, is a circular pigmented area surrounding the nipple. Within the areola are about 18 sebaceous and lactiferous glands known as Montgomery's tubercles. These glands provide secretions to lubricate and protect the areola and nipple during pregnancy and lactation (Inch 2003).

Blood supply

The internal mammary artery (60%) and the lateral mammary branch of the lateral thoracic artery (30%) provide the major blood supply, with smaller sources of arterial blood from the posterior intercostal arteries and the pectoral branch of the thoracoacromial artery (Hirsch et al 1995). The venous supply parallels the arterial supply and bears similar names. Veins end in the internal thoracic and axillary veins and create an anastomotic circle called the circulus venosus around the base of the papilla behind the nipple.

Lymphatic vessels

There is an extensive lymphatic drainage system forming a plexus beneath the areola and between the lobes of the breast with free communication between the two breasts. There are two main pathways by which lymph is drained from the breast and include the axillary nodes and the internal mammary nodes. Lymph from both the medial and lateral portions of the breast drains to the axillary nodes (75%) whereas the internal mammary nodes receive lymph from the deep portion of the breast.

Nerve supply

The breast is innervated primarily by branches from the fourth, fifth and sixth intercostal nerves. The nerve supply to the corpus mammae is sparse and contains only sympathetic nerves accompanying blood vessels. The sensory innervation of the nipple and areola is extensive and consists of both sensory and sympathetic autonomic nerves:

- Somatic sensory nerves convey impulses from skin receptors to the central nervous system.
- Sympathetic (efferent) nerves innervate blood vessels and the contractile muscles of the nipple.

Development of the breast

The mammary gland undergoes three major phases of growth and development before pregnancy and lactation: in utero; during the first 2 years of life; and at puberty. **Embryogenesis** refers to the embryonic development of the organ in utero. **Mammogenesis** refers to the growth and development of the mammary glands. This stage occurs in two phases as the glands respond first to the hormones of puberty and then later to the

GESTATION

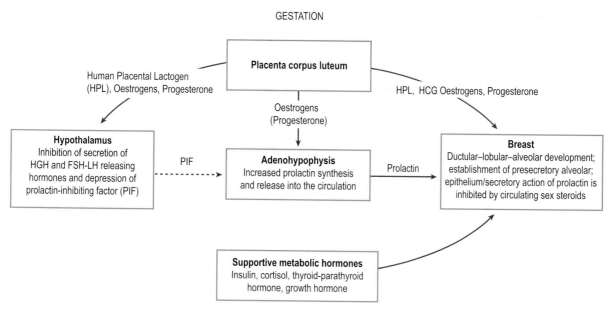

Figure 54.4 • Hormonal preparation of breast during pregnancy for lactation. (Reproduced with permission from Lawrence & Lawrence 2005.)

hormones of pregnancy. **Lactogenesis** refers to the initiation and production of milk.

Early development and puberty

In the 4th week of embryonic life, a primitive milk streak develops from axilla to groin on the trunk of the embryo (2.5 mm long at this stage). This streak becomes the mammary ridge or milk line by the 5th week. The ridge is actually a thickening of epithelial tissue and is accompanied by growth inward at the chest wall, which will be the region of the future gland.

Embryogenesis of the mammary glands begins in the 6-week embryo and proliferation continues until milk ducts are developed by the time of birth. During this time, processes of dividing and branching take place, giving rise to the future lobes and lobules and much later to the alveoli. Specialised cells differentiate into breast structures such as nipple, areola, glands, hair follicles and Montgomery glands. Development is influenced by the placental sex hormones between 28 and 32 weeks to stimulate the formation of channels (canalisation). From 32 to 40 weeks of gestation, lobular–alveolar structures containing colostrum develop. During this time, the fetal mammary glands increase four times and the nipple and areola further develop and become pigmented. After birth, the neonate may secrete colostrum known as 'witch's milk'.

Mammary gland development during childhood merely keeps pace with physical growth. At puberty, oestrogen becomes the major influence on female breast development. Under the influence of oestrogen, primary

and secondary ducts grow and divide and form terminal end buds which develop into new branches and later become alveoli in the mature breast. During each menstrual cycle, proliferation and active growth of duct tissue occurs during the follicular and ovulatory phases, reaching a maximum in the late luteal phase before regressing. Complete development of mammary function occurs only in pregnancy.

Development in pregnancy

The breast reaches its full functional capacity at lactation and, as a result, several internal and external changes occur (Geddes 2007). Changes in levels of circulating hormones result in profound changes in ductular–lobular–alveolar growth during pregnancy (Fig. 54.4). Breasts begin to exhibit changes at about the 6th week of pregnancy and may be useful in confirming pregnancy (Blackburn 2007).

1. Early in pregnancy, the luteal and placental hormones are responsible for a marked increase in the development of the duct system and formation of lobes. Placental lactogen, prolactin and chorionic gonadotrophin contribute to the accelerated growth. Oestrogen is responsible for development in the duct system and progesterone is responsible for lobular formation (Lawrence & Lawrence 2005). This results in the breasts feeling nodular and lumpy and the woman may feel the breasts tender and tingly. Growth continues throughout pregnancy and the breasts increase in size.

2. Prolactin is produced by the anterior lobe of the pituitary gland and this hormone is essential for the complete lobular–alveolar development. It influences the alveolar cells to initiate milk secretion and stimulates the glandular production of colostrum. The prolactin moves through the blood from the central nervous system into the prolactin receptor sites in the lactocytes. Prolactin then transmits a 'message' to the lactocytes to begin production of milk. By the 2nd trimester, colostrum is secreted under the influence of placental lactogen (about 16 weeks). During pregnancy, prolactin is prevented from exerting its effect on milk excretion by the high circulating levels of progesterone.

3. Vascularity increases and the appearance of a network of subcutaneous veins is visible beneath the skin. This network increases in size and complexity throughout pregnancy.

4. By 12 weeks the nipples are now more prominent and the areola develops an increased fullness and brown pigmentation called the primary areola of pregnancy. Montgomery's tubercles further develop and become more prominent and appear as raised projections. The dark pigmentation of the areola may be a visual signal for the newborn baby to find the nipple (Lawrence & Lawrence 2005).

5. By the 24th week, there is further pigmentation around the primary areola known as the secondary areola. This is especially noticeable in dark-haired people.

6. By term the breasts usually enlarge by 5 cm overall and increase by 1400 g in weight.

Maternal nutrition and lactation

During pregnancy, energy is stored in the form of body fat and mainly deposited on the trunk and legs. In women with adequate nutrition, this portion of the weight gain of pregnancy amounts to 4 kg, which is equivalent to an energy store of 35 000 kcal. This will provide for 4 months of lactation and 300 kcal/day for the baby, enough to ensure survival if the mother is deprived of food as may happen in famine conditions. If a woman does not breastfeed, these fat stores may be difficult to remove, contributing to obesity as successive pregnancies deposit their stores (Baker et al 2008). Lactating women are much more likely to regain their figures.

There are two physiological aids to the accumulation of these fat stores:

1. The effect of progesterone and other hormones on the metabolism during pregnancy.

2. The slowing down of energy usage as pregnancy proceeds.

After delivery of the baby, these extra stored calories are converted into milk. The recommendation of an additional 500 kcal/day is now considered to be the upper level for lactating women (Riordan 2005). The conversion of calorie intake to milk is very efficient. Women with marginal nutrition (below 1800 kcal/day), such as those in developing countries, are able to breast-feed for at least 6 months or more. This is due to the enhanced ability to store energy in pregnancy coupled with the highly efficient conversion of food energy to breast milk.

The physiology of lactation

Lactation is the physiological completion of the reproductive cycle (Lawrence & Lawrence 2005). The process of lactation can be divided into three stages during which human milk varies in components, appearance and volume:

1. Lactogenesis I: the initiation of milk secretion.

2. Lactogenesis II: the production of colostrum and transitional milk.

3. Lactogenesis III: the development of milk and the maintenance of established lactation.

Lactogenesis

There are important factors in the initiation of the cascade of events necessary to ensure that a supply of milk is readily available for the baby at birth. These include the preparation of mammary epithelium, the withdrawal of progesterone, the maintenance of prolactin levels and the removal of milk from the breast after birth (Neville et al 2001). This is achieved through the influences and control of the processes involved in lactogenesis (Table 54.2).

Hormonal control of lactogenesis

The four hormones involved in the initiation and maintenance of lactation are **oestrogen**, **progesterone**, **prolactin** and **oxytocin** (Fig. 54.5). An intact hypothalamic–pituitary axis, regulating prolactin and oxytocin levels, is essential for this process.

Oestrogen and progesterone

It is highly likely that the onset and control of labour and the production of milk share the same endocrine trigger. Immediately prior to the onset of labour, during labour and following delivery of the placenta abrupt changes in the hormonal content of maternal blood occur. The pathways remain unclear in humans but it is possible for increasing fetal cortisol levels to alter the

Table 54.2 Stages of lactogenesis

Stage	Developments
Lactogenesis I	
Begins when milk components are first seen in breast tissue and colostrum can be expressed from the breast during pregnancy (normally from mid-pregnancy until day 2 after birth)	A specific milk protein called α-lactalbumin can be detected in maternal blood from mid-pregnancy. During this stage the physical changes in the breasts are accompanied by hormonal changes resulting from the interplay between the pituitary gland, the ovary and the placenta. Differentiation of alveolar cells from secretory. Prolactin stimulates mammary secretory epithelial cells to produce milk. Developments culminate in the initiation of lactation following the birth of the baby
Lactogenesis II	
Begins around days 2–3 after birth when 'milk comes in' and continues until about day 8	This stage is triggered by a rapid reduction in maternal plasma progesterone levels and prolactin levels remaining high. There are rapid cardiovascular changes with an increase in breast blood supply, metabolic processes with the glandular tissue absorbing large amounts of milk substrates from the extra blood supply and secretory changes with the onset of copious milk production There is fullness and warmth in breast and a switch from endocrine to autocrine (local) control The major changes in milk continue until about day 8 after birth when mature milk is established
Lactogenesis III (galactopoiesis)	
Begins around days 8–9 after birth once the mature milk supply is established. It continues until involution of breast milk tissues begins	This involves the maintenance of established breastfeeding through milk production and removal of milk by the baby Control by autocrine supply (supply and demand of milk)
Involution (reduced breast milk production)	
This varies but usually begins about 40 days after late breastfeeding	The baby gets additives of regular supplements There is a decreased milk secretion from the build-up of inhibitory peptides High sodium levels

balance of the placental hormones, increasing the level of oestrogen and decreasing the level of progesterone (Lawrence & Lawrence 2005).

The fall in serum progesterone occurring just prior to the onset of labour may be the lactogenic trigger, releasing the mammary secreting cells from their inhibitory state. The secretory cells can now respond to the circulating prolactin by producing milk. Following delivery, the pituitary gland produces low levels of follicle-stimulating hormone (FSH) and luteinising hormone (LH). The ovaries respond poorly to stimulation by FSH and LH and there is a low level of oestrogen and progesterone production, enhancing the production of prolactin.

Prolactin

Prolactin is a significant hormone of pregnancy and lactation. During pregnancy, concentrations of plasma prolactin rise steadily to term when they reach up to 20 times that of the non-pregnant woman. The **lactotrophs** of the anterior pituitary produce prolactin under the influence of the rising fetoplacental production of oestrogen. This stimulatory effect may be inhibited by human placental lactogen (hPL) as they are of similar activity and biological structure and compete for breast receptor sites. Prolactin (via the anterior pituitary) is also prevented from exerting its effect on breast tissue by the high circulating levels of progesterone (Lawrence & Lawrence 2005). The inhibiting influence of progesterone is so powerful that lactation is delayed if placental fragments are retained after birth (Riordan 2005).

The control of prolactin secretion seems to be controlled by chemical factors, some of which are inhibitory and some stimulatory (Fig. 54.6). The hypothalamus has a stimulating effect on the release of the majority of pituitary hormones. Prolactin is unusual among pituitary hormones because it is inhibited by a hypothalamic

POSTPARTUM

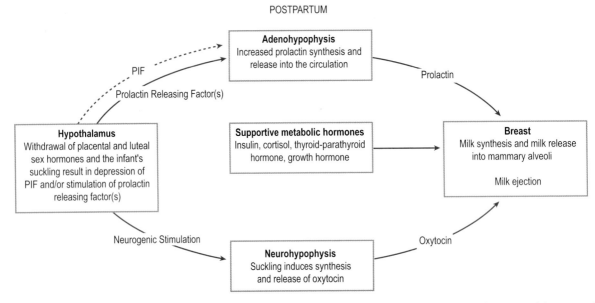

Figure 54.5 • Hormonal preparation of the breast postpartum for lactation. (Reproduced with permission from Lawrence & Lawrence 2005.)

substance. Prolactin-inhibiting factor (PIF), which is thought to be the neuroregulatory substance dopamine, controls the secretion of prolactin from the hypothalamus (Voogt et al 2001). This factor is transported from the hypothalamus along the portal system to exert its effect on the anterior pituitary.

The production of prolactin is supported by growth hormone, insulin, cortisol and thyrotrophin-releasing hormone (TRH). There is also evidence of either serotonin (5-hydroxytryptamine, 5-HT) release of prolactin or catecholamine–serotonin control of prolactin release. Thyrotrophin-releasing hormone is a strong stimulator of prolactin secretion but its physiological role remains unclear as thyrotrophin levels do not rise during normal nursing (Lawrence & Lawrence 2005).

Normally, the production of prolactin varies, following a **circadian rhythm**, with normal diurnal variation in levels in both males and females. Prolactin circadian rhythms persist throughout lactation. Prolactin levels are notably higher at night than during the day (Stern & Reichlin 1990). Increased prolactin levels are influenced by a number of factors that may be significant for lactating mothers. These include psychogenic factors, stress, exercise, nipple stimulation and sexual intercourse (Lawrence & Lawrence 2005).

After delivery of the placenta, progesterone and oestrogen levels fall abruptly and the anterior pituitary gland releases very large amounts of prolactin because it is no longer inhibited by these hormones. The decline in hPL removes any competition with prolactin for breast receptor sites. This also promotes the action of prolactin (Riordan 2005). Prolactin is essential for the production of milk and the amount of prolactin is proportional to

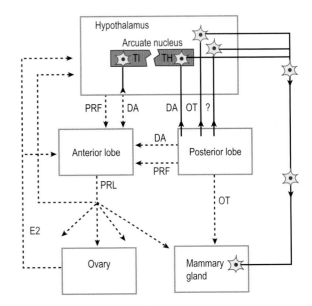

Figure 54.6 • A model depicting the neuroendocrine regulation of prolactin secretion. TH, tuberohypophyseal; TI, tuberoinfundibular; OT, oxytocin; E2, estradiol; PRF, prolactin-releasing factor; PRL, prolactin; DA, dopamine. (Reproduced with permission from Ben-Jonathan et al 1991.)

the amount of nipple stimulation during the early stages of lactation. Nipple stimulation is the only factor influencing the release of prolactin. Therefore other sensory pathways are not involved in the initiation of milk production (Lawrence & Lawrence 2005).

Prolactin levels peak 30 min after a feed and return to a baseline after 3–4 h. As might be expected of a system under the influence of circadian rhythm, suckling-induced prolactin production is minimal in the morning and greatest at night. However, there is no correlation found between the amount of milk produced and the concentration of prolactin.

Oxytocin

Oxytocin is essential for the removal of milk from the breast. The effective removal of milk involves two closely related aspects of breastfeeding:

- The let-down (milk ejection) reflex and the role of the posterior pituitary hormone oxytocin.
- The important role the baby has to play in suckling the breast to remove the milk.

Oxytocin is a peptide hormone produced in the hypothalamus and stored in the posterior pituitary gland. Oxytocin causes contraction of the sensitive myoepithelial cells situated around the milk-secreting glands and also dilates the ducts by acting on the smooth muscle cells lying in the duct wall (Edmonds 2007). Therefore, contraction of these cells has the dual effect of expelling milk from the glands and encouraging free flow of milk along the dilated ducts. This is known as the 'let down' reflex.

The neuroendocrine mechanism or let-down reflex

Oxytocin levels in the blood often rise just before a feed, either due to the baby crying or becoming restless or the mother preparing for the feed (Lawrence & Lawrence 2005). Levels are raised within 1 min of any breast stimulation, and during stimulation the levels remain elevated and return to baseline levels within 6 min after nipple stimulation has stopped (Riordan 2005). Once suckling is initiated, the oxytocin response is transient and intermittent rather than sustained. The nipple and areola have a rich supply of sensory nerves. The afferent fibres terminate in the dorsal horn of the spinal cord, where they synapse on ascending fibres which transmit the messages received from the suckling of the baby to the brainstem. The messages are then relayed to the midbrain and hypothalamus, resulting in the release of oxytocin (Fig. 54.7) from the posterior lobe of the pituitary gland. This hormone contracts the myoepithelial cells and milk is propelled along the ducts. Smooth muscle contraction results in shortening and widening of the ducts to allow milk to flow into the ampullae. Some mothers may feel pressure and a tingling warm sensation during milk ejection. The baby suckling empties the breast and stimulates the release of prolactin.

The effect of higher brain centres

The **neuroendocrine regulation** of oxytocin release and the resulting milk ejection is a complex process which can be inhibited or stimulated by neural influences projected by nerves synapsing on the hypothalamus from higher centres of the brain. These include those parts of the brain involved in emotion, such as the limbic system, and the cognitive interpretation of all aspects of the activity from the prefrontal cortex. The control from higher centres can be more powerful than the nipple–hypothalamic pathway. The let-down reflex can be stimulated by other sensory pathways, such as visual, tactile, olfactory and auditory, or inhibited by emotional states. The mother can and will release milk by seeing, touching, hearing, smelling and/or just thinking about her baby. Anxiety, stress, embarrassment or emotional states can have just as powerful an effect on the inhibition of the release of milk (Lawrence & Lawrence 2005).

Suckling and removal of milk

Encouraging early and frequent breastfeeding is a simple recommendation for the initiation of breastfeeding. Following birth, there appears to be an early opportunity for the baby's suckling to stimulate prolactin receptors (Fig. 54.8), which in turn will enhance milk production. It is essential for babies to be put to the breast as early as possible after delivery, ideally in the first hour, and allow suckling as frequently as the baby demands. Milk production will be affected by factors which interfere with the process of suckling.

The baby needs to actively remove the milk by the process of suckling. The relationship between the tongue and the lactiferous ducts is essential to good feeding and both mother and baby need to learn what constitutes good attachment and efficient removal of milk (see Ch. 55).

Several reflexes enable the baby to play his part in breastfeeding: the rooting, suckling, swallowing and breathing reflexes. Obstetric factors such as medication, particularly pethidine, may have negative effects on the ability of the newborn baby to respond with appropriate behaviour. The reflexes are now considered.

- The **rooting reflex** is elicited when the baby's mouth is touched gently, such as by the nipple. The baby responds by turning the head towards the stimulus and opening the mouth wide. The wider the mouth opens, the easier it will be for the mother to attach the baby to the breast.
- The **suckling reflex** is complex. When the baby feels the mouth is full as far back as the hard palate and the back of the tongue, he will use jaws, tongue and cheek muscles to suckle. During suckling, breast tissue is drawn into the baby's mouth so that an elongated teat is formed from the areola and nipple and the lactiferous sinuses are within the mouth. The lips are closed around the junction of the nipple and areola. The gums are pressed against the areola and the tongue grasps the nipple and presses it against the

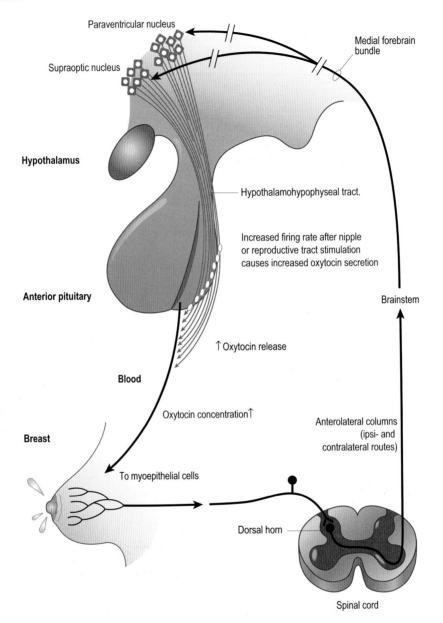

Paraventricular nucleus

Supraoptic nucleus

Medial forebrain bundle

Hypothalamus

Hypothalamohypophyseal tract.

Increased firing rate after nipple or reproductive tract stimulation causes increased oxytocin secretion

Anterior pituitary

Brainstem

↑ Oxytocin release

Blood

Oxytocin concentration↑

Anterolateral columns (ipsi- and contralateral routes)

Breast

To myoepithelial cells

Dorsal horn

Spinal cord

Figure 54.7 • Neuroendocrine reflex in the stimulation of oxytocin (from the posterior lobe of the pituitary) for milk ejection.

hard palate. The muscles of the cheeks create suction and a negative pressure within the mouth.

- The **swallowing reflex** is well developed in the term infant and the baby swallows about 0.6 ml at each mouthful. Oesophageal function is not as developed, with irregular peristalsis.

- **Breathing** is coordinated with swallowing by an **upper airways reflex** to prevent aspiration. Under experimental conditions the introduction of water or milk from another species into the upper airway causes intermittent apnoea. Normal saline or same-species milk does not cause this apnoea. It has been observed that babies fed breast milk from a bottle suck intermittently but breathe continuously. If

the baby is fed formula milk from the same bottle he sucks continuously and breathes intermittently. Breathing appears to be much more regular in babies fed breast milk. Neonates are nose breathers and cannot suckle adequately if their noses are blocked, for instance by breast tissue.

The production of milk

The consistently identifiable stages of human milk are colostrum, transitional milk and mature milk, and their relative contents are significant to nourish the newborns as they adapt to extrauterine life (Lawrence & Lawrence 2005).

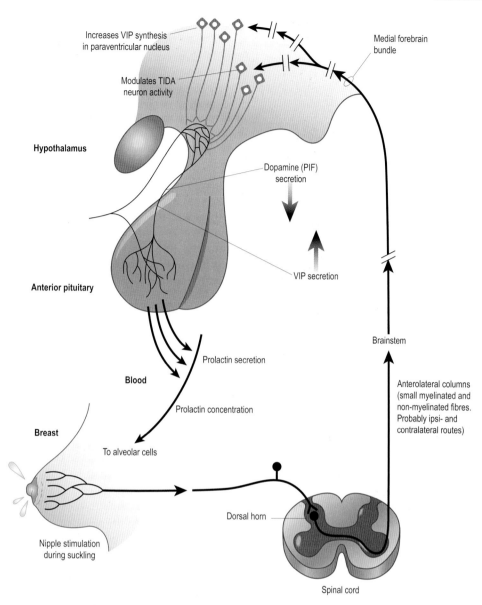

Figure 54.8 • Somatosensory pathways in the stimulation of prolactin (from the anterior lobe of the pituitary) for milk production. TIDA, tuberoinfundibular dopaminergic.

Colostrum, a thick yellow fluid, is synthesised in the breast from around the 16th week of pregnancy and gradually changes into mature breast milk between the 3rd and 14th day following delivery (Fig. 54.9). It is high in density and low in volume, containing more protein, minerals and fat-soluble vitamins (A and K) than mature milk but less lactose, fats and water-soluble vitamins. It also contains more anti-infective agents such as IgA, lactoferrin, lysozymes and leucocytes than mature milk. Colostrum facilitates the establishment of bifidus flora in the digestive tract and facilitates the passage of meconium. It is eminently suited for the newborn baby.

Transitional milk is the milk produced between colostrum and mature milk. The content gradually changes from between 7–10 days and about 2 weeks after birth.

The concentration of immunoglobulins and total protein decreases and the lactose, fat and total caloric content increases. Water-soluble vitamins increase and fat-soluble vitamins decrease to the levels of mature milk.

Mature breast milk is highly variable both within and between women. Its contents change from one feed to another, over the course of a specific feed and as the baby grows and develops. The milk obtained by the baby at the beginning of a feed is called the **fore-milk** and differs from the **hind-milk** obtained towards the end of a feed.

When lactation begins, the mother's metabolism changes greatly and milk may need to be produced at the metabolic expense of other organs (Lawrence & Lawrence 2005). However, milk will continue to be

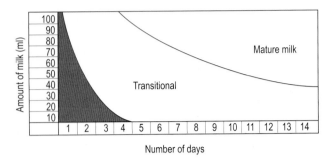

Figure 54.9 • The sequence of milk production. (From Lang S 1997, with permission.)

produced for as long as it is removed from the breast. An autocrine regulator of milk secretion has been identified called the **feedback inhibitor of lactation** (FIL). This factor—a whey protein present in secreted milk—is able to inhibit the synthesis of milk constituents (Wilde et al 1995) and accumulates in the breast as milk accumulates, exerting a negative control on the continued production of milk. Thus milk production slows when milk accumulates in the breast (and more FIL is present) and speeds up when the breast is emptier of milk (and less FIL is present). Removing the milk also removes the regulating protein and milk then continues to be produced. While breastfeeding is not a major factor for the initiation of lactation, it is essential for the continuation of lactation (Riordan 2005).

The contents of breast milk

The main contents of milk include proteins, carbohydrates, fats, electrolytes, minerals, vitamins, enzymes, hormones and anti-infective substances. All mammalian milks differ in the relative quantities of the above contents and have evolved specifically to maximise development of the newborn. Feeding one mammal's milk to another mammal can only be second best, although sophisticated modifications of cow's milk are achieved for human babies.

Protein

The acinar cells (milk-producing cells) are very efficient in removing breast milk precursors from maternal blood. Milk proteins are formed on the ribosomes bound to the rough endoplasmic reticulum from amino acids derived mainly from maternal blood. The protein molecules are then stored in the Golgi apparatus. Vesicles move the protein molecules to the apex of the cell where they are discharged into the lumen of the alveolus.

The main proteins of human milk are casein (40%) and whey protein (60%). These proteins are acidic in the stomach, and form soft curds, which are easily digested

to provide a continuous flow of nutrients to the baby. The chief fractions of whey protein are α-lactalbumin and lactoferrin. In addition to their nutritional function, milk proteins also have specific functions. Casein is an important carrier of calcium and phosphate with which it forms micelles.

The protein in human milk is ideal for the baby and is totally different from cow's milk. Lactoferrin is an iron-binding protein which is low in bovine milk. The total protein content and the balance of amino acids present are essential for the maximum functioning of enzyme systems. The amino acids phenylalanine and tyrosine are present in much lower amounts than in cow's milk, modified or unmodified. The important amino acids glutamic acid and taurine are abundant in human milk but low in cow's milk. Taurine is necessary for the conjugation of bile salts and fat absorption in the first week of life. It is also essential for the myelination of the central nervous system.

Carbohydrate

Lactose is the main carbohydrate in human milk and is formed from glucose or galactose in the Golgi apparatus under the influence of the enzyme lactose synthetase. The enzyme has two components: an 'A' protein called galactosyl transferase and a 'B' protein which is α-lactalbumin. Thus, the regulation of lactose is linked to the production of milk protein, in particular α-lactalbumin. Lactose in turn is linked to the water and mineral content of milk by exerting most osmotic pressure, drawing water from the cytoplasm into the Golgi apparatus. Water makes up more than 80% of milk volume. The lactose content of milk varies between a high 7 g/100 ml in human milk to 4 g/100 ml in the milk of other mammals. Cow's milk is low in lactose.

Lactose is important for brain growth. It is also necessary for the promotion of the growth of the microorganism *Lactobacillus bifidus*, the presence of which leads to increased acidity of the stool.

Several important effects follow the increase in pH of the stools:

- Calcium salts are easier to absorb.
- Lactoferrin binds iron, making it more easily absorbed.
- The growth of pathogenic microbes is inhibited.

Fats

The fat content of human milk provides about one-half of the milk's calories and is the most important component. The lipids found in human milk are mainly globules of triglycerides (98–99%) and are easy to digest and absorb. Long-chain fatty acids are transported directly from maternal blood to the breast as chylomicrons. The acinar cells manufacture short- and medium-chain fatty acids. Although long-chain fatty acids make up most of the fat content of milks, human milk contains more long-chain fatty acids than cow's milk (95% against 83%). In both human milk and cow's milk, 5% of the remaining fatty acids are medium-chain fatty acids and cow's milk also contains 12% short-chain fatty acids.

Arachidonic acid and docosahexaenoic acid (DHA) are two long-chain fatty acids found in human milk that are essential for the development of the brain and nervous system and for vascular tissue. The intake of biologically inappropriate fatty acids could have long-term effects on the growth of nervous tissue. The unavailability of some fatty acids with a corresponding alteration in body tissue composition may be a long-term problem for babies fed on cow's milk. In particular, the formation of the myelin sheaths may be affected permanently.

Arachidonic acid and another fatty acid, linoleic acid, are found in high quantities in human milk. These enable prostaglandin synthesis, which matures intestinal cells, aids digestion and adds to the anti-infective protective effect of human milk. However, the difficulty in achieving a balanced formula in modified milks was illustrated when linoleic acid was added to one infant formula to produce milk rich in polyunsaturated fats. The babies fed on this formula developed a type of haemolytic anaemia. The anaemia, caused by ingestion of large amounts of linoleic acid in the absence of vitamin E, resulted in peroxide formation and haemolysis.

Variations in fat content of milk

Fats are the most variable constituent of human milk, varying in concentration over feeding, from breast to breast, over time and among individuals (Lawrence & Lawrence 2005). The fat content of the hind-milk is significantly increased, especially in late morning and early afternoon. The fat level may reach five times the value of the initial level during the feed. The fatty acid content varies according to dietary source while the fat content varies with calorific intake. High quantities of free fatty acids and cholesterol are present in human milk and act as an important energy source for the baby, providing more than 50% of the calorific requirements. As fat contains 9 kcal/g, the calorific content will vary significantly with the fat content.

Electrolytes

Lactose secretion is directly involved in the transfer of ions across the acinar cell membrane into the milk. The total content of mineral salts is less than one-third of that present in cow's milk with only 0.2% of the sodium, potassium and chloride content. The kidney of the neonate does not cope well with an increased sodium load.

Despite modification in formula feeds, there is a risk of hypernatraemia with dehydration in formula-fed babies if the feed is reconstituted with too much milk powder over a period of time. High solute content leads to thirst and crying. Inexperienced parents may interpret this as hunger and offer more milk, which could predispose to long-term obesity. Although rare, severe hypernatraemia may result in irreversible brain damage. There may be a link between high solute loads and a predisposition to hypertension in later life. The breast-fed baby is less likely to need additional fluid intake except in extreme temperatures.

Minerals

Calcium, phosphorus and magnesium are present in human milk at higher concentrations than in plasma, which suggests active transportation. Absorption in the gut of the neonate depends on the availability of fats and vitamin D. Calcium is more efficiently absorbed from human milk than from substitutes due to human milk's high calcium:phosphorus ratio (Lawrence & Lawrence 2005). Babies fed on unmodified cow's milk are unable to absorb calcium and may suffer hypocalcaemia with tetany. Formula-fed babies tend to have lower serum calcium levels than breastfed babies even when modifications have included the replacement of the fat in cow's milk with a mixture of vegetable and animal fats and vitamin D has been added. Low levels of magnesium may exacerbate neonatal tetany.

Trace elements

The levels of iron, copper and zinc are higher in colostrum than in mature milk. More zinc is present in cow's milk but is not as readily absorbed as that present in human milk. A small amount of zinc is necessary to ensure the baby's health. Other necessary trace elements such as copper, cobalt and selenium are present in optimal quantities. These elements are associated in small amounts with the protein casein, larger amounts with whey proteins and moderate amounts with fats bound to specific carrier proteins (ligands).

Vitamins

The fat-soluble vitamins A, D, E and K are present in breast milk, with higher quantities of vitamin K than previously realised being present in colostrum and hind-milk during the early days after delivery. The need to give vitamin K to neonates is discussed in Chapter 48. All vitamin B complex vitamins and vitamin C are also present in breast milk.

Enzymes

The function of many of the enzymes present in breast milk is unknown. The enzymes lipase, amylase and lysozyme are important. Lipase, the fat-digesting enzyme, is present in breast milk in a form which becomes active in the baby's intestine, making fat digestion easier in breastfed babies. Also present is the starch-digesting enzyme amylase. The presence of amylase may compensate for low salivary and pancreatic amylase activity in neonates. Lysozyme is an important bacteriolytic enzyme present in many body fluids.

Hormones

Hormones present in breast milk include prolactin, oxytocin, prostaglandins, insulin, thyroid-stimulating hormone, thyroxine and growth hormones, specifically epidermal growth factor, which is important for the development of the lining of the gut. Endocrine responses are different in breastfed babies from those who are artificially fed. Growth factor concentration is maximal in the colostrum produced on the 1st day of life.

Anti-infective factors

The following anti-infective factors are present in breast milk:

- A high level of leucocytes is present in breast milk, especially in the first 10 days. These are mainly macrophages and neutrophils whose purpose is to surround and destroy pathogenic bacteria.
- Although immunoglobulins IgA, IgG, IgM and IgD are found in breast milk, the most important is IgA which lines the intestinal mucosal surfaces to protect against pathogenic bacteria such as *Escherichia coli*, *Salmonella* and *Shigella* spp., streptococci and staphylococci and pathogenic viruses such as poliovirus and the rotaviruses.
- Lysozyme is a protein present in breast milk in concentrations thousands of times that of cow's milk. It is bacteriolytic and helps to break down the cell walls of pathogenic organisms.
- Lactoferrin, an iron-binding protein found in human milk, increases the absorption of enteric iron. It provides protection in breastfed babies by inhibiting the growth of certain iron-dependent bacteria such as *E. coli* in the gastrointestinal tract.
- The bifidus factor present in human milk encourages the growth of the Gram-positive *Lactobacillus bifidus*, which in turn discourages the growth of Gram-negative pathogenic organisms.

The transmission of viruses in milk

In the 1990s, women infected with human immunodeficiency virus (HIV) from developed and developing countries were recommended not to breastfeed to avoid mother-to-child transmission of the infection. While feeding infants with formula milk is relatively safe in developed countries, it is very likely to increase morbidity and mortality from other infectious diseases. In light of recent studies and analysis of the situation, it is now recommended that women in developing countries should be encouraged to exclusively breastfeed to maintain the overall benefits of breastfeeding (Coutsoudis et al 1999, Morrison 1999). The World Health Organization has shown that infants in developing countries who are not breastfed and who have received formula or other replacement feed have a sixfold increased risk of dying in the first 2 months of life (Dobson 2002).

In other viral diseases, such as cytomegalovirus, rubella and hepatitis B, the virus may be present in breast milk with no adverse effects on the baby.

Anti-allergic properties

The newborn baby has an immature immune system and gut mucosa and this allows the absorption of large foreign proteins. The IgA and other factors present in breast milk encourage maturity of the gut mucosa to form a barrier against these large proteins. Sensitivity to certain allergens may be inherited, and mothers with known sensitivities may be advised to avoid eating or drinking such allergens as cow's milk for the duration of breastfeeding.

A number of reports have shown a lower incidence of atopic allergic conditions and the degree of symptoms experienced in children who were breastfed (Greer et al 2008, Kull et al 2002, Oddy et al 2004, Rothenbacher et al 2005). Findings are inconclusive at this stage as to whether the predisposing factor is breast milk or the early introduction of weaning foods. The protective effect of breastfeeding may be secondary rather than the primary factor because breastfeeding mothers tend to introduce supplements at a later stage (Edmonds 2007). At present, from these studies, the single most effective measure against children developing allergic tendencies is probably to encourage mothers to breastfeed for at least 4 months and preferably longer.

Main points

- Embryogenesis refers to the embryonic development of the organ in utero. Mammogenesis refers to the growth and development of the mammary glands during puberty and pregnancy. Lactogenesis refers to the initiation and production of milk (three stages).

- Mammary tissue is divided into parenchyma and stroma. The parenchyma (glandular tissue) is the functional component of the breast. The stroma comprises the other supportive tissues, including the skin.

- The glandular tissue contains secretory and ductal tissue within a lobuloalueolar system. Lobes are merged together within a complex network of alveoli, their ductules leading to approximately 9 milk ducts converging at the nipple.

- Each alveolus contains lactocytes which are milk-producing cells. Myoepithelial cells surround the alveoli and ducts.

- The functions of the muscular fibroelastic system of the areola and nipple include decreasing the surface of the areola, producing nipple erection and emptying the lactiferous ducts during lactation.

- Developments of the breast in pregnancy include: a marked increase in the ductal system and formation of lobes; the synthesis of colostrum; increased vascularity; development of the Montgomery's tubercles; pigmentation of the areola; and an increase in size. Montgomery's tubercles lubricate and protect the areola and nipple.

- The four hormones involved in the initiation and maintenance of lactation are oestrogen, progesterone, prolactin and oxytocin. During pregnancy, progesterone inhibits the effect of prolactin on breast tissue to produce milk. Prolactin is involved in milk production (galactopoiesis) and suckling is the main stimulus for its release.

- Stimulation of the areola and nipple initiates the release of oxytocin. This causes contraction of the myoepithelial cells surrounding the milk-secreting cells and propels milk along the duct. This is known as the let-down reflex. The let-down reflex can be also stimulated by sensory factors and inhibited by emotional states. Lactating women require an additional 500 kcal/day.

- Reflexes in the newborn that influence breastfeeding include rooting, suckling, swallowing and upper airways reflexes. Factors interfering with suckling will affect milk production. Feedback inhibitor factor in milk inhibits the synthesis of milk constituents.

- Colostrum is high in density and low in volume and contains more anti-infective substances. Mature milk is highly variable and changes from one feed to another.

- Some proteins in milk form soft curds in the stomach, providing a continuous flow of nutrients to the baby. Fats act as an important energy source for the baby, providing more than 50% of the calorific requirements. The fat-soluble vitamins A, D, E and K are present in breast milk in addition to vitamin B complex and vitamin C.

- Immunity factors present in breast milk include a high level of leucocytes and IgA. Other anti-infective agents include lysozyme, lactoferrin and the bifidus factor. Babies can be infected with HIV during breastfeeding. Exclusive breastfeeding should be encouraged in developing countries.

- Breastfeeding has a protective effect against atopic allergic conditions especially if the neonate is fed for 4 months or longer.

References

Baker, J.L., Gamborg, M., Heitmann, B.L., et al., 2008. Breastfeeding reduces postpartum weight retention. Am. J. Clin. Nut. 88, 1543–1551.

Blackburn, S.T., 2007. Maternal, Fetal and Neonatal Physiology: A Clinical Perspective, third edn. Elsevier Saunders, Missouri.

Coutsoudis, A., Kubendran, P., Spooner, E., et al., 1999. Influence of infant-feeding patterns on early mother–child transmission of HIV in Durban, South Africa: a prospective cohort study. Lancet 354, 471–476.

Czerkas, S.J., Czerkas, S.A., 1990. Dinosaurs, A Global View. Dragon's World, London.

Dobson, R., 2002. Breast is still best even when HIV prevalence is high, experts say. Br. Med. J. 324 (22), 1474.

Edmonds, D.K., 2007. Puerperium and lactation. In: Edmonds, D.K. (Ed.), Dewhurst's Textbook of Obstetrics, seventh edn. Blackwell Science, Oxford.

Geddes, D.T., 2007. Inside the lactating breast: the latest anatomy research. J. Am. Coll. Nurse-Midwives 52 (6), 556–562.

Greer, M., et al., 2008. Effects of early nutritional interventions on the development of atopic disease in infants and children. Pediatrics 121 (1), 183–191.

Heggie, J.C.P., 1996. Survey of doses in screening mammography. Aust. Phys. Eng. Sci. Med. 19, 207–216.

Hirsch, E., Barberis, L., Brancaccio, M., et al., 1995. Structure and differentiation of the mammary gland. J. Cell Biol. 131, 215–226.

Inch, S., 2003. Feeding. In: Fraser, D.M., Cooper, M.A. (Eds.), Myles Textbook for Midwives, fourteenth edn. Elsevier, London.

Jamal, N., Ng, K.H., McLean, D., et al., 2004. Mammographic breast glandularity in malaysian women: data derived from radiography. Am. J. Res. 182, 713–717.

Kent, J.C., Ramsay, D.T., Doherty, D., et al., 2002. Response of breasts to different stimulation patterns of an electric breast pump. J. Hum. Lact. 19 (2), 179–187.

Kull, I., et al., 2002. Breast feeding and allergic diseases in infants: a prospective birth cohort study. Arch. Dis. Child. 87, 478–481.

Lawrence, R.A., Lawrence, R.M., 2005. Breastfeeding: A Guide for the Medical Profession, sixth edn. Elsevier Mosby, Pennsylvania.

Morrison, P., 1999. HIV and infant feeding: to breastfeed or not to breastfeed: the development of completing risks: Part 1. Breastfeed. Rev. 7 (2), 5–13.

Neville, M.C., Morton, J., Umemura, S., 2001. Lactogenesis: the transition from pregnancy to lactation. Pediatr. Clin. North Am. 48 (1), 35–52.

Oddy, W.H., Sheriff, J.L., de Kierk, N.H., et al., 2004. The relation of breast-feeding and body mass index to asthma and atopy in children: a prospective cohort study to age 6 years. Am. J. Public Health 94, 1531–1537.

Ohtake, T., Kimijima, I., Fukushima, T., et al., 2001. Computer assisted three-dimensional reconstruction of the mammary ductal/lobular systems. Implications of ductus anastomoses for breast-conserving surgery. Cancer 91, 2263–2271.

Ramsay, D.T., Kent, J.C., Owens, R.A., et al., 2004. Ultrasound imaging of milk ejection in the breast of lactating women. Pediatrics 113 (2), 361–367.

Ramsay, D.T., Kent, J.C., Hartmann, R.A., et al., 2005. Anatomy of the lactating human breast redefined with ultrasound imaging. J. Anat. 206 (6), 525–534.

Riordan, J., 2005. Breastfeeding and Human Lactation, third edn. Jones & Bartlett, Toronto.

Rothenbacher, D., et al., 2005. Breastfeeding, soluble CD14 concentration in breastmilk and risk of atopic dermatitis and asthma in early childhood: birth cohort study. Clin. Exp. Allergy 35, 1014–1021.

Stern, J.M., Reichlin, S., 1990. Prolactin circadian rhythm persists throughout lactation in women. Neuroendocrinology 51, 31–36.

Voogt, J.L., Lee, Y., Yang, S., et al., 2001. Regulation of prolactin secretion during pregnancy and lactation. Prog. Brain Surg. 133, 178–185.

Wilde, C.J., Addey, C.V.P., Boddy, L.M., et al., 1995. Autocrine regulation of milk secretion by a protein in milk. Biochem. J. 305, 51–58.

Annotated recommended reading

Geddes, D.T., 2007. Inside the lactating breast: the latest anatomy research. J. Am. Coll. Nurse-Midwives 52 (6), 556–562.

This review paper provides an overview of the research findings related to the structure of the breast.

Lawrence, R.A., Lawrence, R.M., 2005. Breastfeeding: A Guide for the Medical Profession, sixth edn. Mosby, St Louis.

This is a very good reference book for health professionals involved with breastfeeding issues. It provides in-depth information, well supported with evidence in the literature and is ideal as a reference book.

Ramsay, D.T., Kent, J.C., Hartmann, R.A., et al., 2005. Anatomy of the lactating human breast redefined with ultrasound imaging. J. Anat. 206 (6), 525–534.

This journal article details the findings of a research study of the structure of the breasts and provides interesting new findings about the structure.

Website: http://www.babyfriendly.org.uk/items/research.

This site provides updates on research findings and other interesting facts about breastfeeding, breast milk and information available for health professionals and parents.

Chapter Fifty-Five

Breastfeeding practice and problems

Introduction

Infant feeding affects every child for life, in many ways known and as yet unknown in other ways (Minchin 1998). Human milk nourishes the newborn, provides protection for child development in early and later life and is optimal for promoting closeness between mother and baby. In mammals, learning about breastfeeding is part of a lifelong process which begins at birth; some is instinctive but a lot is social learning and involves seeing breastfeeding as being a normal and welcome sight, involving shared experiences within the family or community. However, beliefs and attitudes about breastfeeding are very much dependent and influenced by culture, folklore and social context. For example, colostrum is accepted and encouraged as the first food for the baby in many cultures while other cultures believe colostrum to be 'old' milk and unfit for the newborn.

The majority of women are physiologically capable of breastfeeding and when this is not possible then formula milk is available for the baby as an inferior alternative. The art of breastfeeding is a specialised aspect of the science of lactation and is at risk of being lost to future generations because mothers in developed countries may choose to formula-feed in favour of breastfeeding. This is concerning and makes it even more necessary to protect and support breastfeeding practices.

Although breastfeeding is partly instinctive behaviour, mothers will still need support, encouragement and good management to make breastfeeding a success. Breastfeeding is something that has to be learnt. This is true for most new mothers and it is certainly true for midwives and for other health professionals providing care and support. The information in this chapter may help to supply knowledge and information to those involved in helping mothers to successfully establish breastfeeding.

Benefits of breastfeeding

Human milk is easily digested and nutritionally balanced to meet the baby's needs. The benefits of breastfeeding for babies and mothers are well recognised in the current literature and it is useful to consider the benefits of breast milk and breastfeeding separately because the benefits are more than simply the advantages of feeding a baby on breast milk (UNICEF/WHO 2008). Health professionals should share information about the benefits with women and partners when they are making a choice about feeding their baby.

The WHO has recently commissioned a review of the evidence available through a series of systematic reviews to establish the long-term impact of breastfeeding on health. The evidence from two recent reviews suggests that there may be long-term benefits. Horta et al (2007) reported that breastfed subjects experienced lower mean blood pressure and total cholesterol, as well as higher performance in intelligence tests. A review from the USA investigated the effects of breastfeeding in developed countries (Ips et al 2007). The reviewers concluded that a history of breastfeeding was associated with numerous health benefits including a reduction in the risk of otitis media, non-specific gastroenteritis, severe lower respiratory tract infections, atopic dermatitis, asthma in young children, obesity, type 1 and 2 diabetes, childhood leukemia, sudden infant death syndrome (SIDS) and neonatal necrotising enterocolitis. For maternal outcomes, a history of lactation was associated with a reduced risk of type 2 diabetes and breast and ovarian cancer. Early cessation of breastfeeding or not breastfeeding was found to be associated with an increased risk of maternal postpartum depression.

Two other recent studies investigating lung function in children have reported significantly increased lung volume recordings for children who had been breastfed for at least 4 months (Ogbuana et al 2008) and breastfeeding had a favourable influence on lung growth in children (Mahr 2008). A large prospective study (7223 mother–infant pairs) was carried out in Australia over a 15-year period to establish if there was a protective effect of breastfeeding on maternally perpetrated child maltreatment. Findings concluded that breastfeeding, among other factors, may help to protect children against maltreatment by their mothers, particularly child neglect (Strathearn et al 2009).

Breastfeeding may also have a positive effect for babies in relation to interpersonal relationships and sleeping patterns (Renfrew et al 2000). Babies are known to cry less if they stay close to their mothers and breastfeed from birth (Christensson et al 1995). Breastfeeding also helps the mother and baby form a close relationship and is emotionally satisfying for the mother. All of these factors can benefit the whole family emotionally and economically and improve their overall quality of life.

Physiology applied to practice

In Western countries it is rare for a young woman to hold a newborn baby until she bears her own and even rarer for her to closely observe breastfeeding. A primipara is therefore faced with the need to rapidly acquire these two skills without the benefit of prior experience. Midwives must be knowledgeable about the physiology of lactation and apply this to practice if they are going to help mothers to breastfeed. The baby needs adequate nourishment at the breast and the mother must be enabled to develop the necessary skills to feed the baby herself.

In recent years, a number of common breastfeeding practices have been shown to be unhelpful or detrimental to breastfeeding success. These practices were discontinued and included the separation of mothers and babies, restricted feeding and duration of breastfeeding and test weighing babies. The following practices were promoted when they were found to be beneficial in achieving breastfeeding success:

- Early discharge from hospital: women who went home within 48 h were more likely to be breastfeeding at 6 months postpartum (Renfrew & Lang 1999).
- Provision of extra support to breastfeeding mothers increased breastfeeding until the age of 2 months (Sikorski et al 2001).

Antenatal preparation

The decision to breastfeed by women in this society is often made before pregnancy or very early in pregnancy, whereas women tend to make the decision to formula-feed later in pregnancy (RCM 2002). Women are unlikely to change their minds once the decision is made.

During this time, midwives should adopt a sensitive approach with women to help them make their own decision about baby feeding. Women who wish to breastfeed or are undecided should be given all the information and support they require during pregnancy. It may be a bit more difficult to give information to some women who have decided to formula-feed. Women who choose to formula-feed will also be given any information and support needed during pregnancy.

Preparation of the nipples is not necessary other than advising women to keep normal standards of cleanliness and wear a well-supporting bra. Women with nipple problems may find their nipple shape improves as pregnancy proceeds. Breast shells and Hoffman's exercises are ineffective in the preparation of problem nipples (Main Trial Collaborative Group 1994). Teaching pregnant women about breastfeeding physiology and skills may be more important.

The first feed

Mothers should hold their babies with skin contact at birth or within 30 min of delivery and they should be encouraged to give the first breastfeed as soon as the baby is receptive. This should be unhurried as it is important that time is taken to achieve a successful first feed. Health professionals need to know what constitutes good breast attachment to enable them to facilitate mothers appropriately with the initiation of breastfeeding. The mothers need to know how to breastfeed their baby and learn how to hold and position the baby and often they need help with this.

There are several reasons why early and frequent breastfeeding is beneficial for the mother and the baby (summarised in UNICEF/WHO 2008):

- Suckling stimulates uterine contractions, aids expulsion of the placenta and helps to control blood loss.
- The early removal of milk creates the optimum impetus for the development and sensitivity of prolactin receptors, which ensures early milk production.
- The baby's suckling reflex is usually most intense 45 min through the 2nd hour of labour. Initiate soon after birth to prevent any delay in gratification for the baby.
- The baby begins to get the immunological benefits of colostrum.
- The baby's digestive peristalsis is stimulated.
- Breast engorgement is minimised or prevented by the early removal of milk from the breasts.
- Lactation is accelerated and early frequent intake of breast milk lessens neonate weight loss.
- Attachment and bonding are enhanced at a heightened state of readiness for mother and baby.

Positioning

The correct positioning of the baby at the breast is essential to the success of breastfeeding and in the prevention of potential problems for mother and baby (Fig. 55.1). The midwife needs to assess the needs and preferences of the mother and to be flexible in her approach to positioning the baby. Special groups of mothers may need help with positioning such as new or first-time breastfeeding mothers, those with difficulties or previous difficulties with feeding and mothers with multiple births or special needs. Although the mother can adopt different positions to hold the baby, it is wise to offer the baby to the mother in a neutral position so that she can hold him on the arm she prefers for the first attempt (Fig. 55.2).

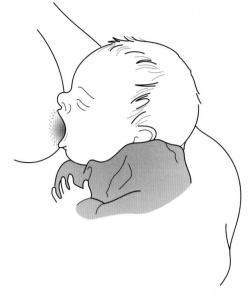

Figure 55.1 • The correct position for breastfeeding. (From Henderson C, Macdonald S 2004, with kind permission of Elsevier.)

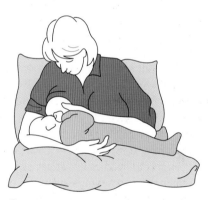

(A) The conventional hold

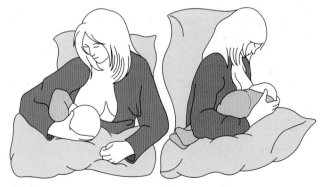

(B) Holding under one arm, dominant hand supports head (C) Holding across the body, dominant hand supports head

Figure 55.2 • Ways of holding a baby during breastfeeding.

Attachment of the baby's mouth to the breast

Attachment to the breast is the most important aspect of breastfeeding and is essential for mothers to achieve success and prevent potential problems occurring (discussed later). Breastfeeding needs to be explained to the mother and she should be taught the basic skills involved. The mother should be given the following information:

- How to elicit the rooting reflex from the baby.
- How to offer the breast to the baby when his mouth is wide open.
- How to recognise when the baby is properly attached.
- How the milk is released by the let-down reflex and begins to flow and how the baby uses suction to hold the breast tissue in the mouth to form a teat (Fig. 55.3) and obtain the milk by the action of the tongue pressing the milk from the sinuses into the mouth. See Fig. 54.1B for up-to-date ductal anatomy of the breast.

Four key points apply to mothers when positioning and attaching the baby to the breast:

1. The baby's head and body should be in alignment.
2. The baby's mouth should face the breast, with the top lip opposite the nipple.
3. The mother should hold the baby close to her.
4. If the baby is newborn, then the mother should support the baby's whole body and not just the head and shoulders.

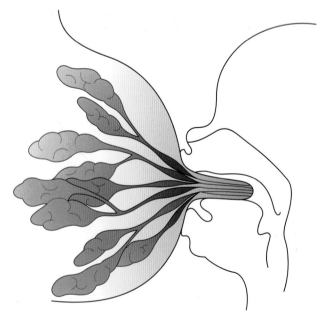

Figure 55.3 • Breast tissue formed into a teat in the baby's mouth. (From Henderson C, Macdonald S 2004, with kind permission of Elsevier.) Please see Fig. 54.1B to review the ductal anatomy of the breast based on recent research findings.

Key signs of good attachment

- More of the areola can be seen above the baby's mouth than below.
- The mouth is wide open.
- The lower lip is turned outwards.
- The chin touches the breast.

Other signs of good attachment are also found during feeding. The sucking pattern is rhythmical and changes from quick short sucks to slow deep sucks. The baby will pause from time to time and then start sucking again without coaxing. The baby can be seen or heard swallowing and is relaxed, happy and releases the breast at the end of feeding. The sucking pattern of babies will now need to be revisited in light of current research findings indicating the absence of the lactiferous sinuses (reservoir for milk) which were previously believed to be behind the nipple (Geddes 2007, Ramsay et al 2005).

Nutritional aspects

The baby must be allowed to obtain both fore-milk and hind-milk from one breast before being offered the other breast. The baby should be encouraged to empty one breast before feeding from the other breast. This will ensure that the baby gets the fat-laden hind-milk and will maximise calorie intake. In addition, the breast will empty of milk and will prevent protein accumulating, which exerts a negative feedback control on milk production (Wilde et al 1995). Removing milk from the breast also removes this protein and milk production is not affected. Both breasts will continue to produce milk if the next feed is commenced on the alternate breast.

Baby-led feeding

Mothers should be assured that there is no need to know how much milk has been taken (one reason for wishing to bottle-feed). The baby will be getting sufficient nourishment if satisfied and sleeping well between feeds. In particular, mothers need to understand that breast milk is not designed to last for 4 full hours between each feed and that newborns do not differentiate night from day. At first, the mother may experience a few problems with tiredness due to frequent feeding but she should be reassured that this will settle down once the baby has developed his own circadian rhythms.

The role of lateral behavioural preferences

Human beings have at least three lateral preferences in behaviour that may influence the establishment of breastfeeding (Stables & Hewitt 1995):

1. The use of a dominant hand for skilled tasks, commonly the right hand.

2. The use of a dominant arm to hold the baby, usually the left arm.

3. A preference by the baby for turning his head to the right.

Right-handed mothers may prefer to hold their baby in the left arm and, if the baby prefers to turn his head to the right, there may be a preference for feeding the baby on the left breast. The mother may feel comfortable with the baby held in her left arm, leaving her dominant right hand to manipulate the breast. The baby who prefers to turn his head to the right will automatically turn to face the left breast. The mother may perceive that feeding at the right breast is more difficult. These lateral preferences occasionally cause transient problems, usually overcome by the 3rd day as the mother and baby develop skills. However, some women who are ambivalent about breastfeeding may feel unable to continue (see Ch. 57).

Taking note of the lateral preferences, the baby may be held across the mother's lap or tucked under her arm (see Fig. 55.3) if it is noticed that the baby consistently turns his head away from one breast (Stables & Hewitt 1995). The mother can be shown how to attach the baby to each breast using her skilful hand.

Breastfeeding problems

The following common situations and conditions often cause difficulties with breastfeeding:

- Insufficient milk supply.
- Abnormal nipples, including flat, inverted, large or long nipple.
- Sore or fissured nipples.
- Full and engorged breasts.
- Blocked ducts and mastitis.
- Breast abscess.

Other problems include breast refusal and the mother and baby with special needs.

Insufficient milk

Almost all mothers are able to produce milk and in many cases mothers can produce more milk than is required. Although the true incidence is unknown, observations in traditional societies suggest that only 1% of women would be physiologically incapable of producing an adequate milk supply (Enkin et al 2000). However, often mothers perceive that they are not producing enough milk for their baby and this is one of the most common reasons why they start bottle feeds or stop breastfeeding.

The best means of preventing insufficient milk from occurring is unrestricted feeding by a well-positioned baby, while giving good practical and emotional support to the mother (Enkin et al 2000). Lactation is a supply-on-demand function and any formula given to top-up or replace breastfeeds will eventually diminish the mother's milk output. If the baby is not correctly positioned on the breast, there may be inadequate emptying of the breast with reduction in milk supply. Often, new mothers lack confidence and may need support and reassurance to overcome their feelings about not giving the baby enough milk. Provided there is good attachment, the most important advice is to encourage the mother to let the baby suckle often to stimulate milk production.

The only two reliable indicators that the baby is not getting sufficient milk are poor weight gain and passing small amounts of concentrated urine.

Abnormal nipples

Sometimes the size and shape of the nipple make it difficult for the baby to attach to the breast. Flat and inverted nipples commonly cause problems (Fig. 55.4), but occasionally large and long nipples cause difficulty for small babies. If the breast tissue is soft and the baby manages to attach to the breast, this will not cause too much difficulty. However, problems can arise when the breast tissue is engorged and the baby just cannot attach to the breast. In these circumstances, it may be necessary to express milk to give to the baby until the breast texture returns to normal.

Sore or cracked nipples

Breastfeeding should be comfortable and pain free. Some mothers may feel the nipples tender for the first

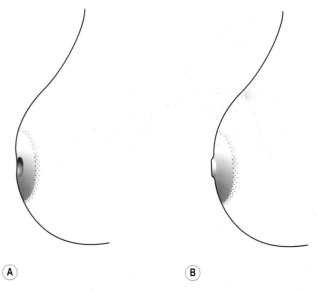

Figure 55.4 • (A) An inverted nipple. (B) A flat nipple. (From Lang S 1997, with permission.)

few days with some discomfort and even pain. During feeding, this usually occurs temporarily at the beginning of a feed only. The most common cause of sore nipples is poor attachment to the breast caused by friction between the baby's mouth and the nipple. This is more likely to occur in women with flat or inverted nipples. Depressing the breast away from the baby's face may also alter the shape of the nipple, leading to friction and abrasion. The only factor that has been shown to both prevent and treat nipple trauma is good positioning of the baby at the breast (Enkin et al 2000). If the nipple is too sore for the mother to continue feeding, she should rest the affected breast, hand express and recommence feeding when the lesion is healed.

Full breasts and engorgement

Normal fullness of the breasts will occur a few days after delivery when the mother's milk is 'coming in'. The breasts may feel heavy, hard and hot and possibly lumpy. The milk will be flowing well and can often be seen dripping from the breasts. During this time, the mother should be encouraged to breastfeed her baby frequently to remove the milk. The breasts will feel softer and more comfortable after the feel and the breasts will adapt to suit the baby's needs within a few days.

Engorgement means that the breasts are overfull, partly with milk and partly with increased tissue fluid and blood. The breasts appear flushed, feel hard and painful and the mother may have a slight rise in pulse and temperature. This will interfere with the flow of milk, and milk production may be affected if the condition is not treated.

Allowing the baby unrestricted access to the breast while properly positioned still appears to be the most effective method of treating and preventing breast engorgement (Enkin et al 2000). The removal of milk is essential to prevent further complications such as reduced milk production, mastitis or a breast abscess. Milk can either be removed by the baby being correctly positioned and attached to the breast or by hand expressing if the baby is unable to attach (Inch 2003). It may help to express a little milk before the baby is put to the breast. The breasts should be well supported and analgesia may be required. The condition may be resolved more quickly if the baby is allowed to empty one breast at one feed and the other breast at the following feed.

Mastitis

Mastitis is an area of inflammation which affects part of the breast, often only one breast. It is often confused with engorgement, which affects the whole breast. Mastitis may develop in an engorged breast or it may follow a blocked duct. In these two conditions, milk stays in part of the breast, called milk stasis. If the milk is not removed, it can cause inflammation of the breast tissue, which can be infective or non-infective mastitis.

Non-infective mastitis

Non-infective mastitis occurs in a substantial proportion of women (Enkin et al 2000). It is probably due to poor drainage of milk and milk leaks into the surrounding tissue when under pressure. Milk contains substances that irritate tissue, causing an inflammatory reaction. Signs and symptoms are rarely seen before the 8th postpartum day. The affected wedge-shaped segment of breast tissue is swollen and painful and the overlying skin is reddened. The woman complains of throbbing pain and tenderness and it is common for her to develop a raised temperature and pulse rate. Aching flu-like symptoms are often accompanied by shivering attacks and rigors.

Good breastfeeding management will help to prevent the development of mastitis. Continued breastfeeding with unlimited feeds gives the best results in milk stasis. It is important to remove milk from the breasts, as milk stasis is an ideal culture for micro-organisms (Inch 2003). Expression of breast milk alone does not have any advantage. The best outcome for women with non-infective mastitis is the continuation of breastfeeding, supplemented with expressed breast milk (Enkin et al 2000). The breast should be well supported and warm compresses or analgesics may be necessary to alleviate any discomfort. Prophylactic antibiotics may be commenced.

Infective mastitis

Breast abscesses may develop in infective mastitis if bacteria, commonly *Staphylococcus aureus* from the baby, enter the breast through a crack in the nipple. The axillary lymph glands will be enlarged. A specimen of breast milk will confirm whether or not infection is present and antibiotics are necessary. Expressing breast milk improves the outcome for mothers with infectious mastitis (Enkin et al 2000). Pain and discomfort may be alleviated with warm compresses and analgesia.

Breast abscess

An abscess is when a collection of pus forms in part of the breast. The breast develops a painful soft swelling. Additional signs include pitting oedema of the overlying skin and a fluctuant swelling under the reddened area (Inch 2003). Simple needle aspiration may be effective or surgical incision and drainage may be necessary (Inch 2003). The baby will not be affected by the abscess and, if possible, should continue to feed from the breast. However, if the abscess is too painful or the mother is unwilling to feed, she should be advised to express her milk until the incision has healed.

Feeding after breast surgery

Nowadays it is not uncommon for women to have undergone breast surgery prior to pregnancy and lactation. Surgery may be performed for pathological conditions and include biopsy and conservative surgery for cancer or for cosmetic reasons. The latter operations include the insertion of silicone breast implants and reduction mammoplasty.

A number of factors will influence the woman's ability to lactate after surgery but success or failure will really depend on the degree to which surgery affected the internal structures involved in lactation. In general, there will be a better chance of breastfeeding if the structures are intact and functioning, but this will depend on the surgical procedure performed. For example, it is most unlikely that breastfeeding would be possible if the nipple was resited. Recent research findings of the co-distribution of glandular and fatty tissue within the breast suggests that it would be difficult to remove fatty tissue and that retention of tissue within the first 30 mm of the nipple would conserve potential lactating (glandular) tissue in women undergoing reduction mammoplasty (Ramsay et al 2005). The ablation of as few as four ducts could completely impair the subsequent lactation potential of a breast.

Women who have had silicone implants or reduction mammoplasty may be able to breastfeed successfully (RCM 2002). Breastfeeding with a silicone implant may have a higher risk of the baby developing autoimmune disease in later childhood, such as scleroderma-like oesophageal disease (Jordan & Blum 1996, Levine & Ilowite 1994). However, the benefits of breastfeeding may outweigh the slight risk of scleroderma (Williams 1994). It is possible for some women to successfully breastfeed after conservative surgery and radiation but it may interfere with milk production (Tralins 1995).

Problems arising with the baby

Congenital abnormalities in the baby

Structural abnormalities of the lip and palate may make a mother feel she cannot breastfeed. In practice, there should be no difficulties if the cleft is only in the lip. The baby with a cleft palate will not be able to form a teat out of the mother's breast tissue and this will prevent the baby from getting the suction necessary to withdraw the milk. Some mothers have expressed their breast milk until the defect has been repaired and then achieved successful breastfeeding. The mother of a

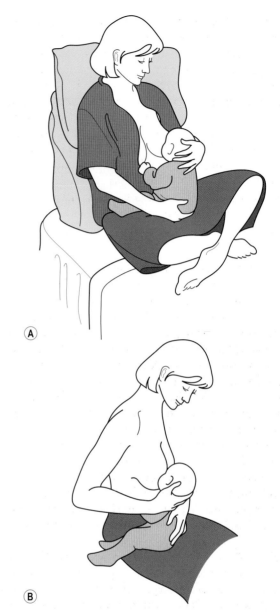

Figure 55.5 • Positions for feeding a baby with a cleft abnormality. (From Lang S 1997, with permission.)

baby with a cleft abnormality may achieve success with breastfeeding if she tries different positions to hold the baby (Fig. 55.5).

Prematurity in the baby

Breastfeeding will be possible with a preterm baby once the sucking and swallowing reflexes have fully developed. If the baby tires quickly at the breast, it may be necessary to use expressed milk to complement his feeding by tube. Preterm babies require a good energy source both for growth and development and to maintain an adequate body temperature. Sometimes, it is necessary to supplement human milk with a nutritional fortifier to ensure adequate growth (Jones & Spencer 2003).

Chemicals in breast milk

In recent years there has been much concern about the amount of environmental toxins that may be present in human breast milk (see Ch. 8). Also, most drugs are of a small enough molecular weight to pass into breast milk and can be ingested by the baby. Substances such as cocaine and nicotine taken as recreational drugs may also have adverse effects on the baby.

Medications

Careful consideration should always be given to any drugs taken by breastfeeding mothers. This is often difficult because of the many factors that can influence the potential effects of the drug for the baby such as the nature, characteristics and the route of administration of the drug and whether the drug appears in the active form or as an inactive metabolite. Other factors to be considered include whether the baby can absorb the drug from the gastrointestinal tract and, if so, whether the drug can be excreted or detoxified normally. A number of sources such as the British National Formulary (2008) and Lawrence & Lawrence (2005) can be consulted for guidance in the use of individual drugs.

Drugs taken in the first trimester may interfere with the development of the fetus whereas if they are taken in the later trimesters they may alter the growth and functional development of the fetus. Any drugs given to the mother during labour may affect the neonate after delivery. Insufficient evidence is available to provide guidance for breastfeeding mothers, and drugs should be avoided. If necessary, the baby should be carefully observed for any possible adverse effects such as changing patterns in feeding and sleeping or skin rashes. Despite this information, lactating women take over-the-counter drugs, other drugs prescribed for family members and the so-called recreational drugs. All women of childbearing age should be reminded that drugs taken for minor symptoms may have adverse effects on the fetus or baby and they should be encouraged to seek advice from their family doctor for more severe illness.

Recreational drugs

Lactating women should be advised to stop or cut down their smoking. Cigarette smoking and nicotine inhalation or ingestion in breast milk can have adverse effects and may be associated with poor infant growth at 1 year (Little

et al 1994) and sudden infant death (Klonoff-Cohen et al 1995). The baby may have colic and breast milk production may be reduced.

Ideally, all mothers should be free of all recreational drugs while breastfeeding. However, this is not always possible and often mothers take drugs such as marijuana, cocaine or the cheaper form called crack and various amphetamines. There is little evidence to suggest that marijuana causes serious harm to the baby and it is probably better for the occasional user to breastfeed rather than wean the baby. Cocaine and crack does harm the fetus and can seriously affect the baby who is breastfed. Cocaine in breast milk can intoxicate the baby and cause convulsions. Amphetamines readily transfer into breast milk, resulting in the baby having three times the plasma levels of the mother, although the baby does not appear to be adversely affected (Riordan 2005).

Environmental toxins

The type of environmental chemicals present in breast milk may include dioxin, organochlorine and methylmercury pesticides, polychlorinated biphenyls (PCBs), phthalates added to polyvinyl chloride (PVC) and heavy metals. The effects of toxins have provoked much discussion and research, especially related to the ongoing motor and mental development of the developing child.

In the meantime, the consensus suggests that women who are anxious about pollution and breastfeeding should be reassured. The advantages of breastfeeding outweigh the risks of the pollutants in breast milk and any effects present in the baby in the early months have disappeared by the age of 18 months (Koopman-Essboom et al 1996). A reduction in the duration of breastfeeding does not have any advantage either, because the milk becomes less polluted as lactation progresses (Odent 2003). Some believe the levels of such pollutants have now begun to fall following publication of popular articles and through the actions of pressure groups.

Taking a wider look at infant feeding, phthalates, which act as environmental oestrogens, appear to leak out of plastics and there has recently been huge concern about their presence in formula milks. The effect on male reproductive development and function is the possible sequel to ingestion by babies (Cadbury 1997).

Suppression of lactation

The suppression of lactation is necessary in a variety of situations such as when women choose not to breastfeed, when there are absolute contraindications to breastfeeding or following the loss of a baby. As breast milk is supplied on demand, there is no need for treatment, as lactation will cease spontaneously. Women are advised to wear a well-supporting bra and although there may be discomfort for a day or two it is rare to find extreme discomfort with engorgement. There is no need to restrict fluids and the woman should not be prescribed a diuretic drug. Drugs used to inhibit milk production and suppress lactation are no longer advised because of the potential adverse effects on the cardiovascular system.

Lactation and fertility

The natural birth-spacing effect of breastfeeding has long been recognised and the WHO has deemed it to be the most effective contraceptive worldwide. The natural contraceptive effect of breastfeeding is not used as a reliable method of family planning in the Western world but it does play an important antifertility role in developing countries.

Natives in hunter–gatherer tribes have long intervals between births. These are healthy well-nourished individuals who nurse their babies several times an hour and wean them for between 3 and 4 years during the next pregnancy. This intensive breastfeeding behaviour keeps the level of prolactin in their blood high enough to block the development of ovarian follicles. Four children is the average number, of which 50% may die before reproductive age and the population remains stable. In the developing world, more pregnancies are still prevented by breastfeeding than all other methods of family planning combined (Edmonds 2007). The current decline in breastfeeding in developing countries could cause the loss of its antifertility effect and will aggravate the increase in population.

The mechanisms of lactational amenorrhoea are complex and not fully understood. The major factor is the frequency and duration of the sucking stimulus which probably inhibits the pituitary–ovarian hormonal cycle (Edmonds 2007). Weight and maternal diet may be important confounding factors. Lactational amenorrhoea may last from 2 to 4 years. Breastfeeding is not absolutely reliable, especially after menstruation returns. Between 1% and 10% of women will conceive during the period of lactational amenorrhoea and most women in developed countries will need additional contraceptive protection (Edmonds 2007). The combined oral contraceptive pill has been shown to reduce breast milk output, an effect not seen in women who take the progestogen-only pill.

Breast cancer and amenorrhoea

There is an epidemic of breast cancer among women of developed countries in the Western world (Edmonds 2007). Breast cancer is a complex disease with involvement of different tissue types. About 5% of all breast cancers are familial, many involving the inheritance of the BRCA1 gene (Leutwyler 1994). Other breast cancers may be associated with environmental toxins (Davis & Bradlow 1995) and the effects of hormones on breast tissue. The relationship between breast cancer and breastfeeding remains unclear but is a question commonly asked. At present, breast cancer is uncommon in countries where breastfeeding is common (Lawrence & Lawrence 2005). Women who have breastfed also have a reduced risk of premenopausal breast cancer and some forms of ovarian cancer (Newcomb et al 1994, Rossenblatt et al 1993, Yoo et al 1999).

The incidence of breast, ovarian and uterine cancer suggests that the probability of female reproductive tract cancer at any age increases directly in relation to the number of menstrual cycles experienced. The highest risk would be an elderly woman, with an early menarche and late menopause, who had never had the reproductive cycle interrupted by pregnancy and lactation (Nesse & Williams 1995). If this is so, it will involve repeated cyclical cellular responses of breast tissue to the changing hormonal environment of the female body. Hormone manipulations may mimic the protective effects of repeated pregnancies and lactation divided by only one or two menstrual cycles. Oral contraception is protective against ovarian and uterine cancer but not against breast cancer.

Modification of cow's milk

Differences between human and cow's milk

All mammalian milks contain water, fat, protein, carbohydrate, minerals and vitamins. The proportions of these nutrients vary in the different milks which have evolved to maximise development of the newborn of the species. Breast milk is an incredibly complex collection of all the nutrients necessary for optimal infant development: metabolically, immunologically and neurologically (Minchin 1998). Relatively few women are physiologically unable to breastfeed but many mothers choose to formula-feed their babies for a variety of reasons. Feeding one mammal's milk to another can only be second best and it is important that a safe alternative to human milk is available. There are now sophisticated modifications of cow's milk available for human babies. The main differences between human and formula milk are now discussed although the constituents of human milk were previously discussed in Chapter 54 and reference was made to some of the differences with formula milk.

Human milk contains other important factors that are absent from formula milks, including hormones, enzymes, growth factors, essential fatty acids and immunological and non-specific factors. The function of most of the hormones and growth factors in colostrum and mature breast milk is unclear. The epidermal growth factor is known to stimulate the growth and maturation of the intestinal villi, which seals the baby's intestine and helps to prevent absorption of large protein molecules without being digested. Undigested cow's milk proteins can pass through the immature gut of the baby and may cause intolerance and allergy to milk protein. The antibodies present in human milk probably help to prevent the development of allergies by coating the intestinal mucosa. Other differences are:

- Lactose readily breaks down into glucose for immediate energy needs. Human milk has a high level of lactose, 7 g/100 ml, while other milks contain about 4 g/100 ml. Cow's milk is low in lactose.
- Fat is the principal source of energy for babies and is very easily digested in human milk due to the combined action of several lipases. Human milk contains essential fatty acids in different proportions to those present in cow's milk and includes some that are commonly absent in formula milk. These essential fatty acids are needed for a baby's growing brain and eyes and for healthy blood vessels.
- The levels of sodium, calcium, phosphorus and magnesium in human milk are ideal for the term baby. While human milk may contain significantly lower concentrations of minerals than formula milk, absorption may be more complete in breastfed babies because of the presence of the specific transport factors of milk. The neonatal kidney does not cope well with an increased sodium load.
- There is a high level of leucocytes in breast milk, especially in the first 10 days, mainly macrophages and neutrophils. The main immunoglobulin present is IgA, which lines the intestinal mucosal surfaces and protects against pathogenic bacteria and viruses.
- Lysozyme is present in breast milk in concentrations thousands of times that of cow's milk.
- Lactoferrin increases the absorption of enteric iron, reducing the amount of free iron. This prevents the survival of iron-dependent pathogenic organisms such as *Escherichia coli*.
- The bifidus factor present in human milk encourages the growth of the Gram-positive *Lactobacillus bifidus*, which discourages the growth of Gram-negative pathogenic organisms.

The manufacture of infant formulae

Manufacturers have achieved a high level of success in modifying cow's milk to match human milk in relation to calorific value and constituents such as electrolytes, vitamins, minerals and fluids. However, it is impossible to match the anti-infective and anti-allergenic properties of human milk, and breast milk will never be totally replaced. The essential composition of infant formulae has been set down in statute and manufacturers must adhere closely to the guidelines.

Formula milk is modified from skimmed milk and whey milk and much of the casein protein is replaced by whey protein. Milks differ in the quantity of protein type: the two main groups are casein-dominant and whey-dominant milks. Although whey-dominant formulae are recommended for the early weeks and casein-dominant formulae for the older baby, there is no evidence to show that one is superior to the other. Lactose is added and some of the milk fat is replaced by vegetable fat. The solute load is reduced. Extra iron is added and the vitamin content is supplemented.

The International Code of Marketing of Breast Milk Substitutes was adopted in 1981 (WHO 1981). This code aimed to protect and promote breastfeeding, to provide safe and adequate nutrition for infants, to ensure the correct use of breast milk substitutes and to control marketing of bottle-milk products. The recommendations for manufacturers of infant formulae include:

- No advertising of breast milk substitutes to the public.
- No free samples to pregnant women or mothers.
- No free or subsidised supplies to hospitals.
- No contact between marketing personnel and mothers.
- No free gifts such as discount coupons or special offers.
- No pictures of babies or idealising images on formula labels.
- Materials for health workers should contain only factual and scientific evidence information.

A global Baby-Friendly Initiative was set up jointly by UNICEF/WHO in 1989 to protect and support breastfeeding. In 1991, the Baby-Friendly Initiative was launched internationally to promote best practice through the implementation of the 10 steps to successful breastfeeding for maternity units, and the 7-point plan for communities. Since the initiative was launched in the UK in 1994, many health professionals have been supported in the implementation of best-practice standards in relation to infant feeding in all health care settings. Since 2008, educational establishments can be accredited if they meet the UNICEF standards for breastfeeding for education (www.bfi.org).

Main points

- Human milk is specially developed to nourish the newborn and provide protection for the child in early and later life. Breastfeeding is optimal for promoting closeness between mother and baby.

- Beliefs and attitudes about breastfeeding are influenced by culture, folklore and social context. In mammals, learning to breastfeed is part of a lifelong process beginning at birth. Some parts of breastfeeding are instinctive but a lot is about social learning.

- The baby should be encouraged to breastfeed as soon as possible after birth. The position of the baby at the breast is essential to the success of breastfeeding and in the prevention of problems. Attachment to the breast is the most important aspect of breastfeeding.

- Insufficient milk is the most common reason given by mothers for discontinuing breastfeeding. Prevention includes unrestricted feeding by a well-positioned baby. The most common cause of sore nipples is poor attachment to the breast.

- Engorgement refers to breasts when they are overfull, partly with milk and partly with increased tissue fluid and blood. Early and unrestricted feeding helps to prevent its onset. Mastitis is an area of inflammation which affects part of the breast. If the milk is not removed, it can cause inflammation of the breast tissue.

- Environmental toxins may be present in human breast milk. Most drugs are of a small enough molecular weight to pass into breast milk. Substances such as cocaine and nicotine may have adverse effects on the baby.

- Breastfeeding has antifertility properties and prevents more pregnancies worldwide than all other forms of contraception.

- About 5% of breast cancers are familial. Breast cancer risks are increased in women who have never had children. Breast cancer may be associated with environmental toxins.

- Formula milk is modified from skimmed cow's milk and whey milk.

- The UNICEF/WHO Baby-Friendly Initiative is a global initiative to protect and support successful breastfeeding.

References

Blackburn, S.T., 2007. Maternal, Fetal and Neonatal Physiology: A Clinical Perspective, fourth edn. Elsevier Saunders, St Louis, Missouri.

British National Formulary (BNF), 2008. No. 56 (September). British Medical Association and Royal Pharmaceutical Society of Great Britain, London.

Cadbury, S.D., 1997. The Feminisation of Nature. Hamish Hamilton, London.

Christensson, K., Cabrera, T., Christensson, E., et al., 1995. Separation distress call in the human neonate in the absence of maternal body contact. Acta Paediatr. 84, 468–473.

Davis, D.L., Bradlow, H.L., 1995. Can environmental estrogens cause breast cancer? Sci. Am. October, 144–149.

Edmonds, K.M., 2007. The puerperium and lactation. In: Edmonds, K.D. (Ed.), Dewhurst's Textbook of Obstetrics and Gynaecology for Postgraduates, seventh edn. Blackwell Science, London.

Enkin, M., Keirse, M.J.N.C., Neilson, J., et al., 2000. A Guide to Effective Care in Pregnancy, third edn. Oxford University Press, Oxford.

Geddes, D.T., 2007. Inside the lactating breast: the latest anatomy research.

J. Am. Coll. Nurse Midwives 52 (6), 556–562.

Horta, B.L., et al., 2007. Evidence on the Long-Term Effects of Breastfeeding. WHO.

Inch, S., 2003. Feeding. In: Fraser, D.M., Cooper, M.A. (Eds.), Myles Textbook for Midwives, fourteenth edn. Elsevier, London.

Ips, S., et al., 2007. Breastfeeding and Maternal Health Outcomes in Developed Countries. AHRQ Publication No. 07-E007. Agency for Healthcare Research and Quality, Rockville, MD.

Jones, E., Spencer, A., 2003. Successful preterm breastfeeding. In: Wickham, S. (Ed.), Best Midwifery Practice. Elsevier, London.

Jordan, M.E., Blum, R.W.M., 1996. Should breast-feeding by women with silicone implants be recommended? Arch. Pediatr. Adolesc. Med. 150 (8), 880–881.

Klonoff-Cohen, H.S., Edelstein, S.L., Lefkowitz, E.S., et al., 1995. The effect of passive smoking and tobacco exposure through breast milk on sudden infant death syndrome. J. Am. Med. Assoc. 273 (10), 795–798.

Koopman-Essboom, C., Weisglus-Kuperus, N., de Ridder, M.A.J., et al., 1996. Effects of polychlorinated biphenyl/ dioxin exposure and feeding type on infants' mental and psychomotor development. Pediatrics 97 (5), 700–706.

Lawrence, R.A., Lawrence, R.M., 2005. Breastfeeding: A Guide for the Medical Profession, sixth edn. Mosby, St Louis.

Leutwyler, K., 1994. Deciphering the breast cancer gene. Sci. Am. December, 18–19.

Levine, J.J., Ilowite, N.T., 1994. Sclerodermal-like eosophageal disease in children breast-fed by mothers with silicone breast implants. J. Am. Med. Assoc. 271 (3), 213–216.

Little, R.E., Lambert, M.D., Worthington-Roberts, R., et al., 1994. Maternal smoking during lactation, relation to infant size at one year of age. Am. J. Epidemiol. 140 (6), 544–554.

Mahr, T., 2008. Effect of breastfeeding on lung function in childhood and modulation asthma and atopy. Pediatrics 112 (Suppl. 4), S176–S177.

Main Trial Collaborative Group 1994, Preparing for breast feeding: treatment of inverted and non-protractile nipples in pregnancy. Midwifery 10, 200–213.

Minchin, M.K., 1998. Breastfeeding Matters. Alma Publications, St Kilda, Victoria, Australia.

Nesse, R.M., Williams, G.C., 1995. Evolution and Healing. Weidenfield & Nicholson, London.

Newcomb, P.A., Storer, B.E., Longnecker, M.P., et al., 1994. Lactation and a reduced risk of premenopausal breast cancer. N. E. J. Med. 330, 81–87.

Odent, M., 2003. Intrauterine pollution and human milk pollution. In: Wickham, S. (Ed.), Best Midwifery Practice. Elsevier, London.

Ogbuana, I.U., Karmaus, W., Arshad, S.H., et al., 2008. The effect of breastfeeding duration on lung function at the age of 10 years: A prospective birth cohort study. Thorax 10.1136/thx.2008.101543.

Ramsay, D.T., Kent, J.C., Hartmann, R.A., et al., 2005. Anatomy of the lactating human breast redefined with ultrasound imaging. J. Anat. 206 (6), 525–534.

RCM (Royal College of Midwives), 2002. Successful Breastfeeding, third edn. Churchill Livingstone, Edinburgh.

Renfrew, M.J., Lang, S., 1999. Early discharge of mothers from hospital. In: Renfrew, M.J., Ross-McGill, H., Woolridge, M.W. (Eds.), Enabling Women to Breastfeed: A Structured Review of Interventions which Support or Inhibit Breastfeeding. Stationery Office, London.

Renfrew, M., Fisher, C., Arms, S., 2000. The New Bestfeeding: Getting Breastfeeding Right for You, the Illustrated Guide. Celestial Arts, California.

Riordan, J., 2005. Breastfeeding and Human Lactation, third edn. Jones & Bartlett, Toronto.

Rossenblatt, K.A., Thomas, D.B.WHO Collaborative Study 1993. Lactation and the risk of epithelial ovarian cancer. Int. J. Epidemiol. 22, 192–197.

Sikorski, J., Renfrew, M.J., Pindoria, S., et al., 2001. Support for breastfeeding mothers. Cochrane Review. Cochrane Library, Issue 4. Update Software 2003, Oxford.

Stables, D., Hewitt, G., 1995. The effect of lateral asymmetries on breast feeding skills: can midwives' holding interventions overcome unilateral breast feeding problems? Midwifery 11, 28–36.

Strathearn, L., Mamun, A.A., Najam, J. M., et al., 2009. Does breastfeeding protect against substantiated child abuse and neglect? A 15-year cohort study. Pediatrics 123, 483–493.

Tralins, A.H., 1995. Lactation after conservative breast surgery combined with radiation therapy. Am. J. Clin. Oncol. 18 (1), 40–43.

UNICEF/WHO, 2008. Breastfeeding Management Course (adapted from Breastfeeding Counselling Training Course.) UNICEF UK. BFI, London.

WHO (World Health Organization), 1981. International Code of Marketing of Breast Milk Substitutes. WHO, Geneva.

Wilde, C.J., Addey, C.V.P., Boddy, L.M., et al., 1995. Autocrine regulation of milk secretion by a protein in milk. Biochem. J. 305, 51–58.

Williams, A.F., 1994. Silicone, breast implants, breastfeeding and scleroderm. Lancet 343 (8904), 1043–1044.

Yoo, K.Y., Tajima, K., Kuroisha, T., et al., 1999. Independent protective effect of lactation against breast cancer. Am. J. Epidemiol. 135, 726–733.

Annotated recommended reading

Horta, B.L., et al., 2007. Evidence on the Long-Term Effects of Breastfeeding. WHO.

This is a very detailed systematic review of breastfeeding studies and provides findings and conclusions related to the benefits of breastfeeding to the mother and baby.

Renfrew, M., Fisher, C., Arms, S., 2000. The New Bestfeeding: Getting Breastfeeding Right for You, the Illustrated Guide. Celestial Arts, California.

This excellent book provides a detailed and clear, well-illustrated step-by-step account of how to breastfeed successfully.

Chapter Fifty-Six

56

The puerperium

Introduction

Traditionally, the puerperium is the time after childbirth, lasting approximately 6–8 weeks, during which the maternal physiological changes, particularly in the reproductive system, resolve and return to the non-pregnant state. At the same time, the woman is going through a transition to parenthood and adapts to take on her new role and responsibilities. The puerperium commences immediately after completion of labour and is considered to be complete with the first ovulation and the return of normal menstruation.

Postpartum is a descriptive term attributed to situations and conditions following birth (parturition). The postnatal period is a social concept occurring after birth and usually involving the baby. In the Midwives Rules and Standards (NMC 2004) the postnatal period is defined as being:

> a period after the end of labour during which the attendance of a midwife upon a woman and baby is required, being not less than ten days and for such longer period as the midwife considers necessary.

The puerperium occurs during a time when the anticipation of pregnancy and the excitement of the birth are over. This period can be a particularly vulnerable time for women as they not only have to deal with the physiological changes to their bodies but also have to cope with any emotional, psychological and social adaptations brought about by their new role.

This chapter will address the physiology of the puerperium and the influences on emotional reactions and mental disorders associated with childbirth. Other aspects of postnatal care, which include family planning (Ch. 6) and interactive aspects of parenting (Ch. 57), are considered in other relevant sections within the book. The main maternal puerperal complications include postpartum haemorrhage, thromboembolic disorders, puerperal infections and mental health disorders. Postpartum haemorrhage can be found in Chapter 45; thromboembolic disorders, including thrombophlebitis, deep vein thrombosis and pulmonary embolism are discussed in Chapter 33. The remaining disorders are considered in this chapter.

Physiological changes

During the puerperium the physiological changes can be divided into:

- Involution of the uterus and genital tract.
- Secretion of breast milk and establishment of lactation.
- Other physiological changes.

The major physiological event of the puerperium is lactation, thus Chapters 54 and 55 are devoted to this important topic. These chapters include the anatomy of the breast and the initiation and maintenance of lactation and breastfeeding.

Endocrine changes in the puerperium

Immediately following delivery of the placenta, there is a profound decrease in the serum levels of placental hormones: i.e. human placental lactogen (hPL), human chorionic gonadotrophin (hCG), oestrogen and progesterone. The removal of the placental hormones initiates reversal of most of the pregnancy-related changes. The rate of removal of the hormones depends on their half-life. Hormones are first removed from maternal blood. Secondary removal occurs as the hormones are mobilised from the tissues. Within 24 h, plasma estradiol decreases to levels that are less than 2% of pregnancy levels. Oestrogen levels return almost to pre-pregnant levels by 7 days. Progesterone levels return to those found in the luteal phase of the menstrual cycle by 24–48 h and to the follicular phase by 7 days (Fig. 56.1). The enlarged thyroid gland regresses and the basal metabolic rate returns to normal.

Resumption of menstruation and ovulation

Most women are relatively infertile during the postnatal period and this may continue during the period of lactation. The return of ovulation is preceded by an increase in plasma progesterone. There is a wide variation in the return to ovulation, irrespective of whether the woman is breastfeeding or not. In most cases, the first menstrual cycle following delivery is anovulatory. However, ovulation may occur before menstruation in 25% of women and pregnancy may result. Anovulatory cycles are more common in lactating women (Blackburn 2007).

Two maternal hormones involved in the initiation and maintenance of lactation will be briefly mentioned here; they are discussed more fully in Chapter 55. **Prolactin** is secreted by the anterior pituitary gland in increasing amounts during pregnancy but its effects are suppressed by progesterone. **Oxytocin** is produced in the hypothalamus and stored in the posterior pituitary gland. This hormone stimulates electrical and contractile activity in the myometrium to aid involution and is critical for milk ejection during lactation (Blackburn 2007).

Involution

The principal change in the pelvic organs is uterine involution and the uterine fundus will have disappeared below the symphysis pubis within 10 days of delivery (Edmonds 2007). Involution is defined as being:

a normal process characterised by a decrease in the size of an organ caused by a decrease in the size of its cells, such as is found in the involution of the uterus in the postpartum period.

During this process, the uterus returns to its normal size, tone and position and the vagina, uterine ligaments and muscles of the pelvic floor also return to their pre-pregnant state. The pelvic floor and subsequent problems that can arise if the ligaments and muscles are permanently weakened are discussed in Chapter 25.

Physiology

During involution there are changes to the myometrium or muscle layer and the decidua or lining of the pregnant uterus (Fig. 56.2). The muscle layer returns to normal thickness by the processes of ischaemia, autolysis and phagocytosis. The decidua is shed as **lochia** and there is regeneration of the endometrium.

- **Ischaemia** occurs when the muscles of the uterus retract at the end of the third stage to constrict the blood vessels at the placental site, resulting in haemostasis. Blood circulating to the uterus is greatly reduced.
- **Autolysis** is the process of removal of the redundant actin and myosin muscle fibres and cytoplasm by proteolytic enzymes and macrophages. Individual myometrial cells are reduced in size with no significant reduction in the numbers of cells.
- **Phagocytosis** removes the excess fibrous and elastic tissue. This process is incomplete and some elastic tissue remains so that a uterus that has held a pregnancy never quite returns to the nulliparous state.

Positional changes

The most marked reduction in the size of the uterus takes place during the first 10 days. The process of involution is not complete until about 6 weeks and the rate at which the uterus involutes varies between women (Edmonds 2007).

Immediately after delivery of the placenta the whole uterus contracts down fully and the uterine walls become realigned in apposition to each other (Coad & Dunstall 2005). The uterus weighs about 1000 g at this

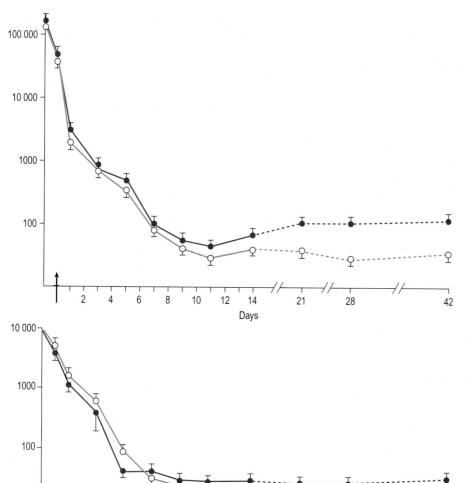

Figure 56.1 • Mean (±SEM) serum concentrations of 17β-oestradiol and progesterone in lactating and non-lactating subjects. Lactating subjects ($n = 10$) ○—○; non-lactating subjects ($n = 9$) ●—●. (From Henderson C, Macdonald S 2004, with kind permission of Elsevier.)

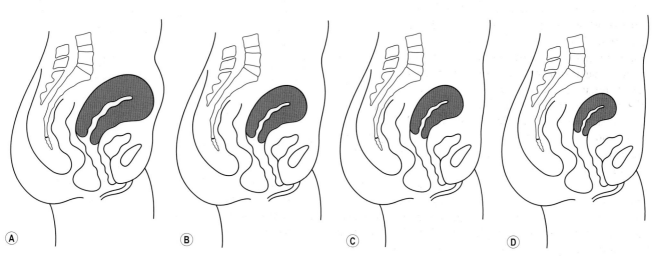

Figure 56.2 • Involution of the uterus. (A) At the end of labour. (B) One week after delivery. (C) Two weeks after delivery. (D) Six weeks after delivery. (From Henderson C, Macdonald S 2004, with kind permission of Elsevier.)

time. The fundus is palpable just below or at the level of the umbilicus which is about 11–12 cm above the symphysis pubis (Edmonds 2007). The muscles are well contracted to aid the process of haemostasis and at this time the uterus feels globular and hard like a cricket ball. Between 1 and 12 h after delivery, the myometrium relaxes slightly, whilst continuing to remain firmly contracted (Coad & Dunstall 2005, Edmonds 2007). Further active bleeding is prevented by the activation of the blood-clotting mechanisms which are altered greatly during pregnancy to facilitate a swift clotting response (Coad & Dunstall 2005).

On average the height of the fundus then decreases at a rate of 1 cm daily. At the end of the 1st week, the uterus has lost 50% of its bulk, weighs about 500 g and is about 5 cm above the symphysis pubis. It has returned to the true pelvis by the 10th postnatal day. By the end of the 6th week after delivery, the uterus should weigh between 60 and 80 g and has returned to its pre-pregnant position of anteversion and anteflexion.

This normal process of involution is slower when there has been overdistension of the uterus due to multiple pregnancy or a large baby or if the pregnancy has been complicated by polyhydramnios. Slow involution may be associated with retained placental tissue or blood clot, particularly if there is an associated infection. There is no evidence to suggest that there is any relationship between parity and the rate of involution.

Uterine contractions

During the first 24 h after delivery, oxytocin leads to uterine contractions with further retraction. The contractions can be quite strong and often result in after-pains, especially in multiparous women. Suckling stimulates oxytocin release. This gradually diminishes over the next 4–7 days and the pain is relieved by mild analgesia.

The decidua

The upper portion of the spongy endometrial layer is sloughed off when the placenta is delivered. The remaining decidua is organised into basal and superficial layers. The superficial layer consists of granulation tissue, which is invaded by leucocytes to form a barrier to prevent micro-organisms invading the remaining decidua. This layer becomes necrotic and is sloughed off as the lochia. The basal layer remains intact and is the source of regeneration of the endometrium, which begins about 10 days after delivery. The regeneration process is completed by 2–3 weeks following delivery, with the exception of the placental site.

Healing of the placental site is complete by the end of 6 weeks. Immediately after delivery, the placental site is reduced to a raised roughened area about 12 cm in diameter. It contains many thrombosed sinusoids. The large blood vessels that supplied the intervillous space are invaded by fibroblasts and their lumen is obscured. Some of the blood vessels later recanalise.

Lochia

The vaginal loss during the puerperium is known as the **lochia** (a plural word). Lochia vary in amount, content and colour as the excess tissue is lost. Women lose between 150 and 400 ml of lochia, averaging 225 ml. Women who breastfeed have less lochia, possibly due to more rapid involution and healing, although flow may increase temporarily during suckling. Three forms of lochia are described: **rubra** (red), **serosa** (pink) and **alba** (white).

Lochia consist of blood, leucocytes, shreds of deciduas and organisms. A summary of the characteristics of lochia is presented in Table 56.1. The lochia may remain red for up to 3 weeks or there may be a brief increase in blood content in the 2nd week. However, lochia remaining heavily bloodstained or a sudden return to profuse red lochia may suggest that placental tissue has been retained. If the lochia are offensive and the woman becomes pyrexial, uterine infection may be present, and she must be assessed by a doctor and appropriate treatment commenced.

Findings from research studies indicate that vaginal loss during the puerperium is considerably more varied in duration, amount and colour than classically reported and described in textbooks (Marchant et al 1999, 2003, Sherman et al 1999).

Other parts of the genital tract

Immediately after delivery, the **cervix** is soft and highly vascular but it rapidly loses its vascularity and returns to its original form and normal consistency within a few days of delivery (Edmonds 2007). The external

Table 56.1 The characteristics of lochia

Type	Content	Average days
Lochia rubra	Blood, amnion and chorion, decidual cells, vernix, lanugo, meconium	1–3
Lochia serosa	Blood, wound exudate, erythrocytes, leucocytes, cervical mucus, micro-organisms, shreds of degenerating decidua from the superficial layer	4–10
Lochia alba	Leucocytes, decidual cells, mucus, bacteria, epithelial cells	11–21

os remains sufficiently dilated to admit one finger for weeks or months (and in some cases permanently) but the internal os becomes closed during the 2nd week of the puerperium (Howie 1995). The **ovaries** and **fallopian tubes** return with the uterus to the pelvic cavity. The vagina almost always shows some evidence of parity. The **vagina**, **vulva** and **pelvic floor** respond to the reduced amount of circulating progesterone by recovering normal muscle tone. Early ambulation and postnatal exercises can enhance this return to normal. Bruising or tears to genital tissues heal rapidly and any oedema is reabsorbed within the first 3 or 4 days.

The body systems

The cardiovascular and respiratory systems

During pregnancy, the increased circulatory volume and haemodilution are needed to ensure adequate blood supply to the uterus and placental bed. Following the withdrawal of oestrogen, a diuresis occurs for the first 48h and the plasma volume and haematocrit rapidly return to normal. The reduction in circulating progesterone leads to removal of excess tissue fluid and a return to normal vascular tone. There is an increase in atrial natriuretic peptide, which may contribute to the well-recognised diuresis that occurs during this period (de Swiet 1998). Cardiac output and blood pressure return to non-pregnant levels.

Delivery of the baby and reduction in uterine size remove the compression of the lungs. Full inflation of the lungs, including the basal lobes, is again possible. With the reduction in cardiac work and circulatory volume and the decrease in metabolism, oxygen demands now return to normal. The tendency to hyperventilation disappears, and blood carbon dioxide levels return to normal, as does the slight alkalosis.

The renal system

There is reversal of the physiological parameters of the renal system to pre-pregnancy levels by the end of the puerperium. During this time, the kidneys must cope with the excretion of excess fluids and an increase in the breakdown products of protein. The dilatation of the renal tract resolves with the removal of progesterone and the renal organs gradually return to their pre-pregnant state. During labour, the bladder is displaced into the abdomen and the urethra is stretched. There may be loss of tone in the bladder and bruising of the urethra, leading to difficulty in micturition.

Because of these features and diuresis, the bladder may become overdistended and retention of urine may occur. This may be missed if the carer fails to notice that frequent small amounts of urine are being passed with the bladder becoming ever more distended. Early ambulation with frequent encouragement to pass urine and ensuring that the bladder is emptied will help to avoid this situation. Catheterisation may occasionally be necessary.

The gastrointestinal tract

Throughout the body, smooth muscle tone gradually returns to normal due to the reduced levels of circulating progesterone. There is a rapid return to normal carbohydrate metabolism and fasting plasma insulin levels return to non-pregnant values between 48h and the 6th week postpartum (Campbell-Brown & Hytten 1998). The minor inconveniences of pregnancy affecting the gastrointestinal tract, such as constipation and heartburn, resolve. Constipation may persist as a problem, possibly due to inactivity or a fear of pain on defecation.

Puerperal infection

At delivery, the normal protective barriers against infection are temporarily broken down, and this gives potential pathogens an opportunity to pass from the lower genital tract into the usually sterile environment of the uterus. Prior to the introduction of aseptic techniques and development of antibiotics, puerperal sepsis was an important cause of maternal mortality. Puerperal pyrexia was then a notifiable disease. Puerperal pyrexia may have several explanations but it is a clinical sign that always merits careful investigation (Lewis 2007). Women are particularly at risk to infection at this time because of the presence of the placental site, the tissue trauma sustained in labour and the decidua and lochia being excellent culture media for the growth of bacteria (Edmonds 2007).

Other sites for infection are the breasts and the epithelial linings of the veins. The possibility that the woman has developed an infection unrelated to pregnancy, such as an upper respiratory tract infection, should always be considered. Infection of surgical incisions is also a significant cause of maternal morbidity. A total of 22 maternal deaths between 2003 and 2005 were recorded as a result of sepsis (Lewis 2007). Of the maternal deaths occurring in the puerperium, 3 were following uneventful vaginal delivery, 10 were following surgical delivery and 3 were late deaths after 6 weeks.

Identification of site of infection

A raised temperature and pulse rate are only indicators that infection may be present. Other signs and symptoms present on clinical examination will help to identify the site of infection. The timing of the onset of pyrexia may also indicate the source of the problem.

Swabs may be taken from all possible sites, and specimens should be obtained for investigations such as organism, culture and antibiotic sensitivity. Depending on the signs and symptoms, these may include high vaginal, perineal, wound, ear, nose and throat swabs, and specimens of blood, urine, stool and breast milk. Antibiotic therapy should commence prior to the results of such investigations if the woman is ill.

Causative organisms

It takes time for invading organisms to multiply sufficiently to cause symptoms, and postnatal infection occurs after the first 24 h from delivery. As in any infection, the severity depends on two factors: the virulence of the causative organism and the resistance of the host. Infecting organisms may originate from the commensal organisms normally present in the woman's own body. These are called endogenous organisms and can cause problems if they invade susceptible sites. Such organisms may come from the vagina, bowel, skin, nose or throat of the woman and include *Escherichia coli*, *Clostridium welchii* and *Streptococcus faecalis*.

Other organisms are transmitted from sites other than the woman's body, commonly from an attendant. These are called **exogenous** organisms and are responsible for the more serious infections. The most dangerous organism is **β-haemolytic streptococcus group A** which leads to intrauterine infection and is currently the main cause of maternal death from sepsis in the UK (Lewis 2007). It may be found in people with a sore throat. *Staphylococcus aureus* is a common organism which lingers in dust and can cause spots, pustules and sticky eyes in babies and breast or wound infections in mothers. A strain of this organism, called meticillin-resistant *Staphylococcus aureus* (MRSA), is resistant to most antibiotics. Overuse and misuse of antibiotics in human disease and animal husbandry has contributed to the mutations of organisms (Coughlan 1996).

Streptococci: Lancefield groups

The genus *Streptococcus* contains a wide variety of species of bacteria with many habitats. Some species are pathogenic to human beings. One group of related species comprises those that cause haemolysis when grown on blood agar, an action referred to as β-**haemolysis**. Streptococci are also subdivided depending on the presence of carbohydrate antigens on their surfaces and are named after Rebecca Lancefield who was a pioneer in the classification of streptococci. These are called **Lancefield groups** and are identified with letters of the alphabet such as A, B and onwards to O (Amezaga & McKenzie 2006).

The most common organism responsible for serious and life-threatening obstetric infections is the β-haemolytic *Streptococcus pyogenes*, categorised as Lancefield group A (Lewis 2007). This organism has the ability to gain access to the circulation via the placental site, causing septicaemia and haemolysis of red cells. This strain was responsible for deaths from childbirth fever and was virulent up to the development of antibiotics, being responsible for the serious childhood illness scarlet fever, as well as for sore throats. This organism caused damage to the kidneys.

Pharmacological interventions contributed to a dramatic decrease in puerperal infections between the 1940s and the 1980s. In the late 1980s, a resurgence of infections was noted as new virulent strains of bacteria emerged, with Lancefield group B being a problem with babies. The Lancefield group B streptococcus can be found in normal vaginal flora and is most commonly associated with neonatal septicaemia and meningitis, particularly in premature infants. Serious maternal infections may also occur with this infection. The Lancefield groups C and G streptococcus may also cause serious clinical syndromes but are less common (Lewis 2007).

Group A streptococci attack people of all ages and are lethal despite vigorous treatment. Scientists are developing new drugs to combat the ability of bacteria to resist antibiotics but it may be some years before these are readily available on the market. It is imperative that vigilance in preventative measures is maintained to protect childbearing women and their babies.

Genital tract infection

Infection of the genital tract may remain localised to the perineum, vagina or cervix or may ascend the genital tract to infect the uterine cavity (**endometritis**). Infection may then spread to the fallopian tubes to cause salpingitis and to the tissues of the pelvic cavity to cause cellulitis and peritonitis.

Postpartum endometritis

Postpartum endometritis is usually caused by an ascending infection from the lower genital tract; about 2% of women experiencing vaginal births and 10–15% of those with caesarean birth are estimated to develop this condition (Walsh 2001). Other factors that may facilitate pelvic infections include prolonged labour, prolonged rupture of the membranes, multiple vaginal examinations, traumatic delivery and manual removal of placenta (Edmonds 2007). Antibiotic therapy is often advised for women with vaginal vaginosis.

Signs and symptoms

- Pyrexia above 38°C occurs about the 3rd postnatal day.
- Pulse rate rises by about 10 beats/min (bpm) for every degree Celsius.

- Pain is present in the lower abdomen.
- The uterus is tender on palpation.
- Headache and rigors may occur.
- Localised infection is sometimes seen in the perineum.
- Lochia may be heavy and offensive, depending on the invading organism.
- Blood cultures may be positive in up to 10% of women.

Spread of infection

The mother's condition may deteriorate rapidly if there is spread of the organism by bacteria such as *Clostridium welchii*. Severe sepsis with acute organ dysfunction has a 20–40% mortality rate (Lewis 2007).

Treatment

The woman should be isolated and examined by medical staff. In the seriously ill obstetric patient where sepsis may be implicated, it is advised that intravenous antibiotic treatment is commenced immediately (Lewis 2007). Bacteriological specimens including high vaginal and wound site swabs and urine and blood culture must be obtained prior to commencing such treatment before these results are available. The most appropriate antibiotic treatment based on the organisms currently identified as being responsible for maternal deaths would be the recently introduced penicillin derivatives piperacillin/tazobactam in combination with the aminoglycoside netilmicin (Lewis 2007). Where appropriate, drugs are changed according to the sensitivity results.

Care is provided to meet the woman's needs, depending on the severity of the illness. Any dehydration should be corrected and analgesics may be required for pain relief. Haemoglobin levels will need to be assessed as anaemia may precede or follow infection. A blood transfusion is sometimes necessary. Any localised wound infections are treated. A light nourishing diet is provided if the woman is well enough to eat. The baby may also require investigation and treatment.

Urinary tract infection

Urinary tract infections are common during the puerperium, especially in women with urinary retention, indwelling catheters, operative deliveries or with a history of urinary infections (Edmonds 2007). Because of the delay in the return to normal in the urinary tract, there is susceptibility for infection for the first 6 weeks and this may present as cystitis or pyelonephritis. The most common organism cultured is *Escherichia coli*.

Signs and symptoms

Most infections take the form of cystitis with the usual symptoms. These include urinary frequency, urgency, dysuria and haematuria. The urine may be cloudy and offensive and there may be a slight rise in maternal temperature.

In the more serious pyelonephritis, the woman may develop:
- Pain and tenderness in the renal angle which may extend along the line of the ureter.
- Pyrexia and rapid pulse.
- Rigors.
- Nausea and vomiting.

The woman will feel ill. On urinalysis, the urine is acidic, opalescent and offensive. Pus and blood may be found on microscopic examination.

Treatment

Diagnosis can be confirmed by culturing the infecting organism on a midstream specimen of urine. A good oral intake of fluids should be encouraged and, if vomiting is present, intravenous fluids may be required to maintain adequate hydration and a good urinary output. Where necessary, drugs will be required to relieve pain, alleviate nausea and to reduce temperature. A broad-spectrum antibiotic is commenced and changed as appropriate, according to sensitivity results. Following completion of the antibiotic treatment, a repeat culture should be performed to ensure the treatment has been adequate to defeat the infection. Following the puerperium, any woman with a history of recurrent urinary tract infections should have further investigations of the urinary tract by cystoscopy and intravenous pyelography to exclude any underlying abnormality.

Other puerperal infections

In the event of puerperal pyrexia, any surgical wound should be examined for evidence of infection. This is particularly important following instrumental deliveries and surgical procedures. Wound infection will present as a reddened tender area and may be oedematous. The wound may have serous, bloodstained or purulent discharge and may be offensive in nature. There may be associated pyrexia and tachycardia with the woman being generally unwell.

Treatment will depend on the extent and severity of the infection. Bacteriology specimens required for culture and sensitivity will include swabs of the wound site for all degrees of infection and blood specimens for moderate to severe infections. Well-localised wound infections may discharge spontaneously and may only require local irrigation with an antiseptic solution. A broad-spectrum antibiotic will be required in more extensive wound infections (Edmonds 2007). In the majority of cases the wound will granulate from its base and heal spontaneously. In rare circumstances, the wound may need to be resutured.

If puerperal pyrexia is present, the legs should also be routinely inspected for any evidence of thrombophlebitis. Breast infections are discussed in Chapter 54.

Emotional states and mental disorders in the puerperium

Behaviour is a complex function influenced by the interaction of biological factors and social, economic and cultural factors (Jessel & Moir 1997). Obstetric factors may also influence the behaviour of women during the childbearing process (Cox & Holden 2003).

Childbirth is generally recognised as being an important life event of great physiological and psychological significance. The events surrounding the birth often leave women both physically and emotionally vulnerable and they commonly experience mood changes in the postpartum period. Mental disorders during the postnatal period can have serious consequences for the health and well-being of a mother and her baby, as well as for her partner and other family members (NICE 2007). Two classes of mental health disorders are the neuroses and the psychoses. In neuroses the individual, although likely to be depressed, remains in touch with reality. In the much more severe psychoses there is a great impairment in the perception of external reality, often with delusions and hallucinations. In most cases women with mental health disorders after childbirth will experience the neurotic disorder of postnatal depression and only a few women, many with a history of mental illness, will suffer from a puerperal psychotic episode of schizophrenia.

The spectrum of 'affective states or disorders' following childbirth is most often divided into three categories in ascending order of severity:

1. The 'baby blues' (emotional state).
2. Postnatal depression (neuroses).
3. Puerperal psychosis (psychoses).

'Baby blues'

The early feelings of elation in the first 3 days after birth are replaced by a normal emotional reaction to childbirth called the 'baby blues'. Over 50% of women experience this emotional reaction, which occurs from around the 3rd day after birth until about the end of the 1st week when women usually return to normal. The reaction is characterised by tearfulness, irritability, forgetfulness, fatigue and inability to concentrate and think clearly. The symptoms have a short impact on daily function and normally it is only a transient and self-limiting emotional change. However, a prolonged, serious episode may be predictive of the onset of postnatal depression (Price 2007).

The cause of the 'baby blues' remains unclear. The physiological changes occurring in the puerperium are thought to be mainly responsible because the reaction is so common at this particular time. The types of changes, which may affect behaviour, include the decrease in oestrogen and progesterone and alterations in the balance of fluids and electrolytes and neurotransmitters. These factors may interact with minor anxieties, attitudes and beliefs about the birth of the child and sociocultural stress to influence maternal mood to a greater degree. The primary treatment is to provide supportive care and to reassure the woman that the feelings that she has are normal and will subside within a few days.

Postnatal depression

Postnatal depression is regarded as any non-psychotic depressive illness of mild to moderate severity usually commencing within 2 weeks of delivery but which may develop at any time in the 1st year following childbirth. For every 1000 live births, 100–150 women will suffer from a depressive illness. This disorder is a serious condition of childbirth and should be distinguished from the brief emotional state called the 'baby blues'. The overall prevalence of postnatal depression is not significantly different from that of depression at other times but there is some evidence of an increased risk of depression occurring in the early postnatal period, being three-fold in the first 5 postnatal weeks (Cox & Holden 2003). A significant number of these women may have developed depression in the antenatal period (Evans et al 2001).

Postnatal depression has an insidious onset, runs a chronic course and is probably the most common complication of the puerperium (Price 2007). Health professionals do not always detect the disorder and usually the women make a complete recovery.

Risk factors

The evidence suggests that risk factors for postnatal depression are no different to the risk factors for non-postnatal depression. Lack of social and psychological support after birth is one of the main reasons that unhappiness after childbirth is such a common problem (Enkin et al 2000). Systematic reviews of sociological and psychological studies have identified factors with a moderate to strong association with postnatal depression (Beck 1996, Hoffbrand et al 2001). These include a past history of psychopathology and psychological disturbances during pregnancy, poor marital relationship, the 'baby blues', social factors such as poor social support and recent life events (Austin et al 2008). Other factors that may also be associated with the risk of postnatal depression include a history of abuse, obstetric complications and social factors such as lower occupational status and low family income (Forman et al 2000). Stillbirth and neonatal or infant death may also affect mental health (Price 2007).

There is no persuasive evidence to support traditional explanations of postnatal depression. No biochemical explanation of women's unhappiness after childbirth has been uncovered, and psychoanalytic explanations cannot be validated empirically (Enkin et al 2000). Researchers agree that the effects of postnatal depression are detrimental and clinical efforts need to be moved towards understanding, recognising and treating antenatal depression.

Screening and early detection

In recent years, health professionals have focused on early recognition and treatment, mainly because it occurs at such a critical time in the lives of the mother and baby and the effect on the woman and her family can be devastating. This can include maternal morbidity, neglect of the child, family breakdown, self-harm and suicide. The more common consequences for children due to maternal mental disorders include emotional and behavioural problems and cognitive delay in the children of depressed mothers (Murray et al 1999, Sinclair & Murray 1998). Overall, psychiatric disorders are known to have caused or contributed to maternal deaths reported in the recent triennium report (Oates 2007). Death by suicide was responsible for around 10% of these deaths.

It is only by close contact with women, observing their behaviour and reactions to events and encouraging them to discuss their feelings and anxieties, that a midwife or doctor may recognise postnatal depression. In the neuroses the individual, although likely to be depressed, remains in touch with reality. Several of the following symptoms may be present:

- Depressed mood, manifesting as either tearfulness or social withdrawal or a change from the usual social functioning. This may include irritability and loss of libido.
- Excessive anxiety about the baby's health and no enjoyment of motherhood.
- Feelings of inadequacy and inability to cope.
- Guilt about their mothering skills and feelings towards their babies.
- Constant tiredness and sleep disturbance, with difficulty in achieving sleep and early morning waking.
- Suicidal thought or fears of harming the baby.

The most commonly used screening tool in the postnatal period is the Edinburgh Postnatal Depression Scale (EPDS). It is a simple and easy-to-use questionnaire and should always be administered by a trained health professional. The EPDS should be used at approximately 6 weeks and 3 months following delivery. There is good evidence for its effectiveness as a screening tool, although diagnosis of postnatal depression does require clinical evaluation (Cox & Holden 2003).

Management

Effective communication between all members of the multidisciplinary team is essential to ensure that the best outcome is possible for the mother and baby within the family unit. Pharmacological and psychosocial therapies are normally used in the management of mental health disorders and this includes postnatal depression. Pharmacological therapies include hormonal and homeopathic therapies and antidepressants, with the additional consideration regarding the use of medication when women are pregnant or breastfeeding. These therapies have been the subject of considerable debate in recent years. The evidence relating to the role of psychosocial interventions in the treatment of postnatal depression focuses mainly on counselling, psychotherapy such as cognitive behavioural approaches in addition to a number of alternative therapies including massage, infant massage and relaxation therapies. In a systematic review of studies, it was concluded that psychosocial interventions do not reduce the numbers of women who develop postpartum depression. However, the provision of intensive, professionally based postpartum support did seem to be a promising intervention (Dennis & Creedy 2004). There is further evidence that women benefit from additional support and counselling, alone or in conjunction with medical therapy (Enkin et al 2000). Women suffering a severe form of depression may need to be referred to a psychiatrist, especially if suicidal.

Puerperal psychosis

Puerperal psychosis is a much less common disorder that affects 1–2 women per 1000 births. In general there is agreement in the literature that this rate represents a significantly increased risk for psychotic illness when compared with other times in a woman's life (Price 2007). The onset is quite often rapid, and typically presents in the early postpartum period, usually within the 1st month. In almost all cases of puerperal psychosis, there is a mood disorder accompanied by features such as loss of contact with reality, hallucinations, severe thought disturbances and abnormal behaviour. A key symptom is insomnia and the woman may also be confused, frightened and distressed and may be disoriented in space and time. Delusions and hallucinations often focus on the delivery or on the baby.

Risk factors

Women with a previous puerperal psychosis are at significant risk of between 25% and 57% of developing a future puerperal psychosis and an even higher risk of developing a non-puerperal relapse (Terp et al 1999). Other risk factors for women developing puerperal psychosis include a pre-existing psychotic illness (especially if it is a severe affective psychosis) and family history of affective psychosis (Schopf & Rust 1994).

Detection and management

Procedures should be put in place to ensure all women are routinely assessed during pregnancy for a history of depression. Psychosocial and biological risk factors for postnatal depression and puerperal psychosis should be routinely and systematically recorded in the antenatal period. During pregnancy, information should be available to women and their partners on the nature of postnatal mood disorders and puerperal psychosis.

Detection of the condition is more readily identified due to the nature of this disorder. Women who are at risk during pregnancy should be referred to a psychiatrist during the pregnancy to ensure early detection and intervention (Cox & Holden 2003). Women who require psychiatric admission following childbirth should ideally be admitted to a specialist mother and baby unit, together with their baby (Oates 2007). Any

decision taken should involve a multidisciplinary assessment, including social workers and family members. In areas where this service is not available, a transfer should be considered if the presence of the baby might hasten the mother's recovery. This should equally apply to mothers with severe postnatal depression and puerperal psychosis and those with a schizophrenic illness exacerbated by the impact of a new baby (SIGN 2002). In general, there are concerns that admission of mothers with their babies to general psychiatric wards may not adequately ensure the safety and security of the baby and the provision of mother and baby units is recommended (Oates 2007). Further research is required to review the effectiveness of mother and baby units in relation to the care of women and their families.

There is limited evidence for the effectiveness of treatment and management specifically for puerperal psychosis. As the nature of puerperal psychosis is essentially affective, treatments used for affective psychoses in general are also appropriate for puerperal psychosis. Such treatments would typically involve one or more drugs from the antidepressant, mood-stabilising or neuroleptic groups. Additional considerations regarding the use of drug treatments will be required for women in pregnancy and when breastfeeding. Prognosis is good; most women recover within 6 months. However, there may be a relapse in a subsequent pregnancy (Austin et al 2008).

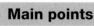

Main points

- The puerperium is the 6–8-week period after childbirth during which time the maternal physiological changes resolve and return to the non-pregnant state. Women also adapt psychologically and emotionally to motherhood.

- After delivery, the subsequent removal of the placental hormones initiates the return of the body systems to the pre-pregnant state. Involution is the main change in the pelvic organs during the puerperium. The process is brought about by ischaemia, autolysis and phagocytosis. Decidua is shed and there is regeneration of the endometrium.

- Fundal height decreases at a rate of approximately 1 cm/day. Slow involution may be associated with retained products or an associated infection. Vaginal loss is termed as lochia. Infection may be present if lochia are offensive and the woman has a pyrexia. The cervix returns to its original form within a few days.

- Following the withdrawal of oestrogen, diuresis occurs and the plasma volume and haematocrit rapidly return to normal. The reduction in circulating progesterone leads to removal of excess tissue fluid and normal

vascular tone returns. Cardiac output returns to non-pregnant levels.

- Delivery of the baby removes any compression on the lungs during pregnancy and ventilation returns to normal. Oxygen requirements return to normal as do carbon dioxide levels.

- A loss of bladder tone and bruising of the urethra may lead to difficulty in micturition. Retention of urine may occur. Constipation may persist as a problem.

- The main maternal puerperal complications include postpartum haemorrhage, thromboembolic disorders, puerperal infections and mental health disorders.

- Women are susceptible to invasion by pathogenic organisms in the puerperium. Puerperal pyrexia always merits medical investigation. Infection of surgical incisions is a significant cause of maternal morbidity.

- Bacteriological specimens for culture should be obtained if infection is present. In moderate to severe infections, the woman should commence antibiotics while awaiting results.

- Commensal organisms normally present in the body can invade susceptible sites and cause infection. The β-haemolytic *Streptococcus pyogenes*, Lancefield group A, is the most common organism responsible for serious and life-threatening obstetric infections.

- Predisposing factors for postpartum endometritis include prolonged labour, prolonged rupture of the membranes, multiple vaginal examinations, manual removal of placenta and traumatic delivery.

- Urinary tract infections are common during the puerperium and recurrent urinary tract infections should be further investigated for urinary tract abnormality.

- Childbearing is associated with three 'affective disorders': the 'baby blues', postnatal depression and puerperal psychosis. The 'baby blues' is a normal emotional reaction to childbirth experienced by over 50% of women. The elated emotions surrounding the birth are replaced with tearfulness, irritability, fatigue and inability to concentrate. It lasts from day 3 until the end of the 1st week after birth.

- Postnatal depression is a non-psychotic illness occurring within the 1st year of childbirth in 10–15% of women. Symptoms include depressed mood, excessive anxiety, sleep disturbances, feelings of inadequacy and guilt. The disorder responds well to counselling, cognitive therapy and antidepressant drugs. Recovery is usually complete.

- The incidence of puerperal psychosis is 2:1000 births and presents within the 1st month after birth. There is a mood disorder accompanied by feelings such as loss of contact with reality, delusions and hallucinations, and abnormal behaviour. Admission to a psychiatric mother and baby unit is usually recommended. Most women recover within 6 months.

References

Amezaga, M.R., McKenzie, H., 2006. Molecular epidemiology of macrolide resistance in beta-haemolytic streptococcus of Lancefield groups A, B & C and evidence for a new mef element in group G streptococci. J. Antimicrob. Chemother. 57 (3), 443–449.

Austin, M.P., Priest, S.R., Sullivan, E.A., 2008. Antenatal psychosocial assessment for reducing perinatal mental health morbidity. Cochrane Database Syst. Rev. 2008 (4) Art. No.: CD005124. DOI: 10.1002/14651858.CD005124.

Beck, C.T., 1996. A meta-analysis of predictors of postpartum depression. Nur. Res. 45, 297–303.

Blackburn, S.T., 2007. Maternal, Fetal and Neonatal Physiology: A Clinical Perspective, fourth edn. Elsevier Saunders, St Louis, Missouri.

Campbell-Brown, M., Hytten, F., 1998. Carbohydrate metabolism. In: Chamberlain, G., Broughton Pipkin, F. (Eds.), Clinical Physiology in Obstetrics, third edn. Blackwell Science, Oxford.

Coad, J., Dunstall, M., 2005. Anatomy and Physiology for Midwives, second edn. Elsevier Churchill Livingston, London.

Coughlan, A., 1996. Animal antibiotics threaten hospital antibiotics. New Scientist 27, 7.

Cox, J., Holden, J. (Eds.), 2003. Perinatal Mental Health: A Guide to the Edinburgh Postnatal Depression Scale. Royal College of Psychiatrists, London.

Dennis, C.L., Creedy, D.K., 2004. Psychosocial and psychological interventions for preventing postpartum depression. Cochrane Database Syst. Rev. 2004 (4) Art. No.: CD001134. DOI: 10.1002/14651858.CD001134.pub2.

de Swiet, M., 1998. The cardiovascular system. In: Chamberlain, G., Broughton Pipkin, F., (Eds) Clinical Physiology in Obstetrics, third edn. Blackwell Sciences, Oxford.

Edmonds, D.K., 2007. Puerperium and lactation. In: Edmonds, D.K. (Eds.), Dewhurst's Textbook of Obstetrics, seventh edn. Blackwell Science, Oxford.

Enkin, M., Keirse, M.J.N.C., Neilson, J., et al., 2000. A Guide to Effective Care in Pregnancy, third edn. Oxford University Press, Oxford.

Evans, J., Heron, J., Francomb, H., et al., 2001. Cohort study of depressed mood during pregnancy and after childbirth. Br. Med. J. 323, 257–260.

Forman, D.N., Videbech, P., Hedegaard, M.D., 2000. Postpartum depression: identification of women at risk. Br. J. Obste. Gynaecol. 107, 1210–1217.

Hoffbrand, S., Howard, L., Crawley, H., 2001. Antidepressant treatment for post-natal depression. Cochrane Database Syst. Rev. (2) Update Software 2003, Oxford.

Howie, P.W., 1995. The puerperium and its complications. In: Whitfield, E.R. (Eds.), Dewhurst's Textbook for Obstetrics and Gynaecology for Postgraduates, fifth edn. Blackwell Science, London.

Jessel, D., Moir, A., 1997. A Mind to Crime, second edn. Signet, London.

Lewis, G. (Ed.), 2007. Saving Mothers Lives: The Seventh Report of the Confidential Enquiries into Maternal and Child Health Report. RCOG, London.

Marchant, S., Alexander, J., Garcia, J., et al., 1999. A survey of women's experience of vaginal loss from 24 hours to three months after childbirth (the BliPP study). Midwifery 15 (2), 72–81.

Marchant, S., Alexander, J., Garcia, J., 2003. How does it feel to you? Uterine palpation and lochial loss as guides to postnatal 'recovery'. In: Wickham, S. (Ed.), Best Midwifery Practice. Elsevier, London.

Murray, L., Sinclair, D., Cooper, P., et al., 1999. The socioemotional development of 5-year olds with postnatally depressed mothers. J. Child Psychol. Psychiatry 40, 1259–1271.

NICE (National Institute for Health and Clinical Excellence), 2007. Antenatal and Postnatal Mental Health. RCOG, London.

NMC (Nursing and Midwifery Council), 2004. Midwives Rules and Standards. NMC, London.

Oates, M., 2007. Deaths from psychiatric causes. In: Lewis, G. (Ed.), Saving Mothers Lives: The Sixth Report of the

Confidential Enquiries into Maternal and Child Health Report. RCOG, London.

Price, S.A., 2007. Mental Health in Pregnancy and Childbirth. Churchill Livingstone, Edinburgh.

Schopf, J., Rust, B., 1994. Follow-up and family study of postpartum psychoses. Part 1: overview. Eur. Arch. Psychiatry Clin. Neurosci. 244, 101–111.

Sherman, D., Lurie, S., Frenkle, E., et al., 1999. Characteristics of normal lochia. Am. J. Perinatol. 16 (8), 399–402.

SIGN (Scottish Intercollegiate Guidelines Network), 2002. Postnatal Depression and Puerperal Psychosis: A National Clinical Guideline. Royal College of Physicians, Edinburgh.

Sinclair, D., Murray, L., 1998. Effects of postnatal depression on children's adjustment to school. Br. J. Psychiatry 172, 58–63.

Terp, I.M., Engholm, G., Moller, H., et al., 1999. A follow-up study of postpartum psychoses: prognosis and risk factors for readmission. Acta Psychiatr. Scand. 100 (1), 40–46.

Walsh, L.V., 2001. Midwifery: Community-Based Care During the Childbearing Year. W B Saunders, Philadelphia.

Annotated recommended reading

Lewis, G. (Eds.), 2007. Why Mothers Die 2003–2005: The Seventh Report of the Confidential Enquiries into Maternal and Child Health in the United Kingdom. RCOG Press, London.

This report provides interesting and informative reading for all health professionals involved in the care of women during and following childbirth. Every case is described in detail and the reader will gain valuable and constructive information from a professional perspective.

Chapter Fifty-Seven

57

Biobehavioural aspects of parenting

Introduction

Besides being responsible for body movements, the brain is the source of a complex set of functions concerning behaviour known as **the mind**. This includes thoughts and language, personality, memories, feelings, emotions and the state known as consciousness. The field is enormous and not well understood. This chapter has been updated to include current research to introduce salient topics on maternal–infant behaviour.

Approaches to the study of behaviour

For thousands of years the brain and mind were viewed as separate entities. Whilst scientists studied the brain, the mind was the realm of philosophers. In the 19th century scientists realised that sensations such as sight were the result of nerve impulses and experiments were devised to explore them. Wilhelm Wundt opened the first psychology laboratory at the University of Leipzig in 1879. Since then other disciplines have been developed to study behaviour, such as:

- **Ethology**: the study of natural behaviour.
- **Cognitive psychology**: the way people process information.
- **Physiological psychology**: the physical brain and its processes.
- **Behaviourism**: observed behaviour (made famous by Pavlov).
- **Psychoanalysis**: how psychological history explains current behaviour.
- **Evolutionary psychology**: the development of species-specific behaviour.

Now, modern techniques are being used to explore the brain. These include **magnetic resonance imaging (MRI)**, **computerised axial tomography (CAT)**, **positron emission tomography (PET)** and **magnetoencephalography (MEG)**. MEG detects the electrical activity in the brain and can spot the site of the activity. The scans cannot tell what a person is thinking but can tell where it is taking place, suggesting the brain consists of functional **modules** or **domains** such as the **Broca's** and **Wernicke's language centres** on the left side of the brain (Smail 2008).

Philosophical roots

The Greek philosopher Hippocrates (460–377 BC) believed that the mind was in the brain and controlled the body. Beginning with Descartes in the 17th century, **dualists** considered the mind and body to be separate. The body was constructed from matter but the mind was not. The soul was located in the brain and controlled the body. Later philosophers, including John Locke (1632–1704), argued that Hippocrates was correct. If the mind can interact with the body then it must be physical, i.e. the mind is a product of the brain. The sense organs send messages to the brain so that the mind can direct the body towards appropriate action. This belief underlies the theory of **monism** (Dennett 1992). There is still no agreement as to whether monists or dualists are correct but most people studying the mind today relate to other sciences such as physics and cannot explain a disembodied mind and therefore are monists.

Smail (2008) says that 'many of the things that we do are shaped by behavioural dispositions, moods, emotions and feelings that have a deep evolutionary history'. These body states have been shown to be physiological in nature, located in specific parts of the brain. They are associated with a range of neurotransmitters and hormones such as testosterone, oestrogen, serotonin, dopamine, endorphins, oxytocin, prolactin, vasopressin, epinephrine and others. These chemicals help to determine how we feel; the role of oxytocin in maternal–infant attachment is discussed later in the chapter. Smail suggests this is firm evidence that the brain generates the mind and that dualism is incorrect.

Meanings and applications

There are two anxieties about psychosocial research findings. First, they may be affected by the biases and beliefs of the researchers' norms (Davis-Floyd & Mather 2002). Secondly, political leaders may use the theories for their own purposes. Hrdy (1999) discusses 'the politics of motherhood', in particular the mother's role in child development. The dichotomy is whether mothers stay at home or go out to work. Governments change their views when women workers are needed. Smail (2008) suggests that, although there are many cultural differences in behaviour, culture is superimposed on biology and there are universal behavioural norms such as parenting.

For example, human societies exhibit multiple ways of thinking which may affect the provision of health care. Davis-Floyd & Mather (2002) describe three paradigms

of health care which influence modern maternity care: the technocratic, humanistic and holistic models.

- The **technocratic model** is dualistic, separating body from mind. The body is an unpredictable machine, likely to need manipulation by machinery and techniques to ensure health: e.g. to ensure that birth is successful. The mind is not the concern of technocratic medicine.
- The **humanistic model** is a monistic approach that recognises the influence of the mind on the body and advocates care that considers both. Partnership between client and carer is essential.
- The **holistic model** stems from Eastern philosophy and arose out of dissatisfaction with Western concepts of health and disease. Body and mind are fully integrated, involving the spirit or soul.

Davis-Floyd & Mather (2002) visualise combining aspects from each model to provide the best care possible. There is evidence that the mind plays an important role in the physical state of the body but more evidence is needed.

The evolution of babies

Human babies are born with some physical and mental attributes. Unlike some species, even other primates such as monkeys and apes, they are particularly helpless and their behaviour mainly consists of sleeping, eating, defecating and seeking comfort. They are **altricial**, rather than those newborns that can run about almost immediately such as deer and most herd animals which are **precocial**. However, humans are secondarily altricial and our ancestors were probably more precocial. Our newborns should probably stay in utero for at least 12 months rather than the 9 months of gestation. There are at least three reasons for this evolutionary pathway (Small 1999):

1. The increase in brain size has provoked early birth and flexibility of skull shape in the development of sutures and fontanelles.

2. Bipedalism has altered the shape of the human pelvis and increased the difficulty of the baby negotiating the birth canal.

3. Human babies are relatively large related to maternal size and their placentae are unable to sustain them in utero for more than the 9 months.

Maternal–child interaction

Instinctive behaviour

Bowlby (1984) wrote:

Behaviour of even the simplest animals is enormously complex. It varies in systematic ways from members of one species to another and in less systematic ways from individual to individual within a species... Yet there are many regularities of behaviour that are so striking and play so important a part in the survival of individual and species that they have earned the name instinctive.

He described four main characteristics of instinctive behaviour:

1. It follows a recognisably similar and predictive pattern in most members of a species.

2. It is not a simple response to a stimulus but a sequence of behaviour that runs a predictable course.

3. Some of its usual consequences are of obvious value in contributing to the preservation of an individual or continuity of a species.

4. Many examples of it develop even when the ordinary opportunities for learning are absent.

In the past there was argument over which behaviours were **innate** (inborn, genetic, natural) and which were **acquired** (learned, environmental, nurtured) but this is a meaningless division. Every biological characteristic, physiological or behavioural, is a product of **gene–environment interaction** (Barrett et al 2002). If a biological characteristic is little influenced by environmental variations it is called environmentally stable and any characteristic that is much influenced by the environment is environmentally labile. Instinctive behaviour is environmentally stable (Hinde 1959).

Some believe that the variability of human behaviour proves that it is culturally driven and nothing is instinctive but Bowlby (1984) disagreed. In higher species instinctive behaviour is not stereotyped but follows a recognisable pattern (characteristic 1) and runs a predictable course (characteristic 2). Mating, child care and the attachment of the young to their parents have survival value for both individual and species (characteristic 3). Despite the immense variety of cultural norms, some behaviours repeatedly emerge (characteristic 4).

Bowlby believed that behavioural attributes contribute to survival and reproduction when they operate within a prescribed environment. Environmentally stable behaviours are controlled by elements he called 'environments of adaptedness': for instance, the range of environmental temperatures the body can tolerate or the altitude at which the cardiovascular system can function.

The human environment of evolutionary adaptedness

Human capacity for innovation has enabled survival in a wide range of environments, called by some the **human environment of evolutionary adaptedness** (Barrett et al 2002, Irons 1998). Also, humans have manufactured safe environments, leading to an incredible increase in world population. In the last 15 000 years a rise in pastoralism and agriculture led to the growth of cities. Unfortunately this led to an increased risk of infection and pollution.

The mother's social surroundings are part of the environment in which childbearing and childrearing take place. The relationship between the sexes is also important as the basis of sexual difference lies in the investment in the gametes. Women produce fewer, larger ova compared to the millions of tiny sperm. Women also provide energy to the fetus in utero and supply milk during infancy (Hrdy 1999). Male parenting is necessary for the support of women and their children during the long human growth to maturity (Small 2002). However, there is no consensus on the biological nature of the human family and it is risky to define evolutionary behaviour in terms of modern hunter–gatherers.

Human childbearing behaviour

Five aspects about childbearing behaviour are discussed below. They are:

- Bonding.
- Tactile behaviour.
- Crying.
- The senses.
- Lateral preferences.

Bonding

The development of theories over time and how they link with culture is interesting. The study of ethology began with Tinbergen and Lorenz in the 1950s. Lorenz believed that if attachment behaviour did not occur within the critical period the opportunity was lost. Hinde (1982) was less restrictive and described **a sensitive period** as 'a given event that can be produced more readily during a certain period than earlier or later'.

Klaus & Kennel (1976)

Klaus & Kennel (1976) developed the concept of a sensitive period or **imprinting** lasting for a few minutes or hours after birth in which **maternal–infant bonding** or **attachment** (and paternal) is ensured. Attachment was defined as 'a unique relationship between two people that is specific and endures through time'. The presence of species-specific behaviour is important to Klaus & Kennel's theory. They were concerned about the effects of separating mothers and their babies for long periods. Rooming-in developed from their research. They believed that a strong mother–infant bond was the basis on which the infant's future attachments are formed and through which he develops a sense of self. If the early opportunity is missed attachment is difficult, but can still develop because it is an ongoing learning process. Therefore adoptive parents can usually form relationships with their children.

John Bowlby (1984)

Bowlby (1984) believed that the immature newborn human infant develops attachment behaviour more slowly than other species do. He did not believe in a sensitive period but did use the term imprinting, suggesting that the infant's focusing on a single figure, although slow to develop, is sufficiently like those of other mammalian species. Maternal involvement in ensuring that infants remain close to them depends on their relative helplessness.

Bowlby talks of 'an evolutionary shift in balance' from the infant taking all the responsibility for keeping contact to total maternal responsibility in humans because of infant immaturity. He suggested that infant attachment behaviour develops over the first 6 months in phases, from response to stimuli to full reciprocal behaviour, in response to parental behaviour. Parental behaviour may depend on a sensitive period and, if this is disrupted, infant attachment behaviour may not develop normally.

He wrote, 'Almost from the first, many children have more than one person towards whom they can direct attachment behaviour'. The young infant is given opportunities to form attachments to other family members, particularly the father. The mother does not usually have to accept total responsibility for child rearing. However, a child constantly surrounded by a succession of stranger-carers may become withdrawn.

Wenda Trevathen (1987)

Trevathen (1987) observed maternal and neonatal behaviour during the first hour after delivery. She believes that there is a **sensitive period** in the first hour which varies markedly across time and between cultures. This cultural variability superimposed on a biological process is emphasized by Small (1998). Trevathen wrote, 'Although the process may not always be perfect, behaviours of mammalian females have been **selected** to complement the needs and capabilities of their young'.

The neonate is **secondarily altricial**, requiring a period of **exterogestation** (gestation outside the uterus) with prolongation of infancy. This is a trade-off between pelvic size and shape and the size of the neonatal brain. The human gestation period should probably be over 12 months compared to other mammals. Human infants, born after only 9 months, do not achieve equality of developmental status with other primates until they are 6 months old. Unlike a **primarily altricial** baby whose eyes are closed at birth, human babies have their eyes open

and can use them to interpret the environment. Bowlby's observation that attachment behaviour equivalent to a newborn gorilla does not occur until about 6 months may support the above theory of shortened gestation length.

However, Trevathen concludes that there is scant evidence that contact between mothers and their babies in the immediate postpartum period is necessary for bond formation. The observed behaviours may be 'relics from the past and have no significant function'.

The role of oxytocin in bonding

Bonding theory has been criticised by stating that early studies lacked scientific methodology and have been difficult to replicate. Lamb (1983) believed it unlikely that a species as dependent on social learning as humans would exhibit such narrow behaviour as sensitive periods. However, events during the first few hours after birth are important.

Modern studies of **oxytocin** are interesting for those caring for mothers and babies. The hormone's role in labour and breastfeeding is discussed in other chapters. In animals oxytocin is called the 'hormone of love and bonding' and it seems it plays a similar role in humans. Oxytocin is released into the brain in response to social contact, especially in skin-to-skin contact (Palmer 2002). Feldman et al (2007) found that social affiliation is linked with changes in serum oxytocin levels. Increased levels were related to 'maternal holding behaviours, gaze, vocalisations, positive affect and affectionate touch as well as attachment-related thoughts and frequent checking of the infant'.

Tactile behaviour

Attendants present at normal births report specific **maternal tactile** behaviour when they are given their infants to handle. Rubin (1963) noted an orderly progression of behaviour. Mothers appeared to take about 3 days to complete their sequence but they had limited access to their babies without clothing. Klaus et al (1970) saw the same behavioural sequence occurring within minutes if mothers were given their naked babies to hold. The others began with finger-tip touching of their baby's extremities. Within 4–8 min they began to massage, stroke and place the palms of their hands around the baby's trunk.

Trevathen (1987) observed 66 women for the first 10 min of contact to examine tactile interactions as a possible species-specific behaviour. Tactile behaviours were observed in all women but varied widely between women. Trevathen sought **endogenous** (from within) and **exogenous** (environmental) factors that might create the differences. She analysed the behaviour in 'Hispanic' and 'Anglo' mothers and in primiparous and multiparous women. Anglo mothers spent less time holding their babies and changed state more often than Hispanic women. Primiparous women spent more time not touching their infants than multiparous women but slightly longer exploring their babies. Trevathen decided that there is a species-specific pattern of tactile interaction. Mothers cradled their baby for the first few minutes after birth with occasional palmar massage. Finger exploration of face, hands and extremities followed soon after.

Kontos (1978) found that when mothers were allowed an hour of skin-to-skin contact following birth they demonstrated more **holding, encompassing** and *en face* behaviour. Their infants cried less and smiled more than those of mothers who were separated from their infants in the first hour. Mothers who hold their infant close provide warmth, stimulation, eye contact and a chance to talk to the infant in a typical high-pitched voice (Kuhl et al 1997).

Crying

According to Brazelton (1961), an American paediatrician who is still writing books, babies have **six states of consciousness**: quiet sleep, active sleep, quiet alert, active alert, crying and drowsiness. **Crying** is an early and very compelling infant signal. The ability to cry has been part of human baby's behaviour for thousands of years as a signal to obtain adult attention and motivate action to relieve distress. The same vocal signals have been found in Rhesus monkeys on separation from their mother. Primate babies shriek when something frightens them (Small 1998). Crying occurs when a baby is hungry, uncomfortable or lonely (Klaus & Klaus 1999).

In the consciousness scale, crying is the highest state of arousal. If a baby is left in contact with his mother for the first hour he remains in the quiet alert state longer and cries less, sometimes hardly at all. In Western societies mothers most often link crying to hunger and may change from breastfeeding to bottle-feeding if a baby cries a lot saying 'he is not getting enough from me'. But in other cultures, where babies are carried most of the time and sleep with adults, babies cry much less often.

Harlow (1965) demonstrated that an unhappy monkey infant will choose comfort rather than food. If parents ignore crying they are not keeping their end of the biological bargain which is to relieve distress and keep the baby safe. If parents feel manipulated by crying they are correct because that is its function.

Babies may stop crying if they are quickly picked up rather than left to cry, soothed and put to the shoulder but it takes detective work for parents to understand why the baby is crying. Infants cannot soothe themselves as they release stress hormones when they cry. If a baby is treated in this way when he cries he will soon learn that his parent is there and will care for him so he can relax.

The problem of colic

Small (1998) defines **colic** in Western minds as 'a pathological reaction of infants to some internal distress that causes them to cry excessively and uncontrollably'. Parents believe that their baby has a physiological problem such as wind or inappropriate feeding causing abdominal pain. Very few babies are milk-intolerant and changing the formula only helps parents feel they are doing something to help. This label is applied to 10–20% of Western babies over the early months and mainly in the evenings. Clinically the diagnosis is applied if the **Wessel rule of three** is present: the crying lasts more than 3 h, over more than 3 days and carries on for more than 3 weeks.

Research has shown that many so-called colicky babies do not cry more frequently than babies whose parents consider them normal. When parents are inexperienced or isolated from family they may be unsure of what to expect. Crying of this intensity may be the upper end of normal (Soltis 2004).

Once a baby has been examined and found to have nothing wrong, parents can be reassured that time will bring the behaviour to an end. Crying follows a definite curve, increasing around 6–8 weeks and then decreasing. It may be a mismatch between what babies ask for and what they receive. It appears that care-taking is the initial cause and the most effective strategy for relief from excessive crying.

The senses

Although the **motor state** of the newborn is rudimentary, neonates have **vision, hearing** and **olfaction** and seem to be capable of differentiating stimuli. Studying neonatal sensory processes relies on using a stimulus to elicit a reflex response. One of the best responses is high-amplitude sucking when infants are presented with visual and auditory stimuli (Siqueland & Delucia 1969). Other methods of study include electrical measurement of brain activity and observation of response to stimuli such as head turning.

Babies left on their mother's abdomen for an hour after birth retain their body temperature (Christensson et al 1992), crawl up the abdomen and find a nipple (Klaus & Klaus 1999) and begin to suckle unaided. They may use their sense of smell (Varendi et al 1994) and sight, as well as the stepping reflex to achieve this.

Vision

Newborn babies do not focus very well and **visual acuity** (what detail can be resolved) is about 20–30 times lower than in the adult. Infants focus best at 30–50 cm (Slater & Findlay 1975), which is approximately the distance between them and the adult face when cradled in adult arms (*en face* position). Infants prefer to look at moving objects and follow them with their eyes and head (Brazelton et al 1966). They prefer three-dimensional objects over two-dimensional, high-contrast to low-contrast patterns, curved contours rather than straight contours and novel objects to familiar ones (Fantz & Miranda 1975).

The *en face* position is part of attachment behaviour between mothers, fathers and their infants. It is the distance that a mother holds her baby when she is breastfeeding, a time for optimal contact between them (Fig. 57.1). Trevathen (1987) found that all her mothers spent time in the first hour looking at their infants *en face*.

Neonates recognise their mother's face from very early in life and will suck faster to see an image of their mother preferentially as early as 4h after delivery. Imitation of facial expressions (Kaitz et al 1987) suggests that the newborn recognises expressions such as sticking out the tongue or open mouth expressions and can copy them.

Hearing

Neonates orient to sound by turning their heads. They show interest in human speech and suck more vigorously in response to their mother's voice as early as

3 days after birth (DeCasper & Fifer 1980). Women and men speak to babies in a high-pitched voice (Lang 1972). The neonatal auditory system responds more readily to higher frequencies of the human voice.

Speech is not one-sided. **Entrainment** is the rhythmic movement made by a baby in response to maternal or any other human speech. Condon & Sander (1974) demonstrated this interactional synchrony as early as 12h after birth. Besides altering the pitch of their voice, adults tend to use repetitive, simplistic language when talking to infants. The baby moves its body and limbs in synchrony with the mother's voice and she responds by continuing to talk, thus prolonging the synchrony.

Olfaction

Babies recognise and distinguish different smells. They may use the smell and taste of amniotic fluid and its similarity to the smell of the oil produced around the areola to locate the nipple (Schaal et al 1995, Varendi et al 1994). Macfarlane demonstrated that young babies turn towards breast pads worn by their mothers rather than those worn by other lactating mothers.

Fleming et al (1995) confirmed that mothers quickly learned to recognise their baby's odour on a T-shirt, especially if there had been an early opportunity for mothers to hold and feed their babies. Vernix provides a source for bacterial colonisation and odour production. This recognition by odour may be important for bonding and it also happens between partners.

Lateral preferences

Maternal holding preference

Salk (1961) discovered that women prefer to hold their babies on the left side of their bodies irrespective of handedness. This has been confirmed by many studies over the last 40 years. Various hypotheses have been put forward to explain the preference, all derived from a belief that **the baby elicits the behaviour**. Salk thought that when the baby is held on the left maternal heart beat sounds soothed it. Ginsburg et al (1979) found that mothers' holding preference was related to their baby's head turning preference; infants who preferred to turn their head to the right (more than 80%) were carried on the left side and vice versa.

Mothers carrying the baby on the left may be monitoring their infant's emotions with the right side of their brain (Hope 2002, Manning & Chamberlain 1991). However, Donnot & Vauclair (2007) in a study of 202 mothers and babies found that holding on the left was supported, there was a perceptual bias in the mothers between the right brain hemisphere and the left side of the body but no significant associations between

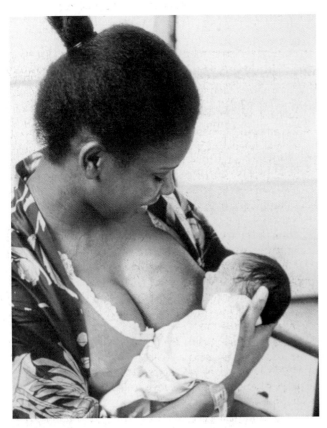

Figure 57.1 • Eye contact during breastfeeding. (From Kelnar C, Harvey D, Simpson C 1995, with permission.)

holding biases and hemispheric specialisation in emotional monitoring. The reason for the behaviour is still not understood.

Neonatal head-turning preference

More than 80% of newborn babies prefer to turn their heads to the right when lying supine (Turkewitz et al 1965). This may be linked to eventual handedness developing out of continued attention to the hand most often in their visual field (Michel 1981). Cornwell et al (1985) found that this right side preference had disappeared by 3 months.

Implications for practice

Attachment theory

If the sensitive period is present in humans, how should midwives interpret the first hour after birth? All mothers should have the opportunity to be with their new babies during this hour. Absence may adversely affect the way that mothers perceive the birth. Although maternal–infant attachment may not suffer, the mother may find the birth less fulfilling. Klaus & Klaus (1999) are adamant that at least 1 h should be set aside for mother and child interaction.

Lateral holding preferences

Mothers often report more difficulty feeding their babies on one breast than the other (Stables & Hewitt 1995). The problem often arises when the woman is right-handed, prefers to carry her baby on the left and the baby turns its head to the right. This makes the left breast much easier to feed from as the woman holds her baby on her preferred left arm, the baby is turning his head to the right and the mother has her dominant right hand to offer the nipple to her baby. When the mother attempts to feed from her right breast she is uncomfortable with the baby on her right arm, he turns his head away from the breast and she has her weaker left hand to manipulate the nipple. Unfortunately, this group included most mothers!

Although mothers and babies adapted after a few feeds, some women gave up feeding because of the initial difficulty. Midwives can use their skills by varying the way the mother holds her baby to ensure that early feeding is successful. The following position can be tried: the baby is tucked under the right arm with his head cradled on her left hand; he can then suckle with his head turned to the preferred right side and the mother can use her free right hand to offer him the nipple. This is not a new strategy. Midwives have used it for decades, but may not have known why it was successful. That is the value of research-based practice.

Main points

- There is still no agreement as to whether those who think the mind is separate from the brain (dualists) or is generated by the brain (monists) are correct. Psychosocial research findings may be affected by the biases and beliefs of the researchers' societal norms.
- Biological characters are products of the interaction between genes and the environment. A characteristic little influenced by environmental variations is environmentally stable and one much influenced by environment is environmentally labile.
- Humans manufacture safe environments within which environmentally stable components of behaviour are found. The social surroundings of the woman are part of the environment in which childbearing and child rearing take place.
- Some believe that pair bonding is part of human ethology. Male parenting is necessary for the support of a woman and her children during the long human childhood. There is no consensus of the family in biological terms and it is risky to define evolutionary behaviour in terms of modern hunter–gatherers.
- Klaus & Kennel developed the concept of a species-specific sensitive period shortly after birth in

- which maternal–infant attachment is ensured. Bowlby believes attachment in humans is slow to develop.
- Trevathen describes the human infant as secondarily altricial, needing a period of exterogestation to complete maturation. The neonate is immature and does not achieve developmental status with other primates until 6 months of age. This is a trade-off between pelvic size and shape and the large neonatal brain.
- There is little evidence that early contact between mothers and babies is necessary for bond formation but when mothers are allowed skin-to-skin contact following birth they demonstrated more holding, encompassing and *en face* behaviours.
- Most infants will form a bond with other family members, particularly the father.
- When first given their infant to handle, mothers began with fingertip touching of their baby's extremities. Within 4–8 min they began to massage, stroke and place the palms of their hands around the baby's trunk.
- Babies have functioning vision, hearing and olfaction and seem capable of differentiating stimuli. A good

stimulus for eliciting neonatal responses is high-amplitude sucking.

- Babies left to lie on their mother's abdomen for an hour retain their body temperature, crawl up the abdomen, find a nipple and begin to suckle unaided. They may use their senses of smell and sight as well as the stepping reflex to achieve this.
- Although the newborn cannot focus well he prefers to look at moving objects in three dimensions with high-contrast colour and curved contours. Novel objects are more interesting than familiar ones. When held in the *en face* position, neonates recognise their mother's face and can imitate facial expressions.
- Women speak to babies in a high-pitched voice and the neonatal auditory system responds more readily to high frequencies. Babies move their limbs and bodies in synchrony with the mother's voice.
- Babies recognise and distinguish different smells and may use their sense of smell to locate the nipple. Mothers recognise their baby's odour, especially if they have had an early opportunity to hold and feed their babies.
- Women prefer to hold their babies on the left side of their bodies irrespective of handedness. Various hypotheses have been developed to explain this, all derived from a belief that the baby elicits the behaviour.
- Over 80% of babies prefer to turn their heads to the right when lying supine. This preference disappears by 3 months.
- Mothers report more difficulty feeding their babies on one breast than the other. Usually it is the right breast which is seen as difficult in right-handed mothers whose babies have right head-turning preferences. This is the majority of mothers. The problem is soon resolved but some mothers give up feeding because of the initial difficulty.
- Midwives can vary the way the baby is put to the breast by tucking him under the right arm with his head resting in the left hand and turned to the right. This leaves the dominant right hand free to help the baby feed.

References

Barrett, L., Dunbar, R., Lycett, J., 2002. Human Evolutionary Psychology. Princeton University Press, Princeton, New Jersey.

Bowlby, J., 1984. Attachment and Loss. Vol. 1: Attachment. Penguin books, Harmondsworth.

Brazelton, T.B., 1961. Psychophysiologic reactions in the neonate: the value of observation of the neonate. J. Pediatr. 58, 508–512.

Brazelton, T.B., Scholl, M.L., Robey, J.S., 1966. Visual responses in the newborn. Pediatrics 37, 284–290.

Christensson, K., Siles, C., Moreno, L., et al., 1992. Temperature, metabolic adaptation and crying in healthy, full term babies cared for skin-to-skin or in a cot. Acta Paediatr. 81, 488–493.

Condon, W.S., Sander, L.W., 1974. Neonate movement is synchronised with adult speech: interactional participation and language acquisition. Science 183, 99–101.

Cornwell, K.S., Barnes, C.L., Fitzgerald, H.E., Harris, L.J., 1985. Neurobehavioural reorganisation in early infancy: patterns of head orientation following lateral and midline holds. Infant Ment. Health J. 6 (3), 126–136.

Davis-Floyd, R., Mather, F.S., 2002. The technocratic, humanistic and holistic paradigms of childbirth. MIDIRS Midwifery Dig. 4 (12), 500–506.

DeCasper, A.J., Fifer, W.P., 1980. Of human bonding: newborns prefer their mothers' voices. Science 208, 1174–1176.

Dennelt, D. C., 1992. Consciousness explained. Lippincott, Williams and Wilkins.

Donnot, J., Vauclair, J., 2007. Infant holding preferences in maternity hospitals: testing the hypothesis of the lateralised perception of emotions. Dev. Neuropsychol. 32 (3), 881–890.

Fantz, R.L., Miranda, S., 1975. Newborn infant attention to formed content. Child Dev. 46, 224–228.

Feldman, R., Weller, A., Zagoory-Sharon, O., Levine, A., 2007. Evidence for a neuroendocrinological foundation of human affiliation: plasma oxytocin levels across pregnancy and the postpartum period predict mother–infant bonding. Psychol. Sci. 18 (11), 965–970.

Fleming, A., Corter, C., Surbey, M., Franks, P., Steiner, M., 1995. Postpartum factors related to mothers' recognition of newborn infant odours. J. Reprod. Infant Psychol. 13 (3–4), 197–210.

Ginsburg, H.J., Fling, S., Hope, M.L., Musgrove, D., Andrews, C., 1979. Maternal holding preferences: a consequence of newborn head turning behaviour. Child Dev. 50, 280–281.

Harlow, H.F., Harlow, M.K., 1965. The affectional systems. In: Schrier, A.M., Harlow, H.F., Stollnitz, F. (Eds.), Behaviour of Nonhuman Primates. Academic Press, New York, pp. 287–334.

Hinde, R.A., 1959. Some recent trends in ethology. In: Koch, S. (Ed.), Psychology: A Study of a Science. McGraw-Hill, New York.

Hinde, R.A., 1982. Ethology. Fontana, London.

Hope, J., 2002. Why women cradle babies on their left. Daily Mail Saturday September 7, p. 41.

Hrdy, S.B., 1999. Mother Nature. Pantheon, London.

Irons, W., 1998. Adaptively relevant environments versus the environment of evolutionary adaptedness. Evol. Anthropol. 6, 194–204.

Kaitz, M., Good, A., Rokem, A.M., Eidelman, A.I., 1987. Mothers' recognition of their newborns by olfactory cues. Dev. Psychol. 20, 587–591.

Klaus, M.H., Kennell, J.H., 1976. Maternal-Infant Bonding. Mosby, St Louis.

Klaus, M.H., Klaus, P.H., 1999. Your Amazing Newborn. Perseus Books, Cambridge, Massachusetts.

Klaus, M.H., Klaus, P.H., Plumb, N., Zuehlke, S., 1970. Human maternal behaviour at first contact with her young. Paediatrics 45, 187–192.

Kontos, D., 1978. A study of the effects of extended mother–infant contact on maternal behaviour at one and three months. Birth Fam. J. 5, 133–140.

Kuhl, K., Andruski, J.E., Christovich, I.A., et al., 1997. Cross-language analysis of phonetic units in language addressed to infants. Science 277, 684–686.

Lamb, M.E., 1983. Early mother–neonate contact and the mother–child relationship. J. Child Psychol. Psychiatry 24, 487–494.

Lang, R., 1972. Birth Book. Genesis Press, Ben Lomond, California.

Manning, J.T., Chamberlain, I.A.T., 1991. Left-sided cradling and brain lateralisation. Ethol. Sociobiol. 12, 237–244.

Michel, G., 1981. Right-handedness: a consequence of infant supine head-orientation preference? Science 212, 685–687.

Palmer, L.F., 2002. The chemistry of attachment. Attach. Parent. Int. News 5 (2) naturalfamilyonline.com/5-ap/38-hormones-in-bonding.htm.

Rubin, R., 1963. Maternal touch. Nurs. Outlook 22, 828–831.

Salk, L., 1961. The effects of the normal heartbeat sound on the behaviour of the newborn infant: implications for mental health. World Ment. Health 12, 168–175.

Schaal, B., Marlier, L., Soussignon, R., 1995. Responsiveness to the odour of amniotic fluid in the human neonate. Biol. Neonate 67, 397–406.

Siqueland, E.R., Delucia, C.A., 1969. Visual reinforcement of non-nutritive sucking in human infants. Science 165, 1144–1146.

Slater, A., Findlay, J., 1975. Binocular fixation in the newborn baby. J. Exp. Child Psychol. 20, 248–273.

Smail, D.L., 2008. On Deep History and the Brain. University of California Press Berkeley and Los Angeles, California.

Small, M.F., 1999. Our Babies, Ourselves. Anchor Books, New York.

Soltis, J., 2004. The signal functions of early infant crying. Behav. Brain Sci. 27 (4), 443–448.

Stables, D., Hewitt, G., 1995. The effect of lateral asymmetries on breast feeding skills: can the midwives' holding interventions overcome unilateral breast feeding problems? Midwifery 11, 28–36.

Trevathen, W.R., 1987. Human Birth: An Evolutionary Perspective. Aldine de Gruyter, New York.

Turkewitz, G., Gordon, E.W., Birch, H. G., 1965. Head turning in the human neonate: spontaneous patterns. J. Comp. Physiol. Psychol. 59, 189–192.

Varendi, H., Porter, R.H., Winberg, J., 1994. Does the newborn finds the nipple by smell? Lancet 344, 989–990.

Annotated recommended reading

Bowlby, J., 1984. Attachment and Loss. Vol. 1: Attachment. Penguin Books, Harmondsworth.

This book is grounded in ethology and lays the foundations for much ongoing discussion and style of care provided for mothers, fathers and their babies.

Davis-Floyd, R., Mather, F.S., 2002. The technocratic, humanistic and holistic paradigms of childbirth. MIDIRS Midwifery Dig. 4 (12), 500–506.

The descriptions of the three paradigms of health care that influence contemporary childbirth in industrialised nations are clear, highly significant for midwives and provide a basis for understanding the many theories that complicate care provision.

Feldman, R., Weller, A., Zagoory-Sharon, O., Levine, A., 2007. Evidence for a neuro-endocrinological foundation of human affiliation: plasma oxytocin levels across pregnancy and the postpartum period predict mother–infant bonding. Psychol. Sci. 18 (11), 965–970.

This scientific article is extremely interesting to those for whom oxytocin is already well known in relation to childbearing. It is also an excellent example of how biology underpins social and cultural behaviours.

Hrdy, S.B., 1999. Mother Nature. Pantheon, London.

Sarah Hrdy is qualified in anthropology, primatology and evolutionary theory and has combined motherhood with an academic career. This book reassesses key assumptions about human evolution and reproduction in the light of human social organisation.

Small, M.F., 1998. Our Babies, Ourselves. Anchor Books, New York.

This is a book on child rearing for parents but written at a level of interest to professionals caring for families. She examines well-known advice passed down generations in the light of current research.

NB: Page numbers in *italics* refer to boxes, figures and tables